Chinese Acupuncture

George Soulié de Morant

Chinese Acupuncture

l'Acuponcture Chinoise
by George Soulié de Morant

Translated By
Lawrence Grinnell
Claudy Jeanmougin
Maurice Leveque

Edited By
Paul Zmiewski

Marvellous points outside the meridians (lower limb)

Library of Congress Cataloging-in-Publication Data

Soulié de Morant, G. (Georges), 1878 to 1955
     [*l'Acuponcture Chinoise.* English]
     Chinese Acupuncture / George Soulé de Morant ; translated by
     Lawrence Grinnel, Claudy Jeanmougin, Maurice Leveque ; edited by
     Paul Zmiewski. -- English ed.
       p. cm.
     Includes bibliographical references and index.
     ISBN 0-912111-31-3:
     1. Acupuncture. I. Zmiewski, Paul. II. Title.
     [DNLM: 1. Acupuncture. WB 369 S723ac 1994a]
RM 184.S6813 1994
615.8'92 -- dc20
DNLM/DLC
for Library of Congress   94-18666
                     CIP

French Edition Copyright © Maloine, Paris, 1972
English Edition Copyright © Paradigm Publications, Brookline, 1994

Paradigm Publications
44 Linden Street
Brookline, Massachusetts 02146 U.S.A.

Printed in the United States of America

Acknowledgments

Many people labored very hard over more than a decade to bring this English edition of George Soulié de Morant's *l'Acuponcture Chinoise* to fruition. In addition to the original translators, Gail Neubert completely revised the punctuation on the original manuscript. Mary Kinneavy retyped the entire manuscript into computer files. Sally Rimkeit and Missa Olatunji edited the larger part of volumes I through III. Diane Putt contributed years of manuscript development, programming and formatting.

One who has written these new truths into the great immortal book of human potentials, thus wresting from the vastness of time a morsel of permanence, cannot be said to have lived and worked in vain.

Professor Paul Mériel

Introduction to the English Edition

George Soulié de Morant

George Soulié de Morant was born in Paris on December 2, 1879. His father, Leon, an engineer who participated in the Mexican War, had met his mother, a French emigrée, while in New Orleans. When still a child, George became acquainted with Judith Gautier, daughter of poet Theóphile Gautier, and learned Mandarin from a highly educated Chinese whom Gautier had invited into his intellectual circle. He completed his early education with the Jesuits, intending to study medicine. However, his father's premature death at sea prevented him from fulfilling this ambition.

Unable to pursue a medical career, but already completely fluent in Chinese, George Soulié de Morant found a position with the Banque Lehideux, which sent him to China at the turn of the century. His almost native proficiency in the Chinese language, his appreciation of Chinese culture and his rapid adaptation to Chinese society soon led to his engagement by the French Ministry of Foreign Affairs. He was appointed French Consul for Shanghai and sent to Yunnan Prefecture. While at this post, he witnessed a cholera epidemic during which acupuncture yielded better results than the Western medicines of the time. It was thus, while still in his early twenties, that George Soulié de Morant first encountered what was to be his life's work.

Although acupuncture was to be his central life interest, Soulié de Morant was not content to study it in isolation; he immersed himself in every aspect of Chinese culture. He became well accepted by the Chinese people, and gained entrance to the highest circles of Chinese society. Between 1901 and 1911, he witnessed the end of the Chinese empire. When he wrote the biographies of the last Empress, Ci Xi, and the revolutionary, Sun Yat-sen, it was as their contemporary. His literary output was voluminous and covered every aspect of Chinese life. Significant works on Chinese art, music, history and literature are among his more than sixty books and articles.

George Soulié de Morant remained in China until 1917, eventually becoming a judge in the French Concession in Shanghai. During his almost two decades in China, he continued to study acupuncture with the most noted practitioners of the time, eventually receiving the highest civilian award, the Coral Globe, for his achievements. He was considered a Chinese doctor by the Chinese themselves, an unheard-of accomplishment for a foreigner, then or now.

His term in China finished, Soulié de Morant returned to France, where he began actively promoting acupuncture among the medical profession. Initially confronted with skepticism and derision that was rooted in the failure of earlier attempts to introduce acupuncture through inaccurate information, he decided to publish articles based on translations of Chinese medical texts. He chose those he thought would be of interest to physicians. He also wrote a series of essays, and then a longer article on acupuncture that was published in *Science Médical Pratique* in 1931. These works attracted the attention of two French physicians, Drs. Flandin and Martiny, who invited Soulié de Morant to work with them in their departments at the Bichat and Leopold Bellan Hospitals. While exact records of their studies have not survived, they obtained remarkable clinical results, and continued to experiment as Soulié de Morant pursued further study and translation.

In 1933, Mercure de France published a short article of his on Chinese pulse diagnosis, and in 1934 the same company published his first book on acupuncture, *Précis de la vrai acuponcture Chinoise (Summary of the true Chinese acupuncture)*. The first two volumes of the present text, *l'Acuponcture Chinoise (Chinese Acupuncture)* were published during 1939-1941. These texts present the culmination of Soulié de Morant's "theory of energy" and its therapeutic manipulation by acupuncture. They stimulated a period of remarkable progress for acupuncture in France, and were the basis for their author's nomination for the Nobel Prize in 1950.

Even though *l'Acuponcture Chinoise* was recognized as an important text by many French physicians, not all welcomed this new information, and some were openly hostile. Soulié de Morant suffered from their hostility, which is said to have adversely affected his health, but he remained in France, refusing a professorship that had been created for him in the United States. He suffered a stroke in the early 1950's that left him partially paralyzed, but he learned to write with his other hand and continued his work. He died of a heart attack on May 10, 1955, just after completing *l'Acuponcture Chinoise*. This monumental work remains today the fundamental European testament to the art and science of acupuncture.

l'Acuponcture Chinoise

This vast text, the result of decades of arduous research and scholarship, demonstrates the extent of the author's intelligence, perseverance and scope of knowledge. The first volume, "l'Energie," was published as a single text by Mercure de France in 1939. The second volume, "le Maniement de l'énergie," again as a single text, followed in 1941. Soulié de Morant completed the third volume, "Physiologie de l'énergie," immediately before his death in 1955. In 1957, a posthumous edition was published by Editeur Jacques Lafitte in which all three volumes were presented as completed and revised by the author.

The fourth and fifth volumes of the present work, "les Méridiens, les points, et leur symptoms," and "les Maladies et leur traitements," required fifteen years of effort by Soulié de Morant's life-long collaborator, Dr. Thérèse Martiny. These sections, derived from Soulié de Morant's notes, translations and records from more than a quarter century of clinical trials, reveal his attempts to associate Chinese and European thought in a manner that in many ways anticipated the modern Chinese synthesis of Chinese and Western medicine known in the West as "Traditional Chinese Medicine." Ironically, while the Chinese chose to fit their indigenous medicine into patterns that could be linked to biomedicine, Soulié de Morant chose to show how Western anatomy, physiology and pathology could be reinterpreted, and in some ways better understood, according to traditional Chinese principles.

These final volumes represent the broadest and most detailed clinical compilation of acupuncture ever published in a European language. That they were compiled without the aid of computers, and yet remain today the richest source of directly translated clinical information about acupuncture, is a testament to the dedication and skill of both Dr. Martiny and Soulié de Morant. More than a simple list of formulae, they are a unique record of decades of clinical experience and cooperation. These last two volumes were finally completed in 1972 when they were published along with the original three volumes by Editeur Maloine. It is this edition upon which this English edition is based.

Technical notes for the English edition

The goal of this effort has been to render in English a practical translation of a work that has already proven to be of immense scholarly and clinical value while preserving its connection to the body of literature it has inspired. What George Soulié de Morant sought to accomplish was the presentation in a European manner of information from three related categories: (1) precise theoretical and clinical information from original Chinese and Japanese texts; (2) theoretical explanations of Chinese and Japanese concepts, again based on authoritative sources; and (3) inferences and explanations based on Western knowledge and clinical experimentation:

> This book is not simply a translation of a Chinese text. My work consists of developing a structure that conforms to European logic. For each part of this design, I have given literal quotations from numerous Chinese and Japanese works. I have compared and commented on the differences, from a Western perspective, that sixty centuries of experimentation have revealed to the Chinese and Japanese, who make up one third of humanity. Finally, for each part, I have tried to throw light upon the extensive experimentation being carried out in France. Conducted under strict scientific control, these experiments have demonstrated the efficacy of acupuncture while offering explanations based on Western physiological concepts. In brief, I have attempted to reveal this ancient tradition in a scientific manner.

l'Acuponcture Chinoise was Soulié de Morant's attempt to teach the acupuncture he knew as a scholar and practitioner to European physicians whose perception and expectations of science and medicine greatly differed from those of the Chinese who had produced the information. Thus, while this text is certainly a reliable source of theoretical and clinical information, it is also the first and most significant attempt to teach the practice of acupuncture to Westerners. It is thus a record of the experience and thought from which many ideas about acupuncture have derived and a record of the cooperative application of acupuncture in a biomedical setting.

When confronted by the vast number of Chinese medical concepts, George Soulié de Morant identified and offered solutions for the same problems that face modern translators of Chinese medical texts. However, as the first to undertake such extensive translations, he was without the advantage of access to current technology, previous scholarly research, experience and critique. At several points in this book he mentions the problems encountered when attempting to translate into modern French the terminology of an alien conceptual process that relied on sensory images developed over two millenia. He chose to confront this problem by consulting both ancient and modern Chinese sources, the classic texts of antiquity, and the most recent reference available at the time, the *Ci Yuan* encylopedia. The *Ci Yuan,* published during the second decade of the twentieth century, was the first Chinese attempt to produce a Western medical encyclopedia and was consequently a hybrid of early twentieth century biomedicine and traditional thought. As a result, George Soulié de Morant related the images of classical Chinese medicine to the most basic concepts of biomedicine.

Although he never explicitly articulated a translational methodology, George Soulié de Morant used different approaches to his sources to accomplish different goals. When translating detailed clinical concepts and observations, he took a denotive approach, maintaining a one-to-one relationship to the Chinese source and selecting French equivalents of Chinese medical terms that matched the definitions provided by Chinese clinicians and literary sources. However, for those major concepts for which his French readers had no conceptual preparation, he took a connotive approach, using ideas he believed would allow his readers to understand the concept within their own frame of reference. In this he was entirely direct, even noting when his choices were ''for want of a better word.'' When attempting to teach, persuade or provide general summaries, the author explained Chinese ideas in his own words, drawing on his decades of study and clinical experience, using quotations from important ancient and modern, Chinese and Japanese sources to support his understanding.

Indeed, recognizing the hybrid nature of his work, the author provided specific references for all his information. Almost every datum is related to a specific source. Although he translated information from seminal Chinese medical texts such as the *Huang Di Nei Jing,* and included many illustrative quotations from these ancient works, he concentrated on references to later compendia, such as *Yi Xue Ru Men* and *Zhen Jiu Da Cheng.* These texts are still recognized as the culmination of Chinese clinical experience. *l'Acuponcture Chinoise* is thus essentially clinical and is supported by references to the fine details required to practice a medicine based on sensory observations accumulated over two millennia. Furthermore, out of concern for authenticity and respect for Chinese tradition, he explicitly labeled that which he had discovered through his own research and clinical experience. Suppositions which he was unable to confirm were noted by question marks, which have been retained in the English edition. Where rigorous translations of clinical indications were obscure, he retained the image inherent in the Chinese language and supplemented it with explicit interpolations or questions.

The number and specificity of the references in the English edition are thus vastly greater than typical of modern English clinical manuals. Although inclusion of references with the text is not a current presentation style, the present edition retains both the full set of references and their placement in the text. In this way, the source of any idea is clearly noted and the intellectual integrity of the author is faithfully preserved. The first three volumes are his own teaching of the acupuncture he knew as a practitioner. Yet, every Chinese source is rigorously documented and clearly distinguished typographically. The fourth volume is an acupoint by acupoint compilation of information drawn from the didactic text of the first volumes and the treatments of the fifth. This information is not referenced datum by datum. However, in the fifth volume where this information is provided as a treatment repertoire, everything is referenced to a specific source.

Some stylistic changes have been made. French editorial style of the period emphasized the collation of related sentences into paragraphs to a lesser extent than does modern English. Where this difference engendered a sense of discontinuity for English readers, paragraphs have been formed where only individual sentences existed in the French original. However, in no case has text been resequenced, added or deleted. The textual organization and headings of the original have been retained, as have the essentials of the original design and typography. Substantive editorial corrections or references to more modern dates or names are noted in editorial notes. All notes, including those original to the French edition, are sequentially numbered within each chapter. Editors' and translators' notes are followed by the abbreviations ''ed.'' or ''trans.''

The English translation parallels the French original so that readers wishing to compare English renderings and expressions with the original French text may easily do so. The exception concerns those chapters that describe meridians and acupoints in sequence. These were originally organized alphabetically, in French, an order that would have proven confusing to clinicians if directly adopted. Therefore these chapters have been rearranged according to current practice. However, the information within each meridian or acupoint discussion is unchanged.

The Bibliography in this edition was translated from the French edition. However, the remainder of the back matter, ''Points de Weihe et points Chinoise'' and the ''Liste alphabétique des organs, parties du corps et troubles,'' has been replaced with a more extensive modern index generated for this edition. The original French ''Table des Matières'' has been expanded and placed at the front of the text as expected by English readers.

The original Maloine edition consisted of two volumes. The first volume is entirely translated in the present text. The second volume contained a collection of Chinese and Japanese illustrations and the author's original drawings, charts representing acupoint locations relative to the gross anatomy of the human body. These illustrations were unique and were an historic contribution to the transmission of acupuncture. While the second volume has not been replicated, the majority of its renderings have been reproduced as volume and chapter illustrations. The French edition also contained a number of photographs, for example, the first electro-acupuncture devices. Because the original photographs are unavailable these could not be reproduced for this edition.

As regards the text itself, there is little that modern scholars or clinicians will find obscure; indeed, many of the author's ideas are still current. Soulié de Morant concluded, as have other sinologists since, that many of the most important ideas in Chinese medicine are essentially untranslatable, because Chinese methods of cognition do not parallel those of Europeans. Thus he began his translation by developing a dictionary of fixed technical concepts drawn from important Chinese texts. The present edition indexes more than a thousand fixed terms exclusive of nomenclature such as acupoint names. He sought specific definitions for these terms from Chinese sources and maintained a consistent relationship between the Chinese originals and their French equivalents. To allow others to reference his decisions, he created a system for transliterating Chinese. To further support the validity of his text, he included numerous references to Chinese clinical definitions from both ancient and modern sources.

Seeking to ''reveal this ancient tradition in a scientific manner,'' Soulié de Morant chose to present central Chinese ideas as concepts that the physicians for whom he wrote would most easily understand. Considering the extent to which acupuncture has become a part of modern French and European medical practice, this must be regarded as a successful strategy. However, the decades that have passed since *l'Acuponcture Chinoise* was written have outmoded some of the author's term selections. For example, he notes that he used ''energy'' to translate *qi* because he supposed that the   *qi* energy would be revealed by science. In this expectation Soulié de Morant reflected the rationale of early twentieth century thinkers in both France and China — ''modern'' science would reveal all things.

At the beginning of the twentieth century concepts like ''human energy'' were referenced in dictionaries and were considered valid matters for scientific inquiry. When the author was writing, Bergson's concept of an *élan vital* was immensely popular in France, indeed in Europe generally. Many nineteenth century ideas of nature were still broadly regarded as truths. Today, however, the scientific era that had just begun when Soulié de Morant chose to use the term ''energy,'' has left that word with new and different associations in both popular and scientific writing.

Regardless, *l'Acuponcture Chinoise* is a source of several ideas like ''energy'' that have played such an important historical role, and become so broadly cited, that they are not necessarily understood as being specific to this text. Thus, their substitution for more modern terms would have isolated this work from its significant historical role. Furthermore, many later authors adopted English renditions of George Soulié de Morant's French terms, making *l'Acuponcture Chinoise* the only link to Chinese sources for many of those texts. Thus we chose to retain the author's interpretations to make the specific context of these now familiar words conveniently available and to help clarify the role *l'Acuponcture Chinoise* has played in the transmission of acupuncture.

However, we did modernize the text as regards access to the Chinese language so that readers who wish to explore Chinese medical concepts, or to investigate its technical terms, may do so with ease. George Soulié de Morant's original transliteration system has been replaced with pinyin. We chose pinyin because linguists and sinologists must deal with a variety of romanization systems, pinyin among them, but clinicians have become accustomed to pinyin. Similarly, while the author's original alphanumeric point numbering system has been preserved, it has been appended when necessary with the acupoint designations currently used in Chinese texts. The acupoint nomenclature used as a base is that adopted by the World Health Organization in 1991; there are, however, some variances. We have used the acupoint label ''PC'' (pericardium) to match the W.H.O. nomenclature, while leaving ''Heart Governor'' in the text. We wanted to preserve the author's original translation, but felt that point numbering using ''HG'' would be foreign to practitioners. On the other hand, while W.H.O. uses ''TE'' (triple energizer), we have used ''TW'' (triple warmer). The abbreviation ''TW'' is familiar enough to clinicians to justify conformation with Soulié de Morant's original French. Furthermore, despite having coined the idea of ''energetics'' for the benefit of his physician readers, he explicitly chose the term *rechauffer* (warmer), not the idea of ''energizer,'' the assumption behind the W.H.O. standard.

Western medical terms have been retained as used by the author. In a few instances, this may require reference to older medical dictionaries. The clinical associations that Soulié de Morant and his colleagues made were to the diagnostic standards of their time, not those of the present. The text provides considerable information concerning the data which are the basis of these associations, defines many medical terms and mentions specific physiological or biological phenomena when such apply. Furthermore, where the author chose to relate Chinese medical concepts to biomedical concepts, he included appropriate qualifications and descriptions, transliterations and precise translations. Also worthy of note are his use of medical terms such as ''lymphatic type'' or ''nervous terrain.'' These are references to French constitutional concepts that are still part of French medical practices such as phytotherapy. However, these ideas only now are becoming known in English-speaking countries.

l'Acuponcture Chinoise is an important part of the intellectual history of acupuncture in the West, not only directly as an authoritative source of information but also indirectly as an influence on how acupuncture has been understood. Therefore, clinicians should be aware that the acupuncture the author studied in China at the turn of the century was the product of a culture that is now irrevocably changed. Acupuncture in China has changed in many significant ways, particularly since the mid-twentieth century. While ideas found in modern English texts are often expressed in English words derived from *l'Acuponcture Chinoise,* these words do not always mean what was meant in the classic works upon which *l'Acuponcture Chinoise* is based. In modern books, for example, the English neologism ''tonification'' that English authors created from Soulié de Morant's French term is used to reference a needle technique or a category of natural drugs. In *l'Acuponcture Chinoise,* it references a much broader set of point selection, stimulation and treatment timing options specifically intended to achieve a relative balance among a patient's pulses. As well, French and English terms that share linguistic roots are not necessarily absolutely identical in meaning, particularly over time. For example, while *nerf* herein must be translated as ''nerve,'' in the author's era *nerf* still carried associations like those of the English term ''sinew.''

The significance of l'Acuponcture Chinoise

Because Soulié de Morant's work has been previously unavailable in English, it has been represented only in abstracts, opinions and reviews concerning its contribution to clinical and scholarly endeavors. The unavailability of the text has led to some inaccurate information becoming common opinion. For example, the author has been criticized for having promoted historical inaccuracies such as ascribing the *Huang Di Nei Jing* to the 20th century B.C. or accepting his Chinese associates' reports of Chinese social and technological advances. However, when he began his work, little historical research had been done either in the West or in China. As a practitioner working in a clinical environment, his acceptance of Chinese tradition was unavoidable. Chinese scholars would only begin to question these traditions in the middle of the twentieth century. The author's perceptions were formed in an elite milieu and his sources' could not possibly represent acupuncture's role in all of Chinese society or through all of Chinese history. While, for example, formulary acupuncture probably played a quantitatively greater role than Soulié de Morant believed, he was nonetheless reporting one of acupuncture's most treasured ideals.

Other scholars have criticized Soulié de Morant's concentration on relatively recent clinical sources, such as the late Ming dynasty compilations *Yi Xue Ru Men* and *Zhen Jiu Da Cheng,* instead of canonical works like the *Huang Di Nei Jing.* What these scholars have failed to realize is that the author was primarily a clinician, not a linguist, anthropologist or historian — the goal he set for himself was not philological or historical documentation, but clinical validity. He wrote *l'Acuponcture Chinoise* to teach acupuncture to working physicians in a Western setting, not to explicate the origins of the art. Accordingly, he chose works that represented the epitome of classical technique, not its conceptual and historical roots.

Soulié de Morant has also been criticized for having failed to develop a formal translational methodology or to provide appropriate philological detail. It is argued that later authors following his work thus failed to retain a precise relationship to the original Chinese and therefore confused clinical concepts and phenomena. Although the author did prepare a dictionary, it was never published, perhaps because of his untimely death. However, the more important point is that *l'Acuponcture Chinoise* was a work of persuasion. The author's goal was to achieve acceptance for acupuncture among French physicians, not to create a model for the development of a technical literature that was by no means certain to follow. His decisions were made in an often hostile climate while he was personally the target of anger and derision. Despite so powerful a need to make his presentation acceptable and persuasive, Soulié de Morant preserved a far larger set of Chinese technical concepts than would many acupuncture works for many years thereafter.

Ironically, Soulié de Morant has also been criticized by some modern Chinese authors for having injected radical ''non-traditional'' ideas into acupuncture. Their opinions, however, have been formed without access to the author's original work. Soulié de Morant was extremely careful to distinguish his original ideas from his classical references. Indeed, when *''GSdeM''* labels a clinical procedure or observation, it represented not only a conclusion from his extensive clinical experience, but also a conclusion that had survived the review of his able French and Chinese peers. While we have been unable to examine the actual records of the clinical trials completed under the supervision of Drs. Flandin and Martiny, we feel that it is fair to assume that these met the standards of the time. Furthermore, although he was a man of powerful intellect who expressed great pride in his observations and discoveries, he did not presume to interpret his sources through his individual clinical experience alone. Instead, he sought the best confirmation available, Eastern or Western.

Regarding Soulié de Morant's own theoretical speculations, most are extensions of classical theory. They are a further development of traditional ideas according to the knowledge of the early twentieth century. As may be noted by many of the *Ci Yuan* quotations, these speculations were not unique to the author, but were part of a general response to the increasing prevalence of biomedicine in China. Chinese medicine has never been a static system, ossified in the books of the distant past. It has always been in development and evolution. George Soulié de Morant's ideas are another step in that evolution, a step that has proven valuable over many years. Readers who are familiar with the modernized form of acupuncture, synthesized with Western and herbal medicine, that is currently explicated in Chinese textbooks produced for export to the West, will recognize some logical parallels between Soulié de Morant's ideas and post-revolutionary developments in the People's Republic of China. However, these readers should also remember that the author's work predates these developments by at least two decades, and while it is influenced by the science and philosophy of the early twentieth century, it is predominantly founded on the classical tradition.

Finally, Soulié de Morant has been criticized for "Westernizing" Chinese acupuncture, for reducing acupuncture points and Chinese medical theory to lists of biomedically-defined illnesses and syndromes. However, even casual inspection of this English edition will reveal that this is another opinion based on subsequent works that have excerpted treatments or ideas without explanation of the traditional concepts. While Western philosophical ideas such as *élan vital* and early twentieth century scientific discoveries certainly contributed to George Soulié de Morant's concept of "human energy," at no time did he fail to acknowledge or attempt to reduce the scope of *qi* in clinical practice. While he did relate Chinese technical terms to the biomedical concepts his readers understood, he also maintained direct connections to the traditional concepts by providing transliterations of the Chinese and rigorous translations of his sources, some of which had already made these associations. Finally, he turned to the strictest means by which such associations may be justified, the clinical trial.

What Soulié de Morant attempted to do, and more often than not succeeded in doing, was to integrate Western medical theory into the theoretical corpus of Chinese medical and philosophical thought, not vice versa. In effect, Soulié de Morant demanded not that Chinese acupuncture be purged of what Western science cannot explain, but that Western knowledge expand to cover all the observations of Chinese acupuncture. Nowhere else has this ever been attempted, before or since.

George Soulié de Morant was the first person to introduce acupuncture systematically to the West. He is legitimately the father of European acupuncture. His place in history will be most probably that of the author of the teaching document that transformed Western fascination with Chinese medical principles into a practical contribution to Western culture. Although it is a rare tribute to a clinical manual that scholars also find it an important contribution, it is rarer still that a book explaining a foreign system can affect anything as deeply tied to culture as medicine. While it is difficult to restrain the use of superlatives in regard to either this text or its author, their place in the intellectual history of the West is already established. Thus only the most important legacy of *l'Acuponcture Chinoise* must not go unmentioned. Without the dedication and perseverance of George Soulié de Morant, millions of people in the West would continue to suffer debilities that are relieved by acupuncture. Their relief is the highest tribute to George Soulié de Morant.

Paul Zmiewski, Ph.D.
Brookline, Massachusetts
August 1993.

Designation

Paradigm Publications is a participant in the Council of Oriental Medical Publishers and supports their effort to encourage explicit statement of the methods and sources used to produce Oriental medical texts in English. George Soulié de Morant followed his sources in a precise manner. He states that he selected French terms that he hoped would be persuasive for contemporaneous readers. For this reason, his most basic conceptual translations are connotive. The French editions of the five volumes contained herein therefore fit the following Council of Oriental Medical Publishers designations: Volumes I, II and III are *Original Documents* containing connotive translations with rigorous source documentation. Volume IV is a reordering of information found in the other volumes; it is a ***Connotive Compilation*** without source documentation. Volume V is a ***Connotive Compilation*** with rigorous source documentation.

The English edition follows the French edition; thus it shares these designations. Because this text is the source of many terms and ideas that have been broadly used in other texts, the translators have attempted to use the most frequently adopted English term translations thus preserving this work's links to the literature it has inspired.

Preface to the Original French Edition

From whatever angle one looks at the Universe, from worlds gravitating in space to the smallest particles of the atom, all is nothing but a perpetual rhythmic movement. Do we not find the essentials in the Hermetic Laws: ''What is above is like what is below. All is vibration; nothing is inert. Everything vibrates; everything is double; everything has two sides, everything has two poles.''

Are not the propagations of force in nature made of undulations in sinusoidal lines, which are reducable to higher and lower parts, which succeed each other according to a more or less rapid rhythm?

Terrestrial life, in its animal and vegetable aspect, has evolved under the same law of alternation of ascension and decadence. Must we not submit to the rhythms of periods of dryness and humidity, of hot and cold seasons, of day and night? Human life, physically as well as mentally, obeys the same rhythmic, universal laws of evolution.

When we consider the perpetual instability of our biological equilibrium in the most favorable conditions of health — the movement of regulation which causes us to oscillate from one position to another; from sleep to effort, from the maximum to the minimum in temperature, from hunger to satiety, from anabolism to catabolism — we understand by what mechanism of constant recovery we are carried along from one extreme to another. The mechanism becomes singularly more obvious when we view it in the light of pathological amplification. In fact, whether it is to stop a pathological crisis or to maintain the physiological rhythm in its most habitual order, the organism must constantly re-establish an equilibrium which all the natural forces of the environment tend to compromise.

Medical science, which has rejected the old idea of ''vital force,'' does not allow us to glimpse how to act on these rhythms of which we more or less feel the importance in a confused way, depending upon the discipline to which we subscribe.

Certainly dietetics, which was recommended by the now deceased Carton, attempts to smooth this inconvenience by adjusting the natural agents of treatment to seasonal and periodic variations, which explained for him why certain treatments always apply in all circumstances, being successively preached, then decried, relating, nevertheless, to the same illness.

We have felt that an effective therapeutic method was needed, a medicine capable of acting on these rhythms to modify them according to the occasion. By this, we could achieve cures which the usual techniques cannot obtain because they do not attack the true cause.

While homeopathy, a medicine for the constitution, had already given us increased therapeutic possibilities, there was still the need to re-establish certain imbalances. Chinese medicine in its symbolic language tried to make exact the principle which governs all phenomena at all levels. As Professor Sakurazawa remarks in his French text, *Yin-Yang,* ''the unique principle of the philosophy and science of the Far East explains the system of the universe in two opposed activities in all physiological phenomena.'' The universe is the oscillation of the two activities, yin and yang. They are both defined only relatively. Their actions and their mutations are constant. It is obvious that a disequilibrium of these two activities can produce illness. But how should we Westerners name this unique principle?

''Energy'' in the literal sense of the word (activity, exercised force) appears to be the best term. Different from the nervous flux, it corresponds to what the Hindus name *Prana.*

It is this energy which George Soulié de Morant, with a benedictine patience, strove to make intelligible and manipulable for us. He opened the way for researchers who will measure it one day, since they are already able to detect its existence. Certainly, there is still much more of the way to go, many ideas being still only hypotheses for research, suggestions more than certitudes. As always in this delicate subject, certain propositions will be shown to be erroneous, while others will be considered truly prophetic. All is far from finished, and it is in this spirit that we must read and meditate upon Volume III, ''The Physiology of Energy.''

What to say about Volumes I and II, for which the proof of time and daily practice has shown the immense value and which all [French] acupuncturists keep like their Bible? Thanks to the needles of gold and silver we are able, according to our liking, and following this time the principles of opposites, to tonify what is empty and to disperse what is full. We finally have it, this medicine of rhythms for which we have aspired. We know now how to manipulate this energy in harmony with the great rhythms of nature. An entire volume is not too much to learn the subtleties of this therapeutic act, which requires for its perfect accomplishment that we know that in order to tonify an organ, energy must be drawn from another organ possessing it in excess; that we should act in a yang period (midnight to midday) on a yang meridian, or in a yin period (midday to midnight) on a yin meridian. How many possibilities of arrhythmia must be known to understand these interrelations among the organs? To crown this work, already so important, an essential part was missing for many years which we incessantly attempted to acquire from the author with an intensity that had no excuse other than the desire for better application of this method in which we felt immense interest. This deficiency is now largely filled by Volumes IV and V of this book, which give all the practical applications. We remain amazed by admiration before such a monument of erudition and conscience.

One who has written these new truths into the great immortal book of human potentials, thus wresting from the vastness of time a morsel of permanence, cannot be said to have lived and worked in vain.

Professor Paul Mériel
Professor of the Medical Clinic
at the Faculty of Medicine of Toulouse,
Doctor of Purpan Hospital

In Grateful Homage

To the ancient scholars of China, who four thousand years ago discovered the principles and practical applications of the science of vital energy.

To all my loyal and faithful friends, who have encouraged me in my research and sustained me in the battle against evil.

To the moral courage, broad scientific minds, exceptional concern and constant helpfulness of Doctors Marcel and Thérèse Martiny of the Foch Hospital.

To the generous and exceptional knowledge of Professor Paul Mériel of the Faculty of Toulouse. He has particularly applied himself to this work, studied and discussed it with me, and has judged it worthy of being submitted as a unique offering from France for review by the Nobel Prize Commission.

To the medical doctors who have begun offering acupuncture consultations in French hospitals on the basis of knowledge gained from my work, thereby pioneering an unprecedented venture in the West.

To the thousands of doctors, my students direct and indirect, who for the first time in France have listed themselves as acupuncture practitioners. In their concern for public welfare, they have supplemented pasteurism and organic medicine, the only methods taught in the medical faculties, with acupuncture. Their numerous achievements rightfully ensure their reputation and success.

George Soulié de Morant

Table of Contents

Table of Illustrations

Volume I

Energy:

Points, Meridians, and Circulation

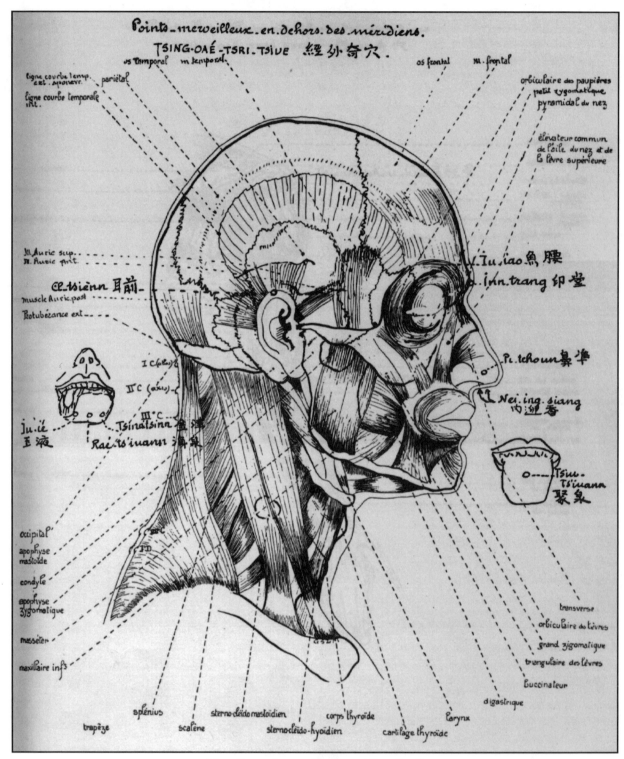

Marvellous points outside the meridians (head)

Introduction

This book is not simply a translation of a Chinese text. My work consists of developing a structure that conforms to European logic. For each part of this structure, I have given literal quotations from numerous Chinese and Japanese works. I have compared and commented on the differences, from a Western perspective, that sixty centuries of experimentation have revealed to the Chinese and Japanese, who make up one third of humanity. Then, for each part, I have tried to throw light upon the extensive experimentation being carried out in France. Conducted under strict scientific control, these experiments have demonstrated the efficacy of acupuncture while offering explanations based on Western physiological concepts. In brief, I have attempted to reveal this ancient tradition in a scientific manner.

Chinese and Japanese sources give brief and imprecise indications for acupuncture point locations, particularly with regard to the respective distances between points. Part of my work has been to determine the precise location of the acupoints through the use of skeletal anatomical references, consistent for all people, and based on a comparison of a large number of individuals.

The description of the syndromes or symptoms cured by each acupoint are scattered throughout a number of Chinese and Japanese works. Therefore, another task, not yet undertaken in China or Japan, has been to list the effects attributed to each point by grouping them according to their associated organs. Acupoints that are reputed to have constant success are specially indicated, as are those that are unique and whose curative effect is not accomplished by any other point. Additionally, other points having a similar effect as the given point are listed. Through this effort I have discovered new effects, often very significant, with the help of modern instrumentation.

Chinese and Japanese drawings of the human body were mainly mnemonic devices, and the development of precise anatomical charts was never highly valued. Hence, I have had to create — not without difficulty — entirely new drawings for Europe as well as for China. Like transparencies, these drawings show skin, muscle and bone simultaneously. They allow the precise placement of each acupoint, even given variations in body size and shape. Consequently, this work exists neither in China nor Japan but has been meticulously extracted from the thousands of works of the Far East.[1]

French medicine, being the first Western system to study acupuncture and put it into practice, may truly presume first place in its scientific elaboration.

In Europe, up to the beginning of the nineteenth century, all scientific books were written in Latin. Therefore, in describing this method in the seventeenth century, the Jesuits of the French scientific mission used Latin to coin the word "acupunctura," from "acus" (point), and "punctura" (to prick). The first books of medicine written in French translated "acupunctura" as "acupuncture," and so it has remained.

In Chinese, its scientific and literary name is *zhen jiu fa* (method of needles and moxa). The layman sometimes calls it *cha zhen* (to stick a needle).

The word "moxa" is derived from the Japanese pronunciation *mogusa*. It was introduced to Europe in the seventeenth century by the Dutch living in Japan.

There are many kinds of acupuncture. One is simplistic and primitive. It consists of puncturing the place of pain without considering any other knowledge. Except for conditions of recent, acute pain, such treatment gives only partial, short-term relief.

Another method, somewhat better, uses points in memorized formulae. Problems are treated with little attention given to the patient or the action of the needles; i.e., in order to tonify or disperse such and such an organ, such and such a point is used; for this particular symptom, that particular point is used. This method allows moderate regulation of the organs, but does not treat the underlying cause of the problem, nor control the vital energy.

The truest form of acupuncture, which we describe here, enables the practitioner to evaluate imbalances of the vital energy, the basis of all functional illness. This is achieved above all through the study of the pulses. True acupuncture is founded on the relationship between the organs, based on the circulation of energy, a system which often differs from the Western anatomical physiological model. The method demands that we locate the exact center of each point, where its action is at a maximum. Although there are failures, these are rare. More difficulties with acupuncture arise in Europe, where the abuses of Western medicine greatly modify natural reactions. For example, when confronted by a soft large intestine pulse of medium amplitude — which it should be — we must always ask the patient if stimulating medications have been taken.

The renowned Yang of the sixteenth century wrote:

*It is obvious that there are channels and pulses. Those who use them are the true doctors (**liang yi**). Those who ignore them are clumsy workers (**zu gong**). (DACH IV, 14v)[2]*

In noting the variations of an illness among individuals, true acupuncture from its beginnings has tended to place greater emphasis on the patient. It is not the microbe that is important, but the terrain. Dr. Nakayama, a Japanese practitioner, thus states: "The illness is not the invasion itself but the weakness that attracts the invasion." Consequently, we are encouraged to treat the patient's vital energy. In an old text it is written:

In the choice of points never forget that each person is ill in his own way. In order to treat disease, the sage must take this under consideration. (DACH IV, 15v)

Although it is necessary to know the pulses, channels, and points, one must also realize, even for true acupuncture, that:

*In order to cure with needles and moxa there are indeed some rules and numbers. But, in truth, the essence of the art lies in the **origin** of the rules and numbers. (DACH IV, 15r)*

Emphasis must be placed on the fact that acupuncture constitutes a physiology of energy that brings to Western science discoveries of great importance. These discoveries have been made through thousands of observations:

Acupoints become sensitive when organs are functionally diseased. The sensitivity disappears with the cure. In the West this observation has escaped us.

Through needling certain points, it is possible to obtain reflex action at the corresponding organ — another discovery for which Western science has only blindly searched.

Channels of energy exist in the body, and the energy circulates continuously in the same direction, another immensely important discovery.

We should be grateful to the Neolithic people who were able to observe these facts, and to the Chinese, who since antiquity have pursued this study and have now transmitted their knowledge to the West. The innumerable patients already cured by this method in France will certainly join us in congratulating French medicine, which has unhesitatingly studied and practiced acupuncture since its arrival in Europe.

What can acupuncture cure?

First, it is advisable to point out that acupuncture can be used with little risk: it does not introduce poisons — foreign elements — into the body; nor does it conflict with any other treatment. In fact, it is often reported to augment the effect of chemical or homeopathic medicines, and dosages may often be reduced. The only risk in these conditions is the possibility of failure that leaves the patient in exactly the original state. Thus, acupuncture can be used with no risk in circumstances where indications for its use are uncertain.

Lesions, defined as physical changes in part of the structure of the organism due to injury or disease, are not directly affected by acupuncture treatment. However, this method may temporarily reduce or nullify the pain or trouble caused by the injury. The seriousness of a lesion may be difficult to evaluate, since its size is not always indicative of the severity of the underlying problem; in some cases, acupuncture effectively treats a small lesion because it has cured a serious underlying condition.

Functional problems constitute the true domain of acupuncture. We must interpret the following directive with this in mind:

To cut the force of an illness nothing is equal to needles and moxa. (DACH II, 19v)

Acupuncture is capable not only of cure but also prevention. The meticulous observers of the Far East have suggested that except in the case of accidents, there are no lesional illnesses that are not preceded by somatic, functional troubles. These problems first manifest in moral or mental changes, so the first changes of personality constitute, in fact, the beginnings of illness. If used at this stage, acupuncture is most effective and is sometimes said to be capable of curing anything. All energetic therapies must be considered as first line, preventive measures which avoid the progression of an illness toward a lesion which is more difficult to cure.

First needle, then moxa, and only third, use medicines. (DACH II, 19v)

Prevention is unquestionably the highest form of medicine. In the fifth century B.C., Bian Que wrote:

> The superior worker (**shang gong**) cures that which is not yet an illness. The average worker (**zhong gong**) cures only when an illness is present. (DACH V, 23v)

This tenet applies to prevention against future development of disease as well as against the repercussions of illness in organs that are still functioning well.

It is impossible to enumerate all the varieties of functional troubles cured by acupuncture in France since I introduced it ten years ago. It is enough to cite some extracts of reports and publications of eminent doctors.

In the article Dr. Ferreyrolles and I published in *Science Médicale Pratique* of June, 1929, our first results are summarized:

> We have tried the method; the results we have obtained are surprising and unexpected. [We observed] the immediate cessation of severe sciatic pain and facial neuralgia for which all other treatments had failed. Asthmatic crises stopped in a few moments. Some crises of spasmodic coryza have had long remissions. Hemorrhoids have yielded to treatment. Some gastric crises have had immediate relief. Constipation and urinary incontinence have been cured.

Doctors Flandin (then physician of the Bichat Hospital) and Macé de Lépinay with Dr. Ferreyrolles have written, in *Bulletin de la Société Médicale des Hôpitaux* of May 3, 1933:

> For one year research has been carried out in our services at Bichat with enough regularity to allow one's attention to be drawn to this simple and effective mode of treatment based on direct action on the skin. . . . We have removed all functional troubles that are connected to hysteria. . . . One group, the algesthesiacs, who by their choice have been cured only with this method, was an effective, easily controllable test. Another group we will only allude to through the various cases we have treated, reserving further comment for later.
>
> We emphasize today the different traumatic and rheumatic arthritic states. The word ''rheumatism'' is taken in the largest sense, that is to say, any articular or muscular pain the etiology of which is for the most part unknown or badly determined, with functional impotence more or less marked.
>
> Case I: Mr. T., 70 years old in May, 1932. Articular rheumatism of the shoulders and hips dating from the first days of January. After a few sessions a complete recovery was obtained.
>
> Case II: Mrs. W., age 51 in October, 1932. Articular rheumatism of the shoulders beginning in March, 1932. Permanent pain so sharp that complete insomnia was induced. As with the preceding patient, Mrs. W. was much improved from the first acupuncture treatment.
>
> Case III: Mrs. C., 42 years old. Rheumatic pain. Left hip and shoulder, beginning many years ago. . . . accompanied by fatiguing headache and insomnia. From the first session and more obviously thereafter, a great improvement was noticed.
>
> These three patients have been chosen from among fifteen or twenty rheumatics whom we have regularly followed for one year. In general the results seem to be better when the pathological symptoms are of recent appearance. We must take note of a number of cases of arthritis of the knee, migraines, femoral nerve neuralgia, lumbago, torticollis and cervicobrachial neuralgia that have generally given us very convincing results. . . . In addition we have studied the action of acupuncture on many diverse syndromes: hiccough, enuresis, deafness, constipation, hemiplegia with contraction, with good results. We have had some failures, but it seems logical to attribute them to defective technique or bad point location.

Dr. Thérese Martiny, physician of Léopold-Bellan Hospital *(Vie Médicale, Nov.10, 1933)* reports on the method and its effects especially on the liver, gallbladder, pancreas, kidneys, etc. Dr. Marcel Lavergne *(Monde Médical, May 15, 1934)* introduces acupuncture and summarizes the cases that are suitable for its use. Our experiences with infants, perfected by him, are now utilized in the maternity wards of several hospitals. Dr. Jules Regnault, famous author of *La Médecine chez les Chinoise,* details possibilities of the method in this book and in an interesting article of the *Lettre Médicale* of January, 1934. Dr. Bonnet-Lemaire utilized our various articles, added his personal experiences and condensed them in his short *Acuponcture Chinoise.*

I am unable to cite here the numerous letters received from French and foreign doctors who, after reading *Précis de la Vraie Acuponcture Chinoise,* have tried this therapy for a large variety of conditions with some remarkable successes.

Some people ask if illnesses treated by acupuncture are really cured; that is, do the patients imagine they are cured while the illness continues its ravages in secret? Others, looking for the cause of the cures they observe, speak of suggestion.

First of all, what is a cure? Important publications in Europe have not yet thoroughly examined the subject. For the Chinese, it is simply a return to the normal condition of the individual with the acquisition of a general immunity against the problem treated, as well as against those problems with the same cause. For example, if migraines are cured using Chinese methods, asthma or varieties of eczema will also be cured, whether or not they have appeared (from a clinical point of view).

As to the hypothesis of a purely imaginary cure, a continued state of illness would be its proof if laboratory instruments could not prove it first. The imagination alone is not able to lower the thermometer reading by one or two degrees in a few minutes nor increase the number of red blood cells by one million in twenty-four hours.

The existence of "suggestion" cannot be denied in any medical modality. In fact, the Chinese have noted that suggestion has the opposite effect; that is to say, success rates may decline due to suggestion. Successes are 100 percent in animals, but rarely more than 80 percent in humans (except for the regulation of recently afflicted organs). Babies give better results than adults. The mental and moral state of the patient at the moment of puncturing is also considered important; e.g., we have observed that infants who fight and cry have the worst results of those groups properly needled. The *Yi Xue* notes:

> The doctor must calm the anxiety of the patient by talking to him. He must repeatedly feign the action of needling, really puncturing only after observing that the patient has no more fear. The breath and appearance of the patient must correspond to his face. His eyes must not shift to the side. The heart rate must be normal and the hands should not be tight as if holding the tail of a tiger or the head of a dragon. If these conditions are met, then one will obtain the best results from needling. (YIX, 2r)

Finally, the texts of greatest antiquity recommend that the patient fix his mind on the needle and recite a sort of prayer, with the idea that anything augmenting the result is useful.

The recent discoveries of European science permit us to explain partially the immediate and powerful effects of acupuncture, but there remains much to be studied. Careful anatomical dissections at the acupoint, done under the direction of Mr. Rouvierre, Professor of Anatomy at the Medical Faculty of Paris, and the surgeon Perretti Della Rocca, have not revealed special structures previously unknown. However, the *British Medical Journal* of February, 1937, published the discovery made by Sir Thomas Lewis, the famous heart and circulation expert. He found a system of cutaneous nerves "until now unsuspected" that seem to have nothing to do with the known sensory nerves or sympathetic system. It does not appear to be a plexus, but a series of channels found in the skin itself. Perhaps these are the meridians of Chinese medicine.

The works of Bonnier are well known under the name of "nasal sympathetic therapy." There seems to be no connection between this method and acupuncture, though the totality of symptoms cured by each Chinese point describes complexes similar to the effects of sympathetic or parasympathetic conditions. (The symptoms treated by each point are not isolated in effect. They form a maximal complex determined by the condition of the individual patient.)

In Volume I, all possible relationships between the Chinese points and similar points known to European science are given, e.g., points of Weihe, points of Valleix, Head's zones. The Chinese points explain the European points, not the reverse.

The phenomenon of pain is not completely understood in Europe. It was only recently noticed that the viscera are insensitive to pain and that the liver, lungs and intestines can be touched or pinched without eliciting pain.

In 1894, Laborde conceived the idea that the bulbar centers can be acted on from a distance. He elicited responses from the respiratory systems and hearts of drowned and asphyxiated subjects by rhythmic traction on the tongue. Indeed, it has been noted (Lichwitz, *Bulletin Médicale,* January 25, 1931) that the effect of injections is sometimes only due to the trauma to the skin, as in acupuncture.

Dr. Martiny, author of the remarkable book *Spécificité Biologique,* believes that acupuncture must utilize ectodermal, circular pathways of excitation. This longitudinal circulation is phylogenetically and ontogenetically much older than horizontal segmentation (which evolutionarily developed as late as the worm). Neurologists have focused on segmentation rather than on longitudinal circulation.

According to Dr. Martiny, we must expand our concept of the human being. We know about individual hydraulic circulation, and its humoral chemistry. We know of the nervous impulse only through the existence of a current conducted along the nerve. Could not the excitation of the appropriate points on the skin create some nervous waves?

Remarkably, acupuncture agrees with the most recent discoveries of our science. Researchers will undoubtedly find in acupuncture important facts that can be utilized immediately or serve as a point of departure for other discoveries.

It is amazing at first glance that a treatment so simple and effective — used by one third of humanity for thousands of years — has been known for so short a time in Europe. Its existence was noticed for the first time in the seventeenth century and reported by Jesuits of the Scientific Mission of Peking in such writings as *De Acupunctura*, by R.P. Cleyer. Much later, several Western travellers were witnesses to surprising cures, but their reports gave only a vague and general idea of this method. Europeans ignored this information altogether, making no use of it. However, around 1810, Dr. James Morris Churchill began applying local acupuncture for pain control. His work was described in his book on surgery translated by Dr. Charbonnier in 1825. In the first quarter of the nineteenth century, Dr. Berlioz of Tours (the father of the musician) was inspired by these reports to invent a method of puncturing which turned out to be completely different from Chinese acupuncture. In an attack on acupuncture, Dr. J. Cloquet, a professor of the Faculté de Paris, published the results obtained from experiments in which he punctured the organs themselves with long needles, totally ignoring the location and even the existence of the Chinese points, channels and pulses. He had several accidents and grave repercussions followed. Medical opinion and the public confused this haphazard method with true Chinese acupuncture, and, through ignorance, true acupuncture was discredited.

It is not surprising, therefore, that the numerous doctors sent to China for the last thirty years, mainly by France, Great Britain and the United States, have closed their minds to the study of this method. Sinologists could have translated the most important texts, but nothing has been done.

Western doctors officially sent to China to teach our sciences and to affirm their superiority cannot easily be educated in the Chinese medical sciences. Many of them, mostly English-speaking, are missionaries and thus even more culturally distant. Almost all ignore the Chinese language or speak it very badly. They commit errors of etiquette that are often inexcusable. Additionally, the great masters of acupuncture, whose time is more valuable than we in Europe can imagine, have never been tempted to teach the whole of their art to our doctors. "Can you see," said a Chinese person to me, "one of your great masters benevolently agreeing to give your whole medical education to a Hottentot who does not understand French and only focuses on the incongruities?"

On the question of translation, one major difficulty in translating Chinese medical texts is that they are full of special terms, particularly for acupuncture, for which our European languages have no precise equivalents. A dictionary explaining the meanings of these terms has not yet been published.[3] Finally, the texts, if completely rendered in the order in which they were published, would disconcert and discourage people by their extensiveness, confusion and phraseology. This is understandable considering that the most important texts in their original form are attributed to the twenty-eighth century B.C.[4] Other texts have been published in their totality, one after the other, without being recast, compared or discussed.

At the beginning of my studies I had to compose a special dictionary, which is still in manuscript form. I have completed but not yet published the first translations of the *Ling Shu*. Thus, this work has yet to be offered to the French public.

A particularly favorable combination of circumstances was necessary to allow me to acquire this protected knowledge. When I arrived in China in 1901, I spoke and read Chinese fluently and was familiar with the complicated etiquette. When visiting the French missions, I was guided by the Bishop of Mongolia, Msgr. Bermyn, who consented to teach me Mongolian, and by the Bishop of Peking, Msgr. Favier. At that time, a great epidemic of cholera broke out in Peking and I saw the deaths of two of my servants in two hours. While passing through several rooms, I saw a Chinese doctor quickly stop the dangerous cramps, vomiting, and diarrhea — whose grave significance I immediately recognized — without using European medicine. Through the favor of the authorities, and through my knowledge of the language and etiquette, I was introduced to this physician, one Dr. Yang. I was then able to obtain permission to study the essential principles of the method, including the most important points and the pattern of the pulses. He found several medical treatises that are now almost unobtainable. Two years later, while acting as judge to the joint French court of Shanghai, I was introduced to an excellent acupuncturist, Dr. Zhang, who was a medical judiciary and secretary to the court. He continued my instruction, helping me to complete my dictionary and to comprehend the profundities of the method. Later, as the delegate consul of Foreign Affairs in Yunnan Fu, I took an active interest in our French hospital and through my friendship with the Viceroy maintained my connections with Chinese acupuncture doctors. I ultimately received official acknowledgement as a Chinese doctor: the Globe of Engraved Coral, which confers the rank of Academician.

During my holidays in France, some of my tentative explanations to doctors met with skeptical smiles: it is scientific to remain in doubt but not to negate that with which we are unfamiliar. I held back publication of all work on this subject. Perhaps I would never have undertaken the heavy task of perfecting and making known what I had learned about acupuncture had not Dr. Paul Ferreyrolles questioned me insistently on the subject. I showed him the acupoints for one illness, then points for another. He patiently and carefully made repeated experiments and presented me to many doctors in hospitals. Aware of the surprising results obtained, they encouraged me to organize my notes and translations of certain comprehensible passages from old texts.

It was thus that Dr. Marcel Martiny, Assistant Chief Physician of the Leopold-Bellan Hospital, and Dr. Thérese Martiny, a physician in the same hospital, studied this method and clarified its application for Europeans. Under strict scientific control, they subjected it to the most rigorous tests on patients with diseases for which the usual therapeutics were without effect or gave only slow and partial results.

For about fifteen years now, under the direction of our best physicians, I have experimented and taught in our hospitals.

Acupuncture, only recently introduced in the Western world, now occupies a growing place in the scientific and medical world as well as with the public. Since the publication of my *Précis de la Vraie Acuponcture,* it has been clinically applied by many doctors. Acupuncture consultancies have opened and have functioned for many years with good results in four Parisian hospitals.[5]

Since then it has been proven that acupuncture gives immediate and complete results in most functional disorders that are generally outside the realm of Western medicine. Along with its other possibilities, it brings an effective and powerful aid to the battle against suffering and disease. It is my hope that this book will allow our clinicians to apply this method with yet more precision and success, and allow researchers to continue their work more easily so that they may finally attain a complete understanding of its actions.

The references throughout this book refer to works recognized as the most important. Abbreviations are given for the following:

(DACH): Zhen Jiu Da Cheng, "Great Perfection of Needles and Moxa," in ten volumes by Yang Gexian of Weijin,[6] published in the Wanli period (1573-1620). The pages refer to the small formatted edition. The plates dating from the eighteenth century (reprinted in Shanghai, 1926) are possible but difficult to procure. The old editions in the large format are unobtainable.

(YIX): Zhen Jiu Yi Xue, "Easy Studies in Needles and Moxa," in three volumes by Li Shouxian, published in 1798. A small edition was published in Shanghai, 1918.

(YIZ): Zhen Jiu Yi Zhi, "Easy Knowledge of Needles and Moxa," by a group of doctors. Published in Shanghai in 1919.

(YXRM): Yi Xue Ru Men, "The Basics of Medical Studies," by Li Chan, published in 1575. An important treatise on general medicine with two volumes devoted to acupuncture.

(JO) [Japanese, Older]: *Zhen Jiu Jing Xue Yi Tian,* "Medical Repertory of Points and Channels for Needles and Moxa," by Dr. Tama-mori No Suke, Tokyo, 1906. Part of the text is in Japanese.

(JM) [Japanese, Modern]: *Tu Xie Jing Xue Xue,* "Studies of the Meridians and Points with Explanations and Drawings," by Dr. Tatse-i, Tokyo, 1908.

Notes

[1] The edition of the text here translated presented the author's charts in a second volume. — ed.

[2] For abbreviations of book titles, see this page (8) above. — ed.

[3] We have used the authors notes and *The Glossary of Chinese Medicine and Acupuncture Points* compiled by Nigel Wiseman and Ken Boss (Paradigm Publications, Brookline, MA, 1990) to confirm and examine terms and their translation in De Morant's work. — ed.

[4] Modern scholarship has dated the earliest complete text on acupuncture, the *Nei Jing,* to approximately 300 - 100 B.C. — ed.

[5] Do not forget that this work was first published in 1939.

[6] The author's contention that the *Zhen Jiu Da Cheng* was written by a "Yang Gexian" comes from a misreading of the last line of the first chapter of that book, which should read, "The *Zhen Jiu Da Cheng* was compiled and corrected under the direction of Jin Xian from Jinyang." Jin Xian was an editor for the first publisher of this book, Zhou Wenbing, but the text itself is credited to Yang Jishi (Jizhou). — ed.

History

High Antiquity

The ''method of needles and moxa'' seems to have been practiced in China since time immemorial. It was perfected by Neolithic man. The *Nei Jing (Ling Shu I)*, attributed in its totality if not in its exact words to the twenty-eighth century B.C.,[1] is a book indispensable to acupuncture. In it we find:

> I regret that all my people must stop paying in taxes and labor because of illness. My desire is that we no longer give them medicines that poison them and that we discontinue use of the ancient stone needles. My wish is that we utilize only the mysterious metal needles by which energy is directed.

This allusion to stone needles takes us into the distant past, for the excavations done in China have yielded copper ornaments in geological strata from the thirtieth century B.C. According to the *Ci Yuan* encyclopedia (the *''Bian Jiu''* article), the name of the method in that ancient period was *bian jiu,* ''stone needles and moxa.'' Information concerning these old instruments is rare and comes from the *Su Wen* (part of the *Nei Jing*).

> The **bian zhen,** stone-point needles, or **bian shi,** points of stone, came from the eastern sea. In that area, a mountain called Gao Feng [High Peak] had stones of a form similar to needles with jade heads. They were naturally long and rounded. They were ground to a sharp point so they could be used as needles in order to effectively cure disease. (DACH III, 29v)

> The territories of the east are where the sky and land begin. It is the land of fish and salt. The people who occupy the seaside eat fish and like salt. The fish causes internal warmth in the people while the salt overwhelms the blood. As a result, all the people have dark complexions. Their most common illnesses are abscesses **(yong)** and pruritis **(yang)**. To cure these ailments it is advisable to use the points of stone. It is for this reason that the stone points come from the east. (DACH I, 2v)

We can only speculate as to whether this refers to Shandong, or perhaps Japan or Korea.

The tradition of these primitive instruments must have continued until much later since a history of the Former Han *(Yi Wen Zhi),* written in the first century B.C., states:

> The Zhou [a dynasty of the thirteenth to third centuries B.C.] used stone needles **(zhen shi)** in order to cure illnesses. This art has been abandoned.

In fact, from that period on, needles of copper were used. However, we can still argue that the ideogram *zhen* was written in the beginning with the elements ''bamboo-above-sharpen,'' referring to the sewing needles that were made of bamboo slivers. From the twenty-eighth century B.C. on, this ideogram has been reserved for sewing needles, and acupuncture needles have been described by the elements ''metal-sharp'' or ''metal-two-fingers.''

Metal needles are said to come from the south, where tradition places the first copper mines (Mount of Copper at the tip of Mt. Qin). At that time the south, for these ancient Chinese, was only as far south as the Yellow River Valley. This information again comes from the *Su Wen:*

> The south is where the sky and earth generate constantly and the yang sun abounds. The lands there are low and the climate debilitating. Fog and dew accumulate. People of the south like sour food. They eat cured meat **(fu)**. This is why they are all delicate and red-complexioned. They mostly suffer from spasms **(luan)** and rheumatism **(bi)**. In order to cure these illnesses it is advisable to use the fine needles. This is why the nine types of needles come from the south. (DACH I, 2v)

Moxa *(jiu),* the ideogram for which is formed from the elements ''fire-extended,'' is said by the *Su Wen* to have come from the north (Mongolia?).[2]

> Moxa **(jiu)** comes from the north, the highland, where wind, cold and ice reign. . . . The cold that prevails generates illnesses of emptiness that the people cure with moxa. (DACH I, 2v)

Several acupuncturists of ancient times are cited in the *Nei Jing* as residing at the court of the Yellow Emperor, Huang Di, who is said to have reigned from 2797 to 2696 B.C. They are Qibo, Leigong, Yu, Fu, Bogao, and Shaoyu. According to the *Nei Jing,* the method of acupuncture had already been completely formed by this time. Indeed, this ancient science must have been developed at this early date. Using astronomical data taken from ancient sources, our scholars have confirmed from the dates and hours of the events described that they are in fact from the thirtieth century B.C.[3]

The *Nei Jing* describes the circulation of the blood, preceding Harvey by forty-five centuries. The spleen is described as "harmonizing the blood and returning it purified to the other organs." The existence of the coordination of respiratory, digestive and genitourinary functions is conceptualized in "an organ that has no form, but has a name" (the Triple Warmer). The weight of the organs, their dimensions, and the length of the vessels are described.

Tradition places the existence of an illustrious doctor Bian Que (also called Qin Yueren) in the fifth century B.C. According to the *Ci Yuan* encyclopedia, Bian Que is an invention of scholars living under the Han dynasty around the third century B.C. Whether from the fifth to the third centuries B.C. there were one or many Bian Que, the important fact remains that there is a work that is always referred to by this name, and this presupposes a doctor of great accomplishment.

The *Nan Jing,* "Classic of Difficulties," is attributed to Bian Que and is still used to this day. It attempts to clarify the most obscure parts of the *Nei Jing.*

Bian Que extracted and clarified the differences between the needles (still meaning the stone points?), which more easily disperse excess energy, and moxa, which more easily tonifies weakness, cold and rheumatism. The *Zi-Wu Jing,* "Rules of Midday and Midnight," was attributed to him around the sixth century B.C., probably apocryphally. It focuses for the first time on the alternating opposition between yin and yang, blood and energy, and night and day. His "Song of the Jade Dragon" *(Yu Long Fu)* is still used therapeutically.

Bian Que *(YXRM I, 29v)* was born in Cheng (present day Xin Cheng), in Henan near Kaifeng. He said happily that he could cure all but six illnesses: wealth that is too heavy for a person too light; pride, which holds reason in contempt; inability to earn a living; insufficiency of yin and of yang; emaciation to the extent that treatment cannot be supported; and, most of all, belief in sorcerers, which doubles the lack of faith in doctors.

The Third Century B.C. to the Third Century A.D.

Han Dynasty

No books about acupuncture have come to us from this long period of history. However, some great names are cited:

Chun Yuyi (between 179 and 156 B.C.) practiced the method of conducting energy *(dao yin fa)* without either tonifying or dispersing.

Wang Mang, who founded the short Xin dynasty from 35 to 8 B.C., carried out anatomical research. He executed three important people, Di Yi, Tang Gong and Sun Jing (among them a regent and a duke), and delivered their bodies to the doctors of the court for dissection.

> We measured and weighed their internal organs. With fine and flexible cane and bamboo, the vessels were traced and their beginning and end precisely determined. Thereafter treatments were improved utilizing the ideas thus perfected. (DACH I, 1v, quoting Zun Zhen Tu)

The genius Hua Tuo (Yuan Hua), born about A.D. 120 or 125, began as a wood cutter in his country of Pei, not far from Kaifeng. This occupation forbade the study of the classics and sciences.

> He practiced the method of conducting energy with needles and perfected the use of pulses. When prescribing medicines, he most often used infinitesimal doses, taking the diluted sweat from one of five domestic animals affected with the same disease as the patient. As for moxa, he applied it to no more than two places and not more than seven or eight times in each place. In needling, two places were sufficient and often only one. When the illness surpassed the action of needles or medicine, he gave a decoction of hemp **(ma fei san)** that made the patient drunk. Then he operated, opening the chest or abdomen and washing and repairing the intestines. He closed the wound and rubbed in an ointment that changed the pain into itching. For four or five days the patient was bedridden; in one month he was in full health. (YXRM I, 30r)

Resections of the spleen, cesareans and other operations were attributed to him. In addition, he wrote a study on medicinal plants, now lost to us. With one puncture of a needle he cured the emperor of Wei of severe headaches, vertigo, and heart trouble. When called upon a second time by the same emperor, Hua Tuo refused to go on the excuse that he was nearly one hundred years old. He was then killed by the messengers.

Zhang Zhongjing (Zhang Ji), whose name is often cited, wrote the *Jin Gui Yao Lue,* "The Essential Prescriptions of the Golden Chest," in the second century A.D.

The Third to Sixth Centuries

The *Jin* and *Wei* Dynasties

Two great advances were made in this period: a first attempt at precisely locating the acupoints, and most importantly, the improvement in diagnosis with palpation of the radial pulse.

Between 256 and 280 Huang-Fu Mi (Shi'an, Yuanyen, A.D. 215 - 282) published the *Jia Yi Jing,* "Rule of One and Five," also called *Zhen Jing,* "Book of Truth." The *Jia Yi Jing* is the first book concerned with the precise location of the points as well as the meridian's total number of points. In this work, the author comments on ancient books that are now lost. His text has been constantly consulted over the years. Its title, "Rule of One and Five," calls attention to the rule studied by the author that draws a correspondence between the organs that have their maximum energy in the first half-day with those that have their maximum energy in the second half-day. (The day was then divided into ten periods.) For example, if stimulated at its time of maximum energy — midnight — the gallbladder acts on the heart, which has its maximum energy at midday. If the heart is stimulated at midday, it then acts on the gallbladder. Huang-Fu Mi developed the rule of midday and midnight from the writings of Bian Que.

Wang Shuhe (fourth century) published his work on the radial pulses under the title *Mo Xue,* "Traditions About the Pulses," or *Mo Jing,* "Rule of the Pulse." It proved to be an essential work for acupuncture, since it perfected the ancient knowledge of the pulses, previously discussed by Bian Que and reputably used by Hua Tuo. The *Da Cheng* (VII, 8r) says: "During the Jin, Wang Shuhe, author of the *Mo Jing,* established the use of the radial pulses at a time when only the left and right carotid pulses were used." The *Ci Yuan* encyclopedia attributes the *Mo Jing* to the Song dynasty (tenth to eleventh centuries).

Ma Siming (Danyang), who lived in the fifth century, discovered several new points *(YIX I, 7v).*

The Sixth to the Tenth Centuries

The *Sui* and *Tang* Dynasties

This period of great national prosperity for China also saw a great development in acupuncture.

Sun Simo (585-682) "was revered . . . he used points for needles and moxa through palpating the pulses." *(DACH I, 2)* He is the author of two books, the *Qian Jin Fang,* "Prescriptions Worth a Thousand Gold Pieces" and *Qian Jin Yi Fang,* "Wings Added to the Prescriptions Worth a Thousand Gold Pieces." These texts include several important discussions: the reasons for not puncturing or burning certain points and the rules for conducting energy without tonifying or dispersing.

Yang Shangshan is often still referred to, although his books are now lost (q.v. bibliography).

Wang Bing, the leading court physician in 762, first became famous for his *Su Wen Ji Zhu,* "Commentaries on the *Su Wen,*" in which he discoursed on the authenticity, origin, substance and form of the *Su Wen.* Most significantly, however, he discovered the "rule of the five vehicles and the six energies," providing an etiology and classification of disease. The five vehicles are wind, dryness, warmth, humidity and cold. The six energies are:

1) Contractions "from shock" associated with the meridians of the liver and gallbladder.

2) The fires (panting, urinary troubles, diarrhea, tuberculosis, eruptions and abscesses) associated with the meridians of the heart and small intestine.

3) Indigestion and distention associated with the meridians of the stomach and spleen-pancreas.

4) Nervous and mental troubles associated with the pericardium and triple warmer meridians.

5) Desiccation and stoppage of function associated with the lung and large intestine.

6) Mucus coming from cold or dampness associated with the meridians of the kidney and urinary bladder.

Wang Tao, of the eighth century, selected 1104 prescriptions of medicine and acupuncture from ancient volumes, the *Wai Tai Bi Yao,* "Important Secrets Outside the Tower."

Zhen Chuan of the ninth century published a new "Rule of the Pulse," *Mai Jing,* which would suggest that the book of Wang Shuhe with the same title should not be attributed to the tenth century as some people presume. Zhen Chuan is also the author of two other books now lost (q.v. bibliography).

Ho Royu of the Southern Tang (937 - 975) in the south is cited for a lost book, *Ze Wu Liu Zhu Zhen Jing,* "The Rule of Needles, Midday-Midnight, Following and Opposing," in which he presents the rule of "following and opposing."

The Tenth to the Fourteenth Centuries

Song Dynasty

A remarkable blossoming of acupuncture occurred under this dynasty. We owe to this period the famous Bronze Man, the founding of a faculty of acupuncture and the printing and distribution of drawings and important works.

In 1027, Wang Weide[4] suggested to the Emperor the casting of a full-sized bronze statue showing all the points and their depths. Some smaller statues were cast for other palaces. (The statue from the Winter Palace is in the possession of the author in Paris.) Drawings were drafted and printed by wood block engraving, which had already been in use for two centuries. Wang Weide then published his "Rule of Needles and Moxa, and Points of the Bronze Man," *Tong Ren Shu Xue Zhen Jiu Jing.*

A university was organized in 1068 - 1086 for teaching acupuncture. Until then study depended on the *Tai Chang Si,* "Court of Supreme Constance," which studied and controlled all religions, researches into the unknown, science and astronomy.

Between 1102 and 1107, the vivisectionist Yang Jie (Jilao), had an opportunity which would have been impossible in Europe. To study the effects of acupuncture, verify the pulses, and so on, he vivisected condemned criminals. The local governor — in the interest of science — sent the criminals to him, instead of to the executioner, to be dismembered. Surrounded by secretaries and draughtsmen, he took notes, exposing a liver, for example, and observing it while puncturing all the points on the liver meridian, and so on. He published his studies in *Zun Zhen Tu,* "Drawings to Keep the Truth," which is still extant.

Hua Shou (Boren), of the thirteenth and fourteenth centuries, was perhaps the most famous of the Song dynasty acupuncturists. Born in Xu Cheng, he lived in Yu Yao, the lower valley of the Yangzi River. He cured mostly through the Triple Warmer meridian. He passed on to us the *Shi Si Jing Fa Hui,* "Sermons on the Fourteen Meridians," and the *Nan Jing Ben Yi,* an elaboration of the *Nan Jing* of Bian Que.

The emperors in those times were good acupuncturists and doctors. A story is told of the Emperor Ren Zong who, while walking with his prime minister met a pregnant woman. "A boy," said the emperor. "A girl," objected the minister. The emperor had the woman come to the palace and punctured her himself. She aborted under the needle; she had twins, a boy *and* a girl.

Chen Wenzhong (Wenxu), of the thirteenth century, was especially interested in the application of acupuncture to infants and noticed that massage of the acupoint almost always gave the same results as the needles. He published *Xiao Er An Mo Jing,* "Rule of Massage for Children," part of which is reproduced in the *Da Cheng.*

Li Gao (Dongyuan), a native of Zhenting, lived at the end of the Song dynasty and the beginning of the Yuan dynasty. A student of Zhang Yuansu, he somewhat surpassed his master. His judgements and indications are constantly referred to by later scholars. He left several works that combine acupuncture and medicine: *Lan Shi Bi Zang,* "The Secret of the Home of Orchids," and the *Pi Wei Lun,* "Dissertation on the Spleen and Stomach."

We still cite Dou Hanqing, who lived at the end of the thirteenth century. He was a critic of the *Su Wen* and author of the *Zhen Jiu Za Shuo,* which discusses the consciousness of man. Another scholar, Wang Shizhong, commented upon constitutional dispositions.

Fourteenth Century

Yuan Dynasty

Under the Mongols of the Yuan dynasty, acupuncture made even more progress.

Between 1314 and 1321, Du Sijing, a Chinese of reknown, published the *Ba Xue* or *Ji Sheng Ba Xue,* "The Graduate Who Helps to Live." In this text he refined the different doctrines, utilizing what had been most successful in his practice.

Houtai Bilie, a Mongol member of "The Forest of Brushes," discoursed on the "rule of following and opposing" *(liu zhu)* in his "Rule Next to the Golden Orchids," *Jin Lan Bian Jing,* published by his son in 1303.

The Fourteenth to Mid-Seventeenth Century

Ming Dynasty

The Ming dynasty is the period of great compilations of acupuncture and medicine, some being as large as 100 volumes. The *Gu Jin Yi Tong,* "Old and Modern Medical Generalities," by Xu Chunfu, in 100 volumes, was published in 1556. It was condensed to eight volumes by Li Chan (A.D. 1575) and published as *Yi Xue Ru Men,* "Door of Entry to Medical Studies." Both works contain many passages on acupuncture.

In the Wan-li period (1573-1620), Yang Gexian of Weijin[5] published the large compendium, *Zhen Jiu Da Cheng,* "The Great Perfection of the Needles and Moxa." This text cites numerous passages from books since the *Nei Jing,* but without sufficient criticism.

Yang Jishi (Jizhou), doctor of the Supreme Court of Medicine in 1573-1620, published the *Zhen Jiu Da Quan,* "Great Compilation of Needles and Moxas," a summary compiled during the Mongol period and already considered a rare treasure.[6]

There was also some private research published:

Chen Hui (Shantong) with his student Liu Jin published the *Shen Ying Jing,* "Classic of Answers from Awareness," in 1425-6. Li Shizhen (Tongpi) published "Examination of the Eight Marvellous Vessels of the Meridians," *Qi Jing Ba Mo Kao,* in 1573-1620. Gao Wu (Meihu of Xiaming) published the *Ju Ying,* "Florilegium," or *Zhen Jiu Ju Ying,* "Florilegium of Needles and Moxa."

The Mid-Seventeenth Century to Our Day

Qing Dynasty and the Republic

This is the period of mnemonic aids and one or two volume summaries. It is also the time of a scientific renaissance, particularly within Japanese scholarship.

In 1798, Li Shouxian published *Yi Xue* or *Zhen Jiu Yi Xue,* "The Easy Study of Needles and Moxa" in three volumes. In 1919, a group of doctors published the *Yi Zhi* or *Zhen Jiu Yi Zhi,* "Easy Knowledge of Needles and Moxa," in one volume. In 1937, Doctor Fang Zun'an of Shanghai published a very interesting book — bound in the European manner — the *Jin Zhen Bi Yao,* "Important Secrets of the Golden Needles." He gives quotations and criticisms of ancient texts, and presents new drawings. He discusses principal symptoms of the points, but does not offer any treatments. Following the style of his master Huang Shiping, he punctured through the clothes, a method also used in Japan.

In Japan

Not to give mention to Japanese studies would be to give an incomplete history. No doubt, Japanese medicine comes directly from Chinese science.

The history of the origin of medicine in Japan is scarce. Only two names of practitioners are given with no fixed chronology of their lives. In A.D. 443, the Japanese Emperor Yinkyo invited several doctors from Korea, where Chinese civilization and thus acupuncture flourished. In 608, the Emperor Suiko sent an official delegation of medical students to the Chinese court of the Tang dynasty. The official introduction of Chinese methods into Japan dates from this period with the introduction into Japan of arts, science and literature. In Japan from the sixth through the eighteenth centuries there is frequent mention of students being sent to China.

However, in this as in all things, the Japanese did not adopt as imitators, but as masters: they adapted Chinese knowledge to their own climate and race. Because of illnesses due to the humidity of Japan and the fish-rich diet, they especially developed the art of moxa. This is in contrast to Northern China, where a dry climate made the use of needles more suitable.

When the Dutch introduced European medicine to Japan in the eighteenth century, the Japanese studied it with lively interest and perspicacity. In a book on European anatomy published at that time by Mitani Koki it was remarked:

> As Western medicine studies more and more detail, it moves further away from the real aim of its research. . . . Their studies of the human body concern only the cadaver. They do not inform us about the living, the only true aim of medical studies.

In 1884, Japan decided to adopt European medical science to protect its own civilization from that of the West. A law established the founding of European-style medical universities that did not include the teaching of Chinese medicine. Oriental medicine, however, remained highly honored, for emperors from the earliest times maintained practitioners of Chinese medicine and acupuncture as their chief doctors.

The students of the Chinese method continued to intern with practitioners who taught traditionally, while the students of the European method learned their lessons at the European-style medical schools. Those first students of the 1884 medical universities became masters of their art. Many of them acquired a world reputation and are referred to in Western scientific texts. Noguchi, Kitazato, Takamine, Nagaoka, Ikeno, Hata and Yoshida are some of the people whose discoveries our students are required to quote. However, the new doctors of the European style observed that their science failed or was slow in many cases that were easily and instantly cured by doctors of the Chinese method. Also, the accidents and problems caused by numerous and varied vaccinations provoked true public fear. The most valued tools of analysis — X-rays, etc. — made many patients recoil. The doctors of the School of the Court (traditional Chinese medicine) saw a new rise in patients and students.

Doctor Nakayama (Tyotoku), who wrote important works on this subject (see *Acuponcture et Médecine Chinoise Vérifiées au Japon,* Trianon, 1934), reports:

> Many doctors of the Chinese style had disappeared in the forty years following the reform. But curiously, the modern doctors who practice the European method — enemies and vanquishers of the traditional doctors — have recently begun to add the two words ''Chinese Method'' or ''Chinese Medicine'' to the words ''Doctor of European Medicine'' on their signboards. In short, we are on the point of recognizing the superiority of the persecuted and suppressed medicine.

From that time onwards, the doctors of the European method used Western laboratory methods to rigorously study the effects of needles and moxa as well as Chinese herbs. The conclusions resulted in an increasingly marked return to Chinese science. Several important books were published.

Among the masters of this renaissance are Dr. Takamori (Mino-Suke), Dr. Nakayama, and Tatse-i, whose books are authoritative. Dr. Hara studied and published the results of his experiments on moxa on humans and rabbits. There is also the illustrious Dr. Sawada.

Modern China

The Japanese studies of the last twenty years, using Western laboratory methods, have caused a considerable renaissance of acupuncture within China. Thus, in Canton, a southern city traditionally known to have a keen interest in medicine and cultural exchange, particularly with India, there were hardly a dozen acupuncturists thirty years ago. A recent investigation counted 1250.[7] Shanghai has become an important center of acupuncture. Dr. Fang Zun'an, a student of Dr. Huang Shiping, has published a book that has served significantly in the dissemination of this method. The north and the northwest, cradle of the first Chinese, have never stopped practicing acupuncture. Even the interest taken by France in this study has had happy repercussions on its rebirth in China.

A collection of 1936 includes four books on acupuncture.

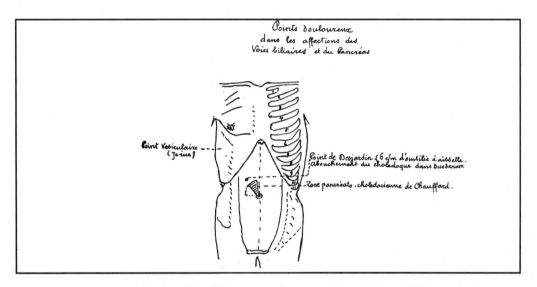

Painful points in afflictions of the biliary duct and the pancreas

Notes

[1] See footnote 2, page 8.

[2] Question marks with or without expressions in parentheses are present in the French edition. These have been retained in this translation. Although the author does not state their purpose, they appear to indicate suppositions about which the author was uncertain. — ed.

[3] As a matter of fact, the phraseology, method of dividing the day into time periods, and system of yearly cycles mentioned in the *Nei Jing* all date it to the late Qin - early Han period, ca. 300 - 200 B.C. There is no evidence that the Chinese had any system of writing at all in 3000 B.C., although there is some archaeological evidence that stone needles were being used at that early date. — ed.

[4] So referred to in the original *Zhen Jiu Da Cheng.* Generally known as Wang Weiyi. — ed.

[5] See footnote 2, page 8.

[6] There was evidently some confusion on the author's part regarding the authorship of the *Da Cheng* and the *Da Quan.* The latter book is generally considered to be the work of Xu Feng, and was written much earlier, ca. 1437.

[7] This information is surprising to many modern readers who are familiar with the widely reported post-revolution renaissance of acupuncture that followed changes in Chinese health care policy in the early 1950's. However, the lack of acupuncturists in Canton is confirmed by other contemporaneous reports. Tin Yao So, for example, reports only one acupuncturist in Canton in 1930. He attributes an increase in acupuncturists to the opening of an acupuncture college in 1934. See the Introduction to: James Tin Yao So, *The Book of Acupuncture Points,* Paradigm Publications, Brookline Massachusetts, 1984. — ed.

Chapter I
The Points

Designation

The word for acupuncture points has not always been the same. In ancient times the ideogram that represented them consisted of the elements "flesh-submission-assent," giving the idea of "command of the flesh." Two pronunciations are given for the old ideogram: The *Nei Jing (Ling Shu I, 1st line),* using the system that takes the first part of one word and the end of the other, gives *q(un)-yu,* or *qi-yu* or *qu.* The *Ci Yuan* encyclopedia gives *sh(u)-yu* or *shi-yu* or *shu.* The modern term, used since the thirteenth century, is *xue,* which means "entry of cavern; hollow," the ideogram in effect suggesting the entry into a cavern. Indeed, all points are at the bottom of a hollow, or pit.

The Japanese often refer to them by two terms, old and modern: *shu-xue.* Sometimes in China they are called *jing-xue,* "meridian points."

The Established Facts

The Chinese texts mention only two important facts, often used and easily observed. The correlations that follow from them seem worth describing as they have also been observed in Paris.

1) The first fact is as follows: Specific organ dysfunctions stimulate consistent reactions in a very limited number of points on the body. This manifests in a sensitivity like a recent contusion, bruise, or black and blue spot, which then disappears when the dysfunction is resolved.

We should add that this sensitivity is generally ignored by the patient and is only revealed by finger pressure on the exact point. Some sensitive patients feel them, however, even without being touched, and call the attention of the doctor to them. Physical types, athletes, and manual laborers rarely feel them. This point sensitivity is greater in patients inclined to be nervous or intellectual, or if the condition is very serious.

The above is a physiological discovery of great importance. Research done in Japan and France has yet to satisfactorily explain this peripheral, cutaneous expression so precisely related to internal troubles.

2) The second fact observed by the ancient Chinese, also very easy to verify, is the following: any action taken on these sensitive points immediately causes a return to normalcy in the function of the organ connected to the point or the part of the body that the point commands. This result may be temporary or permanent and is in proportion to the action taken and the sensitivity of the patient. This physiological discovery, theoretically as significant as the first, has practical importance, for there are many patients who can be immediately relieved of their ailments. This phenomenon can occur either distally on an organ or part of the body, or locally on muscle, nerve or bone.

At a distance, the point acts either on the internal organ or on a group of muscles that are related to a particular meridian. For example, points on the foot or the knee act on the liver, while points in the popliteal crease and on the foot treat lumbar pain that is related to the bladder meridian. The needling of points distal to the problem is considered true acupuncture, since it works systemically to treat the cause. It gives long-lasting, deep effects.

Treating at the area of the problem, whether it be muscles, bones, nerves, pains, inflammations, contractions or weakness, is considered local action. It is generally less effective and more temporary than action at a distance.

The explanations for these two types of actions are necessarily different. For distal action, we cite the work of Rudolph Arndt, which has established that a sick organ reacts to a weak stimulus while a healthy organ remains insensitive. This helps us understand how a stimulus as weak as that of a needle can provoke a powerful response. Dr. Cornelius of Berlin (*Nervenpunkte,* Leipzig, 1909) has observed the heightened sensitivity of points in certain afflictions. He posits that this sensitivity is due to the edema of connective tissue pressing on the microscopic ramifications of cutaneous nervous filaments.

Thus far observed, these points only act directly on the dysfunction, not the lesion. The lesion, however, can be repaired as much as possible by the body itself when functioning properly. Therefore, there is an indirect action on the lesion which may be significant.

Utility of These Observed Facts

Since antiquity the Chinese have observed the above facts. The result of this has been a focus on the study of energy and physiology rather than on chemistry or the microbe. (Nonetheless, the tuberculosis microbe was referred to in a sixteenth century book, deduced or observed by means of a powerful magnifying lens of rock crystal.) Generally, the Chinese medical system has been oriented towards strengthening the body's defenses and perfecting the bodily terrain.

The basis of acupuncture is in the double action of the points: peripheral expression of dysfunctions and centripetal command on the organs or local parts of the body. With knowledge of these points alone, it is possible to obtain a high percentage of cures. But this is only the most material part of the doctrine.

One must have thorough knowledge of the meridians in order to comprehend and differentiate the points and their possibilities. To use the points intelligently, one must study the circulation of energy. Ultimately, this circulation can only be controlled and verified through the knowledge of the pulses. It is irresponsible to judge the possibilities of acupuncture only on the basis of a few points whose actions are learned by heart and used blindly.

Location of the Points

Localization on the surface.

The great majority of failures result from error in locating the acupoint. A difference of one or two millimeters is enough to give a null response, especially where the needle is off the meridian. Therefore, it is of paramount importance to locate the exact center of the point.

In regard to this, we must say that the Chinese indications are imprecise. In fact, they are obviously memory devices. They are based on the Chinese system of measurement, the *cun* (see Appendix II). The length of the *cun* is related to the patient and starts from vague points of reference. Modern Japanese descriptions are slightly more exact and give some references to the muscles.

To take into account the differences seen among human beings, it is critical to describe precisely the anatomical placements of the points. This research has revealed a constant relationship of each point with the bony structure. Thus my drawings show simultaneously the bones, muscles and skin, by means of a formula unknown to anatomists in general.

I have observed four phenomena that allow us to locate the point exactly and to determine its meridian:

1) All the points are at the bottom of a small cupule, hollow or depression. With muscle, the finger first encounters a cupule, then after the finger rests on the point for a moment the bottom of the cupule opens a little. The Chinese assign all hollows on the lateral surface of the limbs to the yang points.

2) When the point is pressed, the patient feels a slight pain radiating at least a centimeter in diameter. This area is much more painful than the surrounding tissue when pricked with the needle. At the precise center of the point, though, there is little or no pain from the tip of the needle. (A worthwhile experiment is to puncture oneself.)

3) When brushing lightly with the finger (particularly the sensitive ring finger) the skin of the surrounding area appears normal; but, at the acupoint, the finger perceives a roughness and stickiness.

4) On repeatedly tapping with the nail on an acupoint, sensitive people (particularly if unclothed) will notice an effect along part of or the whole length of the associated meridian. By pressing on the center of the point an effect can be noticed on the pulse of that organ and within the related organ itself. When first applying this, I used the Chinese method — sliding the dorsal side of the nail along the area and when the patient reports pain, making a line with the nail, then sliding again, making a cross. In this way it is possible to determine the point quite well.

Then the idea came to me to replace the use of the fingernail with a rounded rod about the size of a small pencil. I observed that the tip of the rod slipped to the bottom of the hollow. On crossing again I had only to press the tip of the rod to obtain a mark at the center of the point. From that time on, our successes were more numerous and complete.

The best general advice given by the Chinese is that of the *Da Cheng:*

> *The yang points (on lateral surfaces) are found at hollows and next to the bones. Upon pressing, you find numbness and sensitivity (**suan ma**). This is the true point. All yin points (on the medial surfaces) are over arteries. Press until an artery is felt under the finger. This is the true point. (DACH II, 23; V, 26r)*

Location of depth.

We have also improved upon tradition in locating the depths of the points.

For each point the Chinese have given an exact depth described in tenths of the variable *cun* (see Appendix II). These depths were taken from the ''Bronze Man'' made in the eleventh century. However, all the texts do not agree because of printing errors or other reasons. The considerable differences in individual skin thickness greatly alter the depths of the points. In referencing the ancient texts, these general indications are given as follows:

First, skin thickness varies at different parts of the body:

> *For all the points at the top of the body and close to the bones, it is advisable that the needle enter shallowly and cauterization with moxa be slight. For all the points at the bottom of the body where the flesh is thick, the needle can enter deeply without danger and cauterization can be used generously. (YXRM I, 46v)*

Second, there are differences between thin and fat people:

> *Fat people are empty of energy inside. One must enter deeply. Thin people are full of energy inside. It is enough to needle superficially. (DACH V, 10v)*

Third, the occupation and lifestyle of the patient may alter the needle depth:

> *Sensitive people are frail; one must act superficially and quickly. Ordinary people are coarse and resistant; one must act deeply, strongly, and for a long time. (DACH I, 13r; II, 27v)*

Fourth, the length of the disease:

> *The older the illness, the more deeply one must needle. (DACH)*

The depths given are taken from the Bronze Man, starting from one tenth of a *cun* (about 2 mm. for the average adult) for the fingers to eight tenths (about 1.8 cm.) for the thighs and lower limbs. The depths on the fingers vary little between thin and fat people; those for the thighs vary from a minimum of 4 or 5 mm. to a maximum of 1.8 cm. Given these variations, one may ask in which part of the subcutaneous tissue the point is found.

For a time, Dr. Ferreyrolles attached importance to the ability of moxa to warm superficially and concluded that the points were in the cutaneous tissue itself. But in using needles, we can see that the points are deeper since the needles pass through the derma and the adipose layer (differing in fat and thin people) to reach the subcutaneous tissue.

I have made a few observations that will help to locate the required depth:

In order to stimulate *gaohuangshu* (BL-38, IS BL-43),[1] the Chinese insist on the necessity of separating the shoulder blades by arching the back. In this position the shoulder blades slip between the endoderm and both the subcutaneous tissue and the aponeurosis of the costal muscles. The point is found on the superior surface of the fourth rib and the patient feels a sharp pain on pressure. When the shoulder blade is returned to its natural position, the point is covered over. Now on pressure, the patient feels a diminished pain, although it is still transmitted. Other points can be examined in this manner. Consequently, the points must be in the subcutaneous tissue or more probably the aponeurosis of the muscles, for otherwise the epidermis or dermis itself (although extremely sensitive) would respond to the stimulation.

As mentioned, the dissections done in 1935 by the surgeon Perretti Della Rocca in the presence of Mr. Rouvierre, Professor of Anatomy at the University of Paris, did not reveal any special anatomical formations under the points. It must be a matter of physiology, probably a special function of certain nerve fibers.

Number and Classification of the Points

There are two categories of points: *ding* or *jing xue,* "fixed" or "meridian" points, and *tong zhong xue,* "center of pain points," also called *bu ding xue,* "unfixed points," or *tian ying xue,* "naturally responding points."

The "fixed" or "meridian" points are divided into several groups:

Those of the twelve meridians, which are bilateral. Chinese authors do not completely agree on their total number. Some points are included in other categories. As far as it was possible for me to verify by pressure on the meridian, the total number of points by meridian are as follows:

Heart..............	9	x	2	=	18
Small Intestine	19	x	2	=	38
Bladder...........	67	x	2	=	134
Kidney.............	27	x	2	=	54
Heart Governor..........9		x	2	=	18
Triple Warmer	23	x	2	=	46
Gallbladder......	44	x	2	=	88
Liver..............	14	x	2	=	28
Lung	11	x	2	=	22
Large Intestine.	20	x	2	=	40
Stomach	45	x	2	=	90
Spleen..............	21	x	2	=	42
Total	309	x	2	=	618

Those of the medial line which are by tradition unilateral:

Conception Vessel:	24
Governor Vessel:	27

The points called "extra meridian points" or "marvellous extra meridian points," jing wai qi xue. The *Da Cheng* gives 34 names; however, some of these points are single, others bilateral or multiple, so the total is 88 (see *Da Cheng* VIII).

The new Chinese and Japanese points. The numbers and locations sometimes vary with the author. Some of these points appear to be on meridians. The total number does not exceed 14 bilateral points.

The grand total is thus:

12 Meridians	309	x	2	=	618
	51	x	1	=	51
Extra Meridian Points	34	x	2	=	68
New Points	14	x	2	=	28
Total				=	765

The *Nei Jing* gives a total of 365 points for the twelve meridians and two median vessels, analogous with the 365 days of the solar year. The *Da Cheng* gives 298 points bilaterally for the 12 meridians and the *Yi Xue Ru Men* gives 338. They both agree regarding the total number of points on the median vessels.

As for the "unfixed points" or "center of pain points" or "naturally responding points," they are described as follows:

> *Drive the nail of the thumb into the point. If the patient changes color, groans, grinds the teeth or has an unbearable pain, it is the "center of pain" or "naturally responding" point. The needle will cause "extreme pain." [A note in this passage describes the unfixed points as "places of pain,"* **tong chu.***] (YIX I, 5r)*

The unfixed points show a center of contusion and/or a partial contraction of muscle as from the swelling of a sting. They sometimes overlap with what is considered a fixed point. They are particularly sought for by those who do not practice true acupuncture.

Curative Effects of Points

Some books give a list of problems that can be cured by appropriate stimulation of each point. These lists are very long and astonish Western doctors by the fact that the point not only acts on the organ of its meridian but also on several other organs. Moreover, for a given organ, Chinese medicine observes many more symptoms than does European medicine. Thus, it is rare that a patient presents all the described symptoms for a given ailment. Some symptoms listed by the Chinese are primary for a disease and some are secondary in occurrence.

For example, in cholecystitis — treated by *yangfu* (GB-38) — the bitter taste in the mouth in the morning is a primary symptom while swellings behind the knee in the popliteal crease are secondary and very rare.

Chinese and Japanese texts do not clearly differentiate between primary and secondary symptoms nor do they specifically point out the indications that a single point alone can cure. Identifying these distinctions is another contribution that my book brings to acupuncture, the importance of which is obvious (q.v. Volume IV).

The Name of Each Point

The points have been given names since antiquity. Different names have been used in successive periods and different regions so that certain points are concurrently referred to by several names. Although these names are well chosen, they have never before been cross-indexed to make it possible to identify a given name. I had to do this work in order to facilitate research in the original texts.

Some of these names reflect the anatomical position of the point. For example *hegu* (LI-4), "bottom of the valley," is used because the point is found in the angle formed by the first two metacarpals. Other names suggest the action exerted, such as *fuliu* (KI-7), "arising again," since that point stimulates kidney secretions. Names are also given in reference to the common use of the body part the point is on. Thus, *shaoshang* (LU-11), "lesser bargaining," describes a point situated under the arching phalanx of the thumb which in China was raised to indicate the minimum sum asked for during bargaining.

This book retains the more usual Chinese names and gives their meaning in Volume IV. Use of their translated names within the text would be too lengthy or would appear absurd. I have chosen not to use the numbers assigned to the names since they are not easily memorized.[2] Although the Chinese point names sound unusual, they are the standard used and allow all Europeans to continue my work.

In most of the drawings, certain points bear a special designation along with their name. Thus we find:

1)   The characters *jing, rong, shu, jing, he.* These are the ancient names of the points situated at the extremities of the limbs (see Volume II).

2)   The character *yuan,* "source." This indicates a special action on both the excess and emptiness of the organ (see Volume II).

3)   The indications of the five elements: Wood, Fire, Earth, Metal, Water. Each either creates or controls its neighbor.

4)   The words "tonify" and "disperse." These indicate the dominant action of the point on a meridian's associated organ.

5)   The "crossing and reunion points" *(jiao hui).* These are found on the main meridians and eight marvellous vessels (see Volume II).

6)   The "reunion points." These are meeting points of meridians or parts of the body (see Volume II).

What Do the Points Connote to the Chinese?

The *Ci Yuan* encyclopedia describes the acupoints as being "important, sensitive areas of the human body." The *Da Cheng* qualifies them as "guardians of the frontiers."

> *Whether on the face, the sides, front or back, energy and blood have more than six hundred "guardians of the frontiers." This means that energy and blood circulate in the body through the meridians and secondary vessels by moving across hollow spaces (**kong xue**); this occurs regardless of the position the person assumes. The **rong** (yin energy)[3] circulating inside the vessels passes into more than three hundred "guardians of the frontiers." The **wei** (yang energy) circulating outside the vessels passes into more than three hundred "guardians of the frontiers." (DACH II, 20v)*

It seems that with this as in other areas, the Chinese focus more on practicality than on useless explanation.

Relationships of the Points to European Knowledge

Even though the existence and action of the acupoints have been ignored in Europe, researchers could not fail to observe, at least in small part, what the Chinese diagnosticians observed. On close observation we can see that many acupoints, along with part of their action, were known in Europe. We must distinguish between points that become painful with internal ailments and those stimulated to obtain a centripetal action in an internal organ.

Points becoming painful with an internal problem.

Points of Weihe: In 1903, Weihe, a German homeopath, published a list of points that he had gradually discovered to become painful following an intoxicating dosage of a remedy or poison. Since the symptoms of intoxication from a particular remedy corresponded to those cured by a homeopathic dose of that remedy, he named each point after its associated remedy.

His knowledge of the points came to him from a relative in China, but his genius was in looking for and experimenting with the connections between the points and the homeopathic remedies. This proves that there is an action of the same order in both sciences.

An issue of *Homéopathie Francaise* (October 15, 1932) introduced these points to France. The drawings in that issue were not precise enough to readily allow exact location of the points, and the accompanying text contradicts the drawings in many cases. As a result, it was not possible for me to compare all the locations of the points of Weihe with the Chinese points. However, a large number of the points of Weihe fall so exactly in the same place as Chinese points that one is led to surmise that the others also correspond to the Chinese points.

In 1929 we observed, with Dr. Ferreyrolles, correlations of both the location and the action of certain points of Weihe to the Chinese points. We published our results in *Homéopathie Francaise* (June, 1929). These correlations were later pursued by Dr. de la Fuye and Dr. Bonnet-Lemaire, who published their results in *Homéopathie Moderne* (June 15, 1936).

Certain ailments described in homeopathic symptomatology and unnoticed in the Chinese lists have been treated by needling the indicated points of Weihe and have been immediately cured (generally more rapidly than with the homeopathic remedy).

The third part of this book will list the symptoms of the points of Weihe that seem to correspond to Chinese points. A comparison with homeopathic repertories will then be possible.

Renal points of Guyon, et al. Guyon, Albarman, Bazy, and in particular Pasteau observed that in renal diseases pressure on certain very localized points elicited sharp pain. However, these points were used only for diagnosis. The thought did not occur to the observers to study the reflex action, i.e., to puncture the points.

a)   Intercostal point: at the end of and at the elongation of the tenth rib, immediately in front of and below the costal rim.

b)   Point at the level of the umbilicus or above the ureter: on a horizontal line passing through the umbilicus immediately outside the abdominal muscles; corresponding to the lower abdominal area.

c)   Medial ureteral point: on a horizontal line across the abdomen connecting the anterior superior iliac spines at the level of the third external part, at the places of entry of the ureters into the pelvis.

d)   Lateral sub-iliac point: one centimeter above the middle of the iliac crease. A point with distal effect.

22

e)   The iliac sub-intraspinous point: immediately below and inside the anterior superior iliac spine. Pasteau considers this the most distinctive of the renal points. Pressure on it stimulates the femoral cutaneous nerve and by reflex action indicates kidney disease.

f)   Inguinal point: external orifice of the inguinal canal.

g)   Dorsal costovertebral point: at the angle of the last rib and the vertebral column.

h)   Dorsal costomuscular point: at the level of the angle formed by the last rib and the mass of the sacrolumbar muscles.

Points of Dejardin and Chauffard: Situated on the epigastrium. These points are for diagnosis of biliary or pancreatic disease. Only one point is used in China for the treatment of these diseases.

Painful points of the right hypochondrium, discovered by Martinet: These confirm the diagnosis of different diseases. The connections with the Chinese points are not clearly shown and the European indications are not accurate.

The sciatic points of Valleix: Most are Chinese points for the treatment of sciatica. Valleix noted them only for diagnostic purposes. Only two are unrecognized.

European points used for treatment.

Points of Wetterwald: In his book *Les Nevralgies* (Vigot: Paris, 1910), Dr. F. Wetterwald quotes Dr. Cornelius of Berlin, who published *Nervenpunkte* (Thieme: Leipzig, 1909). They recommend the massage of points that have become sensitive in certain diseases; almost all these points are Chinese points. They posit that the pain may be due from edema of the connective tissue pressing on the microscopic ramifications of the cutaneous nerve nets. According to these authors, since only the skin is sensitive, the treatment consists of cutaneous massage.

These points are different from Chinese points. Although they distinguished some centrifugal points (giving sensitive and sensory effects) and some centripetal points (giving motor, vasomotor and sensory effects) they add that the centrifugal points can only be made evident by the stimulation of the centripetal point to which they are always connected.

Points for electrical stimulation of muscles: Almost all correspond to Chinese points in location and use. The instructions and drawings do not always agree. A work of precise identification would be useful to both acupuncture and electrostimulation. This work would verify whether points of electrostimulation are effective because they are Chinese points and if the non-Chinese points would give an effect when treated with needles and moxa.

Vertebral reflexes of Abrams: Abrams discovered that an action (bump or some other kind) on certain vertebrae stimulated a special reflex. For example, action on the sixth cervical vertebra augments the function of the parathyroids; action taken on the fifth dorsal dilates the pyloric sphincter, etc.

Most of these actions correspond to Governor Vessel points situated between the vertebrae. Some of the points of Abrams do not exist for the Chinese, e.g., the sixth cervical. Interestingly, the stimulation of the sixth cervical vertebra with the needle seems to give results. It would be of great interest to complete each system by the other.

The *Nei Jing* (quoted in *DACH* I, 3v) gives a list of fevers cured by the stimulation of one or the other of the first seven dorsal vertebrae.

Jiujitsu points for knockout or death: Most of these points are Chinese points.

Kuatsu points for resuscitation: The Japanese method of resuscitation depends on the action of certain Chinese points.

a)   For knockout by blow to the throat, sides, abdomen, or the solar plexus: with the patient lying with arms uncrossed, strike several times with an erect palm, sliding from the umbilicus *juguan* (CV-14) and *jiuwei* (CV-15).

b)   For grave knockout, strangling or sunstroke: with the patient lying face down, strike several times with an erect palm, sliding upward over the seventh cervical vertebra and the point *bailao* (GV-13, IS GV-14, *dazhui*).

c)   For a blow to the testicles: give a sharp blow midway between the internal malleolus and the metatarsophalangeal articulation of the big toe at *gongsun* (SP-4). Then, with the patient lying on his back, strike the superior external border of the pubis, at *qichong* (ST-30).

d)   For cerebral stroke: kneel down behind the patient, who is seated on the ground; with the knuckles of the fist strike *jianjing* (GB-21), midway between the neck and the outer tip of the shoulder. Then, with the tips of the fingers drum vigorously on the transverse processes — at *tianding* (LI-17) and *tianzhu* (BL-10) — from top to bottom and back again. Next, press and quickly release the fingers placed on the temples and on the hairline at the level of the eyebrows and eyes — at *hanyan* (GB-4), *xuanlu* (GB-5), and *xuanli* (GB-6).

e)   For attacks of the heart, brain or testicles: with the patient lying face down, strike *mingmen* (GV-4) with the heel of the palm moving upward between the second and third lumbar vertebrae. Then massage with the thumbs on either side of this interval — at *shenshu* (BL-23). If it is serious, strike repeatedly with the middle finger on *mingmen* (GV-4).

f)   For drowning: strike *mingmen* (GV-4) repeatedly between the second and third lumbar vertebrae.

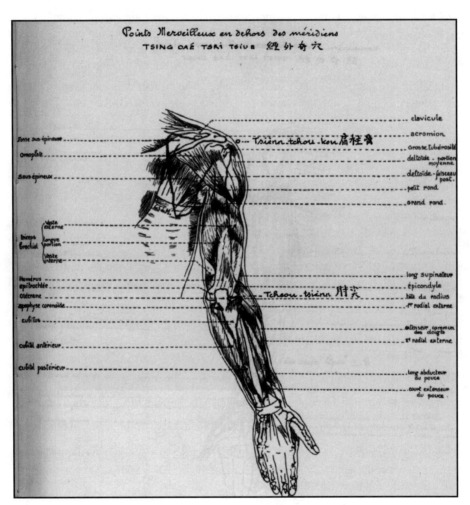

Marvellous points outside the meridians (upper limb)

Notes

[1] ''IS'' indicates the ''International Standard,'' which is the point numbering system in current use. — ed.

[2] The point numbers have been added to the English edition to conform with standard practice. — ed.

[3] The word *rong* was used in the earliest texts to denote yin energy or blood. It is synonymous with, and was later replaced by, the word *ying,* which occurs in later texts. The French edition of this book has *iong,* which is a variant pronunciation of *rong.* — ed.

Chapter II
The Twelve Meridians

Knowledge of the meridians *(jing)*, or lines of points, is an essential foundation for true acupuncture. Without it, it is impossible to understand the circulation of energy. The meridians give us an understanding of the relationships among the organs and help us to classify and analyze the effects of a point. From this knowledge alone, however, deep-seated problems cannot be comprehensively treated; only with the exact management of the vital energy can this be accomplished.

Names of the Meridians

The *Yi Xue Ru Men* explains (I, 1r): "The meridians *(jing)* are the longitudinal paths." The ideogram used to describe these lines of points is formed by the elements "string-line-right-winding-work," the idea being a string connecting a winding alley into a path. From the most ancient times, the term *"jing"* was used in astronomy for the lines of north-south longitude. It is still used in the countryside for the north-south paths of a field.

The pronunciation *jing* has not changed since antiquity. The British transliteration is "ching" while the old French transliteration is "king." Sometimes the name *"jingluo,"* pronounced *"keiraku"* in Japanese, is used.

Observed Phenomena

Although the phenomena described below are not as easily observed as those given for the points, sensitive people always report them. Physical types (manual laborers) do not perceive them as well.

The observations are as follows:

1)   If an organ is dysfunctioning and a specific series of points and no others are sensitive, these points are located on one line.

2)   In sensitive people, the line of points is slightly painful to the touch along its entire length. Sometimes an area is painful enough to mistakenly indicate a point at a place where the meridian only passes over a bone or tendon.

3)   A large number of the sensitive-type patients report the feeling of "something" passing at the moment of puncture. They trace the feeling along a line that is identical to the pathway of the meridian from the stimulated point.

4)   This "something" is always reported as passing in the same direction.

5)   The sensitivity of the line and the points is reduced when the organ returns to normal function.

6)   The respective meridian and points of a healthy organ have a daily two-hour period of maximal activity.

The observations given above are noted in Chinese texts but not in a precise or comprehensive manner. The *Da Cheng* (I, 9r) states: "When the ache is located in the organ, the meridian is ill as a result and becomes painful. All this occurs simultaneously and leaves simultaneously."

Numbers, Names and Groupings of Meridians

A single organ has a right and left meridian, both of which become painful when the organ is troubled. For the single organs, the sensitivity of the two meridians is usually equal. The exception to this is the gallbladder: the left meridian is always more sensitive. In the case of double organs, such as the kidneys, pain in the right meridian indicates disease in the right organ; pain in the left meridian, the left organ. For the liver, the left meridian corresponds to the anterior lobes and the right meridian to the posterior lobes.

Most authors list twelve meridians: those of the ten internal organs, the triple warmer (a command of functions) and the heart governor (which acts on the circulation and sexuality).[1] However, Hua Shou (Boren, thirteenth century), among others, objects to there being only twelve meridians, arguing that the conception and governor vessels have special points of their own and thus form meridians. (The conception and governor vessels are generally grouped with the Eight Marvellous Vessels.) Hua Shou's book is entitled *Elucidation of the Fourteen Meridians.*

In fact, the circulation of energy of the conception and governor vessels is independent of the cyclic course of energy in the organ meridians. Additionally, these vessels do not command any single organ as do the other meridians. Yet, they do have functions. The upper part of the conception vessel acts on the respiratory functions, the middle part on the digestive function, and the lower part on the urogenital functions. The governor vessel is less specialized. These two vessels have points that are specific to them, while the other six marvellous vessels borrow all their points from the twelve organ meridians. In order to keep these distinctions clear, they will be described after the twelve organ meridians. The remaining six marvellous vessels are described in Volume II.

There are two distinct names given to each meridian. One name is derived from the organ to which it is related; for example, the meridian associated with the liver is *gan jing,* ''liver meridian.'' The other name derives from the meridian's position as one of the three yin or yang of the foot or three yin or yang of the hand. In the case of the liver, the name is *zu jueyin,* ''inversion of yin of the foot.''

The three yang of the hand and foot are classified as: *tai yang* (supreme yang); *shao yang* (lesser yang); and *yang ming* (sunlight yang). The three yin of the hand and foot are classified as: *tai yin* (supreme yin); *shao yin* (lesser yin); and *jue yin* (inversion of yin). The twelve meridian names are as follows:

1) On the back of the hand and lateral aspect of the arm up the neck to the head:

    Small Intestine: *xiaochang jing, shou taiyang.*
    Triple Warmer: *sanjiao jing, shou shaoyang.*
    Large Intestine: *dachang jing, shou yangming.*

2) On the palm of the hand and medial aspect of the arm up to the chest:

    Lung: *fei jing, shou taiyin.*
    Heart Governor: *xinzhu jing or xinbao jing, shou jueyin.*
    Heart: *xin jing, shou shaoyin.*

3) From head to foot, posterior, lateral anterior surfaces of the lower limb:

    Urinary Bladder: *pangguang jing, zu taiyang.*
    Gallbladder: *dan jing, zu shaoyang.*
    Stomach: *wei jing, zu yangming.*

4) Medial surface of the lower limb from foot to chest:

    Kidneys: *shen jing, zu shaoyin.*
    Spleen-pancreas: *pi jing, zu taiyin.*
    Liver: *gan jing, zu jueyin.*

The yang meridians of the foot and hand are connected with the yang organs — the *fu* or ''workshop organs'' — which take food from the outside and transform it into energy and blood. They mostly control energy. They are reflected on the superficial, yang level of the radial pulse.

The yin meridians of the foot and hand are in relationship with the yin organs — the *zang* or ''treasure organs'' — which control the purity of the blood and its circulation. They are reflected at the deep, yin level of the radial pulse.

Direction of Flow of Energy in the Meridians

As previously indicated, every sensitive person perceives ''something'' passing along the meridian when they are punctured at a painful point. This feeling always travels in the same direction.

The yang meridians of the hand always flow from the upper extremities to the head. The yang meridians of the foot always flow from the head toward the lower limbs. For the yin of the hand, the energy always flows from the chest to the upper extremities. For the yin of the feet, the flow is always from the lower limbs toward the chest.

The three yin of the hand go from the chest to the hand. The three yang of the hand go from the hand to the head. The three yang of the foot go from the head to the foot. The three yin of the foot start from the foot and go to the chest. (DACH I, 9r)

The specific direction of energy flow in the meridians is considered important, especially for the proper management of the circulation of energy, and for massage along the meridian as well as for puncturing points in a particular order. The *Nan Jing* of Bian Que explains:

> *It is of primary importance to know the flow (**liu-xing**) of the **rong** and **wei** [the yin and yang energy of the body].* *(DACH VI, 7v)*

Dr. Cafford has remarked that in a man with hands raised, the yang descends from the hands to the feet with a connection at the head. The yin ascends up to the chest and from there to the hands.

Localization of the Level of Meridian Flow

It has been demonstrated that the meridians, like the points, are in the subcutaneous tissue or on the aponeurosis. The work of Sir Thomas Lewis confirms that the meridians pass through the subcutaneous tissue. It is clear that the meridians exclusively follow neither arteries, nor nerves, nor veins. The only Chinese text that gives anatomical indications for the level of meridian flow is the *Nan Jing*.

> *Some say that although the yang meridians circulate outside the vessels, all the secondary yang channels circulate in the interior of the vessels. Even though the yin meridians flow in the interior of the vessels, all the secondary yin channels circulate outside the vessels. (DACH VI, 7v)*

Hours of Maximum Activity of the Meridians and Organs

Through careful observation, the ancients discovered that each meridian and its linked organ have a particularly marked activity and sensitivity for about two hours each day. In this two hour period the pulse of each organ is fuller and stronger. In China "noon," or more precisely "midday," is the period between 11 a.m. and 1 p.m. (unlike in the West, where noon is considered the time from 11:59 a.m. to 12:01 p.m.).

The divisions of the day have undergone three great changes in China, the older systems continuing at times to be used with the new.

1) From antiquity to 104 B.C., what we call the 24-hour day was divided decimally into ten *shi*, each of ten *ke*. The *shi* then equaled 2 hours and 24 minutes; the *ke*, 14 minutes and 24 seconds.

2) From 104 B.C. until A.D. 1670, the 24-hour day was divided decimally into ten *ke* and also into twelve *shi*. The *shi* for midday and midnight each included ten *ke* of 14 minutes 24 seconds, each *shi* being 2 hours 24 minutes. The ten other *shi* included only eight *ke*, each being 14 minutes 24 seconds. Midday and midnight thus included 2 hours 24 minutes each, while the other *shi* were only of 1 hour 55 minutes 12 seconds.

3) In 1670, the Reverend Father Verbeist, mathematical advisor to the emperor Kang Xi, had the emperor adopt a division similar to ours — that is, twenty-four half-*shi*, being one European hour divided into four *ke* of a quarter of an hour, or fifteen minutes.

Lung *(shou taiyin)*	*Yin*	hour	3 a.m. to 5 a.m.
Large Intestine *(shou yangming)*	*Mao*	hour	5 a.m. to 7 a.m.
Stomach *(zu yangming)*	*Chen*	hour	7 a.m. to 9 a.m.
Spleen-pancreas *(shou taiyin)*	*Si*	hour	9 a.m. to 11 a.m.
Heart *(shou shaoyin)*	*Wu*	hour	11 a.m. to 1 p.m.
Small Intestine *(shou taiyang)*	*Wei*	hour	1 p.m. to 3 p.m.
Urinary Bladder *(zu taiyang)*	*Shen*	hour	3 p.m. to 5 p.m.
Kidney *(zu shaoyin)*	*You*	hour	5 p.m. to 7 p.m.
Heart Governor *(shou jueyin)*	*Xu*	hour	7 p.m. to 9 p.m.
Triple Warmer *(shou shaoyang)*	*Hai*	hour	9 p.m. to 11 p.m.
Gallbladder *(zu shaoyang)*	*Zi*	hour	11 p.m. to 1 a.m.
Liver *(zu jueyin)*	*Chou*	hour	1 a.m. to 3 a.m.

Lungs (the cycle repeats)

The observations listed above were used by researchers in the study of the meridians. They found it was easiest to disperse strongly and effectively the organ at the exact time of this increased activity. Conversely, greatest tonification of the organ was achieved when acting in the period twelve hours opposite the active period. *(DACH VII, 20r)* Additionally, clinicians have often noted circadian patterns of symptomatology, e.g., hepatic-related asthma patients have their most severe attacks between one and three a.m. (the time of maximum activity of the liver meridian); and over-excitation of the heart and disorders of the circulation become more acute at midday (the time of maximum activity of the heart meridian).

Upon careful observation, we find a pulse of large amplitude and hardness at the position of the given organ during the two hours of greater activity. At present, however, it is very difficult to evaluate the exact significance of this two-hour increase of activity. Precise evaluation and verification will only be possible when an instrument registering the Chinese pulses is developed.

Proportions of Energy and Blood in the Meridians

The ancient works state that the ratio of energy and blood differs for each of the meridians (clearly relating to the meridians, not the organs). The *Da Cheng* (II, 21r) states:

> *The quantity of energy or blood in the yin or the yang is of vital importance. The **jueyin** (heart governor — liver) and **taiyang** (small intestine — urinary bladder) have little energy and much blood. The **taiyin** (lung — spleen-pancreas) and the **shaoyin** (heart — kidney) have much energy and little blood. Additionally, the divisions grouped under **shaoyang** (triple warmer — gallbladder) have much energy and little blood. Those in which energy abounds and which also have much blood are the **yangming** (large intestine — stomach). This means that in the three yang and three yin [divisions] the quantities of energy and blood are not the same. It is very important to remember this when treating.*

Indeed, in the course of this work we will see that certain organs do produce more energy than flesh. In the shaoyang division, the triple warmer is "the father of energy," and the gallbladder, if in excess, may produce feelings of discontent and violence (clearly of energetic origin). In the taiyin, the spleen has been observed to be the source of mental energy, or concentration of mind, and the lungs are a major source of vital energy. In the shaoyin, the kidneys are the source of sexual energy, and the heart, if it is weak, causes melancholy and lassitude.

Conversely, other organs produce more substance (yin or blood) than energy. Of the jueyin, the heart governor is the "mother of blood and yin," and the liver a great purifier of blood. The small intestine of the taiyang adds the ingredient of life to ingested food and allows its integration into the physical being. However, it is difficult to explain the relationship of the urinary bladder (taiyang) and the large intestine and stomach (yangming) to the blood or energy.

European Knowledge of the Meridians

The first anatomical research on the meridians, conducted in Paris by Rouvierre and Perretti Della Rocca, did not reveal any previously known nervous or arterial pathway being used by the meridians. The hypothesis has been offered that it is not a question of anatomy but of physiology; that is, certain pathways have some possibility of nervous transmission not yet observed in Europe.

An extremely important discovery for acupuncture was described by a heart and circulation specialist in the *British Medical Journal* of February, 1937. Sir Thomas Lewis reported the existence — discovered after extensive experimentation — of a cutaneous nervous system unsuspected until now. It appears to be in close connection with the defense system of the body.

Lewis started from the fact that if a point on the skin is injured, many people develop a much greater surface area of painful sensitivity than the size of the injury. This reaches an oval extension of several inches in length after about ten minutes. He studied this phenomenon closely, using different methods of local anesthesia. If a very small area is anesthetized and a slight injury made at the center, the usual oval area of pain is not obtained until the anesthesia wears off. This suggests that it is not the diffusion of substance that produces pain, but an irritation of neighboring nerves. The mode of transmission must be such that the intervention of the sensory or sympathetic nerves is far removed. When the experiment is done on a portion of the skin destroyed by some previous accident, the phenomenon is reproduced. Lewis concluded that this oval extension of pain may be a matter of a particular system "placed in lines on the limbs," and it has nothing to do with the known sensory nerves or with the sympathetic system that controls the blood irrigation of the skin.

Dr. Marcel Martiny has offered the analogy that acupoints are like isolated studs between which a flow of energy could pass without connecting wires. In that case, the points would be where certain fibers emerge, and the flow from one point to another would excite the nerves in its path. But in all its pathways the meridian is most sensitive to its own organ. The heart meridian, which becomes painful in an angina pectoris crisis, is the only well-known meridian in Europe. There is still no satisfactory explanation for this painful zone.

Sometimes ''Head's Zones'' are cited in an attempt to explain the meridians. But these zones are determined by the course of the peripheral nerves emanating from medullary segments. They explain the connection between the sensitivity of certain regions and problems of internal organs. This phenomenon can help us to understand the points but does not explain the meridians.

We must also cite the curious discovery of Dr. Calligaris, professor of neuropathology at the University of Rome (*La Catene Lineari Secondarie del Corpo a Dello Spirito*, Pozzi: Rome, 1930). According to Dr. Calligaris, each internal organ is linked through a fixed law to a cutaneous, axial, interdigital band extending to the hands. Dysfunction of an organ is reflected in hyperesthesia along the corresponding band. This is identified by the patient as unusual sensitivity to pain or touch, and a knowledgeable doctor is able to determine which viscera is diseased by the location of the hypersensitive band. There is certainly some connection here with the meridians.

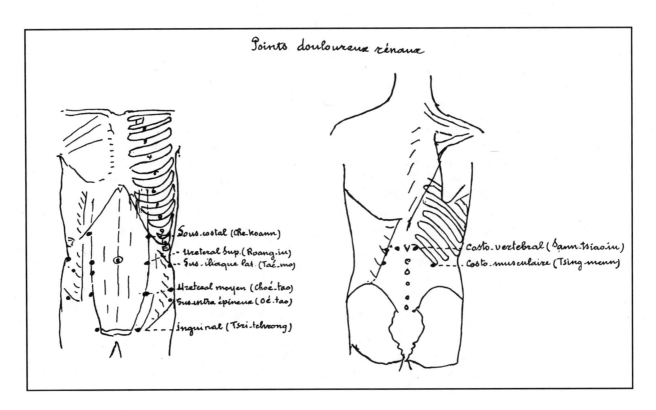

Painful points (thorax)

Notes

[1] Although usually referred to in modern texts as the ''pericardium,'' in acupuncture theory this meridian is only vaguely related to the actual, physical pericardium. ''Heart governor'' is closest in meaning to the author's French, although ''heart-governed'' is a probably a more accurate English translation of the Chinese term, implying a channel that operates under the direction of the heart. We have retained the author's term ''heart governor'' in the text, but for consistency with other texts and ease of reference, we have chosen to adopt the currently used ''PC'' (pericardium) symbol for heart governor point references. — ed.

Chapter III
Description of Each Meridian[1]

Meridian of the Lungs
Fei Jing, Shou Taiyin

The course of the meridian and its branches.

The *Da Cheng* (VIII, 2v) gives imprecise drawings of the lung meridian's course. In contrast, my drawings are based on careful experimentation and give the exact anatomical course.[2] The perceptible branches are as follows:

a)   That which sends the energy of the liver meridian (from *qimen,* LR-14, on the thorax) into the meridian of the lung (at *zhongfu,* LU-1).

b)   That which channels the normal energy of the lung meridian (from *lieque,* LU-7) into the large intestine meridian (at *hegu,* LI-4).

c)   The "secondary vessel" *(luo),* or point of passage sends the excess energy of the lung meridian (from *lieque,* LU-7) into the large intestine meridian.

The less perceptible branches are given below:

a)   A branch from the lesser curvature of the stomach (*shangwan* on the conception vessel, CV-13) to the large intestine organ.

b)   A branch from the large intestine organ upward to the lung organ, and from there to *zhongfu* on the lung (LU-1).

Characteristics of the meridian.

Certain characteristics of the lung meridian must be mentioned since they are important for the proper management of the energy (see Volume II).

a)   The energy flows from the thorax to the upper arm to the hand.

b)   The meridian has much energy and little blood. That is to say, its action is more on the energy and nervous vitality than on blood *(DACH VIII, 2v).*

c)   At the yin period (3 - 5 a.m.) energy abounds here *(DACH VIII, 2v),* and the pulse is more ample. At this time the meridian is most easily dispersed. During the two hours opposite (3 - 5 p.m.), tonification is easiest *(DACH VII, 19r).*

Action of the meridian.

Functionally speaking, the meridian should be called the "respiratory passages meridian" as its action is on the lungs, bronchi, throat and larynx. The meridian first acts directly on the respiratory passages, then indirectly on the related organs (see Volume II). Locally, it acts on the muscles and nerves found along the meridian's pathway.

Meridian of the Large Intestine
Da Chang Jing, Shou Yangming

The course of the meridian and its branches.

The *Da Cheng* (VIII, 4v) gives imprecise drawings of the course of the large intestine meridian. The drawings shown here are based on careful experimentation and give the exact anatomical course.[2] The perceptible branches are as follows:

a)   A branch that brings the normal energy into the large intestine meridian (at *hegu,* LI-4) from the lung meridian (*lieque,* LU-7).

b)　　A branch which sends the energy of the large intestine meridian (from *yingxiang,* LI-20) into the stomach meridian (*touwei,* ST-1, IS ST-8). This branch passes through *shenting* (GV-23, IS GV-24) on the governor vessel.

c)　　The "secondary vessel" *(luo),* or point of passage that sends the excess energy of the large intestine meridian (from *pianli,* LI-6) into the meridian of the lung.

The less perceptible branches are given below:

a)　　A branch from *tianding* (LI-17) to *quepen* (ST-12), from there to the lungs, then to the large intestine organ.

b)　　A branch from *quepen* (ST-12) of the stomach meridian to the maxilla, lower teeth and nostrils.

c)　　A branch from *yingxiang* (LI-20) to the meridian of the triple warmer (*jiaosun,* TW-20).

Characteristics of the meridian.

Certain characteristics of the large intestine meridian must be mentioned since they are important for the proper management of the energy (see Volume II).

a)　　The energy flows from the hand up the arm and neck to the side of the nose.

b)　　The large intestine is a yang workshop organ; its meridian is yang.

c)　　The linked yin treasure organ is the lung.

d)　　At the *mao* period (5 - 7 a.m.) energy and blood abound here. At this time the meridian is most easily dispersed. During the two hours opposite (5 - 7 p.m.), tonification is easiest *(DACH VII, 18v).*

e)　　Energy and blood are equally abundant in this meridian; that is, it acts on vital energy and physical substance equally, as with the stomach meridian.

Action of the meridian.

The meridian first acts directly on the large intestine organ, then indirectly on the related organs (see Volume II). Locally, it acts on the muscles and nerves found along the meridian's pathway.

Meridian of the Stomach
Wei Jing, Zu Yangming

The course of the meridian and its branches.

The *Da Cheng* (VIII, 7r) gives imprecise drawings of the stomach meridian's course. By contrast, my locations are based on careful experimentation and give the exact anatomical course.[2] The perceptible branches are as follows:

a)　　A branch by which the normal energy of the stomach meridian (from *chongyang,* ST-42) flows into the spleen-pancreas meridian.

b)　　A branch by which the stomach meridian (at *touwei,* ST-1, IS ST-8) receives normal energy from the large intestine meridian (through *yingxiang,* LI-20).

c)　　The "secondary vessel" *(luo),* or point of passage which sends the excess energy of the stomach meridian (from *fenglong,* ST-40) to the spleen-pancreas meridian.

No less perceptible branches are given.

Characteristics of the meridian.

Certain characteristics of the stomach meridian must be mentioned since they are important for the proper management of the energy (see Volume II).

a)　　The energy flows from the head down the thorax to the feet.

b)　　The stomach is a yang workshop organ; its meridian is yang.

c)　　The linked yin treasure organ is the spleen-pancreas.

d)   Energy and blood are equally abundant in the stomach meridian *(DACH VII, 7r);* that is, this meridian acts on the vital energy and physical substance equally, as does the large intestine meridian. It is said that the stomach organ is the source of everything.

e)   During the *chen* period (7 - 9 a.m.) energy and blood abound here. At this time the meridian is most easily dispersed. During the two hours opposite (7 - 9 p.m.), tonification is easiest *(DACH VII, 19r).*

Action of the meridian.

The meridian first acts directly on the stomach organ, then indirectly on the related organs (see Volume II). Locally, it acts on the muscles and nerves found along the meridian's pathway.

Meridian of the Spleen-Pancreas
Pi Jing, Zu Taiyin

The course of the meridian and its branches.

The *Da Cheng* (IX, 12r) gives imprecise drawings of the course of the spleen-pancreas meridian. By contrast, the drawings shown here are based on careful experimentation and give the exact anatomical course.[2] The perceptible branches are as follows:

a)   The branch that brings the normal energy of the stomach meridian (from *chongyang,* ST-42) into the meridian of the spleen-pancreas (at *yinbai,* SP-1) *(DACH VIII, 7r).*

b)   The branch that sends the normal energy of the spleen-pancreas (from *dabao,* SP-21) into the meridian of the heart (at *jiquan,* HT-1).

c)   The "secondary vessel" *(luo),* or point of passage through which the excess energy of the spleen-pancreas meridian (from *gongsun,* SP-4) is sent into the stomach meridian.

The less perceptible branches are given below:

a)   A branch from *dabao* (SP-21) to the stomach organ.

b)   A branch from *dabao* to the heart organ.

c)   A branch from *dabao* to the throat, epiglottis and tongue.

Characteristics of the meridian.

Certain characteristics of the spleen-pancreas meridian must be mentioned since they are important for the proper management of the energy (see Volume II).

a)   The energy flows from the foot up the thorax to the axilla.

b)   The spleen-pancreas is a yin treasure organ; its meridian is yin.

c)   The linked yang workshop organ is the stomach.

d)   The meridian has much energy and little blood *(DACH IX, 12r);* i.e., it acts more on vital energy (particularly mental and intellectual energy) than on physical substance.

e)   At the *si* period (9 - 11 a.m.) energy and blood abound here *(DACH IX, 12r)* and the pulse is more ample. At this time the meridian is most easily dispersed. During the two hours opposite (9 - 11 p.m.), tonification is easiest.

Action of the meridian.

Remember that although the meridian is called *pi jing,* meridian of the spleen, it also commands the pancreas. Chinese medicine attributes to the spleen an important role in intellectual work and the faculty of concentration. The experiments conducted in Paris have confirmed this observation (Volume II). The meridian first acts directly on the spleen and pancreas, then indirectly on the related organs (see Volume II). Locally, it acts on the muscles and nerves found along the meridian's pathway.

Meridian of the Heart
Xin Jing, Shou Shaoyin

The course of the meridian and its branches.

The *Da Cheng* (VIII, 19r) gives imprecise drawings of the course of the heart meridian. By contrast, the drawings shown here are based on careful experimentation and give the exact anatomical course.[2] Not all the "branches" and "secondary vessels" of the meridians have been shown in our drawings because of the difficulty in identifying them. The only perceptible, or external branches given are the following:

a) The branch of the heart meridian (from *shaochong*, HT-9) to the small intestine meridian (*shaoze*, SI-1). The normal flow of energy passes through this branch and can be easily perceived by stimulating a point on the heart meridian.

b) The branch that connects the meridian of the spleen-pancreas (*dabao*, SP-21) to the heart meridian (*jiquan*, HT-1). This branch normally brings energy to the heart meridian and is difficult to perceive.

c) The secondary vessel *(luo),* or point of passage, which at the extremities connects the heart meridian (from *tongli*, HT-5) to the small intestine meridian (from *zhizheng*, SI-7). These points of passage are used to transfer excess energy from one meridian to the other. They are very important in this capacity.

Besides the above, the authors of *DACH* (VIII, 15) give pathways of other branches *(zhi)* that have only now been possible to find. These less perceptible, or internal branches are given below:

a)   A root branch from the heart (the organ itself) rising to the lungs, then surfacing at the axilla to become the heart meridian.

b)   A branch from the heart to the throat and eyes.

c)   A branch from the heart following the arteries until reaching the small intestine.

Characteristics of the meridian.

Certain characteristics of the heart meridian must be mentioned since they are important for the proper management of the energy (see *DACH* VIII, 15).

a)   The energy flows from the axilla through the arm to the hand.

b)   Since the heart is a yin treasure organ, its meridian is yin and located on the medial surface of the (upper) limb.

c)   The linked yang workshop organ is the small intestine; the small intestine meridian is yang.

d)   The heart meridian flows into the small intestine meridian (yang) and receives energy from the spleen-pancreas meridian (yin).

e)   It contains much energy and little blood, that is, its dominant action is on the energy. This specifically refers to the energy of morale, of *joie de vivre,* the spirit of enterprise and on the energy of respiration (e.g., if deficient there will be breathlessness after effort).

f)   At the *wu* hour (11 a.m. to 1 p.m.) the blood and energy abound at the heart meridian. At this time the meridian is most easily dispersed. During the two hours opposite (11 p.m. to 1 a.m.) tonification is easiest *(DACH VIII, 19v).*

Action of the meridian.

This will be described in detail in Volume II. Here let us only mention that the meridian first acts directly on the heart organ itself, then indirectly on the related organs. Locally, it acts on the muscles and nerves found along the pathway of the meridian.

Meridian of the Small Intestine
Xiao Chang Jing, Shou Taiyang

The course of the meridian and its branches.

The *Da Cheng* (VII, 17r) gives imprecise drawings of the course of the small intestine meridian. By contrast, the drawings shown here are based on careful experimentation and give the exact anatomical course.[2] The perceptible branches are as follows:

a)   A branch that sends the normal energy of the heart meridian (from *shaochong,* HT-9) into that of the small intestine (at *shaoze,* SI-1).

b)   A branch that takes the energy of the small intestine (from *quanliao,* SI-18) into that of the urinary bladder (at *jingming,* BL-1).

c)   The secondary vessel *(luo),* or point of passage through which the excess energy of the small intestine is taken (through *zhizheng,* SI-7) into the heart meridian.

The less perceptible branches are given below:

a)   A branch from *jianwei* of the small intestine (SI-14) to *quepen* of the stomach (ST-12).

b)   A branch from *quepen* (ST-12) to the heart organ, and from there to the stomach and then to the small intestine.

c)   A branch from the small intestine organ ascends the neck along the entire length of the larynx to the lateral point of the eye (*tongziliao,* GB-1).

Characteristics of the meridian.

Certain characteristics of the small intestine meridian must be mentioned, since they are important for the proper management of the energy (see Volume II).

a)   The energy flows from the hand along the upper arm to the cheek.

b)   The small intestine is a yang workshop organ; its meridian is yang.

c)   The linked yin treasure organ is the heart.

d)   The meridian has little energy and much blood; that is, the meridian produces more substance than energy.

e)   At the *wei* period (1 - 3 p.m.) energy and blood abound here. At this time the meridian is most easily dispersed. During the two hours opposite (1 - 3 a.m.), tonification is easiest.

Action of the meridian.

The meridian first acts directly on the small intestine organ, then indirectly on the related organs (see Volume II). Locally, it acts on the muscles and nerves found along the pathway of the meridian.

Meridian of the Urinary Bladder
Pang Guang Jing, Zu Taiyang

The course of the meridian and its branches.

The *Da Cheng* (VIII, 19r) gives imprecise drawings of the course of the urinary bladder meridian. By contrast, the drawings shown here are based on careful experimentation and give the exact anatomical course.[2] The perceptible branches are as follows:

a)   The branch that brings the normal energy of the small intestine meridian (from *quanliao,* SI-18) into the urinary bladder meridian (at *jingming,* BL-1).

b)   The branch by which the normal energy of the urinary bladder meridian (from *zhiyin,* BL-67) flows into the meridian of the kidneys (at *yongquan,* KI-1).

c)   The secondary vessel *(luo),* or point of passage through which the excess energy of the urinary bladder meridian (from *feiyang,* BL-58) flows into the kidney meridian.

The less perceptible branches are given below:

a)   A branch from the lumbar region to the kidneys and urinary bladder.

b)   A branch from the line of the vertex into the skull.

Characteristics of the meridian.

Certain characteristics of the urinary bladder meridian must be mentioned since they are important for the proper management of the energy (see Volume II).

a)   The flow of energy is downward from the head over the back to the feet.

b)   The urinary bladder is a yang workshop organ; its meridian is yang.

c)   The linked yin treasure organ is the kidney.

d)   The meridian has little energy and much blood *(DACH VIII, 19r);* that is, it acts more on the blood and physical being than on the energy.

e)   During the *shen* period (3 - 5 p.m.) energy and blood abound here. During these two hours the pulse is more ample, the organ more active. At this time the meridian is most easily dispersed. During the two hours opposite (3 - 5 a.m.) tonification is easiest.

Action of the meridian.

The function of the urinary bladder is more complex in Chinese medicine than in Western medicine. It is not merely a container, but more importantly, a regulator of the function of the kidneys (see Volume II). The meridian first acts directly on the urinary bladder organ, then indirectly on the related organs (see Volume II). Locally, it acts on the muscles and nerves found along the pathway of the meridian.

Meridian of the Kidney
Shen Jing, Zu Shaoyin

The *Da Cheng* (VIII, 25r) gives imprecise drawings of the course of the kidney meridian. By contrast, the drawings shown here are based on careful experimentation and give the exact anatomical course. The perceptible branches are as follows:

a)   A branch that brings the normal flow of the urinary bladder meridian (from *zhiyin,* BL-67) into the kidney meridian (at *yongquan* KI-1).

b)   A branch that sends the normal energy of the kidney meridian (according to the Japanese, from *bulang,* KI-22) into the heart governor meridian.

c)   The "secondary vessel" *(luo),* or point of passage, by which the excess energy of the kidney meridian is sent into the urinary bladder meridian (through *dazhong,* KI-6, IS KI-4).

The less perceptible branches are given below:

a)   A branch starting from the meridian at the top of the thigh, following the spine to the kidneys, and then branching to the urinary bladder.

b)   A branch which starts from the urinary bladder and exits into the kidney meridian at *henggu* (KI-11) according to the Japanese.

c)   A branch which starts from the kidney organ "ascending and traversing" through the liver and the diaphragm. It penetrates the lungs, follows the larynx and terminates at the root of the tongue.

d)   A branch from the lungs to the heart.

Characteristics of the meridian.

Certain characteristics of the kidney meridian must be mentioned since they are important for the proper management of the energy (see Volume II).

a)   The energy flows up the lower limb to the thorax.

b)   The kidneys are yin treasure organs; their meridian is yin.

c)   The linked yang workshop organ is the urinary bladder.

d)   The meridian contains much energy and little blood *(DACH VIII, 25r);* i.e., its dominant action is on the energy.

e)   At the *you* period (5 - 7 p.m.), energy and blood abound here and during these two hours the pulse is more ample. At this time the organ is easier to disperse; during the two hours opposite (5 - 7 a.m.), tonification is easier.

Action of the meridian.

The action of the kidney organ is more complex in Chinese medicine than in Western medicine. It is described in Volume II. The meridian first acts directly on the kidney organ, then indirectly on the related organs (see Volume II). Locally, it acts on the muscles and nerves found along the pathway of the meridian.

Meridian of the Heart Governor
Xin Bao Jing or *Xin Bao Luo Jing* or *Xin Zhu Jing, Shou Jueyin*

The course of the meridian and its branches.

The *Da Cheng* (IX, 13v) gives imprecise drawings of the course of the heart governor meridian's course. By contrast, the drawings shown here are based on careful experimentation and give the exact anatomical course.[2] The perceptible branches are as follows:

a)   A branch that carries the normal energy from the kidney meridian (from *bulang,* KI-22, according to the Japanese) into the heart governor meridian (at *tianchi,* PC-1).

b)   A branch that sends the normal energy of the heart governor meridian (from *laogong,* PC-8) into the triple warmer meridian (at *guanchong,* TW-1).

c)   The ''secondary vessel'' *(luo),* or point of passage that sends the excess energy of the heart governor (from *neiguan,* PC-6) into the meridian of the triple warmer.

The other less perceptible branches are given below:

a)   A branch from the heart governor following along the diaphragm to *tianchi* (PC-1) *(DACH VIII, 29r).*

b)   The Japanese indicate that a branch travels from *tianchi* (PC-1) to *shanzhong* (CV-17) on the conception vessel.

Characteristics of the meridian.

Certain characteristics of the heart governor meridian must be mentioned since they are important for the proper management of the energy (see Volume II).

a)   The energy flows from the thorax to the upper arm to the hand.

b)   This functional rather than physical organ (see below) is a yin treasure organ; its meridian is yin.

c)   The linked yang workshop organ (also a functional entity) is the triple warmer.

d)   The meridian has little energy and much blood; that is, it acts more on the blood and physical being than on the energy *(DACH VIII, 29r).*

e)   At the *xu* period (7 - 9 p.m.) energy and blood abound here. At this time the meridian is most easily dispersed. During the two hours opposite (7 - 9 a.m.) tonification is easiest *(DACH VIII, 19v).*

Action of the meridian.

For the action and nature of the meridian see Volume II. The meridian acts on the circulation, the vessels and the blood. It is the mother of yin. A part of this meridian, called *mingmen* (''door of destiny''), acts on the sexual life.

Meridian of the Triple Warmer
San Jiao Jing, Shou Shaoyang

The course of the meridian and its branches.

The *Da Cheng* (VIII, 30v) gives imprecise drawings of the course of the triple warmer meridian. By contrast, the drawings shown here are based on careful experimentation and give the exact anatomical course.[2] The perceptible branches are as follows:

a)   A branch that brings the normal energy from the heart governor (from *laogong,* PC-8) into the meridian of the triple warmer (at *guanchong,* TW-1).

b)   A branch that sends the normal energy of the triple warmer meridian (from *ermen,* TW-23, IS TW-21) into the gallbladder meridian (at *tongziliao,* GB-1).

c)   The ''secondary vessel'' *(luo),* or point of passage that sends the excess energy of the meridian of the triple warmer (from *waiguan,* TW-5) into the heart governor meridian.

The less perceptible branches are given below:

a)   A branch from *shanzhong* (CV-17) on the conception vessel to *quepen* (ST-12) of the stomach meridian, from there continuing to the throat, behind the ears (along the course of the meridian) and ending on the cheek.

b)   A branch from *qimai* (TW-18) on the triple warmer, passing behind and then entering the ears.

Characteristics of the meridian.

Certain characteristics of the triple warmer meridian must be mentioned since they are important for the proper management of the energy (see Volume II).

a)   The energy flows from the hand up the arm to the ears.

b)   The triple warmer is a yang workshop organ; its meridian is yang.

c)   The linked yin treasure organ is the heart governor.

d)   The meridian contains much energy and little blood. That is, its dominant action is on the energy *(DACH VIII, 30v).*

e)   At the *hai* period (9 - 11 p.m.) the energy and blood abound here. At this time the meridian is most easily dispersed. During the two hours opposite (9 - 11 a.m.) tonification is easiest *(DACH VIII, 30v).*

Action of the meridian.

The triple warmer is not a true organ (see Volume II). It commands the important functions of the respiratory, digestive and urogenital systems. The meridian first acts directly on the triple warmer, then indirectly on the related organs (see Volume II). Locally, it acts on the muscles and nerves found along the meridian's pathway.

Meridian of the Gallbladder
Dan Jing, Zu Shaoyang

The course of the meridian and its branches.

The *Da Cheng* (VIII, 32v) gives imprecise drawings of the course of the gallbladder meridian. By contrast, the drawings shown here are based on careful experimentation and give the exact anatomical course.[2] The perceptible branches are as follows:

a)   A branch that brings the normal energy from the triple warmer meridian (from *ermen* TW-23, IS TW-21) into the meridian of the gallbladder (at *tongziliao,* GB-1).

b)   A branch that sends the normal energy of the gallbladder meridian (from foot-*linqi,* GB-41) into that of the liver (at *xingjian,* LR-2).

c)   The ''secondary vessel'' *(luo),* or point of passage that sends the excess energy of the gallbladder meridian (from *guangming,* GB-37) into the liver meridian.

The less perceptible branches are given below:

a)　　A branch (from *tongziliao,* GB-1) on the gallbladder meridian to the stomach meridian (at *daying,* ST-8, IS ST-5). From there the branch descends the neck to join the gallbladder meridian in the supraclavicular fossa near *quepen* (ST-12).

Characteristics of the meridian.

Certain characteristics of the gallbladder meridian must be mentioned since they are important for the proper management of the energy (see Volume II).

a)　　The flow of energy is downward from the head to the feet.

b)　　The organ is a yang workshop organ; its meridian is yang.

c)　　The linked yin treasure organ is the liver.

d)　　The meridian has much energy and little blood. That is, it acts more on energetic and nervous functions than on physical substance and blood *(DACH VIII, 32v).*

e)　　At the *li* period (11 p.m. to 1 a.m.) energy and blood abound here *(DACH VIII, 32v).* At this time the meridian is most easily dispersed. During the two hours opposite (11 a.m. to 1 p.m.), tonification is easiest *(DACH VII, 20v).*

Action of the meridian.

The function of the gallbladder is more complex in Chinese medicine than in Western medicine. It is not merely a container, but more importantly, a regulator that activates or inhibits the liver. Its action on the nervous system is important. The meridian first acts directly on the gallbladder organ, then indirectly on the related organs (see Volume II). Locally, it acts on the muscles and nerves found along the pathway of the meridian.

Meridian of the Liver
Gan Jing, Zu Jueyin

The course of the meridian and its branches.

The *Da Cheng* (IX, 1r), gives imprecise drawings of the course of the liver meridian. By contrast, the drawings shown here are based on careful experimentation and give the exact anatomical course.[2] The perceptible branches are as follows:

a)　　A branch that brings the normal energy coming from the gallbladder (foot-*linqi,* GB-41) into the liver meridian (at *xingjian,* LR-2).

b)　　A branch that sends the normal energy of the liver meridian (*qimen* on the thorax, LR-14) into the lung meridian (*zhongfu,* LU-1).

c)　　The ''secondary vessel'' *(luo),* or point of passage sending the excess energy of the liver (from *ligou,* LR-5) to the gallbladder.

The less perceptible branch is given below:

a)　　A branch from *qimen* (LR-14) on the thorax to the liver organ; from the liver it travels to the lungs, then the throat. Ascending to the ocular artery and then to the cheeks, it travels to the interior of the lips and finally to *baihui* (GV-19, IS GV-20), located on the top of the head.

Characteristics of the meridian.

Certain characteristics of the liver meridian must be mentioned since they are important for the proper management of the energy (see Volume II).

a)　　The flow of energy is up the lower limbs to the thorax.

b)　　The liver is a yin treasure organ; its meridian is yin.

c)　　The linked yang workshop organ is the gallbladder.

d)   The meridian has little energy and much blood; that is, it acts more on the blood and physical being than on the energy.

e)   At the *chou* period (1 - 3 a.m.) energy and blood abound here. At this time the meridian is most easily dispersed. During the two hours opposite (1 - 3 p.m.), tonification is easiest *(DACH VIII, 21r).*

Action of the meridian.

    The relationship of the liver to the other organs is explained in Volume II. The meridian first acts directly on the liver organ, then indirectly on the related organs (see Volume II). Locally, it acts on the muscles and nerves found along the pathway of the meridian.

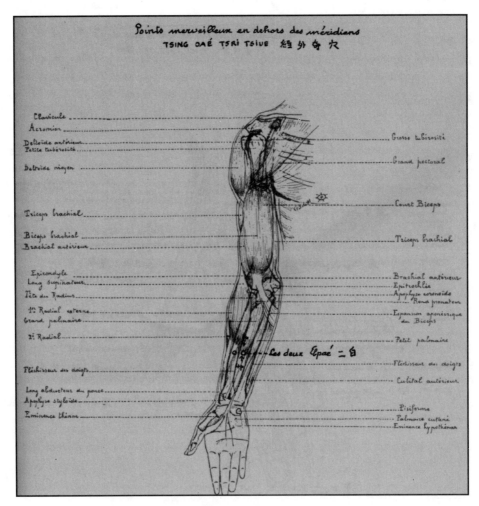

Marvellous points outside the meridians (anterior of upper limb)

Notes

[1] In the French edition, the meridians were listed in alphabetical order. We have rearranged them into traditional Chinese order for the English edition. — ed.

[2] References to drawings are references to the second volume of the French edition. — ed.

Chapter IV

The Two Median Lines

I. Conception Vessel (ren mai) — II. Governor Vessel (du mai)

In addition to the twelve organ meridians *(jing)*, there exist two channels that have special points of their own. They follow the anterior and posterior median lines of the trunk and head and have unilateral points. The line on the anterior surface of the trunk and the lower part of the face is the conception vessel *(ren mai)*. The line on the upper surface of the face, over the head and down the posterior surface of the trunk, is the governor vessel *(du mai)*.

Unlike the organ meridians, the two median lines correspond to a series of complex functions rather than any material organ. Furthermore, while the twelve organ meridians communicate among themselves, forming a continuous circulation of energy moving in the same direction, the two median lines communicate directly only between themselves, both starting at a common point of origin on the perineum and ending at a point on the mouth, forming an independent system of circulation. Hence, from antiquity, the conception and governor vessels have generally not been classified with the twelve organ meridians, but grouped as two of the "eight marvellous vessels" *(qi jing ba mai)*.

However, Hua Shou (Boren) published a book in 1341 which classified the median lines with the organ meridians, giving a total of fourteen meridians. Hua Shou emphasized that all twelve organ meridians do, in fact, communicate with the conception vessel, and that the governor vessel acts on mental and physical strength and consequently the meridians. He postulated that these two lines form a supplementary repository system that becomes active in the case of either excess or insufficiency of energy.

Hua Shou based his ideas on a passage from the *Nei Jing Ling Shu IV:* "The meridians, up and down, right and left, front and back, are twenty-eight in number." This must refer to the twelve bilateral meridians, plus the two median lines twice traversing their course. His ideas were also based on the *Nan Jing,* which recommended using the two median lines when the meridians no longer responded to puncture in an advanced stage of disease.

His ideas were not followed, however. Most Chinese medical texts only recognize twelve organ meridians and classify the two median lines as part of the Eight Marvellous Vessels.

In this text, we have separated the two median lines from the twelve organ meridians. The two lines have also been described separately from the other six marvellous vessels for the following reasons: 1) the other six marvellous vessels seem only to be a group of points having a common effect (see Volume II); 2) the two median lines have points of their own, while the other six marvellous vessels borrow all their points from the twelve meridians; and 3) the two median lines only indirectly communicate with the organ meridians, while the other six marvellous vessels belong directly to the organ meridians.

We have discovered that each point of the conception vessel acts on a given organ meridian. For example, *jiuwei* (CV-15) tonifies or disperses the triple warmer meridian; *juque* (CV-14) acts on the heart; and *zhongwan* (CV-12) and *xiawan* (CV-10) act on the stomach meridian.

Lengthy experiments in Paris have demonstrated the utility of the two median lines for reinforcing the action of an organ meridian when the latter responds poorly. Other uses for these repository median lines have also been demonstrated (see Volume II). Further study is necessary to understand and maximally utilize these special lines of energy.

I. Conception Vessel (*Ren Mai*)

The name.

The ideogram designating this anterior median line is read *ren* and is generally composed of only the elements "man-relation." This combination means "direction," connoting in this case "director vessel." However, several old texts replace the radical for "man" on the left with the ideogram "woman," which gives the sense of "conception," thus "conception vessel." In the treatise *Yi Xue Ru Men* (I, 9r), it is stated: "In reality it is called the 'conception vessel' and not the 'director vessel' because it is the source of birth and growth; it is the ruler of women." The *Da Cheng* (IX, 34v) remarks: "If the *ren mai* of a twenty year old woman is flowing well, she can conceive. It is the sea of all the yin meridians."

The course of the meridian and its branches.

The course of the line is given exactly in the drawings of the *Da Cheng* (IX, 34). Our drawings specify the anatomical location. The branches of the *ren mai* are the following:

a)   A branch that connects the two median lines at the perineum. It starts from *huiyin* (CV-1) and terminates at *changqiang* (GV-1).

b)   A branch that reunites the two median lines at the mouth and which starts from *chengjiang* (CV-24).

c)   From *shanzhong* (CV-17) to the heart governor at *tianchi* (PC-1).

d)   From *shanzhong* to the liver meridian at *qimen* (LR-14) on the thorax.

e)   From *shanzhong* to the kidney meridian at *lingxu* (KI-24).

f)   From *shanzhong* through *quepen* (ST-12) to the gallbladder meridian at *jianjing* (GB-21) .

g)   From *shangwan* (CV-13) through *qishe* (ST-11) to the stomach meridian at *daying* (ST-8, IS ST-5).

h)   From *shangwan* to the lung meridian at *zhongfu* (LU-1).

i)   From *shangwan* and *xiawan* (CV-10) to the small intestine meridian at *tianchuang* (SI-16).

j)   From *xiawan* (CV-10) to the stomach meridian at *qichong* (ST-30).

k)   From *xiawan* to the spleen-pancreas meridian at *fuai* (SP-16).

l)   From *shenque* (CV-8) to the kidney meridian at *huangshu* (KI-16).

m)   From *guanyuan* (CV-4) and *zhongji* (CV-3) to the meridian of the spleen-pancreas at *chongmen* (SP-12).

n)   From *guanyuan* and *zhongji* to the kidney meridian at *zhongzhu* on the abdomen (KI-15).

Additional branches are given below:

a)   The *Da Cheng* cites *lieque* (LU-7) as the point of crossing and reunion of the conception vessel *(jiaohui xue)*.

b)   The point foot-*linqi* (GB-41) of the gallbladder is the point of crossing and reunion of the *dai mai,* the "belt vessel." Action on this point eases the flow of the conception vessel and the *chong mai* and cures difficulties of lactation and menses *(DACH I, 9v).*

Action of the meridian.

The upper third on the sternum predominantly controls respiratory functions; the middle third on the epigastrium, digestive functions; and the lower third on the abdomen, urogenital functions (see Volume II).

II. Governor Vessel *(Du Mai)*

The course of the meridian and its branches.

The posterior line ascends. It starts from the perineum and follows the vertebral column. The points are located in the intervertebral spaces. It then follows the median line of the cranium, forehead and nose to terminate on the upper gum. The branches of the *du mai* are the following:

a)   A branch that is called the "secondary vessel" *(luo)* and which starts from *changqiang* (GV-1) according to one source, and from *huiyang* (BL-35) according to others, to rejoin the conception vessel.

b)   A branch that reunites the two median lines at the lips.

The branches which connect to the other meridians are as follows:

a)   A branch from *bailao* (GV-13, IS GV-14, *dazhui*) between C7 and T1 to the gallbladder meridian at *jianjing* (GB-21).

b)   A branch from *bailao* (GV-13, IS GV-14 *dazhui*) to the triple warmer meridian at *jianliao* (TW-14) and to the small intestine meridian at *bingfeng* (SI-12).

c)   From *bailao* (GV-13, IS GV-14, *dazhui*) to the urinary bladder meridian at *tianzhu* (BL-10).

d)   From *taodao* (GV-12, IS GV-13) to the bladder meridian at *dazhu* (BL-11).

We should also mention that *houxi* (SI-3) is the crossing and reunion point of the governor vessel.

Action of the meridian.

The *du mai* is indicated by the *Da Cheng* as being 1) the reunion place of all the *yang* meridians and 2) the controller and director of physical and mental vitality and actions, primarily in men. (See Volume II and *Yi Xue Ru Men* I, 90r.)

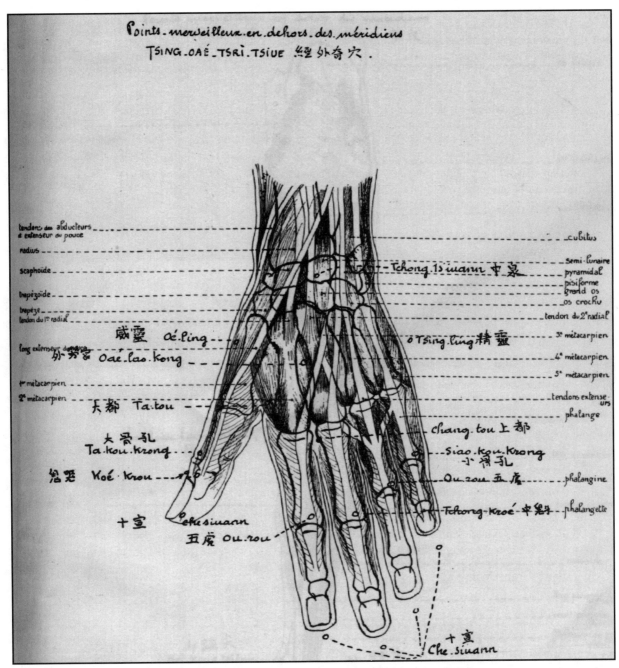

Marvellous points outside the meridians (dorsal aspect of the hand)

Chapter V
The Fifteen Secondary Vessels

The fifteen luo.

From the oldest times authors mention the fifteen *luo* meridians in addition to the twelve organ meridians (*YXRM I, 9r*).[1]

These *luo* or secondary vessels and their points of passage are an important element in the circulation of energy. They are branches that connect the paired meridians; i.e., they send the energy from the yin meridian to its coupled yang meridian and from the yang meridian to its coupled yin meridian. Any given meridian has a point of excitation, or point of passage. When the *jing* (meridians) are functioning normally, the courses of the secondary vessels are not easily perceived.

Of the fifteen *luo*, twelve are located on the twelve organ meridians, two on the two median lines, and one on the last point of the spleen-pancreas (*dabao*, SP-21). The *Yi Xue Ru Men* (I, 1r) explains: "The *jing* meridians are the main pathways, and the secondary vessels are the *luo*." The *Yi Xue* writes more simply (I, 12r): "The *luo* are what run crosswise." A very obscure indication about the secondary vessels is given in the *Da Cheng* (VI, 7v) as follows: "Some say that although all the yang meridians circulate outside the vessels, all the secondary yang vessels circulate in the interior of the vessels. Even though all the yin meridians flow in the interior of the vessels, all the secondary yin vessels circulate outside the vessels."

The luo and points of passage.

From the *Da Cheng* (IX, 11r):

a)   From the lung meridian to the large intestine meridian (*shou taiyin zhi bieluo*). Point of passage: *lieque* (LU-7).

b)   From the large intestine meridian to the lung meridian (*shou yangming zhi bieluo*): *pianli* (LI-6).

c)   From the stomach meridian to the spleen-pancreas meridian (*zu yangming zhi bieluo*): *fenglong* (ST-40).

d)   From the spleen-pancreas meridian to the stomach meridian (*zu taiyin zhi bieluo*): *gongsun* (SP-4).

e)   From the heart meridian to the small intestine meridian (*shou shaoyin zhi bieluo*): *tongli* (HT-5).

f)   From the small intestine meridian to the heart meridian (*shou taiyang zhi bieluo*): *zhizheng* (SI-7).

g)   From the urinary bladder meridian to the kidney meridian (*zu taiyang zhi bieluo*): *feiyang* (BL-58).

h)   From the kidney meridian to the urinary bladder meridian (*zu shaoyin zhi bieluo*): *dazhong* (KI-6, IS KI-4).

i)   From the heart governor meridian to the triple warmer meridian (*shou jueyin zhi bieluo*): *neiguan* (PC-6).

j)   From the triple warmer meridian to the heart governor meridian (*shou shaoyang zhi bieluo*): *waiguan* (TW-5).

k)   From the gallbladder meridian to the liver meridian (*zu shaoyang zhi bieluo*): *guangming* (GB-37).

l)   From the liver meridian to the gallbladder meridian (*zu jueyin zhi bieluo*): *ligou* (LR-5).

m)   From the conception vessel to the governor vessel (*ren mai zhi bieluo or yinqiao luo*): *huiyin* (CV-1).

n)   From the governor vessel to the conception vessel (*du mai zhi bieluo or yangqiao luo*): *changqiang* (GV-1).

o)   The "great *luo*" of the spleen-pancreas (*pi da luo*): *dabao* (SP-21).

Characteristics of the points of passage.

One peculiarity that is difficult to verify is given in the *Da Cheng* (IX, 12r) and the *Yi Xue* (I, 12r): "These fifteen points [which command the secondary vessels] can be easily perceived when they are in excess; but when they are empty, they are sunken and cannot be perceived."

Function of the secondary vessels.

The function and use of the *luo* are not explained with complete clarity. Nonetheless, it has been possible to deduce two functions:

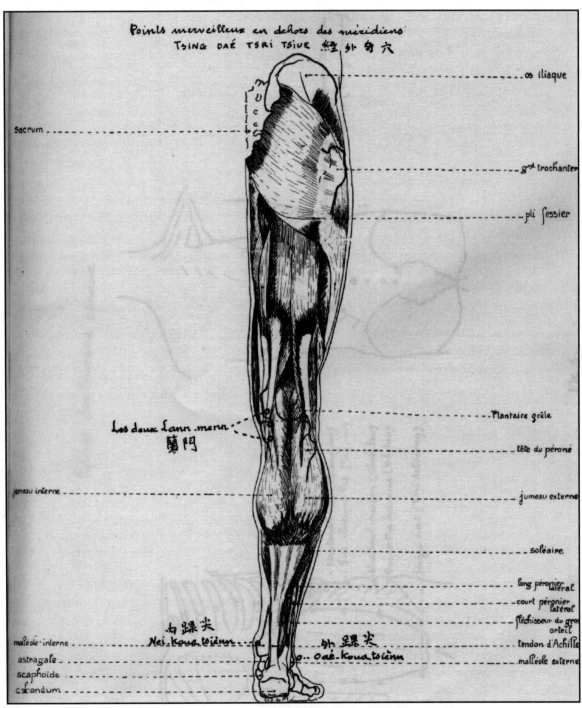

Points merveilleux en dehors des méridiens
TSING DAÉ TSRI TSIUE 經外奇穴

os iliaque
sacrum
g⁺ trochanter
pli fessier

Plantaire grêle
Les deux Lann menn
蘭門
tête du péroné

jumeau interne
jumeau externe

soléaire

long péronier latéral
court péronier latéral
fléchisseur du gros orteil

內踝尖
Nei Koua toiënn
外踝尖
Oaé Koua toiènn
tendon d'Achille

malléole interne
astragale
scaphoïde
calcanéum
malléole externe

Marvellous points outside the meridians (lower limb)

Chapter VI
The Circulation of Energy

The observed phenomena.

The circulation of energy is a physiological finding of considerable importance. The study of acupuncture and the whole of Chinese medicine rests on and is inspired by this discovery. Without it, the impressive successes of acupuncture would be impossible. The circulation of energy, particularly when joined with a knowledge of the pulses, allows us to control the functional intensity of each organ. The ancients arrived at this knowledge through observation of the following phenomena:

a)   The existence of points which become painful when the reflected organ is dysfunctioning, and which are always perceived by sensitive people.

b)   The existence of meridians, which are perceived along their entire length.

c)   When a meridian is stimulated, there is a passage of ''something'' which always flows in the same direction along all or part of the meridian.

d)   The passage of this ''something'' from one meridian to another is always perceived in the same order.

e)   The successive intensity of each meridian is always perceived at the same hour diurnally.

This existence of a circulation of energy through the meridians, independent of the blood and nervous circulation, has been observed from the earliest times in China. The description by the *Nei Jing,* cited in the *Da Cheng* (I, 9r), is as follows:

> *The vessels and the secondary vessels of the meridians transmit the current to each other with rhythmic circularity. It is thus that the vessels of the meridians (jing mai) cause energy and blood to circulate and yin and yang to communicate in the irrigation of the whole body.*

The *Da Cheng* (II, 20v) states further:

> *The human energy circulates in the meridians at the points, describing a circular path throughout the body.*

Order of circulation of the meridians.

The order in which the flow of energy successively passes through the meridians, with the maximum hours indicated, is as follows:

Lung	*Shou taiyin*	about	3 a.m. to 5 a.m.
Large intestine	*Shou yangming*	about	5 a.m. to 7 a.m.
Stomach	*Zu yangming*	about	7 a.m. to 9 a.m.
Spleen	*Zu taiyin*	about	9 a.m. to 11 a.m.
Heart	*Shou shaoyin*	about	11 a.m. to 1 p.m.
Small intestine	*Shou taiyang*	about	1 p.m. to 3 p.m.
Urinary Bladder	*Zu taiyang*	about	3 p.m. to 5 p.m.
Kidney	*Zu shaoyin*	about	5 p.m. to 7 p.m.
Heart Governor	*Shou jueyin*	about	7 p.m. to 9 p.m.
Triple warmer	*Shou shaoyang*	about	9 p.m. to 11 p.m.
Gallbladder	*Zu shaoyang*	about	11 p.m. to 1 a.m.
Liver	*Zu jueyin*	about	1 a.m. to 3 a.m.

During the two hours indicated, the energy is more intense in the meridian and the organ, and they are easier to disperse. During the two hours following, the meridian and organ are more easily tonified *(DACH VIII, 18v).*

Speed of the energy in the meridians.

According to the *Nei Jing Ling Shu* XV (see below), the energy completes the entire cycle through the twelve organ meridians fifty times in 24 hours (one revolution of the sun). This is called the "fifty stages" *(ying)*. The time taken by the energy to complete one revolution of the cycle would be 1/50 of 24 hours, or 28 minutes and 48 seconds. The length of one revolution of the cycle is about 1620 *cun* of about 2.5 cm. each, or a total of approximately 40 meters for an adult of average size. The average speed of the energy through the meridians would thus be about 1 meter 40 cm. per minute, or about 2 cm. 30 mm. per second.

Length of the cycle of energy.

In the *Nei Jing* (see below) a calculation is given for the length of the cycle travelled by the energy in the meridians. The estimation is 1620 *cun* of about 2.5 cm. each, or a total of about 40 meters for the average adult.

The length of the *cun* is determined from the patient himself. It is the length of the medial fold of the middle phalanx on the middle finger, 1/8 of the distance between the nipples, or other bodily indicators (see Appendix II).

Influence of the stars on the energy.

The ancients believed that the universe is an indivisible totality and that man is in no way distinct from nature nor exempt from the laws of nature. They observed connections between the course of the sun in the sky and the flow of energy in the body. In the *Nei Jing Ling Shu* XV, it is written:

> *The turning of the sky has 28 constellations, each of which has 36 divisions [28 x 36 = 1008 celestial divisions]. While the sun goes through these 28 constellations, the energy of man also flows through a round of 1008 divisions [28 meridians x 36?]. Indeed, the vessels of the meridians (**jing mai**) in human beings high and low, right and left, front and back are 28 in number. [6 yang and 6 yin on the right and left is 12 x 2 = 24 meridians, plus 2 median lines traversed twice equals 4, for a total of 28.]*

The circuit made in the body, corresponding to the 28 constellations, is 16 *chang* 2 feet in length (being equal to 1620 *cun* of about 2.5 cm. each). One day and night (24 hours) were divided into a hundred *ke,* during which the water had completely emptied from the water clock (used in China to measure the passage of time). (24 hours divided by 100 *ke* equals one *ke* of 14 minutes 24 seconds.) Each time a person inhales, the pulse beats twice and the energy moves forward 3 *cun,* or about 7.5 cm. With each exhalation, the pulse beats twice and the energy moves forward 3 *cun.* If inhalation and exhalation are peaceful, the energy advances 6 *cun,* or about 12 cm. After ten complete respirations, the energy has progressed 6 feet and the sun has advanced two divisions. The circulating energy returns to its starting point after it has made a complete circle in the body. The level in the water clock has fallen two *ke* (28 minutes 48 seconds) and the sun has advanced 25 of the 1008 divisions. After 270 respirations, the energy will have travelled 16 *chang* 2 feet (1620 *cun* of 2.5 cm. each, which equals 40 m.).

In 13,000 respirations, the energy flows through 50 stages *(ying),* the water has fallen through 100 *ke,* the sun has gone through the 28 constellations, and the energy has travelled through 810 *chang,* or 81,000 *cun* (1620x50 = 81,000).

It appears that the ancient texts have suffered mistakes in transmission. Unfortunately, no indication is made of how it was determined that the energy comes back to its starting point in 28 minutes 48 seconds. The *Da Cheng* discusses the difficulties of observations by the ancient authors of the *Nei Jing (DACH II, 27v):*

> *The **rong** (yin, blood) circulating in the meridians makes a circuit of the body in fifty stages without distinction of day and night. At dawn it reunites itself with the **wei** energy (yang) in the lung meridian (**shou taiyin**). Only the circulating **wei** energy distinguishes between day and night. I have not heard it said that it distinguishes between high and low, male and female, treasure and workshop organ, for the energy and blood which come and go are not usually different. Today, on what basis can we distinguish between morning and evening? This passage has come down to the people of our day; we record it here in order that it be discussed by those who see it.*

Chapter VII

Energy *(Qi)*

I. Human Energy — II. The Yin-Yang Relativity

I. Human Energy

About the name.

Having observed the existence of "something" that passes through a meridian when a point is stimulated, the ancients gave this fluidity, this flux, the name *qi,* which we translate, for lack of a better word, "energy." This is the *prana* of the Hindus.

The ideogram for *qi* is composed of elements representing "the strength of steam lifting up the cover of a pot of boiling rice." It is usually used to express: vapor; strength; respiration, blowing, and by extension, life; anger; nervous influx; in recent times, electricity, and radio waves (see the *Ci Yuan* encyclopedia). The essential idea is of an incorporeal, subtle force.

In ancient and modern texts, the word *qi* is combined with the following qualifying words. These combinations are not adequately defined in any dictionary:

Yuan qi, "ancestral energy:" mostly used in the sense of vitality, strength and resistance.

Zheng qi, "correct energy."

Zhen qi, "true energy:" this and the above term designate healthy or normal energy, as opposed to *xie qi,* which represents the strength of the destructive "perverse energy." The concept here is not one of an invading, foreign force, but of a pathological transformation of the normal energy. This idea is not clearly delineated in most texts. The most descriptive passage is the following:

> *The perverse energy,* **xie qi,** *always follows the healthy energy. If they do not fight, or if the perverse energy does not retreat, or if the healthy energy is not triumphant, then illness returns. (DACH V, 27r)*

Jing or *jing qi,* "energy of the sexual essence": currently used to represent the idea of an extract, or essence; and in medicine, for the idea of sexual power, the instinct of reproduction, libido, sexuality, temperament, sex appeal, and so on. The ideogram is formed from the elements "growth, flesh, " or "the impulsion that governs the flesh." For the Chinese, the *jing* is the source or at least the stimulator of normal energy.

How to observe energy.

Defining *qi* is even more difficult than defining electricity. We will see that in effect the idea of *qi* energy extends to what we call life itself. Even without understanding the exact nature of energy, it is still possible to recognize its existence, appreciate its intensity and to direct it. In the chapter on circulation of energy, it was cited that by stimulating a point on one meridian the sensitive person reports feeling "something" passing into the meridian that follows it; some Europeans describe this "something" as "an electrical wave."

The practitioner needling a patient perceives three general types of sensations:

1) The energy is absent:

> *When the energy does not contact the needle, the needling feels light and slippery as if one punctured into beancurd. (DACH II, 22r)*

> *Light, thus superficial; slippery, thus empty; slow, thus delayed. When putting in the needle, if one encounters these three, the true energy has not arrived. (DACH II, 21r)*

> *If the needle descends [superficially as into a vacuum] with ease and lightness, in a slippery, empty manner, the energy has not arrived. (DACH V, 26v)*

> *When the energy does not arrive, one is as in the silence of an empty house where all is immobile and without sound. (DACH II, 21r)*

If no energy is encountered after puncturing, and if after waiting the energy still does not come, the prognosis is very bad:

If you have punctured as if into cheese, and if after that the energy does not come, then death is certain. (DACH V, 26v)

If one waits for the qi and it does not come, then death is probable. (DACH II, 21r)

2) The energy comes after the entry of the needle. When no resistance is felt after needling, or, if after some time the needle is suddenly pulled as if grabbed by claws, this is a favorable sign. The more quickly the energy arrives the more favorable the prognosis.

When, after needling, the energy arrives under the needle, it is like a fish that takes the bait. Afterwards some tightness and roughness is felt at the needle site. Whether the energy is deep or superficial it takes action. (DACH II, 21r)

Sunk, thus heavy; rough, thus hobbled; tight, thus full. When, after needling, one encounters these three, the correct energy has arrived. (DACH V, 26r)

When slowly inserting and withdrawing the needle it feels as if an artery were beating, the energy has arrived. (DACH VI, 4r)

When the energy comes quickly, the cure will be easy and rapid. When it comes slowly, the cure will be difficult and slow. (DACH II, 21r)

3) The energy is already there. In puncturing, the skin seems hard (firm or rough) like leather; the needle enters only with difficulty.

If the needle sinks into heaviness, tightness, and obstruction on entering, the energy is already there. If the patient feels a dull pain, there is fullness and an excess of energy; if a numbness is felt, there is emptiness; if roughness, there is insufficiency. (DACH V, 26v)

If in puncturing, the needle sinks immediately into tightness, we have directly touched the energy. (DACH VI, 1r)

Without the theory of energy or *qi* it is difficult to explain the fact that needling, which neither adds nor subtracts any substance, instantly normalizes the amplitude and hardness of an excessive organ pulse. There are other signs, not directly related to acupuncture but apparently directly linked to energy, according to the Chinese. Some of these are cited below:

Sight: greater or lesser brightness of the eyes and rapidity of the glance; the power of the look.

Voice: the connection between the sonority of the voice and energy, and between the voice and the strength of respiration; the quality of the energy given by the timbre of the voice. A soft, well modulated voice indicates harmonious, abundant, easy to manage energy; a strong, rough voice indicates gross energy, which is difficult to manage; a weak voice without timbre indicates unstable, weak energy, and so forth.

Complexion:

A grey complexion with thick skin signifies weak energy that is difficult to obtain when needling; a congested complexion with rough skin signifies violent energy, but without duration; a pink, clear complexion with thin skin indicates quick, durable energy, which is easy to displace. (DACH I, 16v)

Circulation:

The blood circulates according to the energy: if the energy circulates, the blood circulates. If the energy is impeded, the blood stops. (YXRM IV, 5r)

And we add that the blood, when deprived of energy, becomes devitalized.

The idea of *qi* extends to that of life. Ancient authors cite the fact that in the passage of life to death, e.g., in cardiac arrest, it is not possible to observe any material change, but only a total loss of energy.

Measurements of energy.

Medical doctors of the Far East, essentially practical, did not attempt to measure the intensity of energy with instruments or numbers. They estimated the quantity and quality of the total energy from the complexion, the appearance, and the voice. They determined the energy of each organ through the intensity and power of the fourteen radial pulses (see Chapter VIII). We can agree that even if some instruments give precise numbers, no instrument has the delicacy of the human finger to perceive the amplitude, hardness, resistance, width, length, placement and regularity of each pulse. In Japan, there exists an instrument for recording each of the fourteen pulses, but it does not give an appreciation of the total energy (see Chapter VIII).

Doctor Dimier, a hospital electrologist who assisted in several acupuncture treatments, offered the hypothesis that human energy is either entirely electric or carried by measurable electric waves. Just before his death he had measured the waves emanating from the body with an ultrasensitive galvanometer. He found the waves intensified along the meridians, particularly at the level of the acupoints. Measurements varied from one microamp (thousandth of a milliamp) in exhausted people to twelve and sometimes fifteen microamps in hypersensitive or tense people. He was unable to determine if the electric wave represented all the energy or if there was another element not measured by the galvanometer.

The scientific radiesthesists, Dr. Leprince, Dr. Savoire, Mrs. Chantereine, and Mr. Turenne, wrote that the body emitted waves of about eight meters in length. Other authors suggest a length of thirty centimeters.

In an experiment done in 1936 by Drs. Leprince and Foveau de Courmelles, two gold needles were inserted into each leg at the important acupoint leg-*sanli* (ST-36). A receiver attached to copper wire joining the needles gave distinctly strong sputtering sounds.

Further research must be carried out in order to measure the energy — the length of the wave and its intensity, and the qualities of smoothness, roughness, power or duration. Also, it is necessary to distinguish the elements carried by the recognized electric wave, if there are any, and to determine if life as it seems is something other than electricity.

Crossing of energy in the meridians.

Among the curiosities of the meridians is the crossing over and same-sidedness of the energy in the meridians. If a point is stimulated with repeated pressure on a sensitive-type person, they will feel a sensation on the same meridian but distal to the point stimulated. For instance, if on the small intestine meridian, either *houxi* (SI-3) or *wangu* (SI-4) (both on the ulnar side of the hand) is repeatedly tapped with the fingernail, the person perceives a passage of energy in the portion of the meridian on the face (from the maxilla to the cheek bone, and from there to the earlobe). One sensitive-type person feels this sensation on the same side that is stimulated, while another feels this sensation on the opposite side.

In many observations, it was found that persons who felt sensation on the same side were left-handed or ambidextrous, and somewhat less nimble in their speech, actions or gestures. Conversely, those who felt sensation on the opposite side were generally right-handed, more sure of themselves, and mentally as well as physically more competent.

The Chinese explain this crossing over of energy through their theory of the opposition of heaven and earth at the cardinal points (see below, ''Yin-yang Relativity''). The crossing over is also cited in discussions of treatments; it is particularly important for the treatment of the illness called ''energy sickness'' (see Volume II, Chapter IV: ''Illness'').

> *When the pain is on the left, it is the right meridian that is ill. When the pain is on the right, it is the left meridian that is ill. (DACH II, 24v)*

Therefore, in migraines on the left side of the head, it is recommended to puncture *lieque* (LU-7) at the right wrist, and vice versa. This gives good results mostly in nervous migraines. This phenomenon has been noted by massage therapists who have cured migraines of the left side by massaging the right thigh, and vice versa. For the gallbladder organ, located on the right side of the body, the gallbladder points on the left leg are more sensitive and active than those on the right.

The variations of energy according to the season, temperature and hour.

Since antiquity, it has been noted that human energy varies in intensity by season, phase of the moon, hour of the day and temperature. Experiments in Paris have confirmed this. In relation to the seasons, humans, like plants, respond to the yearly cycle. In summer, life is at its maximum, in winter at its minimum. Human beings sleep at night; they wake with the sunrise. They are numbed by cold and excited by warmth. Storms bother them.

> *In spring and summer the yang energy is at its highest — human energy is also at its highest. In autumn and winter yang energy is at its lowest — human energy is also at its lowest. (DACH V, 23r)*

Treatments are influenced by cosmological changes. Chronic illnesses are easier to cure at the beginning of summer than in the winter season. May and June are best. At the new moon the yin energy is at its most active level and the yang energy at its lowest. This should be the time of menses for women (ovulation being at the full moon).

> At the waxing of the moon, energy and blood begin to purify one another; the energy begins to circulate. When the moon is full, energy and blood are plentiful; flesh and muscles are firm. When the moon is empty, the flesh is dull, vessels and meridians become empty; energy ebbs away from the body. (Nei Jing, cited in DACH II, 19v)

> At the waxing of the moon, puncture once on the first day; twice on the second day, until fifteen punctures on the fifteenth day. Then thirteen punctures on the seventeenth day, decreasing until two punctures on the thirtieth day. (DACH II, 27v)

Storms upset the response to treatment. Bad weather delays or diminishes the response. Cold weather slows the reactions and certain reactions occur only on the third, fourth, and even eighth day of cold weather, as has been often observed in Paris. With reduced barometric pressure the body is relatively more heavy, the vessels and organs dilate, the arterial pressure drops. The contrary is produced by high barometric pressure. In the *Nei Jing* it is written:

> When the weather is warm and days are sunny, human blood is free flowing and the energy is superficial. At that time, it is easier to promote the flow of energy and disperse the blood. When the weather is cold and days are overcast, human blood is contracted and thick and the energy is deep.

> With cold, energy collects. Cold causes a stoppage of circulation and thus coldness. With warmth, energy dissipates; warmth exhausts itself through perspiration. (YXRM V, 3v)

> On sunny days, energy leads and the blood follows. The meridians reflect this relationship. On cloudy days, blood leads and the energy follows. The meridians ascend to their sources. (DACH VII, 28r)

> On sunny days, the yang workshop organs are especially productive and conduct the energy . . . which leads. (DACH III, 30v)

When the sun shines in a blue sky, the atmospheric electricity is positive; when the sky is overcast, it is negative.

> On cloudy days, the yin treasure organs are especially productive and activate the blood . . . which leads. (DACH)

It is true that on sunny days it is easier to tonify the energy. On cold, cloudy days it is easier to tonify the physical being, the blood, the yin.

Each part of the day favors one action or another. In the morning when the sun rises and the yang, born at midnight, is growing, it is easier to tonify and revive the yang energy. From noon the yang decreases and the yin grows; it is easier to disperse, or calm the yang energy and to tonify the yin energy.

> During the day, the energy leads and the blood follows. At night, the blood leads and the energy follows. (DACH VII, 30r)

Each successive hour of the twenty-four hours is significant for a particular meridian (see "Circulation of Energy"). One school of thought, called "flowing-holding," *liu-zhu,* attaches great importance to this.

> Each day in the body of man the energy moves through a cycle . . . When the organs produce and unite with themselves and are open, stimulate them. When they destroy themselves and are closed, do not stimulate them. During this latter period the points are closed; energy and blood are exhausted either because the circulating energy has not arrived there, or it has already departed from there. If one punctures mistakenly at this time, one introduces perverse energy. (DACH VI, 30r)

Variation of energy according to the emotions and fatigue.

Since antiquity it has been observed that the emotions strongly influence the energy:

> With joy, energy slows down; there is incessant laughter. One is not capable of effort. With grief, the energy melts; there is acidity. With fear, the energy drops; there is a violent descent of clear liquid. With strong emotions, the energy is overthrown; the consciousness has no place to return; stupidity or convulsions result. With unhappiness, the energy mounts until it causes vomiting of blood or thick diarrhea. With obsessive thoughts the energy tightens, but the consciousness has somewhere to return; the mind conserves its energy. (YXRM V, 32r)

Fatigue acts very strongly on the energy, as the following passage suggests:

> *With fatigue the energy dwindles; people have no more sexual energy; women have no more menses; people are sweating and out of breath. (YXRM V, 32r)*

Variations in the placement of energy.

The energy in different parts of the body varies in strength according to the season, the hour and the sex. Each organ has a corresponding low season during which a maximum of ailments and energy failures occurs: the liver at the spring equinox in March (and less strongly at the autumn equinox); the spleen and the pancreas in May; the head and the heart at the summer solstice in June (manifesting such ailments as cerebral congestion or furious madness); the lungs after the autumn equinox; the mind in the month of November (manifesting in depression or sadness); and the kidneys around the winter solstice.[1]

The placement of the energy varies according to gender and time, an observation that has not yet been verified in Europe.

> *Male energy is above in the morning, below in the evening. Female energy, on the contrary, is below in the morning and above in the evening. (YXRM I, 42v)*

However, Yang Jishi *(DACH VI, 4v)* disputes this by writing: "It is not an exact truth that women are the opposite of men."

The ancient texts note that the placement of the energy between the left and right side of the body differs according to the season, but it has not been possible to verify this with certainty. Indeed, it is said in the *Nei Jing (DACH I, 11r)* that the energy in spring dominates the left half of the body. At that time we must avoid dispersing the left side, particularly the left foot, so as not to disperse this energy and empty the body.

In summer, the energy dominates the right side; we must not disperse the right yang meridians, which are fully active. In autumn, the energy is on the right side; we must not disperse the right yin meridians because they are beginning their action. In winter, the energy is on the left side; we must not disperse the yin meridians of the left side, particularly of the foot, because they are in full activity.

In addition, the energy is stronger in certain parts of the body according to the seasons:

> *In spring the energy is in the hair; in summer, the skin; in autumn, the muscles; in winter, the bone and marrow. (DACH VIII, 16v)*

II. Yin-Yang Relativity

Relativity in unity.

Realizing the existence of human energy, the ancients were immediately confronted with perplexing questions: Why the alternations of sleeping and waking? Why hot and cold? What difference between physical strength and mental or moral strength? What is the difference between solids, liquids and solar emanations? and so on.

The ancient Chinese were confronted by the same dichotomy of spirit and matter as Europeans. The latter attempted to resolve the problem through theories of incompatibility and complete opposition in nature: God and devil, good and bad, material and nonmaterial. The ancient Chinese took careful note of natural phenomena which they used in addressing this dichotomy: the evaporation of liquids and the impalpable dispersion of vapor, the burning of wood leaving only a residue of ashes, and other examples cited by Chinese philosophical works. They concluded that there is a universal unity wherein matter is only concentrated, solidified energy, and spirit only vaporized matter returning to its immaterial form, both in a state of movement and perpetual becoming, without any unchangeable, permanent state.

Einstein has written (cited by Dr. Jarricot): "The theory of relativity has demonstrated that mass has no physical significance separate from energy." Dr. Jarricot adds, "To refuse to identify matter with electromagnetic force, we must find arguments other than the difficulty thrown in the face of our old ways of thinking." *(Propagateur de l'Homéopathie, Jan.1938, 13)*

This fundamental unity of energy allowed some apparent temporary oppositions, some alternations, and some relativity in the movement. Lao-zi, in the sixth century B.C., taught: "Up is up only relative to down, and down is down only in relation to up." The names yin and yang were given to represent opposite extremes, conferring only a sense of relativity, not a state.[2]

For the human body, the ancients employed the *rong-wei* opposition; in modern times the *qi-xue* opposition is used.[3]

This vision appears in all things so fully, so practically that not only philosophy, but also medicine and even the sciences have relied on and still continue to rely on it. It is on this vision that the unity of the sciences and the great universal law rests.

> *The way (Tao) of heaven and earth is the yin and yang. All is there. For the human body there is also yin and yang: all is there. Yin and yang are the pivot and the knot of the transformations, the root of differences. (DACH IV, 13v)*

For the modern Japanese, who understand European science, the yin-yang duality is considered in the same light. (In Japanese, yang is pronounced "yong;" in the West we continue to use "yang.") Sakurazawa *(Principe Unique, 35)* writes:

> *Nothing is absolutely yin or yang. Yin and yang are only characterized relatively. All is an aggregate of yin and yang . . . yin produces yang; yang produces yin. All beings are charged with activity: yang at the exterior; yin at the interior. The exterior yang becomes the internal yin, and the internal yin becomes external yang. Activities of the same name repel each other. The force of attraction between two beings is a function of the difference between their respective charges of opposite activities.*

Chinese authors return repeatedly to the ideas of relativity and movement:

> *The root is the Supreme All (**tai ji**). It is divided into two energy forms: rest, which is yin yet contains some yang as its treasure; and movement, which is yang yet contains some yin as its root. Is yang the root of yin? It is then a coming and going without end; a transformation with birth of that which has substance. Is yin the root of yang? It is then an accumulation which at the root transforms itself, is born and goes out. But energy, in truth, is movement. One cannot deny the opposition of rest and action; one cannot deny the opposition of hot and cold. But is there first cold then hot, or first hot then cold? (DACH IV, 16r)*

Yin-yang and the living being.

Yin and yang in humans is relativity and alternation in constant movement, not a fixed condition. Further aspects of yin and yang in man are differentiated as follows:

a) Physical life-energy:

Yang is mental or emotional energy — pure, subtle intelligence, consciousness and conscience. Yin is blood, matter, unconsciousness and the animal instincts with their propensity toward deception and cunning.

b) Workshop and treasure organs:

The internal organs are grouped according to their activities. Those that take energy from the exterior and transform it into human energy are yang: the stomach, large intestine, small intestine, urinary bladder and gallbladder (the latter two organs have a stimulating role on the kidneys and liver, respectively). The organs that control, circulate, and purify the blood are yin: the heart, lungs, spleen, liver and kidneys.

The meridians of the yang organs are on the lateral surfaces of the limbs; their corresponding pulses are located at a superficial level on the wrists. The meridians of the yin organs are on the medial surfaces of the limbs, and their corresponding pulses are located at a deeper level on the wrists.

c) Heat-cold:

Yang tends towards heat, mostly external heat. Yin tends toward cold, mostly internal cold.

> *When yang abounds, there is extreme heat. (DACH III, 30r)*

> *When yang abounds, there is external heat. When there is emptiness of yang, there is external cold. (DACH I, 7v)*

> *When yin abounds, there is extreme cold. (DACH III, 30r)*

> *When yin abounds, there is internal cold. Emptiness of yin gives rise to internal warmth. (DACH I, 7v)*

Thus, in a case of external warmth it is recommended to disperse the yang; in a case of internal warmth, to tonify the yin. In cases of internal cold, one must disperse the yin; in those of external cold one must tonify the yang.

d) Movement-rest; activity-apathy:

Yang is activity, physical lightness, and above all mental lightness; insomnia results from excess yang. Yin, on the contrary, is the tendency towards rest or somnolence; apathy and heaviness result from excess yin.

> *Not being able to sleep is always caused by an excess of yang. Much sleeping is an excess of yin. With an excess of yin during the day one is not able to conquer somnolence. When there is silence and no desire to speak, it is the yin which commands one to rest. (YXRM IV, 20v)*

e) Sensitivity-insensitivity:

Yang gives sensitivity, and when in excess, sensitivity with pain. People who react sharply to feelings or sufferings have an excess of yang. (The gallbladder, a yang workshop organ, is the origin of many pains.) Yin, on the contrary, is insensitivity. The physical, manual people who have an excess of yin react little to emotions and pains.

f) Response to day and night:

The yang correlates to the daytime, the sun, and summer. Normally life, activity, and strength must increase and diminish with the sun. Those who have an excess of yang continue their activities into the evening; they have definite aggravation of discomfort or pain at night. Yin, on the contrary, correlates to night, the moon, and winter. Normally the tendency to rest, to calm oneself, starts towards the end of the day and stops as the day begins. Those who have an excess of yin carry their numbness into the morning. With yin excess, there is aggravation and redoubling of pain or discomfort toward the middle of the day. During the day one must respond to the sun and to yang; at night, to rest and to yin.

Migraines of the right side (which is yang) are generally caused by an excess of yang relative to yin and are normally calmed at the end of the day when the rising yin restores its balance. Migraines of the left side (which is yin) normally get worse in the evening; they are generally from an emptiness of yin relative to yang and are ameliorated towards the middle of the day when there is heat and sun.

It is useful here to further clarify the yin-yang relations of the different parts of the day:

> *In the first quarter after midnight the yang is born. In the first quarter of the afternoon the yin is born. The day is yang; the night is yin. (DACH VI, 4v)*

> *From dawn to midday is the yang within the yang. From midday to twilight is the yin within the yang. From night until cockcrow, the yin within the yin. From cockcrow to dawn, the yang within the yin. This is the cycle to which humans respond. (DACH II, 20r)*

g) Deep-superficial; interior-exterior:

The exterior, superficial, and what is exposed to the sun are yang. The interior, deep portions, and what is not exposed to the sun are yin. The yang meridians are on the external side of the limbs; the yin meridians are on the inner sides of the limbs. They ''flow inside the vessels'' *(DACH VI, 7v).* The anterior surface of the trunk is yin for men and yang for women. The posterior side is yang for men and yin for women. The skin is yang; bones and muscles are yin. Men are yang in relation to women, who are yin.

h) Crossings: left-right; upper-lower:

> *The right side is yang. The left side is yin. (DACH VII, 28v)*

The upper part is yang; it includes the head and the intellect, which are yang. The lower part is yin; it includes the genital system, which is yin.

> *Heaven is insufficient in the north and west [there is less sun]. Thus, north and west are yin. Therefore, [when facing south] the right eye and ear of people of the north and west lack the keenness of the left eye and ear. The earth is insufficient in the south and east [where the islands and the banks of large rivers are higher than in the east or north]. Thus, south and east are yang [the earth is yin]. Consequently, the left hand and foot of people in the south and east [facing south] do not have the strength of those of the right hand and foot. For [those who are] yang, sexual energy tends to rise. The upper part of the body is abundant and the lower part is empty. The left eye and ear are keen while the left hand and foot are without comfort. But for [those who are] yin, the sexual energy tends to descend; the lower part of the body is abundant and the upper part is empty. The right eye and ear lack keenness, but the right hand and foot are at ease. That is why the right side (weaker in yang) is more affected in disorders of both the exterior and upper part of the body (yang). The left side (yin) is more affected in disorders of both the interior and lower part of the body (yin). Thus we cannot change yin and yang, heaven and earth.*
> *(Su Wen, cited in DACH I, 13r)*

One is reminded of the hemiplegics whose lesion is on one side and paralysis of the limbs on the opposite side.

*On examination of the illustrated commentary of the **Nan Jing** and [the works of] Xu Feng, we find: left and right are not identical: chest and back are different. . . . The left side is yin and the right side is yang. For women this state is the reverse. Women are yin; men are yang. The back of woman is yin; the back of man is yang and his abdomen is yin. (DACH V, 28v)*

It has been observed repeatedly in Paris that very nervous but physically weak people have a fuller and firmer pulse on the right wrist compared to the left wrist. Physically strong but apathetic people, on the contrary, have a fuller and firmer pulse on the left wrist.

i) Yin or yang illnesses:

Differentiation between yin and yang diseases is important, yet not always easy. People of a yin nature (male or female) more easily come down with yin types of illnesses. Those of a yang nature more often have yang types of illnesses. One characteristic of yang diseases is that they are quicker, more violent, resolve more easily, and are of a short duration. Those of a yin nature are deep, long-lasting, chronic, and are resolved with difficulty. For example, measles that come out in a violent eruption are yang, whereas measles that come out with difficulty and cause pulmonary congestion or serious bronchitis are yin.

Sometimes there is confusion between diseases of the blood and those of the energy. The *Da Cheng XII, 39r* states: ''All illnesses are either of the energy (yang) or of the blood (yin).'' Illnesses of the energy (yang) are mobile; they generally have long remissions. In the West they are classified as functional or nervous disorders. Illnesses of the blood are localized and constant, without remission. In the West they are classified as organic. In treatment it is important to differentiate between blood and energy diseases:

To casually disperse the energy for a blood disease, or disperse the blood for an energy disease, is to massacre the innocent. Who would pardon such a mistake? (DACH XI, 39r)

j) Deep or superficial pulses; full or imperceptible pulses:

The yang pulses are at the superficial level and reflect the yang meridians. A yang pulse is full, rapid and tense. A yin pulse is situated at the deep level, corresponding to the yin meridians. A yin pulse is sunken, hard and contracted.

Yin-yang and the chemical elements.

Modern Japanese scholars, notably Doctor Nyoiti Sakurazawa, have studied the notion of yin and yang and the chemical elements using modern laboratory instruments. They have proposed that the elements are charged with yin or yang energy. Sodium (Na) is typical of the yang category: the yang radiations of sodium containing and attracting compounds are indispensable for mental and intellectual life. Potassium (K) is typical of the yin category: it is indispensable for vegetal life and for physical development. Between the two extremes of yin and yang are the elements charged with both activities — the halogens and catalysts. Among these are the precious metals gifted with all the ''mystical'' properties.[4]

Colors and flavors are equally charged with yin or yang vibrations. Red is the most yang, highest vibratory color (at 6500 vibrations). Throughout the range of the spectrum, from red to violet, yang activity mixes with yin. Violet (4290 vibrations) is most yin. Pungent is the most yang flavor and corresponds to red (e.g., radish). Next is the sour flavor, which corresponds to orange and yellow (e.g., lemon). Sweet corresponds to green (e.g., sugar cane) and salt corresponds to blue (e.g., the sea). Bitter, which corresponds to violet, is the most yin (e.g., eggplant).

A plant placed in the dark (yin) produces very long, white branches (both yin qualities). When exposed to sunlight (yang), it produces short, colored branches (both yang qualities). The yellow or brown autumn leaves (yang) have a higher sodium content than the pale green (yin) leaves of spring.

Yang and yin produce each other reciprocally. The more opposite they are, the more they attract each other; the closer they are, the more they reject each other. Eggs are always divided into long eggs (yin) and round eggs (yang). The embryo of long eggs are male and those of round eggs are female, because yin produces its opposite, yang, and yang produces its opposite, yin. Women (yin) produce round ovum (yang) and men (yang) produce long sperm (yin). To obtain a female child one eats excessive amounts of yang foods charged with sodium (yang). To obtain a male child one eats excessive amounts of yin foods charged with potassium (yin).

In the treatment of disease, the rule is to give yin elements to cure yang illnesses and yang elements to cure yin illnesses. Yang medicines are stimulants, expectorants, resolvents, substances with a strong smell, and hot decoctions. Yin medicines are astringents, purgatives, emetics, bitters, and infusions.

Origins of yin-yang.

The ancient Chinese, positing that all is active or latent energy, have researched the origins of this dual, alternating energy:

> Yin energy arises from the center of the Earth and nourishes the energy of cereals, the **rong** energy, pure energy, the energy of the stomach, and the original energy. Yang energy first perfects itself from outside. So, what is outside is Heaven. The yang energy flows down and enters the Earth. It brings fire into the yin. (DACH XI, 11r)

According to the *Da Cheng,* there are two poles of energy: Heaven, which is yang and positive; and Earth, which is yin and negative. The yang moves downward, warming the earth, while the yin rises upward and nourishes the vegetation.

The author of the *Yi Xue Ru Men* (V, 38r) presents these concepts in another manner:

> Yang is light and pure. It is the energy which floats up and from which Heaven is formed. Yin is thick and heavy. Yin is energy that has taken form; it solidified to form the Earth. The essence of yang is the sun. The essence of yin is the moon, which hides during the day and appears at night. Vapor tends to condense to form water; this sky-blue energy (water) holds itself up and plants are nourished by it.

In clarifying the passage above, we add that there is probably only one source of energy producing the sun, earth and moon. The lightest part of this energy maintains itself ''on high'' (maintaining the sun), while the heaviest part takes shape and forms the earth and the moon.

Yin-yang, representing relativity and movement, gives rise to constant exchange between the light and heavy: the light becomes heavy and the heavy becomes light. Chemistry demonstrates the transformation between ''heaven and earth,'' or more exactly air and water. The chlorophyll in leaves, with the indispensable action of the sun's rays, reduces carbon dioxide, fixes the carbon in the leaves and releases the oxygen into the air. Carbon enters immediately into combination with the constituent elements of water drawn up from the Earth through the roots. The resulting product is starch (carbohydrates), needed by the plant to form the fats, albuminoids, and so on.

Alternations of yin and yang.

The descriptions of yin and yang above imply that the universe is not in a fixed state but is passing through phases of incessant movement; this is the law of the universe. The energy *(qi)* that circulates in human beings passes from yin to yang and yang to yin without end. In other words, yin becomes yang and yang becomes yin; or, the yin engenders the yang, the yang engenders the yin. A passage out of the *Ju Ying* (cited in the *Da Cheng*) clearly explains this movement:

> Question: What is the rule of the alternation of yin and yang? Answer: This is the idea of mutual overlapping of yin and yang; of how the yang enters into the divisions of yin and, alternately, the yin enters into the divisions of yang. If yin and yang are static, illness results. We must rise to the source, to the cause. Either the **rong** energy (yin) is deficient and weak, or the **wei** energy (yang) is deficient. With the latter case, the **rong** energy (yin) soars to the outside. Consequently, energy and blood no longer keep their place. The energy accumulates in one area creating an excess in that region. The energy expands in one area and makes this region empty. That which is in excess produces pain. That which is empty produces itching. Pain is yin [in excess]. Pain that cannot be reached by pressure of the hand is yin; one must puncture deeply. Pruritus is yang [in excess]; one must puncture superficially. Illness in the upper body is yang; illness in the lower body is yin. (DACH VI, 9r)

Notes

[1] *Qi Bo* states:

> At the first and second moon the energy of Heaven begins to expand, and that of the Earth to produce; the energy of man is in the liver. At the third and fourth moons the energy of Heaven is full of activity and that of the Earth fixes its produce; the energy of man is in the spleen-pancreas. At the fifth and sixth moons, the energy of Heaven abounds and that of the Earth is important; the energy of man is in the head. At the seventh and eighth moons, the yin energy begins to overtake the yang. The energy of man is in the lungs. At the ninth and tenth moons, the yin energy begins to freeze and that of the earth to close; the energy of man is in the heart-spirit. At the eleventh and twelfth moons, ice and the energy of the earth are united; the energy of man is in the kidneys.
> *(Nei Jing, cited in DACH I, 10r)*

[2] Yin is formed of elements which combined give the meaning: "slope covered by the shadow from the clouds." This is equivalent to our "hubac" (French regional dialect), which means the slope of a mountain or hill exposed to the north and always deprived of sunlight. Yin connotes deprivation of light and warmth, and thus gives the idea of cold, immobility, lack of life, obscurity, enclosure, internality, and also water and humidity.

Yang is formed of elements which combined mean: "slope that the sun covers with its rays." It is our "adret," a slope exposed to the south receiving the sun. Yang represents light and warmth, and that which is dry, luminous, warm and also external and superficial.

[3] The yin-yang relativity has been applied to the human body through the following names: *rong-wei, qi-xue*.

Rong is formed from the elements, "flames-enclosed-wood," connoting latent energy in the depths.

> The **rong** energy is sexual energy *(jing)*. It governs the interior. That is why the Book says: It is the sexual energy of food and water. *(DACH VI, 9v)*
>
> The **rong** is the root while **wei** represents the branches. *(DACH VI, 8v)*
>
> That which circulates in the interior of the vessels, the yin, is the **rong** and blood. *(DACH VI, 11v)*
>
> Puncturing at 2/10 of a **cun,** one arrives at the **rong** [at 1/10 of a **cun** it is the **wei**]. *(DACH VI, 7v)*

The ideogram *wei* represents the guard who keeps watch outside the doors of palaces.

> The **wei** energy is the superficial energy. It governs the exterior. It is the life of liquids and food. It does not enter into the vessels, but stays in the epidermis, the dermis, the muscles and the mucus membranes. It spreads over the chest and abdomen. When the **wei** is irritated, illness results. *(DACH VI, 9v)*
>
> **Wei** represents the branches and leaves, the **rong** being the root. *(DACH VI, 8v)*
>
> What circulates at the exterior of the vessels, the yang energy, is **wei**. *(DACH VI, 11v)*
>
> When puncturing at 1/10 of a **cun,** one arrives at the **wei** (at 2/10, it is the **rong**). *(DACH VI, 7v)*

Qi-xue (energy and blood):

> As with all life, humans receive the energy of heaven and earth: the yang energy of heaven is the **qi,** and the yin energy of the earth is the **xue.** *(YXRM, "Shou juan," 41r)*

Chinese texts consistently use *qi* synonymously for yang and *xue* for yin. The treasure organs, which govern the blood, are yin; and the workshop organs, which extract the energy from food, are yang *(DACH II, 20r)*. The role of this opposition is described thus:

> That which moves the pulses is the **qi** (energy). That which gives life to illnesses is the xue (blood). *(DACH VI, 8v)*

First the movement and afterwards the birth.

[4] See *Principe Unique*, 68, by N. Sakurazawa, and the *Revue Franaise d'Homéopathie,* June 1931.

Chapter VIII

The Radial Pulses

I. The Necessity of the Pulses and the Ancient System — II. The System of the Fourteen Radial Pulses

I. The Necessity of the Pulses and the Ancient System

The necessity of knowing the pulses.[1]

The knowledge of pulses is absolutely indispensable for the practice of true acupuncture, which is based on treating the root condition. Using only memorized formulae and treating only visible problems does not constitute true acupuncture.

Only through the pulses can one perceive the functioning of each organ, the intensity of energy — either for each organ or in general — and the proportion of yin and yang. The information derived from the pulses permits the useful questioning of the patient for details not otherwise reported. This information alone allows determination of the meridian in which the equilibrium must be restored and the group of points advisable to use.

> *Each time one uses needles, one must palpate the pulses. One can see the ease of flow or contraction of the energy. Only then can one treat. (DACH I, 14v, citing Nei Jing)*

> *If one wants to know the fullness or emptiness of the organs, one must palpate to feel the abundance or weakness of the pulse. From this one can clearly determine the high and low of the vessels of the meridians. . . . It is evident that there are meridians and pulses. Those who use them are the true doctors (**liang yi**). Those who ignore them are clumsy workers (**zu gong**). (DACH I, 20v)*

> *For doctors, the study of pulses is of primary importance, since through the pulses one can know the fullness and emptiness of the meridians and best determine the treatment strategy and use of needles and moxa. (YXRM I, 21r)*

> *By palpating the radial pulses one perceives fullness or emptiness. One knows the illnesses and in which organs they reside. (DACH I, 17r)*

The pulses give a clear indication of the functioning, vitality, and energetic capacity of each internal organ; moreover, they inform us about the material form of the organ, be it large or small, hard or soft. The pathological state to be discerned necessitates such a delicacy of digital and cerebral perception that Europeans rarely succeed in perceiving it.

The ancient systems.

Through centuries of experimentation in China, many systems were developed which used the pulses of the arteries to diagnose the functioning of the organs. Although differing systems were developed and used in China's various regions, they were all based on years of careful observation — a useful fact is never deliberately put aside in China.

The better known of the ancient systems are mentioned below:

The carotid pulses. Perhaps the oldest system used was the palpation of the pulses of the right and left carotid arteries at the level of the upper part of the thyroid cartilage. (The acupoint *renying,* ST-9, derives its name from one of these pulses.)

> *Hua Shou [thirteenth century] reports that in ancient times both sides of the thyroid cartilage were used as **renying**. The left pulse, indicating the condition of the blood, was called "human meetings"; while the right pulse, indicating the condition of the energy, was called **qi kou,** "mouth of energy." (DACH VIII, 8v)*

The ancient books consistently give the ratio of the strengths of these two pulses (a ratio that may be as great as two or three to one) to verify the emptiness or fullness of each organ. This system, extremely difficult to master, is very rarely used today.

The pulses of the meridians on the four limbs. Many acupoints along the meridians are located above pulsating arteries. Each pulse reflects a special function. Practitioners still utilize the relationship between these pulses and certain disorders for diagnosis. For example, the onset of menses is heralded by agitation of the artery at *chongyang* (ST-42) and *taichong* (LR-3) on the dorsum of the foot. If the pulse under the internal malleolus, *taixi* (KI-5, IS KI-3), beats well, the patient is not in grave danger if diseased.

> *In antiquity, one also used arteries felt by palpation of the meridians. These pulses were divided into three groups, serving each of the treasure and workshop organs. (YXRM I, 21)*

The nine radial guardians. This system, which is different from the actual pulse-organ correlations given in Volume II, nevertheless gives good results through the use of three tension levels of the radial pulse. Each radial pulse is divided into three sections: central, just at the level of the radial apophysis; distal, at the base of the thumb; and proximal, above the apophysis. Each section is divided into three levels: Heaven (superficial), Man (middle), and Earth (deep).

The table showing the relations of the organs to the nine guardians is given below:

proximal section	superficial level	gallbladder
	middle level	triple warmer
	deep level	stomach
central section	superficial level	lungs
	middle level	heart
	deep level	energy in the chest
distal section	superficial level	liver
	middle level	spleen-pancreas
	deep level	kidneys

The descriptions in the texts are imprecise but seem to indicate that the pulses above are bilateral. It has not been possible for us, in spite of all our efforts, to observe any connection between these pulses and the indicated organs. We must suppose that the tradition has been poorly transmitted.

II. The System of the Fourteen Radial Pulses

History and name.

The system of the radial pulses, used since antiquity, was perfected and reported in writing for the first time by Wang Shuhe, who lived during the Jin Dynasty (A.D. 265 - 420). His work, "Law of the Pulses," *Mo Jing,* also called "Traditions on the Pulses," *Mo Xue,* is still extant.[2] These radial pulses are called *guan mai,* "pulses of the barrier," (the barrier being the place over the styloid process where the radial pulse beats). They are also called *cunkou,* "mouth of the thumb" (being the part of the pulse nearest the thumb) (see *YXRM* I, 21r & 28r; *DACH* I, 14r & 17r). The pulses of the left wrist are collectively called *ren-ying,* "human meetings," since the organs reflected on this wrist are easily disturbed by external factors: weather, foods, etc. The pulses of the right wrist are called *qikou,* "mouth of energy," since the organs reflected at this wrist are mostly disturbed by internal factors: the lack or excess of energy, the psyche (emotions), etc. *(YXRM I, 21r).*

Each wrist is divided into three sections, *fen.* The first section (distal) is located in the hollow between the radial styloid process and the base of the thumb. It is called the *cun,* "inch," and is located at one thumb's width from the articulation of the first and second metacarpals. It is also termed the first pulse. The second section (central) is located just at the level of the most prominent point of the styloid process of the radius. Its name is the *guan,* "barrier," because it divides, or rather joins, the yin and the yang (the *cun* pulse is yang and the *chi* pulse is yin). It is also called the second pulse. The third section (proximal) is located in the hollow immediately to the rear of the styloid process of the radius. It is called the *chi,* "foot," because the distance from this pulse to the elbow crease is one foot. It is also termed the third pulse.

Each section is divided into two or three levels. The superficial level is called "Heaven." It is obtained by sliding the finger very lightly on the upper surface of the artery in order to perceive the top of the wave which travels through the mass of blood. We can now say that it corresponds to the Western minimum arterial blood pressure (true diastolic blood pressure). The middle level is called "Man." It is obtained by depressing the artery halfway in order to perceive the quantity of the mass of blood in movement. It corresponds to the Western effective blood pressure (the oscillometric index). The deep level is called "Earth." It is obtained by depressing the artery such that the upper surface touches the lower surface, allowing itself to be raised by the flux of blood. This level measures the force of the impulse. It corresponds to our maximum arterial blood pressure (systolic).

Relations of the pulses to the energy and organs.

All the pulses of the left wrist correspond to physical life, blood and yin. If the whole left pulse is ample and hard, there is an excess of these. If the pulse is hardly perceptible, there is extreme fatigue, weakness, and deficiency of yin.

All the pulses of the right wrist correspond to mental life, energy and yang. If the entire right pulse is harder and more ample than the left pulse, then the mental life, the yang, dominates — the patient acts only by will and energy, not by natural strength. If the right pulses are weaker than the left, the patient is apathetic, but physically resistant. If they are weak and soft, the patient is sad and lacks energy and resiliency; yang is deficient.

On both wrists, all the superficial pulses correspond to the yang workshop organs and the yang meridians. All the deep or middle pulses correspond to the yin treasure organs and the yin meridians. If the superficial pulses dominate, there is excess of yang mental life over yin physical life; excitability and nervous tension may result. If the deep pulses dominate, there is an overabundance of yin physical life, with a tendency toward physical tension or plethora. Each level of each section reflects the functioning and energetic state of an internal organ (or to general functions if referring to the triple warmer or heart governor.)

The following table shows the correspondence between the pulses and the internal organs:

		Left	**Right**
I.	Superficial	Small intestine	Large intestine
	Middle	Heart	Lungs
II.	Superficial	Gallbladder	Stomach
	Middle	Liver	Pancreas
	Deep	High blood pressure	Spleen
III.	Superficial	Bladder	Triple warmer
	Middle	Kidneys-filtration	Heart governor
	Deep	Kidneys-secretion	Sexual organs
IV.	Superficial	Evolved man	Spinal cord
	Middle	Conditioned man	Cerebellum, medulla
	Deep	Primate man	Brain

We have found that it is possible to distinguish between the left kidney and the right kidney: the left side of the artery at the kidney pulse represents the left kidney and the right side, the right kidney. The same is true for the lungs and the heart. This useful discovery is never mentioned in Chinese texts.

Unexplained facts.

It has been noted that there is a connection between the deep level and the organ only at the second and third (*guan* and *chi*) sections of the right wrist. The *cun* section of the right wrist and the *cun, guan,* and *chi* sections of the left wrist have only two levels — there is no significance for their deep levels. However, our modern instruments perceive three levels on both wrists. Volume III expounds on these discoveries. It should be noted, however, that the *cun* pulses, which have only two levels, are actually on the radiopalmar artery, a branch of the radial artery.

Our oscillometers have picked up wave movements lower than the minimal arterial pressure (superficial level), and occurring before the pressure rises. Likewise, beyond the maximum pressure (deep level) and after it rises, there are some additional minimal oscillations. The significance of these small oscillations, which differ from person to person, has not yet been fully appreciated. Some physicians in Paris believe that these oscillations are indicators of mental acuity. They see a correlation between more pronounced oscillations and higher development of emotional or mental sensitivity.

Comparative harmony or discordance of the pulses.

The ideal is that all the pulses are in harmony: ''When all the pulses are in harmony, one says that there is no illness, or if there is illness, it will resolve itself.'' It is best if the superficial pulses are slightly softer and less ample than the deep and middle pulses. Each pulse should have a particular quality, reflecting the functional state of its associated organ.

If there are discordances, then usually these are the same for all the pulse positions. It is rare that a superficial pulse beats at a different speed than the deep or middle pulse of the same section, particularly without the neighboring pulses being equally discordant. In one rare case, however, the right superficial *cun* pulse of a patient beat at 100 pulsations, while the middle pulse beat at 80. The case was observed and confirmed by three doctors, but is difficult to explain given that the levels tested were on the same segment of artery with the same blood-mass flowing through it.

The different qualities of the pulses and their interpretations.

Each pulse can have many different qualities, each indicating a specific problem. Modern instruments give only a few of these numerous qualities. The Vaquez instrument allows the determination of the minimum and maximum pulse oscillations (although without exactness because of the lack of standard technique). With this instrument it is possible to perceive the hardness of the pulse, the resistance to pressure. (It cannot, however, distinguish between the hardness of the artery and an excess blood-mass.) The oscillometers of the Pachon type additionally give the amplitude and energy of the pulse.

The Chinese text *Yi Xue Ru Men* (I, 21r) describes twenty-seven possible qualities for each of the pulses and classifies them as follows:

a)   Seven external, *qi biao,* which the finger can perceive on touching: yang qualities (floating, scallion-stalk, slippery, full, tight, wiry).

b)   Eight internal, *ba li,* which the finger perceives only with pressure: yin qualities (tiny, sunken, slow, retarded, rough, recumbent, soft, weak).

c)   Nine ways, *jiu dao,* qualities of movement (fine, agitated, rapid, empty, hurried, scattered, changing, leather-like).

The pulses are often regrouped according to the European classifications: frequency, intermittence, irregularity, amplitude, hardness, shape, and placement:

Frequency (rapid-slow). Rapidity is always a sign of excess with inflammation. If the pulses are rapid and the temperature is elevated, the pulse of the inflamed organ will be fuller and harder than the others. Slowness is a sign of insufficiency and atonia. If all the pulses are slow, the heart pulse, the heart governor and triple warmer pulses are, as a rule, hardly perceptible.

Rapid *(shuo):* ''More than six times per respiration (instead of four). It is a febrile pulse. It announces an agitation of the heart and can lead to delirium.''

Slow *(chi):* ''Somewhat less rapid than normal (four per respiration). It is an inactivity of the skin. At the extreme, energy and blood do not circulate in the dermis, which is hard, paralyzed and rheumatic.''

Retarded *(huan):* ''Less than three per respiration. There is cold. The blood is empty. Exterior and interior are cold.''

Intermittence (false steps, skipping, stops). Intermittence, i.e., the skipping of a beat, can either be a sign of excess yang if the pulse is rapid with fever, or a sign of excess yin if the pulse is slow.

Accelerated *(cu):* ''The beats are more numerous but sometimes stop; there is extreme heat. Yang abounds; the interior yin is not of equal strength.''

Knotted *(jie):* ''The pulse is slow, comes late and has irregular intervals. It is the pulse of accumulation. The yin abounds and the yang cannot replace it. At the interior or exterior the blood is badly hindered, forming an accumulation.'' Cancer patients have this pulse.

Changing *(dai):* ''After each ten beats there is a gap (or after every twenty or thirty or forty beats). The pulse stops at regular intervals for a little longer than one beat. It indicates an extreme degeneration of energy. For the organs it is the pulse that leads to death.''

Irregularity (sometimes slow and sometimes rapid). Pulses whose beats are not all separated by the same time interval have not been noted by the Chinese. In Europe, it is considered a sign of nervous trouble of the heart or of sympathetic derangement.

Inequality of strength or amplitude. The beats, even and regular in time, are of unequal force, sometimes ample and hard and sometimes tiny and soft.

Rough *(se):* ''The movement is not uniform. It is like a length of bamboo interrupted by knots. It is the opposite of slippery. Sexual energy and yin are injured. Blood is defeated. Men have this pulse through sexual excess, which injures the sexual energy. Women have this pulse when the fetus has little blood or causes pain. Women who are not pregnant have it through reversed or accumulated blood.''

❥ *Amplitude (large and small).* Amplitude is always a sign of excess, mostly the excess of yang (mental life). An ample and hard pulse signifies great nervous tension; an ample and soft pulse, excitability and weakness. Non-amplitude (tiny) is a sign of insufficiency of yin and yang, extreme lassitude and weakness. A tiny and soft pulse is indicative of exhaustion, while a tiny and hard pulse indicates tightness and internal contractions, generally through weakness.

Vast *(hong):* ''With long, full undulations like the sea. It signifies heat, with burning energy and blood. Exterior and interior are hot.''

Fine *(xi):* ''Like a thread, sometimes seeming to exist and sometimes seeming not to exist. Energy and blood are empty and cold. There are cold accumulations under the umbilicus creating pain or laxness.''

Empty *(xu):* ''Without pulses. Nothing is perceived on pressure. It is a serious emptiness.''

Note that the West recognizes *a)* the strong and depressible pulse (ample and soft) of aortic insufficiency; *b)* the depressible (soft) and bounding pulse of mitral insufficiency; *c)* the ample pulse of the alcoholic and high blood pressure; *d)* the tiny pulse of low blood pressure and great fatigue.

Certain Chinese authors add:

Great *(da)* (great and soft): ''Lifts the finger like the vast pulse, but if pressed, it is without resistance. The perverse energy abounds. Energy and blood are empty and cannot act.'' There is nervousness and weakness.

Hardness (hard or soft). Hardness is a sign of excess. A hard and ample pulse is a sign of great nervous tension, whereas a hard and tiny pulse is weakness with tension. A large intestine pulse which is ample and a little soft is a sign of inflammation with diarrhea; ample and hard is a sign of constipation or retention. A kidney pulse which is tiny and soft suggests there is clear and abundant urine; a tiny and hard pulse indicates contracted kidneys with impure and insufficient urine. Softness is a sign of laxity. If the pulse is soft, the organ is lax; if large and soft the organ is inflated and soft. Thus a soft stomach pulse which is large and long is a sign of aerogastry; that which is soft and tiny a sign of slow digestion.

Full *(shi):* ''The more it is pressed, the stronger it beats. It is fullness of energy. It is a pulse representing heat of the blood and energy.''

Leather-like *(ge):* ''Like a very tight drum (full, wide, without beats). Energy and blood are withdrawing or are being disturbed from their normal functioning. Men no longer transform energy into sperm. Women have menor-rhagia or discharge; if pregnant, they will abort. It is a sign of coming emptiness and cold.''

Excess energy is involved in contractions and paralyses.

Wiry *(xian):* ''Like a well-tightened bow string. It is always straight and tight, even if one palpates it superficially or deeply. It represents fatigue or tuberculosis. Energy and blood are both in danger.''

Soft *(ruo):* ''Totally without form whatever the manner of pressing. A light hand lets it come; a heavy hand drives it away. There is abundant and spontaneous perspiration. Frequently found in the aged, it represents the degeneration and weakening of energy and blood. It forecasts a decline in the strength of the aged.''

Weak *(ruan):* ''Seems on the point of stopping, but does not stop. If pressed, it seems on the point of disappearing, and if one lifts the finger, it does disappear. It is a true emptiness of energy; numbness of bone and body. In the elderly, there is no remedy.''

Shape (wide, narrow, long, short, etc.). The West does not currently consider the shape of the pulse important. Our observations, on the other hand, show that the shape can have significance and give very useful indications. For example, a pulse like a grill, like a cross-hatched grating, is regularly found at the lung pulse position when a tubercular lesion is clearly evolving. For the pulse of the stomach, a long, swollen, large and soft pulse is a sure indication of aerogastry. A large intestine pulse with agitation like small ticklings at the base of the thumb is a sign of hemorrhoids or intestinal worms. A long, hard, cutting and wide gallbladder pulse suggests gallstones. A big, swollen, soft liver pulse means congestion of the liver, and so on.

The Chinese make other distinctions:

Slippery *(hua):* "Slow and hard like pearls coming and going. The opposite of rough; it means much mucus; an excess of blood with compressed energy rising and forming mucus.

Turbulent *(dong):* "Like a pea that rolls without coming and going, that seems to roll in place without leaving or returning. If constant, it is a sign of despoiled blood; it is the pulse of tuberculosis, and emptiness. It is caused by emptiness, deprivation, hemorrhage, serious diarrhea or blood disease."

Split *(kou):* "The peak of the pulse is divided into two heads, like an onion stalk crushed in the middle. It signifies emptiness of blood. The blood depends on the yin, the rule of which is constant lassitude."

Squeezed *(jin):* "Like a rope that has just been twisted. It means pain. An evil has taken the blood and energy and overturned them, producing the pain."

The *Da Cheng* (VI, 84) indicates another variety:

Contracted *(ji):* "Giving the sensation of being contracted without reaching true hardness. One must tonify." Perhaps this is a pulse which is small and contracted due to weakness and tension. One must tonify, but at times also disperse the source.

Placement. As in Chinese medicine, Western medical science recognizes the general radial pulses and notes the weakness of the pulse located above the *chi* pulse on the forearm and the excitation of that near the base of the thumb. The Chinese note:

Extended *(chang):* "A pulse that beats beyond its normal placement. It is a sign of excess energy; but energy and blood are well regulated and without trouble. If there is slowness, the hundred diseases are easy to cure."

Unreached *(duan):* "Hardly reaching its place. There is illness or binding of energy, or the energy of the stomach is degenerated, and reduced. In every illness where there is this sign, cure is difficult."

Interpretation of the qualities of each organ pulse.

The following principles are useful for understanding the connections between the quality of each pulse and the function and state of the organ which it reflects:[3]

Small and soft pulse: insufficient organ.
Ample and hard pulse: organ is functionally overactive or congested.
Soft and big pulse: organ is swollen, not functioning.
Small, hard and sharp pulse: organ is in spasm, contracted and painful.

Hua Shou, of the thirteenth century, wrote:

> *People's illnesses have only four aspects: cold or hot, excess or empty. The totality of the pulses may be seen immediately. If the superficial pulses are large and rapid, there is heat; if they are firm and contracted, and at the deep level are small, retarded, and just in advance, there is cold. If the shape has fullness and if all the pulses are slippery and tight like a rope, there is excess. If the shape is soft and if all are empty, rough, and slow, there is emptiness. (YXRM I, 22v)*

The general and practical indications are given by the *Yi Xue Ru Men:*

> *In a general sense, if there is emptiness, the pulse is wiry (**xian**). If the pulse is wiry (**xian**), soft (**ruo**), large (**da**) and without strength, there is emptiness of energy. If the pulse is sunken (**chen**), tiny (**wei**), and without strength, there is serious emptiness of energy. If the pulse is wiry (**xian**) and tiny (**wei**), there is emptiness of blood. Or if it is soft (**ruo**) and tiny (**wei**), there is serious emptiness of blood. If the pulses of the inch (**cun**) are tiny and if those of the foot (**chi**) are large (**da**) and tight (**jin**), it means emptiness of blood. (YXRM V, 7r)*

> *If the pulse is bounding and large, the blood has much fullness; there is swelling and pain. If the pulse is declining and weak, the energy has much emptiness; there is pruritus, paresthesia and laxness. (DACH II, 27v)*

> *A declining and weak pulse indicates much emptiness of energy, pruritus or softness. An abundant and large pulse suggests fullness of blood, swelling or pain. (DACH II, 20v)*

It is difficult to interpret all the qualities the pulse may have for each organ. However, some of the more obvious, common pulses will be used to illustrate and elucidate the tactile language of the pulses. Using the order of the circulation of energy, we can describe each organ's pulse position, depth and possible qualities:

Large Intestine (Section I, Right wrist, Superficial level) — The pulse portion near the thumb, close to the bone, corresponds to the anus. The portion near the second pulse (Section II) corresponds to the cecum. If the pulse is hard and without amplitude: constipation. If hard but ample: inflammation and diarrhea from inflammation. If soft, and hardly perceptible, relaxed (without medication): soft stool. If agitated at the level of the thumb: hemorrhoids or anal pruritus. If very agitated: intestinal worms. If big and hard near the styloid process: fecal retention.

Lungs (Section I, Right wrist, Middle level) — It would be more accurate to use the term "respiratory passages," since the pulse also corresponds to the larynx and bronchi. The end near the thumb corresponds to the base of the lungs. The portion near the styloid process relates to the throat and bronchi. Big and hard pulse: inflammation with constricted respiration. Soft, hardly perceptible: atonia, and exhausted respiration; it can be seen after serious diseases of the lungs. Grilled, like a crosshatched grating: tuberculosis. The pulse should be soft, a bit ample and beat in the center of its location. The part touching the styloid process reflects the bronchi and trachea and may indicate clenched, spasmodic asthma; if swollen, bronchial inflammation. At the first section, right wrist, deep level, there is no known pulse correspondence.

Stomach (Section II, Right wrist, Superficial level) — Big, swollen pulse, soft, long and wide: aerogastry. Stomach swollen after meals: sign of insufficiency of energy or muscle tone of the organ (tonify *gongsun*, (SP-4). Soft, weak, small pulse: atony, slow digestion, insufficient secretions. Small, hard wiry pulse: cramps or burning. An ample, soft and calm pulse indicates good appetite and digestion.

> *A large (**da**) pulse at the stomach position indicates abundance of blood and energy, robustness, and heat.*
> *(DACH I, 12v)*

Pancreas (Section II, Right wrist, Middle level) — Pulse is always large and soft in diabetics, or if the person likes to drink a lot. Small, soft, hardly perceptible pulse: the person does not like meat and takes very little to drink.

Spleen (Section II, Right wrist, Deep Level) — Absent, or weak, soft, small pulse: great fatigue in the morning with amelioration at the end of the afternoon, capricious digestion, difficulty with intellectual pursuits, mostly in concentrating the mind. Big, swollen, hard pulse: swelling or congestion of the spleen, and constant sleepiness. A healthy spleen should have a pulse that is soft, ample and well placed.

Triple Warmer (Section III, Right wrist, Superficial level) — Responds to yang. Wiry, ropy, hard, without amplitude: great tension and nervous irritability, self-control outwardly but inwardly there is tension. Very ample and slightly soft pulse: anger, cannot bear anything. Wiry, but thready: sensitive, discontented, impatient. Soft without amplitude: physical and mental apathy. Pulse without buoyancy: lassitude or great fatigue.

Vessels (Section III, Right wrist, Middle level) — Strong and hard pulse: congested states, high blood pressure, arterial contractions. Soft, imperceptible pulse: hypotension, slow circulation, coldness at the extremities. It responds to the yin.

Sexual Organs ("Gate of Destiny." Section III, Right wrist, Deep level) — Hard and ample pulse: in men, inflammation of the organs or sexual excitement and genital prowess; for women, if occurring one or two days before menses, or between the end of menses and the ninth through the eleventh day after menses, congestion and inflammation of the organ, or sexual excitement. Pulse soft and weak or absent: in men, genital weakness; in women, menses just finishing, genital weakness.

For women this pulse beats with increasing strength from the seventh day before menses until the arrival of menses, when it then disappears. It beats from the ninth to the eleventh day after menses (ovulation) with an average beat like that of the previous seventh day. This pulse also gives information on the state of pregnancy and becomes hard like a small pearl from the second day of the pregnancy. The pulse is sharp if the developing fetus is a boy and round if a girl.

Spinal Cord (Section IV, Right wrist, Superficial Level) — Raised, wiry pulse: the person acts more on reflexes than with reflection. Raised, hard pulse: inflammation. Empty, vacuous pulse: reactions slow or abolished, sluggish thoughts, slow movements.

Cerebellum (Section IV, Right wrist, Middle Level) — Hard, raised pulse: voluntary and involuntary movements are exaggerated. Soft, not raised pulse: movements are weak, poorly coordinated, and imperfectly transmitted to the organs.

Brain (Section IV, Right wrist, Deep Level) — Weak, soft pulse: fatigue or cerebral weakness, finds work difficult and uninteresting. Pulse not present on one side of the artery: anemia or softening of the opposite side of the brain (radial side of the pulse for the left side of the brain: memories and functional relations; medial side of the pulse for the right side of the brain: tradition, instinctive functions). Raised pulse: cerebral agitation. Raised, hard pulse: congestion, serious agitation.

Small Intestine (Section I, Left wrist, Superficial level) — Hard and big pulse: inflammation. Soft and small pulse: atony, lack of strength. Hard, small, sharp pulse: spasm (and if the pulse of the stomach is also small and hard: spasm of the pylorus).

Heart (Section I, Left wrist, Middle level) — Soft, weak or absent pulse: either psychological depression, sadness, or physical breathlessness on effort, e.g., climbing stairs (weakness of the heart muscle). Hard, wiry pulse: pain of the heart, or great shock.

Gallbladder (Section II, Left wrist, Superficial level) — Hard, wiry, long pulse: vomiting, nausea or bitter taste in the mouth on waking, often pain on one side of the head mostly at the temples. Hard and small, with the small intestine pulse small and hard: pyloric spasm (the stomach does not empty). Very hard, big and round: probably a gallstone. Big, soft, long pulse: thick bile. Swelling of the gallbladder often results from lack of tone which causes the same in the liver. We must discern whether the hardness of the gallbladder pulse gives way under light pressure (if so, tonify *xiaxi,* GB-43); or if it resists pressure (then disperse *yangfu,* GB-38). With the latter there are usually joint pains.

Liver (Section II, Left wrist, Middle level) — Ample, firm, lively pulse: liver in excellent state. Soft and big: soft, insufficient liver. Hard and big: congestion or inflammation. Absent or soft and weak pulse: insufficiency. Sometimes the insufficiency affects only certain functions; pruritus, skin eruptions, eczema, bruising at the slightest bump, slow coagulation of blood may result. Generally the digestive functions are injured: there is some difficulty in digesting chocolate, fresh cream, eggs and fats. Constipation and yellow stools result.

High Blood Pressure (Section II, Left wrist, Deep level) — This pulse only appears when the blood pressure is higher than normal, usually between 100 - 200 mm. Hg.

Urinary Bladder (Section III, Left wrist, Superficial level) — Thready, wiry and tight pulse: frequent and urgent urination, cystitis. Wiry pulse in an elderly man: prostatitis. Weak, hardly perceptible pulse: incontinence of urine. The pulse is sometimes wiry simply from nervousness. In that case the pulse of the triple warmer is equally wiry.

Kidney-Filtration (Section III, Left wrist, Middle level) — If low, soft pulse: abundant urine. Swollen, hard: retention of urine. Hard and small: spasm. The radial side of the artery represents the left kidney, the medial side of the artery the right kidney.

Kidney-Secretion (Section III, Left wrist, Deep level) — Indicates secretion of solids. Weak or vacuous pulse: discolored or pale lemon-colored urine. Hard pulse, without striking and deep: red and cloudy urine, hard and sharp pains. Soft and big pulse: swelling, if at the right kidney, prolapsed kidney. The radial side of the artery represents the left kidney, the medial side of the artery the right kidney.

Evolved (Conscious) Man (Section IV, Left wrist, Superficial level) — Raised, supple pulse: presence of mind, observant and attentive, seeing and understanding connections, impartial and without obsession. Absent pulse: absent minded, distracted, not understanding, without insight or deductive reasoning. Hard pulse: obsessions or phobias.

Conditioned Man (Section IV, Left wrist, Middle level) — Radial side of the artery: opposite side of the brain. Robot-like, traditional, conformist. If weak, soft pulse: easily deceived, suggestible, influenced, trusts the newspapers, advertisements, propaganda. Raised, strong pulse: acts by hereditary compulsions — good or bad; not suggestible. Hard and strong: acts blindly through habit. Medial side of the artery: "parrot memory." Pulse not raised: poor conscious memory, memory not present, needs to think before answering. If raised, supple pulse: good student, first at book-learning, brilliant and always prepared to quote with ready-made sentences, citations, references, but seeing only the small side of people and things.

Primate Man (Section IV, Left wrist, Deep level) — Primitive instincts increased to the detriment of other people. If raised, supple pulse: likes to enjoy life, combative, teases to the point of persecution, sly, unscrupulous with weaker people. Weak or absent pulse: no taste for life, without energy, easily discouraged.

Chinese and European pulses.

The existence of various pulse qualities and their connections with the organs seems surprising at first, since Western science does not recognize them. However, if we closely examine our scattered knowledge, we can see that we use the pulses, though in a minimal way that is confused and without method. In order to prove the existence of the pulse qualities we need to review systematically what is taught and used of the pulses, the three types of blood pressure and the arterial segments.

The pulsation. Hédon and Main (in the U.S.) independently teach that the pulsation is caused by sudden changes of arterial pressure at the moment of passage of the wave, which starts at the aorta under the impulsion of the ventricle. This wave spreads to the capillaries with the speed of nine meters per second, and then disappears. We must not confuse the speed of the wave (forma materiae progrediens) with the speed of the liquid mass, which is much slower.

Regarding the wave, if we examine the raised pulse, it is easy to observe that the pulsation does not pass successively at all the points of the artery; it always beats at the same places. The Chinese have established this fact and studied it since ancient times (see below, Arterial Segments). Regarding the change in blood pressure, there is confusion between the pulsation and the pressure. The pressure indicated by the gradation of the meter remains constant. The pulsation is generated from the resistance to the pressure. So the undulatory movements must always encounter an obstacle. But which obstacle? The flow of the cubital artery coming from the pulmonary arch? The capillaries, which do not stop the blood but only slow it down?

According to the independent works of Carrel and Professor Leriche, the pulsation is caused by contractions of the artery under vagosympathetic control, propelling the blood through the artery in order to maintain and reinforce each separate contraction by the ventricle.

For the Chinese *(YXRM, 28r)* the pulsation is "the bump perceived by the finger pressed on a beating artery." Studying the cause of these pulse qualities is left to researchers and not to the medical art, which consists only of curing. The ancient Chinese have closely observed all variations of the pulse and all its different aspects in correlation with patient disorders. From this collected knowledge, they have been able to diagnose the problems by palpating the pulses.

The pressure. The arterial pressure represents the resistance of the artery to blood flow. The ancient Chinese have made a thorough study of the different forms of resistance. Until recently, the West has generally attributed the arterial pressure to the large mass of blood. The experiments of Prof. Leriche have shown that it is due rather to the contraction or dilation of the artery under autonomic control.

The three blood-pressures. The ancient Chinese describe the three pressures of Western medicine by the name "levels." In the West, the sphygmomanometer was devised, as the name implies, to measure the pressure and strength of the pulse. Surprisingly, the existence of three distinct pressures was observed, along with their independent qualities and variable strengths. The three levels of the pulse in Chinese medicine have thus been instrumentally proven.

What is their cause? How can there be three pressures on the same point of the artery? The first published works on this question revealed great uncertainty. However, more recent works, particularly those of Prof. Leriche and Prof. Mériel, were more elucidating. They found that the minimal pressure is caused by the sympathetic tone of the vessels; the middle tension by the power of the cardiac impulse (the force of the heart under autonomic control); and the maximum pressure by the quantity of the blood-mass. This quantity is relative to the dilated or contracted size of the vessel, which depends on the autonomic system, and on augmentation of salt (and therefore of water) kept in excess by the adrenals, which are also under autonomic control.

The arterial segments. The ancient Chinese observed that the arteries are divided into segments of about 15 mm. each. A segment is able to beat with a force, or quality, or speed (in very rare cases) very different from another segment and quite variable for the same segment. This fact was not recognized by Western science until the recent discoveries of Prof. Leriche. His experiments have demonstrated the existence of these segments and their mutual independence under constant autonomic control.

The independent pulsation of each segment, and its fixed location on the wrist, can be seen as pulsing movements controlled by the autonomic system representing very slight time intervals at fixed distances between the heart and the capillaries.

Pulse-organ connections. The predictable correspondence between the organs and the arterial segments at the three levels of tension has great physiological significance. When acupuncture was first taught in France, I was unable to suggest an explanation for this phenomenon. Today, thanks to the studies of Alexis Carrel and Prof. Leriche, it seems that the autonomic system, which is the great motor and regulator of organs, can imprint on the pulses the same sort of *elan* that it imprints on the organs. The variety and number of pulse qualities can thus be comprehended.

The West attributes the varieties of the pulses to changes in pressure, or rather to raised or lowered pressure, without generally knowing what the usual blood pressure of the patient is. The deviation from this *usual* pressure is the overlooked, all-important fact. There are people having either very low or very high blood pressure who live healthy lives. There is no "normal" blood pressure. My book, *Diagnosis by the Radial Pulses,* will give the history and findings of Western studies of the pulses (from more than twenty-five years of testing some ten thousand patients) as well as the bulk of traditional Chinese observations.[4]

The instruments. In Japan, Doctor Morita constructed an apparatus that separately registers each pulse segment at the three levels. However, under the pretext that the apparatus was not yet perfected, the inventor never consented to sell one. In Paris, instrument manufacturers have declined to study or improve existing equipment because of the small number of possible sales. Instruments measuring the amount of the energy at each of the pulses, the points, and along the meridians have nevertheless been designed and developed by individuals. In addition, two recorders, one pneumatic and the other electrical, have been produced.

Doctors Allendy and Maury have reviewed these instruments (*Revue Francaise d'homéopathie,* June 1952):

> All these exploratory instruments, sphygmomanometers, oscillometers, as rigorous as they may be, seem to us in the last analysis to be quite clumsy because they only inform us of what can be called the exterior aspect of the pulse . . . They simply allow the approximate determination of a maximum and minimum. But as to registering the delicacy and infinite variety of pulsations, they are completely useless . . . They will always lack the exquisite sensitivity of the cutaneous nerve-endings on the fingers of those who palpate for this sensation. Without this sensation, clinical investigation is only a distortion of the truth.

The pulses in Indian medicine.

Information on the pulses in Indian medicine is virtually unobtainable. What I have been able to gather was kindly given to me by Doctor Filhiosa.

The pulses are not mentioned in the Sanskrit medical treatises of ancient India, the *Susruta* and the *Caraka-Samhita.* Yi Jing, a Chinese pilgrim in ancient India, observed the use of them in the seventh century A.D. (*Takakusa: A Record of the Buddhist Religion,* 133). The pulses were perhaps first described and borrowed from tantric medical texts. The doctrine seems well established and is described in a similar manner in both the *Nadivijnana,* used in Bengal (Edition Haridas Pal: Calcutta, 1887), and in the *Shivaguligai,* a brief, modern, Tamil medical treatise (Madras, 1901).

The pulses are numbered in six or eight groups. The pulse positions are located as follows: one at each wrist, one at each ankle, one at each side of the head *(Nadivijnana);* or one at each wrist, each ankle, one on each side of the neck, and on each side of the nose (a total of eight points) *(Shivaguligai).*

The doctor takes the hand of the patient, right for men and left for women, and palpates the wrist with three fingers of the left hand. The pulse palpated by the index finger, closest to the thumb, corresponds to the principle of movement in the body, the wind *(vata).* The pulse palpated by the middle finger represents the fire principle *(pitta)* and is usually translated as "bile." That palpated by the ring finger corresponds to the water principle *(slesman)* and is translated as "phlegm."

In the *Shivaguligai,* indications for the pulse positions are as follows — at the wrist: fever, or lessening of the digestive fire; at the neck: thirst, fatigue, sexual impotence, fear, sadness, anger; at the nose: life or death, amorous desire, eye problems, headache, earache, oral problems.

In Sanskrit, the pulse is called *nadi,* a name referring to the vessels of the body. The Tantras made numerous speculations about the pulses because they believed that through them one could cause the energy of the body to pass in the form of breath. Through yogic practices, energy can be made to rise towards the top of the body and be exhaled through the skull into the emptiness of the "Absolute Being."

I will add a comparison of Chinese and Indian pulses to the information given above by Doctor Filhiosa. The radial pulses in India are the same as those of China at the left wrist only. The pulse nearest the thumb, which in Indian medicine corresponds to movement in the human body, are the Chinese pulses of the heart and small intestine. The central pulse, relating to the fire principle, or bile, is the Chinese liver and gallbladder pulse. The pulse furthest from the thumb, the water principle, is the Chinese urinary bladder and kidney pulse. The pulses of the neck *(ren-ying)* have been used both in China and India since antiquity. In both India and China, the name referring to the pulse is used synonymously for the arterial and venous vessels. These are understood as simultaneously transmitting energy and blood.

It appears that the study of the pulses in India and China have started from a similar base, but that China has succeeded in carrying its observations and doctrines much further than its southern neighbor.

Notes

[1] On the necessity of knowing the pulses:

> *The ideogram that signifies pulses and arteries is formed of the elements "flesh-eternal," which gives the idea of incessant action in the flesh. In the past it was formed of the elements "blood-discriminate," meaning that which discriminates between energy and blood. In our day, it is often made up of the elements "flesh-discriminate." (YXRM I, 21r)*

[2] The *Da Cheng* (VII, 8r) attributes this work to Wang himself. However, the *Ci Yuan* encyclopedia cites a thirteenth century author on this subject who suggests that the *Mo Jing* was not written by Wang, but rather by an author of the tenth century. Nonetheless, attributing this book to Wang tends to confirm his fame regarding the pulses. To support this, there exists an additional *Mo Jing* by Zhen Quan of the ninth century, which cites Wang.

[3] *Actions taken according to the qualities of the pulses.* Some qualities of the pulses suggest certain therapeutic actions, such as either dispersing or tonifying. The *Da Cheng* (VI, 8r) gives the following advice:

> *If the pulse is tight (**ji**), puncture deeply and leave the needle in place a long time. If the pulse is slow (**huan**), act superficially and puncture quickly with the needle. If the pulse is large (**da**), let a bit of energy out. If the pulse is slippery (**hua**), enter the needles quickly and superficially. If the pulse is rough, one must be absolutely sure to take hold of the meridian, to follow by supporting or opposing, and leaving the needle a long time; first press the point, then follow with massage, then insert the needle, quickly pressing the point without letting the blood escape when the needle is withdrawn. If the pulse is small (**xiao**), give medicines.*

Unfortunately, this advice is not very clear, being cited from the mysterious *Xuan Ji Bi Yao,* written by Yang Jishi in the sixteenth century.

[4] We have been unable to locate this text. — ed.

Appendix I

The Numbers

There are frequent discussions of numerology in books about acupuncture. To assist researchers who pursue these studies in the original Chinese texts, the following translations of passages explaining the importance and significance of numbers are given.

Several passages of the *Nei Jing* note the mystical significance and practical utilization of the correspondence between numbers and natural phenomena.

The sage considers that the numbers of Heaven and Earth are from 1 to 9. He takes 9 as the master number, 9 + 9 = 18; 9 x 9 = 81. It is the number of the note **huang-zhong.** *The needles respond to the number 9. (Nei Jing, cited in DACH V, 18r)[1]*

When one speaks of 9 it refers to midnight (zi) and yang, which starts at that time. When speaking of 6 it refers to midday (wu) and yin, which starts at that time; 9 and 6 represent much and little and are as different as tonifying and dispersing, following the needle or driving it in.

The First-Number-9 (chu jiu shu) represents 1 x 9. Needle, then after a pause, act on the needle 9 times. Pause again, then act again 9 times. If repeated 3 times the total number is 27; 4 times equals a total of 36. The Number-of-Lesser-Yang (shao yang shu) is 7 x 7 or 49. Just as above, needle, pause, then act on the needle 7 times; repeat 7 times for a total of 49, pausing between each set. The Number-of-Old-Yang (lao yang zhi shu) is 9 x 9 or 81. Act as above, but use the number 27 three times. The First-Number-6 (chu liu shu), is 1 x 6. After needling, pause, then act on the needle 6 times; repeat 2 more times for a total of 18, pausing between each set. The Number-of-Old-Yin (lao yin shu) is 8 x 8, or 64. Each time act on the needle 8 times, for a total of 64, pausing for a short time between each set of actions.

After midnight (zi), use multiples of the number 9 to tonify the yang (meridians). After midday (wu), one must use the number 6 to tonify the yin (meridians). During a yin day (dark, cloudy), to puncture the yang meridians use multiples of the number 6 often; this will tonify the yin. During a yang day (sun shining), for puncturing the yin meridians use multiples of the number 9 often; this will tonify the yang.

That is the correct rule. But when you see symptoms of warmth, disperse. When you see symptoms of cold, tonify. Act according to the circumstances: that is the law of life. (DACH V, 26r)

For the numbers always stimulate by multiples of 9. Why? 9 is the number of Heaven and Earth. Yang 9 governs life. Yin 6 governs death. 9 is the number of old yang (lao yang zhi shu); one uses it to create life and prevent death. That is why the sage stimulates the needles using the idea of numbers. (DACH IV, 17v)

According to the *Nei Jing*, the numbers 1 to 9 each have symbolic meaning:

One *is Heaven; it is the yang. The yin treasure organ that corresponds to Heaven is the lung; it is the flowery covering of the treasure and workshop organs. The skin is linked to the lungs, and is the yang of man. That is why in treating the skin the needles have a large head and a point; to avoid releasing yang energy they should not enter deeply.*

Two *is the Earth. In man the flesh (rou) corresponds to the Earth. In treating the flesh, the needle has a round body in order to avoid injuring the tissue. If there is a lesion, the energy will be exhausted.*

Three *is Man. What perfects life in man are the blood and vessels. In treating blood and vessels the needle has a round point in order to press on the vessels without creating a passage so that when arriving at the energy, only the evil energy comes out.*

Four *represents the seasons and the eight winds of the seasons. These winds, lodging in the meridians and secondary vessels, form the series of illnesses. In treating these diseases, the needle has a sharpened point in order that the warmth can be dispersed by letting the blood to thus end chronic illnesses.*

Five *represents the sounds (yin); it also symbolizes the division between winter and summer, between midnight (zi) and midday (wu), between yin and yang, the fight between cold and heat, and the encounter between the two energies which unite in order to form abscesses and pus. To treat these, the needle has a point like a spade in order to drain purulence.*

Six *represents the notes of music (lü). The notes harmonize yin and yang and the four seasons; they join the twelve vessels of the meridians, and pathogenic emptiness may lodge in the vessels of the meridians to form rheumatism (bi) there. To treat them, the needle is sharp and round; it enters very delicately into the body and removes the violent energy.*

Seven *represents the stars* **(xing)**. *The stars are the openings of man. The evil lodging in the meridians causes painful rheumatism* **(tong bi)** *there. Since it is in the meridians, the needle for treatment has a point like the dart of a mosquito. The needle enters slowly and unobtrusively; because it is thin, it may remain in place a long time; the normal true energy of the body follows it and the evil is driven out.*

Eight *represents the eight winds of emptiness and the eight joints of the thighs and arms. The eight winds injure man, lodging in the interior and the bones, narrowing the spaces between the vertebrae, the areolae of the lungs and the articulations, forming deep rheumatism* **(shen bi)**. *To treat this, the needle is long in order to reach the deep rheumatic evil.*

Nine *represents the formless* **(ye)**, *the nine openings of man. By the formless, the gaps of the epidermis and dermis tighten one another at the articulations of man. If it has the appearance of wind and water, it flows into but cannot pass through the great articulations. To treat this, the needle is pointed, stiff, and a little rounded in order to stimulate the energy without reaching the articulations.*

One is Heaven; Two is Earth; Three is Man; Four, the seasons; Five, the sounds; Six, the notes; Seven, the planets; Eight, the winds; Nine, the formless terrain. Man's form responds to these correspondences, and needles used to treat his illnesses must be in relation to them. That is why there are nine needles.

The skin responds to Heaven (1). The flesh, to the Earth (2). The vessels, to man (3). The muscles, to the seasons (4). The voice, to the sounds (5). The union of yin and yang, to the notes (6). The teeth, face and eyes, to the planets (7). The breath, to the wind (8). The nine openings and the 365 secondary vessels, to the formless (9). That is why each needle has its particular utility. (DACH V, 18r)

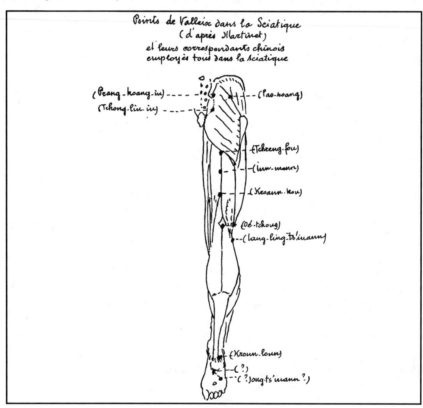

Sciatic points of Valleise (afer Martinet)

Notes

[1] The [Chinese] scale comprises notes composed by an ascending scale mathematically determined by the capacities of the pitch-pipes producing their sound. One pipe gives 9, the descending fifth would give 6, etc. (see *La Musique en Chine*, by G. Soulié de Morant, Ed. Leroux, 1911).

Appendix II

The *Cun:* A Variable Measurement

The ancient medical writings of China note the extreme variety of anatomical shapes, particularly in relation to establishing the placement and depth of the points. The malleolus of some people, for example, is about ten centimeters above the ground; that of others is located barely five centimeters above the ground, even when there is little difference in height. In some people, the thorax in the region of the epigastrium is very narrow, the costal pinions hardly five centimeters from one another; in others, the thorax at this region is very wide, the costal pinions being more than ten centimeters apart. The abdomen of an obese person is at least twice as large as that of a truly thin person of the same height.

To write that an acupoint is, for example, two centimeters from a place of reference, may be quite erroneous for certain people. The Chinese sought to resolve this problem by means of a variable measurement determined from the individual being measured. This variable measure was given the name *cun,* "inch," and divided into tenths called *fen.*

There are many procedures for measuring the length of the *cun* of an individual. The *Da Cheng* (V, 18r) gives the simplest and most widely used method:

> For men, use the left, and for women, the right middle finger, second phalange, medial side. The distance that separates the heads of the two folds forms one **cun**. Mark this length with a stick of bamboo or a thin reed, easily broken but not easily stretched. A string that stretches is not accurate.

Sun Simo (seventh century A.D.), determined another standard which he believed to be more in relation with the rest of the body. Bend the thumb and measure the length of the internal fold formed by the distal phalangeal articulation and the mid-phalange. This measurement is taken as one *cun.* There is generally little perceptible difference between the above two standards.

For finding points on the face, other authors *(Yi Xue I, 2)* have used the length of one eye from the internal to the external canthus as one *cun.* There are eighteen *cun* from the midpoint between the eyebrows over the vertex down to the seventh cervical vertebra. For men's bodies, the standard is 1/8 of the distance between the nipples.

Using the above, the *Da Cheng* (V, 17v) gives measurements for various parts of the body:

Head: From the midpoint between the eyebrows to the hairline — 3 *cun.* From the front hairline to the back hairline — 12 *cun.* From the back hairline to the seventh cervical vertebra — 3 *cun.*

Back: From the "great vertebra" (seventh cervical) to the tip of the coccyx — 30 *cun.* The seven upper vertebrae (C7 to T6) — 1 *cun* 41 *fen* each. The seven central vertebrae (T7 to L2) — 1 *cun* 61 *fen* each. The seven lower vertebrae (L3 to the coccyx) — 1 *cun* 26 *fen* each. The width of the vertebrae — 1 *cun.*

Thorax: Between the nipples — 8 *cun.* From the middle of the suprasternal notch to the middle of the line connecting the nipples — 8 *cun.* From the middle of the line connecting the nipples to the tip of the xiphoid process — 1 *cun* 6 *fen.* From the sternum to the umbilicus — 9 *cun;* 8 from the xiphoid process. (*YXRM I, 8v,* gives 8 *cun* for the first distance, and 7.5 for the second.) From the umbilicus to the pubis — 5 *cun.*

Below are some measurements collected from different chapters:

Arm: From the axillary fold to the elbow crease — 8 *cun.*

Forearm: From the elbow crease to the wrist fold — 10 *cun.*

Thighs: From the middle eminence of the greater trochanter to the superior border of the patella — 13 *cun.*

Legs: From the anterior tuberosity of the tibia to the top of the eminence of the external malleolus — 14 *cun.*

Unfortunately, this *cun* standard cannot give great precision. In practice, since it is very rare to have to puncture a point that is not sensitive to pressure, it would appear more accurate to use an approximate measurement along with the anatomical description of the point. Additionally, by finding the hollow above the acupoint and using the sensitivity of the patient, many errors in point location can be corrected.

Appendix III

Numbering the Vertebrae

Every doctor understands the difficulty of finding a particular vertebra without error. A prominent surgeon told me that in order to avoid error, he would attach an opaque marker to the particular vertebra and make an X-ray.

Usually, the first prominent vertebra at the base of the neck is the seventh cervical; however, it sometimes is found to be the sixth cervical or the first thoracic. The cervical vertebrae, not being apparent, are not counted in the Chinese system. The system counts twenty-one vertebrae: seven superior, seven central, and seven inferior.

The count starts from the first thoracic vertebra, so in the normal person there are twelve thoracic, five lumbar and four sacral prominences. In fact, the five sacral vertebrae, being fused, have only four prominences. The first thoracic vertebra, called *dazhui,* "great vertebra," is often confused with the seventh cervical, as it can also be very prominent. The bones of the coccyx (*wei de gu,* "tailbone") are counted as only one.

Some authors, notably those from the *Yi Xue Ru Men,* do not number the vertebrae, but the interspaces of the spinous processes *(jie).* They take the number from the vertebra above the space and assign it to that space; i.e., the space between the dorsal spines of the fifth and sixth thoracic vertebrae is called the fifth space.

> *From the great vertebra (**dazhui**) to the coccyx totals twenty-one vertebrae (**ershiyi zhui**). The total length is three feet; this is why it is said that humans have a three-foot torso. For the seven superior vertebrae, each vertebra measures 1 **cun** 4.1 **fen**, totaling 9 **cun** 8.7 **fen**. For the seven central vertebrae, each vertebra measures 1 **cun** 6.1 **fen**, totaling 11 **cun** 2.7 **fen**. For the seven inferior vertebrae, each vertebra measures 1 **cun** 2.6 **fen**, totaling 8 **cun** 8.2 **fen**. (DACH V, 17v)*

The Japanese say that the twenty-one vertebrae are formed of twelve thoracic, five lumbar and four sacral prominences. In practice, there are prominent landmarks which vary, only in abnormal persons:

The second to third thoracic space is at the level of the medial superior angle of the scapula.
The fourth to fifth thoracic space is at the level of the middle of the inferior medial tip of the spine of the scapula.
The seventh to eighth thoracic space is at the level of the inferior angle of the scapula.
The second to third lumbar space is at the same level as the umbilicus, with the individual standing upright.
The fourth lumbar space is at the level of the top of the superior iliac crest.

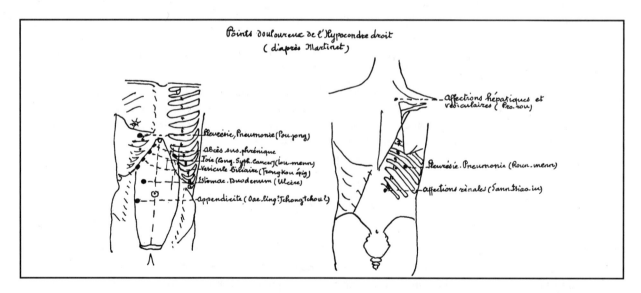

Painful points of the right hypocondrium (after Martinet)

Appendix IV

The Energy *(Prana)* of Indian Hatha Yoga

Indian Yoga is divided into four degrees: Hatha Yoga, Raja Yoga, Karma Yoga and Jnani Yoga.

Hatha Yoga is a practical energetic physiology. It is based on observations made in India thousands of years ago. Yogis believed that the real and final aim of nutrition and respiration is to emit and accumulate cosmic vital energy *(prana)*. This form of yoga teaches one how to derive the maximum energy from food and air while building energy reserves. This energy improves the functions of the mind and body and can be transmitted externally to help renew those lacking it.

It is extremely important to understand these doctrines when discussing Chinese medicine. There is no doubt they have been propagated in China with Buddhism from the third or fourth century A.D. This explains many Taoist practices not previously understood. For example, the gymnastic movements executed by the Boxers in 1900 and 1901 were ridiculed, although they were performed to increase strength and vitality and to develop an insensitivity to wounds and illness.

Jiu-jitsu (Japanese pronunciation of the Chinese ideograms meaning "the art of fighting") was taught in the monasteries of Longmen in eighth century China.

The Chinese may have even surpassed their mentors, since they believed that through intense rhythmic yogic breathing one could concretize the surplus energy and thus obtain a renewed being. The origin of Taoist *gong-fu* is surely yoga. Research into this subject is difficult, since few authoritative texts can be procured from China, Mongolia or Tibet. The only information I have has been taken from those books which the few centers of traditional Taoist culture wished to give me.

Energy does not exist without the physical body, at least for living beings. The first teaching of Hatha Yoga is thus the art of masticating food until it is transformed into a cream and disappears from the mouth without notice. This act, which Europeans believe is only for very good digestion, allows, in Indian thought, the tongue and buccal mucosa to absorb "the energy of the food." From this thorough digestion the food is transformed into blood and tissues by the stomach and intestines. Food is considered dead matter to which life and individualization is given by previously accumulated energy.

The second teaching concerns the use of water by the body. Like food, water has two destinations. If taken little by little into the mouth and rolled on the tongue, it releases energy absorbed by the mucus. The liquid itself is used to hydrate the entire body.

The quantity of water ingested must vary according to the task at hand, life style, climate, season, and the individual concerned. Many problems can be traced to incorrect liquid intake. For example, how, ask the Yogis, can a dehydrated body keep sufficient liquids to maintain unhardened stools when the dried out body requires all the liquid that it has? Some people must drink as much as two liters of water per day to stay well hydrated. The Yogis say that in cases of dry constipation one must follow this procedure: the first evening have an enema of one liter, then rest for one day; the third evening, an enema of one and a half liters; stop for one day. The fifth evening an enema of two liters is taken.

The most detailed and original teaching is that of rhythmic breathing. Indians have observed that all is movement and vibration. Nothing is truly quiescent in nature. All vibration, all movement is composed of a rhythm. To act in rhythm augments the strength of the vibration; to act against it annihilates it. A troop rhythmically marching over a bridge can set up a vibration that could destroy the bridge; if the marching is in broken rhythm there is no danger.

The human body is dominated by rhythms. Each body has its own rhythm of heartbeats, of effort, and so on. To act in accord with the rhythm of the heart augments strength and life; to act contrary to the rhythm weakens the heart. Respiration also has its rhythm. Yogis have studied different ways of breathing:

1) Low or abdominal breathing — considered the best because it empties the bottom of the lungs. (The Chinese count one complete respiration for four heartbeats; each person must adjust his heart rhythm to that of the breath.)

2) Middle or thoracic respiration — less beneficial, but nonetheless develops the chest.

3) Upper respiration, or of the shoulders — tiring and not efficient.

For inhalation, it is recommended to first fill the abdomen (low respiration), then by letting the air rise, to fill the thorax (middle respiration) and last, to fill the top of the lungs (upper respiration). For exhalation, begin by emptying the bottom of the lungs by pulling in the abdomen, then the thorax, and finally letting down the shoulders.

Yoga recommends inhalation through four heartbeats, pausing with full breath during two beats, emptying the lungs through four beats, and pausing with emptied breath during two beats. As one exercises, respiration should increase to six beats, then eight, until fourteen, pausing with full or emptied breath between respirations.

Inhalation sends the *prana,* the cosmic energy, into the body. Exhalation spreads the energy throughout the body. We can learn to direct the energy to a certain point by concentrating deeply. Let us recall that inhalation, by putting pressure on the thoracic vessels, expels the arterial blood towards the periphery and draws the venous blood towards the internal organs. Exhalation, by putting pressure on the abdomen, empties the blood from the internal organs and pushes the venous blood toward the heart. This so-called complete rhythmic respiration is not the only one used by yogis. Other methods are given:

1) *Purifying respiration.* Deeply inhale, then exhale forcefully as if blowing out a candle placed at a distance. Do this once only. The effect is to tonify and to relax the lungs (especially after strenuous effort, such as singing, speaking, etc.). This also stimulates the cells and purifies the lungs.

2) *Vitalizing respiration.* While standing, inhale deeply and extend relaxed arms in front of the body; tighten the fists and vigorously contract and extend the arms several times in front of the chest; exhale and lower the arms. The effect will be to tonify strongly the body and the muscles.

3) *Respiration for the voice.* Inhale very slowly, hold for a few seconds, then exhale brusquely, mouth wide open, and finish with the ''purifying respiration.'' The effect will be to develop the vocal cords. It is recommended to sing while performing the above with the mouth pursed as in whistling; this gives a greater resonance.

4) *Respiration for stimulation of the brain.* Close the right nostril with the thumb and breathe in through the left nostril; then close the left nostril with the index finger and breathe out through the right nostril. Breathe in through the same right nostril, close it and breathe out through the left. The effect will be a feeling of rejuvenation after tiring mental activity, since this exercise directs energy toward the brain.

The art of relaxing, of letting go, is cultivated in Hatha Yoga so that reserves of energy are not exhausted. (The great central reservoir for the storage of energy is the solar plexus.) One must lie down, concentrate on each muscle and imagine it slackened, so that the whole body is loose, without tension. The energy leaves the limbs, which begin to feel heavy like lead. One must feel as if sinking into a soft couch. Intense concentration from limb to limb is often necessary to obtain good results. The effect is to produce a complete calm, to ease away irritations and worries (at the base of which is fear), and to gain full access to one's reserve of energy.

All the physical and physiological methods recommended by Hatha Yoga have as their aim:

1) Obtaining the greatest possible quantity of energy *(prana)* from air and food, this energy considered as originating from the sun.

2) Distributing this energy into consciously chosen parts of the body, either to establish some reserves or to repair some loss, or to supplement the normal outflow of energy.

3) Developing the power of the will over automatic movements of the organs and the body in order to correct imbalances producing illnesses.

Each cell has the necessary intelligence for its work. In the same sense, each group of cells, each organ, or each part of the organism has the intelligence, comprehension and reactions necessary to carry out its complex efforts. An instinctive intelligence, the unconscious perhaps, governs all these cells and organs, yet the consciousness can control the instinctive intelligence after years of yogic training.

The differences between Chinese and Indian breathing exercises are noteworthy. The Chinese system activates normal functions through the respiratory rhythm of four heartbeats per one complete respiratory cycle. Using the rhythm of six, fifteen, eighteen, and thirty beats per breath, Yogis succeed in suspending respiration and the heartbeat, that is, the appearance of life. This has been documented by Dr. Brosse. I have never heard that Indians have attempted, like the Chinese Taoists, to create a new being through surplus *prana*.

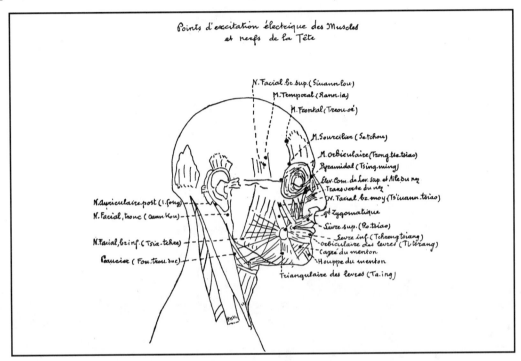

Points of muscle and nerve electrical excitation on the head

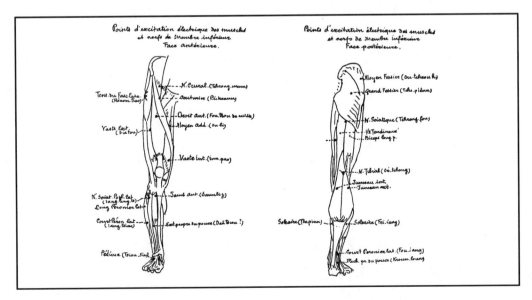

Points of muscle and nerve electrical excitation, lower limb

Volume II

The Management of Energy

There is as much error in seeing what is not, as in not seeing what is.
— *Confucius*

Meridian of the heart (GSDM)

Introduction

To fight off disease successfully by manipulating the energy of the body, one must fully understand the differences between the three methods grouped under the name of acupuncture. The Chinese cite only two, but in reality there are three.

The first method, which could be called local acupuncture or even primitive acupuncture, is rather simplistic and consists of puncturing the center of the pain indicated by the patient. It is used by people who do not know the location of the points, their effects, the pulses, or the circulation of energy. It does not require any study. This method is used for pains, swellings, or local inflammation, without taking into consideration that in Chinese medicine pain is recognized as a sign of dysfunction of a neighboring meridian or of the associated organ. True acupuncture occasionally uses this method after treating the root problem to remove what is called "the branch," the symptom. Even without using this method, the branch disappears some time after the underlying problem is resolved by true acupuncture.

The second method consists of treating the dysfunctioning organ through its main meridian. This method does not take into consideration energetic balances, interactions of the organs, or even the pulse. It is, in fact, "door-bell" acupuncture. It is also called "the rule of the main meridian." It is recommended for curing illnesses said to derive from the blood, having a fixed location and constant intensity. The Europeans call these disorders "organic illnesses."

This form of acupuncture attracts European doctors, mostly specialists whose training focuses more on the organ itself than the interdependence of the organs. Many of these doctors are content to study the tonifying and dispersing points of each organ, using Western diagnosis without concern for the circulation of energy or the pulse. This type of acupuncture is a very useful adjuvant requiring only a short period of study and mostly memorization. Like medication, this method acts directly on the organ, almost immediately but without toxicity. It relieves the condition of the moment and seems to cure it, but does not actually cure the patient of the underlying cause, i.e., an energetic problem that has not been redressed. Thus, some medications that cure asthma leave the root disease to manifest as another problem, such as eczema.

In China, the "superior workers" also use this method, but only after having completely resolved the energetic imbalances, the root cause. "The branches" (resultant pains) are mostly removed in acute cases where every moment counts.

This second method of acupuncture cannot confer immunity against illnesses or epidemics. Real immunity comes from perfect circulation of energy; from an energetic balance within the organs and body; and from an internal yin-yang rhythm in perfect consonance with the day and night, the waxing and waning of the moon, and the summer-winter cosmic rhythms.

The third method, which requires comprehension as well as study, consists most importantly of adjusting the yin-yang balance and the circulation of energy. It is said in the *Da Cheng* (V, 22r): "When the six meridians are in harmony, there is no sickness; or if sickness is present, it will quickly end by itself."

In true acupuncture, the pulses are examined with care to move the blocked or sluggish energy from one meridian to another until there is perfect harmony among the fourteen pulses. For the ancient masters, only this method could re-establish the harmony of the human and cosmic rhythms so as to benefit from the universal vital *elan*. This method is the most subtle and complex form of acupuncture, since one must clearly understand the passage of energy from one organ to another as well as the ascendant and descendent rhythms of the day, the moon, and the seasons. We must cure what is ill by using what is well: the yin by the yang, the yang by the yin, the pain of the head by the feet, the pain of the feet by the hands or the head, the right by the left and the left by the right.

This method successfully treats all functional diseases. It is most useful in curing energetic problems which are mobile in location and appearance, and intermittent in intensity with long or short remissions (such as the migraine-asthma-eczema cycle, or so-called nervous troubles). Through this method, it is often possible to renew one's vitality, activity, and *joie de vivre*.[1]

* * * * * * * * *

In order to manage human energy optimally, it is essential to guard against certain errors. Errors made by the practitioner explain all failures. The most frequent error lies in locating the points to puncture; a difference of one or two millimeters may reduce or eliminate the desired effect.

1) Errors concerning the domain of acupuncture. Acupuncture can do nothing against lesions themselves, even though it can temporarily relieve the problems caused by the lesions. The domain of acupuncture is functional disorders, and the more recent the onset of the disease, the better the result. For pain, inflammation, contractures, weakness, and other ailments of recent origin, acupuncture gives immediate relief. It acts very quickly in insufficiency or congestion of each internal organ. The curing effects are slower, but equally predictable in physical exhaustion or even mental depression. It also successfully treats microbial illnesses, such as influenza.

If the effect obtained from acupuncture is of short duration, and all possibilities of error in treatment have been eliminated, then a lesion or an unobserved organic problem must be present, or the disease is due to severe poisoning by excessive medication, lack of air, poor nutrition, or total exhaustion.

2) Errors regarding the goals of treatment. For the acupuncturist, the goal of the treatment is threefold: first, a return to a normal, healthy state; second, adequate resistance against recurrence of the same illness; third, development of the maximum possible strength and vitality, given the hereditary constitution and environmental background of the patient.

The first goal can be obtained in one session in cases of recent onset. The second goal requires a longer treatment period. The third requires great care and expertise.

3) Errors in evaluating the patient and potential reactions. "Each one is sick in his own way. The sage must always consider this." Even before diagnosing the illness, one must evaluate the potential reactions of the patient. One must not forget that acupuncture adds no energy from the outside but makes use only of the patient's energy. Thus, the patient must have available energy reserves. If the patient is too exhausted, he must first be tonified with energy from air and food before acupuncture can be used to attack his illness.

One must also consider that the same treatment does not give the same result for all people. Nervous people, intellectuals, and city-dwellers have easily manipulable energy but few physical resources. Athletes, manual laborers and country people, on the other hand, have strong physical resources, but their energy is difficult to mobilize; they need large needles and prolonged action. The first group is yang, the second is yin.

Thin people are yang and must be punctured superficially, since their subcutaneous layer contains less adipose tissue and the acupoint is quickly reached. Fat people are yin; the needle must pass through more adipose tissue to reach the acupoint.

4) Erroneous view of the disease itself. For the acupuncturist, the illness is not a fixed entity existing outside of the patient. The terrain of the body may or may not be favorable to the external pathogen: "the sickness is not the invasion; it is the weakness that allows the invasion." Some people are resistant to the most virulent epidemics, while others are vulnerable. Nonresistance is always due to an imbalance of energy that leaves the body powerless to an external attack or upsets the harmony of one or more of the internal functions. The particular imbalance determines the nature of the disease, and is unique to each patient.

Thus, from the perspective of Chinese medicine, there are no illnesses but only complexes of individual expressions reflecting already established energetic imbalances. To limit oneself to the diagnosis of the present illness is realizing only one-third of a possible cure. It is understanding the effect, but not the cause.

5) Erroneous view of the cause of the illness. After recognizing symptoms of disease, we must then search for the deep, underlying (root) cause. What energetic imbalance is present? Is it a question of blockage or emptiness at one point in the circulation of energy? Which is the troubled organ? Which organs are functionally related to the troubled organ and can exacerbate or ameliorate the imbalance?

The interrelatedness of the organs often explains the state of the troubled organ. The symbols of mother and child, husband and wife, etc., which we shall explain later, are important for understanding these inter-organ relationships. The relationship and the functioning of the organs have an importance greater than their states as single organs.

6) Errors in determining the nature of the cause. After determining the root cause, i.e., which organ is imbalanced, it remains to be determined if the illness is due to an excess or an insufficiency of energy. On this point the study of pulses gives precise information, which no other examination can give as completely or as quickly (see Volume I).

An error of diagnosis leads to an error in treatment. Careful diagnosis must be made before tonifying, calming, or dispersing treatments are given.

7) Errors in tonification or dispersion. In principle, tonification provokes trophism, vasoconstriction, augmented activity, increased movement of energy and blood, formation and repair. Dispersion causes vasodilation, diminution, slowing down of energy and blood. In practice, one must tonify emptiness, cold, and lethargy. One must disperse fullness, heat, pain, excess energy, vasoconstriction and contractures.

A single symptom can be yin or yang. Nearsightedness with protruding eyes is yang. One must use a dispersing treatment. Nearsightedness with sunken eyes is yin; tonification is used. Intellectuals are principally yang; one must tonify the yin. Rural people are principally yin; one must tonify the yang. For external influences, one must augment their action: in a yang season or yang weather, tonify the yang; for yin weather or a yin season, tonify the yin.

8) Errors in choosing the favorable moment for treatment. The circumstances which dictate whether or not to use acupuncture are either of an internal or external nature.

Influences of an internal nature: abstain from using acupuncture when the patient is too weak to be capable of a reaction. First give tonics and appropriate hygienic regimen. If he has some strength, use only tonifying points and daily moxa. Abstain from using acupuncture when the energy is either exhausted or in great agitation, since fainting may occur. Do not use acupuncture with the following: fasting, intoxication, extreme fatigue, after a large meal, during extreme anger, after loss of blood or great perspiration, or after recent childbirth.

Influences of an external nature: these influences depend in large part on the cosmic rhythms of the seasons and lunations, of day and night, and hot or cold weather. The energy, like tree sap, comes to the surface and circulates easily in the summer, or with warm weather, a rising sun, a waxing moon, or any other yang condition. The energy is deep and circulates with difficulty in winter, or with cold weather, a descending sun, a waning moon, on dark days, or any other yin conditions. In this respect, one must follow the course of nature in not dispersing the rising yin or yang, but tonifying them; and not tonifying the decreasing yang or yin, but dispersing them. Good results come from waiting for the favorable moment.

9) Errors in selecting points. Through palpation of the fourteen pulses, one can compare the function of all the organs and determine the meridian(s) that must be treated. This action may be taken directly or through the circulation of energy and the relations of the organs. Next, one or more points on the meridian(s) must be selected. For this, one must understand the characteristics of the points, the special uses of particular points, and the subtle differences between forms of the same illness. Herein lies the great art of the acupuncturist — both keen memory and profound comprehension are required for selection of points suitable for curing the patient.

Unfortunately, the Chinese texts have never clarified the special effects of each point nor explained the relationships between points of different segments on the same meridian. From the beginning of my acupuncture studies, the necessity of the above work was apparent. The results of my efforts can be found in Volume IV. I believe it is an important contribution to this science.

10) Errors in point location. Error in point location causes the great majority of failures. A difference of one or two millimeters off the point is sufficient for the effect to be nullified, made temporary or largely diminished. Even when the center of the point at the bottom of its small hollow has been found, it is often difficult to avoid a small movement either of the patient or of the hand that punctures, or a slight displacement of the skin while searching for the subcutaneous point.

My failure rate has greatly diminished since using a small, round-tipped rod for finding and marking the point. By sliding it along the alcohol-moistened skin, the tip of the rod stops at the bottom of the cupule. The center of the acupoint can then be marked by putting slight pressure on the round tip.

With the incredible diversity in sizes and shapes of individuals' bones and muscles, it can be argued that point location is too imprecise using only the Chinese *cun* measurement. We must also know the anatomical location of the acupoint and use the sliding rod described above. The sensation of soreness felt by the patient at the acupoint is useful confirmation and can correct small deviations caused from movement of either of the needle or the hand.

11) Erroneous choice of method. The chosen point can be stimulated using needles, moxa, massage, or electricity. These methods have different effects, and an error in choice or application can be cause for failure.

Comparatively speaking, the most energetic method is needling. Needles give a very strong shock to babies and weak, elderly people and should be used cautiously. Very exhausted people feel like fainting, although this is usually not dangerous. Moxa is gentler than needles; one must use it repeatedly day after day for quite a long period to receive any real benefit from it. It is appropriate for weakened people, the elderly, and in chronic cases. Massage is very gentle; it is sufficient for babies or very nervous people, but must be used repeatedly.

We have tried several types of electrical methods. One technique uses a high frequency, shortwave instrument developed by Leroy. The electrical discharge is quite violent, but the therapeutic result is similar to that of moxa. We have also tried negativization of the body using an electrical device developed by Laville, either by connecting it to a needle at the acupoint, which reinforces its power, or direct contact on the point. Electricity has the drawback of introducing another variable element into the human body and unnecessarily complicates the treatment, one reason for less predictable results.

Electricity is surely an element of the body's nervous fluid, energy, vital influx, or whatever name is given to it. A galvanometer indicates the passage of a current that varies between 1 and 12 to 20 microamperes. However, electricity seems to be only one of the elements of energy, perhaps the transporting medium, or the by-product of the degradation of the energy of digestion or muscular effort. The most important aspect of energy still escapes measurement.

* * * * * * * * * *

We must not forget to mention a cause of failure that is not limited only to acupuncture. It results from a mental attitude derived from our system of instruction, which is not always "educational." The importance given to verbal memorization, quick dictation, exclusive problems of the course, and the necessity of pleasing the professor, stifles individual judgement. The spirit of scientific observation and understanding yields to blind submission and dogma. Rote memorization becomes the foremost concern of students. The ideal student becomes a "parrot-sheep," and realities and facts must bow to the reigning theory of the day.

Here are some remarks we have heard personally:

One patient said with conviction, "Me? Homeopathy has done nothing for me." He then added, in spite of himself, "I must say that after the consultations, I never bought the remedies."

A young intern who had just assisted in a series of cures through acupuncture exclaimed, "After seeing one thousand successes out of one thousand attempts by this method, I would still not believe in it."

Others say, "I shall not try; I have no faith."

It is quite common to meet people suffering many years from serious and ill-defined troubles who have consulted numerous specialists and ingested quantities of active and dangerous medications without, however, obtaining relief. In spite of being told the contrary, they expect immediate results from acupuncture. Experiencing only slight amelioration of the problem after the first session, they do not continue and declare the method to be without value.

Still more numerous are those who, suffering for years and yet cured after the first treatment, do not understand that they still need to follow precautions (as for a recently set leg). They stop all regimes, indulge in excesses not engaged in even before their illness, and then accuse the method of being weak and responsible for their relapse. Many of them even say, "Why start again, since I was cured only for a year or two?"

Others, who could not be cured in one session but who have shown much improvement, note this with regret and add, "My troubles stopped after the treatments, it is true. But I have decided that it was a coincidence and I haven't gone back. And indeed, some months later my troubles started again . . . although before the treatment I had never had such a period of calm."

We must ultimately recognize that certain chronic patients, more numerous than one thinks, benefit from their troubles. Whether or not they undergo psychoanalysis, they do not actually want to be cured. Without alluding to neurotic self-punishment, there is a deep unconscious satisfaction in feeling important, scolding one's spouse, avoiding unpleasant work, and enjoying doing nothing. This is coupled with the unconscious thought that one can rapidly remove these troubles once one tires of them.

This book does not constitute law or literal dogma. When we are discussing life and most of all human beings — deformed and complicated by civilization and artificial foods, it is absurd to speak of uniformity.

The book contains not only a refinement and clarification of the Chinese traditions, but also what has been verified in France and Japan through experimental techniques. The book also discusses the discoveries we have made which add to the centuries-long tradition of ancient China. It is not possible for me to give adequate recognition to science or to the patients on the one hand, nor to the ancient Chinese on the other. Nor can I adequately express my debt to all the modern physicians who have been so willing to guide me in this immense effort, clarifying for me their knowledge and allowing me to help in the treatments and experiments which they suggested. The Introduction to Part I gives their opinions.

My hope is that this book will serve as a starting point for new research, more and more precise, more and more extensive, until the day when our knowledge is complete, if not of nature itself, then at least of the management of energy.

Notes

[1] The following quotes from both ancient and modern texts, although sometimes vague, provide useful advice:

First palpate the pulses of the left wrist and right wrist to determine if the yin (on the left) or the yang (on the right) are in excess or insufficiency. Then examine the entire length of the meridians and secondary vessels. Feel for heat or cold in the upper region and note any abnormalities of the pulses. Press the arteries; look at the color and shape of the blood vessels. If not in excess, they are normal. If in excess, they are abnormal. If the pulses are contracted, there is activity. If they are large and weak, then a strong desire for rest exists. Note the strength of the muscles or their laxity from fatigue (DACH VI, 9v).

Examine the nature of the illness and determine which meridians and points are affected. Keep these in mind and constantly verify them. Ask yourself the questions: is the illness related to the patient's thinness or fatness, height or size? Is the illness in the skin, the muscles or the bones? Seek the source (the root) of the illness before occupying yourself with points. (DACH II, 22v)

See if the illness is high or low, then choose the points and their depth. (DACH II, 27r)

*In order to choose the points for the different illnesses, examine the symptoms, then unite the source point (**yuan**) with reunion point (**he**) according to the Rule of Eight (the eight points of the marvellous vessels on the meridians). Examine the meridians, the secondary vessels, the source points of the twelve meridians, eight reunion points, and the divergent points. (Commentary) The source points of the twelve meridians and the eight reunion points are all points where the blood flowing into the meridians meet. The divergent points are the linking points of the yang.*

*Carefully begin with the assent points and the herald points of the organs. (Commentary) The assent points are all on the two inner urinary bladder lines on the back; the assent point of the heart, **xinshu**, is lateral to the fifth vertebra, etc. The five herald points of the treasure organs are on the anterior surface of the body; the herald point of the heart is **juque** (CV-14) on the abdomen, etc. (YXRM I, 38v)*

The following are very important general laws:

If there is emptiness of the yin organs, it is sufficient to regulate the heart and kidneys and tonify the spleen-pancreas and stomach. Then the food penetrates; sexual energy and consciousness, as well as energy and blood, are born of themselves. (YXRM V, 7r)

The *Nei Jing* says further:

*If the lungs are attacked, increase the energy of the lungs. If the heart is attacked, tonify the **rong** (yin) and the blood. If the spleen-pancreas is attacked, harmonize the food. If cold or hot have damaged the liver, calm the interior. If the kidneys are troubled, make the sexual energy abound. (YXRM V, 7r)*

Chapter I

The Possibilities of Acupuncture

To ask from any method more than it can give leads to sure failure, and to ask less of it is to deprive oneself of possible successes. It is therefore important to know the scope of acupuncture.

Acupuncture cannot be used to treat any lesion or material pathological transformation of a part of the body. It is possible to reduce or temporarily cause the disappearance of the pain or aggravation due to a lesion. More often, acupuncture rebalances the general state so that the lesion may heal on its own. A prolonged treatment is necessary in the case of serious toxicity of the body, either by excessive medication, lack of pure fresh air or bad food, or in cases of prolonged fatigue or sadness.

The true domain of acupuncture is the functional problem, the dysfunction of the organs, the glands, or any other part of the body. Cure and even prevention against future illness can be obtained when there is no lesional cause for these disorders. As soon as there is a material modification, we must expect only a temporary amelioration. The lesion is an indication of less positive prognosis, particularly with treatment by acupuncture. The general state or vitality of the body definitely can be improved with acupuncture, enough to confer protection against future disease.

Acupuncture is most successful for the following:

1)   Problems arising from insufficiency of either physical, emotional or mental energy: weakness, laziness, cold, numbness, certain paralyses, sadness, discouragement, mental depressions, noncancerous and noninfectious anemias, hypotension, organic insufficiencies, etc.

2)   Problems arising from excess physical, emotional, or mental energy: the congestion and excess of organs (lungs, liver, etc.), hypertension (without arteriosclerosis), fever, heat, itching, urticaria, eczema and certain other skin diseases, pains, arthritis, arthralgia, contractures, convulsions, certain stutterings, agitation, mental over-excitement, hallucinations, bizarre ideas, etc.

3)   Women's problems: retarded, advanced, painful, excessive or insufficient menses; vomiting during pregnancy; difficulties with slow or painful childbirth.

4)   Infectious diseases (acupuncture works on these through strengthening the body's immune system): inflammations, influenza or colibacillosis, furunculosis, and the beginning stages of tuberculosis. Our personal experience is still not sufficient to determine its efficacy against typhoid.

5)   Genetic or congenital illness: certain points during pregnancy may block the transmission of bad heredity traits and distinctly improve the vigor of children.

Li Chan, author of the great medical treatise *Yi Xue Ru Men* (I, 38v) wrote: ''The practitioners with needles are without rivals in the relief of rheumatic pain, neuralgia, paresis, hemiplegia right or left. They also have the power to cure internal maladies and even typhoid.'' The *Da Cheng* (II, 19v) indicates: ''To cut the strength of an illness, nothing is equivalent to needles and moxa.''

The possibilities of acupuncture are greater when the illness is in its beginning stages. This motivated the search for the earliest signs of disease. In Chinese medicine, it is taught that there are no lesions (except, obviously, traumas) or infections that are not a consequence of functional disorders. These functional problems are always announced by afflictions of the emotional or mental personality.

Bian Que, the famous doctor of the fifth century B.C., wrote:

> *''The superior worker (**shang gong**) cures those who are not yet ill. The mediocre worker (**zhong gong**) only cures those who are already ill.''* (DACH V, 23v)

Acupuncture gives promising results in treating the chronic and poorly-defined problems labeled as ''autonomic'' by Western medicine. It is evident that since it does not introduce any poison into the body, acupuncture cannot contradict any other form of treatment, and can have no subsequent ill effects. By tonifying the vitality of the body, it increases the effect of allopathic or homeopathic medicines, which can then be used in lower dosages.

Acupuncture is also useful as a means of diagnosis. If the pain or problem returns just a few hours after treatment, the disorder is not a functional one. There must be a small lesion or material deposit that has gone unnoticed.

For example, simple sciatica is immediately relieved by acupuncture and does not return. Sciatica which returns causes us to suspect sacroiliac arthritis which, being of a material nature, cannot be dissipated in a few moments. Nonetheless, some lesional problems, such as hemorrhoids, do yield to the needles.

The border between the lesional and the functional is not very clearly defined. For instance, with varicosities, those veins that are not distended definitely, can for the most part be returned to normal, while the distended ones stay swollen. Prostatitis presents the same situation: those cases declared operable are congestive if they yield in one session to acupuncture. Those that only improve slightly are probably tumorous.

Constipation caused by an enlarged or soft colon does not improve much with acupuncture. However, if it comes from a condition of spasm or from an insufficiency of the liver, it immediately yields to the needles. Atonic colons are slower to respond. Asthma with sudden onset of crisis but without incident between crises is easiest to cure. On the contrary, asthma accompanied by mucus and chronic bronchitis is the most resistant.

In China, they say that yang illnesses yield easily, but yin illnesses are cured more slowly.

The Introduction to Volume I gives reports presented by scholarly societies on the effects of acupuncture.

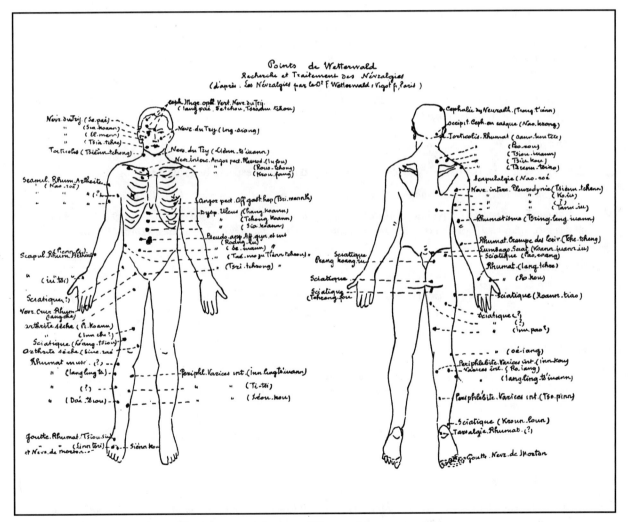

Points of Wetterwald

Chapter II

Contraindications and Precautions

I. Precautions Against Acupuncture and/or Moxa — II. Precautions Against Using the Dispersing Method

I. Precautions Against Acupuncture and/or Moxa

When the patient is exhausted.

Since it is the energy of the patient that is used in acupuncture, it is logical not to depend on energy reserves that are diminished or nearly empty.

> *When the pulse is small, one gives medicine (DACH VI, 8r).*

> *When the energy and blood are both insufficient, do not stimulate; harmonize with the needles and give some gentle medicine (DACH XII, 39r).*

> *When the energy that has form (yin, blood) is insufficient, and the energy of the illness itself is insufficient, yin and yang are equally insufficient. Do not puncture. Through this insufficiency, yin and yang are both exhausted; blood and energy are finished; the five treasure organs are hollow and empty. If one punctures, one increases the insufficiency; muscles, bones, the marrow become dehydrated; old people become completely exhausted; robust ones will not be cured. (DACH V, 22r)*

However, in practice it is possible to act, but only at the points tonifying the general condition (*sanli* of the leg, ST-36; *qihai*, CV-6) by daily moxa rather than by needles.

When the patient is fasting.

During a fast, there is a risk of syncope, or of prolonged malaise (especially during morning fasts).

> *Puncturing when fasting risks fainting. One must eat or drink before the treatment. (DACH II, 25r)*

> *For moxa (and needles), it is always forbidden to act at dawn when one is emptied of all food energy. This causes mental confusion. However, in cases of sudden contractions, this rule may be disregarded. (DACH XI, 16v)*

After a full meal.

> *Do not puncture those who have just had a full meal. And moreover, after needling, discourage the eating of a full meal. (DACH I, 10v; IV, 12v)*

After intoxication.

> *Do not puncture during heavy inebriation. It disturbs the energy and the meridians. Do not puncture immediately after drunkenness. And moreover, after the puncture, discourage the patient from drinking alcohol. (DACH I, 10v)*

In practice, to sober up the patient from drunkenness while preventing a hangover, needle *shuaigu* with dispersing method (GB-8).

During great unhappiness.

> *Do not puncture during a period of great unhappiness. It causes a counterflow of the energy. Do not puncture immediately after a period of great unhappiness. Moreover, after needling, advise the avoidance of unhappy situations. (DACH I, 10v)*

During great fatigue.

> *Do not puncture during great fatigue or immediately after great fatigue. Moreover, after the puncture, advise the avoidance of overfatigue. (DACH I, 10v; II, 26r; IV, 12v)*

After a recent conception.

> *Do not puncture someone newly pregnant. Moreover, after being needled, dissuade acts of conception. (DACH I, 10v)*

When the complexion and pulse do not agree.

> *When the complexion and pulse do not agree, do not puncture. (DACH II, 26r)*

This indicates a serious energetic imbalance that must first be corrected. A florid complexion with no pulse, or a pale complexion with excessively strong pulses require hot drinks, silence and rest.

During unfavorable times or weather.

> *In the evening and at night, never stimulate except in urgent or acute cases of illness. If there is a storm or heavy rain, never stimulate in acute illness; wait for clear and hot weather for chronic and slow illnesses. It is then that the energy is easiest to move. (YXRM I, 32v)*

> *In heavy rain or heavy wind, do not puncture. (DACH IV, 21v)*

II. Precautions Against Using the Dispersing Method

After the loss of blood, diarrhea, sweat, etc.

> *One must not disperse after one of the five despoilments: when face and form are already despoiled and empty; after the loss of blood; after great sweat; after profuse diarrhea; after recent childbirth. (DACH I, 11r)*

At certain times and lunations.

> *One must not disperse at the time of the rising of the sun nor at the time of the waxing of the moon. (DACH II, 25v)*

During the rising of the sun, before noon and the waxing of the moon (from the first to the fifteenth day of the lunar cycle), tonification is more efficient; the yang energy rises with the sun until midday and descends with it. Dispersing would be contrary to the natural course of the energy.

In grave illness.

In all serious illnesses, where the trouble is transmitted from one seriously injured organ to another organ, and when death seems to be imminent, do not puncture the meridian corresponding to the organ that can cause death, although the other meridians can be needled (see *DACH I, 11r & v*).

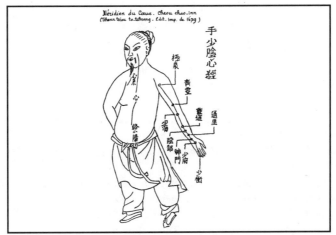

Meridian of the Heart (DACH)

Chapter III
The Patient — The Personality

I. The Patient — II. The Personality: shen, hun, po — III. Decision. Imagination

I. The Patient

The *Nei Jing* states:

> *Everyone is ill in his own way. The sage must take this into account.*

Similarly, according to the *Da Cheng I, 2v:*

> *For the same illness, the treatment for each person is different.*

The individualization of an illness is due to the patient's characteristic energetic imbalance producing susceptibility to disease. The patient's particular state and constitution determine his particular symptoms and their degree of manifestation. The presentation of symptoms and their relative strength will be different for each patient.

Guided by the pulses, one can determine the specific energetic disharmonies which produce the illness and lead to other illnesses if not redressed. In the *Da Cheng III, 31v*, it is remarked:

> *The 404 varieties of illness cannot be described. Their modifications are too numerous. But it is enough to care for the meridians to remove all illnesses.*

However, even if each person is sick in his own way, it is possible to distinguish large groups of patient types. It is not a question here of physical types but of similar reactions from the point of view of energy. It is consistently a question of:

1) "High-placed" people (gui) and "common" people (jian). The former generally describes intellectuals and city people. In China, from the third century onward, "high-placed" people formed a select group, since in order to aspire to state positions it was necessary to present three generations of letters from both the paternal and maternal side of the family.

> *The high-placed are frail. One must avoid acting brusquely. It is advisable to act quickly and superficially. (DACH I, 13r)*

> *When it is a matter of cold or rheumatism for the high-placed people, one must calm them and give tonifying drinks (while common people require heated needles).*

> *High-placed people, also called the "Great Ones"* **(daren),** *are yang and have very developed yang energy. Therefore, it is good to tonify the yin. Commoners, also called "cloth-shirts," are the physical, country people, the manual workers whose minds are less exercised than the body. They are yin and have very developed yin energy. It is advisable to tonify the yang. (DACH I, 13v)*

> *The commoners are resistant and rough. One must act strongly, deeply and for a long time. (DACH II, 27v; I, 13r)*

> *When there is the problem of cold or rheumatism, the "cloth-shirts" require the needles warmed by fire. (DACH I, 13r)*

The physical aspects of each type are opposite:

> *People slim in appearance, with white, thin skin, angular flesh, fine lips, and soft voice, have blood which is pure; it is easy to exhaust their energy or weaken their blood. Puncture these people lightly and with short duration. They are the great ones; puncture slowly and with caution.*

> *People with wide shoulders, thick necks, thick flesh, dark skins, and thick lips have thick, black blood. Their energy is rough and slow. These people of materially large appearance have abundant blood; their dermis is hard like leather. Their illnesses are from abundance. Puncture deeply and leave a long time. (DACH I, 13r)*

2) Thin and fat people. If, as experiments conducted in France seem to prove, the acupoint is in the aponeurosis or under the connective tissue, there is a significant difference in depth location between thin and fat people. It is in this sense that we should interpret this passage: "For fat people, act slowly and deeply, as in autumn and winter; for thin people, act quickly and superficially, as in summer." The following passage concerning fat and thin people is more obscure:

Fat people are empty in the interior; first tonify, then afterwards, disperse. Thin people are full in the interior; first disperse, then afterwards, tonify. (DACH IV, 10v)

In fact, fat, pale people are yin; it is necessary to tonify the yang. Thin people are yang; it is advisable to tonify the yin.

For thin people, some precautions must be taken:

*For puncturing thin people we must warm the needle a little in order to better link **rong** and **wei** (yin and yang). The introduction of yang energy tonifies thinness and weakness. (DACH II, 2v)*

Cold metals, such as steel, make the skin contract, increase pain, and do not allow easy insertion of the needle.

3) Children and the aged. For different reasons, children and the elderly have special responses to the different methods of acupuncture.

Children have delicate flesh, less blood, and weak energy. Consequently, in puncturing them, very fine needles should be used. Puncture superficially and quickly. However, if there is an outbreak the same day, one can puncture again. (DACH I, 13r)

The elderly are generally devitalized; it is particularly necessary to tonify them. Repeated moxas are thus recommended. The needles must not disperse the energy or be used often.

4) Men and women. In theory, men are yang, women yin. In practice, nervous tension and overstimulation of yang are more noticeable in women (in whom yang must not abound). The lack of yin physical strength is more noticeable in men (in whom yin, lassitude, and rest should not abound). Men are more sensitive to pain than women. Conversely, women often have more violent internal reactions, fatigue, or fainting.

It is recommended (for use with steel needles):

*For men, first press the point lightly, push the needle in a little, wait for the **wei** energy (yang) to spread. For women, press heavily on the point, puncture deeply, wait for the **rong** energy (yin) to spread. (YXRM I, 34v)*

One other remark has been made, which has not been possible to verify:

The energy of men is above in the morning and below in the evening, while the energy of women is below in the morning and above in the evening. (YXRM I, 42v)

II. The Personality *(Shen, Hun, Po)*

It may be useful to explain here certain terms linked to the personality, which we see appearing frequently in medical texts. These terms have no direct correspondences in Western languages.

First, we must note that although Indian Buddhism spread the idea of the division between spirit and matter, it was not able to extirpate the ancient Chinese notion that no spiritual or emotional function is separable from the organs. Kong-zi (Confucius) wrote in the fifth century B.C., "What makes the blade is the edge; no edge without a blade, no blade without an edge."

The medical texts depict man as being composed of three elements: *shen, hun,* and *po.* A passage of the *Nei Jing Ling Shu* (VIII, sixth line) explains the relationships of these elements to man:

*When **hun** and **po** are injured, there is depression, and poor memory. When there is no more **shen,** one is no longer fully human.*

Shen.

The ideogram for this word is formed of the elements: "that which drops from the sky; passing through the body"; that is to say, the ethereal element of cosmic energy; the cosmic force that animates form and gives it reason. *Shen* represents the intelligence, or reason guided by principles and morals and not by instincts or needs.

The *Ci Yuan* encyclopedia ("*Shen*" article) explains: "The *shen* can be measured in the yin-yang energy." The *Nei Jing Ling Shu* article further states: "The shen is the sexual energy in the yang." And in the *Hun* article: "The *shen* linked to energy forms *hun.*"

The term *shen* is often found in descriptions of remarkable beings: the geniuses, the guardian-spirits of a region, the gifted. Idiots and deranged people are said to be without *shen.*

Shen is stored (has its lodging) in the heart. It can be compared with our concept of consciousness: the external world and its possibilities are analyzed, and the realization of internal impulses sought. But it also includes a cosmic element specific to man; it must be combined with reason and moral inspiration, without which, it is said, we are not yet fully human.

Hun.

The ideogram is formed of ''speech; ghost.'' Speech and the breath are indications of the strength of energy, and the energy is what animates the ghost of the physical body.

The *hun* represents physical vitality, as opposed to the mental and emotional energy of the *shen*. The *hun* is instinctive intelligence, not guided by the principle of reason, as is the *shen*. Conniving behavior, instinct, and instinctive needs are all ruled by the *hun*. The *Ci Yuan* encyclopedia (*''Hun''* article) explains: ''The *shen* linked to sexual energy forms the *hun*.''

The *hun* is stored (has its lodging) in the liver *(YXRM I, 11v)*. It is known to have a marked influence on the sexual life and its lodging place is at *tianshu* (ST-25).

The term *hun* is used in the sense of the subconscious and can be seen as representing the collective life of the organs. In India, it is considered to be the intelligence animating each organ and assuring their functions. It may be formed of the collective intelligence of the cells.

Po.

The ideogram is formed of the elements: ''whiteness (an abbreviated form describing oneself) and ghost,'' that is to say, the shadow of oneself, the unconscious part of the ego.

The *Ci Yuan* encyclopedia (*''Hun''* article) states:

> *Man just being born, beginning to modify himself, is the **po**. Life (**sheng**) and the immaterial (**ling**), linked to the form, constitute the **po**.*

And in the *''Po''* article of the *Ci Yuan* we find:

> *The **po** is the principle constituting the body. By analogy, we call **po** the dark silhouette of the moon, as opposed to the luminous crescent.*

The *po* is stored (has its lodging) in the lungs *(YXRM I, 11v; DACH VIII, 1v)*. Its ''lodging place'' is at *tianshu* (ST-25).

Chinese doctors often use this expression in the sense of the animal material life, as opposed to the mental *shen*, and the instinctive and organic *hun*.

The wondrous tales about apparitions imply that after death, the *shen* is the first to leave, then the *hun*, and always last, the *po*. If the *po* stays too long in the body, it impedes the decomposition of the corpse and can animate it, turning it into a bloodthirsty, evil vampire.

III. Decision, Imagination

To *shen, hun*, and *po* we add incontestable qualities which have their lodging in certain organs, one mental and the other emotional: the *zhi* and the *yi*.

Zhi.

The ideogram is formed of the elements ''heart; minister.'' In other words, the strength of character of the leader. This word is consistently used in the sense of decision, firm purpose, strength of character.

> *Its lodging is in the kidney with the sexual energy. (YXRM I, 11v; DACH VIII, 1v)*

Yi.

The ideogram is formed of the elements: ''The sun (or speech) which rises above the heart-spirit.''

> *Its lodging is in the spleen-pancreas. (YXRM I, 11v; DACH VIII, 1v)*

Yi is often translated as ''imagination,'' but the term also implies ideation, the concentration of mind, or the faculty of understanding. Children who have a deficient spleen often perform poorly in school and have difficulty concentrating. However, when the spleen is correctly tonified these same children perform very well, particularly with subjects requiring concentration and analysis, such as mathematics.

Chapter IV

Illness

I. Illness Itself — II. Energy, the Origin of Illness — III. Yin and Yang Illnesses — IV. Heat (Yang) or Cold (Yin), Internal or External, Upper or Lower

I. Illness Itself

With the exception of homeopathy, since the time of Pasteur, disease has been seen in the West as a foreign entity defined as an invasive microbe. In China and Japan, disease generally was not viewed as having a microbial origin (although microbes were at least suspected since the question of the "animalcule of tuberculosis" was raised in a book of the sixteenth century.) Doctor Nakayama elucidates the Far Eastern view on the etiology of disease when he writes: "The illness is not the invasion, but the weakness that calls in the invasion."[1]

The several stages of disease are: the period of low resistance; the incubation period; the appearance of major symptoms; lesions or convalescence with lesions. In Europe, lowered resistance is never considered a part of the illness. In China, it *is* part of the illness and even constitutes the true disorder.

The incubation period in Europe is scientifically studied, but only in terms of the length of time passed since the contagion; the symptoms which allow its recognition are ignored. In China, the slightest sign of incubation, perhaps as yet only psychological or emotional changes (representing energetic imbalances), are described and categorized. Treatment is then immediately given to arrest or attenuate the full development of the sickness.

The major symptoms, with or without lesions, are considered in Europe as the "true" illness. In China, these symptoms are seen as the end of the illness; it is then only a matter of stopping the damage from spreading.

In Europe, a problem which may be chronic but which is not microbial, organic, or accompanied by physical symptoms, is considered of little importance, or due to psychological problems. The solution is to give sedatives. In China, great importance is attached to these emotional, mental or physical changes — they are seen as the manifestations of a disequilibrium of energy that will sooner or later lead to lowered resistance of an organ, a part of the body, or the entire organism.

To grasp the importance of Chinese diagnostic and treatment theory, a clear understanding of the differences between European and Chinese views of illness is necessary.

II. Energy, the Origin of Illness

All illnesses come from energy. (Nei Jing, cited in YIX I, 12v)

*Hundreds of illnesses begin [by attacking] the **rong** (yin) or **wei** (yang). They then invade the skin, muscles and the vessels of the meridians. (DACH VI, 8v)*

These initial attacks on the energy, described in the chapter, "Fullness or Emptiness," always manifest through excess or insufficiency.

The study of the vital energy and the pulses has been of extreme value in determining slight functional problems often hardly noticed by the patient, but representing the beginnings of disequilibrium and loss of health. The concept that all emotional and mental disturbances precede health crises has come to China from both a knowledge of energy and medical subscription.

Medical subscription was traditionally a common practice in China. Yearly payments to the doctor were interrupted when there was illness, and the doctor was then obliged to provide medical care without charge until the patient recovered. The attention of the practitioner was consequently focused on the very first premonitional signs of illness, particularly the insufficiency or excess of energy. This method of medical subscription also encouraged the study and use of the most efficient therapies. Further, medical subscription motivated the clinicians to search for the causes of the insufficiencies and excesses of energy observed at the origin of all the subscribers' illnesses.[2]

Two groups of causes were observed: internal and emotional causes, and external and physical causes.

Internal and emotional causes.

An excess of the seven emotions — joy, discontent, sadness, emotional agitation, fear, obsession, and lassitude — give rise to yang illnesses.

The *Da Cheng* (II, 31r) indicates that illnesses due to the above result in emptiness: "From sadness and many cares the blood of the heart weakens; the illness at the interior is the evil of emptiness." However, not all authors agree that an excess of any of the emotions causes emptiness.

Discontent, worry, obsession, and sadness cause a fullness wherein "the fire abounds, heating the fluids and forming mucus accumulation and knots of energy." This fullness must be dispersed. Joy, fear, apprehension, emotional agitation, and lassitude "spread the original energy and cause an internal emptiness" which must be tonified.

The influence of the emotions on the energy is described:

> *From joy, the energy is slowed down; it causes unceasing laughter.*
> *From discontent, the energy rises; it causes vomiting or diarrhea.*
> *From sadness, the energy fluctuates less; it causes acidity in the nose.*
> *From emotional agitation, the energy overflows; consciousness has no place to abide.*
>   *The consequence is stupidity or convulsions.*
> *From fear, the energy descends; it causes sudden descent of fluids, like clear water.*
> *From obsession, the energy is knotted; the heart is contracted and consciousness cannot rise.*
> *From lassitude, the energy is leeched away; men have less sexual energy;*
>   *women lose their menses; there is panting breath and profuse sweating.*
> *(YIX I, 12v)[3]*

The yin, however, is also damaged through the emotions. Many emptinesses of yin (aside from sexual fatigue) come from worry and obsession, which injure the heart and kidneys.

> *Sexual fatigue, or worries and thoughts damage the heart and kidneys; emptiness of yin and blood results.*
> *(YXRM V, 7r)*

If the emptiness of yin comes from the liver and kidneys, it is recognized by muscular discomfort with excessive sweating:

> *In liver and kidney problems, if the form is paretic with considerable sweating, it indicates emptiness of yin.*
> *(YXRM V, 7r)*

In practice, all disorders coming from excessive emotions can be improved by one point, leg-*sanli* (ST-36):

> *In all illnesses which come from disorders of one of the seven emotions, the stomach energy functions improperly. There is fatigue, relaxation and derangement of digestion to such a point that the ancestral energy becomes insufficient. One must stimulate leg-**sanli** (ST-36, the union point of the stomach) to revive and tonify the ancestral energy. This is called "starting from the yin in order to act on the yang." If no cure is achieved, one must stimulate the herald points of all the organs. (DACH VIII, 10v)*

Physical and external causes.

These are mostly yin diseases. Generally speaking, illnesses coming from the exterior result in fullness. Cold or hot wind, dryness and humidity are the most frequent causes.

> *From external cold, the energy collects in the interior [is driven back to the interior]. This causes internal cold [from excess of yin]. From external heat, energy is dispersed; its violent exit causes perspiration. [If yang is driven out this way, then there remains fullness of yin.] (YIX I, 12v)*

> *Cold damages form, and attacks the yang. The antidote is heat. Heat damages energy, and attacks the yin. The antidote is cold. (DACH XI, 20r)*

> *When one is attacked by wind, cold, heat or humidity, the attacking evil is that of fullness. (DACH II, 31r)*

III. Yin or Yang Illnesses

The concept of yin-yang relativity led the ancients to clearly differentiate symptoms as well as treatments. All illnesses fall into groups of yin or yang and can be differentiated as follows:

Illnesses of energy (yang) or illnesses of blood (yin).

Illnesses of energy (yang) are mobile and intermittent. One must treat them by means of the opposite extremity. The illnesses of blood (yin) are fixed and constant. One must treat the disorder directly.

The *Nei Jing* as cited in the *Da Cheng* states:

> **Question:** *There are some cases when the illness is in the energy, others when it is in the blood. How do practitioners differentiate between energy and blood?*
>
> **Answer:** *the practitioners must know that if the illness is in the energy, it moves and is not fixed. When it is in the blood, it is deep and does not move. (DACH XII, 39r)*

Yin or yang illnesses by their external aspect.

All illnesses of deficient blood and flaccid swellings qualify as yin, as do those illnesses accompanied by cold, weakness, flaccidity, and depression. All illnesses with contraction and spasm or pain are yang, as are those accompanied by fever, heat, redness and inflammation. For example, myopia with big, prominent eyes is yang. Myopia with retracted, sunken and blinking eyes is yin. Nephritis with an enlarged kidney is yin; that with a small, contracted kidney is yang. Hemiplegia with aphasia and contractures is yang; that with flaccid paralysis is yin. Eruptive illnesses are yang. Disorders of the lungs or kidneys are yin (see *DACH* XI, 1).

Ancient Chinese and Japanese texts are not very precise in classifying these disorders, as the following passage from the *Nei Jing* shows:

> *In spring, when yang energy is growing, the sap rises in the small branches. The eruptive yang [external] illnesses are numerous. In summer, yang is at its peak, causing disorders of the head, which is the most yang part of the body. In autumn, when the yin begins to dominate, one sees the breakout of numerous lung illnesses, which are yin. In winter, when yin dominates, illnesses of the kidneys are prevalent since they are the most yin part of the body.*

IV. Heat (Yang) or Cold (Yin), Internal or External, Upper or Lower

The internal temperature is governed by the yin and the external skin temperature by the yang. The upper body is governed by the yang and the lower body by the yin.

Excessive yin gives rise to internal cold. Some symptoms are heaviness, desire for rest, and sunken, thin pulses. One must disperse the yin (or tonify the yang). Emptiness of yin results in internal heat. Symptoms are insomnia, over-excitations or pains. One must tonify the yin (or disperse the yang).

Excess of yang results in external heat; one must disperse the yang (or tonify the yin). Emptiness of yang gives rise to external cold; there is somnolence and apathy. One must tonify the yang (or disperse the yin).

When the upper part of the body is hot and the lower part cold, an excess of yin exists which must be dispersed. When the upper part is cold and the lower part hot, yang is empty and must be tonified.

The original sources comment:

> *If there is excess of yin, there is internal cold. If there is emptiness of yin, there is internal heat. If there is emptiness of yang, there is external cold. When yang abounds, there is external heat. (DACH I, 7v)*

> *Great cold entering into the interior must be dispersed. Great external cold must be tonified. If the upper body is cold and the lower body is hot, tonify and the energy will rise. If heat is in the upper body and cold is in the lower body, disperse and the energy will descend. (DACH VI, 9v)*

> *The internal fire resulting from emptiness of yin is perceived through the abundant need to urinate and weak, deep pulses. (YXRM V, 36v)*

> *In all illnesses originating from external cold, the end result is external heat [yang]. One must treat these illnesses by using the assent points of the organs on the back [yang]. (YIX, 4v)*

Notes

[1] For the [Chinese] public, illnesses were divided into two groups: those which cured themselves, for which it was enough to have patience and a bit of rest; and those which worsened if they were not treated from the beginning. The elderly — the experienced advisors of this race of precise observers — guided families on this point armed with faithful memories.

The great medical treatises group illnesses according to their potential cause:

1)   External causes: wind (neuralgia, swellings, pains, headache, eruptions, rheumatism). Cold (cough, abdominal pains, pains of the heart, cholera). Heat (diarrhea, dysentery, jaundice, diabetes, intestinal fermentations, beriberi, etc.) Fire (loss of semen, retention of urine, etc.).

2)   Internal causes: nutritional problems (accumulations, intestinal wounds, etc.). Energy (non-circulation of energy). Blood (hemorrhages, hematemesis, intestinal hemorrhages, etc.) Mucus (asthma, bronchitis, vomiting, indigestion, epilepsy, insanity, etc.). Emptiness (fevers, sweats, tuberculosis, syncopes, paralysis, etc.).

[2] The notion of ''medical subscription'' in China seems to have become very popular in Europe during the early part of the twentieth century and in the United States in the last three decades. However, because evidence of medical subscription of any form has not been found, this reference must be to a system Soulié De Morant witnessed during his years in China. — ed.

[3] The action of the emotions on the organs holds an important place in the etiology of disease in Chinese medicine:

Joy injures the heart and through it the lungs. Its antidote is fear. Discontent damages the liver and through it the spleen-pancreas. Its antidote is sadness. Sadness damages the lungs and through them the liver and the heart. Its antidote is joy. Emotional agitation damages the heart and mind. Its antidote is habit. Fear damages the kidneys and through them the heart. Its antidote is obsession. Obsession damages the spleen-pancreas and through it the kidneys. When there is excessive obsession, the energy of the spleen-pancreas becomes exhausted. Its antidote is discontent. Lassitude damages the sexual energy. (DACH XI, 20r; see also YIX I, 13r)

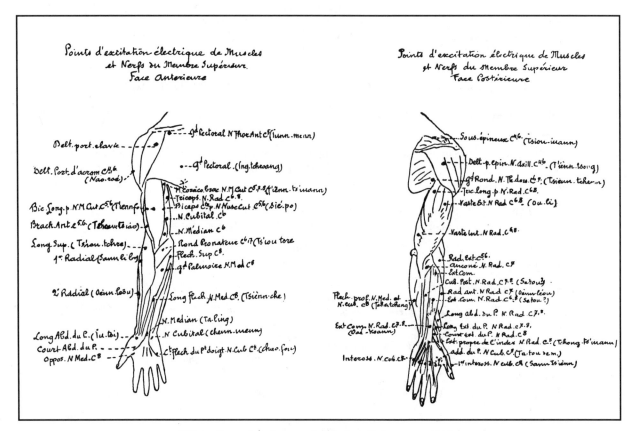

Points of muscle and nerve electrical excitation, upper limb

Chapter V

Excess or Insufficiency

I. The Meaning of the Terms — II. Excess or Insufficiency of Both Yin and Yang — III. Excess or Insufficiency of Either Yin or Yang — IV. Excess or Insufficiency of Each Organ or Function — V. Excess or Insufficiency of the Local Energy

To arrive at a successful treatment plan, it is imperative to clearly differentiate between excess of energy (more than normal fullness) and insufficiency of energy (to the point of emptiness).[1]

The *Nei Jing* states:

> *The hundreds of illnesses which come to exist are all manifested through fullness or emptiness . . . In the use of needles nothing is more important than the necessity of differentiating between fullness or emptiness (cited in DACH V, 20r and 22v).*

Indeed, a mistake can exacerbate the disease instead of curing it. Healthy organs hardly respond to the weak stimulation of the needle, whereas dysfunctional organs are very sensitive to it.

I. The Meaning of the Terms

The *Nei Jing* clearly defines the opposition between fullness (excess) and emptiness (insufficiency) in this passage:

> *Fullness is to have energy. Emptiness is to have no energy. (DACH V, 21r)*

Another description from the *Nei Jing* is less clear:

> *Fullness or emptiness is to have or not to have; it is before or after; it is to conserve or exhaust. (DACH V, 20r)*

One school of thought has even extended the sense of these words to the relation between the resistance of the patient and the virulence of the illness:

> *It is also said that fullness or emptiness is emptiness of the correct energy or fullness of the evil energy. (YXRM V, 36v)*

Fullness is thus an abundance of energy. Emptiness is an insufficiency of energy. However, authors rarely make the important distinction between what is a normal, healthy fullness of energy and an excess of energy leading to illness. Significantly, insufficiency and emptiness of energy are always dangerous abnormalities.

What exactly is in excess or insufficiency, and how can we perceive or measure the extent of deviation from normalcy? Excesses or insufficiencies are, from all descriptions, of the energy *(qi)*. But as explained in Volume I, energy is always presented under a yin or yang aspect, and the disequilibrium of this relativity always causes an excess of one aspect and an insufficiency of the other. A reference from the *Ju Ying* (sixteenth century) clearly expresses this concept of equal alternation of yin-yang, of the fullness or emptiness caused by the disequilibrium:

> *This is the idea of mutual overlapping of yin and yang — how the yang enters into the divisions of the yin, and how yin arises in the divisions of yang, alternating. If they remain [stagnant], illnesses results.*

> *One must go to the source, to the cause. Either **rong** energy [yin] is deficient, and the energy of the **wei** [yang] invades the interior; or, the **wei** energy is deficient, and the **rong** energy springs to the outside. In consequence, energy [yang] and blood [yin] no longer keep their place. In another area, the energy spreads and this place has emptiness. (DACH VI, 9r)*

The *Nei Jing* states this in another manner:

> *When the energy and blood are completely balanced, yin and yang mutually act [on the other alternatively]. But if the energy is disturbed in the envelope of the vessels or if the blood is in counterflow in the interior of the vessels, energy and blood separate from each other. One is full, the other empty. (DACH I, 7r)*

Finally, we should remember a fact not clearly indicated in the ancient or modern texts: the whole person can present fullness or emptiness as well as yin or yang. Excess or insufficiency of energy can be presented in two different aspects: yin and yang simultaneously, or of either yin or yang.

II. Excess or Insufficiency of Both Yin and Yang

It is possible to observe an excess or insufficiency of both yin and yang in the entire body; in a part of the body, such as a limb (yang contracture or yin flaccidity); in double organs; in yin and yang associated organs; or in nervous (mental, emotional, activity) or physical (blood, form, yin) life.

The signs of emptiness of both yin and of yang are the following: at the two wrists, the superficial and deep pulses are both equally nonexistent. The patient is prostrate, without strength. The stomach and the heart and all the other yin and yang organs function poorly. The case is serious — one should immediately give tonics and daily moxa, but not use needles.

The following are signs of excess of both yin and yang: the pulses of the two wrists are ample, hard and big at both superficial and deep levels. The complexion is red and congested. The patient complains of headaches, exhibits irascibility and great nervous agitation, and has high blood pressure. One should quickly disperse the yang energy through the triple warmer point *tianjing* (TW-10), and the yin energy through the pericardium point *daling* (PC-7). Then, through the pulses, one should determine which yin or yang organs are still in excess.

The coupled treasure workshop organs, one yin and one yang (heart and small intestine, etc.), can present excess or insufficiency concurrently.

A part of the body, one limb for example, can have cold and contracture, or heat and great swelling at the same time. Cold represents an excess of yin and contractures an excess of yang; heat represents an excess of yang while swellings are excesses of yin.

This equal rising and descent of yin and yang is not considered really serious. It is more serious when there is disequilibrium of one over the other.

> When there is fullness of energy, there is fullness of form. When there is emptiness of energy, there is emptiness of form. This is normal. The contrary is illness. When there is fullness of the pulses [yang], there is fullness of blood [yin]; when there is emptiness of the pulses, there is emptiness of blood. This is normal. The contrary is illness. (DACH I, 5v)

It is true that excess is accompanied by hyperactivity, which can develop into congestion, but the consequences are not severe. Total insufficiency is the cause of great fatigue and lack of strength, but again, the resulting illness is not very serious.

The principal passages which describe the emptiness-fullness or excess-insufficiency oppositions are given below:

> Signs of excess: scarlet red cheeks; constipation; urine generally red; energy rising to the upper part of the body; rapid panting; accelerated pulses and respiration.

> Signs of insufficiency: white face with obvious tints of blue-black; empty or greatly swollen intestines; frequent vomiting; slightly blue sclerae; small (wei), sunken (chen), and fine (xi) pulses; tendency toward cold mucus and episodes of fever. (DACH XII, 38v)

> When there is heat, there is fullness. When there is cold, there is emptiness. (YXRM I, 43v)

> When the energy and breath through the mouth is abundant, there is fullness. When there is no energy or breath, that is emptiness. (Nei Jing Ling Shu III, 8th line)

> Excess (you yu) is swelling or pain. It is called fullness (shi). Insufficiency (bu zu) is pruritus or flaccidity. It is called emptiness. (DACH II, 27r)

> Whether the body is thin or fat, has pains or swellings, pruritus or flaccidity; whether the illness is in abundance or decreasing; whether under the points there is tightness or relaxation — these are symptoms of fullness or emptiness. (DACH VI, 8r)

III. Excess or Insufficiency of Either Yin or Yang

With regard to the pulses, normal health is indicated by equality of all aspects. However, the superficial pulse levels (yang) are slightly less important than the middle and deep levels. The two wrists are almost equal, although the pulses on the left side should be slightly stronger than those on the right. Other inequalities are signs of disequilibrium.

Normalcy is fullness of energy and the physical aspect — the form, but without excess. Emptiness or insufficiency of energy is accompanied by emptiness or insufficiency of form. If there is disequilibrium of fullness and emptiness, illness may arise.

When forming a treatment strategy, it is important to determine the nature of the disequilibrium. In a general table, we will compare the signs of yang excess to those of yin insufficiency, and those of yang insufficiency to those of yin excess. If this kind of disequilibrium is involved, the disharmony is more complicated. If, on the contrary, there is an excess of yang with an excess of yin, or an insufficiency of yang with an insufficiency of yin, treatment consists only of raising or lowering the yin or yang aspect.

Excess of yang (energy)	Insufficiency of yin (blood)
Right pulses stronger than left	Left pulses less strong than right
Superficial pulse levels more wiry, ample and hard than the middle or deep levels	Middle and deep levels less strong, hard or ample than the superficial level
First pulse section ample, strong; third pulse section normal	First pulse section thin; third pulse section only slightly perceptible
All pulses beyond their place	All pulses thin, small
Voice too sonorous, too resonant	Pale complexion with blue-black hue
Eyes too bright, too alive	Shape is puffy, soft, thin
Movements too rapid	Physical weakness
Speech too excited	Lassitude, laziness, lack of resistance
Excess of gaiety, singing, laughter	Tendency toward fainting
Agitation, external heat	
Pain at the acupoints on pressure	
Local pain, contractures, convulsions, spasms	

Insufficiency of yang	Excess of yin
Right pulses weaker and softer than the left	Left pulses stronger and harder than the right
Superficial pulse levels weaker than the middle and deep levels	Deep and middle pulse levels harder than the superficial levels
First pulse section weak; third pulse section strong	First pulse section ample and strong; third pulse section equally strong
Pruritus	
All the pulses before their place	
Form without firmness; soft, white complexion	Red complexion; solid shape, well nourished
Voice without sonorance; eyes dull; movements slow	Tendency toward congestion, inflammation, abscess
Difficulty in speech; sadness, tears	Internal cold
Subject to cold coughs or excess heat	Swellings
Intestines empty or greatly swollen	
Great heat with much sweat	
Numbness under pressure at the acu-points	

These signs, as with everything in life, are not obligatory and certain. They are not all equally marked.

The *Nei Jing* commented centuries ago:

> When there is swelling or pain, there is fullness — such is the general idea. Yet, there are fat people [normally a sign of internal emptiness] who are prosperous, hard, firm, and who have pain [sign of excess of yang] and swellings [sign of excess of yin]. When there is pruritus or flaccidity, there is emptiness — such is the rule. However, there are thin people [normally a sign of internal fullness] who also have pain and swellings but who are empty. Consequently, one must still discern the origin of the evil; that is, if it comes from the exterior or the interior. (DACH II, 31r)

Chapter VI, ''Illness,'' discusses the cause of disease. Note that the external influences, wind, cold, heat, and humidity, cause excess. Joy, fear, emotional agitation, and internal influences all cause insufficiency.

The principal passages concerning the excess or insufficiency of yin or yang are given:

> In a general sense, if there is emptiness, the pulse is wiry **(xian)** like a cord (without amplitude). It is an emptiness of energy if the pulse is wiry **(xian)**, soft **(rou)**, large **(da)** and without force. It is a grave emptiness of energy if it is sunken, thin and without amplitude. It is emptiness of blood if the **cun** pulses are thin **(wei)**, and the **chi** pulses are big **(da)** and tight **(jin)**. (YXRM V, 7r)

> It is emptiness of yang if there is fire with much sweat, and the shape is fat and the face superficially white. It is emptiness of yin if the shape is thin and the face blue or black. (YXRM V, 7r)

> The blood has much fullness if the pulse is abundant and big. The energy has much emptiness if the pulse is decayed and weak. (DACH II, 20v)

> When the yang abounds, there is external heat. When the yin abounds, there is internal cold. (DACH I, 7v)

IV. Excess or Insufficiency of Each Organ or Function

The notion of excess or insufficiency applies to the energy animating each organ, to functions, and even to some aspects of the emotions.

For the organs, it is possible to cause an immediate decongestion of blood, an increase in functional activity, or the return to the normal state through nervous motor, vasomotor and trophic commands. The *Nei Jing* conceived of fullness or emptiness as dependent on the five treasure organs:

Energy-respiration depends on the lungs. Fullness: panting, cough. Emptiness: respiration without profit, little energy.

Consciousness depends on the heart. Fullness: laughter without stopping. Emptiness: chagrin; shivering in the bath; energy and blood inequal.

Decision depends on the kidney. Fullness: swollen abdomen; diarrhea after eating. Emptiness: withdrawal.

Blood depends on liver. Fullness: discontent. Emptiness: fear.

Form depends on the spleen-pancreas. Fullness: swollen abdomen, menses without result. Emptiness: the four limbs are without strength. (DACH V, 22v)

Below is a table of excess-insufficiency oppositions for each of the organs. The pericardium and triple warmer, the two great regulators of yin and yang energy, are cited first along with their mental and emotional characteristics. The pulse relating to the organ is always hard and ample for fullness, and soft or nonexistent for emptiness.

Triple warmer: "Father of the yang energy"	
Excess	**Insufficiency**
Chagrin, without joy, irritable	Mental and physical lassitude
Desire to sleep, with insomnia	Everything an effort
Non-localized pains from wind	Sadness, ennui; limbs do not obey
Shortness of breath, cannot speak	
Lack of appetite; outflow of urine	Insufficiency of urine; cold

Heart Governor: "Mother of the yin energy"	
Excess	**Insufficiency**
Oppression, anger	Emotional depression
Agitated heart with dull pains	Lack of awareness
Rapid panting from joy or laughing	Fatigue; lack of joy
Congestive headache	Sexual vigor without orgasm
Bad breath	Tightness of the larynx

Heart (yin organ)	
Excess	**Insufficiency**
Easy laughing or disordered sobbing	Sadness; does not laugh
Red face	Pale face
Agitation of the mind; hyperexcitability	Depression, fear, anguish
Pain in the heart and arms	Breathlessness from effort

| Lungs (yin organ) ||
Excess	Insufficiency
Panting, cough	Lack of breath
Pain in the shoulders, back and sides	Cold shoulders and back
Sweating	Changing complexion
Frequent urination	Insomnia
Yawning and sneezing	Pains in the supraclavicular fossa

| Liver (yin organ) ||
Excess	Insufficiency
Discontent; anger	Fear
Ashen or yellow complexion	White, waxy complexion
Difficult or painful micturition	Constipation
Menstrual problems; priapism	Yellow or gray stools
Pain in the lumbar area and genitals	Impotence, frigidity
	Pains in the thigh, lower pelvis, throat
	Easily bruises
	Blood coagulates slowly

| Spleen-pancreas (yin organ) ||
Excess	Insufficiency
Excess flesh; large but weak abdomen	Insufficiency of flesh
Less productive bowel movements	Abundant bowel movements
Painful joints	Fatigue from morning until 5 p.m.
Great sighs, sadness, obsessions, nightmares	Aerogastry, bad digestion

| Kidneys (yin organ) ||
Excess	Insufficiency
Excessive decision making	Indecision, confused speech
Dreams of difficulty unfastening the belt	Dreams of inundated trees
Feeble, colored urine	Frequent urination; colored urine with unusual odor
Heavy, hot, painful feet	Cold lower legs and feet
Dry tongue	Abundant sweat
Headache	

Stomach (yang organ)	
Excess	**Insufficiency**
Cramps, pains in the stomach	Slow digestion
Acidity; hyperchlorhydria	Vomiting up fluids after meals
Cracked mouth; cracked lips	Red face; painful brows
Nightmares	Emotional tears, sadness
Eruptions, acne	Cold feet

Large Intestine (yang organ)	
Excess	**Insufficiency**
Constipation	Diarrhea
Dry mouth; burnt-looking lips	Eruptions, pruritus
Cold body	Cold and warmth slow to return
Ameliorated by pungent flavors and warmth	Ameliorated by sour flavors and coldness

Small Intestine (yang organ)	
Excess	**Insufficiency**
Scarlet face; dry mouth	Blue lips with white edges
Abscesses of mouth and pharynx	Thinness
Feeble urine	Frequent, abundant urine
Joy and laughter	Violent sweats

Gallbladder (yang organ)	
Excess	**Insufficiency**
Excessive sleeping	Insomnia
Great sighs; irritability	Non-localized pain
Bitter taste in the mouth in the morning	Pain in chest and sides
All the joints painful	Swelling of cheek and chin
Numb knee and lower leg	Swelling of the nipples

Urinary Bladder (yang organ)	
Excess	**Insufficiency**
Agitation, fullness	Troubled mind
Excessive erections; prostatitis	Without sexual vigor
Retention of urine	Colorless, abundant urine
Frequent and pressing need to urinate	Incontinence; gets up at night
Painful head when defecating	Many intestinal worms

V. Excess or Insufficiency of the Local Energy

The energy can be in excess or insufficiency in only one part of the body. The symptoms are then local. This disequilibrium of energy in one region or part of the body is only perceived through the pulses with great difficulty. It is therefore deduced indirectly from the fact that the muscles and nerves along the meridian are only overly sensitive or painful when the meridian and the organs themselves are not disordered. The exception to this is pain due to trauma.

The local signs of this disequilibrium are the following:

Excess	Insufficiency
Pain	Insensitivity
Heat	Cold
Contracture	Numbness
Spasms, cramps	Pruritus
Convulsions	Flaccidity
Inflammations	Pale swellings

Notes

[1] The Chinese terms used:

For fullness, the ideogram *shi* is used. It is formed from the elements ''a string of cowries'' (money), and ''under a roof.'' The ancient commentaries define *shi* as: ''to be truly rich, to have a well-filled treasury.'' Usually this term is used for ''truth, authenticity, that which is as it should be.'' Medically, it is used to indicate either a happy state of fullness of energy and strength, or a dangerous excess of energy for which the expression *you yu,* ''to have too much,'' is more correctly employed.

For emptiness, the ideogram *xu* is used. The ancient commentaries say *xu* represents ''a man standing on a vast, uncultivated desert plateau, where nothing is visible in the four [all] directions.'' This term is often the designation for insufficiency going to complete exhaustion. When the quantity of energy is simply under the normal average, the term used is *bu zu,* ''not enough.''

Chapter VI

Tonification — Dispersion

I. The Meaning of Tonification and Dispersion — II. Tonifying or Dispersing through the Circulation of Energy: Favoring, Opposing — III. Beginning by Tonifying or Dispersing — IV. Tonifying or Dispersing Too Much, Not Enough, or Wrongly — V. Choice of the Means of Tonifying or Dispersing

The ancient Chinese observed the existence of points, meridians and the circulation of energy. They noted that disease always develops from an energetic dysfunction, manifesting through fullness (excess) or emptiness (insufficiency). Following through on their observations, they created a system of re-establishing the energy to its normal state in order to correct the dysfunction.

> *When there is emptiness, tonify; when there is fullness, disperse.[1] (DACH V, 23r)*

As all Chinese medicine, particularly acupuncture, is based on this double directive, it is an extremely important concept to understand.

I. The Meaning of Tonification and Dispersion

At first glance, the meaning of ''tonification'' and ''dispersion'' seems very simple. From the text cited at the beginning of this chapter, one understands that to tonify is to remove, or fill the emptiness; to disperse is to take away, or empty the fullness. Such is the general idea. But as soon as we depart the plane of generalities, we will see that the problem can be very complicated.

First, to clearly understand the differences between European and Chinese definitions of these terms, one must review the scientific and medical visions held in these two distinct cultures.

In Europe, the written languages are purely phonetic, and thus arbitrary and dogmatic. Why, for example, do we call a tree by this sound instead of another? And why must we accept without discussion the authority of this tradition as an unchangeable dogma? This sound and its configuration represent nothing to the mind; they are only addressed to the verbal memory.

In China, writing is a pictorial form, which, we can say, borrows only a little from phonetics. (Most of the approximately 53,000 ideograms are not used often in the spoken language.) The Japanese, for example, pronounce the ideogram representing ''mountain'' as *yama,* while the Chinese of the North pronounce it *shan;* both, of course, look at the same sign — a diagram of three summits. This pictorial representation of reality passes into the brain directly from vision without using the pathways of sound. This results in the development of astute observation of the complexity of things and also of their profound composition. Thus, the sign ''tree'' is diagrammed by a vertical line for the trunk, one horizontal line for the branches, two lines away from the trunk and down for the roots. The idea and the vision are mixed without using anything of the sound.

Through the action of the written language, Europe bases instruction on learning, while China does so on understanding. ''To learn'' is only to know one aspect of a question and by hearsay. ''To understand'' is to perceive for oneself the moving interaction of all things.

The triumph of Europe is the state, the abstraction, the admirable blossoming of mathematics and analysis. The triumph of China is the vision of the apparent and hidden reality, synthesis, the profound vision of incessant movement.

In Europe, the existence of specialists for each organ implies the acceptance of the independence of each organ. In China, the interdependence of the organs is so well understood that one labels ''the inferior worker'' the one who cures only a sick organ and ''the superior worker,'' the one who cures those who are not yet sick.

Coming back to the sense of the words ''to tonify'' and ''to disperse,'' Europeans, mostly anatomists, look at the resultant action on the whole body, one part of the body, or on one organ, to see if there is material change. For Europeans, to tonify and to disperse is to activate and restrain, respectively, the following:

Trophism, growth, repairs.

Irrigation and alimentation of blood (congestion, inflammation).

Functional activity (absorption, secretions, excretions, filtration, assimilation, movements, strength.)

Activity of the senses (perceptions, pains).

Cerebral activity.

In Chinese medicine, with its physiological perspective, the words ''to tonify'' or ''to disperse'' express action on the energy represented by alternate aspects of yin and yang. This energy can manifest as vitality, immunity, heat, activity, etc. (see Volume I). We tonify to fill an emptiness and disperse what is in excess. We do this by acting directly on the energy.

> *For all those who use the needle, the aim must be to harmonize the energy. When the six meridians are in harmony, one says that there is no illness. And even if there is illness, one says that it will soon finish by itself. (DACH V, 22r)*

(The six meridians mentioned are the six of the hand and the six of the feet, which in reality are twelve.)

In Chinese medicine, to tonify is to increase the insufficient energy. To disperse is to reduce the excessive energy and to continue until the harmony is re-established among all pulses, and thus between yin and yang.

> *In puncturing excesses, one must obtain emptiness. Keep the needle in until the yin energy floods and arrives; then remove the needle. When puncturing emptiness, one must obtain fullness. The yang energy must first arrive and flood and there must be heat under the needle; only then remove the needle. (DACH V, 20v)*

To tonify, then, is to fill an insufficiency of yin or yang, one of which is abnormally weak in relation to its opposite. To disperse is to evacuate the excess of the yin or yang aspect which is abnormally strong in connection with its opposite.

The yang, also called the *wei,* represents heat, life, pain; it also signifies the exterior of the body, the skin, the right side and the upper part of the body. The yin, also termed the *rong,* represents cold, weakness, insensitivity, the interior of the body, and most importantly, the blood and the internal organs.

Since tonification fills insufficiencies, in principle it gives life and heat. By clearing away excesses, dispersion produces relaxation, calm, and freshness. Using this reasoning, most scholars have posited that to tonify is to excite or activate the yang, giving life and heat. Dispersing, on the other hand, is to excite or activate the yin, augmenting calmness and freshness. Those who tend to oversimplify thus advise action on the yang in order to tonify and action on the yin in order to disperse.

> *To tonify is to start from the **wei** (yang) in order to activate the energy. To disperse is to start from **rong** (yin) in order to quiet the energy. (DACH VI, 8v)*

> *To tonify: after obtaining yang energy under the needle, push the energy in with the needle thus driving the energy in. This is what we call warming the interior. To disperse: After leaving the needle in until the yin energy abounds under the needle, puncture the fullness, taking it out with the needle. (DACH, 10r)*

However, since antiquity, other scholars have noted that by acting on either yin or yang, they acted at the same time on its opposite — as when pressing on one side of a scale we cause the other side to rise. They observed that by acting in this way the results obtained were superior and more durable.

> *Those who are skillful in the use of needles start from the yin in order to manage the yang and from the yang to manage the yin; they use the right to cure the left, the left to cure the right, the exterior to treat the interior, and the interior to treat the exterior. (DACH I, 13v)*

> *For the illnesses of yin treat the yang and vice versa. (DACH. XI, 11r, quoting Li Gao, twelfth century)*

In effect, to re-establish the equilibrium, it is possible either to raise the low side or reduce the high side. Consequently, tonifying the yang would be to disperse the yin at the same time; i.e., to increase heat and life activity, and through that to reduce cold, numbness and insensitivity. In the experiments carried out in Paris, it was constantly reported that for the coupled organs, one yin and the other yang, tonifying the weaker dispersed the stronger.

At a superficial glance, since to tonify is to activate the yang, we would never have to disperse the yang. Likewise, we would never have to tonify the yin. Many texts, however, advise the contrary, these passages among others:

> *When there is heat in the upper part of the body, with cold in the lower part of the body, see which pulses are empty and hollow and among them tonify one lower yin meridian. The energy will descend. (DACH V, 22r)*

> *When the yin energy is insufficient and the yang energy is in excess, first tonify the yin and afterwards disperse the yang. (DACH., 24r)*

In conclusion, we can define the two words as follows: to tonify is to activate the vitality, and consequently increase strength, trophism and functions, through the yang or the yin; to disperse is to calm, to relax, to slow down the vitality, trophism, and functions, through the yang or the yin.

The yang meridians primarily transmit energy for functions of revitalization. They are generally treated to increase heat, life, and activity. The yin meridians transmit energy for functions of maintenance and circulation of blood. They are treated to reduce heat, mental activity and agitation.

In general, to tonify yang, one disperses the yin, and vice versa. But before entering into the particularities of yin and yang, we will discuss generalities relative to the action of tonifying and dispersing — using the rhythm of the circulation of energy recommended by the school of "favoring and opposing"; the rule of beginning by tonifying or dispersing; and the possibility of acting too much or not enough, or mistakenly.

II. Tonifying or Dispersing through the Circulation of Energy: Favoring and Opposing

"Favoring and opposing" *(sui-ying)* [2] is a school of thought that teaches a special technique of enhancing the effect of tonification or dispersion. The theoretical idea is that one must favor the flow of the energy in order to tonify and support, and go against the flow in order to disperse. Three practical applications have come from this idea:

1) Puncture with the needle tilted, with the point facing against the flow in order to disperse (this is "opposing"), the point going with the flow in order to tonify (this is "favoring").

2) Puncture or stimulate several points on the same meridian by following the flow in order to tonify and by going against the flow to disperse.

3) To disperse, oppose the energy of the meridian by treating at the beginning of its two hour daily maximal period. To tonify, favor the energy by treating at the end of the two hour period.

The general idea is described in the *Da Cheng*:

> To tonify is to favor. With the point of the needle, favor the flow of energy of the blood and urge it on. To disperse
> is to oppose. With the point of the needle, confront the flow of energy of the blood and act against it.
> (DACH I, 21r)

Recall that the flow of energy is as follows (with the upper limbs at the sides of the body):

> In the yang meridians of the hand, the energy ascends the upper limb to the head and descends to the feet through
> the yang meridians of the feet. The energy then pours into the yin meridians of the feet and mounts to the chest
> from where it descends to the hand by the yin meridians of the hand. (YXRM I, 42v)

The three practical applications are described again in more detail:

1) Puncture by tilting the needle towards the source (counterflow) in order to disperse; tilt downstream (in the direction of flow) to tonify.

> To oppose with the point of the needle, face the source; that opposes. In order to favor, follow the flow with the
> point of the needle; that favors. (DACH I, 21r)

This technique can only be applied with needles. It is difficult to confirm that this gives better results.

2) Stimulate the first point of the meridian, beginning at its source. Or stimulate in succession several points on the same meridian, by following the flow to tonify; going against the flow to disperse.

> To oppose, to take out, is to disperse the child [that which comes after]. Thus, in an illness of the heart, disperse
> the **shu** point (**daling**, PC-7) of the heart governor; this is to oppose and take out. To favor, to support, is to tonify
> the mother [that which comes before]. Thus to tonify the **jing** point (**zhongchong**, PC-9) of the heart governor is to
> favor, to support. (DACH V, 24r)

Other texts advise stimulating successive points going with the flow for tonification and going against it for dispersion.

3) One interpretation of favoring and opposing is based on the fact that the energy in each meridian is at its maximum for two hours each day. To favor is to activate the departing energy at the end of the two hours. To oppose is to block the entrance of the energy at the beginning of the two hours of maximum activity. Recall that the flow of energy has its maxima of two hours in the following order:

lungs	3 - 5 a.m.
large intestine	5 - 7 a.m.
stomach	7 - 9 a.m.
spleen-pancreas	9 - 11 a.m.
heart	11 a.m. - 1 p.m.
small intestine	1 - 3 p.m.
urinary bladder	3 - 5 p.m.
kidney	5 - 7 p.m.
heart governor	7 - 9 p.m.
triple warmer	9 - 11 p.m.
gallbladder	11 p.m. - 1 a.m.
liver	1 - 3 a.m.

It has been noted that the critical hours of illnesses of each organ generally coincide with these two hours when the energy is at its maximum.

*At the **yin** hours (3 - 5 a.m.) the energy is found in the lungs. At the **mao** hours the energy is found in the large intestine. When the energy is there, lung and large intestine abound. One disperses them, one purges them, by opposing the energy that comes to them. However, at 7 a.m., the energy is going to pass into the stomach; the lungs and large intestine then empty themselves. One tonifies by favoring the energy which is departing. (DACH VI, 10v)*

To tonify is to favor the energy at the moment when it is going away and to add an impulsion to it. To disperse is to oppose the energy at the moment when it abounds and to constrict it. (YXRM I, 42v)

III. Beginning by Tonifying or Dispersing

It is sometimes difficult to know if we should begin by tonifying or dispersing. The authors have extracted some rules which can be summarized in this manner:

One must first tonify insufficiencies of energy, then disperse excesses. Such is the general rule. But when there is acute inflammatory illness, trauma or contracture, we must first disperse the "perverse energy," that is, directly combat the evil; then, tonify the insufficiencies of organs and parts of the body related to the affected area.

First tonify, then disperse.

First tonify, then disperse. (DACH V, 23r)

When yang energy is insufficient and yin energy excessive, first tonify the yang, then afterwards disperse the yin. When the yin energy is insufficient and the yang energy excessive, first tonify the yin, then afterwards disperse the yang. (DACH)

Fat people are empty in the interior. First tonify, then disperse. (DACH, VI, 10v)

But for all these passages, we must not forget the many exceptions of yin and yang, and the fact that to tonify the yin in order to make it rise into the yang is often called "dispersing the yin." Under the name "guiding the energy," *dao qi*, some authors mention an action which is clearly a succession of tonifying and dispersing.[3]

To guide the energy, enter slowly [tonifying] and leave slowly [dispersing]. (DACH XI, 10v)

This action is particularly recommended for *qihai* (CV-6), used for acute lumbar pains. (The action must be repeated three times with an interval of twenty-five respirations.) We have not yet confirmed the efficacy of this method.

First disperse, then tonify.

This is generally used in three types of cases — thin people, acute cases, and contractures with spasms.

Thin people are full in the interior; first disperse, then tonify. (DACH VI, 10v)

First disperse the perverse energy, then tonify the true energy. Indeed, if the eyes are red, the complexion colored, the perverse energy is hot; disperse it. Then, tonify or disperse the rest. (DACH V, 24v)

If the energy of the body is insufficient, and the energy of the evil abundant, quickly disperse the latter. If the energy of the body and of evil are both abundant, yin and yang are in excess: quickly disperse the energy of evil. (DACH 22r)

When there is internal fullness or contracture, disperse first. Likewise, when there is constipation or urinary insufficiency or stopping of functions, increase the functions by first dispersing the contractures or internal fullnesses. (DACH II, 23r)

IV. Tonifying or Dispersing Too Much, or Not Enough, or Wrongly

Four types of errors are indicated: to tonify or disperse wrongly — that is, to tonify excesses or disperse emptiness; to act on an organ that should be left undisturbed; to exaggerate the correct action; or not to act strongly enough.

Tonifying excesses or dispersing emptiness.

This is the most serious and least pardonable error. It could only occur by ignoring the pulses or signs of excess or insufficiency. One must be singularly inattentive or ignorant to make this mistake.

Each time one disperses what is already insufficient or tonify what is already too full, there is a risk of death. If one disperses an emptiness or tonifies a fullness, then awareness leaves its home. Evil continues until the normal is abandoned. The correct cannot be re-established. The physical body disintegrates. Destiny is accomplished. (YXRM I, 43v)

Although not always as grave as described above, the danger is real. The experiments in Paris have demonstrated, for example, that a simple coryza tonified by moxa at *shangxing* (GV-22, IS GV-23), instead of being dispersed as usual, can quickly become a serious congestion.

Acting on a well-functioning organ.

This mistake is not very grave because healthy organs are not notably disturbed by such a weak method. It is necessary, according to the law of Arhndt, that the organ be disordered in order to respond to weak stimuli.

Exaggerating the correct action.

In principle, the dysfunctional organ, stimulated by the correct point, returns to normal without surpassing it. One would have to make repeated and strong actions to go beyond that aim. Such an error is possible only from those who act without consulting the pulses and only on theoretical conceptions.

Do not disperse too much emptiness. Do not tonify too much fullness. Equilibrium is the goal. (YXRM I, 43v)

If by accident such an error had been committed, it would be enough to use some points with opposed action in order to re-establish normalcy. (DACH V, 25v)

The action is insufficient.

Sometimes it happens that the desired effect is not obtained. The cause can be an underestimation of the evil or an overestimation of the energy of the patient. We must recall then the old saying: ''When ten is necessary for the cure and we have given only nine, it is necessary only to add one.''

In fact, when the treatment has been insufficient, the patient feels little improvement, but a careful comparison of the pulses before and after this session always shows a change, a sign that the next treatment will have a marked effect.

V. Choosing the Means for Tonifying or Dispersing

In summary, to tonify is to support, to amplify the normal flow of energy responding to the alternatives of day and night, summer and winter, the waxing and waning moon; to generally treat the yang (yang meridians, right side and upper part of the body) in the morning, in spring and on clear and sunny days. To disperse is to constrict, slow down, and restrain the normal flow of energy following the same alternatives as above; to treat the yin (yin meridians, left side and lower part of the body) in the afternoon, at the waning moon, in autumn and on cloudy, cold days.

In practice, in order to tonify, it is best to treat the tonification and herald points, the points at the extremities of the limbs, and those of the meridians that precede in the circulation of energy. To disperse, it is best to treat the dispersal and assent points, the points at the mid-length of the extremities, and those of the meridians that follow in the circulation of energy.

In order to tonify with needles, it is preferable to use the colored metals (gold, copper, brass, etc.). If the metal is neutral, insert by successive levels; after agitating the needle up and down, ask for inhalation while withdrawing the needle without stopping, then close the point taking a long time. (This is useful also for the colored metals.)

In order to tonify with moxa, make at least seven, or better ten moxas on each point each morning.

In order to disperse with needles, it is preferable to use white metals (particularly silver and zinc); insert without stopping and withdraw by successive levels, turning the needle while withdrawing. With a neutral metal (platinum, iron, steel, etc.), insert during expiration and leave the point open after withdrawing the needle.

In order to disperse with moxa, do not make more than five moxa cones on each point; it is better to act in the evening.

(See techniques of needles, moxa, massage, electricity. See also Volume I, Chapter VII, ''Energy.'')

Notes

[1] The ideograms invented by the ancients to indicate the idea of these two opposed actions have no exact equivalence in our European languages. Having no closer equivalent, we have adopted the words, ''to tonify,'' and ''to disperse.''

The ideograms are given as:

To tonify: *bu.* The sign is formed on the left by ''the hand,'' and on the right by ''the man becomes father.'' The commentaries explain that this ancient term means: ''To respond to the needs of the family, supplying their lacks.'' *Bu* implies that one acts like a good father of the family; one supplies the needs of honest people. [*Editor's note:* the ideogram the author describes means ''to seize, to catch, to apprehend.'' The ideogram used in Chinese medical texts to mean ''to supply, to fill (a deficit),'' etc., has the ''cloth'' radical, not the ''hand'' radical. Its original meaning was ''to patch a garment.'']

To disperse: *xie.* Formed of the elements ''to make flow by lifting up the lid of a closed receptacle on the fire,'' meaning to cause the excess vapor to escape from the receptacle on the fire. The term is used for all deliberate purges: to rout an army, to drain a field, to empty an intestine, etc.

[2] ''Favoring'' *(sui)* is to walk following behind another, pushing the other in front before oneself. ''Opposing'' *(ying)* is to go counter to, confronting and stopping.

[3] Guiding the energy, *dao qi,* is represented by ''a thumb acting at the head,'' the ideogram used to indicate the guides in an unknown country; figuratively, to guide the mind in a search. *Qi* is the energy described in Volume I.

Chapter VII

Where to Tonify or Disperse

I. Local Acupuncture — II. Acupuncture Through the Impaired Meridian — III. True Acupuncture: Yin by Yang and Yang by Yin — IV. Simultaneous Action on Both Yang and Yin

The choice of where the practitioner tonifies or disperses varies according to the three kinds of acupuncture: local; that of the impaired meridian; or that of yin by yang, and yang by yin. The last method has the greatest potential and gives what the other two cannot — a certain immunity against a recurrence of the illness along with a more general immunity. It constitutes true scientific acupuncture.

I. Local Acupuncture

This primitive method, purely empirical, requires no knowledge of the points, the meridians, the circulation of energy, yin-yang or the patient. In brief, it is not necessary to learn or understand Chinese medicine. It gives some immediate results which are not, however, long lasting. It can be used without risk for external local pains, inflammations, muscle weakness and contractures.

For pains that are due to excesses of energy, one must disperse at the center of pain. Those who have studied acupuncture always recognize that this center is an acupoint, and action at this point is much more powerful than that on the surrounding area. Some physicians not familiar with acupuncture remark that there is often a small nodule at the center of pain, which they attribute to cellulite (?).

For inflammations that are also due to excesses of energy, one must disperse around and particularly above and under the inflammation. Swellings are treated in the same manner. For example, for swellings due to an ankle sprain, *shenmai* (BL-62), just under the external malleolus, gives immediate, excellent results.

For muscle weakness caused by insufficiency of energy, the most effective points are close to the insertions or just in the middle of the muscle. One will always find a sensitive point in these places. Since the weaknesses are insufficiencies of energy, one must tonify them. For contractures due to excess of energy, the point at the center of the muscle gives the best results with dispersion.

In China, local acupuncture is particularly used by the "inferior workers." But it is also used by the "superior workers" in order to quickly remove the "branches" after they have treated the root condition.

The points utilized, called "center of pain" *(tong zhong)* or "not fixed" *(bu ding)* points, are not necessarily points on the meridians. Their locations do not have the absolute precision of the meridian points. A difference of several millimeters does not decrease their effect much.

II. Acupuncture Through the Impaired Meridian

This form of acupuncture, which in China is called "of the direct meridian" *(zheng jing),* only requires knowledge of the pulses and tonification and dispersal techniques. It does not demand an understanding of yin and yang or of the circulation of energy. It is clearly more scientific and active than the local form, but does not give the deep and durable results or the marked general immunity derived from the method utilizing yin and yang. It consists of treating only the two channels of the impaired organ meridian, both in the same manner. Thus, when the liver is disordered, one tonifies or disperses only the liver meridian on both sides in the same manner.

This analytic and simplistic form is particularly tempting for European physicians, mostly organ specialists who do not recognize clearly the interdependence of all the parts of the body. This form of acupuncture is conceived by them as "pasteurian medicine" directed to an isolated organ.

Excellent results are obtained by the *zheng jing* method. It is particularly recommended for acute cases of organ dysfunction when immediate results must be obtained. In addition, this method is invaluable for hypo- or hypertensive people, since one avoids the risk of causing the blood pressure to be higher or lower on one side.

We must take into consideration, however, that each of the double organs (kidneys, ovaries, etc.) respond only to the excitation of the meridian channel on its side. When it is a question of a double organ, one first must be sure there is equilibrium between the two symmetrical organs (or in the case of the heart, its two sides); if there is not, this disequilibrium would continue since it could not be resolved by this method.

When treating the yang meridians with this method, it is recommended that the needle be inserted obliquely so as not to reach the yin depth. For the yin meridians, the needle must be implanted deeply and perpendicularly so as to cause the yin to pass into the yang and vice versa. Finally, the needle must be inserted and removed by successive levels (see chapters on needle technique).

This method of treating directly through the meridian is recommended in China for illnesses termed "of the blood" (thus of yin), described as having a fixed location with constant pain, which we can classify as organic disease.[1]

This technique is recommended in numerous passages describing the "rule of root and branches." The root is the true energetic cause of the disease and is considered here within the yin — the interior of the body — and the yin treasure organs, those elements touched first by the illness.

In principle, the root must be cured first. The branches are the secondary problems and will fall down by themselves or can be easily cured. The single exception is in the case of general insufficiency. Here, one must first treat the branch (build up the patient), then the root (attack the evil).[2]

Li Gao (Dong Yuan of the twelfth century) gives the following example:

> In cases of foul-smelling genital organs, one must recall that the genital system depends on the liver; the foul smell depends on the heart. First, disperse the liver at **xingjian** (LR-2) to cure the root. Then, stimulate the heart at **shaochong** (HT-9) to cure the branch. Such is the method of the most celebrated physicians. (DACH XI, 1v)

Finally, different texts recommend treating the meridian directly, whatever the trouble:

> When the illness is in the three yang, be sure to aim at the energy in the yang divisions, and puncture. If the illness is in the three yin, be sure to aim at the energy in the yin divisions, and puncture. (DACH I, 10r)

> If the illness is in the **yangming**, and one attacks it in the **jueyin**, or if it is in the **taiyang** and one attacks it in the **taiyin**, one will not be able to conquer the disease. (DACH 20r)

This form of acupuncture is said to be the most effective for treating the point of entry of the illness, analogous to the law of the root and branches.

> When the illness begins in the yin, the rule is to first treat the yin. When the illness begins in the yang, the rule is to first treat the yang. (DACH VI, 9r)

III. True Acupuncture: Yin by Yang and Yang by Yin

This third type of acupuncture is not only the most subtle and complex, but also the most efficacious for the management of the energy. To apply this method, we must know the points, meridians, excesses or insufficiencies as shown by the pulses, as well as the circulation of energy and the relations of the organs. Most of all, we must understand yin-yang, their constant reciprocal movements, and the action on the energy that these cosmic rhythms can produce.

There is a special needling technique used to invoke communication between the interior and exterior. (Here we speak of stone, copper or iron needles; the use of gold to tonify or silver to disperse render the following actions superfluous.)

To tonify, insert the needle by successive levels to move the superficial yang into the deep yin, and remove the needle without stopping to prevent yang from re-exiting; finally, block the hole so the energy cannot escape. To disperse, insert the needle in one movement to reach the yin without exciting the yang; withdraw it by successive levels to bring the deep yin up and propel it into the yang; lastly, leave the hole open to let the energy escape. (Recall that to treat the impaired meridian directly, when needling for the yang energy, the needle must be put in obliquely so that yin is not reached; for the yin, it must be put in perpendicularly with one movement.)

This method is indispensable for illnesses which are mobile in location, intermittent, and are termed "energetic." It is also recommended for certain yang illnesses that must be cured through the yin, such as myopia with protruding eyes, nephritis with a contracted kidney, spasms and pains; and yin illnesses that must be treated through the yang, such as myopia with sunken eyes, nephritis with an enlarged kidney, and paresis.[3]

In order to understand fully this method of dispersing or tonifying, we must first review the yin-yang concept relative to humans, and then its dependence on the cosmic rhythms.

The human yin-yang.

The yin-yang aspects of humans have been discussed in Volume I. Below is a brief summary.

To tonify is to replenish insufficiencies of energy; to disperse is to empty excessive energy. This energy presents itself under yin or yang, a relativity representing proportional relations of movements rather than a fixed condition or state. Yin only exists as the opposite of yang. The middle of the body relative to the lower portion is yang; the middle relative to the upper portion is yin. Yin-yang is either relativity of position (interior-exterior, down-up, left-right, etc.), or relativity of activity (rest-action, sleeping-waking, cold-heat, weakness-strength, numbness-pain, slow-quick, flaccidity-contracture, etc.).

This yin-yang relativity is always moving and changing, constantly and ceaselessly transforming into one another. Stability is an artificial reality viewed by the mind; true reality is alternating rhythm and constant interchange, where movement is unceasing.

For humans, this yin-yang rhythm is manifest in the circadian cycle: yin corresponds to night, the need to rest and sleep; and yang to the sun, the day, the need for activity.

If activity continues when evening comes, there is excess yang relative to the yin, which is insufficient. And if there is sleepiness not only in the night but also in the day, there is excess yin, thus insufficiency of yang. Pains increasing at midday are an excess of yin not transformed into yang. Pains increasing at sunset and at night are excesses of yang not transformed into yin.

It is possible to have an excess of yang with normal and compressed yin, or with insufficient yin; excess of yin with normal and compressed yang, or with insufficient yang; or equality of both aspects in excess or insufficiency.

The relationship between the human rhythm and the cosmic rhythm is such that, for example, by tonifying leg-*sanli* (ST-36) of the stomach in the morning (yang), one obtains a notable increase of strength, better digestion, and more restful sleep. Tonifying this point at night (yin) will normally cause digestive upset, insomnia and marked malaise.

The cosmic rhythms and the human yin-yang.

To live by the natural, cosmic rhythm is to improve and augment one's strength. Denying this rhythm or rebelling against it is to waste away one's strength.

The aim of the highest form of acupuncture is to synchronize the human yin-yang rhythm with the cosmic rhythm, so that the normal flow of alternating energy is favored. To achieve this it is necessary to tonify the human yang when the cosmic yang is rising and to disperse it when the cosmic yang is diminishing. The same is true for the yin. It appears that action by any means on yin or yang during cosmic rising is tonifying, and action during cosmic decrease is dispersing.

In general, yang increases with the sun, the moon, summer, and heat (with yin decreasing proportionally). Yin increases with the decrease of the sun, the diminution of the moon, winter, and cold (with yang decreasing proportionally).

Indeed, as with humans, the norm in the universe is not constant equality of yin and yang, but cyclical, varying proportions of the one to the other. During the day, yang rises and descends with the sun; yin increases and diminishes with the night. From midnight to midday, the yang rises with proportional diminution of the yin; from midday to midnight the yang diminishes with proportional increase of the yin. To follow the rhythm is to tonify the yang until midday, and then the yin from midday on; to disperse the yin until midday and the yang from midday on.[4]

These are the most important rhythms for human beings. Health, especially mental health, is based on an alternating response of the body to the daytime yang and the nighttime yin. Sleep depends on it.

The phases of the moon have an importance that civilized people, living artificially, do not notice. Birth clinics have observed that the greatest number of births are grouped first around the new moon and second around the full moon. Very few births take place around the periods of the quarter moon. Furthermore, human intestinal parasites reproduce themselves and are most active at the new moon. It is traditional to cut the hair at the new moon; this gives it growth and better vitality. Winegrowers take careful notice of the moon.

For the Chinese, the yang increases from the new moon until the full moon, and decreases from the full moon to the new moon. When the yang is in ascendency, the yin decreases and vice-versa in the lunar cycle.[5]

It is said that while one puncture is sufficient at the new moon, on the second day one must puncture twice, on the third day thrice and so forth, until with the full moon one punctures fifteen times; the number diminishes each day thereafter until the next new moon. It is expressly recommended to tonify, not disperse, on the waxing moon; and conversely, to disperse, not tonify, on the waning moon in order to profit from the lunar rhythm. It is obviously a matter of yang energy.

The rhythm of the seasons has distinct importance. The response to the needles is much less rapid and less profound in winter than in summer. In winter, several days may pass after treatment before the patient is cured; in summer, the response is immediate. It has been observed in Paris that in the treatment of deafness, improvements are only slight in winter, but very marked in summer.[6]

The yang is born at the winter solstice (December 21st) and grows until the summer solstice (June 21st). The yin during this time decreases. The yin is born at the summer solstice and grows until the winter solstice. The yang decreases during this period.

In the spring, until June 21st, tonify the yang and disperse the yin in order to coordinate with this rhythm. In autumn and in winter, disperse the yang and tonify the yin. If in spring the yin is too weak, it is often possible to tonify it by tonifying the corresponding yang and vice versa. For illnesses "of blood," act directly on the insufficient yin-yang aspect.

Given that the left side is yin and the right side is yang, it is recommended that at the first, second, and third moons (January through March), we must not disperse the yang of the left leg because the yang has already been born in the yin. At the fourth, fifth, and sixth moons (April through June), the energy is in the right side, and we must not disperse the yang of the right leg because the yang is fully developed. At the seventh, eighth, and ninth moons (July through September), we must not disperse the yin of the right leg because the yin has already been born in the yang. At the tenth, eleventh, and twelfth moons (October through December), we must not disperse the yin of the left leg because the yin is fully developed.[7]

There is also a seasonal rhythm for the corresponding blood circulation. For example, cerebral congestion (yang) is more frequent and more dangerous in summer (yang). Congestion of the kidneys is more severe in winter (yin). The liver empties its energy at the equinoxes, and so on.

Temperature and weather constitute another natural rhythm: rain in spring, heat and high temperature in the summer, snow in autumn, ice in winter. But in our epoch, this rhythm has been obscured by central heating and cooling. We live with the paradox of winters of more than 20° C. and summers of less than 18° C.

Yang days, clear and sunny, activate the yang; the workshop organs work on these days to "conduct the energy." Yin days, dark, rainy and cold, activate the yin; the treasure organs then work to "activate the blood."[8]

During hot and sunny weather the blood is fluid; the energy is superficial. The blood is easy to disperse, causing the energy to flow. One must not puncture too deeply. On cold, cloudy, wet days, the blood is cooled and contracted; the energy is deep. It is necessary to puncture deeply.[9]

For chronic illnesses, it is recommended to delay treatment until sunny days.[10]

True acupuncture (yin by yang, yang by yin).

In principle this method consists of curing the yang by the yin and the yin by the yang, but given the multitude of variation of the yin-yang expression, it allows for flexibility in application. It is possible to distinguish the following methods:

a) Treatment of the main meridian of the dysfunctional organ, acting in an opposite manner on each of the two channels of the meridian. The channel on the right is yang while that on the left is yin.

b) Treatment of the main meridian of the dysfunctional organ, acting only on one channel of the meridian, on the side opposite the impaired side.

c) Treatment of the feet (yin) by the head (yang), or the head by the feet; the interior by the exterior; and so on.

d) Treatment of the workshop organs (yang) by the treasure organs (yin) and reciprocally.

The great principles which govern true acupuncture are the following:

First, the rule itself:

Those who are skillful with the needles start with the yin in order to conduct the yang, start with the yang to conduct the yin, utilize the right to cure the left, the left to cure the right, the exterior to cure the interior, the interior to cure the exterior.
(DACH I, 13v, citing the Nei Jing)

For illnesses of the yin, treat the yang. For illnesses of the yang, treat the yin. (DACH XI, 11r)

From this rule, one can understand the significance of the oppositions: yang for yin, yin for yang, exterior for interior and vice versa, right for left and the reverse, etc.

What action must be taken on the opposite aspect is not specified. Yin or yang can be disturbed by excess or insufficiency, and the opposite action would not be the same in opposing cases. The only indications collected to date are the following, which direct us to first always tonify the insufficient aspect:

If the yang is gone and one tonifies the yin, or if the yin is gone and one tonifies the yang, this is what is called filling the fullness and emptying the emptiness. One exhausts the insufficiency and makes the fullness abound. If there is death in such a case, it is the doctor who has killed. (DACH I, 14v, citing the Nei Jing)

Acting rashly, either dispersing the energy for an illness of blood or dispersing the blood for an illness of the energy, is called the massacre of the innocent. Who would pardon such a fault? (DACH XIII, 39r)

We must tonify the insufficiency; thus, never disperse the yang for a yin insufficiency illness, nor the yin for a yang insufficiency illness (only the pulses can differentiate the two types). For an excess of yin, tonify the yang, etc.

The goal to reach is a balance between the yin, the physical being, the ''form,'' and the yang energy, the mental life, activity, heat. There is trouble if the body is robust but without activity or heat, or if the body is weak and puny with too much energy.

When form and energy mutually hold together, one lives. If they are not in harmony, there is illness. If they mutually separate, death. (DACH II, 20r)

The following principle, stated previously, dominates all aspects of Chinese medicine.

The superior worker treats what is not yet ill. The mediocre worker only treats what is already ill. Thus, for example, the superior worker will treat the organs not yet affected by a disordered liver. The mediocre worker will only treat the liver. (DACH V, 23v)

The directive for the superior worker demands a thorough knowledge of the succession of organs in the circulation of energy, the dominance of the husband organs over the wives, and all other relationships between yin and yang organs (see Chapter VIII, ''The Interactions of the Organs'').

This principle of treating that which is not yet ill prevents an illness from extending into healthy areas. The treatment harnesses the strength of other related organs to aid the diseased organ, and even if the illness is not yet cured, it is prevented from extending to other organs.

Experiments have shown that dispersing a point on one side of the head tonifies the extremities of the opposite side; likewise, tonifying the same point disperses these extremities. To disperse the left side, tonify the right. To tonify the left, disperse the right.

Acting in an opposing manner on the two channels of the same meridian is as follows: if the right channel is empty, first tonify it, then disperse the left channel; this action will cause the yin excess to pass into the yang insufficiency, since the right side of the body, including its channels, is yang, and the left side, yin. If the left channel is empty, then disperse the right channel; the yang excess will pass into the yin insufficiency. In effect, we tonify the insufficient aspect, calling on the excess energy of the fullness.

Ancient texts detail cases of heat or cold:

When the illness is of heat, then stimulate a yang meridian. Tonify those of the left and disperse those of the right. When the illness is of cold, then stimulate a yin meridian. Tonify that of the right and disperse that of the left. (DACH VI, 6v)

I have confirmed that the double organs are distinguishable through the pulses. With this diagnostic technique, one can then apply the above method in cases where the illness of double organs is opposite in nature. It is rare that double organs function at exactly the same levels; more often, one is either normal or in excess while the other is insufficient. This is particularly true of the kidneys and the lungs. Even the two ventricles of the heart can show functional inequalities, particularly after troubles of the respiratory tract.

For single organs, it seems that the channel of one side acts primarily on the opposite part of the organ. For example, the right channel of the large intestine meridian acts mostly on the rectum and descending colon. The left channel acts mostly on the cecum and ascending colon. For the small intestine, the left channel of the meridian seems to command the duodenum and the right branch of the jejunum and ileum. For the spleen-pancreas meridian, the right channel of the meridian corresponds to the spleen and the left to the pancreas. For the gallbladder and the liver, it has been observed that the left channel is always the more painful of the two.

Action on a single channel of a meridian often gives good results. It is said that the least painful channel of the two is always the healthy one and that action on this one channel is often sufficient.

> *The fuller of the two channels is always the healthy one; it is often sufficient to treat only that.*
> *(DACH I, 9r,* citing the *Nei Jing)*

In practice, being able to distinguish between the double organs, we can now follow two possible treatment strategies: 1) puncture the channel on the same side as the impaired organ; 2) puncture the opposite channel.

When one of the double organs is diseased, one must act on the channel of the same side — the right channel for the right kidney, right lung, right ventricle, right ovary, etc.; the left for the left organs. For external diseases affecting only one side, one must, on the contrary, act on the channel of the opposite side, which is always healthy.

> *Use what is not sick and what is the master; what is sick will respond. First puncture the master, then what is sick. Since the energy already flows in the master, after the puncture it will circulate in all that is sick. For chronic illnesses, such as hemiplegia and serious contractures, one must act in this manner. (DACH II, 21r)*

It is true that this procedure clearly benefits flaccid hemiplegia, weaknesses or insufficiencies of a limb or of one side. There is less benefit when there is contracture or pain. It seems that for weakness, dispersing the opposite, healthy side first sends energy to the sick side. In conditions of excess, such as contractures or pains, puncturing the opposite side does not draw off rapidly or clearly the excess of the sick side.

Although the ancients did not distinguish between one or the other of the double organs, they recommended the above procedure for all energetic disorders and made the important observation reported in the sixteenth century by Yang Jishi: one must differentiate between energetic disorders not accompanied by any changes in the pulse and those which manifest changes of the pulse. The former disorders are not due to functional disturbances of organs, while the latter clearly are. For the latter, he recommends what he calls the "great punctures," which he explains as action on the channel opposite the pain.

Pains, contractures, weaknesses, etc., of one area can only be produced if the vitality of the muscles and nerves of that area have been diminished by disorders of the meridian that traverses it. Thus, for example, the pain of the anterolateral part of the shoulder can only be produced if the large intestine meridian that traverses it has been disturbed, either directly or through a poorly functioning liver. Yang Jishi writes:

> *For the great punctures, which are the punctures of the meridians, if there is pain on the left, the right channel is impaired: use a great puncture. Pain on the left, puncture the right channel; pain on the right, puncture the left channel. (DACH II, 24v)*

Treatment by the opposite extremities consists of treating the head or the hands for problems of the feet and the reverse. The hands are yang relative to the feet, but yin relative to the head; therefore, for problems of the head the hands can be used. This system would logically include action on the opposite meridian, spoken of above. But we will see that it extends to other meridians besides the single impaired one. Treatment by opposite extremities applies uniquely to energetic disturbances causing pain, heat, cold, weakness, contractures, trembling, etc.

> *One must know this: for illnesses of energy, if the evil is above [yang], stimulate below [yin]. If it is below, stimulate above. If it is on the right [yang], stimulate the left [yin]; if it is on the left, stimulate the right.*
> *(DACH XII, 39r)*

Innumerable passages recommend this.[11]

It has been explained above that for conditions that affect the pulse and are related to organ disharmonies, Yang Jishi recommended treating the channel opposite the painful side. However, for pains or weaknesses situated on the course of a meridian that are not reflected at the pulse, Yang Jishi suggests using points of passage on the channel opposite to the painful side.

*When the body is painful without the pulse indicating the malady, then use the "intersecting puncture" (**jiao ci**) on the secondary vessel [point of passage]. For these intersecting punctures: Disease on the left, stimulate the region of the right. Pain on the right, puncture the left. Illness at the head, puncture the feet. The meridians of the three yang go from the head to the feet. That is why it is said: when the head has an illness, one must puncture the points of the feet. (DACH II, 24v)*

The choice of the meridian and point for treatment by this rule of opposition is often difficult, even when using the directive of always tonifying the insufficient aspect.

A first general rule of treatment is given:

For the head [yang] stimulate the three yang meridians of the feet and the hands. For the chest and the abdomen [yin], stimulate the three yin meridians of the hands and feet. (DACH V, 27v)

Experiments have shown that for cerebral congestion, which is a yang illness, excellent results have been obtained by dispersing leg-*sanli* of the stomach (ST-36) and *shenmai* of the urinary bladder (BL-62), both points on yang meridians. For pulmonary congestion and fullnesses of the lung (yin illnesses), amelioration is obtained by dispersing at the wrist *lieque* (LU-7) and *taiyuan* (LU-9), both points on the yin lung meridian.

The following passages of recommendations constitute a second rule completing the first:

*Cold above with heat below — first tonify the urinary bladder meridian at the vertex [**tongtian**, BL-7 or **qucha**, BL-4]. Retain a long time [tonify] and it will finish. The puncture will warm the vertex and the rest will go to the spleen-pancreas. Heat above and cold below: see which pulses are empty and hollow and tonify from among the lower yin meridians [**sanyinjiao**, SP-6 or **fuliu**, KI-7]. The energy will descend. (DACH V, 22r)*

For treatment of facial or cerebral congestion, one can either disperse a yang meridian at the extremities as indicated above, or tonify a point on a lower yin meridian (although *sanyinjiao*, SP-6 and *fuliu*, KI-7 should be used with caution since they may increase the blood pressure). *Dadu* (SP-2) seems to give the best results, above all for heating the legs and feet.

Headaches at the temples and parietal regions, accompanied by neck tension, come from gallbladder and liver disorders. Dispersing the gallbladder at *yangfu* (GB-38) on the leg and tonifying the liver at *ququan* (LR-8) at the knee almost always assures a cure. Here the two general rules are applied together.

In summary, for excess energy and pains of the head, treat at the legs by dispersing the yang and tonifying the yin. For excesses and pains of the feet and hands, in principle, treat at the head, dispersing a yin meridian and tonifying a yang meridian (the latter is less well documented).

The yin-yang comprises a complex relationship within Chinese medicine, a fact exemplified by unilateral headaches. Because headaches are painful, they are yang, but they must be differentiated further. If localized over the right temple and eye, they are from an emptiness of yang; if over the left temple and eye, an emptiness of yin and blood. The emptiness of yang type is soothed at the end of the day with the return of yin; it is thus an excess of yin relative to yang. Conversely, the emptiness of yin type is aggravated at the end of the day when the yin returns; it must therefore be an excess of yang relative to yin. These two types of headaches must not be treated in the same manner.

Treatment of the workshop organs by the treasure organs, and the reverse, is primarily accomplished through the points of passage (see Volume I, Chapter V, "The 15 *Luo*"). This method is most effective for the yin-yang coupled organs (see this volume, Chapter VIII, "Interactions of Organs").

In Paris, it is noted repeatedly that for patients exhibiting sadness and panting after effort with a just perceptible heart pulse, but ample and hard small intestine pulse, tonification of the heart at its point of passage (*tongli*, HT-5) is sufficient treatment. The abounding energy of the small intestine then goes into the heart. The two pulses are balanced and the indicated troubles disappear.

When the liver and gallbladder pulses are clearly discordant, if the gallbladder is enlarged (with nausea in the morning, etc.) and the liver insufficient (stool without color, etc.) it is sufficient to tonify the appropriate point of passage. The two pulses then balance themselves and the condition improves.

For the latter two organs it has been remarked that the season has great significance. In the first six months of the year the best results are obtained by tonifying *guangming* (GB-37), from gallbladder to liver, yang to yin. In the latter six months, the point of passage *ligou* (LR-5), which sends the energy from the liver to the gallbladder, from yin to yang, gives the best effect. In short, at the beginning of the year one must tonify the yang; at the end of the year one must tonify the yin.[12]

The influence of the weather has its importance in all cases where one must move yin into the yang and vice versa. Rapidly tonifying the yang meridians in cloudy and cold weather tonifies the yin. On sunny and hot days, lengthy tonification of the yin tonifies the yang.

> *On a yin day, if one punctures the yang meridians by many manipulations and by six [tonify, but quickly], the yin is tonified. On a yang day, if one punctures the yin meridians by manipulations and by nine [tonify and retain a long time], the yang is tonified. (DACH VI, 26r)*

IV. Acting at the Same Time on Both Yin and Yang

When the whole body is either exhausted or in excess, one must act on both yin and yang. This is used in cases where yin and yang are both too weak or too strong. There is either physical and mental exhaustion, weakness and sadness; or physical and mental hyperexcitability, plethora and redness.

For total physical, mental and emotional exhaustion, it is recommended not to use needles, since the reserves of the patient are not strong enough for immediate mobilization of the energy. Daily moxa is necessary to lift up the tone gradually by regulating the heart and kidney and by tonifying the spleen-pancreas and stomach. For serious cases, one should use medicine.

> *When the pulses are small, one gives medicine. (DACH IV, 8r)*

> *When the [yin] energy of the body is insufficient, so that even the energy of the illness is insufficient, yin and yang are equally insufficient. Do not puncture. (DACH V, 22r)*

> *For what is empty, even all the organs, it is sufficient to regulate the heart and kidneys and to tonify the spleen-pancreas and stomach. Then foods penetrate: sexual energy and awareness, energy and blood are born from themselves. (YXRM V, 7r)*

When physical and emotional exhaustion are obvious, but not extreme, it has been observed that great improvement can be obtained by tonifying the yin and yang at the same time. Use *shaochong* of the heart (HT-9), *zhongchong* of the pericardium (PC-9), *zhongzhu* of the triple warmer (TW-3), and *houxi* of the small intestine (SI-3) or *hegu* of the large intestine (LI-4).

In cases of anemia and depression, the best results are obtained by tonifying *gaohuangshu* of the urinary bladder (BL-38, IS BL-43), leg-*sanli* of the stomach (ST-36), with *qihai* of the conception vessel (CV-6) and *sanyinjiao* of the spleen-pancreas (SP-6).

On the contrary, for cases of general plethora, redness, feeling of internal fullness, agitation, hyperexcitability or tension, good results are obtained by dispersing both yin and yang at the same time: leg-*sanli* of the stomach (ST-36), *sanyinjiao* of the spleen-pancreas (SP-6), *daling* of the pericardium (PC-7), *tianjing* of the triple warmer (TW-10), *shenmen* of the heart (HT-7), and *xiaohai* of the small intestine (SI-8).

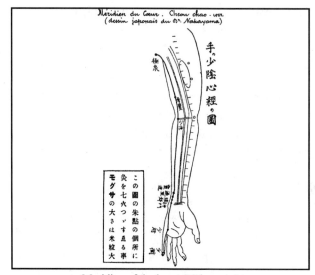

Meridian of the heart (Nakayama)

Notes

[1] *"But if the illness is in the blood, see what has been touched in the blood by the illness and stimulate it."* (DACH XII, 39r) *"If the blood has fullness, disperse it. If the blood is empty, conduct it."* (DACH XI, 11r)

[2] The explanation of the terms "root" and "branches" is as follows:

> *Root (gen) and branches (biao) are of several types. There are those of the meridians, heaven and earth, yin and yang, and the transmission of illnesses. For the human body, the exterior represents the branches; the interior, the root. The yang, the branches; the yin, the root. The yang workshop organs are the branches and the yin treasure organs are the roots. For the meridians there are roots and branches. The root of the urinary bladder meridian is on the foot where the meridian begins; the branches are in the eyes where it ends. For illnesses, what is affected first is the root. What is affected after is the branch. (DACH II, 23r)*

The texts comment on the order of treatment as follows:

> *When the illness comes first and the troubles later, cure the root. And when the troubles come first and the illness later, cure the root. When the cold comes first and generates the illness later, cure the root. And when there is illness first which later generates cold, cure the root. When there is first diarrhea and afterwards other illnesses, cure the root; and when this is calmed, cure the other illnesses. (DACH I, 12v)*

> *First cure the root, then later the branches. (DACH II, 23r)*

This law of starting with the root has some exceptions:

> *If there is internal fullness, for example of urination and defecation, there are no roots or branches; cure the evil itself. When there is first illness and later central fullness, cure the branches. When the illness is manifest through insufficiency of the branches and roots, first cure the branches and then the root. Closely examine what goes together and what goes alone. (DACH)*

[3] There is even a more subtle differentiation of illnesses: "yin of the yang" and "yang of the yin":

> *It is necessary to cure "yin of the yang" illnesses, which are due to cold evil in the internal organs [yin] generating an external fever [yang], by the assent points [yang] of the yin treasure organs. It is necessary to cure "yang of the yin" illnesses, which are from upsetting emotions [yang] causing internal disorders [yin], by the herald points [yin]. (DACH XI, 11v)*

[4] In the *Da Cheng* it states:

> *From the first quarter after midnight the yang is born. From the first quarter after midday the yin is born. The day is yang, the night is yin (DACH VI, 4v).*

> *During the day the energy leads, the blood follows, and the meridians accompany. During the night the blood leads, the energy follows, and the meridians return to their sources (DACH VII, 28r).*

[5] The *Da Cheng* states:

> *That is why when the moon grows, do not disperse, but tonify. When it is full, do not tonify, but disperse. When it is empty, do not treat. Dispersing the yin during a waxing moon increases the emptiness of yin, thus weakens the yin. Tonifying the yin when the moon is full increases the fullness of the yin (the yang becoming yin). To cure when the moon is empty is to disturb the meridians and act wrongly on the yin and yang; health and illness can no longer be distinguished. (DACH II, 19v)*

> *Do not disperse during the waxing moon. Do not tonify during the waning moon. . . . Before the full moon, life increases; after the full moon, death increases. . . . When the moon comes to birth: first day, one puncture; second day, two punctures . . . fifteenth day, fifteen punctures. But at the sixteenth day, fourteen punctures; the seventeenth day, thirteen punctures . . . the last day, two punctures. (DACH, 25v)*

[6] Again, the *Da Cheng*:

> *In spring and summer the yang energy is highest — human energy is also highest. In autumn and winter the yang energy is lowest — human energy is also lowest. (DACH V, 23r)*

[7] The *Da Cheng* states:

> At the first, second, and third moons [yin beginning to decline, yang reborn], the human energy is in the left side. Do not puncture [disperse] the yang of the left foot because the yang has already been reborn in the yin. At the fourth, fifth, and sixth moons [yin at its greatest decline, yang at its apogee], the human energy is in the right side. Do not puncture [disperse] the yang of the right foot because the yang is in full development. At the seventh, eighth, and ninth moons [yin reborn, yang beginning to decline], the human energy is in the right side. Do not puncture the yin of the right leg because the yin begins to be reborn in the yang. At the tenth, eleventh, and twelfth moons [yin going towards its apogee, yang going toward its lowest], the human energy is in the left side; do not puncture the yin of the left foot because the yin has reached its apogee. (DACH I, 11r)

[8] *Da Cheng VII, 30v* states:

> On sunny days, the workshop organs are working and conduct the energy. On cloudy days, treasure organs are working to activate the blood.

[9] The *Da Cheng* states:

> When the weather is mild and the days sunny, the blood is fluid and the **wei** energy is superficial. That is why the blood is easy to disperse, causing the energy to circulate. When the weather is cold and the day dark, the blood is cooled and contracted; the **wei** energy is deep. (DACH II, 19v)

[10] Again, in the *Da Cheng*, it says:

> For slow or chronic illnesses wait for clear and hot weather; the energy is then easy to move. (DACH V, 26r)

[11] The *Da Cheng* states:

> If the head is troubled, stimulate the feet. For the left, stimulate the right; for the right, stimulate the left. For the hands, the feet; and for the feet, the hands. If the two hands are flexed and contracted, then use the two feet to get a response. As soon as you have punctured below, the two hands respond. (DACH V, 27v)

> When the energy abounds at the top, guide it by [acting on] the bottom; [if there is] insufficiency in the upper part, make the energy rise. With cold in the upper part of the body and heat in the lower part, puncture the upper part only [tonify the insufficient aspect]. Great heat above, puncture only below. When the top is hot and the bottom cold, one should act through the bottom [tonify the insufficient aspect]. (DACH VI, 9v)

> Above hot, below cold: it is thus that the yin illness acts on the yang. Start from the yang to guide the yin; decide by the pulses. (DACH, XI, 11r, quoting Li Gao)

[12] The sense of this passage is confused, and was evidently misprinted in the French original. According to the previous paragraphs, tonifying the passage-point *guangming* (GB-37) would tonify the gallbladder, i.e., from yin to yang, not the reverse, as the text states. Likewise, tonifying the passage-point *ligou* (LR-5) would send energy from the gallbladder to the liver, from yang to yin, not the other way. This would then accord with the last sentence of the paragraph: ''At the beginning of the year one must tonify the *yang* [here, the gallbladder]; at the end of the year one must tonify the *yin* [here, the liver].'' — ed.

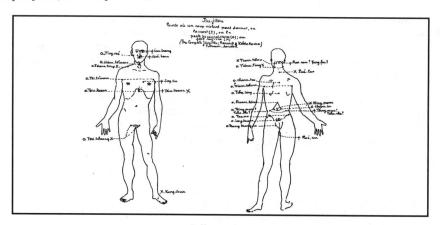

Jujitsu points

Chapter VIII

The Interactions of the Organs

I. Yang Workshop Organs and Yin Treasure Organs — II. Yin-Yang Coupled Organs; Points of Passage — III. The Flow of Energy (Mother-Child Rule) — IV. Midday - Midnight Rule — V. Husband - Wife Rule — VI. Creative and Destructive Cycle of the Five Elements — VII. Diverse Relations of the Organs — VIII. Rule of Liu-zhu, Following and Obstructing — IX. Relations of the Organs with Parts of the Body

From the greatest antiquity, the energetic view of medicine has enabled the Chinese to observe organ interactions not noted in Europe, such as relations between the functioning of the organs and disturbances in certain parts of the body. These observations have been of great significance for treatment with acupuncture. Pasteurian or homeopathic treatments have also given interesting results when using these principles.

The principles are the following: differentiation of the internal organs into two groups — yang workshop organs and yin treasure organs; the link between a yin and yang organ; the rule of mother and child by the flow of energy; the rule of midday-midnight; the rule of husband-wife; the diverse relations between organs; and finally, the action of the organs on the sensitivity or immunity of the region crossed by their meridians.

I. Yang Workshop Organs and Yin Treasure Organs

From the energetic point of view, the internal organs have been observed since antiquity as being either yang or yin and have thus been classified into two groups, termed ''workshop organs'' and ''treasure organs.''

The workshop organs, yang (fu).

The Chinese name, pronounced *''fu,''* is formed by the elements ''flesh'' and ''man working under a roof.'' It is thus named because the workshop organs transform the materials they receive from outside the body into energy and blood. Since they are in relation with the exterior and produce the energy, they are yang.

The stomach, small intestine, and large intestine are workshop organs which transform food into energy and blood. The gallbladder and urinary bladder, also workshop organs, are considered in Europe primarily as containers; the Chinese, however, see them as important initiators and regulators of their associated yin organs. The gallbladder regulates many of the functions of the liver, particularly the biliary function. It also has a frequently observed connection with pain, emotions and courage. The urinary bladder regulates the kidneys, which, in turn, have an effect on the sexual life. The triple warmer is also considered a workshop organ. Although it is not a material organ, it acts energetically on the respiratory, digestive and genitourinary functions as well as on all the yang energies.

These organs are all reflected at the yang superficial radial pulses. They have an obvious relation with the temperament: the superficial pulses and workshop organs are tense in cases of hyperexcitation or nervous tension, and flaccid and without action in cases of depression. These organs are active mostly in the daytime and in good weather.

> *On yang days, the workshop organs are at work to conduct the energy. (DACH VII, 30v)*

If they function in excess the patient will search for coldness and the company of others:

> *If the patient looks for coldness and wants to see people, the illness is in the workshop organs; these organs are yang, and patients with yang in excess search for coldness and want to see people (for using their excess yang). (DACH I, 16r)*

The description of these organs is given thus:

> *The six workshop organs: **Fu,** ''workshop organ'' (formed of flesh-workshop) comes from **fu** ''workshop.'' They transmit the impure energy (from the exterior) to the treasure organs. That is why they are also called the ''store of transformation and transmission.'' They empty themselves without accumulating. That is why they can be **shi** (have an excess of energy) without being **man** (materially full). When, for example, liquid and food have entered the mouth, the stomach is full **(man)** while the intestines are still empty. After the food has descended, the intestines are full and the stomach is emptied. This is why one must not confuse fullness of energy with material fullness. (DACH VIII, 1v)*

The treasure organs, yin (zang).

The treasure organs preside over the purification and the circulation of blood. The Chinese word, pronounced "*zang,*" is formed of the elements "flesh" and "treasure."

> *The treasure organs: **zang** comes from **zang** "treasure" (same sound without the "flesh" radical). The heart stores the evolved consciousness **(shen)**. The liver stores the subconscious, the conscious "parrot" memories, and unconscious "automaton" (the intelligence of the cells, the primitive, animal instincts: **po**). The spleen-pancreas stores the ideation **(yi)** and knowledge **(zhi)**. The kidneys store decision **(zhi)** [and the sexual energy, **jing**]. (YXRM I, 11v) That is why one calls them treasure organs. Together they store sexual energy. (DACH VIII, 1v)*

In the very ancient texts, only five treasure organs are mentioned; from the first century, however, there are six mentioned with the addition of the heart governor. This treasure organ is not a material organ but one that acts functionally on all the yin energy, particularly on the circulation and blood pressure.

In the following, their role is described in a very general manner:

> *Among these organs there are two which relate the interior with the exterior; these are the lungs and heart. Others are exclusively internal; these are the kidneys and liver. (DACH VIII, 1v)*

They are called yin in nature because they control the internal life (yin) and the blood (yin). However, the heart and lungs are called "yang in the yin" because they make the energy circulate (heart: the blood; lungs: the energy drawn from the air) (see *YXRM* I, 10r).

On the radial pulses they are all represented at the middle and deep levels (yin). Their activity is dominant at night and on cold and dark days (yin):

> *On yin days the treasure organs are at work and activate the blood. (DACH VII, 30v)*

> *If the patient looks for warmth and does not want to see people, wants to close his door and live alone, the illness is in the treasure organs [from an excess of yin]. These organs are yin in effect. The yin patients look for warmth [yang] and want solitude [where the yang is remade]. (DACH I, 16r)*

The troubles of yin are also recognized by unproductive heat in the head with cold feet.

> *When the six yin hold evil, one arrives at a point where the top is hot and the bottom is cold. (DACH IX, 13v)*

Thousands of observations have allowed us to notice what is useful and what is harmful to each of the treasure organs, as well as the planet that governs them and the element to which they respond. The relation of the element with the organs is described later on.

The table of what benefits and harms the five organs is as follows (see *YIX* I, 13r):

	Liver	Heart	Spleen-Pancreas	Lungs	Kidneys
Harmful season (1)	Spring	Summer	Late Summer	Autumn	Winter
Harmful climate	Wind	Heat	Humidity	Dryness	Cold
Harmful emotion	Discontent	Joy	Obsession	Worry	Fear
Harmful flavor	Sour	Bitter	Sweet	Pungent	Salty
Beneficial cereal	Wheat	Millet	Rye	Rice	Beans
Beneficial meat	Chicken	Mutton	Beef	Horse	Pig (sow)
Emitted odor	Rancid	Scorched	Perfumed	Fleshy	Putrid
Beneficial color	Azure blue	Red	Yellow	White	Black
Emitted fluid	Tears	Sweat	Saliva	Sobs (2)	Spittle (3)
Sense commanded	Sight	Speech	Taste	Smell	Hearing
Number	Eight	Seven	Five	Nine	Six
Nourishes	Muscles	Vessels	Flesh	Skin	Bones
Flourishes in	Nails	Complexion	Lips	Body hair	Hair
Harmful direction	East	South	Center	West	North
Dominant element	Wood	Fire	Earth	Metal	Water
Dominant planet	Jupiter	Mars	Saturn	Venus	Mercury
Linked yang organ	Gallbladder	Small intestine	Stomach	Large intestine	Bladder

These observations, while valuable for the northern hemisphere, have not been verified for the southern hemisphere.

The knowledge of the seasonal illnesses of the organs suggests some remarks:

1) At the spring equinox — maximum troubles of the skin, migraines, asthma, and constipation, which depend on the liver and gallbladder. At the summer solstice — maximum congestion, hypertension and insanity, which depend on the heart and the vessels. At the autumn equinox — a second bad period for the liver (always linked to the spleen-pancreas). In autumn — trouble of the respiratory passages. At the winter solstice — troubles of the kidneys and urinary bladder.

2) Phlegm?

3) Evidently urine.

II. Yin-Yang Coupled Organs; Points of Passage

The name given in Chinese to these yin-yang coupled organs is "linked and direct meridians," *jiao zheng mo.* A constant relationship has been observed between the internal organs, where a yin treasure organ is always coupled to a yang workshop organ, each one having an important action on the other. There are few passages; the clearest one is given below:

Thus, in the case of an illness of the heart, be sure to stimulate the small intestine meridian at the same time. Such is the rule of linked and direct meridians. (DACH II, 24v)

The interacting couples are as follows: heart and small intestine; liver and gallbladder; kidneys and urinary bladder; lungs and large intestine; spleen-pancreas and stomach; pericardium and triple warmer.

It is true that the relationship between the heart and small intestine, which has not been noted in Europe, is constantly commented on in acupuncture. Action on the small intestine is immediately noticed on the heart.

I should mention that these coupled meridians follow one another in the flow of energy. Sometimes the yin meridian is first, the mother; and sometimes the yang meridian precedes the yin. This observation, made in ancient times, led to another discovery. Besides the channel, which allows the current of energy to overflow from one meridian to another, there is another branch, not located at the extremity of the meridians, that causes the coupled meridians to communicate between themselves: it is the *luo* (see Volume I), which we translate here as "secondary vessel" for want of a better term. *Luo* is also the name given to the veins.

Hence, each of the secondary vessels is commanded by one of the points of the meridian. In Chinese, these points are also termed *luo.* We call them "passage points" for greater clarity. The list is as follows:

Heart to small intestine	*tongli*	(HT-5)
Small intestine to heart	*zhizheng*	(SI-7)
Lungs to large intestine	*lieque*	(LU-7)
Large intestine to lungs	*pianli*	(LI-6)
Liver to gallbladder	*ligou*	(LR-5)
Gallbladder to liver	*guangming*	(GB-37)
Spleen-pancreas to stomach	*gongsun*	(SP-4)
Stomach to spleen-pancreas	*fenglong*	(ST-40)
Kidneys to urinary bladder	*dazhong*	(KI-6, IS KI-4)
Urinary bladder to kidneys	*feiyang*	(BL-58)
Heart governor to triple warmer	*neiguan*	(PC-6)
Triple warmer to heart governor	*waiguan*	(TW-5)

A fifteenth *luo* is indicated in the texts: it is called "the great *luo* of the spleen-pancreas." The point of passage is *dabai* (SP-21). It may reunite all the other secondary vessels, but its role has not yet been fully clarified. Tonifying this point appears to tonify all the yin meridians, the internal body, the left side, the lower body; tonifying it also acts to disperse the yang meridians, the right side, the upper body and the skin.

For the other *luo,* experiments carried out in Paris have resulted in the observation of a very useful fact: when, for example, the pulse of the heart is weak (indicated by labored breathing with little exertion, or emotional depression) and the pulse of the small intestine hard and ample, it is sufficient to tonify the passage points of the heart to the small intestine (*tongli,* HT-5). The pulse of the small intestine then loses its amplitude and hardness to the benefit of the heart, the symptoms of which decrease proportionately. A similar result is obtained by dispersing the passage point of the small intestine (*zhizheng,* SI-7). These mutual reactions of the coupled organs are of great utility, as they allow equilibrium between yin and yang.

In principle, it is better to tonify the passage point of the insufficient organ; then, if the result is not satisfactory, to disperse the passage point of the excess organ.

III. The Flow of Energy (Mother-Child Rule)

A discussion of the circulation of energy gives occasion to make two remarks which experiments in Paris have allowed us to verify:

1)   It is easiest to disperse a meridian during the two hours of maximum energy of that meridian. All dispersing action is more active than at any other moment. When the action of the waning moon is added to that of the descending sun, the effect is augmented.

   During the two hours which follow the maximum of each meridian, it is easier to tonify and the tonifying action is stronger, particularly if it coincides with the waxing moon and the rising sun (see *DACH* VIII, 18v).

2)   Each meridian receives the energy from the meridian preceding it in the circulation of energy. The preceding meridian is called "the mother." Each meridian transmits its energy to the meridian following it, which is called "the child." This is the mother-child rule.

Let us recall that the flow of energy is as follows:

From 1 to 3 a.m.	liver
From 3 to 5 a.m.	lungs
From 5 to 7 a.m.	large intestine
From 7 to 9 a.m.	stomach
From 9 to 11 a.m.	spleen-pancreas
From 11 a.m. to 1 p.m.	heart
From 1 p.m. to 3 p.m.	small intestine
From 3 to 5 p.m.	urinary bladder
From 5 to 7 p.m.	kidney
From 7 to 9 p.m.	heart governor
From 9 to 11 p.m.	triple warmer
From 11 p.m. to 1 a.m.	gallbladder

The text that recommends the utilization of this yin-yang alternation is difficult to comprehend unless its point of reference is understood.

> *When the organs generate themselves and mutually unite, they are open. Stimulate them at that time. When they destroy themselves, they are closed. Do not stimulate them at that time. When the yang grows, the yin begins to die. As one gives me birth, I grow, I communicate, I unite myself. During this time, energy (yang) and blood (yin) generate and prosper, and we can easily differentiate fullness and emptiness. Stimulate then. As one destroys me, I diminish; that is the time when the points are closed. Energy (yang) or blood (yin) are full of weakness and decline. Either the energy that flows has not arrived, or it has already gone. If one punctures wrongly at that time, one introduces perverse energy; one injures the healthy energy; one fills the fullness and empties the emptiness. The damage is not small. (DACH VII, 30v)*

In fact, even if one does observe a stronger pulse at an organ's maximal time, it is questionable whether there is any significant difference between the results of action taken within or outside the recommended hours. Moreover, in practice, it is difficult for the doctor or the patient to consider this rule.

The mother-child rule can be understood in several ways. However, the idea is always the same: the organ that gives the energy is called the mother and the one that receives the energy is the child.

> *That which gives me life is my mother. That to which I give life is my child. (YIX II, 1v)*

The rule governing these connections is that of the mother and child *(mu-zi fa)*. It is formulated thus:

To say that the child gives energy to the mother is to say that the child, which has excess, does not nourish itself at the expense of its mother. One must disperse the child and take energy away from it in order again to cause it to nourish itself from its mother. To say that the mother can give emptiness to the child is to say that the mother, having some insufficiency, cannot give milk to the child. One must tonify the mother; but one must also add to the energy of the child so that it does not nourish itself too much at the expense of its mother. (DACH V, 23v)

If a meridian is empty, tonify its mother; if it is full, disperse the child. (YIX II, 1v)

Among the different interpretations of this rule, let us cite:

a) The Circulation of Energy.

The energy, flowing ceaselessly in the closed circuit of the meridians, passes from one meridian and thus from one organ into the other in the following order: lung, large intestine, stomach, spleen, heart, small intestine, urinary bladder, kidney, heart governor, triple warmer, gallbladder, liver, lung, etc.

For example, to tonify the heart properly, one must tonify the mother, the spleen-pancreas. In addition it must be noted that the child, the small intestine, must not be over-nourished at the expense of the mother, the heart.

b) The Points of the Same Meridian.

The *Da Cheng* (III, 31v) explains the application through the five elements. Each point is governed by one element that generates or destroys another.

*For emptiness, tonify the mother upstream. For fullness, disperse the child downstream. This is the secret of following and opposing. So for the heart meridian (yin, centrifugal), puncture the **shu** point (shenmen, HT-7); this disperses the child. Puncture the **jing** point (shaochong, HT-9); this tonifies the mother. (YXRM I, 43v; see also DACH II, 20v)*

When empty, tonify the mother, which is insufficient. If full, disperse her child, which has an excess. First tonify, then afterwards disperse. (DACH VI, 4v)

IV. The Midnight-Midday Rule *(Zi-Wu)*

The name of this rule in Chinese, *zi-wu,* is based on the naming of the twelve divisions of the day *(shi),* adopted in 104 B.C. and still used in our time. *Zi* represents the two hours around midnight (11 p.m. to 1 a.m.) and *wu* designates those around midday (11 a.m. to 1 p.m.). This rule must be even more ancient since it is mentioned in texts which use the older system of dividing the day into ten hours, abandoned in 104 B.C. It is attributed to Bian Que of the fifth century B.C., the epoch called Jia-Yi.

Since this rule is based on the yin-yang opposition, let us first review the following:

1) ''The yang is born at midnight and declines from noon. The yin is born at noon and declines from midnight.'' *(DACH VII, 28r)*

2) The yin meridians are more active during the yin period; the yang meridians during the yang period.

3) Each meridian has a two-hour period of maximum activity.

4) A yin meridian having its maximum between midnight and noon relates to the yang meridian having its maximum between noon and midnight at the same hour. For example, the liver (yin), which has its maximum from 1 to 3 a.m., corresponds to the small intestine (yang), which has its maximum between 1 and 3 p.m. Action on the liver (yin) at 2 p.m. (yang) also acts on the small intestine (yang), while action on the small intestine (yang) at 2 a.m. (yin) also acts on the liver (yin).

5) A moderate action on the yin in a yin period acts on the yin, but if the action is strong, it also acts on the yang.

In summary, the midday-midnight rule can be specified as follows: all action on the yin meridian in a yin period, if it is moderate, acts on the injured meridian; but if the action is strong, it acts on the corresponding yang meridian. This holds true for the injured yang meridian in a yang period; if the stimulation is strong, it also acts on the corresponding yin meridian.

*On yang days, at yang hours, the yang meridians. On yin days, at yin hours, the yin meridians. The yang open makes the yin closed. The yin open makes the yang closed. For what is closed, based on the **tian gan** (division into ten hours), puncture the associated meridians. On the yang days, during the yin hours, the meridian being closed, stimulate its associate. For example, at the hour of **jia** (midnight) the gallbladder is the master, the other meridian is the guest. First puncture the master, then the guest. When the meridian is not open, puncture the associate.[1] (DACH VII, 30v)*

Some illnesses respond particularly well to this rule:

*For all illnesses which are only on one side, when the exterior and interior respond to one another, use the rule of midnight-midday (**zi-wu**). Tonify or disperse the left or the right. (DACH VI, 10v)*

The table of midday-midnight relations of the internal organs is as follows:

From 11 p.m. to 1 a.m.	gallbladder	From 11 a.m. to 1 p.m.	heart
From 1 a.m. to 3 a.m.	liver	From 1 p.m. to 3 p.m.	small intestine
From 3 a.m. to 5 a.m.	lungs	From 3 p.m. to 5 p.m.	urinary bladder
From 5 a.m. to 7 a.m.	large intestine	From 5 p.m. to 7 p.m.	kidney
From 7 a.m. to 9 a.m.	stomach	From 7 p.m. to 9 p.m.	heart governor
From 9 a.m. to 11 a.m.	spleen-pancreas	From 9 p.m. to 11 p.m.	triple warmer

V. The Husband-Wife Rule

The rule of husband and wife represents another order of organ interrelations that can be profitably studied.

Each organ reflected on the left wrist (husband) dominates the corresponding organ reflected on the right wrist (wife); that is to say, the "husband" organ gives its counterpart life and is particularly essential to its proper functioning. Conversely, each organ reflected on the right wrist (wife) endangers its correspondent on the left wrist (husband); that is, the "wife" organ places its counterpart under the burden of performing abnormal efforts, surpassing its force at the risk of producing a lesion in that "husband" organ. The husband must be robust and the wife supple. Sick husband: soften the wife. Sick wife: tonify the husband.

Thus, at the left wrist, the heart (husband) is essential to the functioning of the lungs (wife), and nourishes them; there is panting if the heart is weak. On the right wrist, the lungs (wife) of the right wrist endanger the heart (husband), e.g., prolonged asthma causes deformations in the left ventricle and cardiac ailments.[2]

The table of the husband-wife rule is given below:

Left Wrist Husband (blood, yin)	Right Wrist Wife (energy, yang)
small intestine	large intestine
heart	lungs
gallbladder	stomach
liver	spleen-pancreas
urinary bladder	triple warmer
kidneys	heart governor, genitals

The following is an example of this rule:

The liver conquers the spleen-pancreas. If the liver is ill, it will give the illness to the spleen-pancreas. In this case, the sage who cures what is not yet ill gives fullness of energy to the spleen-pancreas so that it does not receive the illness of the liver. (DACH III, 31v)

In practice, the same advice is given for illness of an organ reflected on the right wrist (wife): tonify the husband.

The famous Yang has even written:

Weak husband, robust wife; then there is destruction. Robust husband, weak wife, then there is security. (DACH III, 32v)

VI. Creative and Destructive Cycle of the Five Elements

The five elements and their interaction, as well as the interactions of treasure organs dominated by each of the five elements, are discussed frequently in both ancient and modern texts. The action of an element and its organ on another can either be beneficial or destructive. For that which is beneficial, the image used is "mother, generates."

The creative cycle is as follows:

Wood (liver) → Fire (heart) → Earth (spleen) → Metal (lung) → Water (kidney) → Wood (liver), and the cycle recommences.

The destructive cycle is as follows:

Water (kidneys) → Fire (heart) → Metal (lung) → Wood (liver) → Earth (spleen) → Water (kidney), and the cycle recommences.

Note that the creative cycle is precisely the order of succession of the deep (or middle) radial pulses in descending order from proximal to distal:

On the left: kidney → liver → heart.

On the right: (heart governor) heart → spleen-pancreas → lung.

In practice, for example, if the heart is weak, one must tonify its mother: the liver. If it is over-excited or painful, one must disperse its child: the spleen-pancreas (which in the daily flow of energy precedes the heart).

> *Thus, when the illness of the heart (fire) is emptiness, tonify the liver (wood) . . . Wood can generate fire . . . If there is fullness of the heart (fire) disperse the spleen-pancreas (earth) . . . Fire can generate earth.*
> *(DACH II, 20v)*
>
> *If the illness of the liver is fullness, then disperse the heart, which is the child. If the illness of the liver is emptiness, tonify the kidneys, which are the mother. Then, the meridian of the liver will be able to function by itself. This follows for all the five treasure organs. (DACH III, 31v)*

On the opposite side, in the destructive cycle (see *DACH V, 26r*), heart (fire) insufficiency or excess endangers the lungs (metal), which must be supported immediately to prevent lung ailments. In turn, ailing lungs endanger the liver, and so forth.

The destructive cycle corresponds exactly to the husband-wife rule; that is, the organs represented on the left wrist endanger the organs represented on the right wrist. The order of the destructive cycle is seen when moving in a zigzag fashion from distal to proximal on the wrist. The table is as follows:

Endangers:	
Left:	**Right:**
heart	lungs
liver	spleen-pancreas
kidneys	(heart governor) heart

VII. Various Organ Relations

Lastly, it has been observed that there are other relations among the organs which do not correspond to any of the rules elucidated above. Many relate to observations made in Europe; others can be related to the midnight-midday rule, etc.

The *Da Cheng* (II, 18v) gives the following table:

Heart*	if disordered (anxiety), tonify the gallbladder.
Gallbladder*	if disordered (derangement or depression), tonify the heart.
Liver**	to facilitate its function, disperse the large intestine.
Large Intestine**	if disordered, tonify the liver.
Spleen-pancreas**	if disordered, disperse the small intestine.
Small intestine**	if disordered, disperse the spleen-pancreas.
Lungs*	if disordered, purify (disperse) the urinary bladder.
Urinary Bladder*	if disordered, clarify the sexual energy, tonify the lungs.

Kidneys*	if disordered, harmonize (tonify) the large intestine.
Large Intestine*	if disordered, tonify the kidneys.
Heart Governor*	if disordered, tonify the stomach.
Stomach*	if there is emptiness, strongly tonify the heart governor.

Here it is the midnight-midday rule. For example, the heart is at its maximum at midday, the gallbladder at midnight. They act on one another.

**The relations between the liver and large intestine, and the small intestine and pancreas are recognized in Europe. This is not true of the other organs, which all relate to the midnight-midday rule.*

VIII. Rule of *Liu-zhu:* ''Flowing and Obstructing''

When the illness is in the three yin and the three yang [that is, the twelve meridians], use the rule ''cause to flow or obstruct''; tonify or disperse the blood. (DACH VI, 10v)

*To cause to flow (**liu**) is to go (**wang**). To obstruct (**zhu**) is to stop. The hours (**tian-gan**) are ten; the meridians are twelve. **Jia,** gallbladder; **yi,** liver; **bing,** small intestine; **ding,** heart; **wu,** stomach; **ji,** spleen; **geng,** large intestine; **xin,** lungs; **ren,** urinary bladder, **gui,** kidneys. There are still the triple warmer and the heart governor. But the triple warmer is the father of energy and of yang. The heart governor is the mother of blood and yin. These two meridians, although in principle added on as the last two, in reality flow with the ten others. (DACH VIII, 30r)*

According to this rule, the organs are ordered in terms of the coupled meridians, section by section at the pulses.

This rule of *liu-zhu,* which must be very old since it rests on the division of the day into ten hours, revived by Huang-Fu Mi (215-285) in his *Jia-Yi Jing.*

IX. Relations of the Organs with the Parts of the Body

Since great antiquity, medical scholars noted the relationships existing between disorders in particular parts of the body and specific meridians. The *Ling Shu* advises that with disturbances of a certain region, one should first be concerned with the meridian that commands it; determine the problem, whether there is excess or insufficiency in the meridian; and choose points on this meridian relating only to that problem.

For a particular illness, stimulate its related meridian without first being overly concerned with the points. For those who want to stimulate according to the meridian, the rule is as follows:

For illnesses of the upper part of the body — stimulate above all the large intestine meridian.

For illnesses of the central part — the meridian of the spleen-pancreas.

For illnesses of the lower part — the liver meridian.

For illnesses of the front, the chest — the stomach meridian.

For illnesses of the back — the urinary bladder meridian.

Then, according to the illness of the meridian, stimulate a particular point on the meridian.

Such is the most important secret doctrine. (Ling Shu)

Notes

[1] The name of the hour is given here by the older division of the day into ten hours (see Volume I).

[2] The left (East when looking South) is the place of honor. The apartments of the master are to the East. The husband is often poetically called ''The Easterner'' *(dong jia).*

Chapter IX
Various Actions of the Meridians

I. Lungs — II. Large Intestine — III. Stomach — IV. Spleen-Pancreas — V. Heart — VI. Small Intestine — VII. Urinary Bladder — VIII. Kidneys — IX. Heart Governor — X. Triple Warmer — XI. Gallbladder — XII. Liver — XIII. The Two Median Lines: 1. Conception Vessel 2. Governor Vessel

The human being forms a totality with mutual reactions of all parts on one another. Thus, the action of each meridian is not restricted to the single organ it represents. Moreover, as each organ has an action on one or many other organs, it is difficult to know if one meridian acts directly on an organ other than its own, or if it acts indirectly through the intermediary of its own organ. In practice, it is sufficient to know that by stimulating a certain meridian it is possible to modify the functioning of many organs.

All points on the same meridian do not have the same effect either on the represented organ or on other organs. Each point responds to a group of disorders, all of which some patients will have, and only a small number of which other patients will have.

In ancient times, the study of the actions of the meridian on the external body led to an interesting physiological discovery: the pains and problems on a particular meridian are always preceded and accompanied by dysfunction of the organ represented by this meridian. It is recognized in China that pain and disturbances occur only after the region through which the meridian of the represented organ passes has been sensitized by prolonged distress. A long-term illness of the large and small intestine leads to pain in the front and back of the shoulders; illness of the kidney and urinary bladder results in lumbago and sciatica.

For each meridian we have indicated those actions which are cited within the Chinese and Japanese texts, as well as others discovered in our own research.

I. Lungs (Respiratory passages): *Fei Jing, Shou Taiyin*

This meridian responds to the tonsils, the larynx, the trachea, and bronchi, as well as to the lungs themselves.

The functions of the respiratory organs are more numerous than is yet realized in the West. The most important is the assimilation of the energy of the air, which does not only mean the absorption of oxygen and the release of carbon dioxide, but also the development of a personal vital energy comparable to the acquisition of energy from the digestion of food.

The lungs [and the heart through the blood] link the interior with the exterior. (YXRM I, 14v)

The skin depends on the lungs (as well as on the spleen-pancreas); poor respiration leads to a bad complexion, and uneven or dull skin.

The body hair (and hair on the head) is connected to the lungs: too much in cases of inflammation, too little in cases of insufficiency.

The lungs are the "home" of the *po* (unconscious, primitive instincts; see Part V, Chapter VI; also *DACH* VIII, 1v).

They are the root of energy (along with the stomach) . . . the minister of the great chief. (DACH VIII, 2r)

The lungs are the flowered cover of the five treasure organs. It is through the lungs that sound can come out and that the skin is smooth and supple. Injury by the seven feelings or at the exterior by the six climates is enough to cause irregularity of inhalation and exhalation, entry and exit. The meridian of the lungs, then, is no longer pure. To purify it, one must harmonize the respiration, then the troubles cease and the fire of the heart is calmed. In this way, one calms the heart, extends the body, and calms the energy of thought. (DACH 3r)

The lungs command the skin; they flourish in the body hair and hair of the head. (DACH 2r)

Full: the pulse is full. The top of the body is hot, respiration is heavy and presses on the nose. Disperse through pungency. Empty: the pulse is empty. The breath is insufficient for respiration, which is weak and low. Tonify through acidity and warmth. Respiration and the ability to make sound depend on them. Worries injure the lungs. Oranges and sugar make the mucus descend and are the recipe of the spirits. Ginger, which disperses nervous cough, is the medicine of the sage. (DACH 2v)

The lungs are particularly active during the yin (dark) days and during the night when they work and activate the blood. (DACH VII, 30v)

They are tonified and congested by violent perfumes, strong drugs, nutmeg, and ginseng. (DACH VIII, 2v)

Their pains are . . . cramps and pains of the arm. In excess — accumulation in the lungs, contractions of the ribs, and even spitting blood. (DACH IX, 13r)

Worry injures the lungs. Warmth and pungency injure the skin and body hair. (DACH VIII, 2v)

The connections with other organs are given below:

Large Intestine — follows the lungs in the circulation of energy and is the yang coupled workshop organ.

Liver — precedes the lungs in the circulation of energy.

Urinary Bladder —

Disordered lungs: purify the urinary bladder; disordered urinary bladder: clarify the sexual energy of the lungs. (YXRM I, 18v)

Heart — the husband which dominates the lungs, but which is put in danger by them.

Kidneys —

The root is in the kidneys, the branches are in the lungs. (DACH I, 6v)

II. Large Intestine: *Da Chang Jing, Shou Yangming*

Experiments in Paris have confirmed certain functions of the large intestine that are unrecognized by Western physiology: neuralgic pains, particularly of the shoulder and upper limbs and of the anterior shoulder and the edge of the radius, are always connected with a diseased condition of the large intestine, very often related to parasites or inflammation. Furthermore, the diseased state of the large intestine itself is often related to poor functioning of the gallbladder.

The general energy is linked with healthy functioning of the large intestine. (Diarrhea can result from sudden emotions, and lack of courage is often found in people with diarrhea and dysentery.) The point that commands the energy of the whole body is the source *(yuan)* point of the large intestine, *hegu* (LI-4).

It is possible to differentiate the following types of constipation: **1)** Constipation from atony with a completely flaccid intestine due to lack of contractures. This is generally accompanied by nonresistance to parasites. Tonify through *quchi,* LI-11. **2)** Spasmodic constipation with an intestine that is constantly hard or with colic and pains. Disperse through *sanjian,* LI-3. **3)** The absence of secretions or dry stools in balls. Disperse at *hegu* LI-4, *sanjian* LI-3, or *erjian,* LI-2. **4)** Inflammation (big and flaccid pulse).

The large intestine is the minister of transmissions and roads. (DACH VIII, 4v)

The connections with the other organs are as follows:

Respiratory passages (yin) — the large intestine is the coupled workshop organ (yang). Inflammation of the rhino-pharynx is always linked to the state of the large intestine; use *hegu* (LI-4).

Liver —

Dispersing the large intestine helps to cure a liver malady. When the large intestine is disordered, equalize the liver. (YXRM I, 18v)

Small Intestine — When it is disordered, tonify the large intestine.

Stomach — It follows the large intestine in the circulation of energy. Empty the large intestine, tonify the stomach. Large intestine excess: disperse the stomach.

The large intestine is dispersed by pungency, by tepidness. It is tonified by acidity and freshness. Troubles from cold produce songs in the intestines, diarrhea and pains. Troubles from warmth produce fullness of the intestines without pains. (DACH VIII, 5r)

III. Stomach: *Wei Jing, Zu Yangming*

Chinese physiology considers that the digestive action of the stomach, even while being sound, may produce two extremes: mostly flesh and fat as in fat people who eat little, or mostly energy without flesh as with thin people who eat a lot.

The Chinese differentiate between excess and insufficiency of energy, which is manifested either by insufficient or excessive secretion, pains and burning sensation, or by swelling, cramps or atony.

The stomach meridian commands the energy of fermentation and the heat of liquids and foods. The triple warmer utilizes it while traversing the twelve meridians. Thus, the triple warmer is the workshop organ that impels the energy and blood to act. (YXRM I, 18v)

However, energy and blood have their root in the energy of the stomach:

*The conception vessel, the governor vessel and the **chong mai** originate at qichong (ST-30), which is the source of the stomach, demonstrating that the stomach is the source of all. (YXRM I, 9r)*

Digestion has the principal role of extracting from food the energy that is assimilated into human energy; it also extracts that which becomes blood and the body. But the latter live only through the energy.

When the energy of the stomach is equal and harmonious, the five treasure organs are peaceful and firm. If there is fullness, then the pulse is full; the lips and mouth are dry. Under the armpit there is pain and swelling; the face is full and hot. One must disperse the stomach. If there is emptiness, the pulse is empty; the belly is painful; there are sounds in the intestines; the face and eyes are empty and superficial. One must tonify the stomach and also encourage joy, activity and warmth. (DACH VIII, 7r)

The stomach is the minister of the granary. The five flavors come from it. (DACH, 7r)

The stomach has a close connection with the other organs.

All organs —

The stomach meridian is the sea of the five treasure organs and six workshop organs. (DACH I, 12v)

Spleen-Pancreas — the coupled treasure organ (yin) that follows the stomach in the circulation of energy. If the one is empty, it can be improved by tonifying the other.

Heart Governor (and Gate of Destiny) —

The stomach and the Gate of Destiny have a connection. When there is emptiness of the stomach, it is advisable to strongly tonify the heart governor. By tonifying the stomach one improves the heart governor. (YXRM I, 1v)

Gallbladder — the stomach is the wife; it is dominated by the gallbladder but can endanger it.

*The stomach meridian is the sea of the five treasure organs and the six workshop organs. If the pulse is big **(da)**, there is a lot of blood, the energy abounds; robustness and heat results. (DACH I, 12v)*

IV. Spleen-pancreas: *Pi Jing, Zu Taiyin*

Today, the name of the organ corresponding to the meridian indicates only the spleen *(pi)*. However, the pancreas also responds to this meridian and to no other. In ancient texts, an ointment made from the fat of pork pancreas is mentioned as a facial protection against cracks. Today this is still made under the name *"pi sao"* (the name given to European soap). The functions attributed to the spleen *(pi)* are in great part those of the pancreas. Was the pancreas, which is sometimes joined to the spleen in Europeans, normally so in the ancient Chinese? (From the sixteenth century onward the pancreas has been called *"cui."*) In any case, we must translate *pi* as spleen-pancreas, and leave to the physiologists the task of defining what applies to one or the other of the observed functions.

We have discovered that the branch of the left meridian acts on the functions known in the West as being pancreatic — digestion of starches and flour, of sugar, etc. The meridian of the right corresponds to the European spleen — action on the purity of the blood, hence influence on intellectual work.

The *Nei Jing* comments:

> The spleen-pancreas harmonizes and transforms the blood in order to give it to the other organs.
> *(DACH VIII, 11v)*

> It is the home of the blood. *(DACH 12v)*

This action on the blood is the primary one that we recognize as being from the spleen itself. Its digestive action is recognized and attributed by us to the pancreas.

The *Ci Yuan* encyclopedia (*"Pi"* article) states:

> Ancient medical scholars maintained that the spleen helped the stomach in the digestion of food.

In addition to and depending on this digestive action is the influence of the spleen-pancreas on the skin and flesh, a function not known in Europe. If the function of the spleen-pancreas is full, the flesh and skin are supple, smooth, and alive. If insufficient, the skin is dry, and the flesh badly nourished.

> The spleen-pancreas flourishes in the lips and commands the flesh. *(DACH VIII)*

> When the right "barrier" pulse (superficial: stomach; middle: pancreas; deep: spleen) is full, then food and drink are digested. The skin and the flesh are shining and smooth. When the pulse is empty, then the body thins out; the four limbs do not rise. The navel protrudes; the limbs are superficial. It is difficult to live. With the lips blue-black, it is easy to die. *(DACH 12r)*

> When one can trust that it functions, one can eat and drink without limit. But from excess fatigue **and** exhaustion, the energy of the spleen is injured. And when the stomach and spleen are injured, then food **and** drink are not assimilated; the mouth does not know the flavors; the four limbs are tired; the epigastrium is full **and** accumulates; there is diarrhea and expectoration; there is accumulation in the intestines. *(DACH 12v)*

An action on growth, on the "form," is equally indicated.

The meridian of the spleen-pancreas has an intellectual action that has been verified on numerous occasions in Paris: children at the bottom of their class are observed as having an insufficiency of the spleen. From the first acupuncture treatment, they rise to the first level gaining at least fifteen or twenty places, working faster and more easily. This treatment allows a better concentration of attention and mind, particularly in mathematics.

In China the spleen-pancreas is called the "treasury of ideas (or imagination, *yi*) and knowledge *(zhi)*." *(DACH VIII, 11v and 1v)*

It also has an action on awareness and emotions since, as the *Nei Jing* says:

> It is the minister who shows faults and speaks of equity. Total knowing comes from it.

The spleen-pancreas is troubled by obsessions. It is injured by the excess of sugar. Pains related to the spleen-pancreas are cited in the *Da Cheng (IX, 12v)*:

> Pains of the big toe and of the medial malleolus, cramps, pains of the medial surface of the knee and thigh, the two sides of the thorax and the umbilicus, pains at the interior of the spinal column radiating into the thorax.

> Its illnesses are in the root of the tongue . . . its flavor is sweet; its beneficial meat is beef; its cereal is rye; its fluid is saliva. *(DACH 11v)*

In general, its relations with the other organs are the following:

Heart — follows the spleen in the circulation of energy. If it is full, it will tonify the spleen-pancreas; if it is empty, it will disperse the spleen-pancreas.

Stomach — precedes the spleen-pancreas in the circulation of energy; the corresponding workshop organ (yang).

Small Intestine —

> If the small intestine is disordered, make the spleen-pancreas smooth (tonify). *(YXRM I, 18v)*

> If the spleen-pancreas is disordered, act upon the small intestine (disperse). *(DACH XI, 10r)*

Kidneys — If the spleen-pancreas is disordered, there is danger to the kidneys, which must then be tonified.

Liver — The husband that dominates its wife, the spleen-pancreas. The wife may then endanger the husband.

V. Heart: *Xin Jing, Shou Shaoyin*

The heart corresponds to two functions — the circulation of blood and the feeding of the brain. (In Chinese, the ideogram for the heart organ also represents the mind and the intelligence, just as in Europe ''heart'' may connote moral qualities and goodness.)

The heart is the great master of the five treasure organs and the six workshop organs. It is the home of awareness and of vitality. When this organ is firm and solid, perversity does not easily enter. (DACH VIII, 15r)

It governs the blood and blooms in the face. It is from the heart that clarity of awareness comes forth. It is the transformer of awareness, the minister of the master and lord. (DACH 14v)

It acts directly on the temperature of the body:

Its fullness gives heat; its emptiness, cold. (DACH VIII, 15r)

It gives *joie de vivre* and assurance.

When it is empty, there is timidity, fear, false ideas, clear urine. When there is fullness, there is mental hyperexcitation, incessant speech, bright red cheeks, easy laughter. (DACH VIII, 15v)

It has been observed that certain feelings, and certain spices and foods have an action on the diverse function of the heart:

Salt tonifies and stimulates the heart and mind. The sweet flavor, on the contrary, weakens and slows them. Mutton and wheat [millet?] strengthen the heart. Fright stimulates it; joy prolongs the emptiness of energy. Summer and heat are bad for it. Illnesses of heart and circulation are always aggravated in the summer. (DACH VIII, 15v)

Li Gao (Dong-Yuan) of the twelfth century attributes foul body odor to the heart meridian.

*The stench depends on the heart. Disperse **shaochong** (HT-9). (DACH I, 15v)*

The heart's emitted smell is burnt. (DACH VIII, 14v)

The organs in special relationship to the heart are as follows:

Spleen-Pancreas — precedes it in the circulation of energy.

Small Intestine — follows it in the circulation of energy; the corresponding workshop-organ (yang). In the case of emptiness of the heart, tonify the small intestine and the passage point *tongli* (HT-5).

Liver and Gallbladder — tonify them in cases of emptiness of the heart and disperse them in cases of excess energy. Troubles of the gallbladder can give pain along the meridian of the heart. To tonify the heart, tonify the liver.

Lungs — as the wife of the heart, they are dominated by it and endanger it.

Kidneys — endanger the heart by their illnesses; thus, tonify the heart in cases of kidney illness.

Heart Governor — the illnesses of the heart come from it. It can increase or decrease the cardiac function.

VI. Small Intestine: *Xiao Chang Jing, Shou Taiyang*

Precise details are given on its anatomy: the duodenum is the lesser small intestine *(shao xiaochang);* the jejunum, the half small intestine *(ban xiaochang);* the ileum, the left small intestine *(zuo xiaochang).* Its weight, length, etc. are given. ''It is the minister who receives the harvest.''

Besides the functions known in the West, the Chinese attribute two additional ones which are extremely important:

It presides over the division of solids and liquids. (DACH VIII, 16v)

It makes the separation between the liquid residues directed to the kidneys and urinary bladder and the solid residues directed to the large intestine.

Its most important function is the incorporation and individualization of digested food into the living being. The food is transformed into vital and personal elements, or these are extracted and assimilated from the food.

It governs the separation of the pure and the impure. It sends the pure into the blood and the impure into the urinary bladder and large intestine. (DACH VII, 16v)

It is true that tonifying the small intestine at *houxi* (SI-3) or at its herald point, *guanyuan* (CV-4), gives a distinct sense of vitality and a marked rejuvenation.

Troubles of the small intestine are given in the following quotes:

> *With an illness of this organ, there is a white face; warmth in front of the ears; bitter cold; the shoulder and the edges of the arm (interior and exterior) are swollen and painful. If there is emptiness of the small intestine: remorse; blue lips with white edges; swollen chin that cannot be turned; liquid mucus; descending fire; broken lumbar; difficulty of moving and walking. Urinary needs are pressing and numerous, or the sexual energy is not strong. (DACH VIII, 17r)*

> *Pains which depend on this meridian are those of the fork of the little finger, the posterior side of the elbow, the internal face of the arm entering into the axilla, and the posterior side of the armpit around the scapula and mounting to the neck. If the pain radiates into the ears, there is buzzing; if it radiates to the chin, the eyes are darkened for a long time. (DACH IX, 13r)*

The connections with the other organs are as follows:

Heart — precedes it in the circulation of energy. If the small intestine is empty, tonify the heart.

Urinary Bladder — follows the small intestine in the circulation of energy. Disperse the urinary bladder if the small intestine is in excess; tonify it if the small intestine is insufficient. Tonify the small intestine if the urinary bladder is insufficient; disperse it if the urinary bladder is in excess.

Spleen-Pancreas —

> *Tonify it, make it smooth, if the small intestine is disordered. If the spleen-pancreas is disordered, disperse and calm the small intestine. (YXRM I, 18v)*

Large Intestine — The small intestine is the husband. It dominates the large intestine, but the large intestine endangers it.

VII. Urinary Bladder: *Pang Guang Jing, Zu Taiyang*

The urinary bladder is not considered as merely a container. It also has the role of exciting and regulating the kidneys, and this is its most important action. It precedes the kidneys in the circulation of energy and gives them force and vitality. Moreover, it has a role on the psyche that is ignored in Europe.

> *Fullness: pulse full; through the illness the urinary bladder is twisted, one cannot urinate; oppressive fullness; internal agitation; fullness; difficulty in bending forward or backwards. Use cold or coolness to make it communicate and facilitate conduction. Emptiness: insufficiency of energy, sadness, flaccidity; there is incontinence; the pulse is empty; pains of the intestines radiate to the lumbar; difficulty in bending forward and extending; muscles of the feet tight and contracted; difficulty hearing. (DACH VIII, 19r)*

> *It is the minister of the capital of the valleys. The transfused fluids are stored there. When the energy is transformed they go out. (DACH 18v)*

The pains due to the urinary bladder follow the meridian:

> *Pains accompany swelling of the fifth toe and of the heel. Contracture of the popliteal crease; broken vertebral column; muscles of the neck contracted; cannot lift the shoulder; tight pain of the axilla; cannot bend to the right or left. (DACH XI, 12r)*

If the pulse of the urinary bladder is very tense, long and hard, like a steel thread, it indicates in both sexes either colibacillus or cystitis or simply pressing needs to urinate.

The connections with the other organs are given below:

Kidneys — the yin coupled treasure organ; follows the urinary bladder in the circulation of energy.

Small Intestine — precedes the urinary bladder in the circulation of energy.

Triple Warmer — wife of the urinary bladder, dominated by it, but endangers it. It has often been remarked that when the triple warmer is in excess, the urinary bladder is also very tight and its pulse relaxes as soon as the dispersing action on the triple warmer has had its effect.

Lungs —

> *If the urinary bladder is disordered, one must purify the energy of the lungs. If the lungs are sick, one must clarify and encourage the urinary bladder [midday-midnight rule]. (YXRM I, 18v)*

VIII. Kidneys: *Shen Jing, Zu Shaoyin*

The functions of the meridian of the kidneys (without adrenals) correspond to what we recognize in the West:

Filtration — that is, the expulsion of water (quantity or volume of urine) — is assured by dispersing *yongquan* (KI-1) and *rangu* (KI-2). However, a point of the conception vessel, *shuifen* (CV-9), also gives a strong discharge of water. *Rangu* (KI-2) stops saliva, sweat, diarrhea with colic, all symptoms of vagotonia. (Does it encourage the activation of the sympathetic system on the splanchnic nerves?)

The excretion of solid dilute residues in the water (colored urine, leaving of deposits) is activated by tonifying *fuliu* (KI-7). (*Fuliu* acts on edema and watery swellings, the retention of water in the tissues being in this case more due to an excess of unevacuated solid residues and the retention of water than to an insufficiency of filtration.)

Certain qualities of character and cleverness (not intellectuality, which depends on the spleen-pancreas) are increased by very well-functioning kidneys: decision *(zhi) (DACH VIII, 1v)*. "astuteness, or guile and seductiveness" *(zhi qiao) (DACH VIII, 25r)*. It is certain that indecision is ameliorated by tonifying the kidneys. Force of character (vitality, enthusiasm, "pep": *jing-shen*) is improved by the kidneys, which are its home. *(DACH VIII, 25v)*

Some physical qualities unknown in Europe are linked to good kidney function: Sexual energy (force of reproduction, procreativity more than sexuality, but both to some extent) depends mainly on the left kidney for men; mainly on the right kidney for women.

> *The left is named* **shen** *(kidney). Males store sexual energy there. The right is called* **mingmen** *"gate of destiny." Women keep the ovule there. Both are the root of the original energy. (DACH VIII, 25v)*

The vital force: "It is the minister that makes robustness." *(DACH VIII, 25r)*

Hair: "The kidneys flourish in the hair (of the head)." *(DACH)*

The bones: "The kidneys take care of the bones; they produce the bone marrow." *(DACH)*

The adrenals are mentioned in Chinese anatomy, but their actions were not studied. It seems possible to link them to the emotional and intellectual qualities attributed to the kidneys and stimulated by the same points which act on the kidneys, e.g., *fuliu* (KI-7), which often makes the blood pressure rise and which stimulates decision, etc., and seems to act on the adrenals.

The pains of the meridian follow its course (posteromedial aspect of the lower limb), but also are reflected on the urinary bladder meridian as the latter extends from the lumbar region up to the neck. There are also cramps under and on the medial side of the foot, sometimes with contractions. It is indicated that in yang illnesses (contractions) of the kidneys, one cannot bend in front; in yin illnesses (swellings), one cannot straighten up. *(DACH IX, 12v)* Pains going to the lumbar region are from the kidney. Those going to the ribs are from the urinary bladder. *(YXRM I, 17r)*

Fear is said to inhibit the kidneys. *(DACH VIII, 25r)*

The salty flavor stops filtration more than excretion; cold stops excretion, but increases filtration.

> *Its flavor is salty; its beneficial meat is pork. (DACH)*

> *Fullness: pulse full; lower abdomen swollen, full; lumbar and back stiff and contracted; colored urine; dry tongue. Empty: pulse empty, energy cold, yang paralyzed; confused and troubled speech; colorless, abundant urine. When the energy of the kidneys is not harmonized there is dull pain of the lumbar and sides. What one burps has a strange smell; there are pains of the shoulder and back. Chronic accumulations of the kidneys cause asthmatic crises and shallow breathing. When this problem reaches to the bone marrow, the marrow becomes weak. (YXRM I, 17r)*

> *The kidneys are a female treasure organ* **(pin zang)**. *The energy of the earth, which rises, depends on the kidneys as well as the production of water and liquids. That is why it is called* **zhi-yin,** *"supreme yin." (DACH I, 6v)*

The connections of the kidneys with the other organs are as follows:

Urinary Bladder — precedes them in the circulation of energy; the coupled workshop organ (yang). The urinary bladder functions not only as a reservoir but has an excitatory and regulating action on the kidneys. Dispersing the urinary bladder increases the filtration function of the kidneys (not the excretion) and disperses the kidneys; tonifying the urinary bladder inhibits filtration and tonifies the kidneys by increasing excretion.

Heart Governor and Door of Destiny (mingmen) — follows the kidneys in the circulation of the energy; "wife" of the kidneys. The kidneys dominate the heart governor and are endangered by it. In cases of congestion of the kidneys, disperse the heart governor (*daling*, PC-7); in case of emptiness of the kidneys, tonify the heart governor (*zhongchong*, PC-9).

IX. Heart Governor: *Xin Zhu, Xin Bao Luo, Ming Men; Shou Jueyin*

There is no physical organ involved here, but a command over functions.

It is no more a physical treasure organ than the triple warmer is an actual workshop organ. Both have a name, but no form. (YXRM I, 17v)

The heart governor is the mother of blood. (DACH VI, 30r)

To give an understanding of this meridian, we must point out that it is reflected on the right wrist by two pulses: the middle and deep pulses. The middle pulse seems to correspond to the circulation: one finds it tight, hard and ample in cases of hypertension, usually from an excess of blood-mass; it is hardly perceived in hypotension. It is also reflected in the deep pulse, which corresponds to the genital organs: it is almost absent in women from the last day after menses to the ninth day and from the twelfth to the twenty-first day, but strong and agitated at the time of ovulation, and increasingly so from the seventh day before the period. The lateral side of the artery corresponds to the right ovary and the medial side to the left ovary. In men or women with permanent excitation or inflammation of the genital organs, the pulses are big and firm on both sides of the artery.

Its names indicate two different functions which are linked and react on one another: circulation and sexuality, or rather procreativity.

By its use, it is called "heart governor" — it is useful to relate it to the vessels of the heart. Traditionally, it is related to all the points. (DACH VIII, 29r)

*It is the **xinbao**, "the envelope of the heart," and **mingmen,** "gate of destiny [this name is also given to the right kidney]." (YXRM I, 17v)*

The Buddhists have adopted the ancient name of the "entry into life" in order to indicate the exit door of the lower regions by which souls are expelled into the world to be reincarnated.

*Fundamentally, the **mingmen** is the first minister of the kidneys; its fibers circulate in the gap of the urinary bladder. One says that it exists and it circulates. But in fact the **mingmen** is not an actual organ. It is the passage of exit of the sexual energy. The **mingmen** is the minister of unions. Through it men form sperm and women release the ovum and have menses. It forms the energy and the sexual energy. Its disorders are as follows: from emptiness-fatigue — weakness of the four limbs, vertigo, pains of the ears, sexual vigor without orgasm; from extreme cold of the meridian — atony of the genital organs, weak and paralyzed limbs; from warmth — oppression, melancholia, easy laughter, difficult urination; from excess energy — the chest and diaphragm are tight and the ribs are uncomfortable. (YXRM)*

Let those who touch it be circumspect; it has many connections with the consciousness. (YXRM, 18v)

On this subject let us note that *zhongchong* (PC-9), which tonifies this meridian, increases daring. This point will dissipate fear of the night in infants. It augments the amplitude of the pulses in general without raising the blood pressure and gives the body greater strength and vitality. *Daling* (PC-7) causes the blood pressure to decrease (except in hardening of the arteries and blockage of the kidneys) and gives a certain indifference or surrender to destiny.

The organs with which it is particularly linked are the following:

Kidneys — precede it in the circulation of energy; the husband that dominates the heart governor, which endangers it.

Heart —

The heart is the great master of the five treasure organs and six workshop organs. It is the home of consciousness and vitality. When this organ is firm and strong, the evils do not easily enter. This is why all the heart's illnesses come from the envelope of the heart, whose meridian is the heart governor. (DACH VIII, 16r)

Triple Warmer — follows it in the circulation of energy and is its workshop organ (yang).

Stomach — For empty stomach energy, strongly tonify the heart governor. If the latter is empty, strongly tonify the stomach (midday-midnight rule).

X. Triple Warmer: *San Jiao, Shou Shaoyang*

The triple warmer is the father of energy and yang. (DACH VIII, 30r)

It is not a physical organ, but relates to physiological functions, especially to the respiratory, digestive, and genitourinary functions. (In this sense, it is comparable to the conception vessel, mother of the yin meridians.)

It has a name, but no form. The upper warmer commands the yang energy which goes out (respiration) and which circulates in the space between the muscles and the skin. The middle warmer commands the transformation of food, liquids and flavors, the immaterial essence of which rises to the lungs and mixes there with the blood, irrigating the organs. The lower warmer commands the formation of urine and its evacuation. (YXRM I, 18r)

The *Nei Jing* comments:

The triple warmer is the minister of canals of irrigation and drainage, the passages of liquids and their exit. (DACH VIII, 30r)

It is the store for the interior purity. It radiates and guides yin and yang. It opens and causes communication, or closes and stops communication. (DACH)

In Japan, Dr. Sawada, who has studied the triple warmer in detail, writes that this meridian can cure most illnesses.

Numerous studies in France have demonstrated the action of this meridian on the intensity of nervous charge (nervousness, or nervous excitation). When the subject is very tense, tight and irritable, the triple warmer pulse is notably tense, ample, and hard. It is enough to puncture *tianjing* (TW-10, in the olecranon fossa) with a silver needle to obtain a quick response of abatement or relaxation, as after a long bath. Sometimes there is even a small crisis of tears. This relaxation extends to the contracted internal organs and can cause a drop in the blood pressure.

Conversely, when the whole being is flaccid, without spirit, the triple warmer pulse is then either nonexistent or small and soft. It is then sufficient to puncture *zhongzhu* (TW-3, back of the hand) with a gold needle to obtain revitalization and *joie de vivre*. This rejuvenated spirit is always perceived immediately by the patient; on the pulses, it is first marked at the triple warmer pulse, then at the other pulses.

To obtain a profound action on one of the three related functions one must often use the additional command points of each of the three warmers.

*The upper warmer responds to **shanzhong** (CV-17). The middle warmer responds to **zhongwan** (CV-12). The lower warmer responds to **xuehai** (SP-10). (Also to **yinjiao** of the abdomen, CV-7.) The herald point (general) is **shimen** (CV-5). The triple warmer is commanded (nourished) by **qichong** (ST-30). (YXRM I, 18r)*

This passage elucidates the role of the triple warmer:

The meridian of the stomach commands the energy of fermentation and heat from food and drinks. The triple warmer uses this energy by traversing the twelve meridians and causing it to rise and fall. It commands the circulation, energy and blood. It is thus that this workshop makes energy and blood act. But the energy and blood have their roots in the stomach. One must understand these concepts well. (YXRM I, 18v)

The problems attributed to this meridian are as follows:

Fullness of energy of the abdomen; lower abdomen hard; urination difficult or impossible; exacerbation leads to contracture, overflowing, liquid flows. Such are the effects for the abdomen. If there is emptiness, the energy is conducted to the lungs. In the middle, cold or congestion and swelling result. When the case is extreme, there is serious exacerbation, urinary insufficiency, ''singing in the ears'' [tinnitus] due to a branch of the meridian that courses behind the ear and then enters into it. Additionally, the limbs no longer obey. By heat: fullness of the chest, extreme melancholia, thirst and swelling of the pharynx. By wind [neuralgia]: chest as if tight and closed. Little finger, ring finger, elbow, arm, shoulder, outside of the ribs all painful. When the energy is very agitated, at one moment blocked and at the next overflowing, there is pain in the front of the chest, behind it, and at the external canthus. (YXRM I, 18r)

Li Gao (Dong Yuan) comments on the energy of the triple warmer:

If the energy of the upper warmer is insufficient, the brain has no fullness, the ear has harsh buzzings, the head feels topsy-turvy, vision is obscured. If the energy of the middle warmer is insufficient, defecation changes, the intestines are oppressively full and tight. If the energy of the lower warmer is insufficient, then there is slothfulness, emptiness and intermittence of the heart [arrhythmia]. (DACH XI, 11v)

One passage insists on the capital importance of this meridian:

Ah! To contemplate the admirable usefulness of the triple warmer is to know as a consequence that the treasure organs and the workshop organs are linked although different. Divided, they are twelve; linked, they form the triple warmer. To recapitulate, the triple warmer is one warmer; the warmer (jiao) is the origin (yuan). The energy of the origin and only that. (YXRM I, 18v)

*When the human heart is firm and pure, when desire and thoughts are not excited, then the energy of the sexual essence spreads into the triple warmer and the blood flourishes in the hundreds of vessels. When the fire of desire is ardent and when it embraces the triple warmer, the energy of sexual essence flows and overflows, mixes itself with the **mingmen** (part of meridian of the heart governor, or the right kidney) and leaves by flowing out. (DACH VIII, 30r)*

The connections observed with the other meridians are as follows:

Heart Governor — the treasure organ (yin) linked to the triple warmer (yang). It precedes it in the cycle of energy. Tonifying it will tonify the triple warmer. To disperse it, disperse the triple warmer.

Gallbladder — follows the triple warmer in the cycle of energy.

Urinary Bladder — the husband. It dominates the triple warmer, and the triple warmer endangers it.

Kidneys —

Sick kidneys, harmonize the triple warmer. Sick triple warmer, tonify the kidneys. (YXRM I, 18v)

Heart and Spleen-Pancreas —

To remove the heat of the middle warmer (digestive function), disperse the heart and spleen-pancreas. (YXRM I, 18v.)

Lungs and Stomach —

To fortify cold of the middle warmer (digestive function), tonify the lungs and stomach. (YXRM I, 18v.)

XI. Gallbladder: *Dan Jing, Zu Shaoyang*

The gallbladder is considered more than just a receptacle; it has an excitatory and regulatory role on the liver. This role is undoubtedly related to the nervous network that commands the opening or the closing of the Oddi's sphincter at the opening into the small intestine. In cases where the gallbladder has been removed, it has been observed that the command points of the gallbladder still have an action, though much weaker.

In the cycle of physiological action, the gallbladder receives bile from the liver and thus comes after it; however, it comes before the liver in the circulation of energy and transmits energy to the liver.

The pulse of the gallbladder indicates whether the organ is materially swollen by either hypotonia, in which case one must tonify (to increase liver function); or contracture or spasm of the sphincter, in which case one must disperse (to decrease the action of the liver). The distinction is not always easy to make. One should note if the pulse, although big, gives way to pressure; if so, one tonifies. If it is hard and big, one must disperse. However, a hard and big pulse can indicate the presence of stones if it is felt to be more round than long. The bigger the stones are, the bigger the pulse. In this case, action taken on the gallbladder can cause expulsion of the stone, resulting in either acute pains if the stone is of average size, or more dangerous results if the stone is too large. Thus, before acting on the gallbladder when this type of pulse is evident, one should first X-ray.

The gallbladder has an important psychological action unnoticed in Europe. Courage, audacity, intrepitude, timorousness and combativeness are proportional to its activity and fullness. Consequently, in Chinese, the most intrepid and combative soldiers are called the "grand gallbladder" *(da dan)*. It is the organ of courage and combativeness (as the kidney is the organ of character and shrewdness and the spleen-pancreas of intellectuality).

The gallbladder holds audacity, courage. All the other organs rely upon the gallbladder for their decisions. (DACH VIII, 32)

It is also the organ of pain, as has been observed. There are few neuralgic people who have no retention in the gallbladder through atony or spasm. Many neuralgias have been cured simply by dispersing or tonifying the gallbladder.

It is the minister of the interior rectitude. Decisiveness and cutting come from it. (DACH VII, 32v)

If there is illness of the gallbladder: tightknit eyebrows, bitter taste in the mouth in the morning, nighttime vomiting of fluids, frequent deep sighs, fear of being caught by people.

*Fullness: full pulse; character is without control. The best is to disperse and to give a decoction of **banxia** [according to different authors, Serpentina or Aurum tribolatum or Arizaema triphyllum or Pinellia ternata]. If there is fullness and warmth, one sleeps a lot. (DACH VIII, 32v)*

Emptiness: empty pulse; interior agitation; worries; insomnia; the eyes are foggy. If one injures the gallbladder from vomiting, one sees things while lying down. (DACH VIII, 32r)

The connections with the other organs are as follows:

Triple Warmer — precedes it in the circulation of energy.

Liver — follows it in the circulation of energy; its coupled yin treasure organ.

Stomach — the wife dominated by the gallbladder, which endangers it.

Small Intestine —

The gallbladder nourishes [enlivens] the small intestine. (YXRM I, 18v)

Large Intestine — makes an appeal on the gallbladder and is greatly helped by it. Disperse it in case of troubles of the gallbladder.

Urinary Bladder — nourishes the gallbladder.

Heart —

If the gallbladder causes derangement, depression, or hyperexcitation, always tonify the heart. (YXRM I, 18v)

XII. Liver: *Gan Jing, Zu Jueyin*

To the numerous functions of the liver known in Europe (bile, glycogen, sugar, fixing of iron, hematopoiesis, coagulation of blood, etc.), the Chinese add still others:

It is the minister of the leaders of the army; strategies and combinations come from it. . . . If it is ill, there is emotional agitation and excitability. . . . If it is empty, there are torrents of tears. . . . If it is full and hot, the mirror of wisdom (the mind) generates dust; one is capable of burying and destroying. (DACH IX, 1r)

Tears are its external humor. (DACH IX, 1v)

*It is the palace of the **hun** (subconscious, the three memories). (DACH IX, 1r)*

Certain observations have been made:

It responds to the energy of spring. (DACH IX, 1r)

In fact, insufficiencies of the liver are always aggravated around the spring equinox. It is said, ''it responds to the east.'' (In spring, it is the east wind that usually blows in the north of China.)

Dissatisfaction injures the liver:

What is necessary most of all is to avoid quarrels and dissatisfaction as well as excessive silence. One must make the form sleep but not let the awareness sleep. (DACH IX, 1v)

In order to tonify the liver:

*One must borrow the fire of the heart in order to tonify the liver. Lie uncovered under the sun, rise and fly in the light to pacify its lasciviousness. What tonifies the liver is Asarum sieboldi (**xixin**), oranges, ginger, chicken, wheat. (DACH IX, 1v)*

In order to disperse the liver use:

*The acid flavors, angelica (**xiong**), the root of peony (**shaoyao**) rhubarb, legumes. (DACH IX, 1v)*

Experiments carried out in Paris have confirmed the importance of correcting spleen insufficiencies in order to treat liver insufficiencies.

The odors of the body come from excessive or diseased functioning of the liver:

> *Its odor is rancid. (DACH IX, 1v)*

Dan Xi dispersed all bad smells at **xingjian** (LR-2). *(DACH, explaining xingjian)*

Sexual energy comes from good functioning of the liver. Most liver acupoints on the leg have a special action on the genital organs.

> *The sexual energy collects in the liver. (DACH 1r)*

The hematopoietic role of the liver was known:

> *It generates the energy of the blood. (DACH 1r*

Sleeping is partially dependent on the activity of the liver.

> *If the liver is cold (with emptiness of the gallbladder), one does not sleep. If the liver is full and warm, one sleeps too much. Disharmony of the liver and gallbladder is the way of evil spirits who disturb you in sleep. (DACH 1v)*

It has an action on the nails:

> *It flourishes in the nails. (DACH X, 1r)*

Tonifying the liver improves the condition of the nails; it also stops nail biting.

The muscles depend on it for their nourishment:

> *It satisfies the muscles. It makes them live and the muscles make the heart live. Wind and acidity injure the muscles. (DACH IX, 1r)*

> *Its pains are of the great toe and in front of the internal malleolus; the medial side of the knee; the genital organs; cramping. Impotence of the genital organs comes from the liver. If it is disturbed, there are no more erections. If it is troubled by cold, there is retraction of the genital organs and they move inside. If, on the contrary, it is troubled by heat, there is excitation and erection without control. The cure is in the energy of running water and pure sounds. (DACH 13r)*

It acts on vision:

> *It opens an outlet to the eyes. (DACH 1r)*

The connections with the other organs are as follows:

Large Intestine —

> *If there is fullness of the liver, it facilitates the function of the large intestine. If the large intestine is sick, calm the liver. (YXRM I, 18v)*

Tonify it for constipation.

Heart — Tonify the heart if the liver is empty; disperse it if the liver is full.

Spleen-Pancreas — Tonify when the liver is disordered, since the spleen is its wife and is dominated by the liver. The spleen endangers the liver.

Kidneys — If disordered, there is little danger to the liver; however, tonify them.

> *To tonify the kidneys and liver for an external emptiness is to fill the fullness and empty the emptiness, it is to kill instead of cure. [Kidneys and liver are yin, while the external emptiness comes from an emptiness of yang]. (DACH I, 14v)*

Lungs — If they are disordered, there is danger to the liver; tonify or disperse the liver according to the excess or insufficiency of the lungs, which come after it in the circulation of energy.

Gallbladder — precedes the liver in the circulation of energy. It becomes swollen either by atony or by irritation; it restrains and curbs the liver. To empty it through *yangfu* (GB-38) gives good results. Tonifying it through *chongyang* (ST-42), or *xiaxi* (GB-43) sometimes gives better results.

XIII. The Two Median Lines

The conception vessel, ren mai.

This line (one of the eight marvelous vessels) follows the medial line on the anterior surface of the trunk. Its points can be divided into three groups:

a) From the pubis to the umbilicus. Particularly commands the genitourinary functions. *Yinjiao* (CV-7) of the abdomen is the herald point of the lower warmer (genitourinary functions).

b) From the umbilicus to the sternum. Particularly commands the digestive functions. *Zhongwan* (CV-12) is the herald point of the middle warmer (digestive functions).

c) From the bottom of the sternum to the bottom lip. Particularly commands the respiratory functions. *Shanzhong* (CV-17) is the herald point of the upper warmer (respiratory functions).

Certain points, as observed by sensitive people in experiments in France, cause response in particular meridians and can change the pulse corresponding to these meridians. Thus:

Xiawan	(CV-10)	responds to the stomach meridian.
Jianli	(CV-11)	responds to the gallbladder meridian.
Zhongwan	(CV-12)	responds to the stomach meridian.
Shangwan	(CV-13)	responds to the spleen-pancreas meridian.
Juque	(CV-14)	responds to the heart meridian.
Jiuwei	(CV-15)	responds to the heart governor meridian.
Shanzhong	(CV-17)	responds to the lung meridian, etc.

In general, the *Nan Jing* of Bian Que recommends use of the conception vessel (and the governor vessel) when the meridians, through excess evil, do not respond to the needles. In principle, the conception vessel is the vessel of women. *(YXRM I, 9r)*

> When the illnesses are the seven spasms, the eight accumulations **(jia)**, heat that does not harmonize, abscesses generated on the mouth and tongue, and pains of the head and neck, it is the conception vessel that generates these diseases; puncture **chengjiang** *(CV-24)*. *(DACH IX, 9v)*

> In women, the conception vessel and the **chong mai** do not reunite at the level of the lips and mouth; that is why they have no beard. *(DACH IX, 10r)*

> **Lieque** *(LU-7)* is the crossing and reunion point of the conception vessel. It activates the pulmonary arteries. It has a response at **zhaohai** *(KI-3, IS KI-6)*. *(DACH: **lieque**)*

> **Linqi** of the foot *(GB-41)*, crossing and reunion point of the **dai mai,** causes the conception vessel and the **chong mai** to flow easily and cures diseases of lactation and menses of women. *(YIXI, 9r)*

> The illnesses of the conception vessel are swellings and fullnesses of the abdomen with lassitude in the lumbar area; also spasms of men and illnesses of women. It is the course of birth and growth. It is the master of women. *(YXRM I, 9r)*

> The conception vessel is the sea of the yin meridians. *(DACH IX, 3v)*

The governor vessel, du mai.

> It acts on the physical and mental strength, particularly for men. *(YXRM I, 9r)*

It does not divide so clearly into groups of action as the conception vessel. However, *changjiang* (GV-1) under the coccyx acts on the anus, rectum, hemorrhoids, etc. *Mingmen* (GV-4), between the second and third lumbars, acts on the vitality and sexual vigor. The points between the first five dorsals have a strong psychological action. The *Nan Jing* recommends using it (with the conception vessel) when through excess evil the meridians do not respond to the needles.

> The illnesses of the governor vessel are stiffness of the spinal column and lack of strength. *(YXRM I, 9v)*

> When the illnesses are stiffness and pain of the vertebral column, insanity and epilepsy, heat in the middle of the back, deranged running, hallucinations, pains in the eyes, acute pain at the seventh cervical, it is the governor vessel which generates these diseases. Puncture **suliao** *(GV-24, IS GV-25)*. *(DACH IX, 9v)*

> The governor vessel is the reunion of the yang meridians. *(DACH I, 7r)*

> **Houxi** *(SI-3)* is the crossing and reunion point of the governor vessel. It has a response in **shenmai** *(BL-62)*. *(YXRM I, 9r)*

Chapter X

Special Points of Each Meridian

I. The Dangerous Points — II. The Tonifying Points: Tonification, Herald — III. The Dispersing Points: Dispersal, Assent IV. Regulating Points: Sources, Reunions — V. The Points Acting on Many Meridians at the Same Time or on Many Parts of the Body: Reunion of Organs or Reunion of Meridians — VI. The Sixty-six Antique Points — VII. The Eight Points of the Eight Marvellous Vessels — VIII. The Eight Marvellous Vessels

After a particular meridian has been indicated through the direct or indirect rules cited in the previous chapter, one must choose one or more points on the meridian for treatment. For that, one must verify which functions of the related organs are disturbed and choose points with an understanding of the action of each point on these functions. This will be described in detail in Volume IV, ''The Meridians, Their Points and Symptoms,'' where we provide information to allow immediate recognition of the point or points most effective for the case under consideration.

In this chapter, we will cite points which give the same tonifying, dispersing, or regulating effect on each individual meridian. The general groupings of points are listed below:

I.   The dangerous points.
II.   The tonifying points: tonification, herald.
III.   The dispersing points: dispersal, assent.
IV.   Regulating points: sources, reunions.
V.   The points acting on many meridians at the same time or on many parts
        of the body: reunion of organs or reunion of meridians.
VI.   The sixty-six antique points.
VII.   The eight general points of the eight marvellous vessels.
VIII.   The eight marvellous vessels.

I. Dangerous Points

These points are not always and infallibly dangerous. We need to be aware of their potential side effects only in cases of low resistance or when stimulated in a particular manner.

Ancient texts cite many points which are forbidden to moxa, needle or both; however, little rationale is given in these works and the validity of many of these claims cannot be proven by modern experimentation.

One must remember that the whole of the tradition from earliest antiquity has been retained. Hemorrhages and other injuries were undoubtedly produced by the ancient stone needles; this is in contrast to the fine needles used today (particularly Japanese or European), which are unlikely to cause similar injury. For moxa, the same holds true. Without question, there is great difference between the rapid touching with a hot shaving brush, a spoon soaked in boiling water, or the small moxa of mugwort placed above a coin with a hole in it, and the severe scarifications of antiquity, perhaps with a red-hot brand or a needle red from the fire.

Out of respect for tradition, we have indicated for each point the interdiction which has been conserved by tradition, as well as those for which caution is required. In brackets, we have commented on whether the quote applies only to the ancient stone needles.

Dangerous points of the face.

On the face, in general, puncturing a displaced artery can cause blindness.

Puncturing a sublingual artery with prolonged bleeding: muteness.

Kezhuren (GB-2, IS GB-3 *shangguan*): Puncturing the artery causes internal hemorrhage, deafness, and incessant yawning. *(DACH I, 10v)*

Sizhukong (TB-21, IS TB-23): Puncturing an artery and causing bleeding results in blindness. Moxas make the eye smaller *(DACH VIII, 32r)*.

Quanliao (SI-18): Risks causing deviations of the spinal column. If so, puncture *yuji* (LU-10). *(DACH VI, 11v)*

Hanyan (GB-4): Puncturing too deeply causes deafness *(DACH VIII 33r)*.

Tianyou (TB-16): Moxas cause the face to swell and the eyes to close up. If so, needle *yixi* (BL-40, IS BL-45), *tian-rong* (SI-17), and *tianchi* (PC-1).

Lianquan (CV-23): Puncturing deeply can cause deviations of the spinal column. To cure, needle *yuji* (LU-10) *(DACH VI, 11v)*.

Dangerous points of the chest and abdomen.

Quepen (ST-12): Needling in dispersion causes fits of coughing and gasping.

Shanzhong (CV-17): Puncturing too deeply causes the lungs to gasp in rebellion; one sighs trying to hold oneself erect. *(DACH I, 10v)*

Jiquan (HT-1): Puncturing too deeply causes coughing.

Ruzhong (ST-17): Moxa provokes phagedenic ulcers; needling causes deviation of the spinal column (cured by *yuji*, LU-10) *(DACH VIII, 9v and II, 11v)*.

Yuanye (GB-22): Moxa causes erosive swellings.

Dangerous points of the arms and hand.

Yuji (LU-10): Moxa causes swelling. *(DACH I, 10v)*

Laogong (PC-8): If one punctures more than two times, it causes emptiness. Moxa causes the tonsils to enlarge from day to day *(DACH VIII, 30r)*.

Lieque (LU-7): To puncture deeply causes vertigo and can cause fainting. *(DACH XI, 4v)* [This has been observed in Paris.] To take out much blood: death. *(DACH I, 10v)* [The point is between the radial artery and the radius; thus, it would be dangerous using the ancient stone needles. Modern needles, even if they puncture an artery when it is slightly displaced, will only let a few drops of blood.]

Jingqu (LU-8): Moxa injures the clarity of the consciousness.

Chize (LU-5): To puncture too deeply into the artery causes the energy to be seized. One can neither bend nor extend the arm. *(DACH I, 10v)* [This must apply only to the ancient stone needles, since nothing of this nature has been observed with the thin needles.]

Dangerous points of the lower limbs and feet.

Yongquan (KI-1): If the artery is touched and blood does not come out, the sole of the foot swells and gnaws. *(DACH I, 10v)* [Internal inflammation from puncture of unclean feet.]

Taichong (LR-3): With a puncture into the artery, if the blood does not stop — death. *(DACH I, 10v)* [This cannot happen with fine needles.]

Chongyang (ST-42): Same remark as for *taichong* (LR-3).

Taixi (KI-5, IS KI-3): Puncturing the artery increases the emptiness. Letting blood causes the tongue to form words with difficulty. *(DACH I, 10v)*

Yanglingquan (GB-34): Puncturing until fluid comes out causes lameness. *(DACH I, 10v)* [Inexplicable; infected puncture?]

Yinlingquan (SP-9): Same remark as for *yanglingquan*.

Xuehai (SP-10): Puncturing too deeply results in incontinence of urine. *(DACH I, 10v)* [Acts effectively on incontinence.]

Jimen (SP-11): If one punctures the great artery and the blood does not stop — death. *(DACH I, 10v)* [This refers to the ancient stone needles.]

II. Tonification Points

Tonification points (bu xue):

For each meridian there exists a single point that most strongly tonifies the organ related to the meridian. This action is such that if tonification is necessary, yet one attempts to disperse, the point will still have a tonifying effect. Of course, the point will give optimal results with a tonifying action.

The two median lines do not have special tonifying points.

The list of points is as follows:

Lungs	taiyuan	LU-9
Large intestine	quchi	LI-11
Stomach	jiexi	ST-41
Spleen-pancreas	dadu	SP-2
Heart	shaochong	HT-9
Small intestine	houxi	SI-3
Urinary bladder	zhiyin	BL-67
Kidneys	fuliu	KI-7
Heart governor	zhongchong	PC-9
Triple warmer	zhongzhu	TW-3
Gallbladder	xiaxi	GB-43
Liver	quguan	LR-8

Herald points (mu xue):

Each of the herald points acts on a particular organ; they are recommended in all insufficiencies of original energy (yuan qi) and in yin illnesses (i.e., those accompanied by cold, weakness, flaccidity, depression) originating from the emotions or emotional shock.[1]

Li Gao (twelfth century) wrote:

> All the illnesses cured by the herald points are insufficiencies of the original (yuan) energy. Beginning thus from the yin and conducting it into the yang, one cannot commit an error. (DACH IX, 13v)

At that time, only the herald points for the five yin treasure organs were acknowledged, all located on the abdomen.

The Nan Jing states:

> The illnesses of the yang act in the yin; that is why the herald points are all in the yin. The abdomen is yin; that is why the herald points are on the abdomen. (YIX 8v)

Around the thirteenth century, Chinese scholars began to question why there were no herald points corresponding to the workshop-organs. It appears that detailed observation expanded their conceptions, and today there is a herald point given for each of the twelve organs.

An interesting connection has been observed between leg-sanli (ST-36) and the herald points of the (yang) workshop organs:

> When the organs malfunction because of illnesses coming from damage of the seven emotions (DACH III, 23v), the energy of the stomach does not act. There is fatigue and disturbance of nutrition or excretion to the extent that the original energy is insufficient. One must then begin by stimulating leg-**sanli** (ST-36). But if there is no recovery, one must then stimulate the abdominal herald points of all the workshop organs. (YIX I, 8v)

> In illnesses of muscles, skin, bone, flesh, or blood vessels, wrongly stimulating leg-**sanli** certainly endangers the herald points of the abdomen. (DACH I, 13v)

A complete list of herald points follows:

Treasure organs (yin)		
Lungs	*zhongfu*	LU-1
Spleen-pancreas	*zhangmen*	LR-13
Heart	*juque*	CV-14
Kidneys	*jingmen*	GB-25
Liver	*qimen*	LR-14

The heart governor has no herald point. However, we have observed that *jiuwei* (CV-15) reacts as the herald point of the sexual organ, and *qihai* (CV-6) as the herald point of the blood vessels.

Workshop organs (yang)		
Large intestine	*tianshu*	ST-25
Stomach	*zhongwan*	CV-12
Small intestine	*guanyuan*	CV-4
Urinary bladder	*zhongji*	CV-3
Gallbladder	*riyue*	GB-24
Triple warmer	*shimen*	CV-5

III. Points of Dispersion

Dispersal points (xie xue):

Each meridian possesses a point that disperses the organ of the meridian better than any other point. When the organ is truly in need of it, even a tonifying action will disperse it. A dispersing action naturally acts with more strength.

The list is as follows:

Lungs	*chize*	LU-5
Large intestine	*sanjian*, LI-3; also *erjian*	LI-2
Stomach	*lidui*	ST-45
Spleen-pancreas	*shangqiu*	SP-5
Heart	*shenmen*	HT-7
Small intestine	*xiaohai*	SI-8
Urinary bladder	*shugu*	BL-65
Kidneys	*yongquan*, KI-1; also *rangu*	KI-2
Heart governor	*daling*	PC-7
Triple warmer	*tianjing*	TW-10
Gallbladder	*yangfu*	GB-38
Liver	*xingjian*	LR-2

Assent points (shu xue):

For each organ these points serve to calm excitation, fever, inflammation, or congestion (yang illnesses) coming from an external cause (cold, heat, wind, dryness, damp, etc.).

Li Gao of the twelfth century wrote:

> *To cure the diseases of wind or cold, one must treat through the assent points of each treasure organ. In effect, the illness enters through the yang and flows through the meridians. If it originated as an exterior cold pathogen, it will finish by returning to the exterior as heat. For illnesses produced by wind or cold coming from outside, puncture the assent points of the treasure and workshop organs. (DACH IX, 13v)*[2]

*For all heat, dampness, dryness, or fire, stimulate the assent point on the back. For wind: stimulate **fengfu** (GV-15, IS GV-16). For heat that has penetrated: **xiaochangshu** (BL-27). For dampness that has penetrated: **weishu** (BL-21). For dryness that has penetrated: **dachangshu** (BL-25). (YIX I, 8v)*

*According to the **Nan Jing,** the illnesses of yin act in the yang. That is why the assent points are on the back, which is yang. (YIX I, 8v)*

All the assent points of the organs are found on the urinary bladder meridian.

The ancients utilized only the assent points of the five treasure organs, which govern the blood. Later they used those of the workshop organs. They even added subsidiary assent points located elsewhere than the back.

The list of assent points is as follows:

Lungs	*feishu*	BL-13
Large intestine	*dachangshu*	BL-25
Stomach	*weishu*	BL-21
Spleen-pancreas	*pishu*	BL-20
Heart	*xinshu*	BL-15
Small intestine	*xiaochangshu*	BL-27
Urinary bladder	*pangguangshu*	BL-28
Kidneys	*shenshu*	BL-23
Heart governor	*jueyinshu*	BL-14
Triple warmer	*sanjiaoshu*	BL-22
	weiyang	BL-53, IS BL-39
Gallbladder	*danshu*	BL-19
Liver	*ganshu*	BL-18

We also add: *Fengfu* (GV-15, IS GV-16) for shock, and hip-*wushu* (GB-27), assent point of the large intestine, urinary bladder and kidneys.

IV. The Regulators: The Twelve Source Points *(Yuan Xue)*

Each workshop organ *(yang)* possesses a *yuan* (source) point. Additionally, the treasure organs each have a source point, but these are the same as the *shu* (assent) points. The latter should not be confused with the assent points of the back. (See the list of the antique points below.)

These source points are described as ''taking out the fullness or emptiness of the organs.'' Through them one treats poor circulation of energy in the meridian caused by atony or internal cold. It appears that the source point brings the organ back to normal functioning and even strengthens the active cells. The author of the *Da Cheng* (VIII, 17) recommends adding them each time one wants to tonify or disperse. The *Nan Jing* adds:

When the five treasure organs and the six workshop-organs are ill, always stimulate the source points. (DACH VII, 18v)

With a needle one can, for example, either tonify the liver at taichong (LR-3) or disperse it at the same source point. (DACH VII, 18v)

When meridians and secondary vessels are obstructed, one must approach the source points and the reunion points in order to separate the yang or unite it with the yin; that is, when the blood and energy of the meridians and the secondary vessels are frozen and tight and do not communicate well, one must always stimulate the source point, which separates and unites. (DACH II, 23v)

Thus, these source points are similar to the reunion points. The latter, however, are related to parts of the organism or to specific functions.

The twelve source points are commanded by the ''four barriers'' *(si guan)* which are the two *taichong* (LR-3) for the yin and the two *hegu* (LI-4) for the yang (see *DACH* II, 22r):

The twelve source points are as follows:

Lungs	*taiyuan*	LU-9 (also the tonification point)
Large intestine	*hegu*	LI-4
Stomach	*chongyang*	ST-42
Spleen-pancreas	*taibai*	SP-3
Heart	*shenmen*	HT-7 (also the dispersing point)
Small intestine	*wangu*	SI-4
Urinary bladder	*jinggu*	BL-64
Kidneys	*taixi*	KI-5, IS KI-3
Heart Governor	*daling*	PC-7 (also the dispersing point)
Triple warmer	*yangchi*	TW-4
Gallbladder	*qiuxu*	GB-40
Liver	*taichong*	LR-3

V. Points Acting on Several Meridians
(The Reunion Points: *Hui Xue*)

This name applies to two different groups of points: the points which command a part of the body and those which act on many meridians.

The reunion points — either of an organ, a part of the body, or a function.
Also called "the eight reunion points" (ba hui xue).

These eight points are used for all illnesses of the region or group that they govern.

> *The term ''reunion'' means, for example, that all the illnesses of the five treasure organs are reunited at* **zhangmen** *(LR-13), or that all the muscles of the body reunite at* **yanglingquan** *(GB-34). (YIX I, 8v)*

They also command illnesses due to internal heat:

> *For illnesses from internal heat, stimulate the point of energy of reunion. (YIZ, 5v; YIX I, 8)*

Another quotation related to the source *(yuan)* point comments on the internal organs:

> *When meridians and secondary vessels are obstructed, one must approach the reunion points (and the source points) in order to separate from the yang or unite with the yin; that is, when the blood and energy of the meridians and the secondary vessels are frozen and tight and do not communicate well, one must always stimulate the reunion and source points, which separate and unite. (DACH II, 23v)*

The eight reunion points are:

Zhangmen (LR-13): reunion of the six treasure organs (yin) controlling the blood. (Also, herald point of the spleen-pancreas.)

Zhongwan (CV-12): reunion of the six workshop-organs (yang) controlling the energy. (Also, herald point of the stomach and of the middle warmer, i.e., the digestive function.)

Shanzhong (CV-17): reunion of the breath-energy. (Also, herald point of the upper warmer, i.e., the respiratory function.)

Yanglingquan (GB-34): reunion of the muscles.

Taiyuan (LU-9): reunion of the blood vessels. (Also, source and tonification point of the lungs.)

Geshu (BL-17): reunion of blood.

Dazhu (BL-11): reunion of bones.

Xuanzhong (GB-39): reunion of bone marrow.

To these reunion points the *Da Cheng* (VIII, 9v) adds a ninth: *Futu* of the thigh (ST-32) — reunion of the arteries and veins.

Points acting on several meridians.

The reunion points of the second variety are the points which act on several meridians and organs at the same time. The list is not given in the Chinese texts, but it seems to us quite useful to include. (The first meridian mentioned is that on which the point is located.)

Point	Name	Meridians
BL-1	*jingming*	urinary bladder, stomach, small intestine, *yinqiao, yangqiao*
BL-11	*dazhu*	urinary bladder, gallbladder, spleen-pancreas, lung
BL-33	*zhongliao*	urinary bladder, gallbladder, liver
BL-36, IS BL-41	*fufen*	urinary bladder, small intestine
CV-12	*zhongwan*	conception vessel, stomach, triple warmer, lungs
CV-13	*shangwan*	conception vessel, stomach, small intestine
CV-17	*shanzhong*	conception vessel, small intestine, triple warmer, spleen-pancreas, liver
CV-2	*qugu*	conception vessel, liver
CV-24	*chengjiang*	conception vessel, governor vessel, stomach, large intestine
CV-3	*zhongji*	conception vessel, spleen-pancreas, liver, kidneys, stomach, gallbladder, urinary bladder, small intestine, triple warmer, large intestine
CV-4	*guanyuan*	conception vessel, spleen-pancreas, liver, kidney
CV-7	abdomen-*yinjiao*	conception vessel, gallbladder, heart, *chong mai*
GB-10, IS GB-14	*yangbai*	gallbladder, stomach, large intestine, triple warmer, *yangwei*
GB-15, IS GB-9	*tianchong*	gallbladder, urinary bladder
GB-16, IS GB-10	*fubai*	gallbladder, urinary bladder
GB-17, IS GB-12	head-*wangu*	gallbladder, urinary bladder
GB-18, IS GB-11	head-*qiaoyin*	gallbladder, urinary bladder, triple warmer
GB-2	*shangguan*	gallbladder, triple warmer, stomach, large intestine
GB-20	*fengchi*	gallbladder, triple warmer, *yangwei*
GB-1	*tongziliao*	gallbladder, small intestine, triple warmer
GB-4	*hanyan*	gallbladder, stomach, triple warmer, large intestine
GB-5	*xuanlu*	gallbladder, stomach, triple warmer, large intestine
GB-6	*xuanli*	gallbladder, stomach, triple warmer, large intestine
GB-7	*qubin*	gallbladder, urinary bladder
GB-8	*shuaigu*	gallbladder, urinary bladder
GV-1	*changqiang*	governor vessel, liver, gallbladder
GV-12, IS GV-13	*taodao*	governor vessel, urinary bladder
GV-13, IS GV-14	*bailao (dazhui)*	governor vessel, small intestine, triple warmer, large intestine, urinary bladder, gallbladder, stomach
GV-15, IS GV-16	*fengfu*	governor vessel, urinary bladder, *yangwei*
GV-16, IS GV-17	head-*naohu*	governor vessel, urinary bladder
GV-19, IS GV-20	*baihui*	governor vessel, conception vessel, small intestine, triple warmer, large intestine, urinary bladder, gallbladder, stomach
GV-23, IS GV-24	*shenting*	governor vessel, urinary bladder
GV-25, IS GV-26	*renzhong*	governor vessel, stomach, large intestine
GV-27, IS GV-28	gum-*yinjiao*	governor vessel, conception vessel, stomach
LI-20	*yingxiang*	large intestine, stomach
LU-1	*zhongfu*	lungs, spleen-pancreas
LU-7	*lieque*	lung, conception vessel
LR-13	*zhangmen*	liver, gallbladder
LR-14	*qimen*	liver, spleen-pancreas,
PC-1	*tianchi*	heart governor, triple warmer, liver, gallbladder
SI-10	*naoshu*	small intestine, *yangwei, yangqiao*
SI-12	*bingfeng*	small intestine, large intestine, triple warmer, gallbladder
SI-18	*quanliao*	small intestine, triple warmer
SI-19	*tinggong*	small intestine, triple warmer, gallbladder

Point	Name	Meridians
SP-13	*fushe*	spleen-pancreas, liver, kidneys (see SP-6)
SP-6	*sanyinjiao*	spleen, liver, kidney (see SP-13, CV-4)
ST-1, IS ST-8	*touwei*	stomach, gallbladder
ST-4, IS ST-1	*chengqi*	stomach, conception vessel, *yangqiao mai*
ST-6, IS ST-3	*juliao*	stomach, large intestine, *yangqiao mai*
ST-7, IS ST-4	*dicang*	stomach, large intestine, *yangqiao mai*
ST-9	*renying*	stomach, gallbladder
TW-15	*tianliao*	triple warmer, gallbladder, *yangwei mai*
TW-17	*yifeng*	triple warmer, gallbladder
TW-20	*jiaosun*	triple warmer, small intestine, gallbladder
TW-22	ear-*heliao*	triple warmer, gallbladder, small intestine

VI. The Sixty-six Antique Points

The ancients gave special names to sixty-six meridian points located on the extremities of the four limbs. For all the meridians each of these points have similar symptomatology, i.e., an organ dysfunction accompanied with fullness, fever or heaviness of the body, weakness, spasm, a crisis of energy, or panting.

There are sixty-six of these points, six for each yang meridian and five for each yin meridian. The antique points seem to group the effects of many others.

The 360 points of the whole body have their command in the sixty-six points of the feet and hands. (YXRM I, 37v)

Thus, the antique points are of great importance and are indeed very powerful. They are described as follows *(DACH VI, 16v and 18r; YIX I, 3v):*

1) *Jing:* "Well," "where it pours." At the extremities of the fingers and toes, next to the base of the nails. The *jing* points are indicated for curing illnesses of the organ accompanied with "fullness under the heart."

2) *Rong* : "Blood," "like the bend of the water." The point that comes second (or penultimate). For each organ indicated as curing illnesses accompanied by fever or warmth.

3) *Shu:* "Assent," "that which guides." Generally, the third from the extremity. For each organ, indicated when the illness is accompanied with heaviness of the body or pains of the joints.

4) *Yuan:* "Source." Each of the six workshop-organs (yang) has a unique source point, but the treasure organs use the *shu* as the source point. The source points re-establish order.

5) *Jing:* "Meridian," "that which causes circulation." The illness of the organ is accompanied by coughs or panting, or cold and warmth.

6) *He:* "Union," "like the return of the water, that which comes back." For each organ, the disorder is coupled with a crisis of energy or diarrhea.

Each season acts more strongly on one of the series:

In spring, puncture the "well" (jing) point — everything starts. In winter, puncture the "union" (he) point — everything returns, all finishes. (DACH VIII, 16v)

In spring, "well" (jing) points; in summer, "blood" (rong) points; at the end of summer, "assent" (shu) points; in autumn, "meridian" (jing) points; in winter, "union" (he) points. (DACH I, 20v)

Hua Shou states:

*When tonifying the **jing,** one must also tonify the **he**. (DACH VII, 16v)*

The table of these sixty-six points is as follows:

Points / Meridians	Jing "Well" fullness	Rong "Blood" fever, heat	Shu "Assent" heaviness or arthralgia	Yuan "Source" re-establish order	Jing "Meridian" cough, panting	He "Union" crises of energy or diarrhea
Lungs	shaoshang LU-11	yuji LU-10	taiyuan LU-9	taiyuan LU-9	jingqu LU-8	chize LU-5
Heart governor	zhongchong PC-9	laogong PC-8	daling PC-7	daling PC-7	jianshi PC-5	quze PC-3
Heart	shaochong HT-9	shaofu HT-8	shenmen HT-7	shenmen HT-7	lingdao HT-4	shaohai HT-3
Spleen-pancreas	yinbai SP-1	dadu SP-2	taibai SP-3	taibai SP-3	shangqiu SP-5	yinlingquan SP-9
Liver	dadun LR-1	xingjian LR-2	taichong LR-3	taichong LR-3	zhongfeng LR-4	ququan LR-8
Kidneys	yongquan KI-1	rangu KI-2	taixi KI-5, IS KI-3	taixi KI-5, IS KI-3	fuliu KI-7	yingu KI-10
Large intestine	shangyang LI-1	erjian LI-2	sanjian LI-3	hegu LI-4	yangxi LI-5	quchi LI-11
Triple warmer	guanchong TW-1	yemen TW-2	zhongzhu TW-3	yangchi TW-4	zhigu TW-7, IS TW-6	tianjing TW-10
Small intestine	shaoze SI-1	qiangu SI-2	houxi SI-3	wangu SI-4	yanggu SI-5	xiaohai SI-8
Stomach	lidui ST-45	neiting ST-44	xiangu ST-43	chongyang ST-42	jiexi ST-41	leg-sanli ST-36
Gallbladder	qiaoyin GB-44	xiaxi GB-43	linqi GB-41	qiuxu GB-40	yangfu GB-38	yanglingquan GB-34
Bladder	zhiyin BL-67	tonggu BL-66	shugu BL-65	jinggu BL-64	kunlun BL-60	weizhong BL-54, IS BL-40

VII. The Eight Points of the Eight Marvellous Vessels:
Ba Mai Ba Xue

These are also called the eight laws or the eight "means" (*ba fa*) or "points of crossing and reunion" (*jiao hui xue*). They are considered to be points of extreme importance.

> *The 360 points on the body are commanded by the sixty-six points of the feet and hands. [See the listing of the sixty-six antique points above.] In turn, these sixty-six points are commanded by the eight points. That is why they are called the marvellous points of the meridians. (YXRM I, 37v)*

Four are yang and respond to the shoulder, back, lumbar, thighs — to external illnesses. Four are yin and respond to the heart, sides, ribs, abdomen — to internal illnesses (see *DACH* II, 22v).

The *Nan Jing* compares the twelve meridians to large rivers which drain and irrigate their valleys at regular times. The eight marvellous vessels are the canals and drains constructed to guide the water during floods. The eight points assure the flow of the flood of illness in these drains.

> *The meridians are twelve; the secondary vessels, fifteen. Energy and blood continue their course in them like water in large rivers . . . But when the rain of the sky is too abundant, all the large rivers suddenly swell and overflow, filling canals and drains. That is what one wishes to express when saying that the illness penetrates and fills the marvellous vessels. If one treats these conditions using the twelve meridians and there is no response, one must use the master points of the eight marvellous vessels. This causes the so-called canals and drains to circulate. (YIX I, 9r)*

These eight points respond to each other like "host and guest" and "calm the pains of one another." One yang of the hand with one yang of the foot, and one yin of the hand with one yin of the foot are used. One school recommends beginning with them for all treatment, each one having an action on a group of illnesses. They are all borrowed from the twelve meridians. They are as follows:

The four yang:

Houxi (SI-3; of the small intestine, which it tonifies): Point of crossing and reunion of the governor vessel *(du mai);* coupled with *shenmai* (BL-62) of the *yangqiao mai.*

Shenmai (BL-62): point of crossing and reunion of the *yangqiao mai;* coupled with *houxi* (SI-3) of the *du mai.*

Waiguan (TW-5): passage point to the heart governor. Point of crossing and reunion of *yangwei mai;* coupled with foot-*linqi* (GB-41) of the *dai mai.*

Linqi of the foot (GB-41): point of crossing and reunion of the *dai mai;* coupled with *waiguan* (TW-5) of the *yangwei mai.*

The four yin:

Neiguan (PC-6): passage point to the triple warmer. Point of crossing and reunion of the *yinwei mai;* coupled with *gongsun* (SP-4) of the *chong mai.*

Gongsun (SP-4): passage point to the stomach. Point of crossing and reunion of the *chongmai;* coupled with *neiguan* (PC-6) of the *yinwei mai.*

Lieque (LU-7): passage point to the large intestine. Point of crossing and reunion of the conception vessel *(ren mai);* coupled with *zhaohai* (KI-3, IS KI-6) of *yinqiao mai.*

Zhaohai (KI-3, IS KI-6): point of crossing and reunion of the *yinqiao mai;* coupled with *lieque* (LU-7) of the *ren mai.*

Under the title "Rule of Eight," the famous Yang Jizhou of the sixteenth century wrote:

> *These eight points are the "conducting threads." For the rule of eight, first puncture the point [among the eight] that is applicable and follow the illness right or left, up or down. Then puncture all the points which respond. Follow, press, drive, according to the rule. If the illness is not finished, always use the coupled point. Leave the needle in and wait for the energy. Cause the top and bottom to communicate, ease without sharpness. Then take out the needle. If you want to use moxa, you may. But after that do not return to the needles. (DACH VIII, 34v)*

The illnesses for which each of these points must first be used are as follows *(DACH VIII, 25v and 31v):*

The four yang (pains of the lumbar, back, vertex, external illnesses):

Houxi (SI-3) for the governor vessel; *du mai,* coupled with *shenmai* (BL-62). Neuralgia of forehead and eyebrows; neuralgia of drunkenness. Motor troubles of the extremities; contractures of the nape of the neck, throat, jaw; tetanus. Red eyes, crying. Tonsillitis. Raging toothache. Cough and mucus. Deafness.

Shenmai (BL-62 of the *yangqiao mai*), coupled with *houxi* (SI-3). Contractures, hemiplegia, paralysis, aphasia. Pain of the nape of the neck and back. Lumbago.

Waiguan (TW-5 of the *yangwei mai*) coupled with foot-*linqi* (GB-41). Emptiness, exhaustion, expectoration of blood. Headache, pains or troubles of the eyes and ears. Pains and swellings of the front and nape of the neck; ganglions of the nape of the neck; mumps. Abscess of the mouth; pain of the lower molars. Arthritis of fingers or toes.

Linqi of foot (GB-41 of the *dai mai*), coupled with *waiguan* (TW-5). All emptiness and exhaustion. Sharp articular rheumatism; arthritis of the heel. Redness and swelling of the wrists, knees or external malleolus. Flaccid paralysis, trembling or contractures of feet and hands. Pains of the back, shoulder, arm or outside of lower limb.

The four yin (internal organs, internal illnesses):

Neiguan (PC-6 of the *yinwei mai*), coupled with *gongsun* (SP-4) (heart and mind, circulation). Amnesia, loss of words, anxiety, troubles of the brain, disordered epilepsy. Indigestion, internal fullness, spasmodic constipation, hemorrhoids.

Gongsun (SP-4 of the *chong mai*), coupled to *neiguan* (PC-6) (digestive organs). All heart pains. Stomach problems: hiccough, bad digestion, aerogastria, aerocolic. All tropical fevers. All types of jaundice.

Lieque (LU-7 of the conception vessel, *ren mai*), coupled with *zhaohai* (KI-3, IS KI-6) (respiratory organs). Troubles of respiratory passages, coryza, sneezing, bronchitis, asthma. Heat stroke. Meningitis in children. Paresis from fear in children. Diabetes. Food poisoning.

Zhaohai (KI-3, IS KI-6 of the *yinqiao mai*) coupled with *lieque* (LU-7) (genitourinary organs). Lower pelvis, spasms of the urinary bladder, thick, frequent or bloody urine. Constipation in women. Exhaustion in old people. Exhaustion in women. Seminal loss. Women who cannot hold the fetus. Menstrual pains in virgins. Intoxication of women. Abdominal pains after giving birth; inflammation of the uterus.

VIII. The Eight Marvellous Vessels of the Meridians:

(Qi Jing Ba Mai)

This name indicates eight groups of points whose command points have been described above. Two of these, the conception vessel *(ren mai)* and governor vessel *(du mai),* have been described in Volume I and possess points of their own. The six others borrow their points from the twelve organ meridians — we have not yet found a separate existence for these other than the similar actions of the points which compose them. The authors, however, attach great importance to these vessels. Future research may further elucidate their existence and use.

In the ancient literature *(YIX I, 9v; DACH VI, 5v),* the eight marvellous vessels are compared to the canals and drains provided for the excess of floods (the fifteen *luo).* In ordinary times the waters flow in the streams and rivers (the twelve meridians), but when the waters and illnesses overflow, the marvellous vessels begin to fill. At that stage, since the twelve meridians will not respond, it is advisable to use the points of crossing and reunion.

It is curious that it is advised to use the points of crossing and reunion and not the points which form each marvellous vessel.

The marvellous vessels respond to specific disorders rather than to specific organs.

> Among the eight marvellous vessels there are four yang, which respond to the shoulders, back, lumbar, thighs and disorders of the exterior. They are **yangqiao mai, yangwei mai, dai mai** and **du mai**. In addition, there are four yin, which respond to the heart, abdomen, sides, ribs and illnesses of the interior. They are **yinqiao mai, yinwei mai, chong mai** and **ren mai.** *(DACH II, 22v)*

> When the yin and yang energies are no longer mutually reactive, the **wei** *[yangwei and yinwei]* are disturbed. One loses his will and cannot hold himself, nor control his body. If the **yangwei mai** is sick, much cold and heat is produced. If the **yinwei mai** is sick, many pains of the heart arise. *(YXRM I, 9r)*

1) The four yang act on the shoulders, back, lumbar, thighs and external illnesses:

Governor vessel, du mai (described in volume I).

The points of the governor vessel are located in the spaces between the vertebrae and on the median line of the head to the mouth. It is the reunion of the yang meridians and corresponds to physical and mental strength, particularly of men. Its illnesses are stiffness of the spinal column and lack of strength, depression, epilepsy, heat of the back, hyperexcitation and hallucinations, eye pains, sharp pain of the seventh cervical vertebra, and so on.

Point of crossing and reunion: *houxi* (SI-3), coupled with *shenmai* (BL-62 of the *yangqiao mai).*

Yangqiao mai: "vessel of the hollow under the external malleolus."

> The illnesses of the **yangqiao mai** are agitations of yang and mental hyperexcitation. *(YXRM I, 9r)*

> Excess energy in the **yangqiao mai** with emptiness of the **yinqiao mai** causes insomnia. *(Ling Shu XXX, 20th line)*

> The illnesses of the **yangqiao mai** cause the yin to slow down and the yang to contract. The two vessels of the hollows under the malleoli are at their origin a division of the **yangqiao mai**. United in the **yangqiao mai**, the energy rises and acts; it is balanced and mutually exchanged; the eyes are bright. If the energy does not exchange, the eyes are not united. Men count their yang; women count their yin. What is used for counting are the meridians. What is not used for counting are the secondary vessels.

> Its points are **shenmai** (BL-62); **pucan** (BL-61); **fuyang** (BL-59) hip-**weidao** (GB-30, IS GB-28); **jianyu** (LI-15); **jugu** (LI-16); **naoshu** (SI-10); **dicang** (ST-7, IS ST-4); cheek-**juliao** (ST-6, IS ST-3); and **chengqi** (ST-4, IS ST-1). Its point of crossing and reunion is **shenmai** (BL-62), coupled with **houxi** (SI-3) of the **du mai.** *(DACH IX, 10v)*

Yangwei mai: "chain of yang."

Wei, chain, is to hold. The **yangwei mai** holds all yang. It reunites the **zu taiyang** (urinary bladder), **shou taiyang** (small intestine), **zu shaoyang** (gallbladder), and **shou shaoyang** (triple warmer). (DACH IX, 10v)

The **yangwei mai** links all the yang energies. If these cannot circulate, there is much fever. Its illnesses are serious cold and heat. (YXRM I, 9r)

The **yangwei mai** cures neuralgias, cold and illnesses of the skin, as well as joint pains and swelling of the heel. (YXRM I, 10v)

This vessel starts at the reunion of all the yang; with the **yinwei mai**, it links all the secondary vessels of the body. If the yang cannot be linked with the yang, confusion results; one cannot hold oneself.

Shou taiyang (SI) and the **yangqiao mai** are reunited at **naoshu** (SI-10). **Shou shaoyang** (TW) is reunited at **naoshu** (SI-10). In addition, **shou** and **zu shaoyang** are reunited at **tianliao** (TW-15), and with **zu yangming** (ST) at **jianjing** (GB-21). On the head, **zu shaoyang** (GB) is reunited at **yangbai** (GB-10, IS GB-14).

Its points are **yamen** (GV-14, IS GV-15); **fengfu** (GV-15, IS GV-16); **fengchi** (GB-20), **naokong** (GB-19); **chengong** (GB-14, IS GB-18); **zhengying** (GB-13, IS GB-17); **muchuang** (GB-12, IS GB-16); head-**linqi** (GB-11, IS GB-15); **benshen** (GB-9, IS GB-13); **yangbai** (GB-10, IS GB-14); **jianjing** (GB-21); **tianliao** (TW-15); **naohui** (TW-13); **naoshu** (SI-10); **yangjiao** (GB-35); and **jinmen** (BL-63).

Its point of crossing and reunion is **waiguan** (TW-5), which is coupled with foot-**linqi** (GB-41) of the **dai mai**. (DACH IX, 10v)

Dai mai: "belt vessel."

The **dai mai** links all the meridians like a belt. It cures fullness and swelling of the abdomen and makes the conception vessel and the **chong mai** flow easily. That is why it also cures the diseases which come from lactation and menses in women. (YXRM I, 9v)

The **dai mai** treats illnesses with fullness of the abdomen and sensation in the lumbar area as if one were sitting in water. (DACH IX, 10v)

Its points are daimai (GB-26); hip-wushu (GB-27); and weidao (GB-30, IS GB-28).

Its point of crossing and reunion is foot-linqi (GB-41) which is coupled with waiguan (TW-5) of the yangwei mai.

2) The four yin act on the heart, chest, axilla, sides and internal illnesses:

Yinqiao mai: "vessel of the hollow under the medial malleolus."

The **yinqiao mai** begins under the medial malleolus and rises to the pharynx and throat. It is a vessel that separates yin and yang at the foot. It goes up to the throat where it reunites with the **chong mai**. Its illnesses are contractions of the yin and stiffness of the feet. (YXRM I, 9r)

Its illnesses are the slowing of yang and the excitation of yin. It is said to be a division of **shaoyin** (heart-kidney). When it is united with **taiyang** (urinary bladder-small intestine), women use it as a meridian; men as a secondary vessel. (DACH IX, 10v)

Sleepiness comes from an excess of **wei** (yang) in the **yinqiao mai**. (Lingshu LXXX, 10th line)

Its points are zhaohai (KI-3, IS KI-6) and jiaoxin (KI-8). It finishes at jingming (BL-1).

Its point of crossing and reunion is zhaohai (KI-3, IS KI-6), which responds to lieque (LU-7) of the conception vessel (ren mai).

Yinwei mai: "chain of yin."

The **yinwei mai** links all the yin energy. If it cannot circulate, problems with blood circulation result and pains may be felt in the heart. Its illnesses are acute pains in the heart. (YXRM I, 9v)

The **yinwei mai** begins at the crossing of all the yin. If the yin cannot link with the yin, indecisiveness and disappointment result. (DACH IX, 11r)

Its illnesses are pains of the heart. Its points are *lianquan* (CV-23), *tiantu* (CV-22), *qimen* (LR-14), *fuai* (SP-16), and *fushe* (SP-13). Its point of crossing and reunion is *neiguan* (PC-6), used "for the general unification of the lower body, and to cure emptiness and depressions." It is coupled with *gongsun* (SP-4) of the *chong mai.*

Chong mai: "vessel of attack."

> It treats energies in counterflow and internal contractions. Along with the conception vessel and governor vessel, it starts from the genital organs. *(DACH IX, 10r)*

> It starts from the genital organs and goes around the lips and mouth. It is cut in the eunuch, thus the absence of a beard. *(Ling Shu LXV, 9th line)*

> In women, the conception vessel and **chong mai** do not reunite at the lips and mouth, thus the absence of a beard. *(DACH IX, 10r)*

> It is the house of blood for women who have their menses. It controls the illnesses of the heart, abdomen and the five treasure organs. *(YIX I, 9r)*

Its points are those of the kidney meridian on the abdomen: *henggu* (KI-11), *dahe* (KI-12), *qixue* (KI-13), *siman* (KI-14), *huangshu* (KI-16), *shangqu* of the epigastrium (KI-17), *yindu* (KI-19), *tonggu* of the abdomen (KI-20), and *youmen* (KI-21). Its point of crossing and reunion is *gongsun* (SP-4), which is coupled with *neiguan* (PC-6) of the *yinwei mai.*

Ren mai: "vessel of conception" (described in volume I).

> **Ren mai** and **chong mai** start from the groin. **Ren mai** is the sea of meridians and secondary vessels. When energy and blood abound there, the flesh is hot. When the blood alone abounds, the skin is slippery and produces hair. Women, with their numerous menses, may exhibit an excess of energy and an insufficiency of blood when the **ren mai** and **chong mai** are disordered. In women, the **ren mai** and **chong mai** do not reunite at the lip, thus the absence of a beard. The **ren mai** is the sea of the yin vessels. If it ties itself up in the interior, men have the seven spasms and women have contractions and pains **(jiju)**. *(DACH IX, 10r)*

Notes

[1] The name given to this category of points is explained thus:

> "Herald" **(mu)** comes from "to tie" **(jie)** and "to call on" **(mu)**. That is to say, the energy of the meridians accumulates there. *(DACH VIII, 3, explaining zhongfu, LU-1)*

[2] The name "assent" evoked through the element of the ideogram relates to the idea of the tribute paid by dependent nations.

> **Shu** comes from the tribute **(shu)** which supports the envoy. That is, the energy of the meridian is carried from here to there. *(YIX I, 8v)*

> The word comes from **shu,** "tribute" [with the "flesh" radical]. That is, the energy of the meridian sends presents from one to another. *(DACH IX, 13v)*

Chapter XI
Needle Technique (I)

I. Effects of the Needles

Most books on acupuncture are modest reproductions of the ancient texts. In their discussions on needles, it is difficult to determine whether they refer to the antique stone needles, or exclusively to the fine needles of copper discovered in the 18th century, or those of iron, or gold. (Let us not forget, out of respect for tradition, that stone needles were still in use, at least occasionally, up to the end of the Zhou dynasty in the fourth century B.C.), It is with this reservation that one should study these books.

Research carried out by numerous French doctors in hospitals equipped with the latest scientific instrumentation, or by careful and informed clinicians, show that one can tonify or disperse with needles of any metal type, and at all hours and seasons. But the effects are clearly more precise, deep, and durable if one keeps in mind the hour, season, lunation, metal, etc., as cited in the ancient texts.

The ancient authors realized from the earliest times that the effects of needles were not the same as those of moxa. It has been observed in Paris that it is possible to repeat moxa each day for many months on many points with continued benefit. However, if one keeps puncturing with needles the same points every day without waiting for the expected amelioration to be obtained and become established, a contrary effect is often produced. In one case, a blood count of 2,800,000/cu. mm. before the puncture changed to 3,700,000/cu. mm. three days after the puncture. At the insistence of the patient, who wanted to return home, a new puncture was made the same day. The next day the analysis showed 2,750,000/cu. mm. It was only three weeks later that the number of blood cells again started to increase, reaching 4,000,000/cu. mm. after one month. The increase obtained on average is one million blood cells per cubic millimeter the week following puncture. We can assume from this that the body may experience shock from repeating the treatment too soon.

It is in this light that we can understand the following passage:

> The needle is energetic, but it does not have the security of moxa. (YIX I, 12r)

There are numerous discussions, in special treatises, on the effects of needles as compared with those of moxa. The *Yi Xue Ru Men* (I, 45v) states:

> For that which medicines cannot reach, for that which needles cannot effect, moxa is necessary.

It must be noted that in descriptions of the nine antique needles (directly succeeding the stone needles), the dispersing effect is always cited while the tonifying effect is not mentioned at all.

Bian Que always advised puncturing when dispersing and using moxa when tonifying. The *Yi Xue Ru Men* (I, 45v) records this opinion:

> Certain authors assume that puncturing with needles can only disperse, not tonify.

Chen Wenzhong of the twelfth century wrote:

> It is often asked if the needles can only disperse and not tonify. The ancients used them to guide the energy (**dao qi**), and what they cured thereby were the illnesses of excess. Contemporaries who now use needles either know that they can tonify, but do not use them in this way, alleging that the reaction of the original energy is frequently very slight; or they have caused problems when using them this way, and have had to make the excuse that they are not skillful in their use in order to pardon themselves.

> The Classics say that for those with yang insufficiency, one must warm the energy; and for those whose sexual energy is insufficient, one must tonify and use the nature of the metal.

> [Metal] needles are the successors of stone needles. The latter did not have their own energy because of the nature of the material. They broke the skin and damaged the flesh; they made holes in the body through which the energy escaped. How would they be able to tonify?

> When energy and blood, yin and yang are all insufficient, one must not excite with the needles but fortify with sweet drugs. When the energy of the body is insufficient and the energy of the illness is also insufficient, the yin and yang are both deficient; one cannot puncture. If one punctures, then the energy will be seriously exhausted; old people will be dulled and robust people will not recover.

After what has been said, one can see why the needles disperse and do not tonify. (Cited in the DACH XII, 39r)

Nowadays, moxa is especially recommended for old people and children, for coldness and weakness, i.e., for tonifying. The needles are always recommended for warmth, pain, contractures; i.e., when one must disperse. In Japan, a yin and humid country, moxa is mostly used. In the north and northwest of China, a very dry and yang country, moxa is rarely used; on the other hand, the needles are used very often. In the Yangzi valley, a cold and humid country in the winter, moxa is frequently used.

It has been suggested that moxa, which acts on the epidermis in a rapid and superficial manner, would only be able to excite a reflex, while the needles, put into the dermis and left for a relatively longer time (for many minutes), cause a long, strong excitation which would inhibit the reflex.

This hypothesis accords badly with the recommendation of leaving the needles in for a long time to tonify and acting quickly to disperse. But in such a hypothesis, one must keep in mind individual reactions. The stimulation inhibiting the reflexes of a thin, sensitive person is insufficient to excite those of a tough, coarse person — thus the necessity of measuring the fineness of the needles and the depth and duration of puncture according to the sensitivity of the patient. For babies, soft massage with the tip of the finger gives effects comparable to the strongest stimulation with needles on physical and athletic people.

The hypothesis of eliciting a response with slight stimulation is discussed symbolically by the author of the *Da Cheng:*

> *If water is blocked in its course and cannot flow, effort can make it flow freely. Likewise, when the energy and the blood do not circulate, the effort of the needle can make them circulate in the pulses and the meridians.*
> *(DACH II, 21v)*

Recall the phenomenon of ionization. Pure water is a very poor conductor of electrical current; however, it will conduct electricity well if there is an acid, base, or salt (electrolytes) in solution. Certain substances, such as sugar, are not electrolytes. Now, with electrolytic molecules, when the current passes through, the molecule dissociates into two fragments or ions carrying opposite charges, which are then transported to the electrodes where they discharge themselves. The one charged positively goes to the cathode (cation) and the other charged negatively goes to the anode (anion). Thus HCl is dissociated into a cation, and an anion, H+, Cl−. This dissociation pre-exists in the solution. The current has no effect other than to transport the ions to the electrodes.

It has been observed that an electric current passes through the needle into the body. We can ask if the needle in fact affects the blood-electrolyte by causing a certain dissociation of albumin molecules into positive cations, yang, carrying themselves to the yin pole of the body, and negative anions, yin, carrying themselves to the yang poles of the body.

The entire art of tonifying or dispersing with the needle rests, in fact, with the precision (place, number of needles, depth, duration, etc.) with which one harmonizes the action to the possible reaction of the patient; the impact should be proportional to the necessary and possible reaction.

It is certain, however, that the effect is not linked to the pain. Punctures well done and giving good results can hardly be felt. Others, badly done and causing intense pain, may have no effect. Moreover, the pain of the puncture is essentially a personal matter. Each person has his own degree of cutaneous sensitivity. Very sensitive people are rare; insensitive people are somewhat more numerous. The average person ranges from a weak to a marked sensitivity, men always being more sensitive than women. The angle of the needle with respect to the point is also of importance for pain while being punctured.

II. The Instrument

From extensive experimentation in France it seems that of the different elements one can distinguish in a needle (metal type, thickness, form, length, temperature), the most important are metal type and thickness. The form and the length are of interest primarily to the doctor. The temperature of the needle in our temperate climate (and in the pockets of doctors) is not important enough to take into consideration.

In China there is no ''official'' model for acupuncture needles. It is a country of personal experimentation, with neither school nor dogma but with a respect for past experience. Each person uses whatever gives him the best results — or whatever he can afford to buy. Thus, many types of needles are seen in the hands of practitioners, ranging from the luxurious gold needles with two points bound by a spiral, to the humble needle of the tailor.

The name "needle" should be reserved for thin rods with a hole in one end; thus it would be more exact to call the type used for acupuncture "pins."

The thinnest are used for hands, the head and all places where the skin is thin, or for infants and sensitive people. They are .5 or .6 mm. thick and about 2.5 cm. in length, not counting the short handle, and are either polished (which consequently retains fewer possible microbes), crosscut (more practical for holding and manipulating the needle), or with a rounded head. The length of the handle is from five to six mm. with a thickness of about .8 mm.

The thickest needles are used for physical, less sensitive people, in winter, or in the fleshy parts of the body where the skin is thick. They have the true round head of a pin (without which it is difficult to push them in). Their thickness is from .9 to 1.0 mm., with a length of 2.5 cm.

After long trials, we have found that the best results are obtained with two different models of needles with the following composition of metals:[1]

For tonification: 60% to 70% pure gold and 40% to 30% red copper.

For dispersion: 66.6% pure silver and 33.4% pure zinc (this last alloy is very difficult to make: a few thousandths of silver more and the pin is too flexible; a few thousandths of zinc too much and the pin breaks, unable to bend).

The *Nei Jing* describes a set of nine needles which replaced the stone needles of ancient China.[2]

The nine antique needles are thus described:

1) **Chan** — *Length of 1.6* **cun,** *flat, .5* **cun** *wide. Large head and dull point. Also called "arrowhead." Used to disperse the yang energy and to puncture fevers.*

2) **Yuan** — *Length of 1.6* **cun,** *round body, point like an egg. Used to massage the muscles.*

3) **Di** — *Length of 3.5* **cun,** *point like a grain of millet. Used for emptiness and insufficiency of the energy of the meridians.*

4) **Feng** — *Length of 1.6* **cun,** *triangular blade. Now called "triangular needle." Heavy punctures against established illnesses.*

5) **Pi** *or* **Fei** — *Length of 4* **cun,** *2.5* **cun** *wide, point like a saber. It was used to cut abscesses and swellings and to remove great amounts of pus. Today called "spade-needle."*

6) **Yuan li** — *Length of 1.6* **cun,** *round and sharp, like a horse hair. The point is a little long. It was used to puncture children, also to treat rheumatism.*

7) **Hao** — *Length of 3.6* **cun,** *sharp point like the stinger of a mosquito. Used to treat pains, rheumatism, and cold.*

8) **Chang** — *Length of 7* **cun,** *sharp point. Used to treat deep rheumatism, entering in the internal gaps of the lumbar vertebrae or into articulations. Also called "the needle that makes you jump"* **(tiao zhen).**

9) **Huo** — *Length of 4* **cun.** *Also termed "needles to grill"* **(fan zhen).** *Used for swellings from emptiness or shock, when poison invades the flesh; disperses poison. (DACH V, 18v)*

Evidently such needles no longer exist. The descriptions do not allow us to reconstruct them. Those that can be found, with great difficulty, through the intermediary of pharmacists, can hardly be considered authentic.

The *Da Cheng* gives the following advice for making good needles:

First, stretch an iron wire over a hot fire until red. Then cut it into two, three, or five strands; length or shortness is not important. Next, put some clay and "earth passed by a cicada" on the needle and again put it into the fire, this time heating lightly without going to redness. Take it out, change the clay and warm a second or even third time. Still warm, plunge it into three bowls of water heated to boiling, then put it into flesh and fat. Then boil it until dry by leaving it in the water and waiting until it is cold. Next, take the needle and puncture it more than a hundred times into the yellow earth to make it shiny and respectable by removing the faults of the fire. Finally, bind it with a thread of copper, leaving a point that is ground until round. Do not use a sharp instrument. (DACH V, 19r)

For bleeding, the *Yi Xue* advises taking a copper sewing needle and a triangular iron needle and binding them together with a thread of copper to 7 mm. from the point (see *YIX* I, 1v).

Once made, the needles must be used only after certain preparations which vary according to the school.

If they are not clear and brilliant, one must puncture them several tens of times into the earth; then they are polished. For new needles, first warm them in the mouth and then puncture. After having punctured several people, they are "ripe." They no longer need to be heated. (YIX I, 11v)

Other schools use prolonged boiling: first in a bath of sheep's brain and marrow and mother's milk; then of sulphur, cashew, marsh celery, coreopsis root, or sheep's brain and marrow, oliban, myrrh, origanum and mother's milk (see *YXRM* I, 45v; also *DACH* V, 19r).

The different elements which constitute a needle and its use — form, thickness, metal, length, temperature — are worth studying in detail.

The form:

This is only of use to the doctor. The needle must be long enough to be held easily, yet not so long or heavy that it will tug at the flesh when inserted. It must have a head or point so that it is easy to insert even into tough skin without harming the fingers or sliding between the fingers instead of penetrating.

For the patient, only the point of the needle is important. It should be long and without protrusions so the puncture will be without pain. A short point produces more pain.

In practice, Chinese authors advise taking an ordinary sewing needle and inserting a copper thread into the hole which one then wraps around the needle, leaving only 5 or 6 millimeters of length for the puncture. The "triangular needle" with cutting edges, designed to open abscesses or to bleed, is frequently in question as it is an instrument of surgery, not acupuncture.

In France, for large needles of .9 to 1 mm., we use true pins with quite a thick handle; for thin needles of .5 to .6 mm., we use a handle in the form of a casing that is either polished or crosshatched. If one presses on the ball-like head of a needle that is too fine, there is risk of the needle bending or breaking when the skin is particularly tough. One must resist the temptation to make the needle penetrate by any means other than holding the sides of the handle with two fingers, since the casing can puncture the finger.

Some doctors use hypodermic needles, but, being hollow, they are a haven for microorganisms. This often causes abscesses.

A doctor in Paris has needles with a ball in the middle, both extremities being sharpened. He also has some very short needles (3 mm.) like drawing pins, which he covers with a plaster and leaves inserted in the patient for a day or two.

The thickness:

The only directions given for the thickness by Chinese authors is the following:

> Over thirty years old, for **sanli** of the leg (ST-36), it is useful to use thicker needles. (DACH VIII, "sanli")

Experiments in Paris and other parts of France show that thickness has notable importance. For physical and manual people, a thickness of .9 to 1 millimeter is necessary. If less, the effect is less deep or durable. The pain, however, is minimal. For refined people, this thickness causes true, if only slight, pain except in the fleshy parts. It is useful, however, in winter. For the hands and feet, a thickness of about .5 or .6 mm is more suitable.

In Japan, for women, children and even intellectual men, needles of hardly .1 millimeter in diameter are guided in by a tube. If pressed strongly, the end of the tube anesthetizes the point. In general, Europeans feel only a very short and not very perceptible effect from these needles.

Mr. Souteyrand has invented and produced a small apparatus marking a great improvement upon the Japanese system.

The metal:

The importance of the nature of the metal by no means escaped the ancient Chinese:

> For those with insufficiency of yang, one must warm the energy; for those with insufficiency of sexual energy, one must tonify, using the nature of the metal. The metal needles are the successors to the stone needles, but the stone needles did not have their own energy due to the nature of the material. (DACH XII, 39r)

The metal has an importance that is often undeniable. For example, a double lumbar neuralgia punctured on the left with a silver needle and on the right with a gold needle disappeared immediately on the left (silver) and was hardly diminished on the right (gold). The gold needle was taken out and replaced by the silver one in the same hole, and the neuralgia disappeared immediately.

The difference between the metals is often clearly appreciable. The skin, which grips the needle at the moment of puncture and then relaxes after one or two minutes, almost always holds gold needles longer than silver needles. If we had to quantify the difference, we could say that gold tonifies from ten to twenty percent more than a neutral metal (steel, platinum) and that the silver disperses from ten to twenty percent more than the neutral metals.

If one does not have two different metals, one for tonifying, the other for dispersing, one is reduced to depending on either treatment of special points on the body or manipulation of the needle in order to produce a difference in effect. Why not utilize the benefits of two different metals?

The oral traditions of China and careful experiments made in Paris agree on several points: **1)** The colored metals, e.g., red copper and gold, are tonifying. In China they are considered yang. **2)** The white metals, particularly silver, are dispersing. In China they are considered yin. **3)** The grey metals, such as iron, steel, and platinum, are neutral.[3]

The different action of each metal indicates that the body either absorbs an infinitesimal amount of the needle or that the nature of the metal gives it a special radiation. It appears that the effect of this homeopathic or radiant action increases proportionate to the body's needs.

The effects of pure metals studied individually have given the following results, which will undoubtedly be perfected with future technology. The most tonifying of metals is red copper, but it oxidizes instantly in the skin. Gold comes immediately after this for tonification. Silver is the most antifebrile, antineuralgic and decongesting of all. Zinc has a calming action that is very marked in nervous states. Iron seems truly neutral and acts only by the type of puncture (unless its action on the blood is only perceived long-term). Platinum, besides its calming action (particularly on female genital organ problems), seems neutral. Nickel seems neutral although slightly calming.

Despite the medicinal quality of the metal, one still must take into consideration that the needle must be hard enough to penetrate the skin easily, but not so brittle that it breaks if the patient makes an unexpected movement. It should be a metal that remains polished, not oxidizing easily when exposed to the air.

Many alloys of gold and silver possess these three qualities above, plus a microbicidal capacity that is very important for asepsis. A rod of silver or gold plunged into a virulent microbial culture will quickly kill all the microbes.

Passages from the ancient texts concerning metal type are not very exact:

> *The form — that is the needle. In principle it is made of **jin** [at the beginning indicating copper, the only known metal; later it indicated gold]. Formerly, stone (**bianshi**) was used. Today iron is used instead. (DACH II, 21v)*

> *The **Ben Cao** states: "Iron from the bit of a horse is without defect." The **Ri Hua** states: "In antiquity those made of the old iron of arrows were good." Following the **Ben Cao**, needles for doctors were made with soft iron or burnt iron (steel), but there were defects. That is why the bit of a horse, which was without defect, was used. Moreover, the horse depends on the ox, which depends on fire. Fire conquers metal and dissipates its defects. That is why it was used for the needle.*

> *The ancients said that the needles of gold (**jin**) are also precious. But **jin** [which means both metal and gold] is a general name: it refers to copper (**tong**), iron (**tie**), gold (**jin**), and silver (**yin**); they are all used. If one uses gold (**jin**) needles, it is more respectable. (DACH V, 19r)*

The length:

The minimum penetration depth of the needle is about one millimeter — this is for puncturing the fingers. The maximum depth is in the fleshy part of fat people, whose skin and subcutaneous tissue often reach two centimeters. It is enough to use needles of 2.5 to 3 centimeters in length. If the needles are too long, they will bend when inserted and pull on the skin, causing needless pain.

The temperature:

Cold needles cause the skin to contract; one cannot insert them. Tepid needles (at body temperature) facilitate the circulation of energy and blood. Very hot needles (60-65° C) act on paresis and rheumatism. Needles heated to redness are used to open abscesses.

> *Cold needles make the skin contract. One cannot easily put them in. The needle must be tepid. One thus avoids the fight between warmth and cold. One can then harmonize energy and blood. (DACH V, 19v)*

> *To puncture thin people, always warm the needle slightly either in the mouth or in fire. Tepid needles make the **rong** and **wei** mutually follow each other. (DACH II, 21v)*

> *Always keep the needles on the body so that they keep their warmth. (YXRM I, 45v)*

*For paresis (rheumatism-**bi**) which has neither pain nor itching, burn four or five cones of moxa as large as grains of rice on the point of the needle. When pain is noticed, stop. These punctures are also used for paralytic illnesses. (YXRM I, 40r)*

*Most often, "fire needles" (**huo zhen**) or "warmed needles" (**wen zhen**) are those that have been plunged into castor oil and heated by a lamp until they become completely red. This preparation is effective. If there is no redness, it does not remove the illness, but on the contrary exhausts and depletes the patient.*

When warming the needle, keep its tip down so that the oil does not burn your fingers, or have someone else heat the needle. These needles of fire are very difficult to manage. Use them with care . . . most importantly, avoid putting them in too deeply for fear of injuring the meridian. Inserting them too superficially, however, will not remove the illness. The pain of the fire-needle does not last. Just after puncturing, take out the needle; do not wait. With the left finger press the hole; that stops the pain.

These needles of fire can be applied on the whole body, except on the face, where they are to be avoided. Do not use them against beriberi; it will increase the swelling and pain [the swelling should be dispersed, not tonified]. They are used especially to open deep abscesses in order to take out the pus. Make three punctures. Do not press directly on the swelling but come from the two sides and drive out the pus. (DACH V, 19v)

Notes

[1] Made by the expert jeweler, Mr. Souteyrand, 23 rue Racine, Paris, following long research on alloys.

[2] The ideogram used today for the needles is composed of the elements: metal-two-fingers-holding-a-needle or metal-thinned. In the old texts it was composed of the elements: bamboo-thinned. This last composition leads us to believe that the first needles were slivers of bamboo, used with the stone stylus (see *DACH* IV, 15v and V, 19v).

[3] It is of interest to summarize here the recognized effects of several metals as used in homeopathy.

Gold — Antiscrofulous. Antisyphilitic. Ideas of suicide. Exostosis. Tooth decay. Congestive palpitations. Arteriosclerosis. High blood pressure. Sexual hyperesthesia.

Copper — Antispasmodic. Cramps. Convulsions. Trismus. Whooping cough.

Zinc — What iron is to the blood, zinc is to the nerves. Difficulties from growths on the skin; illnesses which will not go away. Cannot expectorate. Difficulties of menstruation with improvement when it comes. Aggravation from stimulants.

Silver — Special action on articulations, bones, ligaments, cartilage. Capillary contraction; tooth decay. Acts especially on the larynx. Pains of the left side, sensation of expansion. Emaciation and gradual drying-up.

Platinum — Mostly a medicine for women. Spasm; trembling. Paralysis, anesthesia and local numbness.

Iron — Paleness of the skin and excess mucus; anemia; iron-deficiency anemia (chlorosis) of young people. Easy blushing. Cold extremities. Weak with appearance of strength.

Recall the tonifying effect of gold salts, and the anti-inflammatory action of colloidal silver in fever, influenza, and infections.

Chapter XII

Needle Technique (II)

I. Before the Puncture — II. Preliminary Massage of the Points

I. Before the Puncture

Before the puncture, the patient must meet certain physical and mental requirements.

> *The patient must be lying down or sitting. If he is standing during the puncture, there is a possibility of syncope. (DACH I, 10v)*

There must be a state of physical repose:

> *Those who have come a long way by wagon should lie down and rest. Then, after a light meal, they can be punctured. Those who have come from nearby on foot should sit down and rest. (DACH I, 10v)*

Some conditions which forbid puncture are described previously in Chapter II. In principle, it is better not to puncture on an empty stomach as this may lead to vertigo. In practice, however, this does not often happen; what does seem to happen is that the energy does not circulate as well on an empty stomach.

> *If one punctures on an empty stomach, one will always cause vertigo. Before puncturing, locate the points and mark them so they are not lost. After the patient has had some food, have him sit straight or lie down, then puncture. (DACH V, 26r)*

These preparations having been made, the doctor must dissipate the apprehension of the patient through calming speech and attitude so that the patient relaxes emotionally and physically.

> *At the moment of puncturing, the doctor, through his speech, will dissipate the excitability of the patient. He will cause the energy of the patient to correspond to the appearance of his face. Thus, his eyes will not look to the sides. His heart will not have any supplementary beats. His hand will not be tight as if it were holding the tail of a tiger or the neck of a dragon. Then he will obtain the best effects from the punctures. (YIX I, 2r)*

> *The breathing of the doctor and patient should be regular and calm. The energy, which responds to the breath, will also be calm. (DACH VI, 1r)*

> *Profound awareness must appear and be maintained. (DACH VI, 22r)*

II. Preliminary Massage of the Points

Before puncturing, it is recommended to massage the point with the nail of the left thumb (the right hand holds the needle):

To tonify: one cross. To disperse: three crosses.

> *To tonify, firmly make one cross on the point with the nail of the left thumb. To disperse, firmly make three crosses on the point with the nail of the left thumb. (DACH VI, 6r)*

Oral tradition says that to tonify is to activate the passage of external energy to the yin interior. Making one cross excites the skin slightly and calls on the yang energy around the point. The puncture pushes this yang into the deep yin. On the other hand, to disperse, push heavily three times. This causes the yang energy to leave, to spread out. Before it returns, the puncture reaches the yin energy and attracts it to the exterior.

For some other authors, making crosses is not enough. One must press, pat and massage. The *Da Cheng* (V, 23r) explains that to puncture the yin without troubling the yang (thus dispersing), one must massage the point to push away the yang energy.

> *Those who know trust their left hand [which indicates and massages the point]. Those who do not know only trust their right [which holds the needle]. Before puncturing, press and massage the point to be punctured with the nail of the left thumb, patting and playing. When the energy comes, it feels as if there is an artery beating — puncture then. (DACH V, 24r)*

Press with the nail on the four sides of the point to excite. That makes blood and energy circulate. Then press on the point with the nail of the left hand and make the patient cough ten times. On the tenth, the needle enters the epidermis. (YXRM I, 43v)

Press above, below and on the four sides of the point to be punctured. This forces the blood and energy to spread. (DACH V, 26v)

If the pain is old, massage the painful point; this spreads the pain. Then put in the needle by agitating three times; that will remove the pain. "Massage" also refers to closing the needle hole after the puncture. (DACH V, 26v)

It has been observed in Paris that, for more sensitive people, massaging the point before the puncture considerably lessens the pain of needle insertion.

There does not seem to be any clear difference between marking with one cross for tonifying or three crosses for dispersing, or for that matter not marking at all. As for pressing around the point before puncturing, this increases the rapidity of the response at the pulses in a noticeable way.

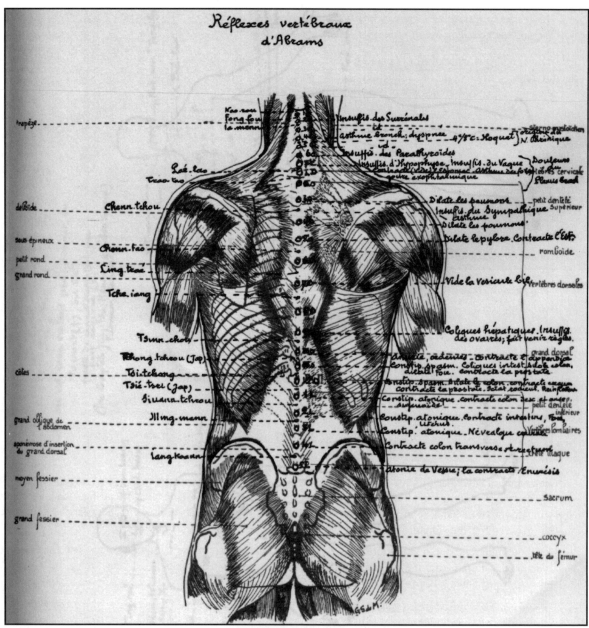

Vertebral reflexes of Abrams

Chapter XIII

Needle Technique (III)

I. The Puncture — II. To Tonify or Disperse by Respiration — III. Depth of Puncture — IV. Duration of Puncture — V. Movements of the Needle — VI. Massage During Puncture — VII. Removing the Needle

I. The Puncture

It would seem that the action of puncturing is very simple and can only be accomplished in one way. However, the word "puncture" has three meanings: the action of puncturing, the excitation produced by the puncture, and the trace produced.

Each of the necessary actions has been analyzed, differentiated and studied in order to obtain the maximum effect through the needle. Details on needling technique have been elaborated throughout the ancient history of acupuncture: during the time of the stone needles, which injured and dispersed; then at the time of the copper needles, which tonified; and lastly for the needles of iron or steel, which were neutral. The use of metals with opposite effects (gold for tonifying and silver for dispersing) allows most of these recommendations to be dispensed with. Nonetheless, knowledge is useful for increasing insufficient effects.

The method of inserting the needle into the skin is determined by the following factors:

1) Whether or not the needle is inserted to the required depth, either in one motion (with horizontal insertion, the yang is tonified; with straight insertion, the yang is dispersed); or by successive levels (with straight insertion).
2) The position of the needle: either perpendicular or oblique, and in which direction.
3) The manner of holding the needle for producing the least pain.

It has been noted in Paris that for the round-headed, thick needle, it is possible to put it in more quickly, more cleanly, and less painfully if the needle is held between the thumb and the index finger with the index finger pressing on the head. For thin needles or handles, there is risk in holding them like this for they may bend or break, or the head of the needle may be pushed into one's finger. For this one should follow the Chinese advice:

Guide the tail of the needle [the head] with the index finger of the right hand while the thumb and the middle finger grip the waist [shaft] and the ring-finger supports the head [the point]. (DACH V, 24v, 26r)

For short needles, hold one side with the thumb and the other with the index and middle fingers. (However, to feel the special vibration in the needle, the needle must be held between the thumb and ring-finger.)

Entry to the required depth either in one movement or by successive levels gives different effects which have not yet been clearly understood by Europeans. Inserting the needle to its required depth by successive levels tonifies by making the yang pass into the yin. The idea is that the skin is superficially charged with yang energy which is attracted to the point of the needle; the needle then carries the yang to the deep level, the yin. When the needle is inserted to its final depth in one motion, it reaches the deep yin level immediately. The needle drives the yin energy to the surface yang, and the action is dispersing.

It is also recommended (see Chapter VII) to enter in one "shot," but with the needle horizontal, acting on the yang without touching the yin.

To insert slowly and take out quickly gives great warmth. To insert quickly and take out slowly renders cold as ice. (DACH V, 26r)

To tonify, puncture first superficially then push deeply. To disperse, first puncture deeply, then come back superficially. (DACH VII, 10r)

*To tonify, first enter a little deeply; the needle first excites the **wei** energy (yang); then push it from behind and assist, filling the emptiness. To disperse, go in at one time deeply; then the needle excites the yang energy (yin), drives it, and takes out its fullness. (YXRM 43v)*

Inserting the needle in one movement disperses and creates cold. Pushing the needle slowly tonifies, reheats. (YXRM 42v; YIX I, 2)

The time necessary between successive advances in order to tonify is not fixed: in principle one must wait for the energy to ''bite'' at each level. The *Yi Xue Ru Men* (I, 43v) advises to wait ten respirations at each level before advancing further.

Three levels are differentiated: the superficial, which is in reality the epidermis, called Heaven *(tian);* the middle level, the dermis, called Man *(ren);* the deep level, the subcutaneous tissue, called Earth *(di).*

The difficulty preventing the use of these indications in Europe is that entering in three successive levels renews the pain of the puncture (or at least the annoyance) three times. Furthermore, it is difficult to distinguish the true clinical differences between insertion in one single movement or by successive levels. It would only be through a series of analogous cases that a judgement could be established. What has been shown is that for contractures, the effect is better with insertion to depth in one movement (dispersal) than by successive advances (tonification).

The perpendicular or oblique entry of the needle is governed by different conditions. First, the location: where the skin is very thin, for example on the finger, it is better to hold the needle obliquely, while in thick muscles it can be put in perpendicularly.

> *Where there is tendon or bone, puncture obliquely. Where there is neither tendon nor bone, puncture through.*
> *(DACH IV, 12v)*

There is also the distinction between yang and yin. When we want the yin to enter the yang or the yang to enter the yin, we must insert straight in and take out by successive levels as has been described above. But when one acts on only the yin or yang, one should insert horizontally for the yang and perpendicularly for the yin:

> *To puncture the yang meridians, lay the needle down so that it does not injure the **rong** [yin]. To puncture the yin divisions, raise the needle straight up in order not to injure the **wei** (yang). (DACH V, 23r; VI, 5r, 23r; II, 21v).*

> *To puncture the yang, lift and insert by laying down the needle, then turn it; the energy will respond. To puncture the yin, press in order to spread the yang energy and go in perpendicularly. (DACH VI, 9v)*

II. To Tonify or Disperse by Respiration

Making the patient cough or inhale or exhale forcefully while the needle is entering by successive levels at the moment of puncture produces effects which generally have been verified in Paris.

To cough just at the moment of puncture alleviates the pain to a great extent. Nurses and doctors who have adopted this method for their hypodermic punctures have observed that their needle enters more easily and causes less pain. This recommendation is made in Chinese books, but no comment is given on the diminution of the pain. One author even recommends making the patient cough ten times and puncturing only on the tenth cough *(YXRM I, 43v).*

> *To tonify [and to disperse], order the patient to cough one time while the needle enters into an area of the skin.*
> *(YIX I, 2r)*

> *To tonify, make the patient cough and drive the needle in at this moment; then, during the following exhalation, make it enter progressively up to .3 **cun** [about 5 mm.] at the maximum. To disperse, put the needle in during the cough in one movement, inserting it to .3 **cun**. (DACH VI, 6r)*

Let us add that for the points of the abdomen, if one punctures at the moment when the patient inhales brusquely, the pain is very much diminished, and the needle goes in more easily.

Inhalation or exhalation have several different effects acknowledged in Europe.[1] Europeans note that inhalation compresses the viscera and empties them of blood; likewise, the ancient Chinese commented:

> *To inhale is to disperse the interior, the yin of the five treasure organs. (DACH VI, 7v)*

Europeans recognize that exhalation increases the pressure on the peripheral vessels. The ancient Chinese commented:

> *Exhalation tonifies the yang of the triple warmer at the exterior. (DACH VI, 7v)*

The following clarifies the type of respiration in question:

There is natural respiration and forced respiration. The respiration made at the entrance and removal of the needle is forced respiration. In coma, where one cannot obtain a forced respiration, wait for the natural respiration. If at the time of exhalation you close the nose and mouth of the patient, his energy will beat like a drum. (DACH V, 25v)

It is explained that breathing is the means of harmonizing yin and yang. The *Nei Jing* states:

When one exhales the yang exits. When one inhales the yin enters. Though respiration is thus divided into yin and yang, it is in truth a single energy that animates the body. This energy is distributed in the interior to the five treasure organs [yin]. At the exterior, it follows the triple warmer, circulates throughout the body, follows and circulates in the meridians, flowing in all the points.

What enters and comes out of the five treasure organs responds to the four seasons. What circulates in the meridians and secondary vessels responds to the movement of heaven. All that is yang is superficial in the meridians and secondary vessels. All that is yin is deep in the treasure organs or workshop organs.

To exhale three times at the most is to tonify the yang and the triple warmer at the exterior. To inhale three times at the most is to disperse the yin of the five treasure organs at the interior. (Nei Jing, cited in DACH VI, 7v)

Given the above, one would think naturally of utilizing the differences between exhalation and inhalation to increase the tonifying or dispersing action. But here the authors are divided into three groups: for some, there is no marked difference; for others, exhalation at insertion augments the tonifying effect, while inhalation augments the dispersing effect; for still others, there is difference of effect according to male and female, right and left, morning and evening.

There is no marked difference. Experiments in Paris confirm the opinion that the effects are minimal although sometimes useful.

To tonify or disperse, it is not critical to exhale or inhale while putting in or taking out the needle. (DACH V, 25v)

Exhale to tonify; inhale to disperse. No difference has been clearly observed in Paris.

To tonify, order the patient to inhale through the nose and [at the puncture] to exhale through the mouth. The heat will come of itself. To disperse, order the patient to exhale through the nose and [at the puncture] to inhale through the mouth. The cold will come of itself. (DACH VI, 5r)

To exhale is to follow [to tonify]. To inhale is to go contrary to [to disperse]. (DACH V, 25r)

To tonify, make the patient exhale forcefully. The chest must be empty at the puncture. To disperse, inhale deeply; the breath should abound at the moment of the entry of the needle. (DACH V, 21v)

Make the needle enter the pore at the end of an exhalation; wait for the inhalation, then push the needle in slowly; this is to tonify. To make the needle enter the pore at the end of an inhalation without waiting for the exhalation, advance the needle in one movement and leave it; this is to disperse. (YXRM I, 42v)

To tonify, tell the patient to strain [to exhale] by closing the mouth. To disperse, tell the patient not to strain, and to inhale naturally. If the energy has come, it is of no use. (DACH V, 26v)

To tonify, insert the needle when the breath is just going out. To disperse, insert the needle when the breath enters. (DACH VI, 7v)

Since forced exhalation increases the pressure in the peripheral vessels and tonifies the yang, driving the superficial yang to the interior, it would be logical to make the patient cough or exhale for tonifying. On the other hand, since forced inhalation compresses the viscera, empties them of blood, and disperses the internal yin, thereby driving the excess yin to the exterior, it would be logical to make the patient strongly inhale at the moment of the puncture in order to disperse.

There is a distinction between men and women, morning and evening, and right and left:

Nothing of this sort has yet been observed in Paris.

In order to tonify or disperse, the ancients differentiated between right and left. Contemporaries make a distinction between men and women, although both are similar in that their blood circulates day and night in the same manner.

Before midday, when puncturing a yang meridian in a man, to exhale is to tonify and to inhale is to disperse. On the other hand, for the yin meridians, to inhale is to disperse. After midday, all is reversed.

In women, before noon, to inhale is to tonify the yang meridians; to exhale is to disperse them. To exhale is to tonify the yin meridians; to inhale is to disperse them. After midday, this is reversed. (DACH V, 25v)

III. Depth of Puncture

The depths should be fixed for each point. Texts which cite point locations also give point depths in *cun*. (Recall that the *cun* differs according to the individual.) These depths had apparently been determined in the twelfth century of our era, when a life-sized statue of bronze bearing all the points was made by order of the Emperor.

These depths are obviously debatable. Moreover, they are indicated as varying between adults or infants, fat or thin people. And if one concedes as probable that the point is under the subcutaneous tissue, the thickness of fatty tissue makes a great difference.

For understanding the depths, it is important to remember the three levels spoken of by the authors:

*When the needle arrives in the skin, that is the region of Heaven (**tianbu**). When it passes through the skin and enters the flesh, it is the region of Man (**renbu**). When it arrives in the gap of muscle and bone, it is the region of Earth (**dibu**). (DACH II, 27v)*

For other authors, it is a question of epidermal, dermal and subcutaneous tissue. However, it is certain that in proportion to size and stoutness, the more deeply one enters, the more marked, prolonged and certain is the effect.

The effects obtained vary according to the depth. In practice, the superficial (epidermis in summer, dermis in winter) is yang, life, warmth, and movement. The deep (dermis in summer, internal surface of the subcutaneous tissue in winter) is yin, cold, and immobility.

The yang region governs movement. The yin region governs immobility. (DACH VI, 9v)

When yang abounds, there is external warmth. If there is emptiness of yang, there is external cold. Excess of yin, internal cold; insufficiency of yin, internal warmth. To puncture superficially [yang] makes the disease go out to the external part. To puncture deeply [yin] makes the disease go out from the interior. (DACH I, 7v)

Yang excess causes excitations, agitation, spasm, external warmth. Yang insufficiency produces mental depression, weakness, flaccid paresis. Yin excess produces internal cold and atony. Yin insufficiency causes internal heat and congestion.

Because the two terms are relative, if there is excess yang (thus insufficiency of yin), one must make the yang pass into the yin; this is called "tonifying." In fact, tonifying the yin disperses the yang. If there is excess yin (thus insufficiency of yang), one must cause the yin to pass into the yang; this is called "dispersing." In fact, one should disperse the yin and tonify the yang.

Puncturing superficially removes the perverse energy and makes the energy of yang arise; that is, to puncture only through the epidermis makes the perverse energy go out of the yang exterior surface. Puncturing more deeply reaches the perverse yin energy. That is, to penetrate beyond the dermis without penetrating into the flesh makes the perverse energy of yin go out. Puncturing very deeply causes a descent into the energy of food. That is, entering into the muscle makes the energy of food go out.

Epidermis and dermis is the region that responds to the lungs and heart where the yang energy circulates. The flesh [muscle] is the region which responds to the liver and kidneys and where the yin energy circulates. (DACH VI, 9r)

To puncture the yang regions, start from the superficial. This is the division that responds to the heart and lungs. Starting from the superficial, needle obliquely, follow [along the meridian] and press, pushing slowly, tapping and making an effort. This causes the energy to abound and prosper. Afterwards turn the needle; the energy then spreads and expands by itself. Through the yang region one controls movement.

To puncture the yin region, start at the depth. It depends on the kidneys and liver. Those who desire to act on the yin must first press with the nail in order to spread the yang energy. Puncture straight and deep to the interior. Having obtained the energy, take out the needle. The energy harmonizes by itself. Through the yin region one controls immobility. (DACH VI, 9v)

Direct entry to the correct depth is not always easy. Difficulties may arise when the skin contracts from the rapid afflux of energy. If this occurs, put the needle first into the pore, then penetrate deeply at the moment the patient inhales or coughs.

To push the needle in, make it first penetrate slightly into the pore. Then at the moment when the patient inhales [to disperse] push softly. One can then enter into the depths. If not, the energy encounters the needle; one cannot enter. (DACH VI, 10v)

The place of puncture determines the depth, which is relative to the thickness of the skin and flesh. Near the nails on the fingers, the authors indicate .1 *cun* (hardly 2 mm.); needle horizontally. In fact, 1 mm. is sufficient. In the fleshy parts, particularly at *sanli* of the leg (ST-36), between the anterior tibial muscle and the extensor, the "certain" depth would be .8 *cun* (1.6 cm.). In fact, five or six millimeters is completely sufficient.

The general rule is well-defined, and is confirmed by the depths indicated for each point in Volume IV:

At the place where the flesh is thick, one enters deeply; where the flesh is thin, one stays superficial. (DACH VI, 10v)

The age and the nature of the patient determine the depth.

For thin people, and those who are thin-skinned, white complexioned, thin-lipped, light-voiced, the blood and energy are pure and easy to displace; the blood is easy to exhaust. Stay superficial and act quickly . . . This is also true for children and young people with weak energy.

For robust people with abundant energy and skin like leather, and for fat people, or those with thick skin, dark complexions, or pinched lips, their blood is black and thick, their energy rough and slow. Puncture deeply and leave a long time. (DACH I, 13r)

Fat people, being empty at the interior: tonify first, then follow by dispersing. Thin people, being full in the interior: first disperse, tonify after. (DACH VI, 10v)

The seasons alter the effects of each depth. Indeed, in winter when the energy retires to the interior like the sap and when the cold makes the skin and flesh contract, one must puncture more deeply than in summer in order to obtain the same effect. It has been observed in Paris that the reactions are slower in winter.

*The depth has some importance. It varies according to the seasons. In spring and summer, since the yang energy and the sun are higher, one must puncture less deeply: .5 **cun** [about 1 cm.] is to sink to the bottom; one must never go there. In autumn and in winter, the yang energy and the sun are lower, thus one must puncture deeply: .3 **cun** [about 6 mm.] is to stay superficial; one must always go beyond. (YXRM I, 43v)*

In spring and summer and for thin people, puncture superficially. In autumn and in winter and for fat people, puncture deeply. (DACH I, 20r; V, 25v)

Spring, summer, autumn, winter: each has its rule for the depth of the puncture.

In spring, if one punctures to the level of summer, one will cause diminished appetite and little energy. At the level of autumn, one will cause fear and often tears. At the level of winter, one will cause fullness and swelling without cure, and an incessant need to talk.

In summer, if one punctures at the level of spring, one will cause laziness. At the level of autumn, one will cause reticence and apprehension of being taken and held. At the level of winter, one will cause diminished energy and occasionally unhappiness.

In autumn, if one punctures at the level of spring, one will cause inquietude; and if there are desires, one forgets them upon arising. At the level of summer, one will cause the desire to stretch out and the capacity to dream. At the level of winter, one will cause shivering in the sun.

*In winter, if one punctures at the level of spring, one will cause insomnia. At the level of summer, one will make the energy rise; one will cause all the crippling pains [rheumatisms, **bi**]. At the level of autumn, one will cause thirst. (DACH I, 10r, citing the Nei Jing)*

Modern experiments have yielded no verification of these curious assertions.

In spring, the illnesses are in the body hairs. In summer, the illnesses are in the epidermis and dermis. In spring and summer, the yang energy is light and swimming on top. Flesh and muscles are thin and slim. The energy of blood does not abound. It is best to puncture superficially.

In autumn, illnesses are in the internal vessels. In winter, illnesses are in the muscles and bone. In autumn and winter, the yang energy concentrates and hides. The flesh thickens and fattens. The energy of blood is dominant and full. It is best to puncture deeply. (DACH I, 29r)

The type and chronicity of the illness also vary the depth.

Superficially: coldness with fever. At the middle level: illnesses of the vessels. Deeply: ankylosis, paralysis, rheumatism; also pain that cannot be aroused by pressing the finger on the place or on the point.

In each of these illnesses, the older the illness, the more deeply one must puncture.

> *For all illnesses of cold or warmth, make the energy circulate at the level of Heaven [superficial]. For the illnesses of vessels, act at the level of Man [middle]. For ankylosis, paralysis, rheumatism and pain, act at the level of Earth [deep]. (DACH V, 26v)*

> *Pain that cannot be reached by pressing with the finger is yin; one must puncture deeply. (DACH V, 26v.)*

> *If the illness is old, the perverse energy has entered deeply. One must puncture deeply. (DACH VI, 9v)*

> *In a general way, if the illness is in the skin, puncture it without injuring the flesh. If the illness is in the flesh, puncture it without injuring the muscles. If it is in the vessels, puncture it without injuring the skin. And if in the muscles, puncture these without injuring the bones. (YXRM I, 43r)*

The *Nei Jing* (quoted in *DACH II, 20r*) contains a long text on this subject (see also *DACH I, 5v*).

The type of meridian needled dictates the depth:

> *When the illness is in the three yang meridians [or in one of the three?] be sure of this and then puncture into the yang. When the illness is in the three yin meridians, be sure of this and then puncture into the yin level [or the yin divisions?]. (DACH I, 10r)[2]*

IV. Duration of Puncture

The length of time the needle is left in the flesh is said to have great importance, as it is considered to determine the tonifying or dispersing action.

> *To keep the needle a long time tonifies, whether or not there is emptiness. To act quickly disperses, whether or not there is fullness. (YIX I, 1v)*

What is meant by the vague terms "long time" and "quickly"? For some authors, "long time" and "to tonify" is a maximum of three inhalations and five exhalations. For other authors it is given as twenty-four respirations for puncture at the hands and during the spring and summer seasons; for the feet and for autumn and winter, thirty-six respirations is cited.

> *To tonify, do not keep the needle in more than three inhalations and five exhalations. (YIX I, 2v, citing Ba Cui of the sixteenth century)*

> *To tonify the meridians of the hands, keep the number for spring and summer at twenty-four respirations. For the meridians of the feet, the number for autumn and winter: thirty-six respirations. (DACH VI, 6r, quoting Yang)*

It has not been possible to determine whether these prescriptions were compiled for using the ancient stone needles or the iron needles that both tonify and disperse.

Using gold needles to tonify and silver to disperse, extensive experimentation in Paris has shown that almost immediately after their insertion the needles are gripped by the skin and often with such force as if held by metal pincers. Then, after a variable amount of time (from one to fifteen minutes), the skin relaxes and the needle can easily be taken out. During the entire puncture, the pulse of the organ related to the point continues to amplify and strengthen. When the skin is relaxed, the pulse ceases to amplify, no matter how much longer the needle is left in place. In general, gold needles are kept in for a longer time than silver needles.

It appears that the point holds steel or platinum needles longer when tonification is needed. The body thus makes its own choice. Gold needles are retained longer because the metal is used to tonify.

The collaboration of the organism plays an important part. When an organ is in perfect equilibrium, tonifying or dispersing it is difficult. Conversely, the more disordered an organ, the better it responds to the needles.

The *Da Cheng* recommends:

> *Verify that the energy is exhausted [that is, relaxed] before taking out the needle. If it is not exhausted, keep the needle at the door. (DACH VI, 8v)*

The pain under the needle is an indication of the duration:

> *If there is pain upon insertion, remove the needle the moment the pain stops. (YIX I, 2v)*

Heat and cold also give information:

> *For heat, one must wait for cold: retain the needle. When the yin energy has come abundantly, then, at the exhalation, remove the needle slowly without closing the hole.*

For cold, one must wait for heat. When the yang energy arrives abundantly, the energy at the needle will surely be hot. Then, upon exhalation, remove it quickly, immediately pressing on the hole. (DACH II, 21r)

Contractions or contractures also give an idea of how long to retain the needle:

If contraction occurs at insertion, remove the needle the moment the contraction stops. If no contraction occurs at insertion, remove the needle the moment there is contraction. (YIX I, 2v)

The constitution and vitality of the patient alter the duration because of the variation in the movement of the energy:

Puncture quickly for thin people with thin skin, pale complexion, thin lips, light voice . . . [and for] children. Retain a long time for fat, large shouldered, thick-skinned, dark complexioned people. (DACH I, 13r)

The age or strength of the illness also alters the duration:

For illnesses which resist cure, retain the needle a long time. Take the needle out quickly for illnesses which leave quickly. (DACH VI, 10v)

To tonify great cold, retain a long time. (DACH I, 12v; V, 25v)

The seasons have their importance. It has been observed in Paris that in winter improvement is slow to come; sometimes the effect is felt only after many days. In summer, on the other hand, the effects are immediate or very rapid and longer lasting.

In summer and spring, retain during twenty-four respirations; in winter and autumn, for thirty-six respirations. (DACH VI, 4r, quoting Bian Que)

V. Movements of the Needle

Both ancient tradition and modern experiments confirm that certain manipulations of the inserted needle markedly increase, even double, the tonifying or dispersing effect of the puncture.

These movements can be divided into three groups:

1) Rotation, or twirling back and forth.
2) Agitation up and down.
3) Agitation or inclination to the side.

Rotation, or twirling back and forth. It is possible either to make the needle turn in place without changing level (*dong*, to shift), or to rotate while advancing (*tui*, to push). To enter by twirling clockwise tonifies and is a yang movement. To take out by twirling counterclockwise (*yin*, to conduct) disperses and is yin.

Rotating too slowly does not remove the illness. Rotating too quickly causes considerable pain.

To enter, rotate as if twisting a thread, but not so tightly as to cause acute pain. Making the needle turn by pushing the thumb ahead makes the energy rise; this tonifies. (DACH VI, 4v; V, 26r)

Dong *is to rotate in place.* Tui *is to rotate while advancing. Twisting too quickly causes pain. Twisting too slowly does not remove the illness. One divides the movement into yin by rotating to the left and yang by rotating to the right. (DACH V, 26v)*

Driving the needle in by twirling [clockwise] to the middle level tonifies. Removing the needle from the middle level by twirling [counterclockwise] disperses. (DACH VI, 1v)

To tonify, twirl the needle nine times [see ''Numbers,'' Volume I, Appendix I]. (DACH VI, 6r)

Enter slowly by twirling clockwise (tui); *the energy will progress by itself. Removing [the needle] by twirling counterclockwise is called* fei, *to fly. (DACH VI, 8r)*

Agitation up and down. It is possible simply to agitate up and down (see *DACH VI, 5r*):

Yao, to agitate, is to agitate up and down and to the right and left; that can dissipate all shock. (DACH V, 28r)

To tonify, put the needle in 1/10 **cun,** *make the patient exhale once by the mouth. Withdraw three times and insert three times. The heat will come by itself. To disperse, insert the needle to 1/10* **cun,** *make the patient inhale, insert it three times and withdraw it three times. The cold will come of itself. (DACH VI, 5r)*

Even without this positive agitation it is possible to obtain a similar movement by tapping the needle lightly with the tip of the finger or with the nail; that is called *tan* (this also means "to pinch above or below the needle" (see *DACH V, 26v*, and *DACH VI, 5r*). The word *nu*, "to make an effort," seems to have the same meaning:

> *Tan and **nu** mean to use the nail for tapping **(tan)** with the finger and waiting for the energy to arrive. One must take it bit by bit, first superficially, then deep, and from the outside push to the interior; this is the means of tonifying. (DACH VI, 5r)*

The movements of agitating up and down and rotating can be combined. The name of this complex movement is *fei*, to fly.

> *To agitate up and down, from the right to the left, by twirling and "flying" the needle like the beating of wings, is **fei**, to fly. (DACH V, 28r)*

> *Twist the needle between the thumb and index finger and agitate it three times up and down, making it tremble. (DACH V, 26v)*

The action thus described greatly increases the action of the punctured point, but it is somewhat painful. Its use is recommended for all cases where the pulse of the organ is modified quickly enough by the puncture.

> *To incline the needle* is called *zhuan*, "to lean."

> *Incline the needle upward, and the energy will rise by itself. Incline the needle downward, and the energy will descend by itself. Incline the needle toward the left, and the energy will go to the left. Incline the needle toward the right, and the energy will go to the right. (DACH VI, 8r)*

> *To disperse or to tonify, turn the head [the point] of the needle towards the area of the illness. (YIX I, 2r, citing Ba Cui)*

These effects have yet to be verified.

VI. Massage During Puncture

Certain kinds of massage are useful for attracting the energy to the needle, or to make it circulate along the meridian. This can be observed when puncturing areas which are slow to respond, or when puncturing apathetic or tired people, whose energy may be massed in certain regions with local fullness.

The *Da Cheng* states:

> *If there is fullness, then follow **(xun)**, massage **(men)**, pinch **(tan nu)**. This will conduct the energy. (DACH II, 21r)*

One must distinguish between massaging the point before the puncture, already described in the preceding chapter; massaging along the meridian; and pinching with the nail.

1) *Massage along the meridian:*

> *To follow **(xun)** is to go up or down by following [the meridian] with the hand. This causes going and coming [of energy and blood]. (DACH II, 21v; 25v)*

> *If, when one punctures, the energy is obstructed and does not move, follow the track of the meridian by pressing it with the nail of the thumb; the energy will communicate. (DACH VI, 1r)*

The effect, based on the flow of energy, is different depending on whether one directs the needle towards the place of the illness or follows the course of the meridian.

> *To tonify, follow the meridian [from the point] to the area of the illness. The energy follows the hand and circulates. To disperse, follow the meridian by pressing towards the needle from the area of the illness and drive the energy past the location of the needle. (DACH VI, 4v)*

This has been verified on occasion and is a potential aid which must not be forgotten in cases which require it.

2) *Pinching with the nail:*

> *Tan is to pinch between the nail of the thumb and the index finger. Now up with the nail of the thumb when the illness is up, now down with the nail of the index finger when the illness is down. This makes the energy circulate and it arrives more easily. (DACH VI, 26v)*

VII. Removing the Needle

The method of removing the needle is said to vary the pain, the effusion of blood and the effect. In fact, this aspect of removing the needle is not very obvious.[3]

However, if one waits for the skin to relax around the needle, the removal causes no pain; the brusque removal from the skin when it is still tight causes acute pain and bleeding.

It has been shown that a skillful puncture with a needle with a slightly rounded point very rarely causes bleeding. A few drops of blood will appear if there is a misplaced venule under the point (which is not a usual occurrence) or if the puncture has not been made at the center of the point.

> *Take out the needle slowly. Taking it out too fast injures the energy. (DACH VI, 6r)*

> *Take the needle out slowly two or three times and make it turn; then no blood will come. (DACH II, 26r)*

Removing the needle quickly after having inserted it slowly is supposed to have a warming effect. Removing it slowly after having inserted it quickly has a cooling effect.

> *To remove quickly after having inserted slowly gives great heat. To remove slowly after having inserted quickly causes cold like ice. Before midday, taking out until the level of Heaven favors the yang and thus warms again. After midday, this favors the yin and thus causes cold again. For men, taking out before midday gives heat, and in the afternoon, cold again; for women, it is the reverse. (DACH V, 26v)*

These assertions have yet to be verified. The editor of the *Da Cheng* even adds:

> *Each time one takes the needle out quickly without waiting, the illness will come back at dusk. (DACH II, 28r)*

Another author, however, writes:

> *To implant slowly, to take out quickly [to tonify] gives great heat. To implant quickly and take out slowly [to disperse] causes cold like ice. (DACH V, 26v)*

One should distinguish (see Chapter VII) between: 1) treating only the yang (horizontal insertion) or only the yin (needle inserted in one movement and slowly taken out); and 2) making the yin pass into the yang and vice versa (to tonify, insert by successive levels and remove in one movement; to disperse, insert in one movement and remove by successive levels.)

One should not be confused between taking out slowly and taking out many times; the latter is said to bring to the surface the compressed yin energy which is not transforming itself into yang. It is written:

> *To disperse, take out the needle level by level [Earth, Man, Heaven] stopping for three respirations at each. (DACH VI, 1v)*

> *To disperse the heat, take out in three levels, first deep, then more superficial. One obtains energy each time. (DACH V., 2r)*

For tonification, it is recommended to take the needle out slowly, but not by successive levels:

> *To tonify by removing, take the needle out one level; stop and twirl; wait one inhalation before removing; withdraw slowly. (DACH VI, 6r)*

Opening or closing the exit hole when the needle has been removed can have different effects for energy and blood.

> *If, with the belly of the index finger, one rushes to press on the eye of the point, the energy does not escape and the blood does not come out. If, in addition, one presses on the point with clay and massages a great deal, it is admirable. (YIX I, 2v)*

> *If the blood is abundant, massage surely stops it. It is the means to stop the blood. Order the patient to continue to massage for some time. After that there will never be any difficulties. (DACH II, 21v).*

Hence, for tonification it is recommended that after taking out the needle one closes the punctured point with the tip of the finger and massages and compresses the place. Conversely, to disperse one should leave the point open.

These prescriptions probably date from the time of the stone needles. Closing the exit hole prevents blood flow. Opening the point favors blood flow which, like all bleeding, is dispersing. With modern needles, which do not cause bleeding, it has not been possible to observe these distinctions.

However, the theory speaks of energy. Thus, for tonification of the external yang energy pressed towards the internal yin, the energy must be contained within. To disperse the internal yin energy, bringing it to the surface by dispersion, its passage outward must be free and unrestrained.

To tonify, close the door of the point in order to keep the energy of awareness at the interior . . . To disperse, do not close the hole. (DACH V, 28v)

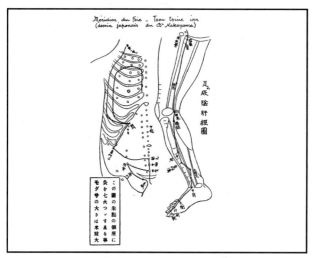

Meridian of the liver (Nakayama)

Notes

[1] According to Hédon *(Physiology, 263)*, brusque exhalation compresses the heart and thoracic vessels and partly empties them of blood. A venous stasis follows. The pressure increases in the peripheral vessels. On the other hand, forced inspiration by thoracic suction attracts the venous blood to the heart; by the lowering of the diaphragm the abdominal viscera are compressed and the portal vein, vena cava, and the internal organs are thus emptied of blood.

[2] Each depth corresponds with an organ according to the ancient observations. This has yet to be verified.

When reading the Nan Jing, I always noticed that the most virtuous masters of the needle commented that the skin and flesh of man has some thick places and some thin places. In actuality, the yang energy circulates at the surface of the skin in the region of the heart and lungs. The yin energy circulates under the skin in the region of the liver and kidneys.

However, through insightful examination, the Qian Jin Fang of Sun Simo says: "The needle enters at 1/10 of a **cun** *to meet the energy of Heaven and Earth. The needle enters at 2/10 to determine what expires and inspires, the entry and exit of energy from above and below, from water and fire. The needle enters to 3/10 to determine now if the energy of the four seasons, five elements, five treasure organs and six workshop organs are harmonized or in counterflow.*

By contrast, the **Xuan Zhou Mi Yao** *says: "At 3/10, one reaches the region of the heart and lungs where the yang energy circulates. If one enters in the skin at 5/10, it is the region of the kidneys and liver where the yin energy circulates. . . ."*

These rules are different from one another; they do not clarify each other. (DACH VI, 9v, citing the Ju Ying)

[3] Taking out the inserted needle is indicated by *ti*, to bring, or *shen*, to extend.

Shen *is [the same as]* **ti**. *Ti is to take out from the level of the Earth [deep] until the level of Man [middle] or of Heaven (superficial). (DACH V, 26v)*

Chapter XIV

Needle Technique (IV)

I. Number of Punctures — II. Number of Sessions — III. Risks and Possible Accidents

I. Number of Punctures

For the number of punctures in a single session, one must distinguish between the number of punctures on the same point and the total number of points punctured in the same session.

Several consecutive punctures on the same point are recommended for tenacious pain and for lightning-like lumbar neuralgia.

The *Yi Xue* states:

> *For pain like lightning in the lumbar area, puncture **qihai** (CV-6), leaving the needle in for three respirations; take it out and wait twenty-five respirations. With the left hand, strongly press the point. Then puncture again during three respirations. Puncture like this three times with tonification and three times with dispersal. (YIX I, 43v)*

Experience shows that we can extend this method to all pain and contracture with good results, the rule being to stop when the pain or contracture has ceased.

For the organs, there is risk of delayed reactions, particularly in wintertime, adding to the immediate effect and going beyond the aim. It is always wiser to see the patient again two or three days after the first puncture and to add what is needed. In acute and serious cases it is beneficial to treat again every half-hour until the symptoms are relieved.

The number of punctures in the same session is determined by the state of the patient.

> *For the number of punctures, first examine the meridians; decide according to the illness; see where there is fullness or emptiness; harmonize. (DACH I, 9v)*

As each puncture has an effect on one organ or region, it is obvious that the number of punctures is proportional to the number of disordered organs or regions. This is true unless it is possible to treat both the root and branch of the problem with one puncture.

> *Illnesses do not always affect only one organ and meridian — it may be necessary to treat many. (DACH VI, 11, quoting Li Gao)*

> *Finally, there are roots and branches. One puncture can cure the branches without taking out the root, or can remove the root without touching the branches; then many punctures are necessary to cure the roots and neighbors. (DACH V, 28r)*

The state of the patient and his nervous resistance are also important factors to take into account:

> *The number of punctures depends on the abundance or degeneration of the energy . . . when the illness is stopped, do not puncture further. (DACH I, 8v)*

Another factor involved in determining the number of punctures is the lunar cycle. (This has been possible to verify, but not with Chinese precision.) It is true that at the new moon the needles have a much livelier action than at the full moon, and the patient feels the puncture more strongly.

> *If one punctures more than the number of days [of the moon], then the energy is drained. If this number is not reached, then the energy will not be dispersed. Do not forget: one puncture the first day of the moon with progressive augmentation until fifteen punctures on the fifteenth day [full moon]; then with a progressive diminution until one puncture at the last day of the moon. (DACH I, 8v)*

The seasons also have their importance: in summer, it is possible to cure the secondary disordered organs ("branches") if one discerns the primary disordered organ ("root"). In winter it is much more difficult to obtain such a result. The climate of the north of China, enlivening, dry, and especially bright, explains the more intense action of the needles. In Japan, a humid country, it is necessary to use a great number of moxas in all seasons. The north of France is the same.

The seriousness of the illness and how chronic it has become are also elements to take into consideration.

For several reasons, it is better to keep the number of punctures to a minimum. First, the patient does not suffer as much. Second, since his energy is utilized without adding anything to it, it is better to direct all the strength he possesses to the illness and to act in the same direction. Finally, the real effects of each point can be better appreciated while reducing the unpredictable variables each additional point adds.

However, Europeans, who take a lot of medicine, need to be punctured in more points, since they respond less sensitively.

> For each patient choose one or two points. (DACH 4r)

> A single puncture can make hundreds of illnesses disappear. Make at the maximum four punctures. Those who riddle the whole body with needles are detestable. (YIX I, 28v)

II. Number of Sessions

The number of sessions is always proportional to the seriousness and the age of the illness. Although one session generally suffices for recent problems, many more are needed for illnesses of long duration.

> One puncture [session] suffices for tonifying or dispersing slight illnesses. But if the illness is more serious, two or three sessions will be necessary. (DACH VI, 8v)

> When the illness is recent and less deep, one session should be enough to cure. When it is deep and entrenched, many punctures are necessary to begin to cure . . . Moreover, illnesses do not always exit from a single meridian. With one needle, even if the branches are cured, the root is not removed. (DACH VI, 11r)

Of clinical and diagnostic interest is the observation that if two sessions do not give even a weak, noticeable result, there is a material obstacle, an unperceived lesion, which an attentive search always reveals. In such a case, the illness may not be within the scope of acupuncture.

A second session the same day is permissible for children. There must be very serious reasons to allow this for adults. One must not forget, however, that the effects of the needle are not always immediate, particularly in winter. By puncturing again the same day one risks going beyond the goal or reversing the effect. Therefore, if many sessions must be condensed into a shorter time period, it is wiser not to use the same points but to use alternative points (mother and child, husband and wife, midday-midnight, etc.). For acute and serious cases, it is sometimes necessary to repeat the sessions every half-hour.

> Children, having very tender flesh, must be punctured very superficially. However, they can be punctured a second time the same day. (DACH I, 13r)

The interval between sessions varies according to the season, the age and strength of the patient, and the desired effect. In general, it has been observed in Paris that we get the best effects by waiting until the end of the resultant amelioration before recommencing. Except for acute cases, if there has been only slight immediate improvement, it is best to wait two days in summer and eight days in winter before repeating the treatment. Frequently, sudden improvement has been noted over these intervals.

In China, these intervals can be shortened, due perhaps to the climate, or the fact that less medicine is taken there, or even perhaps because the race is more receptive.

> Children can be punctured a second time the same day. (DACH I, 13r)

> In chronic illnesses, puncture with an interval of one day [first, third, fifth, seventh day]. (DACH VI, 9v)

> When the evil is lodged in the gap of the five treasure organs, the meridians are sick and painful . . . One session every two days. If with one session there is no cure, five sessions in all. (DACH I, 9r, citing the Nei Jing)

III. Risks and Possible Accidents

The pain of the puncture is the first possible risk. However, for the same individual all points are not equally sensitive. The skin is naturally more sensitive on the sides of the fingers than on fatty areas of the thighs or the forearm. Likewise, sensitivity varies greatly from one individual to another. We know of some children who puncture themselves or who say they have felt ''merely the fingernail'' when even a sensitive spot has been punctured. On the other hand, we know some robust and courageous men who speak of true pain. However, most patients speak about the puncture as only disagreeable or irritating, and compare it more to a mosquito bite without the itch.

The condition of the needle, dexterity of the hand, and accuracy in finding the center of the point (which is nearly insensitive, even though the region one centimeter in diameter around the point is hypersensitive) are undoubtedly important for puncturing without pain:

> If there is pain under the needle, the hand is too rough. The "loins" of the needle must be supported and stabilized with the left hand while the right, according to the case, tonifies or disperses. If, in spite of this, there is still pain, do not take out the needle. Ask the patient to inhale deeply, and during the inhalation twirl the needle while withdrawing it one step; then there will be no pain. If there is still pain, withdraw it a little again. And if there is still pain, insert another needle, which commands [higher on the meridian]; that will surely stop the pain.
> (DACH V, 28r)

This directive has been verified many times and is beneficial when dealing with hypersensitive people.

Syncope under the needle is extremely rare. Of the means cited, those which give the best results in preventing fainting or reviving a patient are the following: make the patient lie down on a flat surface, massage *sanli* of the arm (LI-10) and *shaochong* (HT-9) firmly with the nail; add *renzhong* (GV-25, IS GV-26) if needed.

The author of the *Yi Xue* of the eighteenth century wrote:

> Nowadays, practitioners with needles are less numerous; those with poisons are more numerous. This is because of the patient's erroneous fear of fainting from the needle.
>
> Fainting is an emptiness of the energy of awareness. So, the ancients said: "When the vessels are not in a favorable state, do not puncture." Also avoid puncturing during great wind, great rain, great snow, and cloudy weather [storms]; also during drunkenness, great fatigue, menses, fear, fasting, and great grief.
>
> Of the three thousand patients that I have punctured, I have seen only sixteen men and one woman faint. (YIX I, 2v)

It is somewhat curious that in Europe also men are more susceptible to syncope than women. It is possible to say that of the more than three thousand patients seen in Paris, there have not been more than five cases of fainting.

> If this happens, press at the flesh 2 mm. above the nail of each of the ten fingers; the person who has fainted will then be revived. Nowadays one also presses with the nail under the nose of the patient in the flesh of the midline (philtrum). But the preceding action is more rapid.
>
> It should be noted that people who faint under the needle always obtain a great effect [from the treatment] because of the effective vigor of their energy and blood. (YIX I, 3r)

The *Da Cheng* indicates one other method:

> If there is fainting under the needle, tonify **sanli** of the leg (ST-36) or at **shuigou** [middle of the lip, also called **renzhong** (GV-25 IS GV-26)]. Fainting in general comes from the heart. If the patient has no fear, one can see it in the unchanged color of his face: he will surely not faint. If there is syncope by puncturing a point on the liver channel, puncture **xingjian** (LR-2); as soon as the needle is put in the patient will revive. (DACH II, 28r)

The *Yi Xue* again states:

> The celebrated Li of Nanfeng gives this advice: in case of fainting under the needle, do not take it out; puncture alongside it with another needle. When the patient wakes up, give him a hot beverage to drink. Wait a long time before giving the puncture again.
>
> In serious cases, puncture at the hand and arm, above and on the sides, in the interval of the ribs, on the flesh of the belly, at the epigastrium, at the "point that revives" [arm-**sanli**, LI-10]. His malaise will disappear. But if the needle is removed, it will cause some pain for the patient. (YIX I, 3r)

For needle breakage, which can occur only with instruments of steel or brittle and non-pliant alloys, the advice is as follows:

> When a needle is broken, immediately puncture very near it with another needle. Tonify [put in slowly] and the broken bit will come out. Or have a magnet which draws the bit out. Or apply a wet plaster which will make the broken bit come out little by little. (DACH V, 28r)

The *Yi Xue Ru Men* gives additional advice along with an herbal formula in cases of inflammation.

Chapter XV

Moxa Technique

I. Description — II. Effects — III. Tonifying or Dispersing with Moxa — IV. Order of Succession of Moxa, Hours, Times — V. After Moxa

I. Description

The French word ''moxa'' comes from the Japanese *mogusa* and was transmitted to us by the Dutch living in Japan during the sixteenth and seventeenth centuries. The Chinese name is *jiu.* The ideogram is composed of the element ''fire — reclining man.'' The pronunciation of this character in Japanese is *kyu.* The word ''moxa'' also indicates very rapid touching, with the body itself being burned. (The burn, if there is one, is called *chuang.*)

In China, moxa consists of a small ball called *zhu,* ''candle'' (thickness of a large pea or a chickpea), made of desiccated leaves of artemisia (*ai, Artemisia sinensis* or *Artemesia urens,* commonly called mugwort). The little ball is put on the hole of a coin (like our coins of nickel) and ignited, burning to red without flaming like tinder.

Authors emphasize the fact that no other plant can give results as good as artemisia. Indeed, this plant — similar to absinthe — contains a stimulating ingredient which when heated suddenly is projected with the burning gas, penetrating the skin. This accords with the traditional theory on moxa's penetrating qualities.

> *Dan Xi states: The nature of artemisia is its extreme heat. The moxa makes the fire enter, rise and circulate. If it enters by the mouth with medicine, it descends and circulates . . . The flavor of artemisia is bitter. Its energy is heat. Through it, yin and yang have no more poison. (DACH XI, 17r)*

The best artemisia is cultivated and harvested on the fifth day of the fifth moon (beginning of June) in Qizhou (northeast of Hubei on the Yangzi in the lower part of Hankou). It is quickly dried, crushed finely in a mortar, and when separated from the dust, is ready. If used during great drought, its effects increase. Wild artemisia is equally good (see *DACH* XI, 17r).[1]

The little balls of artemisia, called candles (*zhu*), sometimes contain other substances:

> *For moxa at **juquan** [Extra point 8 on the tongue]: if the cough is hot, take only the tips of **xiong-huang** [natural sulphur of arsenic] and burn with artemisia. If the cough is cold, take the tips of **kuan dong hua** [coltsfoot] and burn with artemisia. (YIX II, 22v)*

The thickness of the ''candles'' is given according the *Nei Jing:*

> *Either the size of a grain [similar in size to a chickpea] of azedarach [Melia azedarach], or for infants up to one year, the size of ''the dropping of a little bird.'' The **Ming Tang** requires at least 3/10 of a **cun** [7 mm. in diameter]; if not, the fire will not penetrate. For intestinal spasms, angina of the chest, or accumulations of the heart, large candles are necessary. On the face, use very small ones; on hands and feet, a little larger. (DACH XI, 17r)*

For igniting:

> *In antiquity one used a lens, probably of rock crystal (**huo zhu,** ''pearls of fire''). If not this, then a wick put into hemp oil, or an iron rod heated to redness. (YIX I, 12v; DACH XI, 17v)*

In fact, one should light the moxa from underneath through the hole of the coin so that it is consumed slowly, rising with all the heat directed to the skin.

Japanese practitioners use a stick of artemisia tinder that burns to redness without flame. The burning end is touched rapidly on the point protected by several thicknesses of note-paper; the number of papers depends on the sensitivity of the patient, the place touched and the seriousness of the illness.

In Europe, we have experimented with separating the heat element from the other elements. For this one of the following is used:

1)   A tube of metal full of boiling water giving dry heat. The tube should not be too small lest the acupoint be missed.

2)   A spoon dipped in boiling water and rubbed rapidly against the point. Many patients choose this method.

3)   For humid heat, a plug of cloth about a centimeter in diameter soaked in boiling water (cotton-wool absorbs too much and burns) or a hot shaving brush soaked and shaken.

In all three cases, one should touch very quickly without resting the instrument on the skin in order to avoid a burn, since the contact is made at about 70° C.

Although dry or wet heat alone gives very good results, it is undeniable that artemisia tinder has a more tonifying effect and activity. Thus, it would seem that artemisia adds a special tonifying element. However, the above warming techniques by themselves are complicated enough to administer, not to mention the even greater difficulty of obtaining artemisia tinder.[2]

The origin of artemisia moxa is attributed to two different places:

The *Nei Jing* suggests that it could have been used first in the north of China or Asia:

> *The north is the territory where the inhabitants hide themselves between heaven and earth. The land there is elevated and mountainous. They stay there in the wind, the cold and the ice. They like the wild and nourish themselves with dairy products. From the cold the organs create illnesses of fullness. To treat, moxas and firebrands are preferred. That is why moxa and firebrands come from the north. (Su Wen, cited in DACH I, 2v)*

Regarding the prehistoric firebrands, the ancient texts state that burns cause redness and activate the blood, whereas an injury causes paleness and weakness.

On the other hand, a passage in a book from the seventh century A.D., the *Qian Jin Fang* by Sun Simo, indicates that moxa was used in the valley of the Yangzi.

In the third century B.C., numerous people from the Korean peninsula had been transported into the lower valley of the Yangzi. The Japanese, who borrowed their medicine first from the Koreans, still have a preference for moxa. Could the mountainous and cold region of the north mentioned in the *Nei Jing* be Korea or Mongolia?

> *The **Qian Jin Fang** reports: The civil servants travelling to the countries of **Wu** and **Zhou** [lower and upper Yangzi] always bear two or three partially healed moxa scars. Miasmas, tidal fevers and poisons cannot reach them. That is why in the countries of **Wu** and **Zhou**, moxa is used a great deal. (YIX I, 12r)*

II. Effects

Moxa is rightly considered as having a different effect from needles. Moxa is softer, smoother, and has much less risk of causing shock. It is possible to use it every day, which one could not safely do with needles. Moxa is recommended for the aged, infants and weak people. As it can be used repeatedly, its continued action gives results which would not be possible with needles. Moxa is recommended for cold, emptiness, and rheumatism, for which its continued action is unequaled.

After one session of needles, daily moxas are excellent.

> *The needle is energetic but does not have the reliability of moxa. Moxa is reliable but does not have the energy of the needle. When energy and blood are lacking at the same time, either in old people or infants, or when treating the throat, the chest, the abdomen or the back, the needle does not have the reliability of moxa. What the needle cannot affect, moxa gives. (YIX I, 12r)*

> *When the yin and yang are empty, the fire fills them. When the meridians are hollow and low, the fire fills them. (DACH XI, 17r)*

When comparing the action of needles and moxa, one should not forget that many traditions come from the time when the stone needles were used only for dispersing and moxa was necessarily used for tonifying. It is true, however, that the needles bring only their metal to the body in contrast with moxa which, besides the light shock caused by the sudden heat, brings the heat itself, and if one uses artemisia, the additional bombardment of stimulating ions.

The *Yi Xue Ru Men* (I, 45v) even comments:

> *For what medicines have not been able to affect, for what the needles cannot reach, moxas are necessary.*

Bian Que, the illustrious practitioner of the fifth century B.C., always recommends the use of moxa for tonifying, although for needles he indicates means of tonifying as well as dispersing. In fact, it has been observed in Paris that hot compresses relax spasms and cause the blood to circulate. It seems that moxas have a similar action for the energy.

In Paris, when treating exhausted or chronically diseased patients, the best results have been obtained through the daily use of moxa on the point responding to their condition.

Whatever the means used to give moxa, it is best if the patient is not burned deeply. A simple redness gives adequate results, particularly if it is necessary to repeat the moxa every day for one or two months. However, in China, an important school says that moxa has an effect only if it provokes a water-blister (*chuang,* ''injury''). Perhaps this is an ancient tradition.

> *According to the* **Zi Sheng,** *each time that one obtains a blister, the patient is cured. If one does not get it, the illness is not dissipated. The* **Jia Yi Jing** *states: ''If the moxa has not produced a blister, repeat and burn deeply so that the heat fries — in three days there will be a blister.'' This text gives prescriptions on making moxas over red onion (with a three to five day old stem, without the green part) mixed with cinders and applied ten times; the blister will appear on the third day. (DACH XI, 18r)*

The cure attributed to the blisters makes one think that they were trying for a truly derived abscess:

> *The ancients did not anoint the blisters and did not cover them with drugs or fat. It must be that pus came out abundantly; then disease was suppressed. It is better to wait to anoint. If one closes too soon, one cures too soon. It is to be feared that the root of the disease will not be completely removed. (DACH XI, 18r)*

The same passage even gives prescriptions for irritating ointments to ''guide the disease towards the mouth of the blister and to make it come out,'' which recalls our cauteries.

The preference for moxa over needles is governed by three different considerations: the site of burning, the illness, and the patient.

The site:

> *Moxa is only useful on the four limbs. (DACH IX, 14r)*
>
> *For all points which are close to bone, for the top of the body, where the needle enters a little deeply, one can burn a lot and without danger. (YIX I, 12v)*

The illness:

> *What cannot be done by the needle can be done with moxa. (YIX I, 12r)*
>
> *When the energy is empty, when yin and yang are both empty, the fire cures by itself. When the pulses are hollow and low, fire supports them; tonify with fire. When energy abounds, when pulses and vessels are firm and hard, disperse with fire. However, when the meridians are empty and the secondary vessels full, use moxa for the yin and needles for the yang. And when the meridians are full and the secondary vessels empty, use moxa for the yang and needles for the yin. (DACH XI, 17r)*

Recall that the secondary vessel passage points make the yin communicate with the yang and vice versa.

Moxa is not advisable in certain congestive or inflammatory illnesses.

> *Do not burn a lot in fires of the chest or diaphragm. It is not at all wise to burn when there is fire [inflammation]. Indeed, that would be to tonify a fullness.*

The patient:

Moxa is especially advised for the aged, infants, or weak and exhausted people. In practice, it is indicated as adding much to the effect of the needle when it is used at the point immediately after the needle is taken out. For people having a tendency toward hypotension, repeated moxa at leg-*sanli* (ST-36) can raise the blood pressure considerably.

III. Tonifying or Dispersing with Moxa

When the stone needle was still used, it was thought that moxas were only for tonifying, needles for dispersing. Later it was recognized that it was possible to tonify or disperse with moxa as well as with needles. Furthermore, it is often advised to use one method on the yin, for example, and another on the yang.

The difference between tonifying and dispersing is thus revealed:

In order to tonify with fire, do not blow on the burning artemisia; wait for it to go out. Then press the point [with the finger]. And if there is a blister, that is perfect. To disperse, quickly blow out the fire and open the point. (DACH XI, 17r)

In Paris, experiments have shown that the difference between tonifying and dispersing relates particularly to the number of moxas: three or four moxas in succession made each day (particularly in the evening) disperses. Seven to ten moxas on the same point each morning tonifies.

The combining of moxa with needles is given:

If the meridians are empty and the secondary vessel passage points full — moxa to the yin and needles to the yang. If the meridians are full and the secondary vessels empty — moxa to the yang and needles to the yin. (DACH XI, 17r)

The number of moxas (zhuang) can be counted either by those made following one another on the same point or by the total distributed over many days. It depends on how chronic the illness is, the age of the patient and the points chosen.

Experiments in France have shown that the number in one day must not go beyond three or four to disperse and seven to ten to tonify. More than five on the same point tonifies instead of disperses; more than ten gives the risk of a burn which can cause suffering and leaves an unsightly scar.

The ancient texts do not clearly distinguish between the daily number and the total number, a distinction of very great importance. However, the aim is to cure. The celebrated Li Gao (Dong Yuan, twelfth century) wrote:

*For moxa at leg-**sanli** (ST-36), if seven does not give a result, make five more and there will be a result. (DACH IV, 14v)*

In Japan, the principal numbers are from five to seven by day and by point, repeated each day during fifteen days per month until the cure. As for the length of the treatment, it is written:

Mencius states that an illness of seven years demands three years of moxa. (YIX I, 2r)

*The hundred meridians of the **Ming Tang** states: needles 6/10 **cun** [1.5 cm.] maximum; moxas, three at most. But that is not enough to cure. This is why from that time onward we have evaluated the exhaustion of the patient and the seriousness of the illness. For the head, up to seven moxas; for accumulations, seven times seven moxas.*

*According to the **Qian Jin Fang**, for a strong man, or with an illness having deep roots, one can double the number of moxas in the prescription. If it is a matter of old people or infants or thin or weak people, one can diminish this amount by half.*

*In his Rule of Moxas, Bian Que gives up to 300 or 500 times; 1000 times, that is too much. Zao, in his Rule of Moxas, talks of 50 to 100. The **Xiao Bing Zhu Fang** (''All Prescriptions for Small Sicknesses'') quotes the same number.*

*The guide to the **Tong Ren** [Bronze Man of the Twelfth Century] states: for curing neuralgias **(feng)** burn at **shangxing** (GV-22, IS GV-23); **shenting** (GV-23, IS GV-24); and **baihui** (GV-19, IS GV-20), up to 200 moxas on the abdomen and up to 500 moxas on the back.*

*At **juque** (CV-14) and **jiuwei** (CV-15), it is not wise to burn a lot because the four limbs would be without strength. At **sanli** of the leg (ST-36) the Qian Jin Fang speaks of 300 times at most. **Xinshu** (BL-15) is forbidden to moxa except for apoplexy, where one burns rapidly up to a hundred moxas. One sees that the rule of the seriousness of the illness is observed.*

There is no fixed rule; it would not respond to the variety. (DACH XI, 17v)

The *Da Cheng* (IV, 15v) indicates that one should never use too much moxa at *gaohuangshu* (BL-38, IS BL-43); *zhongwan*(CV-12); *tianzong* (SI-11); and leg-*sanli* (ST-36). After some months or years too much moxa at these points results in a constant elevated blood pressure with headache, etc. The difficulties commented on in the following text have not been verified:

*At **juque** (CV-14) and at **jiuwei** (CV-15) not more than four or five moxas and small candles. On the vessels, too many moxas would remove the strength of the heart. On the hand, many moxas cause the loss of vitality and enthusiasm **(jingshen)**. On the back and the feet, it causes the vessels to dry up. The four limbs weaken and we lose the vitality **(jingshen)** of our awareness. At the fine articulations it shortens existence. (DACH XI, 17r & 17v)*

IV. Order of Succession of Moxa, Hours, Time

The order of succession has its importance.

> *For moxa, according to the **Ming Tang** one should first burn the top and then the bottom; first a little, then a lot. Never burn first the bottom and then the top. The **Zi Sheng** says: "First the yang, then the yin." That is, first the right [certain texts say the left by mistake] of the head, then one descends. Then the left of the head and one descends. First up, then down. (DACH XI, 17v)*

This order is rationalized by the ancient idea that moxa can only tonify; as for the needles, one should first approach the yang, and use the yang to tonify the yin.

The hours of moxa change the effects. For example, it is true that for *sanli* of the leg (ST-36), moxa in the morning at the rising sun tonifies and makes the digestion active and assimilative. Moxa in the evening prevents sleep and troubles the digestion. Although such a large number of patients have mentioned this that it must be valid, this condition is not reproduced in all patients every time.

Moxa certainly has a tonifying effect, hence it is logical that there be more action until midday, since after midday it is easier to disperse.

Some texts, considered as apocryphal, advise the contrary of the observations made in France:

The *Qian Jin Fang* says:

> *After the **zheng wu** hour (11 a.m. to 1 p.m.) one can then apply moxa. It is said in effect that before the **wu** hour in the morning [the yin energy having not arrived], moxa cannot be used. The food-energy is empty; people will become depressed or agitated. Neither needles nor moxa are necessary at that time. This rule, however, is not used in acute and sudden cases. (DACH XI, 16v)*

We fear that these recommendations of the *Qian Jin Fang* are not in accord with the oral tradition of its author, the seventh century sage, Sun Simo.

The temperature has as great an importance for moxa as for the needles.

> *If there is dark fog, great wind, snow, or rains, the heat of moxa adds to the electric fire of the lightning. Wait for calm weather for moxa, except in cases of acute difficulties. (DACH XI, 16v, citing the Nei Jing)*

> *In great dryness, there is unparalleled increase of effect. (YIX I, 12r)*

> *In hot weather do not apply moxa [but use needles]. Do not tonify what is already in excess. (Nei Jing)*

V. After Moxa

> *After moxa, do not drink tea; that would risk undoing the energy of the fire. The energy of the meridian would also be held up by food. Wait two to four hours; return home and rest in solitude, avoid sex, and desires; calm the spirit and focus the energy; shun great anger, fatigue, hunger or large meals; avoid fruits; do not have hot or cold in the stomach. Take only light food, in order to make the energy and blood circulate; fish and chicken, and that for more than ten days. If not, it might provoke mucus, which would block the exit of the evil. (DACH XI, 18v)*

Notes

[1] Let us recall that the essence of absinthe (Artemisia absinthium) is formed of three ingredients: 1) an oil of unclear identity; 2) a hydrocarbon $C_{16}H_{10}$; 3) a type of camphor, $C_{16}H_{10}O$. The derivative of potassium carbonate has long been called "salt of absinthe" and was prepared by the incineration of absinthe. Our medicine uses the flowers of armoise (Artemisia vulgaris) to encourage menstruation and as an antispasmodic. In homeopathy, artemisia is used to treat alcoholism.

[2] Moxa was undoubtedly difficult to obtain in France at the time thus the need for substitute methods. It is now widely available. — ed.

Chapter XVI

Massage and Electricity

I. Massage — II. Electricity

I. Massage

Massage of the meridians *(mo jing)* and even more so on the points can give good results. However, it is much less effective than the needles, less even than moxa. Additionally, the sensitivity of the points often makes massage painful, for some people even more so than either needles or moxa. But massage causes less fear and for that reason is better accepted.

In fact, it gives marked results only in children or for nervous and extremely sensitive people. However, by doing it every day, it can be a great help, for example, in treating constipation, even when the patient is not hypersensitive.

This procedure, which certainly goes back to great antiquity, was studied in depth and perfected during the Song Dynasty (eleventh to twelfth centuries A.D.). A children's doctor, Chen Wenzhong (Wen Xu) from Xu-zhou in Siming Fu, has left two books: "Massage of Meridians for Children" *(Xiao Er An Mo Jing),* and "Discourses and Prescriptions on the Origin of Illnesses of Children" *(Xiao Er Bing Yuan Fang Lun). Da Cheng* (XII, 26r et. seq.) reproduces the most important passages of these works. The complete study of this method would form an entire volume in its own right.

Experiments in France have proven that massage on the points for children up to seven years is more than sufficient to obtain the desired result. One session of massage at the beginning of the illness stops the illness as well as a puncture. For adults, who are not as sensitive, it is recommended to repeat the massage each day, many times per day.

The simplest procedure consists of pressing firmly with the nail of the thumb or index finger on the active points indicated by the pulse and the nature of illness. Then one moves using friction from the top down and from the right to the left, so that although the skin is not scratched, the nail presses to the level of the subcutaneous tissue.

By this procedure mothers can quickly stop tonsillitis in their children at the beginning of the illness, as well as treat coryza, vomiting, and hiccoughs. After many sessions, they can correct constipation, nervous anger, etc.

Massage has only one inconvenience: the slight pain it causes. Even though it does not upset infants as much as needles or moxa, rubbing the relatively sensitive point can produce acute pain. Chen recommends rubbing until the pain produced by the massage disappears, which he says cures the problem that initially increased the sensitivity of the point.

II. Electricity

French doctors who have studied and applied acupuncture have reasoned that it is possible with our modern arsenal to find new methods of stimulating points that are sensitive due to internal disorders. Experiments with electricity have been most common.

The simplest application is electric moxa made with a spark at high frequency. Although not very strong, this is a true electric puncture. Its advantage is that it does not terrify the patient. Its fault is that it slightly cooks the skin and lessens the sensitivity for the following session. The action is somewhat crude and lacks predictability, sometimes being very strong and at other times inadequate. Like moxa, it is particularly tonifying, even if one makes only one or two sparks. Ten sparks clearly hardens the skin.

We have also tried massage on the point with a bulb that emits high frequency without sparks. This gives much gentler results than that of the spark method above. It does not damage the skin and thus allows us to continue every day if necessary.

A galvanic or faradic current put in contact with an inserted needle seems to remain on the surface without reaching the point of the needle or the deep acupoint. In our experience, this method does not seem to substantially increase the action of the needle.

We have also tried the apparatus called "Negativation," invented by Mr. Laville, and which Dr. Aubourg has studied at length. This apparatus is based on the measure of the electrical energy emitted by the human body. Instruments have recorded this as being from one to three microamperes (thousandths of a milliampere) for exhausted people and from twelve to fifteen microamperes for hyperexcited people, contracted limbs, etc. Experiments have been conducted in three different ways: 1) A carbon washer connected to the apparatus is put on the point. An action at the point takes place but is hardly superior to that of massage with the nail. 2) A rounded point connected to the apparatus is pressed but not pushed into the point. The action is clearly superior to that of moxa. It adds energy and can be repeated every day. It is very useful, for example, for the points around the eyes which can neither be punctures nor treated repeatedly with moxa. 3) The apparatus is connected to the needle, which is put into the point. The action of the needle is certainly strengthened, but not to a major degree.

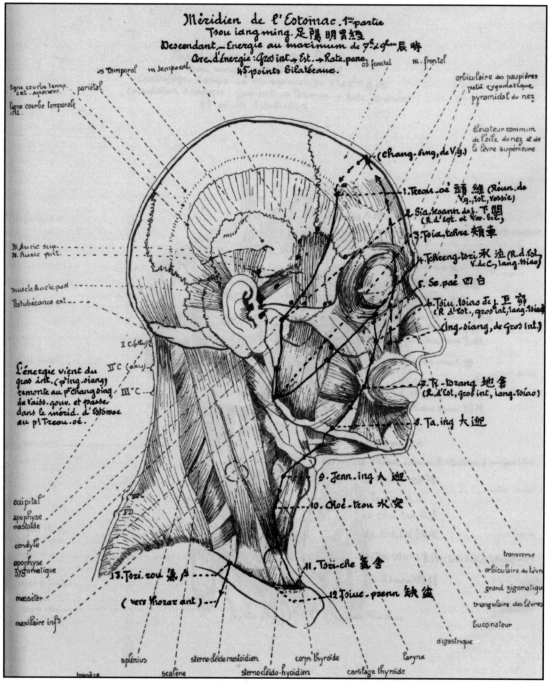

Meridian of the stomach (part 1) (GSDM)

Volume III

The Physiology
of Energy

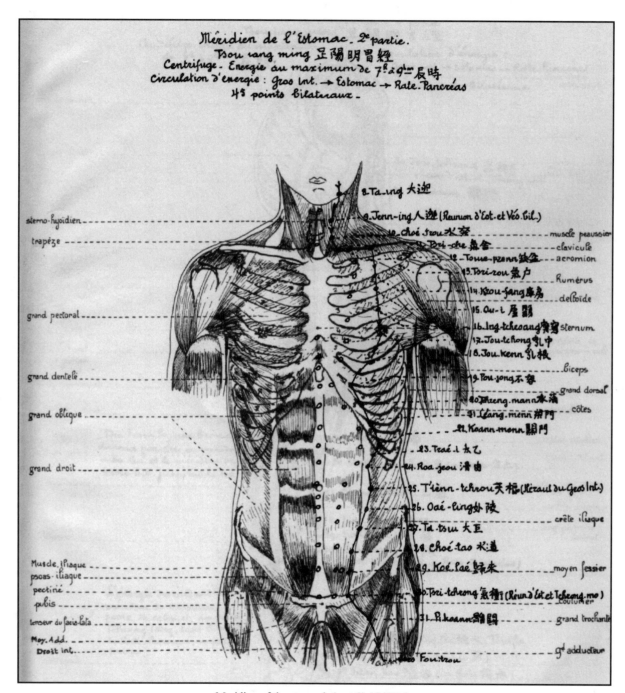

Meridian of the stomach (part 2) (GSDM)

Introduction

Personal happiness in the family and peace in the world are based as much on mental health as on physical health. The discoveries made through testing and verifying the traditions and teachings of ancient China have great importance for public health, human reason, and peace in the world. Among these discoveries, we have found that it is possible before birth to halt the transmission of weak hereditary traits passed on through many generations. We have also found that from infancy it is possible to develop moral consciousness, reason and judgement, and to assure the full development of the individual.

The practical study of the all-powerful vital energy is the subject of this section, ''The Physiology of Energy.'' This study includes the continued maintenance of a harmonious supply of energy in all parts of the body as well as the correction of any affliction. It is essentially the science of the practical synthesis of the human being.

Having been immersed in the Chinese doctrine for three decades of textual research and extensive observation of a variety of maladies, we have been able to enrich the fundamental, ancient discoveries of the Chinese, particularly with respect to the following: the existence and circulation of vital energy, the existence of its command points, the measure of this energy through the pulses, and its practical utilization.

Through many centuries the Chinese have studied and brought to maturation the significance of the first three pulse segments of the radial artery (see Chapter III). My research, in full accord with their rationale and methodology, has led me to discover three new radial pulse segments.

It seems that the Chinese did not recognize the independence of each side of the radial artery. This discovery, which I believe is mine, will allow independent verification of the functioning of one or the other of the double organs; control of the action on each side of the single organs; control over each lobe of the cerebrum, cerebellum, medulla oblongata and each part of the spinal cord; and determination of the relative strength of each level of the psyche. These affirmations can be further evaluated by the clinician. I believe that these discoveries will lead to many others, and that a new path of investigation has been opened.

After carefully documenting the effects obtained after action on a point, I have concluded, as the Chinese believe, that it is impossible to modify the function of an individual organ without modifying that of many others.

Extensive observation has led me to redefine important laws of interaction: I would postulate that any action on an individual organ, even by medication, has the same effect on two others and an opposite effect on two more.

Having proved the above, I believe as well that certain points have effects on a number of organs, some points even acting on all the organs and the entire body. This knowledge of the plurality of command points, essential for the master acupuncturist, permits us to use one point in place of many, thus avoiding the conflicting effects between points that may occur.

This corollary has led to another, even more important discovery: the hierarchy of command points.

The command points are graded by their effects on increasingly numerous groupings, from the lowest level of command points, acting on only a single organ, limb, part of the body, muscle, etc., to the highest level, acting directly on the force that ensures perfect equilibrium of all functions. This force provides a defense system that prevents external influences from penetrating; in the interior, it ensures the proper distribution, perhaps to the hundred-millionth part, of indispensable substances which the body makes and stores.

These discoveries could constitute a scientific and clinical superstructure for the great tradition of Chinese antiquity. In addition, they make it possible to better understand and utilize the unbelievably all-powerful vitality of our being, both psychological and physical.

This new vision of human energy has been conceived only after direct study of the enormous collection of observations and explanations of ancient China. These traditions have come to us in their original texts, thanks to the permanence of Chinese written thought. (The Chinese ideogram fixes the thought and not the sound of the language.) I have been able to translate the eighty-one chapters of a work attributed to the twenty-seventh century B.C., ''The Immaterial Axis,'' or *Ling Shu.* (This text is the second part of the lengthy ancient compilation, the *Nei Jing,* the first part being the *Su Wen.*) This book is the most ancient text in the world dedicated to the study of human energy, even though some passages from later centuries have been inserted into the work. The West is still ignorant of this subject.

My continuing explorations and the rationale for my discoveries, verified by many of our great specialists, have perhaps more than doubled the initial amount of knowledge of the tradition. I have revealed and rediscovered this tradition through the numerous popularized books and reprints of the ancient texts.

My vision is to provide the first scientific and clinical work on the description and utilization of human energy. Certain very specific elements have already been published in the brilliant and very instructive work of Niboyet. This author, uncompromising in his scientific honesty, acknowledges that I am one of the sources of his information. Acupuncture has taken wing, although some still practice the simplistic type that the Academy of Medicine has wisely rejected. Fortunately, my fellow researchers are exploring the true science of energy and intelligently use the Asian tradition on which my published works are based. Acupuncture consultancies now exist at Beaujon, Cochin, St. Louis, Foch de Paris, and in Lyon at St. Luc Hospital.

The following experiments have been carried out by Dr. Niboyet in Marseille and by many members of the faculty under the direction of Dr. Heckenroth. Electrocardiograms have been made on sixty-five cardiac patients before and after acupuncture sessions. Important changes have been recorded when the puncture is made at the correct point.

Innumerable blood samples analyzed before and after puncture have shown that after stimulation of the appropriate point there is infiltration into the blood supply of 50,000 to 1,500,000 developing red blood cells per cubic millimeter. Their great number has allowed us to follow their development every two hours until maturity is obtained fifteen to eighteen hours later. It is not a question here of contraction of the spleen, but rather a true, accelerated mechanism of hematopoiesis.

New instruments have been invented to measure the forms of energy in the body. The Pouret-Niboyet apparatus, based on a cathodic oscillometer using domestic current, measures the resistance of the body to the flow of electric current along the meridian and at the command points. The apparatus of Loch, improved by Leplus and Pompon, is based on a microampere meter connected at two poles; the needle measures the intensity of current flowing between two points located either on one side of the body, along the meridians, or at command points before and after the appropriate stimulation.

Other instruments have been fabricated, namely the Leplus Sonopunctor and the Leplus Moxator. Upon publication of this work, we are sure that other devices, even more advanced, will see their day and bring to conventional physiology a dazzling demonstration of the reality of Chinese acupuncture. The science of energy is in full development.[1]

Notes

[1] *Editor's note from the French edition:* Dr. R. Brunet and Mr. L. Grenier have recently perfected an apparatus allowing the precise localization of points. (Recall that the surface area of most points does not exceed one square mm.) As with other instruments of this kind, it is based on the heightened conductivity of the body at the Chinese point, but it has the advantage of recent electronic advances. This "punctometer" is able to detect the minimal amount of energy necessary for the production of an observable phenomenon. The apparatus is safe, simple and works rapidly, and is thus very suitable for clinical use. The instrument has a ballistic galvanometer designed specifically to retain both sensitivity and the necessary simplicity. It consists of a sturdy but sensitive electronic relay assuring the amplification of extremely weak currents by which the machine is activated. The design principles have been drawn from that of the Wheatstone bridge. The threshold of conductivity of each individual is taken by reading the dial, then the Chinese point located either by the quick movement of the needle or flash of the indicator light. The apparatus allows us to stimulate the located point with a precisely measured quantity of electrical energy, giving a kind of "electric moxa" that the authors have named "galvanopunctometry."

Contrary to what we would think in electrophysiology, it has been observed that as soon as the general threshold of the individual is determined, the distance between the detected points and the return electrode does not influence this threshold. This is also true of the surface area of the contact electrodes — there is no change in the general threshold even if one of them is reduced to a fine point. These phenomena can be explained only by taking the totality of the meridians into consideration. This circumstance constitutes a very important element of proof of their existence.

Part I

Vital Energy

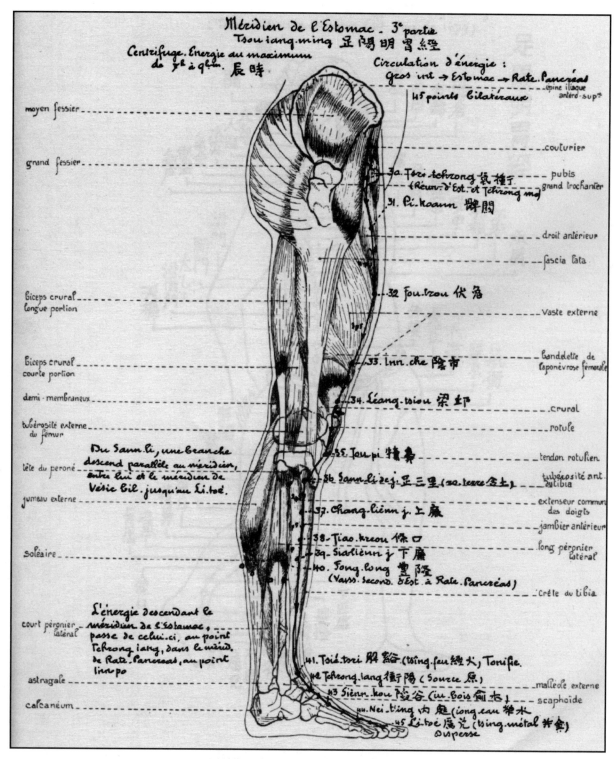

Meridian of the stomach (part 3) (GSDM)

Chapter I

Vital Energy (I)

I. Evidence and Names — II. Evidence and Instrumental Measurements of the Energy: 1. The Vital Force 2. The Resistance to Outside Forces 3. Quantity of Energy 4. Variations of Energy 5. Nature of the Vital Force — III. Unity and Relativity — IV. Diverse Forms: 1. Universal Physical Forms 2. The Proper Forms for Thinking Beings 3. Transformation of the Energy

I. Evidence and Names

There appears to be something in us that is all-powerful, though it may be inaccurate to call it "the vital force." It animates and forms us to the smallest detail. When it weakens, we decline; we lose all resistance, all activity. When it turns off in an area of the body, this part dies; the chemical elements which form the cells dissociate. If it leaves the body, we die.

Our scholars first began to discuss the existence of this force at the beginning of the nineteenth century. In 1809, Magendie noted in his *Memoire Physiologique* at the Academy:

> *Why invent a specific force for each phenomenon of the living body? Instead, could we not be satisfied with acknowledging a single force termed the "vital force" that gives rise to different phenomena following the structure of the organs and the tissues which function under its influence?*

Some years later, in his *Organon* (paragraph 9), the genius Hahnemann underscored for the first time the extreme vital power of this force:

> *In a state of health, the vital force, dynamically animating the material part of the body, exercises an unlimited power.*

Chinese science, ever based on the study and practical utilization of reality, has known for more than four thousand years of the existence of this force. The Chinese have termed it "energy," without the bias of conventional speech of latter-day physics. They have unceasingly pursued its practical application. Yet our books on physiology give it only a few lines. In the West, its existence is still in question, the subject of experimentation by only a few researchers. The most lucid work, that of American biologist R.J. Main *(Synopsis of Physiology),* is far from popular. He explains:

> *That protoplasm is not a simple aggregate of these substances [proteins, carbohydrates, lipids, salts and enzymes], all laboratory reproducible, is demonstrated by the fact that it maintains a basal metabolism utilizing oxygen and liberating carbon dioxide with heat. If that is prevented, the protoplasm "dies."*

> *These constituents remain unchanged, yet the protoplasm is no longer living and consequently is no longer protoplasm. Thus, its constituents must form a flexible structure which requires a constant supply of energy in order to subsist.[1]*

Hence, vital energy is not inherent in chemical aggregates: vital energy is the life of these aggregates but is independent of them. Confucius knowingly wrote: "The cutting edge taken from a blade leaves only a piece of iron."

For R.J. Main, this energy was produced and maintained by the metabolism; for the Chinese, it was maintained by the Earth and the stars, food, drink, air and the environment.

Today, the word "energy" replaces the words "life" and "vital force" and connotes all the various forces, be it electrical, hydraulic, mechanical and so forth.

The word comes from the Greek "en-ergon," meaning "of activity." The *Larousse Dictionary* defines "energy" as:

> *Power [e.g., military energy], virtue, efficacy [e.g., energy of a remedy]. Figuratively: force, firmness [e.g., energy of the soul]. Physically: faculty possessed by the body in order to provide work.*

According to *Webster's Dictionary:*

> *1) Power. 2) This power when it is exercised. 3) Power inherent or internal; capacity to act. 4) Power used with force and efficiency. 5) Capacity to accomplish work.*

When applied to the vital energy, these definitions give only a very general idea. We propose ''intensity of manifestation of life.'' By ''life'' we mean the force that can be transmitted only from one living being to another and that radically distinguishes organic, animate matter from inorganic, inanimate matter, the living from the dead.

Yet, we must further differentiate between active energy, which manifests itself, and latent energy, which does not manifest itself but becomes active with the appropriate stimulus (R.J. Main). Thus, wood does not manifest any energy until it is ignited and its latent energy becomes active. A Chinese proverb says: ''Power exists only on the condition that it is exercised; one must think of power-bondage.'' Therefore, we use the word ''energy,'' either active or latent, in the sense of intensity of life, that which animates the being; that is, the vital force.

The written language of China is not arbitrary, as are all the spoken languages. It describes the idea by its essential trait — the tree by a trunk, some branches and schematic roots. The ideogram for energy is its definition: it represents a cauldron on the fire with the cover half-lifted by the pressure of the escaping vapor. The immaterial force is emitting the material— water; latent energy is transformed into active energy. This ideogram is used for all immaterial force: the life force of man, animals, and plants; the force that animates the muscles; a flash of lightning or, in our day, electricity; astral energy and cosmic rays; and the favorable or noxious energy of a particular terrain, climate or person.

The omnipotence of this force has been demonstrated in China, Japan and now the West by suppressing and manipulating it and at times instantly causing the most varied disturbances to appear.

Since 1925, I have been lecturing on this force, experimenting with it and verifying its existence in the hospitals of Paris. It has been shown that for all disorders, microbial or not, by approaching the force directly it was possible to arrest asthmatic crises, violent pain, contractures and so forth. These results were immediate in cases of recent onset, or very rapid in chronic cases. An abscess reabsorbs overnight; typhoid is sometimes cured in three to five days, as with antibiotics.

II. Evidence and Instrumental Measurements of the Energy

Special instruments have been invented and constructed for measuring the vital energy. The apparatus of Pouret-Niboyet uses industrial electricity while that of Loch, further developed by Leplus and Pompon, does not. Technical breakthroughs are close to being realized in this area.

All measurements are based on nomenclature borrowed from electrical science. Different apparatus use distinct yet properly standardized scales of measurement. The relative results have proven to be consistent.

The following are various factors that should be considered when dealing with the question of energy: 1) the force produced by the body; 2) the resistance of the body to foreign forces and influences; 3) the quantities of energy; 4) the variations of energy; and 5) the nature of the energy.

The vital force.

Vital force detected and measured by instruments without external energy sources:

The ultra-sensitive galvanometer with a mirror. In 1929, Dr. Dimier, a hospital electrologist, experimented with existing devices with which he was already familiar. He used only the subject and the galvanometer (with no external energy source), permitting the detection and measurement of the force emitted by the subject.

These instruments gave the idea that what was measured was electrical force. But Dr. Dimier remarked to me that aside from electrical waves, the apparatus detected another wave. His death prevented the pursuit of this research and the construction of a device that could distinguish the two forces.

The Loch apparatus (further developed by Leplus) also has no external energy source. It consists of a microamperemeter. The two contacts or electrodes are made of different metals, a copper-silver alloy and aluminum. The indicator scale is divided into one hundred parts, each part a tenth of a microampere (millionth of a milliamp). The indicator scale of the Leplus apparatus has divisions of five microamperes, a halving which allows the measurement of ten microamperes. (A scale gives the division in 100ths of five microamperes.)

There is a maximum of ten microamperes, which is very rarely exceeded. When the two electrodes are placed in dry contact, the needle is deflected according to the thickness and humidity of the skin; a finger wet with salt water gives the standard measure. It is estimated that the electricity generated by the two different metals and salt water is just enough to counterbalance the inertia of the needle. In consequence, the energetic potential (or electroenergetic) of the body is detected by putting one hand on each contact. The needle falls if the subject holds the contact for too long; the length of time varies according to the energetic reserves of each person.

Wide variations in measurement are obtained from different locations on the same person: between the command points; the meridians and the rest of the cutaneous surface; the upper and lower, left and right parts of the body; anterior and posterior surfaces of the limbs; between the fingers, i.e., the thumb— reflecting cerebral intensity, the index finger— digestive intensity, middle finger— physical vitality, ring-finger— nerve vitality, little finger— circulatory intensity. Finding these differences is one aim of this work.

The measurements from these instruments prove the existence of the vital force and its manifestations of varied intensities in different parts of the body. We can observe the independence of body parts through such disorders as hemiplegia, local edema, and other localized problems. Only ideally is the vital intensity equal throughout the whole body. One fact remains to be explained: the physical force of the dynamometer does not necessarily follow the energetic potential. It is possible to have a period of great physical weakness with a high potential and vice versa. Yin (blood, physique) and yang (energy, nerves) are independent.

The resistance to outside forces.

The resistance to outside forces is detected and measured by instruments with a cathodic oscillometer using domestic current, typified by the Pouret-Niboyet apparatus. The electrical "puncture" is strongly felt. The dial is divided into fifty divisions corresponding to ohms, from which microamperes can be deduced. The needle set at fifty, for example, drops with contact on the body and even more so if the subject is tired. A cadaver makes it fall maximally. Resistance is therefore a vital phenomenon; it is exactly equal to the outside force. This is analogous to the sphygmomanometer — the higher the "pressure," the stronger the arterial tension, the measure being that of the force used to overcome the resistance.

Mr. Pouret has written to me:

> When we puncture electrically, we inject energy inversely to the resistance of the point. Following the work of Stohl, Denier, Dausset, etc., it is well accepted that an organism is a resistance-capacity system. A resistance of around 1000 to 8000 ohms is encountered beginning at the cutaneous and corneal layers; at the levels corresponding to the viscera and non-homogenous areas, another resistance is encountered, this time a very weak one of about 250 ohms. When we puncture with the detector, the current is shunted past the resistance due to the relatively weak resistance of the impulse and is dissipated there in the form of the Joule effect, that is, heat giving the sensation of a puncture.

Some researchers arrive at much greater numbers (up to 800,000 ohms) for the cutaneous resistance of the individual potential to the pressure of outside forces.

Quantity of energy.

Even with the various instruments and their measurements, we still cannot give any exact numbers. It is only possible to cite some data obtained.

On the ultra-sensitive galvanometer of Dr. Dimier, the quantity was around one microampere for a fatigued person, from eight to ten for a person feeling well, and from twelve to fifteen for hyperexcited people.

On the Loch apparatus, the following data has been recorded: 3/10 of a microampere for a hemiplegic shortly after the stroke, and from five to seven microamps for fatigued people. Healthy people feeling well give nine to ten microamps, often surpassing the limit of the dial.

On the Pouret-Niboyet apparatus, which does not use a microampere meter, the needle falls to zero for a cadaver. The fall of the needle is quickest for tired people. It is a quarter of the dial for people who feel well.

There are significantly different readings from the same person, depending on contact with: 1) a command point of the energy (see Points); 2) the course of the meridian; 3) a part of the body far from a meridian and any point. Finally, considerable variations are noted on the same point according to thoughts, the weather, etc. It is not a question of mathematical measures, a "norm" for everyone, but one of relativity.

Variations in the energy.

The variations observed on the Loch-Leplus instrument have been attributed to three causes (for those taking place on the same day):

1)   Psychological: Having the patient recount sad and emotional stories of his past makes the potential drop by 10 to 15/100 microampere. If happy stories are recalled immediately after, the drop in potential is regained and the level further rises to more than 5 to 10/100 microampere.

2)   Atmospheric: After thunder or rainstorms, there is sometimes a drop of 30/100 microampere in depressed people. By contrast, the readings of hyperexcited people rise from 20 to 30/100 microampere. Heat causes a rise; cold causes a fall; wind can cause either.

3)   Physical: tired people show a great drop before eating and a strong rise after eating; tea causes a rise.

Wearing certain substances can produce momentary action. A pearl necklace worn by a sensitive person, for example, can cause a fall of fifteen divisions in the Loch instrument. Necklaces and bracelets of gold cause the potential to rise.

Certain colors also influence the readings: a vivid red coat lining causes a rise of 10 to 20/100 and more than doubles physical endurance (for walking, and so forth.) A clear blue sky causes a drop.

Leplus comments:

> It is rather curious to observe the considerable variations (of about 300,000 ohms) in the resistance of the body without apparent reason.

It has been reported (Lorgeril: *Presse Médicale,* Oct. 3, 1928) that listening to music produced a variation in patient readings on the mirror galvanometer. Veragut of Zurich related forty years ago that for patients listening to emotionally moving, ideological speeches the luminous rays of the mirror galvanometer were modified, while for those listening to indifferent ideas no change was elicited. Herlitzka writes that an unconscious, fleeting emotion provokes a deviation in the galvanometer. Our instruments measure the differences of potential according to our thoughts. Lazareff even writes:

> In principle, it should be possible to capture the material emanations which accompany physical phenomena in exterior space in the form of electromagnetic waves.

Nature of the vital force.

Muller, director of the Salus Institute of Munich, attributes the action of the vital force to a kind of emanation he calls Anthropoflux R (the letter R indicating the radiation modifying the electrical resistances). His approach to ascertaining its nature was to test the conductivity of certain substances (e.g., air, silk, hair-lacquer) through the body. Anthropoflux R comes out most abundantly at the palmar surface of the phalanges of the left hand (Cazamalli: *Quaderni de Psychatria,* Gences, no. 5 - 6, 1929).

What has been called the power of magnetism has been the object of extensive experimentation. Dr. Locard, a forensic surgeon, has not denied its action in stopping microbial fermentation or in sterilizing water.

Professor Cazamalli writes:

> There is no reason to attribute special qualities to the energy in question or to particularly consider it of a mechanico-humoral nature. It is better to think of it as electrical and electromagnetic in nature.
>
> In my experience, it appears that the human subject radiates electromagnetic waves of the radio-electric type in close correlation with certain metapsychological and psychosensorial phenomena of the brain . . . Some radio-electric waves emitted by the brain have been recently discovered.

Is the vital energy of an electric nature, or is human electricity a form of the vital energy?

III. Unity and Relativity of Energy

It is generally accepted that energy cannot be lost, destroyed or created apart from the phenomenon of atomic disintegration. Energy is recognized as unique but is presented under two great relative quantities: latent energy, known only through calculation until a stimulus transforms it into active energy; and active energy, which can be detected and measured.

In the Far East, energy is also considered a singular entity, yet again presents under two broad categories: yang energy of activity (heat, etc.) corresponding to our active energy, and yin energy of rest (cold, etc.) corresponding to our latent energy, or energy becoming latent (see Volume III, Part III, Chapter III, Section I: ''Law of Relativity''). In reality, these two terms are relative, representing excess or insufficiency of universal and vital energy.[2]

The yin nocturnal and yang diurnal relativity in its alternating relative rhythm is the most easily observable manifestation. All nature obeys this alternating and relative rhythm. During the night: need of rest, slowing down of all the functions, except the sexual function. Vegetables, trees, and leaves give off carbon dioxide. All nature sleeps. During the day: need of activity, activation of all the functions. Vegetables, trees, and leaves give off oxygen and take in carbon dioxide. All nature is active. The temperature of the body is lowest at 5 a.m. (sunrise, local) and rises 0.5° C by 5 p.m.

The facts are there. The Far East has verified and utilized them and has given them great importance. The West, while necessarily observing these facts of nature, has not attempted to research all their implications, such as the daily cycle of temperature change of the body.

The presence of the sun and light disturbs sleep and rest while their absence disrupts activity and promotes sleep. Yet these are not the only causes for this daily rhythm, since the 0.5 degree difference in body temperature between the evening and the morning is identical for the night-worker who sleeps during the day.

Note also that there are animals of all kinds who live and hunt during the night and sleep during the day. Hunters more easily surprise their sleeping victims. (To better defend themselves, why are these victims sleeping rather than active during the day?)

According to the ancient Chinese, the sun spreads its rays over the earth, giving waves of heat activity and cerebral stimulation. This constitutes the diurnal ''yang'' energy, positive and activating. At night, the moon, particularly when hidden and not reflecting the sun, emits waves of cold, rest, cerebral sluggishness and fear. This constitutes the nocturnal ''yin'' energy, negative and inhibiting.

It is written that ''the new moon is death,'' and ''the full moon is life.'' All is reborn and waxes with the full moon, which sends out a mixture of its rays and those reflected from the sun. With its waning, all begins to decline. Acting in accordance with and enhancing these rhythms is of great importance.

This day-night opposition has served as a solid basis for the study of man's response to the two categories of energy, yin and yang.

IV. Diverse Forms of the Vital Energy

The human vital energy can manifest and present itself in numerous forms. These can be divided into two groups: 1) Those that are also external to man: electricity, force-movement, heat-cold. 2) Those that are proper to thinking beings and specific to man: internal psychology, thoughts, feelings; or external energetics: personal and magnetic waves, sexuality, mental or emotional emanations, authority, etc.

Universal physical forms.

Electricity. Two needles connected by a copper wire were placed by Drs. Dimier and Foveau de Courmelles into bilateral points, most significantly at leg-*sanli* (ST-36), the most important point for the energy. When a telephonic receiver was put in contact with the wire, a ''taca-taca'' sound representing an intermittent discharge of electricity was distinctly heard. When ultrasensitive galvanometers were put in contact, in addition to the electric waves, another type of wave occasionally appeared. Unfortunately, Dr. Dimier passed away before he was able to construct an apparatus to clearly separate the two waves.

Is this electricity a form of energy? Or is the vital energy a form of electricity?

The Far East instructs us that the energy of the interior of the body, and the anterior and medial surfaces of the limbs is of a negative nature (yin); while that of the external surface of the body, the dorsal surface, the lateral part of the body and the lateral surface of the limbs is of a positive nature (yang).

Recall that the wavelength recorded by the radiesthesist varies according to the vital force. Are these waves, if we can call them that, of the electric sort, purely energetic, or electromagnetic? Recall also that when some people comb their hair they cause sparks, and that the phosphorescence of the body can be observed. In total darkness, the face can be faintly seen.

The Loch apparatus gives almost no response when the two electrodes are on the same yin or yang surface; it gives the greatest response when a yang surface is connected with a yin surface. This indicates that there may be two positive and negative poles on the two sides of the body and on the lateral and medial surfaces of a limb, according to the yin-yang relativity. There might also be a current emanating from the body.

The following are explanations that modern science puts forward, beginning at the cellular level. Quoting R.J. Main *(Synopsis of Physiology):*

> *All living cells at rest show a difference in electrical potential between the inside (negative) and the outside (positive). The membrane of the normal cell acts as an insulator preventing the flow of current.*
>
> *If a cell's membrane is destroyed, the cell becomes negative relative to the uninjured cells. If a completed circuit is made with the injured cell by a conductor such as a galvanometer, a flow of current takes place— the current of the lesion.*
>
> *The fact that this difference of potential disappears when the cell dies indicates the necessity of the metabolic process to provide energy in order to maintain and produce this potential. This possibly consists of the orientation of more anions towards the interior of the cell and of cations towards the exterior.*
>
> *When the permeability of the cell membrane is increased, as happens when an adequate stimulus is applied, a movement of ions and a flow of current results; this is the current of activity. This stimulates the surrounding area so that the excitatory process results. Lastly, a contraction-like response takes place. . . .*
>
> *All stimulation of the cell produces first a discharge and then a recharge; a period of activity and one of rest.*

Movement-immobility-force. The force of movement is an expenditure of energy; it is measured in kilogram-meters by the resistance overcome. Immobilization and the maintenance of immobility also consists of an expenditure of energy which can be very great in certain cases, e.g., in agoraphobia, when the patient is riveted to the spot. The force necessary to move the person from his immobility has not yet been measured.

Heat-cold. The heat is measured in calories. Correct stimulation of certain command points can make the body temperature rise or fall. We do not yet know if these acupuncture points act through the autonomic system on the centers of heat and cold, or if they regulate the quantity of energy necessary for the transformation of energy into heat or cold.

We know that a heat center exists in the posterior hypothalamus (center of the sympathetic system), and a lesion there (thus a cessation of the function) causes hypothermia which can reach 28° C. A cold center exists in the anterior hypothalamus (vagal center), and a lesion there produces hyperthermia reaching 43° C. (We have seen 52° C.)

The daily changes in body temperature are not explained. Is it merely a question of the diurnal rise of .5° C by 5 p.m. or a lowering by .5° C during the night? This change in body temperature is the same for individuals who work at night and rest during the day and those who work during the day and rest at night. Far Eastern thought explains this in terms of the response of the whole organism to the diurnal activity and nocturnal inactivity of energy.

The heat of the body depends on many conditions. The most thoroughly studied is the heat from digestion. The caloric value of different groups of food and drink has been studied, measured and specified, most notably by Rubner. He established that man can only survive and maintain his structure through a constant supply of energy furnished by the combustion of food. In an organism at rest, heat fully represents the energy liberated in the using up of the substance, the food reconstituting the material substance. The centers of heat and cold in the hypothalamus ensure the constant elimination of excess heat or cold, sweat being an important means.

Heat also comes from inhaled air, as has been demonstrated by Lavoisier. He states:

> *Air passing through the lungs shows a decomposition analogous to the combustion of carbon. . . . The flame of life is lit at the time of the infant's first breath and is extinguished at the time of death.*

He demonstrated that oxygen is removed from inhaled air; and also that it fixes into certain metals or metalloids during combustion (tin, lead, sulphur, phosphorus, etc.), thus increasing their weight. Organisms are like thermic warmers continually producing heat by the fixation of oxygen onto carbon (eliminated as carbon dioxide).

The heat that suffuses the body during sexual excitement is perhaps due to accelerated internal combustion and excitation of the sympathetic system.

According to the science of energy, the three sources of heat are 1) air, 2) food and drink, and 3) an excitatory sexual hormone. For the Chinese, heat from these sources is distributed by a special meridian, the triple warmer (the Chinese ideogram for which depicts ''the body of a small bird over a fire'').

The heat from fever is not a source of heat, but an expenditure, a discharge.

Cold of the body is generally considered an insufficiency of energy. But in certain cases, a true cold energy (the energy of yin inactivity) takes hold, and after passing leaves the body fatigued, demonstrating an expenditure of energy.

Proper forms for the thinking being.

Thought, feelings. Their intensity is in proportion to one's psychological sensitivity and vitality. Thought represents an energy expenditure of significant qualitative importance: concentration, imagination, intense intellectual work, prolonged meditation, etc. On the contrary, the exercise of memory, such as that of good students of the parroting kind, fatigues little; gossip relieves.

Feelings such as hatred, indignation, or anger may provoke an abrupt internal or external discharge of energy, while those of affection, love, respect, and good news, etc., may replenish the energy.

Confucius teaches:

> *What we call feelings in man are seven in number: joy, unhappiness, regret, fear, love, hate, and desire. We are capable of these seven feelings without learning them. But desire or repulsion greatly rule the heart-spirit. They are buried to such an extent that they can be distinguished from one another only with difficulty.*

Freud teaches that love and hate are paradoxical and can suddenly transform into one another. Yet experience shows that love characteristically gives energy, the *elan* in life, while hate uses energy, drying the face and body and inciting violent action. Fear paralyzes or causes flight.

Human magnetism. This term is used to denote the human energy directed outwardly to the exterior. Some forms of human magnetism are natural and unconscious, e.g., aura, authority, emotional and spiritual emanations, seduction or sex appeal, or repulsion. Others are cultivated and directed — our energetic power is directed inwardly through the will to influence an organ or part of the body, or outwardly, even at a great distance, to act on material objects or persons.

This magnetism will be proven primarily through instrumentation and analysis of results. In a series of hearings on people who use human magnetism (all science that is new is persecuted by Western narrow-mindedness), Dr. Locard, the famous medical lawyer, gave certain proofs of the effects of human magnetism, notably the sterilization of water and the imbuing of it with curative energetic properties. Charcot has reported the effects of what he calls ''suggestion,'' which is in fact obtained by the magnetism of the person making suggestions. He and his students, particularly Dr. Regnault, have exposed and described some experiences of suggestion over physical and other functions. Christian Science is based on magnetism from a distance directed through prayer. Church prayers for sick people use the same force.

It is in the ancient tradition of India that we find a systematic and practical study of this force and the best means of utilizing it either on oneself or on others. The science of yoga has been made the object of scientific research, notably by Dr. Thérèse Bross around 1933. She brought instruments for recording the activity of the lungs and heart into India. The resultant graphs show that true yogis (not charlatans) can voluntarily stop the function of their heart and lungs for more than an hour and even, she says, for more than a year. If the voluntary arrest has not gone beyond many months, they can start the organs again voluntarily; longer than that and the help of other yogis is required. The existence of this considerable force is also denied in the West and those claiming its existence are persecuted. In some sense this is perhaps wise, since it would undoubtedly be used more for bad than good.

The unconscious force of magnetism, the aura, has many forms:

Through *authority.* We should note the force of authority that allows a new professor entering the class to obtain silence and work without word or gesture, while another upon entering arouses general uproar. I have studied this force in depth since discovering a point on the kidney channel (*dazhong,* KI-6, IS KI-4) which gives a demeanor of authority to those who lack it. These persons immediately see the difference in the impressions they make. The effect of this point is statistically verifiable.

Spiritual, moral and physical emanations. A person is present and only sublime thoughts come to mind; before this person was present, no one would consider speaking of these elevated topics. These emanations do not require ecclesiastic trappings. Without this emanation, the uniform only gives the impression of a puppet.

Certain people empty us of our potential while others recharge us by their presence.

Charm evokes the impression of tenderness, or sweetness, and is very different from sex appeal, which arouses the sexual appetite. But both depend on a function of the kidney, acting through *dazhong* (KI-6, IS KI-4). As with all forms of attraction, both seem to come from the sexual energy. Since life can be reproduced only from life, this attraction no doubt comes from the blind impulse towards the communal reproduction of all living beings; it is perhaps the primary cause and aim of all things here below.

Men and women do not have the same kind of sexual energy. The role of the woman is to attract; that of the man, to conquer, to annihilate even the idea of resistance. But for both, the sexual energy animates the entire being, changes the physiognomy, disturbs the brain and the reason: the emanation is modified and greatly intensified. Sexual stimulation is dangerous for people with congestive conditions.

Transformation of energy.

The transformation of energy into these different forms and from the one to the other is controlled by the nervous centers.

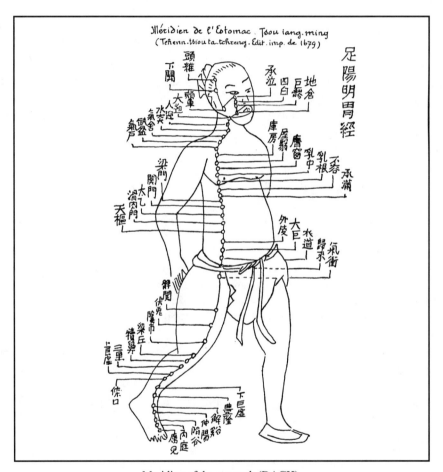

Meridian of the stomach (DACH)

Notes

[1] As this book is long out of print, this is a retranslation of the French translation of the English quotation — trans.

[2] Ancient Chinese texts differentiate between the *rong* energy in the meridians and the *wei* energy outside the meridians. Our instruments measure a potential at the meridians and a weak potential outside the meridians — without doubt the *rong* and *wei*.

Chapter II

Vital Energy (II)

The Human Form, The Unique Individual

I. Uniqueness, the Form — II. Growth — III. Repair — IV. Old Age — V. Death — VI. Form and Heredity

The force or vital energy imprints both our psychological and physical being while maintaining our life and health. It creates our way of being, our "form," a plan that is absolutely unique to each person and rigorously, unceasingly maintained throughout life. It assures growth and repair exactly in the same way and not otherwise. It is the general order of being. "The form is solid. What animates the solid is the energy that gives dimension to matter."

Claude Bernard exposes this fact with his characteristic clarity of thinking and style:

It is not a chance meeting of physiochemical phenomena that constructs each being on a plan following a fixed design. It is seen in advance and directs the wonderful coordination and harmonious concert of life processes. The animated body has an arrangement, a kind of order, which we must bring to light as it is truly the most outstanding characteristic of living beings.

The renaissance of biotypology under the impetus of Marcel Martiny reflects the new attraction of researchers to the uniqueness of life's order to the smallest detail and with all its significance.

Since antiquity, the Far East has observed and utilized this uniqueness of being as much for structure as for reactions. It is written in the *Nei Jing:* "Each one is sick in his own way; of this the sage cannot but take notice." The *Da Cheng,* or *Great Compilation,* of the sixteenth century, states: "For treatment of the same illness, each one is different."

I. Uniqueness, the Form

It is indeed true that no two individuals on earth are exactly alike in appearance and reactions. This law extends to all living beings. At conception, each individual receives his uniqueness, which will be sustained until death. His psychological and physical personality has certain potentialities absolutely unique to him. These can be cultivated and developed, but can be neither altered nor surpassed. Each one is predestined, favorably or unfavorably. No two individuals react exactly in the same degree or the same manner to the same stimulation. Even probabilities of longevity are unique.

We are left dumbfounded by the incredible power of the organism to maintain such uniqueness throughout all the assaults of life, moment by moment adapting its actions to meet these challenges. Facts observed in China and explained by European science illuminate the origin of this uniqueness and how it reveals itself throughout the body.

This individuality, this personality, may be due to the cells of the central nervous system. Bogomoletz writes,

It is they [these cells] which sustain the unity of the psychological personality and its development during the entire life.

He does not address himself to the physical unity linking the biological specificity of all tissues composing the body, a unity despite the heterogeneous supply of food.

The Chinese observed this in the action of the small intestine and specifically of the duodenum. A short but significant passage from the *Nei Jing* states:

The small intestine receives the dead food from the stomach and adds to it a life absolutely correct for each individual.

With this passage in mind, the following discovery of modern physiology has greater significance. It is now known that action in the small intestine causes the large protein molecules of albumin to burst. From the debris, a live molecule of albumin absolutely specific and differentiated for the tissues and blood of that individual is reconstituted. This represents the most developed stage of the vital function's uniqueness.

It has been observed clinically that if the small intestine is insufficient in energy (mostly from the duodenum), the individual recuperates very slowly and poorly from fatigue or effort; healing is slower. He has clearly less psychological and physical vitality. Hence, the command point that tonifies the small intestine allows the immediate correction of these disorders.

These operations depend on a general command point and particular points of the small intestine. It is possible to act either through the points of the small intestine or through those of the governor vessel, all of which are in relationship to the small intestine. The tonification point of the small intestine is in fact the point of command of the governor vessel (*houxi,* SI-3); all act on the nervous centers.

II. Growth

Within the limits of each person's plan, it appears that growth can be activated or retarded by the spleen-pancreas command points that act on nerve centers. It appears that through heredity, retarded people develop to their maximum potential of body size by an accelerated rhythm. The development of the body thus depends on heredity and on the vital energy that must actualize the form.

We think that psychological development, particularly that concerning moral consciousness and synthesis of thought, is also induced by the spleen-pancreas meridian. For this development to be realized, must we call in the action of the pancreas to intervene by providing the brain with its fuel, glucose, since the brain has no reserves of its own?

Note that several elements act on growth:

The growth hormone of the pituitary gland acts mainly on skeletal bone. Excess secretion of growth hormone before closure of the epiphyses causes giantism; excess secretion after closure causes bony plates such as the maxillary bone or the hand and foot bones to enlarge, resulting in acromegaly.

A point discovered by us at the superior edge of C-7 (see Volume IV, GV-13b) on the governor vessel seems to regulate and normalize this hormone. It appears to act on repairs of bone and periosteum.

Vitamin A is closely related to growth. It is formed and distributed by the liver. The lack of it results in retardation of growth in young people, and in dryness of skin and hair, often with diarrhea or genital disturbances.

All points that are able to activate the thyroid gland are also of importance here.

The tonification point of the liver has demonstrated its action on these problems of deficiency, above all when accompanied by an appropriate diet. However, we have observed no effect on growth.

III. Repairs

Lecomte du Nouy has studied and demonstrated the relationship between the rapidity of healing and the exact measure of age, that is, the degree of power of the vital force on the form. Healing depends on this force.

A command point of the gallbladder meridian, *xuanzhong* (GB-39) above the external malleolus, reduces by more than half the time of bone suturing, the healing of wounds and problems of the mucus membranes. It combats with great efficacy septicemia and resolves abscesses which are not yet at the point of bursting. It seems to activate the leukocyte defenses. In addition, it appears as one of three points which increase the capacity and quantity of the vital energy. What the Chinese call the gallbladder is in reality the entire biliary reflex with all its mechanisms — gallbladder, cystic canal, bile duct (Oddi's sphincter, etc.) which connects the liver to the duodenum.

IV. Aging

Aging and old age are very far from being synonymous. Aging appears inevitable. However, it is far from being equal for all in onset or intensity. It has been noted that there is great resemblance between the signs of aging and those of scurvy (Walter Eddy, *The Vitamins*).

Alexis Carrel has shown that some organs separated from the body can go well beyond their normal longevity without aging if kept in adequate conditions. The determination of "adequate conditions" has not been made, for the good reason that we are all different. A transplanted vegetable can revive or die. When questioned, each centenarian attributes his great age to different conditions of life. Each person must determine the conditions which give him the greatest vitality and health; it is very difficult to realize these conditions.

It is incontestable that heredity is of very great importance. There are families in which great age is often reached; in others, they are white-haired at twenty and bent at fifty.

It has not yet been verified in Europe if *zhubin* (KI-9) of the kidney meridian, tonified during pregnancy, assures a particularly beautiful child and prevents aging. The oldest infants for whom the mother was thus treated are now twenty years old; their vital force is exceptional as is their immunity to illnesses.

Roland J. Main writes:

The cause of senility is unknown, since in vitro the cells seem to be immortal. Senility seems inexplicable unless we postulate the accumulation of toxic products of metabolism.

This would explain why growth and reproduction of protozoa diminish in a limited and non-renewed area; and also why some rats forced onto a regime deficient in calories live longer than those receiving the maximum regime.

Each person is aware of the general signs of aging. But some signs do not adequately explain aging. R.J. Main questions:

Why is hypertrophy of the prostate produced instead of atrophy? This fact has not been explained, particularly as it does not happen in eunuchs or eunuchoidism.

Gerontology is a complex science. It is easy to observe, however, that certain signs of aging are due to excess of the parasympathetic and insufficiency of the sympathetic systems. We do know that the young are more quickly sympathicotonic and old people clearly vagotonic. However, even after extensive experimentation, we cannot yet say whether or not this fact is utilizable.

Voronof's experiments with grafting have proven the part of gonadal hormone deficiency in aging. Strong tonification of this gland by the science of energy must give, and moreover does give, renewed strength and regression of aging. This is our absolute conviction.

Bogomoletz has written:

It can be considered that senile atrophy is caused by the starvation of the cells. This starvation does not come from insufficiency of food, but from diminished ability of the cells to assimilate this food.

For Bogomoletz, the endocrine system plays a primary role in stimulating specific functions of the cells, among them assimilation. He adds:

The study of the sympathetic system increasingly confirms that its functions consist of maintaining the activity of the cell, physiological tension, the tonus. . . . On the other hand, we cannot doubt the influence of the sympathetic nervous system on the psyche. . . . The influence exercised by cortical nervous activity and psychological states on the general state of the body is undeniable.

V. Death

Death by simple extinction of life often is not clearly distinguished from organ disorders which can put an end to life.

The gradual weakening of the heart and arteries can always be detected and corrected through the science of energy. The West lacks this refined system of diagnosis. The synthesis of Chinese pulse diagnosis and Western medical technology will undoubtedly help to resolve this problem.

As a final note, we add that the Sequoia gigantia in California reach six thousand years and more without aging or dying. What hereditary factor gives them more vitality than other conifers?

VI. Form and Heredity

In summary, as this chapter points out, whether it be a question of uniqueness, growth, repair, aging or death, heredity plays a very important role. The Far East has been so impressed by this fact that the word ''form'' is often used in the sense of ''heredity.''

Is it necessary, as Martiny believes, to consider the duration of life in accordance with the notion of space-time, with the form being four-dimensional?

For the West, heredity is transmitted by chromosomes, which have a limited and known number. Their combinations are extremely numerous. But at present it is only a question of the transmission of characteristics; there is no mention of a hereditary transmission of a vital force. The totality of both characteristics and energy forms the wholeness of the individual and, in fact, the intensity of energy does seem to vary between families.

It is justifiable to say that the vital force (vital energy) and the form, with all its vital attributes, are hereditary gifts. The breeding of all animals rests on this concept. But there are also acquisitions and mutations. Hence, the goal is to improve heredity, to purify it. This can be accomplished through the science of energy and by the maintenance of the best personal conditions— pure air and natural, living food.

Chapter III

Vital Energy (III)

Measurements of the Energy, the Radial Pulse:
Existence, Explanations

I. Various Measures — II. The Pulses: Problems, Explanations 1. Pulsation 2. The Blood-Pressure 3. The Three Blood-Pressures 4. The Segments of the Artery 5. The Pulses of Organs 6. Organ-Pulse Relations

I. Various Measures

Apart from the instruments already described for measuring energy, there are instruments in the West which measure the various forms of vital energy: for electricity — the galvanometer; for heat — the thermometer; for strength — the dynamometer. We have no instruments as yet for personal or sexual waves, however powerful they may be.

For thousands of years, humanity has used a sensitive, thorough and dependable instrument to ascertain the state of the total energy, its strengths and weaknesses, its diverse and local forms, as well as forms of heat and fever: the finger. It has been used with great precision to differentiate the various aspects of the radial pulses.

Our oscillometers (the sphygmomanometers are less complete), invented barely three quarters of a century ago, only give us numerical measures for each wrist as a whole. They have confirmed what the Chinese learned long ago: there are three blood pressures on each arm, all variable through their connections with one another. The variations for each blood pressure have their own significance. They can often be different at each wrist; thus, in reality, without being particularly discriminating, one can detect six pulses, each one having its significance and measure. Without instrumentation, the Chinese of antiquity had already registered the existence of the three blood pressures and the significance of their variations.

Our instruments and electrocardiographs have allowed us to assign definite importance to the qualities of the arterial pulsation as a whole. However, attention has not yet been focused on the mutual independence of the segments of the artery which have been perceived, studied and utilized in China since ancient times. No instrument in either Japan, China or the West has been developed to register and measure these pulse segments. An instrument designed in Japan by Dr. Moritani only a few decades ago has not yet been marketed, as it is still in the testing stage.

Since 1925, when I began to teach acupuncture in hospitals, French researchers have addressed themselves to designing instruments for measuring the pulses of the organs. Several models exist but are not satisfactory enough for their inventors to assume the cost of public promotion. The sphygmomanometers of Mr. Pouret and Dr. Nogier exemplify this.

Throughout human history, with the present no exception, the finger has been the most thorough and sensitive instrument for the perception of all that can be revealed by the radial pulses. Until recent times, doctors always palpated the pulses, not only for evaluating fever, but for ascertaining the resistance of the patient and the adequate dosage of the appropriate medicine. This custom, I should say this art, is now disdained and forgotten. At present, taking the blood pressure is a routine procedure, giving only one indication without any connection with the older system of palpation.

What useful scientific and clinical information have we lost from this great disdain for our ancients? (What would we know without them?) Hippocrates (440-360 B.C.) formed a diagnosis from certain qualities of the pulses naturally perceived with the finger. Charicles, doctor of Tiber, is famous for having determined the state of health and troubles of the emperor by taking his wrist to kiss his hand at the end of a meal. Galen (A.D. 130 - 201) has left two works on diagnosis by pulse-taking. In later times, Strutius, Baillou, and Bellini have all contributed works on this subject.

In seventeenth century Spain, Solano de Luque perfected a method of diagnosis which had considerable influence. In 1732, Sénac, Principal Physician to the King of France, gave this method an excellent appraisal, followed in 1756 by Th. de Bordeu and in 1767 by Fouquet.

Evaluations of the total energy, its diverse forms, and the energy of local areas were made by these illustrious ancients through palpation without instrumentation or arbitrary numbers. Our instruments have only relative measures: their readings give different numbers according to their type, and even samples of the same type are not always in agreement. It is rare to meet two doctors who use the same method for taking blood pressure and arrive at the same numbers. The source of uncertainty lies in the numbers themselves, in what is expected from the instrument, and in the interpretation that must be given to the numbers found.

The discovery of the Chinese pulse system holds great importance for physiology and even more so for every person. Illumination of the ideas transmitted from Far Eastern tradition and comparisons with modern European knowledge are necessary in order to encourage further study which will undoubtedly lead to useful, new discoveries on the measurements of the total, diverse and local energy of the body.

For the significance of different aspects of the radial pulses, see Volume III, Part III, Chapter IV: ''Significance of the Radial Pulses.'' What follows below is a discussion of the meaning and explanation of the pulses.

II. The Pulses: Problems, Explanations

Important discoveries would no doubt follow from scholarly investigation of the facts I have pointed out regarding Chinese pulses. These discoveries would more than doubly enhance the tradition from the East and would require modification of the Western concepts of pulsation itself, the unity of the radial artery, and its singular circulatory significance.

The pulsation.

The Chinese of antiquity observed the fact that pulsation is always perceived at the same places on the artery (the ''bumps''), and that between these segments there is no beat (the ''knots''). This concept is apparently in contradiction to the Western notion that the pulsation moves throughout the whole artery.

Several complementary explanations have been given for the pulsation itself:

The pulsation is produced by the tendency of a distended or flattened artery to resume its natural form. (Dastre, Doyon)

The pulsation is due to a temporary hypertension produced by the cardiac systole, without dilation of the vessel. (Marey)

The rapid augmentation of the aortic blood pressure passing from the diastole to the systole creates the waves of pressure of the pulses during systolic discharge. This is rapidly transmitted through the arterial system (at the rate of 2 to 20 m. per second according to the diameter of the vessel). This wave is much more rapid than the ejected blood (eight seconds from head to foot, 25 cm. per second). (Main)

The speed of the wave is 9 m. per second until the capillaries; that of the blood is 45 cm. per second in the aorta and 36 cm. per second in the radial artery. (Hédon)

The pulsation is due both to the systole and to the elasticity of the artery. (Larousse)

The pulsation is due to an autonomous modification of the caliber of the arteries, which are commanded by the nerves of their muscular envelope. (Alexis Carrel)

Professor Mériel and Professor Leriche believe that the nerves involved are autonomic, reacting under the stimulus of the passage of the wave and blood. Professor Leriche's experiments on arterial segments, cited below, are material proof of the independence of the segments and the effects of autonomic action on them.

As early as 1826, Laënnec wrote (*Auscultation Médiate*, Chapter ''Du pouls''):

*The actual impulsion increased. This phenomenon is one of those that best proves, contrary to the opinion of some physiologists, that **the arteries have their own action, independent from that of the heart.** There even exists a notable difference in the state of health between the beats of one of the radial arteries and the other. The right pulse is almost always stronger than the left.*

The Chinese of antiquity have written: ''The blood is at the interior of the arteries and the energy is at the exterior.''

In this conceptualization, pulsation is due to the blood and the contraction of the vascular envelope. The ancient Chinese also taught that the right pulse represents the energy, the nervous life, and the left pulse the blood, the physical life. The tubercular patients examined by Laënnec were obviously more nervous than physically strong.

Blood pressure (not the "pressure" necessary to overcome resistance).

According to Professor Mériel, the different pressures of the artery are equally due to the autonomic nerves, as is shown by experiment:

> *If the muscles of the arteries are in a hypotonic state, the pulse will be ample and soft; if hypertonic, the pulse will be hard and contracted. Hence, their tone depends totally on the autonomic system.*

Clinically speaking, when the arteries are contracted, without palpitation, and with elevated pressure, it suffices to rebalance the tone of the autonomic system. This is accomplished by dispersing with a precise point and tonifying with another. The artery becomes supple and ample and the pressure decreases.

The contraction of an artery from autonomic imbalance results in the relative increase in blood volume; consequently, it is necessary to consider the balance between the peripheral and visceral circulation.

R.J. Main sees several factors relating to the maintenance of the pressure:

> *The primary factors involved in regulating arterial blood pressure are ejection by the heart, venous return, the blood volume, the elasticity of the vessels, the resistance to flow (caliber of the vessels, viscosity of the blood, interstitial pressure, gravity, capacity of the circulatory system, and the volume of the blood).*

In summary, the volume of blood, its nature, the power of ejection of the blood by the heart, the venous return, and the contraction of the vessels by themselves or by their surroundings are the main factors.

The three blood pressures.

Western science recognizes and measures with instruments three different levels of the artery. Each level has a quality, character, and beat different from the other two. Additionally, the same level cannot be identical for both wrists.

From antiquity, the Chinese observed the existence of these three levels under the names of superficial, middle, and deep. They discovered the correlations between aspects of each level and the functional qualities of the organs and large areas of the body. Important physiological information was extracted from this before writing was developed.

Oscillometers permit the measurement of each of the three pressures. Sphygmomanometers, used by most doctors, give some information on two levels, the diastolic and systolic. Let us repeat that not all instruments are adjusted to the same scale, that they very easily go out of adjustment, and that it is rare for two doctors to give the same numbers even when using the same instruments. One must also remember that the blood pressure varies according to the hour, the position, the barometric pressure, the emotions, whether or not a meal has been eaten, etc.

We must point out that our physiology books do not explain the full import of each of the different aspects of the three blood pressures. They teach neither the organic disorders which cause them, nor the linked organ particular to each of the modifications, nor even the autonomic function that activates them.

Minima pressure (superficial; diastolic. Superficial pulses): perceived by lightly touching the surface (superficial edge) of the artery. R.J. Main states:

> *Augmented by excessive ejection from the heart, rapidity of the heart, peripheral resistance, and non-elasticity or contraction of the vessels. Diminished by vasodilation, decreased blood volume, diminished cardiac ejection, a slow heart, nonresistance of the peripheral vessels.*

In brief, excess or insufficiency of the heart, vessels or blood can augment or diminish the pressure.

The practice of the science of energy permits us to observe that an elevated diastolic pressure always corresponds to nervous excitation resulting from weakening and irritating chronic pain, to an excess of yang energy. The diastolic is lowered by dispersing the triple warmer at *tianjing* (TW-10), after calming the pains using *kunlun* (BL-60). An elevated but hard diastolic pulse indicates an excess of the kidneys (disperse *yongquan*, KI-1) or of the vessels (disperse *daling*, PC-7).

Intermediary pressure (dynamic; middle; useful; efficacious. Middle pulses):

The middle pulse is seen on oscillometers as the largest oscillation between the diastolic and systolic. It can be close to one or the other according to the case. Sphygmomanometers used by doctors do not register it. If jerky and near the diastolic, it is attributed to the irritability of the autonomic system accentuating the abrupt contraction of the arteries. It depends on the triple warmer.

In practice, an excessive intermediary pressure is usually seen in highly nervous people, and an insufficient pressure is seen in lymphatic people. It is nearer the diastolic in nervous people and nearer the systolic in depressed people. If elevated and jerky, it drops and softens when the triple warmer is dispersed at *tianjing* (TW-10). If insufficient, one must tonify the triple warmer at *zhongzhu* (TW-3).

Maxima pressure (deep; systolic. Deep pulses): Perceived by pressing the finger on the artery to the bottom, yet without arresting flow. R.J. Main states:

> *Increased by the energy of the systole, the rapidity of the heart, or vasoconstriction. Diminished by sympathetic vasodilation, weakness of the systole, or slowness of the heart.*

Vasoconstriction, which augments the systolic pressure, produces a relative excess of blood volume. This may be due to an excess absorption of salts or liquids, an excess of adrenalin leading to retention of salt and consequently water, or most significantly, to insufficient filtration (excess of the middle kidney pulse).

In practice, an elevated systolic (not flattened, sunken) is partially lowered by dispersing the vagus at *tianzhu* (BL-10). It follows then that this condition could be caused by an excess of the vagus. Tonifying the sympathetic system in insufficiency using *fengchi* (GB-20) also acts according to the indications of the pulse. If there is an excess of blood, disperse the arteries (*daling,* PC-7), the filtration (*rangu,* KI-2) and the adrenals (*fengfu,* GV-15, IS GV-16).

An excess of the systolic (for deep pulses) can be transferred to an insufficiency of the diastolic (for superficial pulses) by tonifying *waiguan* (TW-5) or dispersing *neiguan* (PC-6). It is clearly evident that the autonomic system holds primary importance for the three pressures, as it is the underlying cause of change in pressure through its direct action on certain organs.

Keep in mind that there is no "normal" pressure. Each person has his "customary" pressure assuring his own balance and can retain good health if this pressure is within the range of 12/6 to 25/12. What must be considered are pressure changes. The diastolic pressure is the most significant since it can indicate blockages in vital organs.

The segments of the arteries.

The Chinese discovery of arterial segments is of the greatest importance, for it allows us to measure the energy in each of the organs as well as in the body. Their existence was unknown in Europe until the seventeenth century, the period in which Don Solano de Luque perfected a method of diagnosis through the pulses that had great popularity. (He used the relative changes in quality of several segments of the radial artery.)

In China, their existence was known and used from greatest antiquity. They have been verified since that time, experimented upon and brought to perfection. In Paris, we have also been able to verify them using modern instrumentation, making the indications precise while adding discoveries of new segments and their significance unknown in China. The experiments of Professor Leriche between 1935 and 1946 have contributed greatly to the explanation and proof of the existence of arterial segments and their mutual independence.

The observed and verifiable facts are these: on an energetic radial pulse we see many points beating at the same time; the beats do not pass from one point to another but are always at the same spots; between them nothing beats. Professor Leriche has observed that after removing the sympathetic enervation from a single segment, it loses its beats and becomes a hard tube while the other segments continue to beat as usual. This indicates that the aligned segments are independent of one another. They form, so to speak, a rosary of small peripheral hearts following the action of the heart.

The pulses of the organs.

The ancient Chinese made a discovery of considerable importance, a discovery verified instrumentally and experimentally beyond all possible doubt, and I hope considerably extended by my own research:

1) For each arterial segment, each of the pressure levels is independent from one another and from all others.

2) Each responds to an organ, and its qualities are modified as soon as the organ is modified.

The tradition of Asia recognizes three segments and two pressure levels at each wrist, totaling twelve pulses, one for each of the ten material organs (yin: heart, lung, spleen-pancreas, liver, kidney; yang: stomach, large intestine, small intestine, urinary bladder, gallbladder) and one each for the yang triple warmer and the yin heart governor.

Our instruments, observations, and experimentation have almost quadrupled the number of pulses. In effect, it has been observed that:

1)   The three pressure-levels (instead of two) have significance.

2)   Three segments on the right and three on the left have been added to the three ancient segments at each wrist. These have been recognized by us as linked to certain organs or functions: those of the governor vessel, nerve centers, and endocrine glands on the right, and those of the conception vessel, psyche, and organs of sense on the left.

Classically, they were perceived as being on the anterior face of the radial eminence, distal and directly proximal to it. The surface-deep coupling on the right is as follows: large intestine — lungs; stomach — spleen-pancreas; triple warmer — vessels-sexuality. Those on the left: small intestine — heart; gallbladder — liver; urinary bladder — kidney. Our modern findings indicate for the right: large intestine — lung; stomach — spleen-pancreas; the three levels of the governor vessel; triple warmer — vessels — sexual organs; spinal cord and medulla oblongata — cerebellum and pons — brain; adrenals — thyroid — parathyroids — pituitary. On the left, small intestine — heart; gallbladder — liver — blood pressure; the three parts of the conception vessel; urinary bladder — kidney filtration — kidney excretion-secretion; psyche: development — automaton (parroting) — primate; eyes, ears, taste, smell.

These three new points are located on the radiopalmar artery, but distal to the large intestine — lung position on the right wrist and the small intestine — heart on the left wrist.

3)   Each edge of the artery (radiopalmar as well as radial artery, radial edge and medial edge) is independent of the other and responds singularly to stimulation of a point located either on the right or the left.

This is an important observation allowing us to recognize modifications of function: *a)* For the double organs, of its left or right member. We have been able to observe which kidney has been removed, which lung was attacked, etc. *b)* For the singular organs, the existence of nervous and motor command for each half of the organ on the same side as the pulse and the stimulated point.

4)   For the trained hand and delicate touch, it is observable that each level of each segment responds only in its upper or lower part to the stimulation on the points acting on the upper or lower part of the organ. Thus, for the pulse of the heart, the upper (proximal) half represents the ventricles and the lower (distal) part, the auricles. For the sexual organs, the upper part responds to the testicles or ovaries, the middle to the fallopian tube or penis, the lower part to the uterus, etc.

The repertoire of pulses is thus considerably extended and developed. It allows a precise appreciation greatly facilitating the discrimination between the left or right, high or low, and disturbances in energy of the same organ.

Instead of the twelve primary pulses, researchers now have sixty-eight. They are the subdivisions of the twelve segments of the radial artery multiplied by three levels, and the two segments of the radiopalmar artery multiplied by two levels.

Organ-pulse relations.

The ancient Chinese physiologists observed the mutual independence of each pulse segment, of each pressure level, and finally the relationship of each pulse with one organ. They thereby made a physiological discovery of great importance for measuring the intensity of the energy in each of the internal organs. Each pulse modifies its beat independently of all others when the function or condition of a certain organ and no other is altered. Each organ is thus represented by one pulse (or, as we have said above, by the edge of the artery at the pulse).

We estimate that it is possible to discern not only, for example, if a kidney has been removed and which one, but also to say if urine is abundant and less colored by loose filtration (in the glomeruli) or by excretion which has not been made (in the tubules). We can also say which part of the respiratory tract and which side of the body is in excess or insufficiency; we can indicate which area of the large intestine is dysfunctioning, if there are intestinal worms or hemorrhoids; and determine if a person has or does not have moral consciousness, if the person easily understands problems of mathematics, etc.

The proof of these claims lies in the data collected from instruments registering the existence of the three independent pressures at each wrist and the experiments showing the correlations between major internal functions and particular radial pressures. These should not go unnoticed, since they form the basis in the West for proof of

Eastern discoveries. They are the result of extensive observations, interpreted according to modern analytic and synthetic thought. Unfortunately, there are also those scholars with excessively analytical, mistrustful, and narrow minds, who confuse caution in learning with wisdom.

The banal objection to the artery not having segments is no longer tenable after the simple observations and published results of experimentation by Professor Leriche. His findings prove the independent functioning of the segments of the superimposed pulse (three pressures) at each segment. However, the mechanism linking each pulse to each organ still awaits scientific explanation. This would allow us to use these discoveries clinically, without mental reservation, and obtain optimal results.

Professor Paul Mériel of the faculty of Toulouse has taken a lively interest in this problem and has devoted himself to a great deal of research and experimentation. I can do no better than to cite his conclusions:

> *The function of the organs is commanded by a corresponding vegetative center, first in the spinal cord, then in the medulla oblongata and finally in the hypothalamus. The changes in organs are accompanied by alterations in their control centers and vice-versa; an alteration in one of the centers provokes in the organ either a functional disturbance or a lesion which can be serious (sclerosis of the liver or kidney, or hemorrhage).*
>
> *It is through the sympathetic or parasympathetic systems that these centers are kept in contact with the corresponding organs.*
>
> *We know that the pulse and its qualities give us information about the arterial tone commanded by the autonomic system, which is itself commanded by the vegetative centers higher up.*
>
> *The pulses, therefore, give us information about the state of the higher vegetative centers. This may explain why, after deterioration or removal of an organ, its pulse is not always modified, since the function continues under the direction of the higher vegetative center. For example, the function of the gallbladder continues in spite of its removal. Hence, serious organic lesion of an organ does not disturb the pulse as much as a functional disturbance, since the latter is under the control of higher vegetative centers.*

A comment is necessary in order for the reader to understand clearly what Professor Meriel writes about the persistence of the pulse after removal of an organ. In effect, the removal of one kidney is perceived and will always be perceived at its pulse. Conversely, for a removed gallbladder, the pulse at first almost disappears, returning after some six months with nearly all its functional aspects. This contradiction is explained by the fact that the pulse of the kidney represents its filtration as well as its reabsorption and excretion; if it disappears, its function disappears. It is not the same for the gallbladder. If it is removed, all the other anatomical and nervous parts still remain which are activated by the biliary reflex: the choledochal canal, Oddi's sphincter, etc. So, in reality, the pulse indicates the biliary reflex, of which the gallbladder is only a part.

Therefore, we can see that the autonomic system explains the pulse-organ relations: the pulses and organs communicate through it with the higher vegetative centers. (For the significance of the pulse, see Volume III, Part III, Chapter IV.)

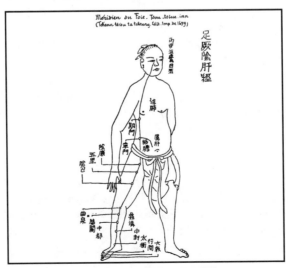

Meridian of the liver (DACH)

Chapter IV

Vital Energy (IV)

Origin and Conservation

I. Origins — II. Conservation — III. Conditions for the Maintenance of Energy — IV. Astral Rhythms — V. Atmospheric Conditions — VI. Accumulation and Reserves

I. Origins

Living organisms can only be produced by other living organisms. The perplexing question of how universal energy transforms into vital energy and when this originally occurred must be left in the realm of metaphysics.

II. Conservation of Energy

Hédon wrote the following before the discovery of atomic fission:

> *The law of conservation of energy in nature (Mayer, Helmholtz) states that nothing is lost or created. The total quantity of matter and energy does not vary; thus, when a certain quantity of energy seems to have been destroyed, it has in actual fact been transformed.*

People of the Far East, in general more discerning, had long before considered that all is energy. Matter was seen as concretized energy, transformed into its latent form.

With this knowledge of the conservation of energy, we must question why there is a loss of vital energy in illness, aging and death, and how it can be prevented. The discoveries and experiments of Alexis Carrel have proven that under certain conditions the vital energy and matter do not age or expire. Some organs *in vitro* can continue to live undamaged, indefinitely longer than their normal life-span, if they are kept in absolutely optimal conditions. Once deprived of these conditions, they deteriorate.

Experiments have not been carried out on living beings. This would be much more difficult, since optimal conditions for living organisms would entail psychological as well as physical components; and as each individual is absolutely unique, ideal conditions would differ from one to the other. To arrive at a basic understanding of these conditions, one must have a thorough knowledge of the physiology of energy. Under ideal conditions, one could speculate that impairments, aging, and death could be postponed in the same manner as in Carrel's isolated organs.

III. Conditions for the Maintenance of Vital Energy

As each individual is unique, we can only consider the most general conditions necessary for the maintenance of energy: air, food and drink; psychological components; astral rhythms and atmospheric influences. *Air* is the most essential factor — no life can continue for more than a few minutes deprived of air.

No existing work fully considers the influence of the differing qualities of air, although each person easily assesses them and declares that for himself one quality tends to improve his condition while another aggravates it. The qualities might be described as light, heavy, pure, thick, exciting, depressing, etc. (see ''Sources of Energy'': lungs). *Shanzhong* (CV-17) increases the intake of air and its assimilation.

Intake of food and drink must be considered in relation to the individual, temperature, season, country, and lifestyle. Those who enjoy, easily digest, and perfectly assimilate particular foods or drinks will nearly be poisoned by others, while these other foods might perfectly suit another person (see ''Sources of Energy'': small intestine, stomach, etc.). We will say only that by starting with a very small quantity and increasing very slowly, it is quite possible to train ourselves to benefit from all food, even that which previously had been injurious. The meridians of the stomach, liver and small intestine regulate assimilation.

Psychological conditions are of greatest importance: a favorable environment expands and fortifies; a hostile environment contracts and atrophies. Good news can revive or kill according to the person who receives it; bad news may deplete a person or incite the will to conquer. We must take into account the action as well as the possible reactions of each individual (see ''Sources of Psychic Energy''). Tonifying the adrenals at *fengfu* (GV-15, IS GV-16) allows us to better support psychological shocks. *Kufang* of the stomach meridian (ST-14) allows us to remove or diminish noxious effects.

These psychological reactions have deep and prolonged effects at the unconscious level of our instinctual being. They may extend to the body and even surface at the evolved conscious level, the latter judging them as signs of weakness.

IV. The Astral Rhythms

The vital rhythm is linked with and strongly influenced by the rhythm of the astral bodies. It would be unscientific not to take this into account. (Modern urbanites often neglect or ignore this influence.) During the waxing of astral bodies, the vital energy of yang activity is also increasing, while the energy of inactivity decreases. At that time, it is clearly easier to tonify the yang energy and disperse the yin energy. When astral bodies are at their maximum decline, it is possible to obtain the greatest, most lasting results by dispersing the yang energy and tonifying the yin energy.

The energy of yang activity precisely follows the ascendency and descendency of the astral bodies. A large proportion of one's energy is transformed to its most active yang state when the astral bodies are in ascendency. During this period, the energy of yin inactivity is at its weakest. The converse is true when the astral bodies are descending.

All astral bodies have an influence on the energy. Cosmic rays, in particular, can be of great importance. Apart from the sun, earth and moon, the influence of the astral rhythms is not easily understood.

The diurnal and yearly solar rhythms are firmly linked with the energy of yang activity. Yang is at its maximum at midday and at its minimum at midnight. Sunshine gives positive electricity to the atmosphere, the increase of which is more evident at the beginning of the day.

Problems arising from a yang insufficiency (thus a relative yin excess) exhibit their maximum at midday, while problems of yang excess (thus relative insufficiency of yin) are maximal at midnight. Hence, there are nervous migraines which rise and fall with the sun and nocturnal congestive headaches which disappear in the morning.

The absence of the sun leaves the moon and earth dominant.

During the year, the seasonal solar rhythm causes the energy of yang activity to increase from the winter solstice, until the summer solstice when the yin energy is at its minimum. The yang energy then decreases from the summer solstice until the winter solstice, when the yin energy is at a maximum.

Each season of the year has its particular illnesses. At the spring equinox, the liver is at its minimum: migraines, eczema, asthma, spasms, poliomyelitis and granular tuberculosis are at their height. In May and June, eruptive disorders such as measles and scarlet fever are seen. At the summer solstice, cerebral hyperexcitation is at its maximum. At the autumn equinox, there may be recurrence of poliomyelitis and liver insufficiency disorders. As we advance towards the winter solstice, we find an increase in cerebral anemias, depression and inflammations of the respiratory passages and kidneys.

This seasonal rhythm is reminiscent of the rhythm of the daily maximum and minimum of each organ (see "Flow of Energy"). We must not consult the inaccurate Western calendar, but use the signs of the zodiac and the precession of the equinox.

The moon has a monthly rhythm which influences the energy just as it does the tides and menses. At the new moon, when sunlight is not reflected, the energy of yang activity is at its minimum; the ancients say, "it is death." This is the time to tonify the yang. One puncture is as effective as fifteen at the full moon.

Most women have their menses at the new moon and maternity hospitals record the largest number of deliveries at that time. Cutting the ends of the hair at this time strengthens its regrowth. It is a good time for planting and doing certain kinds of vineyard work. Intestinal worms proliferate during this period.

"The full moon is life." It reflects the sun; yang energy is at its maximum. It is the time to disperse excesses; however, if tonification is required, fifteen punctures will be necessary where one would have sufficed during the new moon. Yin energy is at its minimum. Lunar rays corrode marble four times faster than solar rays. Intestinal worms have a second period of proliferation at this time.

The Earth is always electrically negative. Each geographical formation has a marked yet unexplained influence on the vital energy. This influence is beneficial for some and harmful for others. It is not just a matter of large regions of mountains, seas, etc., but also of smaller localities. The effects of Berck[1] cease outside of its valley and its beach. Two streets of the same town may have different influences.

Living or travelling in mountainous regions (yin) leads to an increase in the number of red corpuscles, imposing greater effort on the heart. For some, this effect lasts after returning to the plains; for others, despite the healthy exposure to the sun, the return is followed by severe nervous and emotional depression and sometimes anemia.

Valleys, or the shores of lakes or rivers (yin) are favorable for congestive and hypertensive people. This is due to vasodilation which occurs there. These same places are depressing for nervous, anemic, and lymphatic people.

Forests (yin) have differing effects according to the type of soil and wood. Fir trees act on the lungs, oaks are depressants, etc. The oxygen given off during the day by leaves strengthens depressed people, provided they close their windows at night in order to avoid the carbon dioxide given off nocturnally. The green color of the leaves can aggravate sadness.

The great plateaus, viewed as sunny and dry (yang), are where atmospheric electricity is constantly positive. These plateaus stimulate the energy and strengthen the muscles without developing them. They are beneficial to lymphatic, sad people and stimulate nervous people. The vital energy responds maximally to stimulation there.

The sea develops the physical energy through its water (yin), and develops and strengthens the energy of the nervous centers through its salt, which is dynamized by the constant movement (yang). Forcefulness and rapidity of thought and action are increased. The respiratory and digestive passages are hyperstimulated there. *Shiguan* (KI-18) on the right side can counteract the adverse reactions which often follow, from the first sign of improvement and up to fifteen days.

Whatever the nature of the greater region, one should also consider the effects that the specific locality may have on the usual reactions of the person involved.

V. Atmospheric Conditions

Atmospheric conditions affect each person differently according to his or her nature. Wind, humidity, dryness, heat, cold and storms were classified in high antiquity under the name of the "Six Brigands" which disturb one's energy. To these we have added a seventh — atmospheric pressure. Acupuncture is most efficacious on a pleasant, calm sunny day.

Atmospheric pressure is recognized in the West as having a definite action on the body. Increased pressure (high barometric reading) — a yang influence— compresses the body, lightens it, compresses the arteries and increases high blood pressure. As a result, there is aggravation in plethoric people and improvement in hypotensive and lymphatic people. Diminished pressure (low barometric reading) — a yin influence — relaxes the body, makes it heavy, distends the arteries and slows the circulation. Weakened and exhausted people feel heavy and tired. Hypertensive people are improved. Changes in atmospheric pressure may be preceded by aggravations (e.g., headache, neuralgias, rheumatic pain) or by amelioration, depending on the individual. *Waiguan* (TW-5), dispersed or tonified according to the case, alleviates warning symptoms and aggravations caused by barometric changes.

The wind (yang) stimulates and irritates the energy. It stimulates and contracts the gallbladder. People with neuralgia and migraines experience aggravation of symptoms, while lymphatic types and those who are exhausted but not nervous are improved. Wind from the east causes neuralgia; from the south, congestion; from the north, it tonifies; and from the west (from the sea), it calms.

Atmospheric electricity acts powerfully: storms may completely devitalize some people; others may experience irrational terror or overexcitation. *Waiguan* (TW-5) again provides great help in relieving these sensitivities.

Humidity (yin) at saturation and 37° C. prevents sweat from evaporating from the skin and heat from dissipating from the lungs through the breath. It weakens the spleen-pancreas and the yang energy. So also it calms nervous types but tires those who cannot easily expel water from their tissues and who become swollen from water in the air. The kidney is fatigued by humid conditions since it must operate as the only mechanism for evacuating water from the body; this predisposes people to rheumatism. Finally, humidity greatly increases the effects of heat and cold. *Shiguan* (KI-18) prevents problems of humidity, as do *tiaokou* (ST-38) and leg-*sanli* (ST-36).

External heat (yang) causes cutaneous vasodilation, sweating and increased respiration, and if it continues there is hypotension, a tendency to weakness, anemia and dehydration. (At 18° C one liter of water is lost through perspiration at rest.) Hyperchloremia and diminished urine with swollen ankles may result. In Asia, it is said that the exterior is dilated and the interior emptied, that the yin energy is at the periphery at the expense of the interior. Action on the energy gives some immediate results but often fatigues the patient. The sensation of heat is diminished by dispersing *shenmai* (BL-62).

External cold (yin) contracts the exterior (yang) and congests the interior (yin). It causes vasoconstriction which increases the concentration of blood cells by diminishing the volume of blood. "The blood loses its water to the profit of the internal organs, glands and muscles" (Hédon). In Asia it is said, "The sap withdraws from the branches and bark and concentrates itself in the trunk and roots." Clinically, action on the energy is retarded, and in certain cases the effect of treatment is obtained suddenly after eight days. Deafness shows a much higher rate of cure in summer than in winter. Tonifying *guanyuan* (CV-4) diminishes the invasion of cold, while tonifying *shenmai* (BL-62) lessens the sensation of cold.

Dryness (yang) increases evaporation, dries the skin and the lungs and aggravates the intestines, which need moisture. If prolonged, as in certain countries (e.g., the dry season in India), nervous hyperexcitation is produced and even some mental disorders. Lymphatic and hydrogenoid types find a great sensation of well-being and improvement in dry climates.

VI. Accumulation and Reserves of Energy

The facts are as follows: Some people can produce the same amount of work for weeks and months while receiving very irregular quantities of nourishment and keeping irregular eating times. From where do they take the steady quantities of energy that they put out? Conversely, other people ingest a consistent quantity of food daily and keep very regular eating hours, yet feel their potential ever diminishing. What happens to the energy they extract from the food? It should be at their disposal, yet they seem to be deprived of it.

If tonified, certain command points (particularly leg-*sanli,* ST-36) revitalize the entire body — nervous centers, circulation, muscles, etc.— by working on increasing the ability to extract energy from food. All the pulses are increased, as are instrumental readings of energetic strength. No diminution is observed in any other part of the body (as is the rule for all other points). Where does this revitalizing energy come from?

On the Loch apparatus, the needle stays at the maximum in certain cases. For others the needle falls immediately, indicating that there are no reserves.

In brief, we see that the expenditure of energy can be very regular or irregular, even to the point of sudden and considerable consumption. Likewise, contributions of energy from food and drink can be very regular or irregular. The two are without influence on the capacity to expend energy. As for obtaining energy from the air, this is constant, if not regular, in quantity and quality; its arrest for a few minutes necessarily brings death (except for yogis?). It would be of great clinical benefit to precisely understand this phenomenon.

Two possibilities present themselves: 1) The existence of reserves of energy from which it is possible to draw according to need. 2) The progressive transformation of latent energy into active energy according to need.

The hypothesis of reserves of energy leads us to another hypothesis— that of accumulators. We know that the liver stores all the vitamins formed or transformed by the different organs and that it distributes them according to need. Vitamins are considered biocatalyzers. We also know that when the endocrine glands are functioning well they respond to the body's messages by secreting hormones into the blood according to need; occasionally, they are true stimulants of energy. But what does this word "stimulant" mean? Is it a question of bringing energy or exciting its production? Or, as Bogomoletz writes, following Betcherev, is it that "the cells of the brain are accumulators"?

People who increase their work output without increasing their food intake become thin. With equal vitality, energetic fat people can sustain an effort longer than thin people. In effect, flesh, muscle and fat, which increase with rest and diminish with work, are burned up and are combustible accumulators which produce heat. This is not a direct expression of energy, but rather of force, a form of energy.

On the other hand, the blood along with its fluids provides irrigation to the smallest of cells and brings them energy (see "Energy and Blood") as well as indispensable chemical elements. It appears that in addition to being a powerful electrolytic solution, blood is a true accumulator of energy that constantly recharges and purifies the organs.

We cite the following though it has yet to be verified. Tradition places *shimen* (CV-5, midway on the line joining the navel to the pubis) over the "reservoir" of energy and *qichong* (ST-30, at the groin) over the "center of distribution" by the triple warmer.

The hypothesis of the instantaneous transformation of latent energy into active energy is constantly proven by the action of energy. Certain points (notably leg-*sanli,* ST-36) tonify the whole body without our having to determine where it gets its supply. Two others, *shenmai* (BL-62) and *zhaohai* (KI-3, IS KI-6), transform the latent energy (of rest, yin) into active energy (of activity, yang) and vice versa. It is easy to verify this through the pulses and the results.

Most points transfer energy from one part of the body to another in equal quantities: all yin meridians into yang meridians and vice-versa; that of several organs into several others; or, that of one organ to another. The transfer of energy from one side to another is measurable.

Recent discoveries lead us to suppose that these transformations and transfers can be very profound. Recall what R.J. Main writes on this subject:

> *All cells at rest show a difference of electrical potential between the interior (−) and the exterior (+), the cell membrane acting as an insulator . . . All stimulation of cells first produces a discharge, then a recharge; thus, a period of activity and one of rest.*

But if the discharge is greater than the recharge, the exhaustion of the cells is rapid. Furthermore, if the supply of energy for the recharge of the cells is interrupted, the cell dies. It seems that the cells act mostly as transformers.

Present knowledge does not yet allow us to determine the accumulators or magnetos (the brain, according to Betcherev) which assure a constant and regular energy supply, indispensable to the life of the cells. It is only possible to suggest that it is an essential vital function, individual to each person and providing energy according to momentary needs. This function consists of transforming the active energy taken from air and food into latent energy and fixing it in all the tissues, and also transforming this latent energy into active energy when the need arises.

The fact that by tonifying the small intestine it is possible to acquire almost instantaneous recuperation from fatigue and effort inclines us to think that the function of transforming energy may depend as well on the small intestine and the duodenum (see ''Small Intestine''), perhaps through the manufacture of small albumin molecules specific to each individual. Chinese medical scholars would place this accumulator in the brain, since they write: ''When the energy of the body is exhausted, the brain can reconstitute it.''

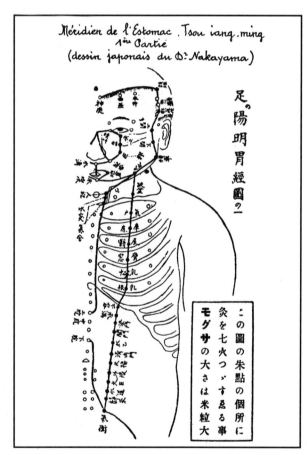
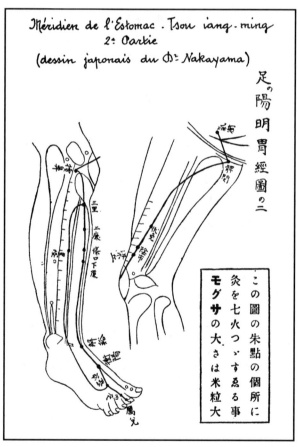

Meridian of the stomach (Nakayama)

Notes

[1] A small northeastern French town known for its good air.

Chapter V

Vital Energy (V)

The Circulation of Energy and Meridians

I. Circulation and Cycles of Energy 1. The Facts 2. The Level of the Body 3. The Speed of the Energy — II. The Meridians: Meridians and Organs (Number, Inequality; Meridian-Organ Relations; Names and Orders) — III. Laws of Meridian-Organ Interaction (Succession of the Flow; Mother-Child; Coupled Meridians; Points of Passage; Maximum-Minimum) — IV. The Two Medial Lines 1. Anterior Medial Line: Conception Vessel 2. Posterior Medial Line: Governor Vessel

I. Circulation and Cycles of Energy

Ancient physiologists made a discovery that has totally escaped the West until now — that of the circulation of energy. It is of the greatest importance, since through it the science of commanding the vital energy has been developed, understood and explained. This science investigates the existence of an additional circulatory system having no relation to the nervous, circulatory or lymphatic systems.

It is no longer a question of theory or opinion, but of reality. I begin by supporting this through the discoveries of the late Sir Thomas Lewis (circulation specialist and Director of the Privy Council's College of Medical Research). In the *British Medical Journal* (Feb. 1937), he announced his findings concerning a "new nervous conduction totally different from what is known." It was "unknown" because he ignored the existence of the Chinese meridians. He defined it as "a new conduction of sensitivity — heat force and life — totally different from all that we know for blood, lymph, and nerves." The numerous experiments he described were carried out only on the anterior part of the thigh and lower leg. Our new instruments register it.

The facts.

A circuit of conduction exists in each lateral half of the body; the energy there always circulates in the same direction without interruption and sustains all the organs, our whole being. A simple galvanometer allows us to detect it along its entire course.

Specially designed dialed instruments (namely, the Pouret-Niboyet, Loch, Leplus, or Brunet-Grenier apparatus) allow measurement of the intensity of the energy flow. If the electrode leaves the line of flow even by one millimeter, the needle drops.

All people with average sensitivity (they are quite frequent even among Occidentals) can perceive them along their entire course. For example, by pressing around the limb with the tip of the finger or the nail, they notice that several lines of particular sensitivity exist. Just by pressing on the line we obtain the sensation of "something," say most people, passing along the line like an electric current. By coincidence, and only for short distances, these lines follow known pathways, such as those of vessels and nerves.

By carefully following one of these lines, we note that it ascends and descends along the limbs repeating for a total of six different but connected lines, three descending and three ascending, before returning to the original starting point. These two circuits of energy, one on each side of the body, do not directly communicate.

For example, when the arm is elevated, we can follow the circuit starting from the hand descending along the lateral surface (yang) of the upper limb to the head and from there on to the lateral surface of the leg to the foot. From the foot it ascends the anterior surface of the lower limb up to the chest, and from there along the medial surface (yin) of the upper limb to the hand. It then descends and ascends again by different lines six times in all before coming back to the starting point. These lines form a closed circuit in which the "something" indicated by the observers always passes in the same direction without interruption or cessation, a true circulatory system of energy.

The level of the body.

The level of the body through which the circuit passes has been determined by the following fact: a very important command point of this circuit, *gaohuangshu* (BL-38, IS BL-43) can only be reached by crossing the arms at the elbows so that each scapula is totally moved to the side. If the scapula is in its usual place, stimulation at the skin gives no result, but with the scapula displaced the result is obtained. This shows that the point and circuit are not at the level of the skin, but beneath the epidermis, dermis and fatty hypodermis, i.e., in the subcutaneous tissue, which the needle reaches by passing through the skin.

The total length of the circuit naturally depends on the height of each individual. We have observed that it is six times the length from finger tip to toe tip (with the hand and foot extended). The ancient physiologists cited their calculation of its length as 162 "feet" or cubits (each of ten *cun*). We do not have a measure corresponding to their "foot" or cubit. Excavations in China have uncovered a "foot" measure dating from the second century B.C.; this "foot" corresponds to 24 cm. If we accept this measure, the length of the circuit would be 38 m. 88 cm., which divided by 6 x 2 would give about three meters from the foot to the elevated hand, already a very great height of nearly two meters. (Much of the population of the Shandong region is taller than two meters. The Lolos of the great Yangzi often reach 2 m. 20 cm.). Our "cubit," from the fold of the elbow to the fold of the wrist, varies according to height, but is around 24 cm.

The speed of the energy.

The speed of the energy in these closed circuits was calculated and discussed by the physiologists of high antiquity. Ancient sources give the following calculations: the energy completes a cycle in the double circuit fifty times between the two passages of the sun at the zenith (38 m. x 88 = 1940 m. divided by 1440 minutes). This would give a speed of about 1 m. 35 cm. per minute.

The ancients compared the fifty daily cycles with the fifty divisions of the zodiac. They also saw a relation between the constellations and the divisions of the circuits of energy. The *Nei Jing* states:

> *The circle of heaven encloses 28 constellations, each having 36 divisions [28 x 36 = 1008]. While the sun makes a round of the 28 constellations, the energy also makes a round of the 1008 divisions of the meridians, those having a number of 28.*

We shall see that there are 12 meridians for each circuit, thus 24, plus the addition of the two medial lines multiplied by their two ascending and descending currents, thus 4 + 24 = 28. The significance of the 1008 divisions of the meridians still eludes us. (There are only 800 points.)

We must point out that ancient Chinese astronomy was very advanced. Details in the ancient works concerning particular aspects of the sky at the moment of an eclipse are used by modern scholars to verify their exact date and hour.

II. The Meridians: Meridians and Organs

Each lateral circuit is divided into twelve meridians; the energy circulates within these divisions, which are of unequal length. Each meridian is in constant connection with its corresponding internal organ: the meridian assures a supply of energy to the organ and reflects the latter's disorders.

The name "meridian" derives from the analogy between these hand to foot lines and the north-south terrestrial lines of longitude. Ancient scholars in China had already measured the globe in degrees of longitude and latitude and knew it to be a sphere. The measures were taken physically on the immense plain of Northern China and correlated with the solar hours measured by the water-clock and by the stars from north to south and east to west.

This division into twelve meridians is not theoretical, but based on observations and experimentation upheld by Claude Bernard. It is based on the connection of each meridian to a single organ.

It has been observed that the lateral surface of the upper and lower limbs (yang) is traversed by the meridians of energy-producing workshop organs (stomach, the two intestines, urinary bladder, gallbladder). The medial surface of the limbs (yin) is traversed by the meridians of energy-distributing treasure organs (heart, spleen, liver, kidneys and lungs). The same division is found on the wrists between the superficial pulses (yang) which reflect the producers of energy on the lateral surface (yang), and the deep pulses (yin) which reflect the distributors of energy on the medial surface (yin).

Each of the twelve meridians has two names; we use the more common name of the organ which the meridian commands. Thus, there is the meridian of the lungs, of the heart, etc. The other name gives its point of departure (hand or foot), its importance in the production or distribution of energy, and its role as producer (yang) or distributor (yin). Thus, there is the "supreme yin of the hand," which is the meridian of the lungs, etc. We give the list as a footnote for researchers.[1]

The *tai yang* contains mostly yang energy. The *tai yin* contains mostly yin energy. The *shao yang* and *shao yin* contain energy and blood in equal quantity. The *yang ming* and *jue yin* contain mostly blood and little energy.

The shortest meridians are those going from the hand to the head (the yang) and from the chest to the hand (the yin). The longest are those going from the head to the feet (yang) and from the feet to the chest (yin).

The meridian-organ connections are as follows:

1) When an organ is disordered, the whole meridian is more sensitive than usual and more so than meridians of the normally functioning organs.

2) When the points of a meridian are stimulated, the corresponding organ responds.

3) When an organ possesses a healthy fullness of energy, very strong stimulation is necessary on the points of the corresponding meridian to obtain a modification of the organ's function, and the change is neither great nor long-lasting.

4) When an organ has excess energy, action on the points of its meridian cannot easily tonify it. On the contrary, it is easily inhibited and dispersed.

5) When an organ's energy is insufficient, stimulation of the points of its meridian easily tonifies it; only with difficulty will stimulation disperse it.

These meridian-to-organ connections have been verified so frequently in both hospital clinics and research studies that we can accept without reservation the laws recorded for millennia.

We know that it is through the autonomic nervous system that the organs communicate with the vegetative centers in the pons, medulla and hypothalamus. We have shown how these centers are linked with the pulses through the autonomic system. It is logical then to see a connection between each organ and meridian via the autonomic system, since such a relationship exists between the organs and pulses. The Chinese explanation is that the circuit of energy possesses branches which connect each meridian to its organ.

Between A.D. 1102 and 1107, a research scholar named Yang Jie (Ji Lao) had the opportunity of vivisecting criminals given to him by the provincial viceroy. His research entailed, for example, exposing the liver and observing the modifications of the pulses. He then tonified the liver through its special point and verified the effect on the pulse and in the organ itself. He was surrounded by artists, painters and secretaries who noted the least change. We still have access to the reports of these observations; they have been a great help in understanding the physiology of energy.

III. Laws of Interaction of the Organ-Meridians

Neither the meridian nor its corresponding organ is singularly modified by any kind of stimulus; other organ-meridians are always modified simultaneously either in a similar or opposite manner (see Volume III, Chapter VI, "Interaction of Organs").

This principle, which we have developed from several ancient Chinese laws, has great importance for correcting energetic disturbances. It explains the differing effects of the same puncture or medicine in similar cases: one case is cured while another is aggravated, depending on the treatment's positive or negative repercussions on other organs. We give the practical utilization of this principle in Volume III, Chapter VI: "Action on the Energy — Interaction of Organs."

Circulation of the energy in the same direction. Always careful observers, the ancient Chinese searched for an explanation of this phenomenon. In an age devoted to astronomical principles, they correlated this phenomenon with known astronomical laws, determining the revolution of the planets around the sun and the rotation of the earth. There is no such Western hypothesis for this phenomenon.

They then deduced several consequences which necessarily follow: *a)* the influence of succession; *b)* the passage from one meridian to another; *c)* the maximum and minimum hours.

The influence of succession.

As in every flow, it is taught that if upstream is empty, downstream will be empty; if upstream overflows, downstream will overflow; if downstream is blocked, upstream will become swollen. The Chinese symbol is that of the mother and child. A satisfied child will not ease the mother. An empty mother will produce a hungry child; an abundant mother, an overnourished child.

Indeed, it is usually observed that if the heart governor (which follows the kidneys in the flow) is blocked, the kidneys will become engorged and the blood pressure (particularly the systolic) will mount. Dispersing the heart governor is sufficient treatment for decreasing the blood pressure; the kidneys are then freed.

The succession of the organ meridians in the flow of energy is as follows (the custom is to take the lungs as the point of departure since they never stop; they constantly bring the astral energy to the body; their cessation for even a few minutes causes death):

Lungs — large intestine — stomach — spleen-pancreas — heart — small intestine — urinary bladder — kidneys — heart governor (vessels and sexual organs) — triple warmer — gallbladder — liver — and then back to the lungs.

The triple warmer is the mechanism for distributing the energy from its various sources to the organs. This is described in the chapter entitled ''Distribution of Energy.''

In this succession all is relative: the mother of ''downstream'' is the child of ''upstream''; the child of ''upstream'' is the mother of ''downstream.'' The mutual influence of mother and child can be modified when ''coupled meridians'' are involved if they are of very unequal intensity.

The passage from one meridian to another.

Regarding the coupled meridians, the passage of energy from one meridian to another is made end to end by a line of linkage that acts on the two meridians and their organs. By pressing along one of these lines of linkage, sensitive people perceive a response in the two meridians and the two organs; continued pressure causes a modification in the two pulses.

Hence, we have seen that the circuit of energy, when the arm is raised, descends from the hand to the head by a meridian that follows the lateral surface of the upper limb (yang); it continues to the feet through the lateral surface of the lower limb (yang). Then it is linked to a meridian that ascends the medial surface of the lower limb (yin) up to the chest and from there it continues by another meridian that follows the medial surface of the upper limb (yin), and so forth.

All the meridians of the lateral surface (yang) have their pulses at the superficial level (yang) — the systolic blood pressure. They correspond to the yang organs, the producers of energy. The meridians of the medial surface (yin) have their pulses at the deep or middle level (yin) — the diastolic blood pressure. They correspond to the yin organs, the distributors of energy. At the wrists these pulses are superimposed on top of each other as yang-yin couples (superficial, deep at each segment). The table is as follows for the couples:

Pulse Postitions for Coupled Organs						
Postition	Left Wrist			Right Wrist		
	Distal	Middle	Proximal	Distal	Middle	Proximal
Superficial	SI	GB	BL	LI	ST	TW
Middle		LR	KI (filtration)	LU	Pancreas	H.G. (Vessels)
Deep	HT	Blood Pressure	KI (reabsorption, excretion)		SP	Sex Organs

Thus, the large intestine and lungs form a yang-yin couple, as do the stomach and spleen-pancreas, etc.

The passages. In addition to the terminal branch of communication between two coupled organs, it is possible to perceive an intermediary canal *(luo)* commanded on each meridian by a passage point *(luo xue),* assuring the flow in cases of excess (see ''The Command Points''). Clinically, this phenomenon is proven by constant and efficacious usage, perception of it by people of even average sensitivity and instrumentation.

This case complicates the application of the mother-child rule. When two organs have similar intensity of energy, the mother-child rule can be applied. On the other hand, when there is strong inequality between two organs, it is enough to tonify the point of passage of the weaker or disperse that of the stronger in order to re-establish equilibrium.

The law of maximum and minimum (midday-midnight).

During the twenty-four hours of the day, each meridian and organ receives a maximum of energy for a two-hour period, and twelve hours later a minimum of energy for a two-hour period. This periodic difference can only be perceived on perfectly harmonious pulses. Organ disorders at particular hours clinically verify this law. This explains, for example, insomnia from 2 to 4 a.m. (liver insufficiency), or migraines which increase during the day and decrease in the afternoon (gallbladder in excess), and confirms these periodic increases and diminutions.

Each of the twelve organ-meridians has a maximum period that corresponds to a minimum period of another organ:

	Maximum	Minimum
Midnight	Gallbladder	Heart
2 a.m.	Liver	Small intestine
4 a.m.	Lung	Urinary bladder
6 a.m.	Large intestine	Kidney
8 a.m.	Stomach	Heart governor
10 a.m.	Spleen	Triple warmer
Midday	Heart	Gallbladder
2 p.m.	Small intestine	Liver
4 p.m.	Urinary bladder	Lung
6 p.m.	Kidney	Large intestine
8 p.m.	Heart governor	Stomach
10 p.m.	Triple warmer	Spleen

The above phenomenon of a maximal two-hour period for one organ with a coinciding minimal two-hour period for another organ is not well explained. However, we do know that when a production (workshop) organ is in its maximal period, a distribution (treasure) organ is at its minimal period, and vice versa. These two are not coupled organs, but their pulses are neighbors and cross between blood pressure levels (one superficial, the other deep). One is a yin organ, the other yang.

This matter should be studied closely, since we have observed that by dispersing one organ at its maximal period, we simultaneously tonify the other organ then at its minimum; when we tonify one organ at its minimal period, we disperse the other organ at its maximum.

That these periods of time are equal poses a problem, for the meridians are unequal in length and number of points. Their maximum and minimum period of activity are equal in time, although the speed of the energy is said to be constant (1 m. 35 cm. per minute), given as two minutes to ascend from the feet to the hands and the same to descend. The meridians of the gallbladder (44 points) and urinary bladder (67 points) are respectively slightly more and slightly less than two meters. They therefore will have half again as much energy at the maximum as the meridians of the heart (9 points) and the lungs (11 points), which are each less than a meter long.

The ancients also observed a seasonal period of maximum activity for each meridian. Around the spring equinox most disorders appear from liver insufficiencies: skin disorders, migraines, asthma, etc. (which can also occur from gallbladder excesses). This is also a maximal time for poliomyelitis and tuberculosis; a lesser maximum occurs around the autumn equinox, the time of spleen-pancreas disorders and stomach excesses (linked to the liver and gallbladder).

We have not yet found an adequate explanation for these phenomena.

Other mutual interactions of the organs exist, though they do not seem to be in direct connection with the circulation of energy (See ''Interaction of the Organs'').

IV. The Two Median Lines
(Conception Vessel and Governor Vessel)

In addition to the two lateral circuits of energy, two median lines also exist, each with its own points. The conception vessel *(ren mai),* the anterior line, is on the abdomen and sternum. The governor vessel *(du mai)* is on the dorsal surface of the body and follows the vertebral column and cranium.

Tradition describes them as both starting from the perineum and finishing at the mouth, consequently having only a rising flow. Only one chapter of the *Nei Jing Ling Shu* considers them as being double.

These two flows, rising from the same point and finishing at the same point, are difficult to interpret. In our investigations of this phenomenon, including the direction of flow and the precise placement of points, we have made the following discoveries:

1) Each line is formed of two currents, with the right ascending and the left descending.

2) Each point is doubled. Those on the conception vessel are separated from one another by less than a millimeter: on the abdomen and epigastrium by the narrow relief of the linea alba; on the sternum by the width of the vertical narrow groove. The points of the governor vessel are separated by the narrow width of the intervertebral medial tendon; and at the head, on the occiput by the width of its hollow, on the top by the width of the groove between the parietal bones, and on the face by the width of its hollow.

3) These two double currents join by crossing and form a special circulation of energy. When a point on the right ascending flow of the conception vessel is stimulated, a descending current is felt on the left descending side of the governor vessel. In stimulating a point on the left descending flow of the conception vessel, one senses the current traversing the junction and then ascending in the right flow of the governor vessel. These two median lines form a circulation of energy between themselves and in this way balance the reception of astral and sexual energy.

They have been perplexing to physiologists throughout the centuries. Some have grouped them with the twelve meridians, giving a total of fourteen. Most physiologists, however, have classified the median lines separately, reasoning that they are not a part of the two circuits of energy. Others have commented that the command point of each median line has a mutual response with the command points of one of the "vessels of the marvellous meridians" (see Volume III, Part III, Chapter VIII, "Hierarchy of Commands").

All authors recommend using them when action on the meridians fails to give sufficient results. They consider that the median lines, rather than the meridians themselves, provide the ultimate source of energy of the meridians.

My discovery of a pulse for each median line allows us to study them more extensively in relation to the meridians. For the conception vessel this pulse is located at the first pulse segment of the left wrist on the portion of the radial artery that deflects towards the dorsal surface of the hand. The pulse for the governor vessel is at the same position but on the right wrist. For each of these pulses, the superficial level (diastolic pressure) reflects the intensity of the lower third of their lines; i.e., the genital and urinary command. The middle level (intermediate pressure) reflects the middle third, the digestive functions; the deep level (systolic pressure) represents the respiratory functions, and in addition, for the governor vessel, the activity of the nervous centers.

We must emphasize here that the two pulses are modified in response to signals from the parasympathetic system (first left pulse position) and the sympathetic system (first right pulse position). Nonetheless, the relationship of these two median lines to the known autonomic system is not an obvious one. Only extensive observation will reveal whether or not the effects of these two lines may be attributed to that system.

The anterior conception vessel has neither been studied nor utilized in the West. However, the posterior governor vessel, with all its points on the vertebral column, has been recognized by an American, Dr. Abrams, whose teachings form the basis of chiropractic. A special diploma of chiropractic is given after two years of study at colleges in America. Instruction is based on the effects of vertebral manipulation on the internal organs.

Yin: median anterior line — conception vessel (ren mai).

This line begins at *huiyin* (CV-1), as does the governor vessel. It ascends along the midline of the abdomen and sternum, terminating under the lower lip. From there a branch encircles the right side of the lips joining the governor vessel at *shuigou* (GV-25, IS GV-26, *renzhong*), where it enters the descending left current of the governor vessel. The ascending right flow of the governor vessel at *shuigou* (GV-25, IS GV-26, *renzhong*) sends a branch around the left side of the lips to the descending left flow of the conception vessel at *chengjiang* (CV-24).

Its name comes from its fundamental importance in reproduction and the taking in of sexual energy. Its use is recommended when the meridians fail to give good results, in cases of emotional disorders, and in disturbances of the psyche accompanied by cold and depression.

The pulse (also that of the parasympathetic system) is on the left wrist, first segment, where the radial artery deflects towards the dorsal surface of the hand. The significance of each pulse level is as follows: superficial level — the lower third of the conception vessel (sexual and urinary functions, general tonification); middle level — the section of the line from the navel to the sternum, (digestive functions); deep level — the upper third of the line (respiratory functions, but also in the lower part, liver and spleen functions).

Most of the herald points of the organs are on this meridian. On the lower third we find the herald point of the small intestine, *guanyuan* (CV-4), which gives heat and strength; the urinary bladder, *zhongji* (CV-3), which also acts on the genitals (sexual function); the lower warmer, *yinjiao* (CV-7); the triple warmer, *shimen* (CV-5); and the sexual organs, *qihai* (CV-6). On the middle third, the herald points of the middle warmer, *zhongwan* (CV-12), which acts on the digestive function; the heart, *juque* (CV-14); and the vessels, *jiuwei* (CV-15). On the upper third is the herald point of the upper warmer, *shanzhong* (CV-17), which acts on the respiratory function.

All points on this line are primarily used for tonifying and vitalizing. It is rare to have to disperse them. They all have a mutual response with *tianzhu* (BL-10), which acts on the parasympathetic.

This median line is said to distribute its energy to all the meridians via the triple warmer. As its pulse is also that of the parasympathetic, a possibility exists that it has a similar contracting and vasoconstricting role and, likewise, that the parasympathetic has a vitalizing role as well as being a vasoconstrictor.

All its points respond in the meridian and pulse of the lungs. Its general point of command is *lieque* (LU-7). *Lieque* has a mutual response with *zhaohai* (KI-3, IS KI-6), which commands the yin energy through the *yinqiao mai*.

Yang: median posterior line — the governor vessel (du mai).

The governor vessel is thus named because, above all else, it governs the physical strength of men and intellectual vitality. Starting from the perineum at *huiyin* (CV-1), the right portion of this vessel ascends the length of the vertebral column, mounts the median line of the cranium and terminates under the nose at *shuigou* (GV-25, IS GV-26, *renzhong*). From this terminal point, a branch circles the lips to the left and joins the left descending flow of the conception vessel at *chengjiang* (CV-24) under the lower lip.

The governor vessel's left descending flow is fed from *chengjiang* (CV-24) by a branch circling the right side of the lips; it traverses the vertex, then descends the vertebral column to pass into the ascending flow of the conception vessel at *huiyin* (CV-1).

As with the conception vessel, it is possible to treat one side of the body by acting exclusively on points of either the right or left flow of the governing vessel. Those bilateral points situated along the vertebral column are located in the angles formed by the inferior border of each vertebra and the lateral borders of the median tendon.

All the points elicit a response in the meridian and pulse of the small intestine. The governor vessel's general point of command is *houxi* (SI-3). *Houxi* has a mutual response with *shenmai* (BL-62), which commands the yang energy through the *yangqiao mai*. Its pulse is on the right wrist, first position, where the radial artery deviates towards the external tendon. The superficial level of the pulse corresponds to the inferior third of the vertebral column and the strength and vitality of the lower part of the body. The middle level corresponds to the strength of the back and the general vitality. The deep level corresponds to the superior third of the vertebral column, the strength of the upper body and arms, and the cerebral line and nervous centers.

There is evidence that the pulse of the governor vessel is that of the sympathetic system, the vasodilator of the yin treasure organs. At present the relationship between the sympathetic system and governor vessel is not clear and needs further study. It is recommended, however, to use governor vessel points in all exogenous disorders accompanied by fever or hyperexcitation — interestingly enough those ailments which are directly influenced by the sympathetic system. (In cases of weakness, the points are not to be dispersed, but tonified.) Furthermore, there is a mutual response between the governor vessel and *fengchi* (GB-20), which acts on the sympathetic system. Most of the governor vessel points also act on the spinal cord and medulla.

We also note here a discovery of ours: a line of points located on the dorsal surface of the thumb, called "outside the meridian," which has a response only in the nervous centers (cerebral line).[2]

Notes

[1] These are as follows:

1)   Lungs: supreme yin of the hand (hand-*taiyin*).
2)   Spleen-pancreas: supreme yin of the foot (foot-*taiyin*).
3)   Heart: middle yin of the hand (hand-*shaoyin*).
4)   Kidneys: middle yin of the foot (foot-*shaoyin*).
5)   Vessels, sexual organs (heart governor): integral yin of the hand (hand-*jueyin*).
6)   Liver: integral yin of the foot (foot-*jueyin*).
7)   Small intestine: supreme yang of the hand (hand-*taiyang*).
8)   Urinary bladder: supreme yang of the foot (foot-*taiyang*).
9)   Large intestine: luminous yang of the hand (hand-*yangming*).
10)   Stomach: luminous yang of the foot (foot-*yangming*).
11)   Triple warmer: middle yang of the hand (hand-*shaoyang*).
12)   Gallbladder: middle yang of the foot (foot-*shaoyang).*

[2] These points have not been studied sufficiently to warrant their inclusion in Volume IV.

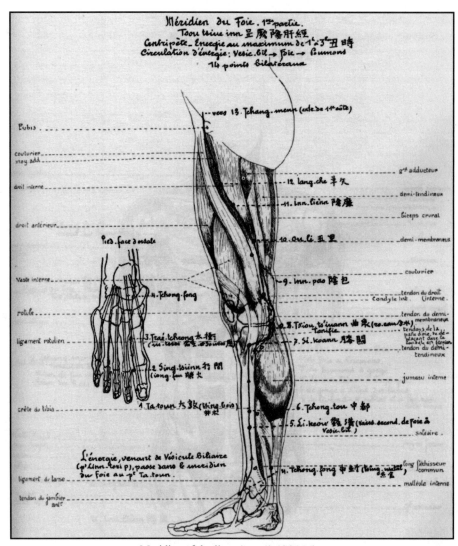

Meridian of the liver (part 1) (GSDM)

Chapter VI

Vital Energy (VI)

The Command Points

I. Existence of Points — II. Location of Points — III. Physiology of Points: 1. Sensitivity 2. Response 3. Effects 4. Double Action of the Points, Centrifugal and Centripetal 5. Hierarchy of Power 6. Specific Actions of Each Point 7. Discharge, Recharge, Inversion 8. Brain-Body Crossing — IV. Explanations — V. Western Points

The discovery of the circulation of energy and the measurement of this energy through the pulses and instrumentation would remain simply theoretical knowledge if a still more important discovery had not provided for its practical use — that of the command points. Through these points it is possible to have control over the energy, to enliven it, to tonify it, to slow it down, to disperse it or to activate its production, distribution or transformation. In brief, we can maintain or increase the vitality of the whole being, re-establish immunity and fully develop all inborn possibilities.

The discovery of the command points makes possible a precise, deep and enduring action on each function of each organ-meridian as well as on the areas which it commands. This knowledge cannot be emphasized enough for its use in physiology and in maintaining the maximum vitality of each individual. In the West, the existence and significance of the sensitivity of some of these points has been noted, but only in relation to their use in diagnosis.

I. Existence of the Points

Observation of the existence of active points goes back to greatest antiquity. Recording the effects obtained through their stimulation has been the work of many generations of observers. For the first time in the West, we have extracted these records from their Chinese sources. In the relatively brief period of our studies, we have verified and supplemented the original findings with effects shown through instrumental analysis.

Scientific proof of the existence and power of the command points was instrumentally demonstrated on September 23 and 24, 1950, at the home of Doctor Niboyet, 11 Castellane Place, Marseille, France. These experiments were carried out in the presence of and in collaboration with Professors Heckenroth and Rimattei, and the medical experts Drs. Lorenzi, Bernard and Béroud. The instruments, an electrocardiograph and energy detecting apparatus, were provided by the engineer, Mr. Pouret.

165 patients were examined under the following conditions:

1) An electrocardiogram before all punctures.

2) An electrocardiogram after puncturing in locations clearly outside the meridian system.

3) An electrocardiogram after puncturing a point of the heart meridian detected by means of the Pouret-Niboyet apparatus.

The results were convincing. A random puncture (no. 2 above) did not influence the graph. A puncture on the tonifying point of the heart (no. 3 above) made it change considerably, proving the effect obtained by the point. The published works of Niboyet cite these numerous recordings.

The instruments designed by Loch, Leplus, and Pouret-Niboyet allow the observation and measurement of differences in energetic potential between surrounding skin areas and the course of the meridians. Through this method, the precise location of the command points can be obtained. These instruments provide us with scientific proof of the existence of the points and confirm what ancient tradition posits and modern experimentation supports.

Some points on the meridians are not truly acupoints — pain from pressure on these points can be misleading. They have only a mild effect on the meridian and fail to rouse a response at the pulses, nervous centers or points up or downstream.

Finally, there are acupoints with special effects that exist outside the meridians (see Volume II).

II. Location of the Points

Since the acupoints alone give the desired effects, it is imperative to know how to find their exact location easily.

Works of the Far East describe these locations by their distance from one or two neighboring reference points, but measures cited and reproduced from the ancient texts are unreliable. The standard employed was the *chi,* the foot or forearm, divided into ten *cun,* inches. The question of what constituted an ancient "foot" is too problematic to go into here. There are only a few references to these measurements in Western books, namely that of Rev. Cleyer, written in Latin during the seventeenth century, and a chapter on acupuncture in Dabry's 1863 book on medications. The lack of understanding in the West of the exact location of the points is perhaps a reason for the dearth of doctors in Europe declaring themselves acupuncturists and the lack of acupuncture consultations in hospitals. This situation is improving since the publication of my work, which gives the precise location of these points.

It has taken me many years of research to discover the precise locations of the more than eight hundred points. Because our Western languages are not always indisputably clear, considerable effort has been made to write detailed descriptions that can be comprehended by doctors who have more often than not forgotten anatomy and scholars who have never studied it.

The center of an acupoint has the dimension of the point of a pin; it is this area alone that gives any complete, deep or lasting result. As we move away from the center, the power decreases. The effect is almost nil to the right or left of the meridian. Only very powerful points still retain their effects some millimeters from the center. In order to stimulate acupoints, we need to know clearly how to find them and determine if we are at the center of the point. Additionally, no two people are alike and the location of points may differ considerably. Some people have malleolae two centimeters from the sole, others at fifteen centimeters; some have six lumbar vertebrae instead of five, etc.

The muscles, which vary from one person to another, and even over the course of time on the same person, are misleading references. The bones, though presenting differences on different people, are the surest references.

As a standard measure, I have kept the less variable (although still unfixed) width of the fingers. So we must briefly compare the width of the patient's fingers to his height, and then to the width of the therapist's fingers.

The point, as well as the meridian, is in the subcutaneous tissue. The surface skin may be displaced over the deep tissue, making it easy to miss the underlying point. It is wise to utilize a small guide that fixes the skin and has a "gutter" along which to push the needle. Use of this guide diminishes the pain of insertion. All points are at the bottom of a small hollow or cupule; the deeper the hollow, the more the point needs to be excited.

III. Physiology of the Points

Various physiological aspects of the points allow us to determine if we are on the correct point or meridian. One cannot rely on the sensation of pain alone, but must seek confirmation through responses in the meridian, organ, pulse, points up and downstream, the nervous centers, and if possible the other organs and in different parts of the body.

People with a fine sense of touch feel that the skin over the acupoint is sticky, rather than slippery. By passing the finger some centimeters above the point, some people feel a current coming out of the point. In raising and lowering the finger there, they feel a tapping as if this current were solid. This important observation, although intriguing, risks being too subjective.

When yang meridian points are pressed with the finger, the surrounding area has a sensation of numbness. The yin meridian points are very often on the sides of arteries. The pulsation of the artery at the point is not felt as clearly as elsewhere.

Besides cultivating this sensitivity, we must advance our understanding of the responses aroused by each acupoint, allowing us to distinguish one point from another.

Sensitivity.

There are fixed points along the circuit of energy and median lines which, when pressed by the finger, clearly appear more sensitive than the channel of the meridian and surrounding areas. When touched with the electrode of a galvanometer, these points deflect the needle far more than does the meridian channel, while the surrounding area remains almost neutral (see "Instrumental Proofs of the Energy"). These points, normally sensitive in most people, are increasingly so in more sensitive, less physical types.

When a functional disorder of a meridian is present, a related acupoint becomes highly sensitive to the point of being painful, and its surrounding area is also slightly sensitized. This sensitivity is very great in cases of contractures, inflammations, and excess pain disorders. It is less intense when the disorders are of insufficiency atonia, but that is always relative to the sensitivity of the person.

Responses.

When touched, the point awakens a response, an echo: *a)* in the pulse of the organ; *b)* along the meridian of the organ; *c)* in the organ itself; *d)* in the point's own pulse; *e)* in the part of the brain and nervous centers concerned; *f)* more weakly, in the overall pulses, the meridians, the organs in relation to it; *g)* in certain parts of the organ or the body, either along the meridian on the same side of the body or along other meridians in relation to it and often on the opposite side to the point touched; and *h)* in the point upstream and downstream along the channel of the meridian. "False" points on the meridian awaken some of these sensations, but never the last, which provides an important verification of the location.

These responses are perceived more easily by persons of a refined heredity and intellectual nature. They are only slightly perceived by physical types, sportsmen, laborers and certain other people. Some rare individuals who are well practiced know they are on a true point by the response they feel on the pulse of the related organ, on the organ itself, and in the muscles, etc. of the meridian. By holding the puncturing needle, they feel the effect produced in their pulse, the organ and those in relation to it, and in their muscles, etc.

Effects.

If an appropriate stimulus is applied to the point, its organ or its region is "reminded" of its normal function. This happens immediately if the case is recent in onset, if the patient is not exhausted, and in summer or in good weather. It happens more slowly and less intensely if the person is intoxicated by tobacco, alcohol, or poisonous medicines, if the case is more chronic, if the patient is exhausted, and in winter or in bad weather.

The double action of the points: centripetal and centrifugal.

All the points can and do act in two opposite ways on their organ:

Centrifugal: A flow passes from the organ to the point. This is in accordance with the level of organ dysfunction, the sensitivity of the point to pressure, the size of its hollow, or the intensity of the waves it emits. These signs are significantly diminished if the appropriate stimulation has been given and if the organ is no longer troubled, or if the centrifugal flow has been diminished or emptied.

Centripetal: A flow passes from the point to the organ. All action taken on the point by needling, moxa, massage, sonopuncture, or other methods of stimulation modifies the organ and the pulse in the same way, and puts the organs and the commanded parts of the organism into action. The more marked the disequilibrium, the greater the effect of this action. It has a very weak effect on organs in complete balance.

In fact, the points fulfill a double role. Centrifugally, they warn of the internal disorder; centripetally, they transmit the action exercised on them. In one direction they are used to discharge the excess energy; in the other, they capture energy in order to supply internal insufficiencies.

Explanation for this double physiological function lies in the acupoint's dual relationship with the circulation of energy and the organs. One is again reminded of the similarities with the autonomic system.

Hierarchy of the power of the points.

All points do not give identical readings on instruments measuring energetic potential. This is true even in people whose pulses are fully balanced. Some points are very powerful while others are much less so. It is therefore possible to classify them according to a true hierarchy of power.

For a person with a mean total average of 4 to 5 microamperes, the most powerful points reach 10 microamperes. Leg-*sanli* (ST-36) and *hegu* (LI-4) exemplify such points.

The secondary points do not elicit much of an increase above mean average levels; the measuring apparatus may show readings of from 4 up to 7 microamperes.

Specific actions of each point.

First, like the meridians and organs, each point has an action on the quantity of energy of an organ, then in the same sense on two other organs, and in an opposite sense on still two other organs. This should always be kept in mind so as not to annul the results of treatment at these points.

Moreover, each point possesses a specific action on either **a)** its entire corresponding organ, or a single function of this organ; **b)** an organ other than that of the meridian the point is on; **c)** many organs; **d)** one of the large groupings of the body; **e)** yang activity or yin inactivity; or **f)** the total energy of the entire being.

Action on the point's entire corresponding organ, or a single function of this organ. The following groups of points are common to every meridian: **tonification point** — increases the energy of the organ more than any other single point; **dispersal point** — decreases the intensity of the organ's energy; **source point** — depending on the stimulation, tonifies or disperses the organ, regularizing it; **passage point** *(luo xue)* — joins a meridian with a coupled meridian (always a yin with a yang) by a branch or secondary vessel *(luo),* allowing the excess of one meridian to pass into the insufficiency of another (see chapter on circulation).

Tradition does not tell everything regarding the *luo* secondary vessels; our own observations have been helpful in understanding their use. The fifteen *luo* may be divided into the following three groups based on their ease of detection:

The first type are clearly detectable through palpation along their entire course; or alternatively, through palpation of one of the paired *luo* points, or overflow valves. The following exemplify this type: the secondary vessel connecting the heart and small intestine, between *tongli* (HT-5) and *zhizheng* (SI-7); the secondary vessel connecting the gallbladder and liver, between *ligou* (LR-5) and *guangming* (GB-37); and the secondary vessel connecting the lung and large intestine, between *lieque* (LU-7) and *pianli* (LI-6).

The second group of *luo* are difficult but possible to perceive by using palpation at the *luo* points, or valves. Some examples are the secondary vessels linking the kidney and urinary bladder, between *dazhong* (KI-6, IS KI-4) and *feiyang* (BL-58); the spleen-pancreas and stomach, between *fenglong* (ST-40) and *gongsun* (SP-4); and the triple warmer and heart governor, between *waiguan* (TW-5) and *neiguan* (PC-6).

The third grouping represents secondary vessels which we have been unable to detect through palpation. Two examples are the *luo* linking the governor and conception vessels, between *huiyin* (CV-1) and *changqiang* (GV-1); and that which connects the spleen-pancreas to all the meridians, the ''great *luo* of the spleen'' *(pidaluo).* The latter is not between two points but commanded by only one point, *dabao* (SP-21), which acts by dispersing or tonifying the upper-lower or right-left balance.

It is clear, then, that the points of the secondary vessels are passage points between two coupled meridians. One is tempted to group them with all points transferring energy from meridian to meridian. However, that would ignore the fact that the *luo* points alone have a secondary vessel linking the coupled meridians, while the other points act in a direct sense on two meridians and in an opposing sense on two other meridians without a channel linking them.

Action on an organ other than that of the meridian the point is on: Each of the **assent points** acts on the excess of energy of one of the twelve organs. These points are all located on the urinary bladder meridian, two finger-widths from the spine. Additionally, each organ has a corresponding **herald point** which tonifies and activates it; all are located on the anterior thorax, either on the meridian of the organ, another meridian, or the conception vessel.

Action on many organs: yutang (CV-18) acts on eight different organs; *zhongwan* (CV-12) acts on the organs which produce yang; *zhangmen* (LR-13) acts on all the organs which distribute yin.

Action on one of the large groupings of the body: yanglingquan (GB-34) acts on all the muscles; *xuanzhong* (GB-39) on the bone marrow and bone; *dazhu* (BL-11) on the bones; *gaohuangshu* (BL-38, IS BL-43) on the blood; leg-*futu* (ST-32) and *shangqiu* (SP-5) on the veins.

Action on yang activity or yin inactivity: shenmai (BL-62) stimulates yang activity, while *zhaohai* (KI-3, IS KI-6) acts on yin inactivity. Alternatively, points may be used to balance out excesses or insufficiencies of yin and yang: *neiguan* (PC-6) acts on yin energy and all the yin meridians, whereas *waiguan* (TW-5) acts on yang energy and all the yang meridians.

The total energy of the whole being: The only point having this effect is leg-*sanli* (ST-36).

Discharge, recharge, inversion.

The following phenomena are regularly observed and should be taken into consideration, especially when acting on points of command:

1) A point is discharged once it has been stimulated by needles or moxa; that is, it has lost its sensitivity and no longer elicits the same response in the meridian, at the pulse, in the organ and related organs, or in an apparatus measuring its energy.

2) When the stimulation is repeated before an interval of several days (this varies with the person, point and season) we often obtain the reverse effect, the opposite of what we want.

3) After several days the point is recharged and regains its usual power.

Brain-body crossing.

In the West it is acknowledged that the nervous centers in the brain command the opposite side of the body. Hemiplegia exemplifies this — a lesion in the right hemisphere of the brain causes disorders in the left side of the body, and vice versa.

The majority of acupoints act in a similar manner: points on the left command all or part of the left side of the body but excite responses in the right hemisphere of the brain, and the reverse. The pulse corresponding to the right side of the brain is on the radial artery of the left wrist, thus on the same side as the point. This agrees with Western knowledge.

However, there are exceptions to this rule:

1) Some points elicit a response on the opposite side of the brain, following the rule, but also act on the entire opposite side of the body and the organ, and on the opposite portion of the pulse: such a point is *houxi* (SI-3), which acts on the opposite side of the spine through the governor vessel. This double anomaly is still poorly explained and poses curious physiological and anatomical problems.

2) There are some points which are even more perplexing. A point of the right arm, for example, acts on the right arm and left lower limb. It seems to us to excite a response in the left mid-portion of the posterior frontal lobe and right arm; and the right superior portion of the posterior frontal lobe and left foot. The response at the pulse of the frontal lobe is on both sides of the artery. All the points of the large intestine, *waiguan* (TW-5) and foot-*linqi* (GB-41) are such points. For the points of the foot, the crossing is felt between the sixth and seventh cervical vertebrae and the second and third lumbar vertebrae. Explanations of these phenomena according to Western knowledge are even harder to find.

Clinically speaking, it is essential to be aware of these anomalies when working with the transfer of energy; a point tonified on the left may disperse the area commanded by the point on the right and vice versa.

IV. Explanations

A satisfactory anatomical and physiological explanation of the existence and double action of the Chinese points has yet to be found. Explanations given in Far Eastern sources suggest that a branch exists connecting each point to the organ. However, as we will see, each point may have a special action on a single function of the organ or on all functions. It may very well be that each function of an organ has a special point of command, since we consistently see a single function of an organ disordered, without the organ's other functions being affected.

Scholars taking great interest in this problem have yet to find a clear solution. In 1929, Professor Rouvière of the Department of Anatomy at the Faculty of Medicine in Paris carefully dissected the various points I indicated. He stated that he was not expecting to find anything previously unknown. However, his work showed evidence that under the acupoint the subcutaneous network of nerve fibers were bound tighter; yet, as he questioned, in this number of fibers how do we know which ones are acting? As they say, all roads lead to Rome: is it a matter of anastomoses or of transmission to other networks? Here anatomy must yield to physiology.

Around this time other researchers suggested the possibility that a fiber of the sympathetic system terminates under each acupoint. However, this does not explain the meridians themselves, which are inseparable from the points.

V. Western Points

The West has discovered, albeit rather recently, the existence of sensitive points in certain circumstances. Curiously, some of them are used only to confirm diagnosis while others are used only for treatment. Very little research has been carried out to elucidate the value of these sensitive points.

Among the points for finding disordered organs are the following:

1)   McBurney's point for appendicitis.

2)   The points of Guyon, Pasteau, Albarran, and Bazy for renal ailments (all located on the kidney meridian and its herald point).

3)   The points of Desjardins for gallbladder or pancreatic affections.

4)   The Chinese points of Valleix for sciatica.

5)   The Chinese points for which Dr. Weihe has verified and noted the correspondence with homeopathic remedies.

Among the points for treatment, we cite:

1)   All the vertebral points of Abrams used in chiropractic medicine.

2)   The points of electrical stimulation of the muscles and nerves.

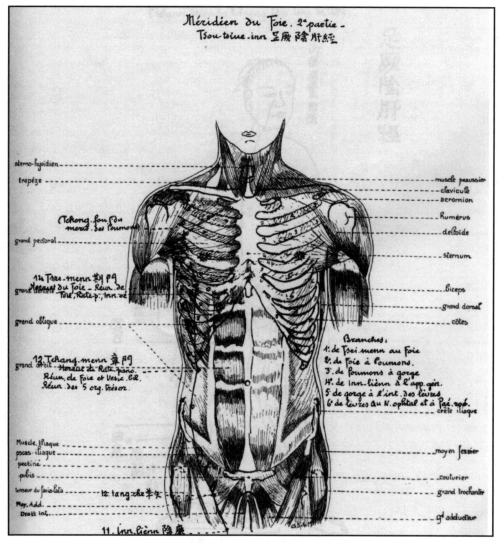

Meridian of the liver (par t2) (GSDM)

Part II

Sources, Transformation, Distribution, and Stimulation of Energy

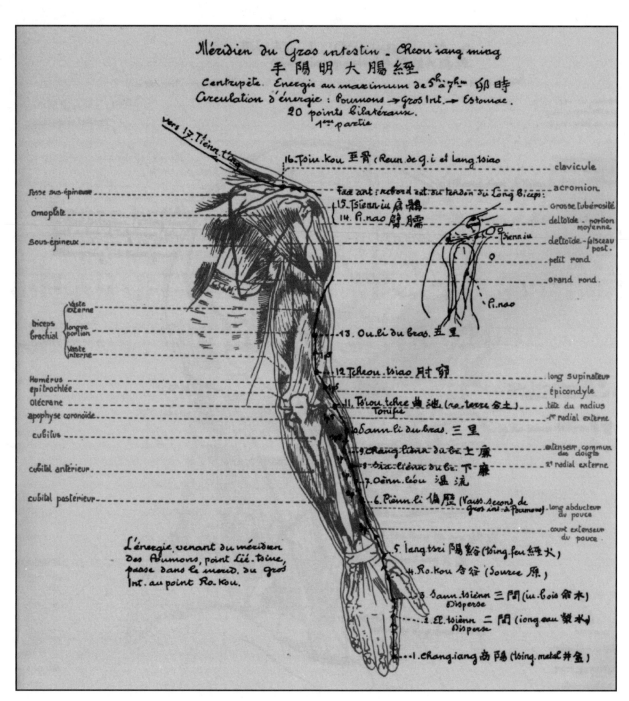

Meridian of the large intestine (part 1) (GSDM)

Chapter I

Sources of Energy (I)

Air, Food, and Drink

I. Sources of Celestial Energy (Lung, Skin) —
II. Sources of Terrestrial Energy (Small Intestine, Stomach, Pancreas-Digestion)

With energy as their primary concern, the ancient Chinese classified the internal organs into the following two groups:

The Yang Workshop Organs: Their meridians are on the lateral, yang surface of the limbs and their pulses at the superficial, yang level. ''Workshop'' here means *producer of energy.* This group consists of the stomach, small and large intestine, gallbladder, and urinary bladder.

The role of the stomach, intestines and gallbladder (taken to represent the entire biliary reflex) in digestion, or the transformation of food and drink into energy, is better understood than the functioning of the urinary bladder. However, evidence of the urinary bladder's influence on the energy is provided by the powerful effects of its channel's dorsal points (see Part II, Chapter II). Western studies have shown the importance of the small intestine in the production of albumin molecules specific to each individual.

The Yin Treasure Organs: Their meridians are on the medial, yin surface of the limbs and their pulses at the deep, yin level. This group consists of the heart, lungs, spleen-pancreas, liver, kidney, sexual organs and the vessels.

In Chinese medicine, the lungs are classified as treasure organs, or distributors. However, they also perform the important function of assimilating air and capturing the solar and celestial energy of activity (yang energy); if this function fails, death follows within a matter of minutes. We therefore place the lungs first among the sources of energy. The dual role of the pancreas in the transformation of sugar and the digestion of fats, meats, and starches will be examined separately.

We shall first look at the sources of solar and celestial energy of activity (yang energy) obtained through the lungs and skin. Then, in their order of importance, we will explore the sources of terrestrial, latent energy (yin energy).

I. Sources of Celestial Energy: Lungs, Skin

Deprived of air, living beings die in a matter of minutes. From this fact, ancient physiologists concluded that through air we capture the energy of celestial activity. Without this energy, we are immediately overpowered by the yin energy of inactivity, of death. The harnessing of celestial energy is accomplished almost entirely by the lungs, and also to a slight extent by the skin.

The electricity of the earth is negative (yin), but a positive atmospheric electricity (yang) prevails in clear, sunny weather. Atmospheric electricity becomes negative when a thick veil of clouds intercepts the solar and astral rays. At present, knowledge of the powerful cosmic rays is so little understood that we can only say that they exist. Given that these rays can penetrate four meters of lead, it is amazing that our bodies are not destroyed by them.

Without sunlight, nothing vital could be produced (Hédon). Plants could not manufacture certain chemical compounds; because of it, they are able to emit oxygen during the day and carbon dioxide at night. In a cave, green leaves become white. The sun of the mountains is dangerous for people with congestive tuberculosis (yang excess) but favorable for people with atonic tuberculosis (yang insufficiency).

By modern conceptions, the respiratory system not only functions to capture oxygen, but also works to maintain a constant level of carbon dioxide in arterial blood and tissue fluids.

In 1948, American scientists discovered a respiratory center the size of the head of a pin in a bilateral cross-section of the medulla. This center is stimulated when oxygen levels in the body become insufficient.

The lungs also excrete water (at rest, about 500 grams at 18° C at mean saturation of air; during exercise and dry heat this is more than doubled). The more water evaporated from the lungs through the breath, the less the kidneys and skin release. Conversely, the more copious the urination, the less water is released from the lungs.

The skin, which absorbs solar rays, celestial waves and other emanations, contributes in excreting water through evaporation of sweat (about one liter at 18° C at rest, much increased with exercise and dryness). Tight, rubber clothing can produce asphyxiation.

In great antiquity it was written: ''The lungs give life to the skin, which in turn nourishes the kidneys.'' The greater the output of urine by the kidneys, the lesser the output of water through the lungs and skin. Likewise, the more the lungs and skin excrete, the less urine there is. But what is this life given to the skin? What is the energy brought to the cells? The maximum period of energy for the lungs (4 a.m.) corresponds to the minimum period for the urinary bladder; and vice versa. Tonification of the one disperses the other.

Texts of the Far East attribute to the lungs the function of ''giving life to the hair.'' Additionally, the lungs represent ''the home of the primate [primitive instincts].'' An old European adage states, *''Homo villosus libidinosus vel phtisicus.''*[1] This brings to mind the long hair of tubercular women, and their need for tenderness.

The relative insufficiency-excess of the lungs is as follows:

Insufficiency	Excess
Troubles of the respiratory passages from weakness, inability to breathe, cold.	Troubles of the respiratory passages due to inflammation, congestion, swelling, fever, spasms, pulmonary edema.
Atonic tuberculosis, waxy complexion, slight fever.	Congestive tuberculosis, high fever, hemoptysis, red face, pneumonic plague.
Sadness, chagrin, anguish.	Agitation, hyperexcitation, excessive laughter.
Insomnia with melancholia.	Insomnia with agitation, heat.
Heart weak, intermittent.	Nervous palpitations.
Hypotension.	Hypertension.
Cold in the back.	Heat in the back. Hot palms.
Shivering, chattering of the teeth.	Sweating from shock, at night. Fever.
Diarrhea from weakness after eating.	Diarrhea and vomiting. Spasms of the esophagus.
	Contracted urinary bladder. Feeble urine.
Abundant urine, frequent at night.	Abundant head and body hair.
Facial paralysis.	Tic and spasms of the face and head.
Paralysis of the radial nerve.	Pain of the back and chest. Rheumatism of the five fingers. Pain of the radial nerve.

The meridian of the lung includes a very important point, *lieque* (LU-7). Below is a list of its main effects:

1) Naturally, it has an effect on the respiratory passages: either weak and rapid respiration with cold in the back, shivering, abundant urine; or congestive tendencies with heat in the back and chest, hot palms, difficult and insufficient urine.

2) It acts on the energy of inactivity (yin energy): for this it is coupled with a kidney point, *zhaohai* (KI-3, IS KI-6). When tonified, it acts on insomnia and abundant urination in the evening.

3) Insufficiency or excitation of the heart.

4) Illnesses of the blood, abscesses of the nipple.

5) Burns.

6) Nervous trembling, nervous shivering.

7) Spasm, tics, paralysis or swellings of the face.

8) Headache on one side or at the vertex.

9) Troubles of the radial nerve.

10) It commands the whole conception vessel (the medial anterior line).

11) It commands the passage of energy between the lungs and large intestine.

All the points of the lung meridian act on respiratory troubles:

With all excesses, inflammation, congestion with fever, pleurisy, pneumonia, and even hemoptysis and fever of congestive tuberculosis, use *chize* (LU-5), the dispersal point.

With paralyzed, contracted or swollen lungs, bleeding bronchioli, or asthma with crises at 4 or 5 a.m. after lying down (edema of the lungs), use *taiyuan* (LU-9), the tonification point.

Contraction of the larynx: *zhongfu* (LU-1).

Suffocating cough with pain in the heart: *yunmen* (LU-2) and *jingqu* (LU-8).

The cough of laryngitis or of tonsillitis: *shaoshang* (LU-11).

Hoarseness or rough voice: *kongzui* (LU-6).

Shaoshang (LU-11), *taiyuan* (LU-9), and *chize* (LU-5) evoke responses in the medulla oblongata.

Amnesia, agitation or despair: *yuji* (LU-10).

Talks to oneself or does not speak: *tianfu* (LU-3).

Cerebral congestion, infantile meningitis: *shaoshang* (LU-11).

Nervous shivering: *chize* (LU-5).

Nervous crisis: *taiyuan* (LU-9).

Slow pulse: *shaoshang* (LU-11).

Disorders of the atrial valves: *yuji* (LU-10), *xiabai* (LU-4).

Contractions of the urinary bladder to the point of incontinence: *taiyuan* (LU-9), *yunmen* (LU-2).

Profuse urine at the beginning of the night: *lieque* (LU-7).

Feeble urine from respiratory disorders: *chize* (LU-5), *lieque* (LU-7).

Alcoholism: *yuji* (LU-10).

Intractable diarrhea or vomiting: *chize* (LU-5).

Back and lumbar pains: *chize* (LU-5).

Facial pains, spasms or paralysis: *lieque* (LU-7).

Pains on one side of the head or vertex: *lieque* (LU-7).

Burns: *lieque* (LU-7).

The lung meridian, with arms upraised, traverses the medial, yin surface of the upper limb, ascending from the chest. A branch starts from the last point of the liver meridian, *qimen* (LR-14), and rises directly to *zhongfu* (LU-1). Another branch proceeds from *shaoshang* (LU-11) to the large intestine meridian at *shangyang* (LI-1) by traversing the finger joint.

Its time of maximum energy is 4 a.m., the minimum for the urinary bladder. Its minimum is at 4 p.m., the maximum for the urinary bladder. The organ upstream, the mother, is the liver; downstream is the large intestine, the child as well as the coupled meridian. The husband organ is the heart. The herald point is *zhongfu* (LU-1). The assent point is *feishu* (BL-13), lateral to T3.

Its pulse is on the right wrist, first segment, middle level.

II. Sources of Terrestrial Energy (Yin)

The small intestine.

The *Nei Jing* summarizes the importance of this organ:

> The small intestine enlivens the dead food coming from the stomach in a manner absolutely specific and proper for each individual.

It has been discovered quite recently in France that in the duodenum of the small intestine a small molecule of albumin absolutely specific to the blood and tissues of each individual is synthesized. In this process, the large protein molecule of albumin is broken apart, an essential transformation as yet not able to be reproduced *in vitro* and which classifies the small intestine as an important producer of vital energy.

This provides evidence of the strict order specific to each individual. This ''order'' governs the organism continually throughout life; it is the *Form*.

It has been suggested that enterokinase (enteropeptidase), secreted by the small intestine, forms the basis of this vital act by catalyzing the breakdown of the large albumin molecule and that of peptones into amino acids.

It follows from the above that by tonifying the small intestine and hence duodenal production, it is possible to rapidly recuperate from fatigue, effort and shocks. No other meridian gives such a result. The stomach, though possessing similar powers, can only dissipate the effects of shock or prevent fatigue.

Perhaps we can also find here an explanation for the action of the small intestine on vision and hearing. This action comes from all its points.

Works of the Far East attribute to the small intestine a role not yet proven by Western physiology: the function of ''separating the liquids from the solids, directing the former to the kidneys and the latter to the large intestine.'' Indeed, observations show that the small intestine creates a balance between the urine and all other secretions, namely sweat, saliva, respiratory mucus and milk. If there is little urine, there are more secretions; much urine, fewer secretions. In Chinese medical thought, its action on energy is exercised mostly through the mediation of the governor vessel (posterior median line). The small intestine acts on the latter through all its points, but especially *houxi* (SI-3), the small intestine's tonification point, which is also the general command point of the governor vessel.

These digestive functions, extensively studied in the West, must also be considered as acting on the energy obtained from food with the other physical elements. Let us review these facts:

1)   Its enterokinase breaks down peptones into amino acids and strengthens pancreatic secretions.

2)   Its secretions stimulate the production of secretions by the pancreas, the latter indispensable for the digestion of sugar, fat, meat and starches.

3)   Its enterogastrone, the production of which is stimulated by fats and sugars, inhibits the motility and secretions of the stomach.

4)   Its cholecystokinin, stimulated by fats and proteins, causes a strong contraction of the gallbladder while relaxing Oddi's sphincter, bringing bile into the duodenum. An acid injection into the duodenum also increases biliary and pancreatic secretions.

The jejunum and the ileum primarily have functions of absorption.

The relative insufficiency-excess of the small intestine is as follows:

Insufficiency	Excess
Poor resistance to shocks and fatigue, slow healing, weak character, weeps easily, always cold.	Joyous, laughs easily. Recuperates quickly from shocks, resists them well. Emotionally strong; easily overexcited, easily angered, always hot.
Heart easily fatigued.	Heart strong.
Colorless complexion, bluish lips, bordered with white.	Colored complexion, easy swelling of mouth and maxilla.
All secretions (sweat, saliva, milk, etc.) increased.	All secretions diminished. In excess, edema of the lungs.
Urine slightly abundant.	Urine abundant, frequent.
Muscles of the eyes and ears easily fatigued to the point of shortsightedness.	Muscles of the eyes and ears energized to the point of farsightedness.
Pancreatic insufficiency. Diabetes. Poor digestion of meats, fats or starches.	Energetic pancreas. Likes and easily digests meats, fats and starches. In excess, pains of small intestine, ulcers of the duodenum.
Stools either shiny or grey-white, with undigested food.	Yellow, pale, golden diarrhea.
Swollen, flaccid gallbladder. Large intestine insufficient.	Hardened gallbladder with cramps. Stimulated large intestine.
Skin supple, wet, cold; night-sweats.	Skin warm, dry. Sweats little, holds water.

The small intestine meridian follows the lateral, yang surface of the upper limb, ascends the posterior surface of the shoulder and scapula, and ends on the cheekbone. It receives the energy of the heart through a small branch on the little finger and transmits its energy to the urinary bladder via a branch crossing the cheek to the first point of the urinary bladder, *jingming* (BL-1).

Its time of maximum energy is 2 p.m., minimum hour of the liver. Its minimum is at 2 a.m., maximum hour of the liver. The organ upstream, the mother, is the heart, which is also the coupled meridian; the child downstream is the urinary bladder. The wife is the large intestine. Its tonification point is *houxi* (SI-3); its dispersal point, *xiaohai* (SI-8); its source point, hand-*wangu* (SI-4). Its right branch acts mainly on the jejunum and ileum, while its left branch acts mainly on the duodenum.

Its pulse is on the left wrist, first section, superficial level of the radial artery. In our studies, it appears that the proximal part, towards the radius, reflects the duodenum; the distal part, towards the thumb, reflects the jejunum and the ileum.

The small intestine is contracted by the parasympathetic system, *tianzhu* (BL-10); it is relaxed by the sympathetic system, *fengchi* (GB-20).

The various effects of the meridian points are as follows:

Recuperation from fatigue, shock, diseases: *houxi* (SI-3), which acts on the governor vessel, spinal cord, medulla, cerebellum and the opposite cerebral hemisphere.

Balance between urine and secretions (sweat, saliva, milk): *houxi* (SI-3), *shaoze* (SI-1), *qiangu* (SI-2).

The eyes, sight, by almost all the points. Farsightedness ameliorated, weakness of sight by age or illness: *houxi* (SI-3).

Ears, hearing: *tinggong* (SI-19), *xiaohai* (SI-8).

Pulmonary edema: *houxi* (SI-3).

Cough with mucus: *houxi* (SI-3).

Lactation: *shaoze* (SI-1), *qiangu* (SI-2).

Motility of the extremities (contralateral): *houxi* (SI-3).

The stomach.

The ancients considered the stomach the most important organ for the production of energy from food and drink. The *Nei Jing* comments:

> *An important point for the general vitality [referring to **qichong** (ST-30)], it is the source hastening both the transformation of food and drink into energy by the stomach and the distribution of this energy to the twelve meridians by the triple warmer; the stomach is the source of all.*

Recall that food cannot be used to maintain life if it is not derived from a living being or plant, which in the final analysis extracts energy from the sun and stars. Those fluids which are energized by movement and irradiated by the sun are superior in effect to those found collected in icy stone pits.

Moreover, since the stomach lacks teeth, it is first necessary for food to be mechanically ground in the mouth, while the first portion of the food's energy is simultaneously extracted by the saliva and absorbed through the mucus membranes. Many medicines produce their effects by being kept in the mouth. An ancient Chinese work gives this recommendation for hygiene:

> *The stomach can only digest what has first been reduced to pulp by the mouth, the latter having already extracted some energy from the food. The stomach has no teeth; what is not received as a paste irritates it, is evacuated, not digested. It poisons the organism as well as wasting food and time. To swamp digestion with quantities of drink during meals is to weaken it until it ceases to function effectively. Most illnesses of the digestive organs come from this serious error in conduct.*

We will not reproduce here the increasingly precise descriptions found in Western texts of the chemical operations accomplished by the stomach. These operations can be reproduced *in vitro* and thus are not truly vital.

Far Eastern texts focus primarily on the relevant production of vital energy. Observations made on this subject in France give support to the claim that by acting on the vitality of the stomach, it is possible to diminish or augment its production of two forms of energy: physical-vital, and psychic-mental.

1)   The total physical-vital energy: Tonification of a point on the stomach meridian (leg-*sanli*, ST-36) in persons lacking strength and spirit and whose pulses are empty or nonexistent will alleviate the lack of vitality and return the pulses to normal. It has been suggested that this is the result of a still unknown substance secreted by the stomach, which is immediately released into the organism.

2)   The mental-psychic energy. In some cases of mental hyperexcitation recognized by neurologists as necessitating internment, it has been observed that by dispersing a point on the stomach meridian, either *lidui* (ST-45), the dispersal point, or *neiting* (ST-44), the delirious mental hyperactivity disappears immediately. To a lesser degree violent nightmares or agitated dreams cease with the same points.

This hyperexcitation, or insanity, either in the waking or sleep states, has been compared to that of alcohol intoxication. It has been suggested that alcohol does not produce such effects by its own qualities, but through the stimulation of a still unknown substance produced by the stomach. Indeed, depression, timidity, and fear are arrested upon tonification of the stomach, while the devitalizing effects of psychological or violent physical shock also cease by acting on a stomach point. The popular French expression ''to have a stomach'' seems to corroborate this empirical observation.

Finally, we have found that the frontal lobes (the centers of reason) are commanded, along with the spleen, by *fenglong* of the stomach (ST-40). The temporal, parietal and inferior occipital lobes are commanded by *xiajuxu* (ST-39), and the superior occipital lobe by *shangjuxu* (ST-37).

On the physical plane, action on the stomach meridian has two other effects. That on the veins, potentiated through leg-*futu* (ST-32), is frequently employed; however, that on cancer of the digestive tract or the genitals has only been rarely experimented with but has given some surprisingly palliative results in cases where the progress of the disease was not too advanced. The West has still not recognized these properties of the stomach.

Spasmodic coughs, whooping cough and night coughs are arrested by the stomach point *yingchuang* (ST-16).

Plantar warts or chilblains, which are beyond Western treatment, are cured and do not recur with *xiajuxu* (ST-39).

The relative insufficiency-excess of the stomach is as follows:

Insufficiency	Excess
Depression, timidity, no taste for life, no desire; ennui, desire for solitude and heat. Restlessness, sadness.	Agitated dreams or violent nightmares to the point of raging insanity, speaks too much and too quickly, walks quickly and for a long time; if extreme, gets up on the table, sings, etc.; oppressed, malcontent, agitated, feels that everyone is wrong.
Red face and cold feet, especially during meals.	Occasional swelling of the body, the limbs or under the arms.
Slow digestion. Stomach swells after meals or fails to empty at night due to weakness; nothing is digested, no appetite.	Painful, hard, burning digestion; stomach fails to empty mostly due to spasm of the pylorus. Nausea; ravenous, excessive appetite.
Bad breath.	Hot or fetid breath. Dry or cracked lips.
Eyes empty, dull.	Eyes red, congested.

The stomach meridian descends on the anterior thorax and anterolateral, or yang, surface of the lower limbs. It starts at the temple and descends down the anterolateral aspect of the neck to the mammillary line, then to the lateral edge of the rectus abdominis muscle. It then follows the lateral edge of the rectus femoris muscle along the anterior thigh to *liangqiu* (ST-34). On the lower leg, the meridian descends along the medial edge of the tibialis anterior muscle. A branch follows the lateral edge of this muscle from *dubi* (ST-35), under the patella, to *fenglong* (ST-40) at the bottom of the muscle.

Its time of maximum energy is 8 a.m., minimum hour of the heart governor, sexual organs and vessels. Its minimum is at 8 p.m., maximum hour of the heart governor. The organ upstream, the mother, is the large intestine; downstream is the spleen-pancreas, the child as well as the coupled meridian. It is the ''wife'' of the gallbladder. Its assent point, *weishu,* is on the urinary bladder meridian on the back (BL-21). The tonification point is *jiexi* (ST-41). The dispersal point is *lidui* (ST-45).

Its pulse is on the right wrist, second section, at the superficial, yang level.

Pancreas-digestion (see sections on spleen-pancreas and pancreas-sugar).

The action of the pancreas on digestion, transformation and assimilation of meat, fats and starches was not well known in ancient times. We now know that it plays an essential part in the digestive process and is thus of great importance for the production of energy of the blood and physique. The production of mental energy is also dependent on this organ, since it plays an equally essential role in the transformation of sugar into glycogen by insulin, sugar being indispensable for the brain. (Its trypsin acts on meat, albuminoid and protein; its amylopsin on starches, beans, chestnuts; its lipase on fat, lipoids and lipids.)

These pancreatic functions are stimulated by secretion of the small intestine which additionally augments the effects of the pancreatic juices through another secretion, enterokinase. The pancreas, like the small intestine, is tonified, or stimulated, by the parasympathetic (*tianzhu,* BL-10), and inhibited, or dispersed, by the sympathetic system (*fengchi,* GB-20).

The pancreas in excess reduces adrenal function. Likewise, the adrenals in excess reduce pancreatic function. Pancreatic insufficiency (an insufficiency of trypsin which aids in the digestion of meat) is accompanied by an elevated percentage of urea in the blood.

The pancreas is seriously weakened by sadness and worry. It acts on the taste.

The relative insufficiency-excess of the function of the pancreas, that of aiding the digestion of fats, meats and starches, is as follows:

Insufficiency	Excess
Debility, depression.	Strength, energy.
Swollen from chestnuts, beans. Meat produces toxicity.	Digests meats, fats, and starches quickly and well.
Thinness with big belly.	Thin with vigorous muscles.

The spleen-pancreas meridian follows the internal, yin surface of the lower limbs. It is said that the left branch is connected to the spleen, hence the left branch commands the spleen, and the right, the pancreas, though its actions may cross over.

Its time of maximum energy is 10 a.m., minimum hour of the triple warmer. Its minimum is at 10 p.m., maximum hour of the triple warmer. The organ upstream, the mother, is the stomach, which is also the coupled meridian; the child downstream is the heart. Its assent point is *pishu* (BL-20); tonification point, *dadu* (SP-2); dispersal point, foot-*shangqiu* (SP-5); herald point, *zhangmen* (LR-13); and source point, *taibai* (SP-3).

Its pulse is on the right wrist, second section, middle level.

Chapter II

Sources of Energy (II)

Secondary Sources of Energy

I. Large Intestine — II. Gallbladder — III. Urinary Bladder

The large intestine, gallbladder and urinary bladder are classified in Chinese medicine as "workshop organs," or producers of energy. Although Western scientists have studied extensively the functions of these organs, they have not yet explored the energetic aspects of organ function. However, as we shall see, each of these organs has an undeniable relationship with the vital energy which must not be overlooked.

I. Large Intestine

Since ancient times, the "source" point of the large intestine, *hegu* (LI-4), has been called the "herald point of the energy" because of the multiple actions of the large intestine on general vitality, excitability, nervous centers, and so forth. The point itself acts on all the workshop-organs and hence on their pulses, all at the superficial, yang level.

The principal energetic relations of the large intestine are as follows:

1)   Stool-energy relations. The West fully recognizes that prolonged diarrhea saps the vitality and weakens the whole person; that purgation lowers the blood pressure and strength; that, on the other hand, a constant state of irritation contracts the whole being and puts the intestine into spasm, encouraging constipation; and that constipation makes one gloomy and tense.

We know very well that strong emotions and great danger produce laxity of the intestine. Intestinal worms irritate the large intestine, provoking in children constant states of nervousness, nervous crises and even convulsions or incontinence. These facts come from Asian observation and experience.

2)   It has been observed and taught since ancient times that by tonifying the large intestine, it is possible to prevent hemorrhages and greatly reduce excessive menstrual bleeding (*hegu*, LI-4). The West has confirmed this through its discovery that the large intestine synthesizes an antihemorrhagic substance, vitamin K. The liver uses this vitamin in its manufacture of prothrombin, the blood coagulator. (A liver insufficiency is accompanied by easy bruising and prolonged, slight bleeding from a scratch.)

3)   By tonifying the large intestine, it is possible to completely eradicate pain, most markedly in cases of eye pain, earache, toothache, headache, throat pain and pains of the skin.

4)   The action on hypertension, mostly through *jianyu* (LI-15), is described as both preventive and curative at the beginning stages of hemiplegia. It possibly acts through dilation of the vessels (tonifying the large intestine disperses the kidneys and vasopressin). Instrumental confirmation has yet to be carried out.

5)   The action on the brain is quite distinct. Problems ranging from serious cerebral fatigue to encephalitis, with its ocular and urinary troubles, are treated by *shanglian* (LI-9). Heat stroke is ameliorated by *xialian* (LI-8), meningitis by *hegu* (LI-4). *Shousanli* (LI-10), when massaged, will revive a person from syncope. Explanations are still hypothetical.

6)   The action of *hegu* (LI-4) on the nose, rhinopharynx, and throat, as well as the eyes and ears, is marked. It has become standard practice these days to treat problems of these regions by first attending to the large intestine. The current explanation is that an infection is involved; this, however, does not account for all the phenomena observed.

The relative insufficiency-excess of the large intestine is as follows:

Insufficiency	Excess
Without enthusiasm, discouraged, heavy; dreams of deserts, of uncultivated land.	Irritable, discontented, agitated.
Atonic constipation.	Spasmodic constipation, pain, colic.
Diarrhea from weakness.	Diarrhea from inflammation. Typhoid.
Air in the colon, gas, fermentation.	Inflammation of the mouth.
Coated tongue, yellow at the base.	Red tongue.
Cold, cannot get warm again.	Prolonged fever. Hypertension.
	Head cold, sore throat. Troubles of the eyes and ears, troubles and pain of the teeth and gums.
	Eruptive illnesses. Illnesses involving dry skin or pus. Problems on the face such as acne, scurf, pruritus.

The large intestine meridian is on the external, yang surface of the arms. A branch proceeds from the last point of the lung meridian, *shaoshang* (LU-11), to the first point of the large intestine meridian, *shangyang* (LI-1), at the tip of the index finger. The meridian then mounts the radial edge of the arm up to the nose. From the last point on the meridian, *yingxiang* (LI-20), at the side of the nostril, a branch rises up to the first point of the stomach through *shangxing* (GV-22, IS GV-23) to *touwei* (ST-1, IS ST-8). The branch on the right acts mostly on the cecum, ascending colon and the hepatic flexure; that on the left acts on the transverse colon, the splenic flexure, rectum and anus.

Its time of maximum energy is 6 a.m., the minimum for the kidney. Its minimum is at 6 p.m., the maximum for the kidney. The organ upstream, the mother, is the lung, which is also the coupled meridian; the child downstream is the stomach. The husband organ is the small intestine. The herald point is *tianshu* (ST-25) on the abdomen. The assent point is *dachangshu* (BL-25) in the lumbar region.

Its pulse is on the right wrist, second section, superficial, or yang level. The distal portion of the pulse, near the thumb, responds to the rectum; the proximal portion, near the styloid process, responds to the cecum.

II. Gallbladder

The gallbladder meridian commands not only the gallbladder itself but also the common bile duct, Oddi's sphincter and the entire group of nerves responsible for the biliary reflex. Resection of the gallbladder weakens the pulse for about six months; it then reappears as a new pocket is formed in the common bile duct. Even with resection of the gallbladder, the points of the meridian continue their action on their related disorders.

The gallbladder is said ''to give *elan* to all the organs.''

Effects on the psyche: gallbladder excess manifests as jealousy, envy, aggressiveness and malcontent. This is recognized in the West. To treat this, disperse *yangfu* (GB-38).

The gallbladder has an effect on courage, strength of character, the enterprising mind, audaciousness. A fighting spirit has been so emphasized in China that intrepid people there are nicknamed ''big gallbladders.'' Apprehension, setbacks to effort and fear of failure can be corrected by *xiaxi* (GB-43), the tonification point.

Yanglingquan (GB-34) commands the cerebellum and acts on all the muscles, reviving them by increasing their strength.

Xuanzhong (GB-39) commands the medulla and augments the production of polynuclear leukocytes necessary for the destruction of inflammation and abscesses, for the healing of bones, and for rapid general healing. This point is also used to treat irritation of the respiratory and digestive mucosa.

Pains extending throughout the whole body yield to *yangfu* (GB-38), foot-*linqi* (GB-41) or *xiaxi* (GB-43). Hepatic migraines of the right temple are relieved by *yangfu* (GB-38), as is eczema, constipation and asthma.

Sight and hearing are much improved by *tongziliao* (GB-1) and *tinghui* (GB-2).

Physically, the gallbladder commands nervous excitability. Lymphangitis, lymphadenitis, ganglia and mastoiditis yield to foot-*linqi* (GB-41).

Depending on their development, arthritic ankle pains are alleviated by foot-*linqi* (GB-41). Arthritis of the shoulder and upper limb (treated by the acupoint on the opposite side) respond equally well to this point.

In Western medicine, it is taught that the gallbladder is primarily used for biliary transit. It stores bile for occasional use and closes itself off in order to resist the back-pressure resulting from distention of the biliary ducts (for example, after resection of the gallbladder). The gallbladder also functions to concentrate bile through a process involving reabsorption of water. (Because of the insolubility of substances such as cholesterol, concretion may result, giving rise to gallstone formation.) Pains from this region are caused by the back-pressure of blocked secretions resulting in distention of the biliary ducts, pyloric spasm, nausea and irregularities of the heart.

Its action on leukocytes, the nervous centers, poliomyelitis, and an aspect of the psyche are my own personal discoveries.

The relative insufficiency-excess of the gallbladder is as follows:

Insufficiency	Excess
Lack of confidence in oneself, inhibition before an effort, lack of courage, insecurity, apprehension.	Aggressiveness, need to act badly, sure of oneself, unhappiness, irritability, envy, jealousy, autocratic behavior.
Insomnia from insecurity, worries.	Migraines particularly on the right temple. Nausea on waking. Bitter or dry taste in the mouth on waking. Asthma. Constipation.
Lymphangitis, mastoiditis, lymphadenitis.	
Agitation over trifles, trembling.	Pains in the whole body or articulations; cutting pains in the shoulder; swelling of the popliteal fossa. Skin troubles.
Hazy vision.	Black circles around eyes; difficulty turning eyes. Otitis, numbness, buzzing.
Colorless or gray complexion.	Earthy complexion.

The gallbladder meridian starts at the temple and zigzags along the side of the head, then descends the anterior side of the thorax crossing several meridians, and finally travels down the lateral, yang surface of the lower limb. It receives energy from the triple warmer through a branch connecting *ermen* (TW-23, IS TW-21) to the first point of the gallbladder, *tongziliao* (GB-1). It flows into the liver from a branch starting at foot-*linqi* (GB-41), moving to the liver at *dadun* (LR-1). The left branch of the meridian is much more powerful in its effects on the biliary passages than the right branch.

Its time of maximum energy is at midnight, the minimum for the heart. Its minimum is at noon, the maximum for the heart. The organ upstream, the mother, is the triple warmer; downstream is the liver, the child as well as the coupled meridian. It is the husband of the stomach. There are two herald points, *riyue* (GB-24) and *zhejin* (GB-23), both on the side of the thorax. The assent point is *danshu* (BL-19).

Its pulse is on the left wrist, second section, superficial level.

III. Urinary Bladder

In Chinese medicine, the urinary bladder plays an important role in the urinary system as regulator of the kidneys, increasing or diminishing their flow according to its nervous stimulation. The urinary bladder is also responsible for the sudden voiding that often results from nervous crisis.

In Western medicine, it functions as a reservoir for urine. When filled, the muscles of expulsion relax and the sphincter contracts. When beyond a certain fullness, the muscles of expulsion contract and the sphincter relaxes.

By contrast, in the Chinese medical system, the urinary bladder has multiple energetic roles: it commands all the organs, the blood, pains, spasms, the yang energy, eyes and more.

We must first examine some of its characteristics. The meridian starts at the root of the nose and traverses the top of the head. The points along this part of the channel seem to act strongly on the eyes, sinusitis, and pains of the face; one point, *tianzhu* (BL-10), even has all the effects of the parasympathetic system. This meridian, however, seems to have only a weak effect on the urinary bladder itself (although responding in the pulse and the organ).

On the back, the effects on the urinary bladder are still not very obvious. Two parallel lines separating at *dazhu* (BL-11) descend from the neck to the buttocks. The line closest to the vertebral column has all the assent points of the organs; these are dispersed in cases of problems of fever or hyperexcitation. The lateral line contains a particularly important point, *gaohuangshu* (BL-38, IS BL-43), capable of inducing an increase in red blood cell production.

The portion of the meridian that traverses the posteromedial surface of the thigh has by itself a strong, direct action on the urinary bladder.

Points along the urinary bladder meridian show a surprising range of effects: there is the point of the parasympathetic system, *tianzhu* (BL-10); the assent points; the point for red blood cells, *gaohuangshu* (BL-38, IS BL-43); for fevers, *yixi* (BL-40, IS BL-45); cramps, *chengshan* (BL-57); physical as well as emotional pains, *kunlun* (BL-60); the point for insomnia with an overactive mind, also furuncles, *shenmai* (BL-62); epileptic troubles, *jinmen* (BL-63); and finally, the point for expelling different varieties of intestinal worms, including tapeworm, *zhiyin* (BL-67).

Such multiple functions demand study and experimentation to substantiate the efficacy of their actions; however, such research has not been carried out, save for *gaohuangshu* at the level of the scapula (BL-38, IS BL-43). Through extensive analysis, we now know that this point induces the formation and introduction into the blood stream of from 500,000 to one million red blood cells per cubic millimeter, which mature only fifteen to eighteen hours later. The point also acts to increase the total immunity of the blood and to maximally harmonize the production of hormones. This suggests an action on the red bone marrow of the sternum (where it awakens a response) and ribs.

Diseases of the bone are all improved by *dazhu* (BL-11).

When the yang energy of activity is in excess, insomnia and heat result; when insufficient, cerebral weakness and coldness develop. *Shenmai* (BL-62) is used to treat these imbalances.

Tenacious furunculosis: *shenmai* (BL-62).

Intestinal worms: *zhiyin* (BL-67).

The relative insufficiency-excess of the urinary bladder is as follows:

Insufficiency	Excess
Lack of character, easily frightened and confused brain.	Excessive character, agitation, oppresssive fullness, and pains.
Sleeps too heavily, somnolence, bad hearing.	Insomnia from an excess of yang (active) energy.
Anemia, pulmonary tuberculosis, or atonic ossification.	All fevers from excess.
Internal cold; suffers from cold.	Internal heat; suffers from heat.
Intestinal worms.	Tenacious furunculosis.
Urinary needs are abounding and frequent. Atony, atonic retention. Incontinence by sphincter atony.	Irritated urinary bladder, cystitis, frequent need to urinate with little result, spasmodic incontinence, spasmodic retention; urethritis.
Epileptoid troubles from insufficiency; absent-mindedness.	Epileptoid troubles from excess; seizures.
	All physical and emotional pains. Internal or external spasms.

The bladder meridian traverses the back and the posterior aspect of the lower limbs. On the back there are two parallel lines, both running from the neck to the bottom of the buttocks; on the sacrum four points form a third line.

The upper part of the meridian reflects the head, top of the back and upper urinary bladder; the middle part reflects the back; the lower part reflects the thigh and the sphincter of the urinary bladder.

The meridian receives energy through the last point of the small intestine, *tinggong* (SI-19), through a branch following the lower eyelid and to the inner canthus (*jingming*, BL-1). It transfers its energy to the kidney through its last point on the little toe, *zhiyin* (BL-67), by a plantar branch to *yongquan* (KI-1).

The numbering of the dorsal portion of the meridian starts with the medial line, then moves to the sacral line and finally to the lateral line, all three from the most superior points downwards. This numbering system has led most authors to believe that the meridian first descends along the points of the medial line, then ascends without points to the first sacral foramen and descends again down the sacrum with points. The flow then moves up without points to the neck to descend again along the points of the lateral line to the gluteal fold. Some Japanese authors, however, in using an uninterrupted numbering system, have depicted the meridian as separating into two parts at the base of the neck with an additional third line on the sacrum. The three lines then rejoin at the gluteal fold. In fact, the medial and lateral lines separate at *dazhu* (BL-11) and the line of the sacral foramen at *dachangshu* (BL-25). The three rejoin at *chengfu* (BL-50, IS BL-36).

Its time of maximum energy is 4 p.m., minimum hour of the lungs. Its minimum is at 4 a.m., maximum of the lungs. The organ upstream, the mother, is the small intestine; downstream is the kidney, the child as well as the coupled meridian. The herald point is on the conception vessel, *zhongji* (CV-3). The assent point is on the urinary bladder meridian itself, *pangguangshu* (BL-28).

The pulse is on the left wrist, third section, superficial level.

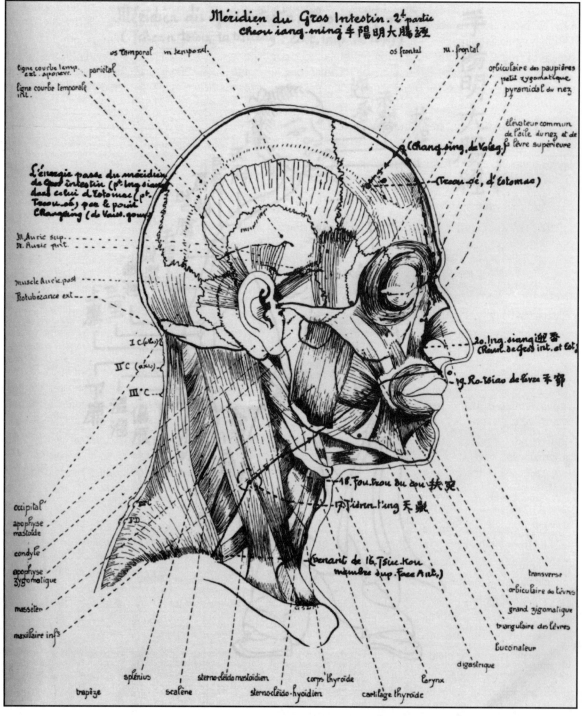

Meridian of the large intestine (part 2) (GSDM)

Chapter III

Sources of Energy (III)

Sources of Psychic Energy

I. The Psyche: 1. The Three Planes 2. The Energy of the Psyche — II. Spleen-pancreas: 1. Spleen 2. Pancreas-sugar — III. The Kidneys: 1. Action on the Psychic Energy 2. Action on the Renal Functions

I. The Psyche

By psychic energy we mean the intensity of feelings and thoughts, ''of that which feels, loves, and thinks — in a word, of the soul,'' as Pascal wrote. In other words, psychic energy connotes the intensity of function of all that feels and thinks in a being. Above all, it reflects the function of the brain and nervous centers which are fed by the organs, and yet command them.

The brain commands our reactions and all our being. Each of the command points awakens a response in part of the brain and nervous centers. (This response is the most accurate means of knowing if point location is correct.) The nervous centers are studied in more detail in Chapter V of this section. Here, we will only look at the sources modifying the intensity of the psyche and the psyche itself, independent of the nervous centers.

Experiments carried out in India in 1920 by Dr. Therese Brosse (published in the *Press Médicale*) have proven that through the ''will,'' thus the psyche, it is possible to completely arrest the movement of the organs for an indefinite period. The recording instruments used were connected to the heart and lungs — two organs which ostensibly cannot stop without causing death. The same ''will'' can make them start again, providing that the period of cessation has not been too long (several months?). Otherwise, the help of an outside ''will'' must be used.

These facts suggest two propositions: 1) The absolute power of the psyche on the physical body, either by personal will or by outside influence. 2) The possibility of maintaining life when the heart and lungs are stopped, the explanation of which is problematic. Here, we will only discuss the power of the psyche over the physical; that is, its action as a source of life or death.

The impressive experiments of Charcot and his students have more than adequately demonstrated this power. Even without such experimentation, numerous phenomena are well recognized: boredom is exhausting, the vitality can no longer sustain itself; bad news or even good news can kill; excess pleasure wears down the heart; unfavorable surroundings atrophy the intelligence and pollute the taste for life, opening the door to all evils. On the other hand, favorable circumstances develop talent, vital force, and activity.

We must distinguish between the reflective will and outside strength in both the experiments conducted in India and the West:

1)   The reflective will, which must be a function of the kidney since it can be developed by *fuliu* (KI-7).

2)   Outside strength, either by hypnotism, shocks or emotions. Hypnotism is recognized as putting in action the unconscious will, conceded as being all powerful for the subject. A point on the thumb, *guiyan* (a nonmeridian point) relieves one from the unconscious impulses and influences of this hypnotizing force. The noxious effects of shock and emotions, even if chronic, are negated by *kufang* (ST-14), particularly on the right side. Pernicious ''complexes'' resulting from outside forces, relieved only slightly by *kufang,* cease with *dazhong* (KI-6, IS KI-4).

The conscious mind strives to defend itself and impose its thoughts. It gives a spirit of synthesis, reasoning, judgment and moral awareness and in doing so impedes the influence of suggestion. It attempts to satisfy its desires while at the same time comprehending the consequences of its actions. Sound operation of the conscious mind depends on the full functioning of the spleen-pancreas (*dadu,* SP-2).

Indeed, consciousness itself and the easy functioning and development of certain faculties have been shown through experimentation to depend on a healthy fullness of energy in the individual as well as in certain organs, particularly the spleen-pancreas. Thus, judgment, good sense, and an understanding of mathematical problems and life problems are clearly enhanced by improving the functioning of the spleen-pancreas. This is a matter of harmonizing that part of the mind that synthesizes and superimposes data while at the same time strengthening the moral consciousness, which strives to understand the consequences of actions with the same intensity as it strives to satisfy desires.

That part of the will involved with decision making — the process of quickly assessing the pros and cons of various actions — and the intensity of the willpower itself depend on the healthy functioning of the kidneys.

Reason depends on the functioning of the anterior lobes of the brain, the suppression of which gives a happy unawareness. The heart and spleen-pancreas command this part of the brain through certain points. Memory is under the function and command of the left parietal lobes, whereas the right parietal lobes act particularly on hereditary talents, good or bad. The reflexes may be quickened or retarded by acting on certain command points of the spinal cord.

The three levels of the psyche.

In devising a system of modifying particular faculties, ancient physiologists created a practical psychology analogous in all ways but one to the psychological concepts of Freud.

Like Freud, the Chinese recognized three planes of the mind:

The inferior plane is dominated by primitive instincts analogous to those of a plant in the process of sprouting — it seizes all that can be taken, breaking it up and making from it its substance. The "primate," egoistic and greedy, develops such characteristics as acquisitiveness, aggressiveness, destructiveness and constructiveness. Its Chinese name is *po,* and represents "what is not seen and which is under the influence of the new moon." Freud also describes an inferior plane, but it relates only to the unconscious, not to the primitive instincts themselves.

This "inferior plane' is reflected on the left wrist, fourth section, deep level.

In truth, this level of mind is the instrument of a horrible law of nature driving us to live only by killing and devouring other life. It is through this inferior plane that nature blinds us with the coarsest instinct of reproduction.

The intelligence of the primate is characterized by cunning and shrewdness. The art of lying or duping through speech or silence gratifies such intelligence.

A complexion that is lacking color and slightly fat gives evidence of the intensity of the "primate." Pasty, dry skin may be a sign of insufficiency, while a prominently large occipital bone may be a sign of dominance.

The tradition teaches us that there is a relationship between the "primate" and the lungs.

The relative insufficiency-excess of the primate is as follows:

Insufficiency	Excess
Pasty complexion, without life, dry.	Fatty complexion, supple skin.
Generosity, disinterestedness.	Greediness, envy, avarice.
Altruism to the point of an inferiority complex and failure.	Egoist, with admiration for himself, looks at himself in the mirror. Sure of himself, always has a reason.
Indecisive, without will.	Cunning, wily, without equity or reciprocity.
Naive, suggestible.	Contradictory, defamatory, persecutory, can lead to paranoia.
Detached. Can lead to schizophrenia.	Servile when confronted with strength, sadistic when confronted with weakness.

The pulses corresponding to the primate and the superior occipital lobe of the brain exhibit the same changes in response to certain points — *shangjuxu* (ST-37), and also *baihui* (GV-19, IS GV-20) and *houding* (GV-18, IS GV-19) of the governor vessel.

The middle plane: The Chinese name is *hun,* "that which remains when the higher faculties, the evolved, are no longer." This is analogous to Freud's "subconscious," but includes memory. From the clinical action taken, it appears that this "middle plane" is twofold:

1) The right parietal lobe seems to command the hereditary memory, the good or bad inborn talents, the totally unconscious memory; it causes action without reflection, with the eyes closed. It forces certain conceptions. Through it our destiny is accomplished. If parts of the psyche or environment are in contradiction and the mental state is unstable, it can bring on neurosis or psychosis. It is the "automaton." If it dominates the left side, the right parietal bone is larger than the left one.

2) The left parietal lobe seems to act on two forms of memory: conscious memory, enabling one to bring to mind images and words at will; and semiconscious memory, registering sensory data but without total awareness. Images, rhythms, or slogans which are heard or seen but not attended to still influence the mind and can, in certain circumstances, reappear in the conscious memory (the "parrot"). If it dominates the "automaton," the left parietal bone is larger than the right one.

The pulse is on the left wrist, fourth section, middle level, radial edge of the artery for the "automaton," medial edge for the "parrot."

The bilateral points act on opposite parts of the parietals. Principally indicated are the points of the heart governor, but *qianding* (GV-20, IS GV-21) and *xiajuxu* (ST-39) are also used.

Good students and "competitive animals" have a very developed parrot. While very bright in ordinary conditions with clear precedent, these types are disastrous leaders in serious circumstances.

The relative insufficiency-excess of the automaton is as follows:

The relative insufficiency-excess of the automaton:

Insufficiency	Excess
Nonconformist. Attracted to unexpected enterprises; no respect for tradition.	Conformist. Led by the family and environmental tradition.
Victim of the occasion.	Acts with eyes closed, by routine.
Obliged to reflect before acting.	

The relative insufficiency-excess of the parrot:

Insufficiency	Excess
No memories for words, dates, pictures or sounds; cannot learn by rote memory, must understand.	Speaks only by quotations, in abundance, with assurance about any subject of their readings or conferences. Memory for words and dates.
Reasons from facts, not from words.	The words replace and conceal the facts.
Independent, researcher.	Takes profit from the work of others.
Mediocre bureaucrat, distracted, but a great leader in case of crises.	Good bureaucrat in second position, dangerous in a high post during serious times.

The superior plane: Stronger when the frontal lobes (and frontal bone) are more developed. The Chinese have studied it well. Several command points act on it.

It is the foundation of all faculties that differentiate actions of the evolved human from those of instinctive animals. This is the moral consciousness which, above all, assesses the consequences of its actions while striving to satisfy desires; notions of good and bad result. The superior plane provides a precise perception of reality, of the facts which words deform or hide. It gives vision of the relationship between these realities and hence is responsible for what we believe to be correct ideas and judgment. In recognizing the consequences of our behavior, we can wisely act on the future. Finally, it gives the ability to rapidly solve mathematical problems and problems of life. All this can be summarized as a talent for observation and synthesis. This is the intelligence that comprehends justice and acts correctly, that is, in harmony with the total reality.

The name "evolved" seems the most appropriate translation of the Chinese *shen,* wherein a being "has become a man and is evolved, no longer an animal." This name is also used for geniuses, sages and the soul.

We see that in addition to consciousness as described by Freud, this plane possesses reason and moral consciousness, the sense of reality. Its pulse is located on the left wrist, fourth section, superficial level. The pulse changes simultaneously with the pulse of the frontal lobes.

Several command points act on the evolved consciousness to increase its function and maximize its potential development. These points have helped young mathematicians understand their problems easily and quickly, and have been used for enhancing the development of moral consciousness in children.

The meridians involved are mostly those of the spleen-pancreas and heart. It is possible that through better assimilation of sugar by the pancreas (indispensable to the nervous centers) and improved blood circulation, the functioning of these lobes is strengthened. Of note are the points *dadu* (SP-2), *shaochong* (HT-9), and *fenglong* (ST-40).

In Japan, the teaching of Zen Buddhism, termed *chan* in Chinese, aims to remove the distorting influence of words and learned notions from the mind; in effect, to transcend automation and parroting. The result is an ability to perceive the complexities of reality and the profound essential relations of things. Through this form of meditation, one can transcend words and their oversimplifications and vagueness. The aim, in fact, is to re-establish the integral primacy of the evolved man.

The relative insufficiency-excess of the evolved man:

Insufficiency	Excess
Unconsciousness. Amorality.	Moral consciousness. Morality.
Does not understand the deep aspects of reality, nor its relations; lack of synthesis.	Immediately superimposes the given facts of a problem and resolves it; able to synthesize.
Obeys without understanding; easily suggestible.	Distinguishes immediately the true from the false; understands all questions easily.
Carefree, happy, sociable; improvident.	Foresightful, preoccupied with the future, brooding.
Reality always distorted.	Balanced view of reality.
Cannot conceive a viable plan.	Organizer, thinks of everything.
Cannot concentrate for a long time, the mind escapes.	Easy and prolonged concentration.

The energy of the psyche.

A specific energy animates these three planes. It is called "color" because its presence is seen in the color of the face and the animation of the visage. It is considered as having as its source the vital *elan* of birth that first animates the primitive instincts of growth, intake, destruction and greed. With the subsequent development from primate into human, the unconscious, traditional and conscious memories are animated. Then, finally, when the being is evolved, the most elevated faculties are enlivened.

The ancients taught that when this "color" is fully developed and animated, the evolved man becomes temporarily depleted in the inferior or middle planes. However, the being can be called back by the evolved man into these lower planes without diminishment of the evolved man.

It is tempting to compare "color" with the libido of Freud, all the more so as the word "color" is often used in the sense of "license." We must, however, consider that the "color" is the growing force of the whole living being, and that its sexual aspect is only one of the forms of its multiple activities in life.

It appears that it is this particular energy that we tonify or disperse by acting on the points commanding each plane of the psyche; as these are linked to each of the great cerebral groups, it would be this energy that animates the cerebral life.

In the last analysis, psychic energy could be considered as a differentiated form of the original vital *elan*.

II. Spleen-Pancreas

The interaction between the spleen and pancreas is confirmed by the following facts:

1)   Professor Mériel has written to me, stating:

> *(Argand's) experimental removal of the spleen in animals leads to hyperfunctioning or a sort of compensa-*
> *tory hypertrophy of the rest of the reticuloendothelial tissue of which the spleen is only a voluminous accu-*
> *mulation. Sometimes, there is even a curious metaplasia of the pancreatic parenchyma. . . . This has*
> *confirmed the spleen-pancreas unity.*

2)   For the spleen and pancreas there is only one meridian; however, each branch acts very strongly on one of the two organs and only weakly on the other. The action is possibly contralateral, i.e., right branch for the spleen and left branch for the pancreas, but unilateral actions are also encountered. There are, however, two distinct pulses — right wrist, second section, middle level for the pancreas; right wrist, second section, deep level for the spleen.

3)   When the spleen is distended and insufficient, the pulse of the spleen is also soft from insufficiency. The digestion of carbohydrates and pastries is difficult and one suffers from acid stomach as well. When the spleen is rebalanced, the pancreas becomes normal again. However, the pancreas as well as the stomach (their pulses vary together) are stimulated by the parasympathetic and slowed down by the sympathetic system. The opposite is true for the spleen.

4)   The small intestine acts directly on the pancreas by activating its secretions and concentrating its juices. The action of the small intestine on the psyche is close to that of the spleen, the former giving quick recuperation from both mental and physical fatigue, and the latter preventing the fatigue from recurring.

5)   Judging from Chinese medical texts, it appears that there has been a high incidence in Asia of congenital joining of the spleen and pancreas. These cases are rare in the West.

6)   In the West, in those few people who have had their spleens removed, the function of the spleen on the blood does not disappear and at most is only slightly diminished. Other functions attributed in Chinese medicine to the spleen-pancreas meridian do not disappear, but again are only slightly diminished.

The salient conclusions derived from these facts are that, first, the spleen and pancreas are closely linked and respond to the same energetic commands; and second, the spleen can possibly compensate for pancreatic insufficiency. Here we must take into account that the removal of the pancreas has not been the object of specific experiments.

Extensive experimentation has been carried out in France to determine the correct action of each branch of the spleen-pancreas meridian. Results clearly show that tonification of the left branch most noticeably modifies the pulse of the pancreas while that of the right branch most noticeably affects the spleen pulse.

We will give an account here of the observations correlating the action of the spleen or pancreas with modifications of their distinct pulses. We will additionally discuss the role of the pancreas in the transformation of sugars and essential functions of digestion, already enumerated in Chapter I of this section, under the heading ''Pancreas-Digestion.''

Some diverse effects are obtained by acting on the spleen-pancreas meridian. Thus far, it has not been possible to attribute the origin to one or the other organ. The following are our own physiological discoveries, previously unknown in the West:

1)   After tonification of *dadu* (SP-2), laboratory analysis has consistently found a notable augmentation in the number of mononuclear leukocytes. These generally abound in skin diseases marked by an overgrowth of staphylococci, namely, pemphigus, psoriasis, eczema, and impetigo (recall that a liver insufficiency is always observable in such cases). For the West, the spleen contains lymphoid tissue that produces lymphocytes; mononuclear lymphocytes are not involved.

2)   Another materially verifiable effect is that by tonifying this double meridian and using daily moxa on it, it is possible for the subject to reach the maximum size and width of the chest, given the limitations of his or her hereditary "form." This is useful in cases of retarded growth, but is not effective after twenty years of age or in people whose parents are small. We must question whether or not this effect involves action by growth hormone liberated by the anterior pituitary.

3)   The synthetic mind allows the immediate superimposition of all data pertinent to a problem, the appraisal of the consequences of an act and the satisfaction of a desire. This function prevents suggestibility arising from making parallels without considering the facts of a problem and gives good sense, judgement and reason. It is possible that this faculty involves both the pancreas and liver, which function to augment the quantity of sugar in the blood, thus stimulating the brain, the frontal lobes particularly.

4)   Prolonged concentration, attention maintained without effort; the possibility of preventing the mind from losing its way during a tiring conversation, or difficult or boring reading.

Besides the physical or psychological functions of the two organs, some points of the double meridian possess specific effects which merit being classified as functions.

Cranky or lazy children. Emptiness of energy in old people: *sanyinjiao* (SP-6).

Pains of the periosteum and the periosteum itself: *shangqiu* (SP-5).

All fevers: *xuehai* (SP-10). If agitated, *taibai* (SP-3).

All abscesses, osteomyelitis: *xuehai* (SP-10).

All troubles of the inguinal glands: *jimen* (SP-11).

Before conception, prevents miscarriage during the course of the pregnancy: *sanyinjiao* (SP-6).

A blow to the testicles: massage at *gongsun* (SP-4).

Inflammation or pain of the spermatic canal or epididymis: *chongmen* (SP-12).

Sphincter of the urinary bladder: *yinlingquan* (SP-9).

Cold of the body or extremities: *sanyinjiao* (SP-6), *fuai* (SP-16).

Rheumatism of the bones or decalcification: *shangqiu* (SP-5).

The spleen-pancreas meridian traverses the medial, yin side of the lower limb and the anterior thorax. It receives energy from the stomach by a branch starting from *chongyang* (ST-42). A branch rises from its last point near the nipple to *jiquan* (HT-1).

Its time of maximum energy is 10 a.m., minimum hour of the triple warmer. Its minimum is at 10 p.m., maximum of the triple warmer. The organ upstream, the mother as well as the coupled meridian, is the stomach; the child downstream is the heart. The herald point is *zhangmen* (LR-13). The assent point is *pishu* (BL-20).

The spleen-pancreas pulse is on the right wrist, second section, middle level for the pancreas, deep level for the spleen.

The spleen.

Cases of physical distention of the spleen, or splenomegaly, have given us the opportunity to observe the following consequences:

1)   The principal function of the spleen in Western physiology relates to the blood. In the above cases, a reduction in the increase of red blood cells and hemoglobin is noted.[2]

In splenomegaly, the spleen pulse is very weak if not nonexistent. R.J. Main *(Synthesis of Physiology)* suggests that the increased destruction of red blood cells may be the result of increased mechanical filtration, augmented by the distention of the filter; that is to say, by the spleen's laxness and greater dimension, not by an increase of its vital activity.

Additionally, the pancreas becomes compressed and disturbed in its function. It is then difficult to say if the modified mental functions come from changes in the spleen or the pancreas.

2)   Often a pronounced fatigue has been noted, beginning in the morning and persisting throughout the day, which is relieved in the evening. Does this come from the spleen or the pancreas?

3)   Swelling of the stomach with sleepiness after the noon meal is also noted, the explanation being that the stomach is compressed between the spleen and liver, the latter always distended at the same time as the spleen.

4)   The expulsion of fecal matter is difficult and slow. The splenic flexure of the large intestine is compressed by the distended spleen and the hepatic flexure compressed by the liver.

5)   The kidneys are compressed, which can lead either to low or high blood pressure, or blood in the urine and sharp renal pains.

6)   Palpitations of the heart which may be compressed by the spleen are noted primarily at night when the spleen swells further. False angina pectoris can mislead some specialists.

7)   Occasionally, breathlessness occurs from walking quickly or climbing stairs, a sign that the lungs are being compressed by the spleen and liver. Distention of the spleen and liver is always a result of severe sadness, physical shocks, great fatigue or prolonged worries.

This ''syndrome of the eight organs'' must depend on a single energy command since one point is enough to put everything right: either *yutang* (CV-18) of the conception vessel, or, when the kidneys are more affected, *taixi* (KI-5, IS KI-3), a point said to act additionally on the spleen-pancreas and stomach. I discovered the action of these two points only a few years ago and cannot yet provide a satisfactory explanation.

Pancreas-sugar.

The extreme importance of the pancreas for digestion, assimilation and transformation of meat (trypsin), carbohydrates (amylopsin) and fats (lipase) into general energy has already been discussed (see Chapter I of this section). All of this is enhanced by the stimulation of secretion by the small intestine and its role in concentrating the pancreatic juices.

One other function, the transformation of sugar into glycogen, is indispensable to cerebral, mental, and physical energy. Glycogen is held in reserve by the liver and muscles and is retransformed into sugar as needed. Without a sugar supply, the nervous centers, particularly the brain, would lack energetic nourishment, since these centers contain no glycogen reserves. All excesses and insufficiencies of this function result in very serious disorders: diabetes, dehydration with excess urine, depression and so forth from hyperglycemia; rage, coma, etc., from hypoglycemia.

Particular command points allow us to moderate or stimulate the pancreas itself, namely those of the small intestine, which stimulate the pancreas and concentrates its juices; those of the stomach (the mother upstream); and those of the heart (the child organ). Dispersing the adrenals may also prove helpful, since excessive adrenal function slows down the production of insulin, encourages the transformation of proteins into sugar, and retards the digestion of meat in the small intestine with a resultant excessive production of urea.

Likewise, pancreatic insufficiency will restrain the adrenals. Since the latter encourages the retention of salt, pancreatic insufficiency leads to less salt retention and consequently more abundant urine.

The pancreas is seriously weakened by sadness or worries. It acts on the sense of taste.

The very close interaction between the spleen and pancreas has thus far impeded our ability to clearly differentiate the effects obtained by tonifying or dispersing one or the other alone. Thus, for understanding the direct or indirect effects of the pancreas, the list given above for the spleen must suffice at present.

III. The Kidneys

The effects of the kidneys on the psyche is little recognized in the West, but traditional Chinese medical theory combined with my own discoveries on this subject hopefully will provide a solid basis for study.

First, with regard to the measure of the physical and mental functioning of the kidneys, the ancients identified only a single pulse for the two kidneys — left wrist, third section, deep level. We think there are two representative pulses: left wrist, third section, deep level, giving a measure of the functioning of the tubules, that is, the color of the excretion; and left wrist, third section, middle level, giving a measure of the glomerular function, that is, filtration. A new pulse technique, the palpation of one particular side of the artery, allows us to determine the functioning of an individual kidney. Using this method, it is possible to verify the removal of one kidney; or ascertain which kidney is filtering excessively or insufficiently, or which one is failing in its excretory function.

The main energetic role of the kidneys appears to be the nourishment of the psyche. We commence by stressing the relationship between action on the psyche and the kidneys' physical function.

Action on the psychic energy.

This action is absolutely specific to the kidneys. This presents particular problems for the field of psychology, since it relates the strength of the personality to the functioning of an organ, as well as to sexual intensity.

The following are the main types of behavior specific to kidney insufficiency: inferiority and failure complexes, lack of authority, misanthropy to the point of claustrophobia, lack of decision-will, emotional agitation, fear, lack of cleverness and guile; and for women, irritability or tears the week before menses; and a lack of charm, seductiveness or sex appeal. All these actions coincide with modifications in the function of the superior occipital lobes of the brain and the lower psychic plane, the primate, in which heredity is dominant.

Note here a discovery of the greatest importance for the family, nation and race, a discovery to which I was led by unexpected, but confirmed results. A point on the kidney meridian, *zhubin* (KI-9), when tonified or dispersed according to need during pregnancy (in the third and sixth months) is sufficient to check the passing on of poor hereditary traits. Mothers testing positive for syphilis, who have been treated using this point, give birth to children who test negative for syphilis, and who have none of the inevitable signs of such heredity. In normal cases where no such diseases are involved, poor hereditary traits are perhaps suppressed since the children maintain a particularly luminous complexion their whole life. Babies sleep at night and smile during the day. When they are older they do not contract illnesses, or, if they do, they have them at the extreme minimum of intensity and duration, some hours or one or two days. This is on the condition that they have not been poisoned by vaccines.

There are various behavior patterns that relate to the energetic functions of the kidneys; how they manifest in an individual depends on the level of functioning. Inferiority or failure complexes, the desire not to see people, and the closing up of oneself, are clear signs of insufficiency of a function which, when operating fully, gives a natural sense of authority. This authority allows, for example, a new teacher to open the door to his classroom and obtain a respectful silence straightaway; if it is lacking, the whole class immediately "catcalls." Thus, on the one hand, we have authority, assurance and personal influence; and, on the other, inferiority, failure, misanthropy to the point of claustrophobia and lack of authority. One point of the kidney meridian corrects imbalances of this function: *dazhong* (KI-6, IS KI-4), which is also the passage point to the urinary bladder meridian.

Another function, when in energetic excess, gives rise to cleverness and guile — the ability to immediately understand and profit from another person's weak side — and such audacity that one fails to worry about rules or obstacles. Insufficiencies of this function lead to mental and often physical clumsiness, emotional agitation and fear. One point of the kidney corrects these imbalances: *fuliu* (KI-7), the tonification point.

Decision-making may also be influenced by an excess or insufficiency of kidney energy. Some people make clear decisions with little reflection, while others are very indecisive and balance pros and cons to the extreme of not knowing what to do. Will is the power of accomplishment coming from the impetus of decision; lack of will comes from having little power of impetus or attraction toward a goal. *Fuliu* (KI-7), the tonification point, corrects insufficiencies. *Rangu* (KI-2), the dispersal point, corrects excess; indeed, there can be a noxious excess of decision or will.

Sexual functions directly related to the kidneys are given below:

For men — sexual authority: when this is in abundance, even an ugly, unattractive man meets no resistance; on the other hand, a man lacking this authority never excites great love though he may ostensibly have everything in his favor. Antiquity links this male function to the left kidney. Healthy functioning of this kidney is also necessary for full vitality of the spermatozoa. A particular strength of character would also be a corollary. The tonification point of the kidneys should produce results in these cases; one must understand, however, that this has not been sufficiently studied.

For women — charm, seductiveness, sex-appeal, as well as fertility and even the vitality of the fetus depends on the right kidney. Insufficiency deprives one of charm and fertility. Here again, observations have not been systematically verified. For insufficiency, use the tonification point, *fuliu* (KI-7). For excess, use *rangu* (KI-2), the dispersal point.

A particular point on the kidney meridian is highly successful for treating mental problems arising for most women during the eight days preceding menses. Hyperexcitation and irritability become marked to varying degrees of severity; occasionally nervous crises result. Sometimes there is inexplicable sadness, tears, and depression, even without motive. *Shiquan* (KI-4, IS KI-5) is the acupoint that corrects these imbalances; it must be tonified or dispersed according to the particular case involved, be it one of excess or insufficiency.

It is not yet possible to specify the mechanisms involved in the phenomena above. It may be a matter of the kidney's hormonal influence on the circulation, of insufficient excretions of toxins, or of hormones in excess.

Note again, for insomnia due to insufficiency of yin energy of inactivity: *zhaohai* (KI-3, IS KI-6).

For loss of memory and vocal force through sadness: *yongquan* (KI-1).

For the malcontent who speaks a lot: disperse *fuliu* (KI-7).

For dreams of being in water, of submerged trees, of being on the edge of a precipice: tonify *fuliu* (KI-7).

For lead poisoning with cephalitis: *zhubin* (KI-9).

Action on renal functions.

In the West (Hédon), two different theories are current, and each is supported by substantial observations:

1) That of Ludwig, taught in the United States (R.J. Main) and increasingly adopted in France: the glomerular capillaries allow all their filtrates, water and solids, to pass through; at the proximal end, only part of the water and salts are reabsorbed by the tubular cells, but towards the distal end, reabsorption of the rest of the water and solids has occurred until the quantity or threshold needed by the blood is reached.

2) That of Bowmann: that the glomerular capillaries allow water to pass in the needed quantity regulated by their vasoconstriction; the tubular cells excrete excess solids up to threshold for those substances having a threshold and all excess for the others. The normal adult glomerular filtration rate is about 125 ml./min. Additionally, they secrete vasoconstrictive renin, colorings and other substances.

According to the science of energy, two points, *jiaoxin* (KI-8) and *rangu* (KI-2), act on the quantity of water. When dispersed they augment it, and when tonified they diminish it. This occurs without modifying the quantity of solids, so that the more they are dispersed, the more the urine is colorless. Two other points, *fuliu* (KI-7) and *yongquan* (KI-1), act on the color and smell. They stimulate excretion and secretion but do not diminish the proportion of liquid, nor do they stimulate the reabsorption of water. When tonified, they increase the color and smell and thus the excretion of solids; when dispersed, they diminish the same. These results would tend to confirm the theory of Bowmann.

Excretion and secretion: both are carried out through the tubule cells, though by different mechanisms. They are purely energetic and vital renal functions. They are both represented by the same pulse reflecting tubule function — left wrist, third section, deep level. The point that commands them is *fuliu* (KI-7), the tonification point of the kidney. *Yongquan* (KI-1) is also useful.

It is taught that the level of reabsorption of water and substances from the blood at the glomeruli depends on a threshold particular to each substance. Such precision in the variety of thresholds is obtained through a mechanism declared by the West as still unknown. Chinese physiology would attribute it to the ''form'' — that force which rules the threshold of healing, growth, etc.

This subject brings to mind some of the other mechanisms for maintaining a balance of fluids or substances: the action of the pituitary gland's antidiuretic hormones on water reabsorption; of the parathyroid on phosphorus retention; and of the adrenocorticotropic hormones on salt reabsorption.

Excretion has nothing to do with osmosis and is indeed renal in function. This function involves the use of various substances, namely colorings, such as phenolsulfonphthalein, urochrome, and urobilin; hippuric acid; aminohippuric acid and creatine. The cells form NH_3 in order to neutralize the acidity of the filtrate; they also retain the necessary bases, Na and K.

Some organic actions are commanded by certain points:

Mouth: *dazhong,* (KI-6, IS KI-4). Contracted throat: *zhaohai* (KI-3, IS KI-6). Saliva: *rangu* (KI-2).

Digestive organs: *shencang* (KI-25). Esophagus: *dazhong* (KI-6, IS KI-4). Lack of appetite: *taixi* (KI-5, IS KI-3). Upset stomach: *zhaohai* (KI-3, IS KI-6); or spasm: *huangshu* (KI-16). Painful spasms of the abdomen: *huangshu* (KI-16). Jaundice with lack of stools and urine: *yongquan* (KI-1); or from food: *zhaohai* (KI-3, IS KI-6); or with fever: *qixue* (KI-13). Diabetes: *rangu* (KI-2); with thirst, impotence: *taixi* (KI-5, IS KI-3).

Respiratory passages (all inflammatory excess): *taixi* (KI-5, IS KI-3), *rangu* (KI-2). Pleuritis, pulmonary congestion: *shufu* (KI-27). Asthma with weakness: *rangu* (KI-2); if elderly: *shufu* (KI-27).

Heart problems (false angina): *taixi* (KI-5, IS KI-3). Hypertension from excess of the kidneys: *yongquan* (KI-1). Hypertension from kidney insufficiency: *fuliu* (KI-7). Fever with profuse sweating: disperse *taixi* (KI-5, IS KI-3) and *fuliu* (KI-7).

Genital system — women: in virgins, troubles and pain during menses: *zhaohai* (KI-3, IS KI-6). All disorders of the ovaries: *qixue* (KI-13); of the fallopian tubes: *dahe* (KI-12); vulva and vagina: *rangu* (KI-2); irritation of the vagina: *rangu* (KI-2). Menses insufficient or do not come: *shuiquan* (KI-4, IS KI-5). Men: excessive erections, pruritus of the penis: *zhaohai* (KI-3, IS KI-6). Impotence: *dahe* (KI-12), *rangu* (KI-2), *yongquan* (KI-1). Sperm insufficient: *qixue* (KI-13), *dahe* (KI-12), *rangu* (KI-2).

Eruptive illnesses (scarlet fever, measles, rubella): *yongquan* (KI-1). Furuncle: *rangu* (KI-2).

Internal cold: *dazhong* (KI-6, IS KI-4), *fuliu* (KI-7); in the chest: *rangu* (KI-2); in the legs and feet: *fuliu* (KI-7) or *yongquan* (KI-1).

Cramps of the feet — at night: *rangu* (KI-2); in the day: *zhaohai* (KI-3, IS KI-6).

Articular rheumatism: *yongquan* (KI-1); knee: *rangu* (KI-2); internal malleolus: *zhaohai* (KI-3, IS KI-6).

Traumas, internal pains: *rangu* (KI-2).

The kidney meridian is on the medial, yin surface of the lower limb. It receives energy from the urinary bladder, by a plantar branch at *zhiyin* (BL-67). A branch starting from the last point, *shufu* (KI-27), descends towards the external side of the nipple to the first point of the heart governor, *tianchi* (PC-1).

Its time of maximum energy is 6 p.m., minimum hour of the large intestine. Its minimum is at 6 a.m., maximum of the large intestine. The organ upstream, the mother as well as the coupled meridian, is the urinary bladder; the child downstream is the heart governor. The herald point is *jingmen* (GB-25); the assent point, *shenshu* (BL-23); the tonification point, *fuliu* (KI-7); the dispersal point, *rangu* (KI-2) and also *yongquan* (KI-1); the source point, *taixi* (KI-5, IS KI-3).

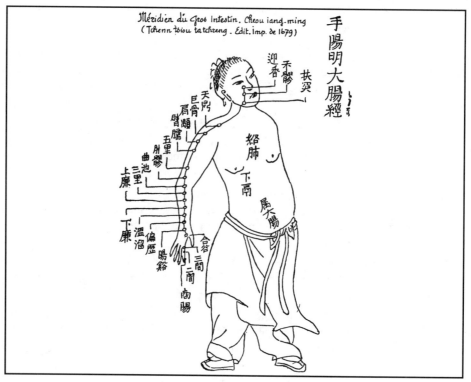

Meridian of the large intestine (DACH)

Notes

[1] This expression reads: "Hairy people are sexy or tuberculor." — Trans.

[2] The *Nei Jing* states: "The spleen takes the blood and sends it purified to the other organs."

Chapter IV

Sources of Energy (IV)

Sources of Sexual Energy

I. Sexual Energy — II. Forms and Sources of Female Sexual Energy: 1. Forms 2. Ovarian Hormones — III. Forms and Sources of Male Sexual Energy: 1. Forms 2. Testicular Hormones

I. Sexual Energy

In the Far East, the manifestations of life have been consistently examined from the point of view of the vital energy. Great importance has been attached to human reproduction and to all that favors this end. Hence, Eastern studies on sexuality, complete with observations, experiments and teachings, have contributed greatly to our own knowledge. This is particularly true as research on reproduction has been hampered in the West by inhibitions not culturally subscribed to in the East.

Through modern physiology, we have become increasingly aware of the personal, familial, social and racial importance of sexual matters. Experiments carried out in select hospital clinics in the West have confirmed the ancient teachings of China on the possibility of improving the various sexual functions through manipulation of the energy. This knowledge enhances the treatment of sexual disorders and confirms the importance of sexual energy as a source of vital energy.

Western researchers have clearly observed this importance. We know that sexual excitement causes an immediate increase in blood pressure and that in hypertensive persons such excitement can cause a stroke. We recognize that sexual excitement gives heightened activity and drive, and that people who are sexually unexcitable have weak reserves of strength and must rely on virtuous or mental activities to sustain them. How many women, just before menstruation, experience great depression or expend themselves physically by walks or hard work, or have negative changes of character as tedious for them as for those around them? And contrariwise, how stimulating are even innocent flirtations and loving friendships?

II. Forms and Sources of Female Sexual Energy

The forms.

The forms of woman's sexual energy are specific, given her role in sexual relations which can potentially end in reproduction. The woman, in effect, must attract, seduce and retain the man; she receives and takes through her art, which is to permit herself to be taken. Curiously, her attractiveness is not in direct relation either to her pleasure or to the possibility of conception. However, her pleasure may have great bearing on conception.

Attraction, seduction, sex-appeal: Until recent times, marriages in China were made by family arrangement, the bride and groom often never seeing each other before the ceremony. In this arrangement, attractiveness was of no value for getting married. Instead, a high sense of morality and culture, perfect politeness of speech, grace in tone of voice, gestures and attitudes, and respect for the husband were the virtues taught to the future wife.

Keen observers in the West will note that a woman mediocre in all respects save for that very special talent — sex-appeal — is assailed with requests, while another woman with beauty, grace and intelligence, but without that sex-appeal, has no effect on men.

Certain command points of the kidney meridian, particularly the tonifying point *fuliu* (KI-7), develop cleverness, astuteness, and decision, and by doing so develop seductiveness itself. Authority is developed by *dazhong* (KI-6, IS KI-4). Is a still unrecognized function of the kidney involved, or perhaps of the renal hormones?

Pleasure: With the goal of conception in mind, China has given its sustained attention to the delicate topic of sexual pleasure. The Chinese have noted the existence of command points which allow for an augmentation or diminution of pleasure in the desired proportion at will. The West acknowledges the difficulty of studying this topic given the lack of standardization in comparative reports on sexual pleasure and the paucity of true statements. Either public lies exist, or there is ignorance of one's own sensations when the sensations are not very strong. Also, pleasure can be nil with one person and intense with someone else.

Two questions are posed on this subject: the nature of sexual pleasure and its necessity for conception.

Numerous experiments carried out in gynecological clinics on the subject of sexual pleasure and conception have confirmed China's ancient observations: if pleasure is completely absent, the internal organ fails to open and conception does not take place, or does so only with great difficulty. A medium level of pleasure favors conception. An intense level of pleasure contracts the internal organ, closes it and blocks conception. This conclusion differs from Western teaching. R.J. Main writes: "The orgasm of the woman is not essential for impregnation."

Some women who call themselves frigid and others who experience strong orgasms also become pregnant. But one must question whether the former group were completely frigid or if the latter actually had only a medium level of sensation.

Excitation caused by caressing the nipples is an important index of temperament. The only evidence, however, lies in the correct stimulation of *shimen* (CV-5), the herald point of the lower warmer (genital function).

Again, R.J. Main writes: "The nature of the orgasm is not clearly known. It begins by an erection of the clitoris, vagina and nipples." But it is said these days that the pleasure comes only through the stimulation of the clitoris in certain cases, while in others it extends into all the interior organs with the slightest touch, even of only the nipples.

The action of sexual pleasure on energy is of great and well-known importance. In the beginning stages, sexual arousal increases the circulation, enriches the complexion, animates the look and vivifies. As the arousal increases, it excites, enervates and makes one tense; the blood pressure rises. When the orgasm comes, the moment of great relaxation, there is a sudden drop of potential commonly called "the little death."

Lack of arousing sexual encounters leads to irritability, malaise, sadness, lack of enthusiasm or lethargy. A harmonious frequency of encounters is warming, vivifying and slenderizing. Too great a frequency is exhausting.

When hormones of the opposite sex were administered to frenetic young people we observed a marked calming and blossoming effect. We therefore propose that on sexual contact there is a real exchange of hormones and that this exchange increases with pleasure. We further suggest that there can also be an exchange of energy.

The ovarian hormones.

During the growth years, follicle stimulating hormone (FSH) elongates the leg and arm bones while hindering the development of the nipples and uterus. If insufficient, menses are blocked. A deficiency of luteinizing hormone (LH) causes sterility or miscarriage; an excess causes problems during menses.

Though the ovarian hormones were unknown in antiquity, observation and experimentation verified the efficacy of certain command points on the genital organs: the ovaries, *qixue* (KI-13); the fallopian tubes, *dahe* (KI-12); the blood, *sanyinjiao* (SP-6). Ancient Chinese physiologists had also discovered acupoints for correcting certain gynecological conditions: premenstrual problems, *shuiquan* (KI-4, IS KI-5) — disperse for irritability and tonify for depression; an imbalance of the antihemorrhagic vitamin K, *hegu* (LI-4) and *taichong* (LR-3); and tendency to miscarriage, *zhubin* (KI-9) and *sanyinjiao* (SP-6). Through use of these acupuncture points, properly functioning sexual organs could be re-established.

The female reproductive organs are reflected at the deep level, third section, right pulse. The distal part reflects the condition of the ovaries and upper portion of the fallopian tubes; the middle part, the fallopian tubes; the proximal part, the uterus. Each edge of the artery describes the ipsilateral aspect. It is possible through this pulse even to have a measure of the capacity for pleasure, of "temperament." It can be used to detect ovulation and the coming of the menses.

III. Forms and Sources of Male Sexual Energy

The forms.

The male forms of sexual energy differ from female forms, just as the sexual roles of men and women differ. If the woman gives the man the illusion of conquest, then the man has indeed conquered. But if there is no physical desire, he finds himself greatly inhibited. Male sexual pleasure is separable from his fecundity and from his erection.

True sexual mastery is an amazing talent, as inexplicable as feminine attractiveness. It removes all inclination to resistance even before the attack has begun. As with those women with sex-appeal, men with true sexual mastery win numerous successes easily, though they may be quite unattractive in the usual sense. Others who appear to ''have it all'' may consistently be repulsed.

Of course, power, money and fame are sure attractions, but other qualities are also important. *Dazhong* (KI-4, passage point to the urinary bladder) helps supply these by acting against inferiority and failure complexes, thus against the lack of authority; in doing so, it indirectly helps build sexual confidence.

Desire in men is of great importance; if absent for even a moment, there is an incapacity to perform. This incapacity is the sure sign of a lack of desire.

Sex-appeal and desire are relative, and of course psychological factors have great significance. Desire can remain bestial or be transformed into loving tenderness or even into loving passion. It can also be sublimated. Some men experience a continuous state of desire, no matter what the object.

The point which commands sexual desire is *qichong* (ST-30), which is described as giving energy to the twelve meridians. The stomach is thus the source of sexual desire, and in fact food and drink, according to their nature, stimulate or reduce desire.

Pleasure can exist with or without an erection or ejaculation.

The command points for pleasure are still unknown for men (perhaps abdomen-*yinjiao*, CV-7?).

The erection depends on several types of energy:

1) Psychological — by thought, in solitude, or from evocative reading, thus pure imagination. Imagination depends on the spleen and the anterior brain.

2) By visual excitation — licentious pictures, still imagination but more material; by direct sight of an embrace, etc.

3) Without contact, by the sight or smell of a particular person and no other — here it is a question of sexual sensitivity, not just psychological suggestion.

4) By contact, also with a particular person and no other.

5) By touching.

The level of energy in general is important for erections. The inability to have or sustain an erection often coincides with the weakening of the vital energy in old age. In addition, psychological inhibitions from the unconscious mind (such as complexes, prohibitions of parents or the environment, or childhood trauma) may influence one's ability to have erections. Psychoanalysis can help remove these.

Impotence may arise from unconscious comparisons, e.g., impossible in bed or easy in bed, etc. An unexpected setback can stop things for a long time. Untreated diabetes can weaken or stop erections.

For the West, it depends, first, on the sacral nerves, through the junction of the splanchnic fibers of the parasympathetic system (q.v. Hédon, Main). The response of the parasympathetic system, *tianzhu* (BL-10), is at the glans; that of the sympathetic system, *fengchi* (GB-20), at the penis. Promising results are being obtained by tonifying the command points of these nerve pathways at *zhongliao* (BL-33) and especially *xialiao* (BL-34). It further depends on the following mechanisms explained by Main (226):

> [The erection] can be a reflex, as by mechanical stimulation of the sensorial terminations of the penis via a nerve center in the spinal cord [opposite lumbar?], with sensorial impulses passing into the sensory cortex [opposite parietal?], or the act can even be of cortical origin. The parasympathetic fibers produce arterial dilation, thus increasing the blood entering the cavernous body. These fibers also constrict the muscular valves in the veins, and with the assistance of contractions of the ischiocavernous muscle, the veins are compressed and the outflow blocked. The stimulation of the sympathetic system probably has the inverse effect.

> Is erection from hanging perhaps due to the suppression of the superior controls on the erectile center in the spinal cord? [Main does not mention exactly what the superior controls are.]

> Erection can be produced in small children and eunuchs, which indicates that testicular testosterone is not essential.

Erections at night and in the morning, called urinary erections, suggest an action of the urinary bladder and kidney.

Why does impotence come with a certain age? Is it from habitual lack of desire? Or the development of a consciousness which sees all the dreariness in our society which this act can cause? Or the feeling that one cannot be loved?

Ejaculation can be immediate (sign of nervousness) or delayed at will. *Diji* (SP-8) clearly increases sperm production and the tone of the ejaculatory mechanism. Experimentation must be carried out to confirm the actions of other acupoints.

The testicular hormones.

Here androgens (testosterone, androsterone) are involved. These are produced by the interstitial cells as well as the corticoadrenal cells.

Insufficiency of testicular hormones causes hypogonadism (by reducing the gonadotropin of the pituitary), thus sterility. This also leads to retarded growth (reduction of growth hormone of the pituitary) and sometimes cryptorchidism.

Their excess causes precocious puberty, secondary sex characteristics, masculine aggressivity, and diminished urinary excretion of salt and water.

Two command points act on the androgens: the command point of the adrenals, *fengfu* (GV-15, IS GV-16); and that of the pituitary, *dazhui,* at C7 (GV-13a, IS GV-14). Also *mingmen* (GV-4).

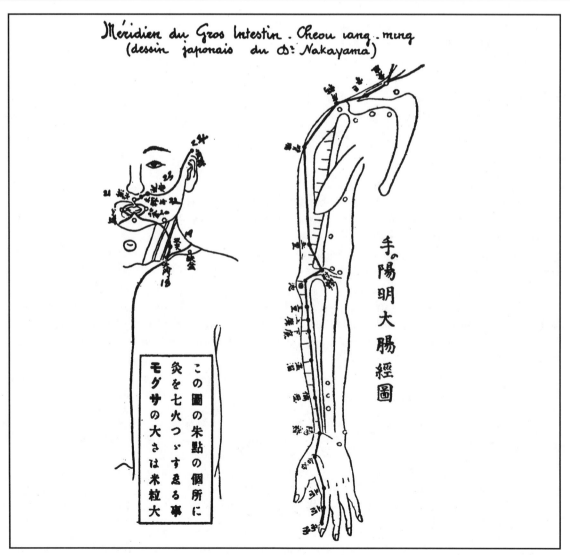

Meridian of the large intestine (Nakayama)

Chapter V
The Transformation of Energy

The Nervous Centers

I. Transformation of Energy — II. The Brain: 1. Frontal Lobes 2. Parietal, Temporal Lobes 3. Occipital Lobes 4. Midbrain — III. Cerebellum, Pons — IV. Spinal Cord — V. Medulla Oblongata

I. Transformation of Energy

A passage from the *Nei Jing* exclaims:

How marvelous is the brain! It transforms images and sounds into thought, speech and movements.

The same can be said of the cerebellum, medulla and spinal cord. In this regard, we now know the role of the nervous centers and their special regions for transforming information into speech, movement, warmth or cold, etc.

The nervous centers are thus transformers of energy. This happens in four phases:

1) Perception of the stimulus (images, sounds, touched shapes, heat, cold, smells).

2) Transformation of these stimuli into thoughts and feelings.

3) Transformation of these thoughts and feelings into forms or immaterial waves (speech, looks, psychological or physical waves).

4) Transformation of the energy into material forms: movements, heat, electricity, etc.

The nervous centers are also accumulators. Professor Cazamalli states:

The fact is that each cerebral center is an accumulator of energy. This allows it to remain inactive until the energy has reached a certain threshold of tension; only then is it activated, simply holding the flow which continues to abound.

One should keep in mind that all the command points elicit a response in a part of the brain and the nervous centers.

The necessary energy comes from the source points described in the preceding chapters. The quality of the blood is another important factor with regard to the energy. Two thirds of this energy comes from sugar, and as the nervous centers cannot make or store reserves of sugar as the muscles can, they constantly depend on a proper supply carried by the blood.

This explains the importance of the spleen-pancreas meridian for cerebral functions, emphasized in the Far East since antiquity. The influence of the heart and circulation, of course, were also recognized as important.

The necessity of sugar for the very life of the nervous centers is highlighted in recent writings on physiology. R.J. Main states:

The cells of the brain, especially of the cortex, depend heavily on this constant supply of glucose since they do not stock appreciable quantities of glycogen like other cells, muscle, liver, etc. Hypoglycemia first affects brain cells with cerebral constraint . . . then it causes unconsciousness.

Let us add that this lack of higher awareness (also caused from an excess of insulin) manifests through violent language or gestures before reaching the comatose stage. Dispersing the spleen-pancreas returns things to order.

The hyperglycemic symptoms of diabetes mellitus are well known: excessive diuresis, dehydration, thinness, signs of intoxication, and cerebral depression. For this condition tonify the spleen-pancreas and disperse the adrenals. A hormone of the latter causes the release of sugar through the breakdown of albumins (neoglycogenase).

The degree of function for the different parts of each nervous center was deduced by the ancients through measurement at the pulses. In the West this was done only a short time ago from the observation of symptoms. The important discovery of their multiple pulses allows us to now perceive every change in the function of each of these parts.

The pulse involved is on the right wrist, segment IV. Each side of the artery reflects the intensity of energy of one lateral half of the center under consideration: the radial side reflects the left aspect of a nervous center; the medial side, the right aspect.

1) Superficial level: spinal cord and medulla. In our judgement, a sensitive hand can detect more than just the condition of the lateral sides of these nerve centers. The lower part of the pulse corresponds to the inferior third of the spinal cord and vertebral column (including sacrum) when the vertebrae, the cord or the nerves of the ''horse's tail'' (cauda equina) are appreciably disordered. The middle part of the pulse relates to the middle part of the cord and column, the upper part to the superior third of the cord and column. The very top portion of this pulse corresponds to the medulla.

2) Middle level. Lower part: cerebellum. Upper part: pons.

3) Deep level: brain. Lower quarter: anterior lobes. Lower middle quarter: temporal and parietal lobes. Upper middle quarter: central lobes. Upper quarter: posterior lobes. (See Part III, Chapter IV).

II. The Brain

Recent operations on the cerebral lobes have greatly elucidated the diverse functions of the brain and the purely physiological, analogous effects obtained on these functions through acupuncture.

From the results obtained above we can make preliminary remarks regarding the brain and the other nervous centers: the pulse and points of one side always act on the nervous centers of the opposite lateral side. Conversely, for the body they act on the ipsilateral part of the body, except the points *hegu* (LI-4) and *houxi* (SI-3), which act contralaterally. These latter actions have not been explained.

Acupuncture can act specifically on different parts of the brain: the anterior frontal lobes, posterior frontal lobes, the parietal and temporal lobes together, midbrain (thalamus and hypothalamus), inferior occipital lobes and superior occipital lobes.

Over many years of observation, I have confirmed that the pulse of the brain as a whole is on the right wrist, section IV, deep level. The radial side corresponds to the left hemisphere; the medial side, to the right hemisphere.

The strongest points on the brain as a whole are the following:

Xinhui (GV-21, IS GV-22) and *baihui* (GV-19, IS GV-20), both consisting of bilateral points separated by a small medial rise on the top of the skull. These bilateral points have contralateral effects. *Shanglian* (LI-9) is also involved.

There is a generally held opinion that the cells of the brain and nervous system no longer multiply after the birth of the child. They disappear and are replaced by neuroglias. The objection has been given that the brain of the child at birth is hardly a third of that of the adult. If the cells of the adult do not triple in number, would the volume triple? Furthermore, if they do not reduplicate, how are lesions repaired? In some cases of hemiplegia, where encephalogram readings showed an apparently irreversible and definitive lesion, the lesion or at least the functional trouble totally disappeared after many months of acupuncture (Dr. Féraud of Marseille).

Frontal (anterior and posterior frontal lobes).

In phrenology, a very prominent frontal bone extending up to the middle of the top of the skull was always correlated with a reflective type of person, conscientious to the point of scrupulousness. A small frontal bone was thought to be found in unreflective people, those who were impulsive, only slightly conscientious, and without great scruples.

In our research, we have found that the points acting on the anterior frontal lobes act also on the posterior frontal lobes, but more weakly. The inverse is also true.

Anterior frontal lobes. Region of the frontal eminence. In the West this region is considered the seat of the most important mental functions. Brain surgery confirms the ancient Chinese observations on the effects of the points and their modification of the pulses.

The pulse of the anterior frontal lobes, which an attentive hand can differentiate from its neighbors, is the distal, lower part of the inferior quarter of the right wrist, section IV, deep level.

In the West (Main, 196), insufficiency of the frontal lobes is accompanied by lack of imagination, social sense, tact, emotional control, perceptive correlations and foresight. After surgery (Houdart, 7-8; Bertagna, 32; Main), there is decreased intelligence, a lack of feeling for the future, indifference to conventions, a feeling of being worry free, loquacity, expansiveness, a tendency to easy playing on words and euphoria. This can lead to mental confusion, physical laziness and apathy. (The posterior frontal lobes act mostly on motor functions.)

Those familiar with the theory underlying acupuncture will note that insufficiency in this area of the brain is manifested by a lack of moral consciousness. (Recall that when moral consciousness is failing or has not developed one cannot distinguish good from bad; the consequences of one's actions are not considered, only the satisfaction of one's impulses.) Additionally, there is lack of foresight and comprehension, especially of connections between notions and images, and of synthesis whereby known ideas are superimposed and mathematical and life problems solved. There is also a tendency toward suggestibility: one accepts everything without making connections to other ideas. This insufficiency is also accompanied by lack of imagination (one fails to see complex images and movements, only perceiving the words and the state); a lack of reason, judgement, attention, concentration and, in fact, intelligence (*interligere:* to connect that which is remembered, to understand, to take together). Also, on the physical plane, there is laziness, morning fatigue and insomnia in the evening.

The effects of the command points and of surgery are the same.

In the West, excess of the frontal lobes is linked to states of agitated, anxious and inveterate depression, and even psychosis. The mind is troubled by an excess of scruples (Bertagna, 15). In Chinese medical theory, this excess manifests in flurries of unpleasant images and thoughts, in excessive worries and anxiety, and in obsessions causing nightmares and incessant dreams.

The points acting on the anterior frontal lobes are:

1)   Insufficiency: tonify *dadu* (SP-2); *taibai* (SP-3); herald point of the spleen *zhangmen* (LR-13); *shaochong* (HT-9); *shenting* (GV-23, IS GV-24); *fenglong* (ST-40); and arm-*qimen* (PC-4).

2)   Excess: disperse foot-*shangqiu* (SP-5); *taibai* (SP-3); and *shenting* (GV-23, IS GV-24).

Posterior frontal lobes. These are a poorly defined band just anterior to the fissure of Rolando at the level of the posterior part of the frontal bone, descending on each side down to the temporal lobe. They regulate tone and motor functions, gross movement of the large muscle groups, and coordination of fine movement (Main, 194).

In the West, insufficiency of the posterior frontal lobes is thought to result in weakness, even flaccidity of the contralateral part of the body, and diminished coordination of automatic movements and fine motor control. (Insufficiency of the pallidum of the corpus striatum results in rigidity.)

 ⱴ A lesion can cause contralateral hemiplegia, spasms, exaggerated tendon reflexes, contracture of the hand, and later, weakness with disability in gross movement and problems with locomotion (Main, 192; Houdart, 4).

The above symptoms are often accompanied by extreme weakness of the pulse of the posterior frontal lobes. In cases of diminished cerebrovascular circulation due to arterial spasm or shock without functional destruction, these symptoms can show improvement or be suppressed if acupuncture is used from the first day of the stroke. Even where lesions are involved, there may be partial, progressive return of motor control after many months of acupuncture treatment, with encephalographic readings confirming the disappearance of the lesion.

Excess of the posterior frontal lobes is described in the West as follows (Main, 191): electrical stimulation causes slight movements of the hands and feet on the contralateral side. It also results in perspiration, stronger respiration and defecation (functions which, however, have their centers in the medulla). The latter results explain the immediate perspiration of the palms (stopped by dispersing the parasympathetic system) and the hypertension and hyperventilation resulting from exercise.

Physical strength in Western medicine is not recognized as depending on the posterior frontal lobes, even though this area commands the tone of gross movement. With acupuncture, it is possible to increase physical strength by about 25 to 30 percent using one of the following three points:

Yanglingquan (GB-34), which acts on the vitality and strength of all the muscles and on the cerebellum and posterior frontal lobes; *shanglian* (LI-9), which acts primarily on the strength of the hands (the flexors) and the contralateral brain as a whole; and *qihai* (CV-6), which augments the strength of all the muscles but clearly less than the preceding two.

The points acting on the posterior frontal lobes:

Yanglingquan (GB-34): posterior frontal lobes and cerebellum.

Wushu (GB-27): posterior frontal lobes, medulla and spinal cord.

Tianzhu (BL-10): posterior frontal lobes, midbrain and parasympathetic system.

Fengchi (GB-20): posterior frontal lobes, midbrain and sympathetic system.

Neiguan (PC-6): frontal, temporal, and parietal lobes.

Parietal and temporal lobes.

In our view, it appears that the ancient observations on what was called the "lateral brain" refer, in fact, to the parietal and temporal lobes taken together. These areas of the brain together have a single pulse and always respond simultaneously to stimulation of their command points. It was only out of prudence that I mentioned just the parietal lobes in my earliest experiments.

Indeed, the interdependence of the parietal and temporal lobes is clear: how would the temporal lobe and the sense organs function without the parietal lobe and the sensitivity of perceptions? What would be the use of this sensitivity without the parietal lobe if it did not animate the temporal lobe and the organs of sense?

The pulse, which we believe to have discovered a few years ago, is at the right wrist, section IV, deep level, inferior middle quarter. The radial side of the artery is linked to the left lobes (present memory, language, the parrot). The medial side is linked to the right lobes (hereditary memory, hereditary talents, the automaton).

Past observations in China have confirmed that the right and left lobes of the "lateral brain" are clearly different and that the two parietal lobes are different in size (the displaced median suture) with a dominance of the left or right.

The left lobes are the site of the conscious, present memory and the subconscious memory, which can be evoked with effort. Western physiologists recognize the predominance of the left lobes for language and sensory functions, both physical (vision, etc.) and psychological (understanding perceptions and memories of visual, auditory, olfactory and taste experiences).

The right lobes are the site of the totally unconscious memory and hereditary talents. Hereditary tendencies, qualities and defects are transmitted here. Young hunting dogs which hunt before any training display this sort of innate talent.

The roles described above for the right lobes are not yet taught in Western physiology. Experimentation to date only reveals a very marked difference of intensity between the right and left temporal lobes (the right lobe, considered "dumb," is weaker and less important for language). Differences between the right and left parietal lobes have not yet been noted.

Here as always it appears that the Chinese have focused on clinically observable manifestations, with little concern for what is not expressed exteriorly (and therefore difficult to know exactly). Through careful observation, Chinese medical researchers have identified the differences between the present memory of the parrot (at the left "lateral brain") and the unconscious memory of the automaton (on the right). (The latter causes action before thinking.)

For convenience, we will examine separately Western knowledge of the parietal and temporal lobes.

Parietal lobes. Covered over by the two parietal bones, these lobes form a band just on the posterior edges of the fissure of Rolando. The parts of the body whose sensations are transmitted there are represented with the feet at the top and the head near the temporal lobes. The impulses are transmitted to the parietal lobe through the mediation of the midbrain (thalamus) (Main, 193).

Insufficiency of the parietal lobes is poorly studied in the West. A slight lesion does not produce anesthesia nor does it greatly alter the superficial sensitivity. It does, however, affect the recognition of shapes, qualities, types, etc. of the deep sensitivity, mostly that of prominence. A posterior lesion can impair the contralateral awareness of the body (Houdart, 5). A lesion can produce epilepsy preceded by a feeling of cold or of prickling (see Excess of the Thalamus). In children it can provoke growth retardation of the part of the body corresponding to the lesion, such as the hand (Main, 193).

Excess of the parietal lobes by electrical stimulation produces vague sensations of stinging as with a lesion (Houdart, 5), numbness, movement or pressure on the contralateral part of the body. Using strychnine on a small area of the parietal lobe provokes hypersensitivity to pressure at the corresponding part of the body (Main, 193).

Temporal lobes. Experimentation in the West has demonstrated that the two temporal lobes do not have the exact same function or importance. The left lobe in right-handed people, or the right lobe in left-handed people, acts in a dominant manner on speech. The opposite lobe remains a "silent region" (Houdart, 6; Main, 194-5).

Chinese medical scholars have noted similar differences. They claim, however, that the left lobe determines conscious, present and subconscious memory (speech, visual, auditory), while the right lobe determines the memory of hereditary talents, tendencies and knowledge and is thus absolutely unconscious.

The difference between the two definitions lies mostly in the fact that the West describes the body in an analytical sense whereas the Orient uses synthetic description.

Western researchers are now beginning to distinguish special centers in the temporal lobes:

Smell-taste. ''What appears to be a taste is in reality a smell.'' (Main 195) This center is located in the upper part of the anterior temporal lobe and the lower and posterior part of the anterior frontal lobe, with support in the medulla, the uncus and the hippocampus around the corpus callosum. The olfactory nerves, in fact, pass through the anterior perforated substance to the medulla, then to the cortex.

Two areas have been differentiated: 1) primary or material, for the perception itself; 2) cognitive, for discrimination and memory of odors and tastes, their relations, etc. (considered by the Chinese as conscious memory).

Insufficiency from a lesion may either inhibit the sensation of odors and tastes or provoke hallucinations of the same (Main, 195). Excess by electrical stimulation produces the perception of unpleasant odors (Main, *idem.*) or provokes smell-taste crises (Houdart, 5).

The pulse is at the left wrist, section V, deep level.

Certain points clearly act on smell and therefore taste:

Yingxiang (LI-20) responds in the contralateral smell-taste area.

Hegu (LI-4) responds in the temporoparietal lobe.

Fengchi (GB-20) responds in several areas: vegetative, sympathetic, and posterior hypothalamus.

Baihui (GV-19, IS GV-20) and *shangxing* (GV-23) act on the temporal, parietal and occipital lobes.

Hearing. Two areas: 1) primary, or physical: the perception of sounds. Located in the superior temporal lobe on the superior edge of the first convolution entering the fissure of Sylvius; 2) cognitive: distinctions and relationships of sounds, and auditory memory. Located under and around the preceding area described. The left temporal lobe is almost always dominant for these two centers.

Insufficiency (Main, 194) can hinder sound recognition and the ability to distinguish specific sounds from a group of sounds. Removal of the non-dominant right side blocks speech but does not cause deafness. A tumor can produce buzzings, tinglings or auditory hallucinations.

Excess caused by electrical stimulation can produce the sensation of rumbling and buzzing noises in the head. It can also make the head and eyes turn and cause vertigo (the vestibule of the ear is hence represented there: Main, 194).

The pulse is at the left wrist, section V, middle level.

Points that act on hearing: *ermen* (TW-23, IS TW-21), *tinghui* (GB-2) and *tinggong* (SI-19). All three have a response in the hearing center.

Language, speech: The most important center (and dominant in right-handed people) is in the left temporal lobe. It is located along the entire length of the first convolution and the superior edge of the fissure of Sylvius. It is inferior, anterior and posterior to the auditory center, behind the olfactory center, and above the visual center on the edge of the occipital lobe. Hence, it is linked to all the sense organs and depends on them for the recall of object names.

Distinguishable areas: 1) A motor area in the posterior frontal lobe coordinating muscular movements necessary for speech. If insufficient or injured, it becomes impossible or very difficult to pronounce familiar words and to coordinate sounds. 2) A primary auditory area for the hearing of sounds and a cognitive area to understand and keep them in memory. 3) A region of visual memory, necessary for learning a language or written words. If insufficient or injured on the dominant side, there is memory loss for names of objects or persons.

A lesion on the non-dominant side causes explosive, emphatic speech (Main, 195-6) and perhaps stuttering.

Influential points are as follows: *yamen* (GV-14, IS GV-15). Those acting on the contralateral hemisphere: *shanglian* (LI-9) and *shenmai* (BL-62). For further points see temporal-parietal lobes below.

Temporal-parietal lobes in acupuncture. Traditional Asian observation and our recent discoveries have demonstrated that for the sensation, action and response to points and pulses, the temporal and parietal lobes form an inseparable combination.

The pulse located at the right wrist, section IV, deep level, second inferior quarter equally reproduces aspects of one or the other lobes without distinction.

Points acting only on one and not the other have yet to be found.

Acupoints acting on the temporal-parietal lobes also act on neighboring parts of the brain vital to the functioning of the sense organs. Examples of such points are *shaohai* (HT-3), *neiguan* (PC-6), *shanglian* (LI-9) and *xinhui* (GV-21, IS GV-22).

Certain points act more specifically on certain centers:

Odor-taste: *yingxiang* (LI-20), *baihui* (GV-19, IS GV-20). Pulse position: left wrist, section V, deep level. Hearing: *ermen* (TW-23, IS TW-21), *tinghui* (GB-2), *tinggong* (SI-19). Pulse position: left wrist, section V, middle level. Language-speech: *yamen* (GV-14, IS GV-15). Also, the points acting on the contralateral half of the brain: *xinhui* (GV-21, IS GV-22), *baihui* (GV-19, IS GV-20), *jiuwei* (CV-15), *taodao* (GV-13). The special pulse is still unknown. Parietal, temporal and occipital lobes: *jianshi* (PC-5).

Occipital lobes.

In Western thought, the occipital lobes are involved entirely with vision. For acupuncture, two regions respond to different points: 1) the superior part, which controls primitive instincts, the primate; 2) the part that acts on vision.

The size of the occipital lobe is proportional to the primitive instincts.

The pulse of the primate is on the left wrist, section IV, deep level (contralaterally). The pulse relating to vision is the left wrist, section V, superficial level.

For the West, the occipital lobes relate only to visual sensations (Houdart, 6; Main, 193). The optic fibers from the eyes cross at right angles at the chiasm and pass into the thalamus. From there, fibers connect into the occipital lobes. Thus the right occipital lobe receives its impulses from the right side of the two retinas (left visual field). The left lobe receives its impulses from the left side of the two retinas (right visual field) (Main, 193). The different areas of the retina are precisely located: a limited lesion of a point on the occipital lobe causes problems in the corresponding visual area. These are kept in memory. The region of primary vision is in the inferior-posterior part of the occipital lobe.

In acupuncture, the primary and cognitive regions of vision in the inferior occipital lobe are elements of the conscious and present memory.

Insufficiency of the occipital lobes: In the West, a lesion in one lobe causes hemianopia of the contralateral visual field in both eyes. A lesion in both lobes produces complete blindness, but does not act on the pupillary response (Main, 193). A lesion in the cognitive region does not cause blindness, but prevents the correct recognition of objects, distances or shapes and can even cause visual hallucinations and the inability to read (alexia). (Main, 194) Problems within the cortex of primary vision impairs the recognition of shape, color and contrast.

Excess of the occipital lobes has not yet been discussed in the Western works consulted.

In acupuncture, the points which act on the primitive instincts (the primate) also act on vision. However, it is possible to distinguish the following:

Active points:

Superior occipital lobe (primate): *shangjuxu* (ST-37); in the cerebellum, the pons: *jiuwei* (CV-15), *zhongfeng* (LR-4) and *yinlingquan* (SP-9).

Inferior occipital lobes: head-*wangu* (GB-17, IS GB-12), *tongziliao* (GB-1), *jingming* (BL-1) and *zanzhu* (BL-2).

Inferior occipital lobe and parietal, temporal and central lobes: *neiguan* (PC-6).

Temporal parietal and occipital lobes: *jianshi* (PC-5).

Midbrain (thalamus, hypothalamus, corpus striatum).

Traditional Chinese texts do not give any indications for points acting on the midbrain; however, extensive observation has allowed us to substantiate the responses and actions of certain points on this area.

Although the midbrain is composed of three parts having distinct functions, it has only been possible to recognize a single pulse: right wrist, section IV, deep level, upper quarter, contralateral side.

Some command points act on the midbrain as a whole. It has not yet been possible to differentiate effects on each part other than by function.

Thalamus. Two separate bodies separated by the third ventricle (the hypothalamus); anterior part connected to the cortex; posterior part (and external geniculate body) relays the optic fibers. Internal part (cupuliform body) linked to the corpus striatum, hypothalamus and anterior frontal lobes; external part linked to the ascending parietal.

The thalamus relays motor impulses from the cerebellum, medulla, and spinal cord to the cortex of the posterior and anterior frontal lobes. In so doing it plays a vital role in the coordination of movements and maintaining muscle tone. In addition, fibers from the thalamus pass into the pons and coordinate the motor signs of emotion, laughing and crying (Main, 197-8).

Its insufficiency or lesion produces intense pains (Main, 198). A lesion causes spontaneous pains, pains from cold, emotions, or from any sensation whatever. It can produce a diminished superficial sensitivity with problems of deep sensitivity (Main, 198; Houdart, 11).

Its excess from electrical stimulation makes the head or the body turn or the head move up or down (see Corpus Striatum below). Strong stimulation of the anterior-medial part (linked to the cortex and the corpus striatum) may cause a petit mal seizure or absent-mindedness (insufficiency of the parietal lobe). Very strong stimulation causes convulsions.

In acupuncture one pulse registers the entire midbrain: right wrist, section IV, upper quarter.

Some points, particularly of the urinary bladder, but also of the triple warmer, heart, and spleen-pancreas act on separate functions of the thalamus and have responses in its different parts.

Pain (response in the thalamus): *kunlun* (BL-60) for all physical or emotional pain; *tianjing* (TW-10) for pain from emotions, nervousness, or cold; foot-*shangqiu* (SP-5) for pains of the bones and periostitis (this point also acts on the bone marrow).

Epileptoid troubles, mental absence (and petit mal?) — response in the anterior thalamus: *jinmen* (BL-63), *shugu* (BL-65), *tonggu* (BL-66) and *shaohai* (HT-3).

Convulsions, spasms: *kunlun* (BL-60), *jinmen* (BL-63) and *yintang* (extra point between the eyes).

Hypothalamus (nucleus particularly related to the vegetative life); also called the floor of the third ventricle. Situated between the two thalami; controls the vegetative, autonomic functions (Main, 200); the affective life, the sexual functions, depressions or psychological hyperexcitation; the metabolism of the carbohydrates, fats, water; the regulation of heat through respiration; vasoconstriction and vasodilation (Houdart, 12-13).

The anterior part contains: the vagal center (parasympathetic, which stimulates all the secretions and contractions of the digestive tract); a center of hunger, which if disturbed can cause excessive gorging or bulimia; a center of response to insulin, with urination from insufficiency of insulin and hypoglycemia from excess; a center of cardiac inhibition, producing bradycardia if disturbed. In acupuncture one should act on all the yin organs.

The posterior part contains: the center for the sympathetic system (which slows movements and secretions of the digestive tract and accelerates the heart and arteries); hyperglycemia, center of heat, of fat, of olfaction (Main, 202). In acupuncture one should act on all the yang organs.

One must maintain an equilibrium within the autonomic system since to inhibit the parasympathetic leaves the sympathetic system dominant and vice versa.

Excess from electrical stimulation of the two parts of the hypothalamus produces: 1) hypertension from vasoconstriction caused by an excess of the parasympathetic system; 2) erection of the body hair, protrusion of the eyes, accelerated respiration — excesses of the sympathetic system (Houdart, 13).

Insufficiencies are not mentioned in the Western works consulted.

In acupuncture, the pulse of the midbrain corresponds to the hypothalamus (right wrist, section IV, deep level, medial upper quarter). Through the pulses it is possible to evaluate separately the intensity of energy in the parasympathetic or sympathetic systems. The parasympathetic system is represented at the pulse of the conception vessel (left wrist, section I) and also by all the superficial pulses and pulses of the vessels. The sympathetic system is represented at the pulse of the governor vessel (right wrist, section I) and also by all the deep pulses and that of the triple warmer.

The point that acts on the parasympathetic, *tianzhu* (BL-10), awakens a response in the anterior hypothalamus.

In cold (tonify) or heat (disperse): *shenmai* (BL-62), which responds to the central, posterior brain. Also *zhaohai* (KI-3, KI-6), which responds to the central anterior brain (but in cold disperse and in heat tonify).

Corpus striatum (motor control) or striopallidum, lenticular nucleus. Composed of the corpus striatum, caudal nucleus, putamen, pallidum. It seems to control involuntary movements through inhibition of impulses. Its pulse is that of the thalamus and hypothalamus of the midbrain: right wrist, section IV, deep level, superior medial quarter. It receives impulses from the cortex of the anterior and posterior frontal lobes and thalamus.

Insufficiency: a lesion in this area produces shaking or St. Vitus Dance (see Excess of Thalamus). Lesions of the pallidum cause hypertonia with weakness and trembling (as in Parkinson's disease). Lesions of the corpus striatum and the pallidum cause Wilson's disease (rigidity, trembling, shaking, uncoordinated movements, dysarthria) (Houdart, 10). Rigidity from lesion of the striopallidum is a characteristic of extrapyramidal lesions; this is in contrast to the flaccidity of pyramidal lesions (Main, 197).

Lesion produces rigidity and trembling at rest due to loss of the inhibitor control. Resection also produces rigidity and trembling at rest. Resection of the frontal anterior lobe relieves the tremblings of athetosis. Paralytic tremors have been relieved through extirpation of either the posterior or anterior frontal lobes (Main, 197).

Excess: The effects of electrical stimulation are not discussed in the works consulted. This kind of stimulus would logically inhibit tonus, as well as involuntary and even voluntary movements.

In acupuncture, experimentation is not extensive enough to be conclusive. However, from the data collected thus far it is possible to suggest that in the case of trembling at rest (Parkinsonism), one must tonify the following points:

Those acting on the midbrain as a whole: *tianzhu* (BL-10), *fengchi* (GB-20), *jinmen* (BL-63), *yintang* (M-HN-3) and *kunlun* (BL-60).

The anterior frontal lobes (with dispersing method): *dadu* (SP-2) and foot-*shangqiu* (SP-5).

The posterior frontal lobes: *yanglingquan* (GB-34).

The entire brain: *shanglian* (LI-9).

III. Cerebellum and Pons

In Western physiology the cerebellum and pons command equilibrium and the coordination and timing of movements.

Insufficiency: Spasms of the throat, internal organs or muscles of the back. A lesion on one side causes a wavering, stumbling walk; hypotonia or asthenia on one side; astasia; incoordination of the eyes; an explosive, jerky voice; awkward movements with trembling; and difficulty with alternative movements. A small lesion has more serious effects than a large one. Movements which are impossible when standing are possible while lying down.

Excess: Causes excessive rotation of the body, head and eyes toward one side. An excess of the anterior part causes the eyes and head to raise upward; that of the posterior part causes the eyes and head to move downward; and that of the lateral part produces excessive rotation of the eyes and head to one side as well as contraction of one pupil (miosis) on the excessive side, then nystagmus.

The pulse that I believe I have located for the cerebellum and pons (right wrist, section IV, middle level) allows one to measure the intensity of the energy in each of their parts. The medial side of the artery responds to the right part of the cerebellum and the right side of the pons. The radial side of the artery responds to the left part of the cerebellum and the left half of the pons. The lower part responds to the cerebellum, the upper part to the pons.

Chinese and Japanese observations and experimentation have not been as elucidating for this area of the brain as for the others.

Our own studies of acupuncture and the pulses have given us an idea of the modifications produced through dispersal or tonification. These effects, which I am probably the first to discover, operate through command points especially on one particular side of the cerebellum or pons.

The results obtained on the cerebellum relate particularly to the coordination of movements, equilibrium and muscular tone. The results on the pons are less clear; primarily it appears that nervous transmission is improved.

The gallbladder meridian seems to have a greater effect on the cerebellum and the posterior frontal lobes, especially through *yanglingquan* (GB-34) and *xiyangguan* (GB-33).

For the pons (and the medulla) the gallbladder is the master, particularly through *xuanzhong* (GB-39).

These command points of the cerebellum and medulla have arrested neuralgic pain in the sequelae to poliomyelitis. These points have also induced redevelopment of the muscles and the affected limb, rapidly in cases of recent onset. In chronic cases, some children have been able to reach their full growth without any trace of the illness. Very chronic cases show only an amelioration of the general state and of the muscles.

IV. Spinal Cord

In the Orient it is possible to act on the spinal cord through all the points of the governor vessel (posterior median line). Additionally, all the points of the governor vessel awaken a response in the meridian and pulse of the small intestine, and the small intestine possesses a marked action on the spinal cord.

I have discovered pulses independently reflecting the function of the spinal cord and governor vessel. Evaluation of modifications related to spinal cord function and verification of the relation between the spinal cord, governor vessel and small intestine has been possible through these pulses.

Spinal cord pulse: right wrist, section IV, superficial level (also reflects the medulla at the superior extremity). Along this pulse it is possible to determine the location of the problem on the spinal cord, i.e., in the upper, middle or lower section. Comparing the spinal cord pulse with that of the governor vessel (right wrist, section I) gives verification of whether or not the energy of the governor vessel is involved. The pulse of the spinal cord indicates where on the dorsal spine the circulation is blocked; vertebral displacements can be diagnosed thus.

From the perusal of age-old observations, we now know all the effects of the governor vessel points at each vertebra and their action at each level of the spinal cord. The understanding of these effects is much more exact and in-depth than those noted by the relatively modern science of chiropractic, although the latter also claims to affect the organs via the vertebrae.

In the West, it is taught that motor and sensory functions depend on the spinal cord and that the nerves at each vertebra command particular organs and certain functions of these organs.

The Orient teaches that the governor vessel brings energy to the nervous centers by acting on the circulation of the spinal cord.

The study of the spinal cord and the effects of acupuncture on its functions have been greatly illuminated by comparison of Eastern and Western teachings and the knowledge of the command points and pulses. However, many questions remain unanswered — experimentation is still greatly limited because of inadequate instrumentation.

Points that affect the spinal cord (see governor vessel, posterior median line):

Spinal cord and medulla: *yinshi* (ST-33).

Small intestine: *houxi* (SI-3), and additionally *fuliu* (KI-7).

V. Medulla Oblongata

The pulse of the medulla, which I believe I have discovered, is felt as a small head at the upper extremity of the spinal cord pulse — right wrist, section IV, superficial level. The radial side of the artery reflects the left lobe; the medial side, right lobe.

In European texts, the following functions are given under the control of various centers within the medulla oblongata:

Vasoconstriction — If insufficient: slow heart, relaxed arteries. The center for vasoconstriction is located on the medial edge of the medulla oblongata (a discovery made at the University of Minnesota Medical School in 1948).

Swallowing, sucking, salivation (see also Hypothalamus).

Vomiting — this center acts on the phrenic nerve and the contractor nerves of the abdominal and diaphragm muscles, the sympathetic dilators of the esophagus and on the cardiac sphincter and salivary glands. Insufficiency leads to the inability to vomit, while excess produces violent vomiting.

Hyperglycemia (see Pancreas).

Defecation (see Large Intestine).

Respiration — at the center of the medulla (Minnesota University Medical School, *N.Y. Times,* July 17, 1948). This center also acts on the voice. If insufficient, one is too weak to breathe (as in poliomyelitis). If excessive, the thorax is contracted.

Movements of the eyes and eyelids — acts on the ipsilateral common ocular motor nerve and contralateral external ocular nerve and facial nerve. If in excess, there is blinking of the eyelids and nystagmus.

In general, if the medulla oblongata is insufficient, the heart and vessels are lax. One cannot suck, swallow, vomit, or breathe deeply. The chest is without strength or paralyzed. There is profuse saliva. The eyes and eyelids move slowly, weakly or the lids remain closed. One has a tendency toward hypoglycemia, and defecation is difficult.

If the medulla is in excess, the heart, vessels and thorax are contracted and there is spasmodic swallowing and frequent sucking. Salivation is reduced and respiration difficult. Eye movements are rapid and the eyes remain wide open possibly with nystagmic involuntary movements (see Cerebellum). There may be a tendency toward hyperglycemia. Defecation is too easy.

Points — medulla: *qiangjian* (GV-17, IS GV-18), *zhangmen* (LR-13), *lieque* (LU-7) and *shenmen* (HT-7). Medulla, cerebellum, protuberance: *hegu* (LI-4). Medulla and spinal cord: *yinshi* (ST-33).

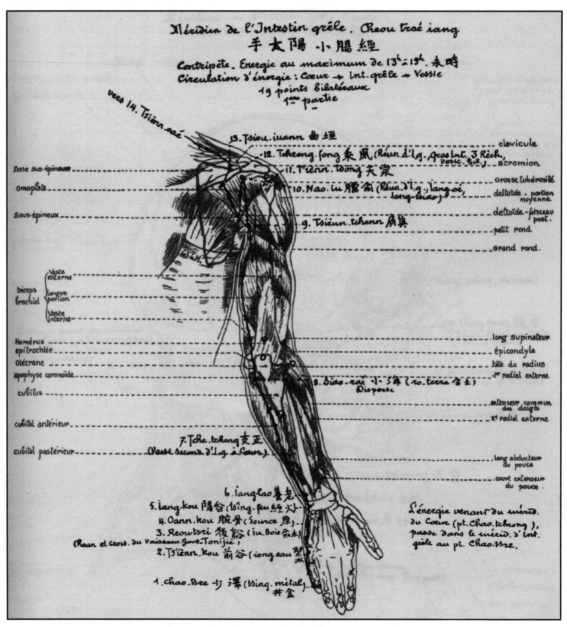

Meridian of the small intestine (part 1) (GSDM)

Chapter VI

The Distribution of Energy (I)

The Liver and Vitamins

I. The Liver — II. Vitamins — III. Varieties of Vitamins

I. The Liver

Among the some thirty-five known functions of the liver, Western physiologists have studied and classified only the physical or chemical ones: bile formation, glycogen formation, antitoxic action, iron metabolism, etc. The discovery of vitamins made it necessary for a new role to be ascribed to the liver, this time energetic.

The role of the liver in vitamin metabolism appears to be threefold:

1) *Formation:* until recently, it was believed that only vitamin A was formed in the liver (from the precursor carotene). Now, however, it is suspected that other vitamins are also formed in the liver.

2) *Storage:* all the vitamins are stored in the liver, those formed in the liver as well as those formed in other organs, particularly the large intestine. The liver of animals and cod liver oil contains them all (as does milk).

3) *Distribution:* the liver is in charge of the distribution of vitamins to the blood and thus to the whole body. The supply is determined by the needs of the moment and is often in homeopathic proportions (e.g., vitamin H at the hundred billionth concentration, corresponding to the fifth or sixth homeopathic dilution).

Hence, the liver must function with constant, absolute precision so that the transport of vitamins to the cells is carried out correctly. The infinitesimal quantities of each vitamin distributed rules out the idea of variable roles for them. Indeed, their importance is very great — the lack of vitamin C, for example, brings death from scurvy.

The liver also acts on energy by transforming certain hormones to less toxic forms. Thus it transforms testosterone into androsterone, estradone into estrone, etc. (Main).

There has been considerable research on the transformation of these stimulants of energy. This research will no doubt be facilitated by understanding the action of energy itself. In the Orient, nothing was known of endocrines or vitamins, and yet the liver was considered to have considerable importance in maintaining the vital energy.

Chinese medical theory places great emphasis on the liver's strong action on the sexual energy, and through this, the vitality and psyche. Indeed, it has been verified that by tonifying the liver, it is possible to correct testicular insufficiencies and insufficient erections; and by dispersing, to correct prolonged erections and inflammations of the testicles, epididymitis and prostatitis. In women, tonification of the liver can cure certain types of sterility, menorrhagia and metrorrhagia (vitamin K), excessive leukorrhea and prolonged metritis. Through dispersal of the liver, we can suppress pains of the lower pelvis and perineum, and treat insufficient or difficult menses (vitamin K). For both sexes, tonifying the liver relieves anxious melancholia, fear and depression with desire to die; using a dispersing method will moderate unhappiness, envy and jealousy.

In addition to the physical and chemical functions ascertained in the West, the Far East recognizes two nervous functions for the liver, one relating to sexual energy and the other to physical energy:

Spasms — general: *taichong* (LR-3); genital: *zhongfeng* (LR-4); those of the perineum: *yinbao* (LR-9).

Pruritus — pacified by tonification of *ligou* (LR-5), therefore caused by an insufficiency of the liver or an excess of the gallbladder.

Inflammations of the skin, swellings — swellings without edema generally disappear very quickly by tonifying *taichong* (LR-3).

Skin problems are always accompanied or caused by a serious insufficiency of the liver. They worsen at the spring equinox and during the hours of minimal energy in the liver, and disappear when the liver has recovered its entire strength and can evacuate all its toxins.

We should mention that the tonification point *ququan* (LR-8) on the left is more sensitive and effective in cases of biliary trouble; that on the right is more useful in cases of intoxication, of poisoning.

The relative insufficiency or excess of the liver is as follows:

Insufficiency	Excess
Liver distended, passive congestion.	Liver hard, painful, active congestion.
Poorly formed, pale yellow stools.	Brown stools, dark to black.
	Bile in the stomach. Vomiting of bile or cold, acidic water.
Atonic constipation.	Constipation with spasms and pains.
Diarrhea from weakness.	Diarrhea from inflammation with pain.
Anxious melancholia, fear.	Unhappiness, envy, jealousy.
Depression, desire to die.	Acute or chronic meningitis.
Spasms of the chest, asthma, bronchitis, pleurisy.	
Palpitations.	Sudden cardiac pains.
Profuse bleeding, slow coagulation. Varicosities, hemorrhoids, easy bruising.	
Intestinal spasms.	
Abundant, prolonged menses.	Insufficient menses.
	Prolonged erections.
Pruritus or genital swellings. Seminal loss, spasms of the vagina.	
Spasms of the genital apparatus.	
White vaginal discharge.	
Urine too abundant.	Insufficient urine with white foam.
Spasms of the gallbladder sphincter.	
Migraine of the right temple.	
Pain of the whole body.	
External spasms, convulsions, cramps.	
Illnesses of the skin, eczema, urticaria.	
Swellings, swollen face.	
Waxy complexion, pale.	Gray-yellow or ashen complexion.

Functions and interactions of the liver meridian are given below:

Any liver excess, active congestion, pain, vomiting of bile or cold, acidic water: *xingjian* (LR-2).

Fever from inflammation of the liver, jaundice with fever: *taichong* (LR-3).

Jaundice with cold and heaviness: *zhongfeng* (LR-4).

Pain at the liver and heart: *taichong* (LR-3).

Pale yellow stools: *ququan* (LR-8).

Atonic constipation: *ququan* (LR-8).

Spasmodic, painful constipation: *xingjian* (LR-2).

Diarrhea from weakness: *ququan* (LR-8); from inflammation: *xingjian* (LR-2).

Anxious melancholia, likes to be in bed, fear, deranged mind: *ligou* (LR-5).

Depression, wishes to die: *ququan* (LR-8).

Unhappiness, envy, jealousy: *xingjian* (LR-2).

Migraines of the right temple: *ququan* (LR-8).

Congestive headaches, bleeding of the nose: *dadun* (LR-1).

Superior occipital lobes, primate, cerebellum: *ligou* (LR-5).

Obstruction, occlusion or putrefaction in the intestine: *zhongdu* (LR-6).

Peritonitis: *zhongdu* (LR-6), *xingjian* (LR-2).

Cessation of functions: *taichong* (LR-3), *zhongfeng* (LR-4).

Intestinal spasms: *ligou* (LR-5).

All swellings (except edema): *taichong* (LR-3).

Edema of the whole body: *xingjian* (LR-2).

Spasms: *taichong* (LR-3), *dadun* (LR-1) and *xingjian* (LR-2).

Arterial and coronary spasms: *taichong* (LR-3), *ligou* (LR-5), *xingjian* (LR-2).

Varicosities, varicose ulcers: *taichong* (LR-3).

All troubles of the respiratory passages from toxins, autointoxication: *ququan* (LR-8), *taichong* (LR-3).

Respiratory spasms: *ligou* (LR-5).

Men:

Testicular insufficiency: *taichong* (LR-3).

Inflammation of the testicles or epididymis: *yangshi* (LR-12, IS *jimai*).

Prolonged, excessive erections: *ligou* (LR-5), *xingjian* (LR-2).

Prostatitis: *zhongfeng* (LR-4), *taichong* (LR-3).

Blennorrhagia: *zhongfeng* (LR-4).

Women:

Sterility; insufficient, difficult menses: *ligou* (LR-5).

Menses too abundant: *ququan* (LR-8).

Metrorrhagia after giving birth or miscarriage: *taichong* (LR-3).

Profuse leukorrhea: *ligou* (LR-5).

Persistent metritis: *zhongdu* (LR-6).

Spasms of the vagina: *zhongfeng* (LR-4), *xingjian* (LR-2).

Spasms of the genital apparatus: *ligou* (LR-5).

Contractions of the perineum: *yinbao* (LR-9).

Pains of the lower pelvis or of the genital apparatus: *taichong* (LR-3), *dadun* (LR-1).

General:

Hernia, violent pain of the abdomen and heart, flowing urine: *dadun* (LR-2).

Spasms at the neck of the urinary bladder: *ligou* (LR-5), *dadun* (LR-1).

All varieties of urethritis: *dadun* (LR-1).

Urine blocked by spasm at the neck of the bladder: *ligou* (LR-5); with pains in lumbar area: *yinbao* (LR-9), thigh-*wuli* (LR-10).

All problems of the skin, eczema, urticaria, psoriasis, impetigo: *ququan* (LR-8), *taichong* (LR-3).

Difficulty walking, weakness while walking: *taichong* (LR-3), *zhongfeng* (LR-4).

Shivering from cold: *zhongfeng* (LR-4).

Cold of the lower limbs: *ligou* (LR-5).

Icy feet: *zhongfeng* (LR-4), *taichong* (LR-3).

Pains of the whole body: *ququan* (LR-8).

Pains of the shoulder and hand: *taichong* (LR-3).

Pain of the obturator nerve: *yinbao* (LR-9).

Metatarsal-phalangial arthritis and pains at the five toes: *xingjian* (LR-2), *taichong* (LR-3).

Rheumatic problems aggravated by humidity: *zhongdu* (LR-6).

Articular rheumatism, particularly of the knee: *xiguan* (LR-7).

Contracture of the muscles of the back and lumbar region: *ligou* (LR-5).

Contracture of the psoas major: *yangshi* (LR-12, IS *jimai*).

All inflammation of the corners of the mouth: *taichong* (LR-3).

Heat of the sole of the foot: *zhongdu* (LR-6).

The meridian is on the anterior side of the tibia and the medial surface of the thigh; it finishes under the nipple. Its maximum is at 2:00 a.m. (from 1-3 a.m.), hour of the minimum of the small intestine; its minimum is at 2:00 p.m. (from 1-3 p.m.), hour of the maximum of the small intestine. The gallbladder is the mother and coupled meridian; the lungs, the son.

Tonification point: *ququan* (LR-8). Dispersal point: *xingjian* (LR-2). Source point: *taichong* (LR-3). Alarm point: *qimen* of the thorax (LR-14). Association point: *ganshu* (BL-18). Point of passage from gallbladder to liver: *ligou* (LR-5).

Pulse: left wrist, section II, middle level, radial side. We believe that we can distinguish the function of the anterior lobes and bile. Medial side: posterior lobes and antitoxin function.

Left branch: acts particularly on the bile; right branch: particularly antitoxin function.

The energy comes through a branch of the gallbladder (from *xiaxi,* GB-43). It passes into the lung meridian through a branch from *qimen* (LR-14) at *zhongfu* (LU-1).

The liver is at its lowest at the March equinox, and to a lesser degree at the September equinox.

II. The Vitamins

Since their recent discovery, researchers are finding a greater and greater role for vitamins in key bodily functions; the lack of just one of them can cause death.

All vitamins are stored in the liver and distributed from this organ in homeopathic quantities according to the body's needs. Through expert command of the vital energy, it is possible to maintain the liver at its maximum harmony.

In addition to storing vitamins, the liver manufactures one vitamin (vitamin A) and perhaps many others. Two of the most essential vitamins, K and B, are made in the large intestine, which depends on the liver for healthy functioning. Both these organ systems must be regulated for optimum vitamin metabolism.

That these vitamins act in infinitesimal quantities (H at a hundred billionth) precludes the notion of a purely chemical action and necessitates ascribing to them a primarily energetic action.

They are not extracted like nutrients from food, yet food is indispensable to their formation by the body — certain foods allow their formation better than others. Future studies will undoubtedly clarify the many complex questions surrounding vitamin research. Indeed, this field of study is relatively recent, dating from the early years of the twentieth century with the work of Eijkmann, Bunk, Javillier and Karrer.

But what are vitamins? It is difficult at present to find a better definition than that given in the *Traité de Biochimie Médicale* of Polonovski, Boulanger, Macheboeuf, Roche and Sannié:

> *In animals, there exists a series of compounds grouped under the name of biocatalyzers that are physiologically analogous though structurally very different. These compounds have the common quality of existing only at very low concentrations. This fact precludes the possibility of their having a plastic role comparable to that of proteins or glucosides or an energetic role analogous to substances such as glucosides or lipids. However, their importance is such that the absence of one of them almost always causes significant disorders in the function of an organ or of the entire body. Their absence can even lead to the cessation of all vital functions and the death of the organism . . .*

We must remain cognizant of the fact that for all vital elements — vitamins in particular — knowledge of only the chemical formula is seriously inadequate since it fails to take into consideration life itself. Even if everything was known about the structure of vitamins, their effect on human beings very much depends on the action-reaction relativity, that is, on the quantity and quality relative to need. The facts are that we know very little about the vitamins themselves, and the observed quantities are often infinitesimal. The quantities vary according to the needs and the reaction of each single individual at each observed moment; hence, we must consider that only the living organ charged with their distribution is capable of giving the necessary quantity and quality.

The liver, which is responsible for this distribution, stores vitamins and manufactures some of them. Other vitamins are produced in the large intestine. Can we not predict that future research will find that the liver and large intestine, by some vital act, transform elements in food into something absolutely unique for the given individual? This process may be likened to that of the small intestine and its action on albumin. The primary role of the liver and large intestine in the physiology of vital energy and conservation of life and youth would thus be further substantiated.

Clinically, it is possible to prevent vitamin deficiencies by acting on the command points of the liver and large intestine. This assures that the vitamins are distributed in constant and harmonious supply and that they are used most effectively. It is also important to eat foods containing the best elements for synthesis of vitamins. Certain foods, such as liver, cod liver oil, and milk, contain all the vitamins. Other foods are essential for the production of specific vitamins: carrots for vitamin A (for vitality); wheat germ for vitamin B (antineuralgic) and vitamin E (for genital function); citrus fruits for vitamin C (prevents scurvy; retards aging); cod-liver oil for vitamin D (irradiated cholesterol); spinach, cabbage and egg yolk for vitamin K (antihemorrhagic); egg yolk and yeast for vitamin H (prevents seborrhea) and vitamin L (promotes lactation); lemons and paprika for vitamin F.

III. The Assorted Vitamins

The recent successes with vitamin therapy have spurred an increase in vitamin research. A number of vitamins have been isolated and their particular effects identified. The many researchers who have written on this subject usually discuss which organ is most specifically responsible for the production, storage and distribution of each vitamin. To date, it appears that the liver and large intestine are most often cited.

The various names given to the vitamins often relate to the country or name of the researcher involved with their discovery. The abridged list that follows gives the role of each vitamin in the maintenance of the vital energy and possibly its production. Also given is the relative importance of the organs which produce, transform, store or distribute the vitamin in question.

1) *Vitamin A:* vitality or growth, antixerophthalmic (liposoluble).

Produced, stored and distributed by the liver.

The more useful foods are carrots, cod-liver oil, liver, fresh butter, milk, green salad, spinach, apricots, mulberries.

Vitamin A deficiency may cause growth retardation in the young. In the adult, signs of deficiency are dry skin and hair, sometimes with diarrhea; excess formation of tartar on the teeth; poor resistance against infection; hemeralopia (diminished vision in bright light); problems of the genitals to the point of impotence or sterility; allergic affections of the mucosa; or the tendency to stones. If serious, dryness of the conjunctiva and cornea can lead to the shrinkage of the eyes (xerophthalmia).

Toxicity from excess vitamin A has not been extensively studied. However, it is observed that with excess the skin thickens and takes on a fatty, damp quality and the hair is often greasy.

R.J. Main states that vitamin A is formed from carotene by the liver.

> The transformation of carotene into vitamin A is effected in the liver under the influence of carotenase, and it is in this organ that the reserves are formed. We thus understand how a hepatic insufficiency can be at the origin of a [vitamin A] deficiency. (Biochimie Médicale)

The daily requirement is from 1 to 2 mg.

2) *B Group:* (F, G, PP) antineuralgic, hair, skin.

This group is subdivided from year to year into increasing numbers, B1, B2, B12, up to B20 for certain researchers; each of these subdivisions has several names. They are considered antineuralgic, protect the skin, prevent pellagra, etc.

The B vitamin complex is naturally dependent on the large intestine. Assuring a regular and harmonious supply of the B vitamins is thus a question of regulating the energy of the large intestine and liver, which store and distribute them according to the needs of the moment.

For all individuals, the more useful foods for formation of B vitamins are, liver, milk, wheat germ; and for many people, fruits, tomatoes, nuts, egg yolks and pig kidneys may be included as source foods.

Signs of deficiency are pessimism, worry, melancholy, insomnia, emotive instability, nervous tension, "nerves just under the skin," muscular spasms, trembling, neuralgia, lack of appetite, emaciation, diarrhea, hypothermia, constipation, large abdomen, gas, excess menses, troubles with menopause with lack of calcium in the blood, perlèche, hemeralopia or graying, thinning hair.

Its excess is accompanied by agitation and heat (insufficiently studied).

The diverse varieties are as follows:

B1: Thiamin, or F. Necessary to the uninterrupted production of energy. (The Far East attributes the command of the energy to the large intestine, at *hegu*, LI-4.) Deficiency: constipation, digestive difficulties, gas, fatigue, nervousness, insomnia. Necessary food: wheat germ.

B2: Riboflavin, lactoflavin, or G. May prolong life. Important for the eyes; prevents cataract, hemeralopia (*hegu*, LI-4). Necessary foods: beef liver, wheat germ, milk.

B3: Niacin. Necessary for the skin, blood digestion. Necessary food: wheat germ, milk, brewer's yeast.

B4: Nicotinamide, Adenine. Assures fluid equilibrium. May help against alcoholism; prevents cancer.

B6: Trembling, nervous troubles.

B12: Used in association with folic acid with success against grave or pernicious anemia. Taken from liver (1 gram per 4 kilograms of liver).

B pantothenic acid: Acts against graying hair (canities). Point *weizhong* (BL-54, IS BL-40) has sometimes given good results. Liver, wheat germ, egg yolk.

B para-aminobenzoic acid (PABA): Also acts against canities (grayness or whiteness of the scalp hair). Liver, grain hulls.

B inositol: May help the growth of hair. Milk, fruits, nuts.

B (see vitamin H): Gives energy, conserves cerebral health. Liver, egg yolks, pork kidney, tomatoes.

B choline: Helps the liver and gallbladder to function and digest fats. Liver, brewer's yeast.

PP or nicotinic acid: Linked to the B complex. Antipellagra. Beef liver, salmon. Deficiency is indicated by lesions of the skin, mostly in the parts exposed to light (first erythema, then blisters, then ulceration). It can be accompanied by mental problems and anemia. It acts on human pellagra, which occurs mostly in areas where corn is a usual food.

3) *Vitamin C*, ascorbic acid: Anti-scurvy, bone development.

The considerable resemblance between the signs of scurvy and that of aging has been stressed:

> *This vitamin is found in abundance in the enamel of teeth, the adrenal cortex, the corpus luteum, and the ovaries, and reinforces their hormones. (Walter Eddy, The Vitamins)*

> *A close connection has been observed between the quantity of vitamin C in the body and susceptibility to infection and intoxication. Finally, it seems that ascorbic acid has a transporting role for hydrogen. (Biochimie Médicale)*

Thus, vitamin C is necessary against old age, infection, intoxication; for the solidity of teeth, good action of the adrenal hormones and female genitalia, and for bones (bone cells).

Its deficiency is marked by wrinkled skin, bleeding gums, loose teeth, easy bleeding, stiff joints, and bones becoming fragile and decalcified. If serious, there may be scurvy with all its symptoms, loss of teeth, decalcification, vomiting, serious diarrhea, cardiac insufficiency. Its excess is not described.

It is stored in the liver.

Necessary foods: acid fruits— oranges, lemons, mulberries, grapefruit.

It is destroyed by desiccation, heat and by air. The optimal quantity is 10 to 30 milligrams per day. Compared with vitamin K: anti-hemorrhagic; vitamin P: anticapillary permeability; vitamin D: calcification.

4) *Vitamin D* (ergosterol): Calcifier, anti-rickets.

> *It has recently been demonstrated that vitamin D (in reality irradiated ergosterol) in small doses favors the deposition of calcium in bones. But in large doses, on the contrary, it causes the calcium to pass from the bones into the blood (Marzetti, Homeopatia 91, 92).*

It is distributed by the liver. Cholesterol becomes irradiated ergosterol from sunlight and is stored by the liver.

Necessary foods: milk, liver, cod or tunafish, liver oil, irradiated yeast.

By acting on calcium, it regulates the phosphorus-calcium equilibrium in the blood, the proportion of which must vary from 5 to 2. It has been suggested that this occurs through the intermediation of the parathyroid gland.

By the action on the energy and through the measure of the parathyroid pulse, it has consistently been observed that parathyroid deficiency corresponds to a relative excess of phosphorus and thyroid function with all the concomitant nervous disorders (spasms, neuralgia, tics, etc.). An excess of the parathyroids (and deficiency of the thyroid) corresponds to a relative excess of blood calcium with flaccid muscles, etc. Parathyroids and vitamin D act in similar ways: with small doses of vitamin D (and by dispersal of the parathyroids), blood calcium is deposited in the bone and there is a relative excess of phosphorus and thyroid function. With large doses (or by tonifying the parathyroid), there is a passage of calcium from the bones to the blood and a relative deficiency of phosphorus and thyroid function. Action on the liver and the parathyroid increases the desired effect.

5) *Vitamin E* (either tocopherol or alpha): For strength and the genitalia. The first one to be called a vitamin. Stored in the liver.

Necessary foods: liver, wheat germ, watercress, green salad, peanut oil. Quantity necessary: about 30 milligrams per day.

It is indispensable for the normal functioning of the genital organs and the muscles. Its deficiency can aggravate the problems of menopause (hot flashes, night sweats, obesity or rheumatism), weakness or atrophy of the muscles, arthritis, asthma and diabetes. *Sanyinjiao* (SP-6) acts against these problems by stimulating the spleen, pancreas, liver and kidney.

Vitamin F: see B1.

Vitamin G: see B2.

6) *Vitamin K:* Antihemorrhagic.

Formed in the large intestine and stored by the liver which, without it, could not form the antihemorrhagic prothrombin.

Necessary foods: pork, spinach, cabbage, cereals, carrots, potatoes, cheese, egg yolk.

> In mammals, the intestinal bacteria are capable of effecting the synthesis of substances endowed with an analogous activity. That explains the independence of numerous animal species vis-a-vis the food supply. (Biochimie Médicale)

The action on the energy allows us to observe that by tonifying the large intestine (primarily through *hegu* LI-4), menses became less excessive and metrorrhagia and hemorrhage ceased; by dispersing, menses and hemorrhage increased. Also, a liver insufficiency which is always accompanied by a slight discharge of delayed blood disappears by tonifying the liver.

7) *Vitamin H* (biotin): Antisebaceous. (See vitamin B antiseborrhea, or X.) Stored in the liver; can be produced by it.

Foods most useful: liver (1 mg. per kg.), kidney, egg yolk, yeast, rice hulls.

Vitamin H activates the cellular metabolism in the concentration of 100 billionth of a part, in between the fifth and sixth homeopathic dilution. (Marzetti, *Homeopatia* 115)

Its deficiency is accompanied by an increase and modification of sebaceous secretions and by a fatty degeneration of the superficial strata of the epidermis (cellulitis), a favorable state for all forms of infectious dermatitis. There are also paresthesias and some modification of the blood *(Biochimie Médicale).* On the whole, it may stimulate the synthesis of body fat by the skin and the liver.

Thyroid deficiency produces cellulite; tonify *huagai* (CV-20).

Its toxic action from egg whites or a diet too rich in fats has been noted. *(Biochimie Médicale)* Tonification of the liver corrects one or another of these sensitivities. The action of the liver on all skin problems is consistently observed energetically.

8) *Vitamin L:* Lactation.

By its regular supply, it assures lactation.

It may be stored in the liver.

The more useful foods are beef, liver, and yeast. *(Webster's Dictionary)*

A restrained small intestine greatly helps lactation by diminishing urine flow and increasing secretions (disperse *shaoze,* SI-1, and *qiangu,* SI-2).

9) *Vitamin P:* Anticapillarity, permeability.

It has not yet been proven to be stored in the liver.

The more useful foods are lemon, paprika and liver.

Deficiency is accompanied by increased permeability of the capillaries with less resistance of their tissues; and hemorrhage at the level of the skin, mucosa, and subcutaneous tissue. Similar symptoms to those at the beginning of scurvy (vitamin C deficiency); also similar to vitamin K deficiency.

The action of the vital energy has allowed us to observe the important relation between a liver and large intestine insufficiency and the tendency to hemorrhage and the consequent possibility of correcting this by tonifying these two organs.

Vitamin PP: see B.

Vitamin X: see H, also E.

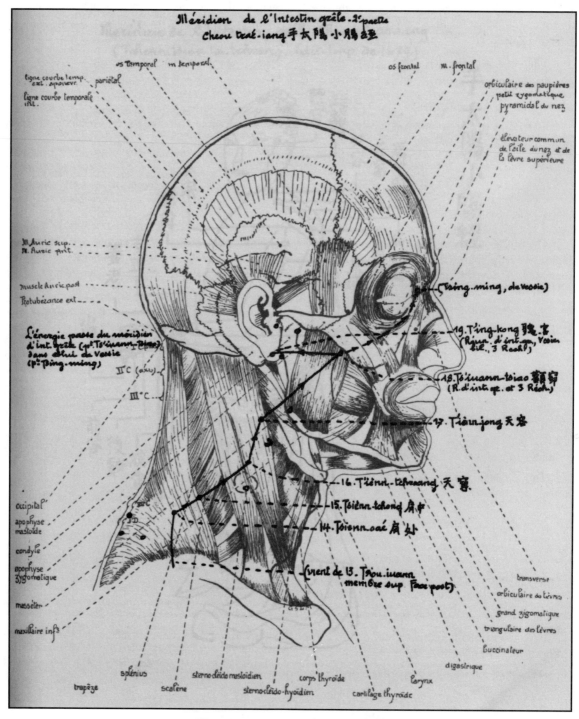

Meridian of the small intestine (part 2) (GSDM)

Chapter VII

The Distribution of Energy (II)

Distributor Organs

I. Triple Warmer Meridian — II. Heart Governor Meridian: Sexual Organs, Vessels, Parasympathetic System — III. Sympathetic and Parasympathetic Systems in the West and in China

I. Triple Warmer Meridian

In Chinese medicine, it is the triple warmer that regulates and distributes energy to all parts of the body. The triple warmer is not an organ but a function; nonetheless, it is represented by the material network of its meridian. Its meridian is yang, traversing the posterior surface of the upper limb from the ring finger up to the tragus, skirting around the ears.

Energy passes to the triple warmer meridian from the heart governor meridian (vessels and sexual organs) at *laogong* (PC-8). It then passes into the gallbladder meridian from *ermen* (TW-23, IS TW-21) to *tinghui* (GB-2).

The pulse of the triple warmer is represented on the right wrist, section III, superficial level, either edge of the artery reflecting one side of the body. Its maximum is at 10:00 p.m. (minimum hour of the spleen-pancreas). Its minimum is at 10:00 a.m. (maximum hour of the spleen-pancreas).

Its name comes from the fact that it commands and nourishes the three great functional systems that give heat and life to the body through the production of new energy — the respiratory, digestive and genitourinary (particularly genital) systems.

The triple warmer meridian receives energy produced by the stomach through *qichong* (ST-30) (for which *shimen*, CV-5, is said to be its reservoir). In addition, it receives energy through the herald points located on the conception vessel, which extracts the energy of sexual vitality. The triple warmer then distributes the energy throughout the entire body.

The triple warmer is considered so important that the eighteenth century Japanese author, Chang Fushen (Chinese pronunciation), wrote a five volume text, *Jie Di Fa Meng* (Diffusion and Explication of the Organism), which explains how to use and maintain all its functions.

Indeed, its role is very complex. Through the herald points, it is closely linked with the conception vessel. Each third of the conception vessel commands one of the three great functions, commanded in turn by the triple warmer. The triple warmer also takes energy from *qichong* (ST-30), closely connected with genital function. If its pulse has the same intensity as all the superficial (yang) organs, it shows the activity of the yang energy. If its pulse has the same intensity as the deep pulse (yin) organs, with the exception of the heart governor, it shows the activity of the sympathetic system. This meridian thus has very variable effects on the vital energy.

Therefore, we must study it under three different aspects:

1) *The triple warmer alone.* The meridian or pulse indicating disorder of the triple warmer function.

2) *The yang energy.* As with the other superficial pulses, it reflects dysfunction in the yang energy and nervous activity.

3) *The sympathetic system.* Except for the heart governor, the deep pulses have similar effects to those of the sympathetic system.

The triple warmer alone.

The triple warmer pulse gives an indication of the intensity of intellectual, moral and mental vitality; decision-will and nervous resilience; nonphysical vital energy; and perhaps some reserves of energy or the capacity to recharge.

The relative insufficiency-excess of the triple warmer from this point of view is as follows: [the table on the following page]:

Insufficiency	Excess
All nervous insufficiency, without resilience. Insufficient function.	All nervous excess: nerves are tense, tight; spasms, nervous crises.
Depression. Depressive distress.	Hyperexcitation: hyperexcited distress; holding back worries. Does not exteriorize, but is upset. Takes everything upon himself. Trembling, tics, agitation.
Sad, discouraged, passive, slow, weak.	
Somnolent, heavy.	Nervous insomnia at the beginning of night.
Deafness from weakness.	Deafness from nervous excess. Tinnitus.
Shivering from cold.	Nervous shivering. Spasms from shock.
Weakness or pain from cold, rain, humidity, snow, slight decreases of barometric pressure.	Congestive headache or disturbance of the vitality brought about by storms, wind, heat or a sharp drop in barometric pressure.
Lifeless pulse, hypotension, diastolic and systolic low.	Tight pulse, particularly the superficial pulses. Nervous hypertension. Systolic high with diastolic low.
Pains in the heart, angina with weakness, anguish.	Pain in the heart, angina of the chest with agitation, tightness, nervous excess.

The principal disorders in the regions where dysfunction of the triple warmer manifests are as follows:

Nervous shivering, nervous crisis, hyperexcited depression, irritability, emotional agitation, distress, nervous insomnia at the beginning of night: *tianjing* (TW-10). Extravagant speech, hyperexcitation: *yemen* (TW-2). Nervous fever: *guanchong* (TW-1), with agitation: *yangchi* (TW-4). Frequent yawning: *yifeng* (TW-17).

Shivering from cold: tonify *tianjing* (TW-10). As if seized by ghosts, incessant melancholia: *zhigou* (TW-6). Emotional agitation, deranged mind, depression, weakness: *yemen* (TW-2).

Heart (and three warmers) — *zhigou* (TW-6), *yemen* (TW-2). Agitation, pain of the vertebrae behind the heart: *guanchong* (TW-1). Angina pain of the chest: *zhigou* (TW-6). Hyper- or hypotension: hand-*zhongzhu* (TW-3). From energy: *tianyou* (TW-16).

Eyes — muddled or troubled: hand-*zhongzhu* (TW-3), *waiguan* (TW-5). Eyes bulging: *xiaoluo* (TW-12). Spasms of vision: ear-*heliao* (TW-22). Acute pain in the eyes: *guanchong* (TW-1), *qinglengyuan* (TW-11). Eyes swollen, pupils red: *waiguan* (TW-5). Scarlet and painful eyes: *yemen* (TW-2).

Ears — all troubles: *ermen* (TW-23, IS TW-21). Tinnitus: *jiaosun* (TW-20), *yemen* (TW-2), *guanchong* (TW-1), *waiguan* (TW-5); if painful: *luxi* (TW-19); if with deafness and headaches, deafness from energy or shock: *tianyou* (TW-16), *tianjing* (TW-10), *luxi* (TW-19). Ears blocked: *luxi* (TW-19); painful: hand-*zhongzhu* (TW-3).

Teeth — inflammation, caries, pain: *ermen* (TW-23, IS TW-21), *yemen* (TW-2). Molars: *jiaosun* (TW-20). Lower molars: *sidu* (TW-9). Swollen gums, inflammation of the mouth: *jiaosun* (TW-20).

Throat — painful, irritated, pruritus: hand-*zhongzhu* (TW-3). Painful, adenitis: *sidu* (TW-9). Tight: *tianjing* (TW-10). Painful larynx: *guanchong* (TW-1). Tired tongue: *yemen* (TW-2), *guanchong* (TW-1). No voice, no speech: *sanyangluo* (TW-8). Cough, cannot speak, bronchitis with pus: *tianjing* (TW-10). Short inhalation and exhalation: *yemen* (TW-2), *sidu* (TW-9).

Contracted stomach: *tianjing* (TW-10). Diabetes, dry tongue, prostatitis, epididymitis, blennorrhagia: *yangchi* (TW-4). Constipation from emptiness or diarrhea, vomiting: *zhigou* (TW-6).

Pain of contracted muscles: *zhigou* (TW-6). Alternating flaccidity and contracture: *guanchong* (TW-1).

Troubles from changing weather, from external temperature, sweat without reason: *waiguan* (TW-5).

Mumps: *waiguan* (TW-5). Ganglia: *tianjing* (TW-10), *naohui* (TW-13). Neck and nape: *yifeng* (TW-17). Tumors or swellings at the nape of neck: *naohui* (TW-13).

In women, poor circulation through the conception vessel, fainting after childbirth: *zhigou* (TW-6).

Tics, trembling, chorea: *huizong* (TW-7), *luxi* (TW-19). Spasms of the face, cheek: ear-*heliao* (TW-22).

The meridian commands disorders along its course. Articular pains, periarthritis: *xiaoluo* (TW-12). Flaccidity of the four limbs or the upper limbs: *waiguan* (TW-5), *sanyangluo* (TW-8).

The yang energy: dysfunction with all the superficial yang pulses.

Here, this is a question of energetic dysfunction of the total yang activity. The yang superficial pulses are all equal but opposite in intensity to that of all the yin deep pulses. Nervous activity is in disharmony with physical activity.

Intervention at the proper triple warmer point, *waiguan* (TW-5), balances excesses of yin and yang on a large scale by channeling an excess of one into the emptiness of the other. Similar results can be obtained by using the heart governor point, *neiguan* (PC-6).

The relative insufficiency-excess of the triple warmer with the yang group is as follows:

Insufficiency	Excess
Sadness, mental depression, discouragement, indolence.	Excitation, nervousness, tight nerves, irritability, does all from will.
Good, slow digestion.	Bad digestion, thin.
Physical strength, but without energy.	Physical exhaustion, but continues to work; tension on top of weakness.

If there is excess, precise dispersal at the dispersal point, *tianjing* (TW-10), will produce an immediate sense of relaxation, sometimes with a crisis of tears, followed by a sensation of well-being and calm. If there is insufficiency and the tonification point, hand-*zhongzhu* (TW-3), is precisely tonified, the sadness, discouragement and indolence give way to a normal need for activity. In both cases, the yin and yang return to a harmonious balance.

The sympathetic system: dysfunction of the triple warmer with deep, yin pulses, except for the heart governor pulse.

Fengchi (GB-20), which modifies this group of pulses, also modifies the pulse of the governor vessel.

In cases of this type, stimulation of the sympathetic system (at *fengchi*, GB-20) or the triple warmer (at the tonification point hand-*zhongzhu*, TW-3), gives results that the table below shows are superimposable — on the left the effects of the Western sympathetic system, on the right those of the triple warmer.

	Sympathetic	Triple Warmer (of Sympathetic)
Vessels in general	+	+
Coronaries	−	
Vessels of general application	−	
Heart: amplitude, rapidity	+	+
Bronchi	−	−
Lungs		−
Smooth digestive muscles	−	−
Internal anal sphincter	+?	
Intestines	−	−
Pancreas	?	−
Liver	+	+
Gallbladder	−?	−
Spleen	+	+
Kidneys		+
Urinary bladder: expulsor muscle	−	−
Internal sphincter	+	+

II. Heart Governor Meridian: Sexual Organs, Vessels and Parasympathetic System

Chinese tradition posits the existence of a single meridian and a single pulse for the heart governor. Our observations have led us to the following conclusions:

1)   The existence of two absolutely independent pulses: a) representing the variations of the sexual organs: right wrist, section III, deep level, right and left sides of the artery (right and left organs); b) representing the variations of the vessels: right wrist, section III, middle level, right and left sides of the artery (vessels of the right or left side of the body; inferior half, arteries, upper half, veins).

2)   Massage of the pulse of the sexual organs elicits a response only at *laogong* (PC-8), *quze* (PC-3) and *tianquan* (PC-2). When massaging the pulse of the vessels, the response is in all other heart governor points except the three mentioned above.

3)   The points of the vessels on the right meridian respond more weakly on the vessels and the heart but more strongly on the sexual organs than the same points on the left side.

4)   When the pulse of the vessels is of the same intensity as that of all the superficial pulses (except the triple warmer), variations of the parasympathetic system are represented. The pulse of the vessels elicits a response at *tianzhu* (BL-10), which acts on all organs commanded by the parasympathetic system. In turn, pressing this point elicits a response at the pulse of the vessels and all the yang superficial pulses except the triple warmer.

The heart governor meridian is indeed complex. For years, Western science has recognized the inseparable link between the sexual life and the tone of the arteries: hypertension may arise from sexual excitation, and conversely, sexual weakness from serious hypotension. Also recognized is the action of the parasympathetic on the arteries and the sexual life.

The heart governor meridian has its maximum at 8:00 p.m. local time (minimum hour of the stomach). Its minimum is at 8:00 a.m. (maximum hour of the stomach). Energy passes to the heart governor meridian via a branch of the kidney meridian, from *shufu* (KI-27) at the top of the sternum to *tianchi* (PC-1) at the lateral side of the nipple. The energy passes from the heart governor at *laogong* (PC-8) into the triple warmer at *guanchong* (TW-1).

We have consistently observed that the tonification point of the meridian, *zhongchong* (PC-9), and the dispersal point, *daling* (PC-7), act only on the pulse of the vessels. In contrast, *laogong* (PC-8) is the ''source'' or ''regulator'' of the sexual organs: when this point is tonified they are strongly tonified; when dispersed, they are strongly dispersed. *Laogong* (PC-8) also elicits a strong action on the general energetic potential, as measured instrumentally. *Quze* (PC-3) and *tianquan* (PC-2), two additional points acting on the sexual organs, act as well on the pulse. The heart governor assent point, *jueyinshu* (BL-14), acts particularly on the vessels. Of the two herald points, one of them, *qihai* (CV-6), acts only on the sexual organs, while the other, *jiuwei* (CV-15), acts only on the vessels.

It is advisable to study individually the three actions of this meridian on the sexual organs, the vessels and the parasympathetic system.

Sexual organs.

This bilateral meridian is also called *mingmen,* ''the door of destiny.'' The name evokes the idea of conception and sexual function — souls are thrown back into existence through the exit from the Buddhist hells.

The pulse of the sexual organs is at the right wrist, section III, deep level. The herald point is *qihai* (CV-6); source point, *laogong* (PC-8). Through the activity of its strength it is possible to understand its action.

The relative insufficiency-excess is as follows:

Insufficiency	Excess
Deficient character, apprehension, insecurity, noncombative. Pity, emotional agitation, fear.	Strong, hard, pitiless character. Subject to repression, obsessions or even hallucinations or insanity.
Hates darkness and night.	Likes darkness and night.
Insomnia from fatigue or emptiness.	Fears nothing, always in movement, agitated.
Weak, tired, distracted.	Worries, malcontent.
Fever from fatigue or nervousness.	
Insufficiency of the inferior instincts of the primate. Passivity.	Hyperexcited primate, aggressive, angry, wicked.
Sexual indifference, frigidity or idealistic love.	Sexual preoccupation and activity.
Impotence, sterility.	Fertility.

Significant aspects of the pulse:

Women — a swollen superior side: increasing from the seventh day before menses; ovulation or congested ovary. Middle part, on one side: congested fallopian tube. Both sides: the whole organ is congested, or pregnancy. No pulse: insufficiency or absence of the organ.

Men — upper part swollen on one side: swollen testicle. If nil, insufficient or absent testicle. Inferior part swollen: swollen penis. If nil, few erections.

Tonification, dispersal and source point of the sexual organs: *laogong* (PC-8). Herald point: *qihai* (CV-6). Assent point: *zhishi* (BL-47, IS BL-52).

Direct and indirect effects of the points of the sexual organs:

Heart — pain with thirst, agitation, pericarditis, myocarditis, endocarditis: *quze* (PC-3); palpitations: *tianquan* (PC-2).

Taste-smell — mouth or throat abscess: *laogong* (PC-8); violent thirst, dry mouth: *quze* (PC-3).

Stomach — vomiting of blood or saliva and blood: *quze* (PC-3); pain in the stomach and heart; jaundice: *laogong* (PC-8); swelling of the epigastrium: *tianquan* (PC-2).

Blood in stool or urine: *laogong* (PC-8).

Eyes — myopia and optic nerve atrophy, tired, weakened vision: *tianquan* (PC-2).

Ears — *quze* (PC-3).

Respiratory passages — cough, chest pains, dyspnea: *laogong* (PC-8); chronic bronchitis, pulmonary tuberculosis: *quze* (PC-3); coughing fits, cough and pain in the back: *tianquan* (PC-2).

Sweat at the head and shoulders: *quze* (PC-3).

Loss of feeling, particularly of the fingers: *laogong* (PC-8).

Bad abscess, measles and German measles, involuntary movements of the upper limb and the hand: *quze* (PC-3); hand contracted, writer's cramp: *laogong* (PC-8).

Vessels (arteries and veins).

The heart governor points which elicit changes in the pulse of the vessels (right wrist, section III, middle level) act principally on the arteries and not the veins. (The arteries are reflected at the inferior half of the pulse while the veins are reflected at the upper half.) The herald point of the heart governor, *jiuwei* (CV-15), also acts on the vessels.

The relative insufficiency-excess is as follows:

Insufficiency	Excess
Insomnia from anemia, emptiness, lassitude, weakness, desire to rest, vertigo, fogginess.	Insomnia from sensation of congestion. Need to spend one's energy. Hyperexcited by all emotion.
Pale face.	Red face, redness after meals.
Lowered blood pressure.	Elevated blood pressure. Tendency towards congestions.
Heart problems from insufficiency.	Heart problems from excess.
Palpitations from fatigue or the night.	Palpitations from hyperexcitation, warmth, or exercise.
Always cold.	Always hot.

The effects of the vessel points of the heart governor meridian determine whether or not the action on the vessels is direct or indirect.

Anterior brain: *ximen* (PC-4). Anterior and lateral arm: *neiguan* (PC-6). Lateral and posterior: *jianshi* (PC-5).

Insufficient consciousness (evolved man, reason, etc.), emotional agitation, fear, fears people: *ximen* (PC-4). Repressing fears, weakness of nerves and brain, apprehension, insecurity: *jianshi* (PC-5). Does not like darkness;

fears the night; cries at night (children): *zhongchong* (PC-9). Indecisiveness, emotional agitation: *quze* (PC-3).

Aggressiveness, combativeness, anger, nastiness: *daling* (PC-7), particularly on the right wrist. Hyperexcitation, hyperexcited sadness and great tears: *daling* (PC-7). Stubborn or hyperactive children, apoplexy, mental unclarity, coma: *jianshi* (PC-5).

Hypotension: *zhongchong* (PC-9). Arterial spasms: *daling* (PC-7). Hypertension, fears the sun, congestive headaches: *ximen* (PC-4), *jianshi* (PC-5), *daling* (PC-7).

Heart — all varieties of pain: *jianshi* (PC-5). Pain of the heart, pericarditis, myocarditis, endocarditis: *daling* (PC-7), *jianshi* (PC-5). Tired heart from emotions: *daling* (PC-7).

Sore throat, fever, cough: *daling* (PC-7), *jianshi* (PC-5).

Bad breath: *daling* (PC-7).

Vomiting and belching from energy: *daling* (PC-7), *ximen* (PC). Vomiting or dry vomiting from cold or cholera: *jianshi* (PC-5).

Swollen stomach from failure to empty itself: *zhongchong* (PC-9). All disorders of the pancreas (left point) or the spleen (right point): *jianshi* (PC-5). Blood in the stools or urine: *daling* (PC-7).

Poor vision in children at night (hemeralopia): *zhongchong* (PC-9). Troubled vision: *jianshi* (PC-5).

Colds, tight chest, cannot breathe: *jianshi* (PC-5).

Night sweats: *jianshi* (PC-5).

Persistent ganglia: *jianshi* (PC-5). Abscess or blisters in the hand: *daling* (PC-7). Scabies: *daling* (PC-7).

Eruptive illnesses: *daling* (PC-7).

Troubles along the course of the meridian, around the line of the median nerve: *daling* (PC-7) if there is excess; *zhongchong* (PC-9) if there is insufficiency. Writer's cramp: *ximen* (PC-4).

Pain of the chest and side: *daling* (PC-7). Swollen armpit: *daling* (PC-7), *jianshi* (PC-5), *tianchi* (PC-1).

The herald point of the vessels is on the conception vessel: *jiuwei* (CV-15). The assent point is on the back, on the urinary bladder meridian: *jueyinshu* (BL-14).

The parasympathetic system: dysfunction of the vessels and all the yang producer organs.

When all the superficial pulses, except that of the triple warmer, are similar in intensity to the pulse of the vessels, the latter can be used to give an indication of the energetic functioning of the parasympathetic system. (*tianzhu*, BL-10, a command point of the parasympathetic, modifies this group of pulses and also that of the conception vessel.)

In such cases, the effects obtained by stimulation of heart governor points are identical to those of the parasympathetic system. Pressing the vessel pulse elicits a response at *tianzhu* (BL-10). Likewise, massaging *tianzhu* awakens a response in the vessel pulse and all the superficial pulses except the triple warmer.

The following table illustrates the parallel functions of the heart governor and parasympathetic system. (The data on the parasympathetic system is provided by R.J. Main.)

	Parasympathetic System	Heart Governor
Vessels in general	0	+
Sweat glands	0	0
Eye: iris	+	+
Salivary glands	+	+
Digestive and respiratory mucus glands	+	+
Heart: rapidity	−	−
Bronchi	+	+
Smooth digestive muscles	+	+
Digestive secretion	+	+
Pancreas	+	+
Spleen	−	−
Liver: bile	+	−
Gallbladder	+	+

Urinary bladder: expulsor muscle	+	+
Internal sphincter....................................	−	−
Genital apparatus, vessels	+	+
Uterus...	0?	+

III. Sympathetic and Parasympathetic Systems in the East and West

The difference between Western and Chinese theory.

Although Chinese antiquity had no knowledge of the autonomic nervous system as we know it, the effects of two command points clearly parallel its dual aspects: the points *fengchi* (GB-20) and *tianzhu* (BL-10) elicit responses analogous to those of the sympathetic and parasympathetic systems, respectively. However, upon close examination we find that there are several exceptions to the otherwise identical effects. These relate to the physiology of the vessels and heart.

First, it is important to discuss the grossly different methods of investigation leading to the findings above. In Europe, conclusions are based on studies using drastic surgical or pharmaceutical techniques. Nerves are cut or very violently stimulated by powerful electrical discharges. Massive doses of potent medicines are injected into the blood, in contrast with natural hormones, which are dosed by nature in infinitesimal quantities. Conversely, experiments in China involve only very weak, distal physiological stimulation on the skin.

The law of Arhndt, reintroduced by Brown-Séquard and Claude Bernard, posits that weak stimulation excites, while strong stimulation paralyzes. The strong stimulation used in European experiments would thus result in paralysis while Chinese methods would cause excitation. However, "strong" and "weak" are relative terms and refer to very different intensities on the two continents.

In Chinese medical thought, weak stimulation (silver needles, massage through ten to fifteen respirations) is far from being excitatory. Rather, it calms, quiets and decongests. European researchers have probably not yet applied such weak stimulus on subjects since there is no mention in their experiments of a calming or decongesting effect. What the Chinese physiologists consider as strong stimulation (gold needles, moxa, massage through thirty respirations) must be in fact equivalent in intensity to what the Europeans consider weak and excitatory.

The strong, paralyzing stimulation of European experiments would be regarded by Chinese physiologists as excessive and inordinate. In acupuncture this level of intensity dazes or tetanizes. Punctures at too great a frequency with large diameter needles might produce this ill effect. Clearly, Chinese acupunctural and Western neurologic perspectives on strong stimuli are vastly different.

Significantly, Arhndt also recognized the relativity between action and reaction: a single stimulus may elicit a response in a weakened organ but not in a healthy one. This phenomenon is most clearly discernible in the science of energy, particularly through the special autonomic pulse discovered by us. In European discussions on the autonomic system there is no mention of this relativity of action and reaction, since researchers have not yet recognized this pulse and have no way of detecting subtle, energetic variations. Also, Westerners confuse the physical nerves with their specific physiological effects. The effects of the autonomic nervous system of the West are equivalent to the effects produced through stimulation of two command points, used by the ancient Chinese for their opposing effects: *fengchi* (GB-20) (sympathetic system) and *tianzhu* (BL-10) (parasympathetic).

The difference between the sympathetic and parasympathetic systems.

Let us briefly recall the profound physiological and anatomical differences between the sympathetic and parasympathetic systems.

The sympathetic is anatomically a true autonomic nervous center. Although connected to the brain, its center is in the posterior hypothalamus. It is linked to the whole body by its centrifugal as well as centripetal fibers and has reactions and functions specific to these fibers.

The parasympathetic system is not an anatomically distinct, autonomic nervous center. Rather, it is a group of cranial nerves: the vagus or pneumogastric nerve (tenth pair), with fibers coming from the common ocular motor nerve (third pair), the facial nerve (seventh pair) and the trigeminal nerve (fifth pair). It is anatomically connected to the fibers of the sympathetic system through the plexes and is intimately associated with the sympathetic system. It has its center in the anterior hypothalamus. A functional antagonism exists between the two systems (Hédon, 777).

While Europeans have studied these two systems primarily through surgical experimentation, Easterners have observed their physiological effects through stimulating points on the skin distal to the area researched. The most significant difference on this subject between the West and China relates to the action of the autonomic nervous system (and points *fengchi* and *tianzhu*) on the vessels and heart. Effects of these two acupoints and the autonomic nervous system on the other organs are exactly paralleled.

The differences between Western and Chinese medical thought: vasomotor effects.

In European medical thought, the sympathetic system is clearly the vasoconstrictor. The only exception to this is its vasodilation of the coronary arteries. In Asian medical thought, however, the point *fengchi* (GB-20), which produces all the other effects of the sympathetic system, rapidly causes vasodilation, increased amplitude of the vessels, increased strength of the heartbeats and lowering of the blood pressure.

The vagus (parasympathetic) system is considered in Western medicine as the vasodilator (with the exception of the coronary arteries, which it constricts). Conversely, in Chinese medicine, the point *tianzhu* (BL-10), paralleling the parasympathetic system, is considered a vasoconstrictor.

Interestingly, the works on this subject in Europe are fraught with obscurity and contradiction, particularly with regard to the "feedback" characteristics of the autonomic system. Hédon states (294):

> The muscular fibers of the arteries are arranged in rings which only allow constriction. The dilator nerves act only by inhibition of the vasoconstrictor in constant tonus. All trauma results in the contraction of the vessels.

Unfortunately, there is still little precision as to which nerves act as vasoconstrictors and which as vasodilators.

It is well known that severing the cervical sympathetic nerves in rabbits causes dilation of the vessels of the head and ears. Here, the sympathetic acts as a vasoconstrictor. Conversely, Professor Leriche observed that after cutting the sympathetic fibers of a segment of the radial artery (about 12 mm. long) this segment became hard, without beat, the other part remaining supple with a beat. Here, the sympathetic fibers caused vasodilation. Hence, there is an apparent contradiction between local and regional effects of resection of a sympathetic fiber. This contradiction is explained by Professor Mériel:

> The sympathectomy frees inhibition of the local arterial tone; the artery thus becomes rigid, without beats. Periarterial sympathetic fibers normally inhibit this tone. Hence what we are seeing here is a local phenomenon.

It appears that local sympathetic fibers act as vasodilators by inhibiting vasoconstriction of the parasympathetic fibers, supporting Hédon's teachings.

The general action of the sympathetic would be the same, but by more complicated interventions. Professor Mériel writes:

> When the sympathetic system is stimulated as a whole, the acknowledged tonic action on the heart is clearly obtained. This reinforcement of the heart, however, is found to be immediately counterbalanced by the depressive action of the carotid sinus, which causes vasodilation with increased arterial amplitude. Without this counter-check, hypertension would be produced following the sympathetic reinforcement of the heart. The inverse action is caused by excitation of the vagus [parasympathetic] system.

The command points of the autonomic system produce a resonance, a clear response in sensitive or trained patients. This response takes place in the respective centers within the nervous system: for the sympathetic system, the response is in the posterior hypothalamus; for the parasympathetic system, the anterior hypothalamus.

For the vessels of the heart, however, there are many causes which increase or block the action of the sympathetic or the parasympathetic. Some of these are the following: an excess or insufficiency of certain hormones, e.g., vasopressin, adrenalin, angiotonin (angiotensin); acetylcholine, some metabolites, CO_2, lactates, histamine, adenosine, ions, potassium; lack of oxygen, blood volume, heat (which dilates) and cold (which contracts). Shock or compression produces metabolites such as histamine. These in turn cause vasoconstriction followed by vasodilation; hence, the paleness and subsequent flushing of the face in shock, or white and then red marking of the skin when pressed.

Finally, stimulation of the carotid sinus through its command point *lingdao* (HT-4) produces dilation of the vessels. Dispersing the same point produces vasoconstriction and blood pressure. (This effect is similar to dispersing the command point of the sympathetic.)

Western and Chinese parallels.

Respiratory system. The actions of the autonomic system and their command points are identical: excitation, inflammation, contraction by the parasympathetic system and its command point; relaxation, decongestion by the sympathetic system and its command point.

Digestive system. Here, equally, the actions of the autonomic system and the command points are identical: contraction, excitation by the parasympathetic system, relaxation by the sympathetic.

Sexual organs. These questions are so complex and at the same time so delicate that it still has been only possible to find some partial similarities.

For women, the motor function of the body of the uterus is commanded by sympathetic fibers arriving along the vessels through the tenth thoracic vertebra. However, for the inferior part of the uterus and for the cervix, it is the pelvic nerves of the parasympathetic which act (Main, 273). The command point of the whole uterus, *qugu* (CV-2), is just above the pubis. The action of the points of the parasympathetic or sympathetic systems have not been studied extensively, but they appear to awaken a response in the point for the uterus and for the organ.

For men: 1) The erection gets its stimulus from the plexus of the 1-4th sacral nerves (with fibers from the parasympathetic and pelvic sympathetic systems). Vasodilation of the erectile tissue has resulted from tonifying the command points of these nerves. Stimulation of the sympathetic has the reverse effect (Main, 266). 2) The ejaculation is inhibited by resection of the sympathetic (L1 ganglion, Main, 266) and even by presacral resection. There are no convincing observations on the dispersing action of L1 by needling, but tonification with acupuncture hastens ejaculation. 3) resection of the anterior nerve of the cord blocks the sensation of orgasm (Main, 267). Observations to confirm this are not yet conclusive. Tonification of L1 and L2 seem to give positive results.

The sympathetic system (*fengchi,* GB-20) and the parasympathetic system (*tianzhu,* BL-10) respond in the organ.

To facilitate comparison, I have borrowed from Main (215) a comparative table of the sympathetic and parasympathetic systems, inserting the effects of the command points for both.

	Symp.	*Fengchi*	Paras.	*Tianzhu*
Vessels in general	+	−	0	+
Coronary vessels	−		+	
Vessels of the genital apparatus	+		−	
The muscles at rest	+		0	
Gastric and salivary glands	+	−	0	+
Pilomotor muscles	+		0	
Sweat glands	+	−	0	+
Eye: radial fibrils of the pupil	+	−	0	+
Circular fibrils of the pupil	0	−	+	+
Circular fibrils of the ciliary muscle	0	+	+	−
Radial fibrils of the ciliary muscle	+		−	
Smooth muscles of the eyelids and orbit	+		−	
Lachrymal glands	−		+	
Salivary glands	−	−	+	+
Thyroid	+		0	
Digestive and respiratory mucus glands	0	−	+	+
Heart: S-A node (rapidity)	+	+	−	−
Auricular (atrial) muscle: force and time at rest	+	+	−	−
Ventricular muscle: force and time at rest	+	+	0	−
Bronchii	−	−	+	+
Smooth digestive muscles	−	−	+	+
Internal anal sphincter	+	+	−	−
Digestive secretions	−	−	+	+
Pancreas: insulin	?	−	+	+
Exocrine glands	?	−	+	+

	Symp.	*Fengchi*	**Paras.**	*Tianzhu*
Liver: glycogenolysis, hyperprothrombinemia ....±....		+	–	–
Bile..	?	+	+	–
Gallbladder..	–	–	+	+
Ureters..	–		+	
Bladder: contractile muscle	–	–	+	+
Internal sphincter......................................	+	+	–	–
Spleen..	+	+	–	–
Adrenal medulla..	+		0	
Vas deferens, seminal vesicles	–		+	
Uterus..	+		0	
Thoracic canal	–		+	

+ stimulation (secretion, contraction).
– inhibition (diminutions of secretions, dilation).
0   no innervation.
? questionable.
No sign: not verified.

Equilibrium of the parasympathetic and sympathetic systems.

There is an important equilibrium between the actions of the sympathetic and parasympathetic systems. The weakness of one creates an apparent dominance of the other but without it being stronger than normal. This creates some difficulty in understanding their effects and in deciding what action to take.

The examination of the pulse alone allows us to differentiate the following combinations: 1) In equilibrium — the two systems being equally normal, equally excessive, or equally insufficient. 2) In disequilibrium — normal sympathetic system with strong or weak parasympathetic system; strong sympathetic with weak or normal parasympathetic; sympathetic weak with normal or strong parasympathetic.

This precise method of differentiation enables us to correct very complex problems. The fact that the sympathetic is dominant does not mean that we want to disperse or reduce it. Rather, it may be necessary to tonify the parasympathetic. Below is a table giving the physiological modifications of people suffering from a dominance of one or the other of the two systems.

Sympathetic Dominant	**Parasympathetic Dominant**
Hyperexcitation from shock, emotion.	Frozen, contracted by shock, emotion.
Brilliant eyes, too open, protruding (muscles of eyelids and orbit stimulated). Pupils too dilated (mydriasis). Ciliary muscles relaxed (farsighted, sees in shadow and at a distance).	Eyes dull, too closed, recessed (muscles of eyelids and orbit relaxed). Pupils contracted (myosis). Ciliary muscles contracted (easy sight, sees in light and close up).
Accelerated pulse.	Slow pulse.
Heat. High, easy fever.	Cold, weak fever, not easily produced.
Sweating difficult.	Easy, abundant sweating of palms and extremities.
Pale complexion, red hands.	Red face. Cold extremities.
Dry mouth, without saliva.	Excessive saliva.
Strongly beating heart, mostly rapid.	Heart contracted, slow or arrhythmic.
Rapid healing and coagulation.	Slow healing and coagulation.
Arteries supple, ample (carotid, epigastric).	Arteries contracted, without beat, hard (carotid, epigastric).
Bronchi relaxed, decongested.	Bronchi contracted or inflamed.

Sympathetic Dominant	Parasympathetic Dominant
Lung decongested, relaxed to the point of atony, cannot breathe out.	Lungs congested, irritated, inflamed, cannot inhale.
Atonic diaphragm. Difficulty in vomiting.	Diaphragm in spasm, hiccups, easy vomiting.
Esophagus, cardiac sphincter relaxed.	Inflammation or spasms of the esophagus or cardiac sphincter.
Stomach slow, atonic.	Stomach spasm, distention, or irritation.
Small intestine insufficiency, grayish stool.	Small intestine spasm, irritation, or inflammation.
Atonic large intestine with contracted sphincter.	Spastic large intestine with relaxed sphincter.
Liver in excess and painful, or contracted and insufficient. Stool brown to black.	Liver insufficient and distended. Waxy complexion; yellow stools.
Gallbladder supple, swollen, empties poorly.	Gallbladder spasm and pain. Migraines; constipation.
Spleen in excess, contracted.	Spleen insufficient, distended.
Pancreas insufficient and swollen. Grayish stool. Pancreatic diabetes. White stool (from relaxed small intestine).	Pancreas in excess and contracted (from small intestine excess).
Kidney contracted, congested, painful.	Kidney relaxed, atonic.
Urinary bladder relaxed; contracted sphincter. Urination infrequent to difficult.	Urinary bladder contracted; sphincter relaxed. Urination frequent or abundant.
Ovaries insufficient; menses insufficient. Contracted cervix.	Ovaries in excess; menses overabundant. Relaxed cervix.
Tendency to obesity.	Tendency to emaciation.
Frigidity, sexual calm.	Sexual overexcitation or obsession; vulvar pruritus.
Testicles insufficient or diminished. Non-erection (mostly daytime).	Testicles in excess or swollen.
Inability to get an erection (mostly daytime).	Prolonged erections (at night).
Rapid ejaculation.	Retarded ejaculation.
Adrenal excess.	Adrenal insufficiency.
Glossopharyngeal nerve inhibited.	Glossopharyngeal nerve hyperstimulated.

The command points are: for the sympathetic, *fengchi* (GB-20); for the parasympathetic, *tianzhu* (BL-10). Both are found at the nape of the neck. Note that the sympathetic system is stimulated by the pituitary, the adrenal medulla (adrenalin), thyroid, testicles and ovaries. It is inhibited by crataegus, and paralyzed by ergotoxin. It stimulates the suprarenals.

The parasympathetic system is stimulated by eserine and pilocarpine, and inhibited by atropine (belladonna). It stimulates the ovaries and testicles.

Chapter VIII

The Distribution of Energy (III)

Energy and Blood

I. Energy and Blood — II. Circulation (Arteries and Veins; Heart) — III. Spleen-Blood

I. Energy and Blood

A constant supply and regulation of energy is indispensable to the life of the organs and the tiniest cells. Circulation of energy through the meridians never ceases; however, if we have proven the energetic relationships existing between the meridians and the organs, as well as those between the parts of the body (muscles, nerves, bones, etc.) traversed by each meridian, it is only by deduction that we might consider that the cells themselves are also irrigated by the meridians.

There is another fluid, however, that also circulates ceaselessly throughout the body, and which has been exhaustively studied in the Occident: the blood, which ensures the nourishment of the tiniest cells and carries away their waste products. Perhaps we should examine whether this is not the agent of distribution of energy to the cells.

It is recognized that the blood distributes, to each cell, the chemical substances and hormones necessary for its function, while carrying away its waste products. But it also transports the albumin A molecule, which is absolutely specific and appropriate to the blood and tissues of each individual.

On the other hand, the Far East maintains that through the lungs the blood takes in the yang energy of activity and distributes it to the whole body. The air which enters the lungs is charged by the energy of the sun and stars. Recall that the lung is the only organ, along with the skin, which captures the energy of activity (yang energy). All other producer organs extract energy of inactivity (yin energy) from food and drink.

In order to understand these assertions, it is necessary again to cite passages from two ancient texts:

> *Humans receive, as life, the energy of heaven and earth. The energy of heaven, energy of yang activity, becomes vital energy (general name: **qi**); while the energy of the earth, energy of yin inactivity, transforms into blood (**xue**). (YXRM I, 41r)*

> *The origin is the Supreme-All which differentiates the two energies. East is yin. However, there is yang included in it as the treasure. Movement is yang. However, there is yin included in it as the root. (DACH IV, 16r)*

We can say that life is an alteration of two forces: rest and activity, cold and heat, etc.

Energy and blood respond to the alterations of two cosmic forces:

> *During the day the energy leads, the blood follows. During sunny days the energy leads, the blood follows it, the meridians accompany them. During dark days, the blood leads, the energy follows, the meridians rise again to their source. (DACH VII, 30r)*

These passages elucidate the true differences and connections between energy and blood. This knowledge is essential for guiding the manipulation of the energy.

The West reports the facts precisely and in great detail, yet does not make conscious connections between energy and blood. However, Western physiology does recognize what no one can help observing — the blood is altered as soon as it leaves the body, coagulating and changing form completely. The blood does not seem to lose its life entirely, though. Recent techniques allow measurement of emanations from the blood specific to each individual. The emanometer of Boyd, radiesthesia, etc., give startlingly precise indications on the functions of the individual from whom the blood has come.

Blood is made up of 45% living cells and 55% plasma. As with all cells, those in blood cannot function without a constant supply of energy. We must ask, then: what happens to a specific molecule with its atoms in perpetual movement when the blood, separated from the body and deprived of its energy supply, dies and disintegrates?

Physicians in the Far East treat the small intestine, spleen-pancreas and stomach in order to give full strength to the blood and increase longevity. The stomach dissolves the food; the small intestine synthesizes specific nutrients; the spleen purifies the blood; while the pancreas plays a digestive and glycogenic role.

The vital energy is carried by the blood to the cells. This energy may be the vital element within the atoms of specific molecules found in the blood. Sodium and potassium transported by the blood are found on each side of the cellular membrane. They play an important role as electrolytes in the complex operations of life.

The energy-blood ratio can be measured by noting the difference between the general pulses of the two wrists: all the pulses taken together on the left wrist represent blood, while those on the right represent energy.

It is possible to measure the intensity of the total energy through the two wrists. In addition, we can surmise the level of yang energy of activity or yin energy of inactivity by their relative proportions. We must further research the influence of the variations of these energies on the material elements which they animate.

Below is an account of the various blood constituents. Variations in their quantity can seriously modify the quality of the blood. This, in turn, will alter the blood's action on the vessels, heart and all that it supplies with energy and products. It will also alter the action of certain acupoints.

As noted above, blood contains 45% living cells and 55% plasma.

Blood cells.

Red blood cells (erythrocytes): about 5 million per cubic millimeter. The active element is not the cell itself, but the amount of hemoglobin within the cell. It is the hemoglobin which fixes oxygen. Iron is an essential element of this molecule although the lack of any one of these elements — protein, iron, traces of copper and cobalt — will produce anemia. The blood cells are formed in the red bone marrow of primarily the flat bones, e.g. the sternum and ribs. A sufficient supply of oxygen to the bone marrow is necessary in order to maintain the number of blood cells. There can be anemia of both quantity and quality of blood cells.

A urinary bladder meridian point, *gaohuangshu* (BL-38, IS BL-43), stimulates a constant increase and later growth in the number of blood cells and the level of hemoglobin. Another point, *xuanzhong* (GB-39), acts on the bone marrow.

The transport of carbon dioxide and the maintenance of its levels are considered important functions of the blood cells.

Erythrocytes survive for 120 days according to Main, for 47 days according to Frédéricq, and 21 days according to Hédon. The authors do not cite the length of time necessary for maturation. After acting on the energy by stimulation of *gaohuangshu* (BL-38, IS BL-43), we have determined through analyses that the blood is inundated with forming corpuscles, the matured state attained after fifteen to eighteen hours. When old and spent, the cells are destroyed in the reticuloendothelial system from which the spleen is largely formed. The fact that *gaohuangshu* acts effectively again only after the interval of a month indicates that the life of the blood cell is about five weeks.

White blood cells (leukocytes): numbered at about 5000 to 7000 per cubic millimeter. Not all have the same origin, and their names vary according to the author. We distinguish among them:

Polymorphonuclear leukocytes originate in the bone marrow. Their function is to destroy bacteria. A gallbladder point, *xuanzhong* (GB-39), stimulates an increase in their numbers. This point is also used to increase their activity in cases of inflammation with streptococcus and pus, septicemia, low fevers and above all abscesses and furuncles. Their life span is about twenty days. They are divided into neutrophils (65-70%), basophils (.5%) and eosinophils. The latter appear in certain diseases such as intestinal worms.

Mononucleocytes are errant cells analogous to reticuloendothelial tumor cells. They represent 3% of the leukocytes and originate in the bone marrow, spleen and liver. They abound when there are problems of the skin, such as psoriasis, eczema and impetigo. Their number and activity are augmented by tonifying *dadu* (SP-2) as well as the liver. (The liver, remember, is important in all skin ailments.)

The lymphocytes are formed in the lymph nodes. They make up about 20% of the leukocytes, yet their function is unknown. Foot-*linqi* (GB-41) has great power over the lymphatic ganglions. *Tianjing* (TW-10) and *jimen* (SP-11) exhibit a great effect on those of the inguinal nodes.

Reticuloendothelial cells: considered to be tumor leukocytes lodged in the bone marrow, liver, lymph nodes and spleen. They clean up the bacteria, foreign matter, used red cells and platelets.

Platelets (thrombocytes): without nuclei. These cells furnish the thrombokinase necessary for coagulation by disintegrating on contact with an injured surface. Removal of the spleen causes an increase in the number of platelets. Their constant excess may be the cause of hemophilia. Coagulation can be made much more rapid by tonifying the energy of the liver and large intestine (vitamin K).

Plasma (55% off the blood) contains many substances dissolved from protein (albumin, globulin, fibrinogen, antibodies, enzymes), some non-proteinic nitrogen (urea, uric acid, creatine, creatinine, amino acids, NH), diverse organic substances (glucose, lactates), some lipoids (cholesterin, lecithin, fat), hormones, some vitamins, gas (O_2, CO_2), and some elements of inorganic salts (Na, Ca, K, Mg, Fe, Cu, Cl, HCO_3, SO_4, PO_4, I, etc.).

Action on the energy can modify certain of these elements, particularly those which can cause problems.

Urea (normal .30 to .40) of which half is nitrogen: If insufficient, tonify the liver and the adrenals; if excessive (hypertension), disperse kidney filtration and the adrenals, tonify the pancreas.

Sugar (about 1.10): If excessive in the blood (diabetes), tonify the pancreas, disperse the adrenals, regulate the pituitary; if insufficient, disperse the pancreas, tonify the adrenals.

Cholesterin (about 1.50): If excessive, disperse the gallbladder, liver, spleen, adrenals; if insufficient, tonify the adrenals and spleen. Irradiated, it becomes ergosterol (vitamin D).

Calcium: Insufficient in the blood, tonify the parathyroid, disperse the adrenals; if excessive in the blood (cloudy urine), disperse the parathyroid, tonify the adrenals.

There is a balance between blood (ionized Ca) and bone (soluble Ca), and between Ca and phosphorus.

Phosphorus: If insufficient, disperse the parathyroid; if excessive (cramps, neuralgia, tics, etc.), tonify the parathyroid.

Potassium: in the case of excess, tonify the adrenals; if insufficient, disperse the adrenals.

Salt: In excess, disperse the adrenals; in insufficiency, tonify the adrenals.

II. Circulation (Arteries, Veins, Heart)

Arteries, veins.

The blood and the energy which it distributes are carried throughout the entire body and to the cells through the vascular network.

Energy is essential to the harmonious functioning of the cardiovascular system. Specific command points can modify the energy directed to the various parts of this system. By studying these command points we have arrived at some useful classifications and have further clarified the role of the vital energy in circulation.

Changes in arterial contraction may activate or slow down blood circulation. These modifications may be obtained by 1) inducing a relative dominance of either the parasympathetic system (contraction) or sympathetic system (relaxation); 2) stimulating or inhibiting the vitality of the adrenals (excess: contraction; insufficiency: relaxation); 3) stimulating kidney excretion (vasopressin: contraction) or by provoking their relaxation.

Naturally, the blood volume is of great significance. Blood volume can be: 1) Relative and proportional to the contraction of the arteries. It depends, therefore, on the energy causing vasoconstriction, either directly via the autonomic system or through the intermediary adrenal hormones or the kidney. 2) Real and due to an excess of salt and ingested liquids. This may depend on hygiene and the aid of diuretics. Manipulation of the energy may be used for correcting the root causes — the desire to drink, or retaining salt (regulate adrenals) or water (kidney filtration).

The special command point of the carotid sinus, *lingdao* (HT-4), adds a useful tool. We ask acupuncturists to confirm this.

The arteries, veins and vessels are commanded by the heart governor meridian, thus named because of its dual action on the circulation through the vessels and sexual organs. They are commanded also through a point of the lungs, *taiyuan* (LU-9). It appears that certain points command more specifically the vessels and others, the sexual organs. Their interaction is marked enough to separate them, though with difficulty.

The pulse of the vessels is one of two pulses of the heart governor (right wrist, section III, middle level), arteries on the interior half, veins on the upper half. (The pulse of the sexual organs is right wrist, section III, deep level.)

The pulse of the vessels is in constant and indisputable relation with the condition of the arteries and veins, be it contraction, relaxation, hardness, suppleness or inflammation. The pulse is modified, as stated previously, by the command points of the parasympathetic, sympathetic, adrenals, kidneys, lungs and its own command points. The pulse of the veins is altered by the command points of the stomach and spleen-pancreas.

We are led, then, to study the energy which animates the vessels themselves, the muscles of their sheath; and the internal energy brought by the blood into the cells. The Far East differentiates these as the external energy of activity, of expenditure (yang) outside of the arteries and the energy of inactivity, of recuperation (yin) carried by the blood. Verification by instrumentation has yet to be carried out.

The heart.

The heart meridian is the only one attracting attention in the West, although not as a meridian per se, but by the fact that the pain of angina exactly follows the length of the upper limb along the course of the meridian. It starts from the heart and ends at the extremity of the little finger, last phalanx, on the ring-finger side.

The pulse which reflects it is on the left wrist, section I, deep level. The radial side reflects the left side of the heart, receiving the blood from the lungs and sending it into the arteries; the medial side, the right side of the heart, receives the venous blood and sends it to the lungs.

The circulatory functions of the heart are known in both continents, but there are differences regarding the energetic and psychological role of the organ. In the West, the heart is synonymous with sensitivity, affectivity, courage. In Asia, it is synonymous with cleverness, and they teach that it is through the heart that the brain is irrigated. In fact, the vigor of the brain does drop at the same time as that of the heart. The *Nei Jing* states:

> *The heart is the home of the evolved man (reason, moral consciousness), of vitality and sexual energy; also, it nourishes speech. When it is firm and vigorous, illness cannot easily invade the body.*

The psychological modifications obtained by tonifying the heart to harmonize fullness are optimism, gaiety, enthusiasm, vitality. The eyes shine, there is an animated complexion and the body is erect. Insufficiency of the heart observed by instruments and pulses is accompanied by sadness, fear, timidity, discouragement, delusions to the point of anxiety and also distraction and boredom. Physically there is lassitude, sudden grey fogs to the point of cerebral anemia and also regretfulness with remorse. If there is excess, there are fixed ideas, hallucinations with violence, hyperexcitation and even insanity.

With inhibitions of the unconscious, treat *tongli* (HT-5). For depressions and encephalitis with headache and diplopia, use *shaohai* (HT-3).

Congestive or nervous crises: *xinxi* (HT-6).

Cold, aversion to cold water: *lingdao* (HT-4). Cold and weakness of the fingers: *shaohai* (HT-3).

Fevers with agitation of the heart, palpitations: *shenmen* (HT-7).

In Western physiology, the sympathetic system increases the heart rate and strength of the beats. It also produces dilation of the coronary arteries. The parasympathetic system decreases the heart rate and its strength of contraction (particularly of the auricle). It additionally contracts the coronary arteries and the peripheral arteries and veins. According to Main: ''The fibers of the left vagus go principally to the A-V node; its stimulation can produce cardiac block.''

The relative insufficiency-excess of the heart can thus be established:

Insufficiency	Excess
Heart weak or slow, arrhythmia, intermittence, irregularities.	Strong palpitations, pains, inflammations, endocarditis, pericarditis, myocarditis.
Hypotension.	Hypertension.
Fear, timidity, emotional agitation with trembling, frozen by emotion, passive phobias.	Energetic, courageous, audacious if in excess, redness and agitation from emotion; mental and physical hyperexcitation.
Sadness, depression, regrets, remorse, anxiety, inhibitions.	

Insufficiency	**Excess**
Cold, aversion of cold; cold hands, white.	Always hot, does not fear cold water.
Muffled voice, dull eyes, sad.	Sonorous voice, brilliant eyes, vital complexion.
Insufficiency of all the organs, particularly liver and spleen.	Activity of all the organs to the point of congestion and excess.
Insufficient menses.	Excessive menses.
Clear, frequent urine, or insufficient.	
Ganglia.	

The meridian is on the internal (yin) aspect of the upper limb. The pulse is found on the left wrist, section I, deep, yin level. The upper part of the pulse reflects the ventricles; the inferior part, the auricles. The maximum time is at noon (minimum hour of the gallbladder); its minimum is at midnight (maximum hour of the gallbladder). Mother: spleen-pancreas. Child: small intestine, which is also the coupled meridian. Herald point: *juque* (CV-14). Assent point: *xinshu* (BL-15). The wife is the lung.

I have discovered that the ventricles respond to *shaochong* (HT-9), the auricles to *yuji* (LU-10) and *xiabai* (LU-4).

III. Spleen-Blood

The spleen and pancreas, we must repeat, together have a single meridian. Although they have two pulses, there are multiple interactions between them.

The action of the spleen-pancreas on the psyche, which the use of command points allows us to observe, is described in Part II, Chapter III of this volume.

The action on the blood, the vehicle of the internal, yin energy, was described by the *Nei Jing* accordingly: "The spleen-pancreas takes the blood, purifies it and then returns it to the other organs."

The ancient Chinese ideogram designates the entire spleen-pancreas. The West does not accept that the pancreas takes part in this purification of the blood.

Extensive research has been carried out on the destruction of the red blood cell and the filtration of foreign matter. It has been deduced (Main) that this destruction is carried out by a lysin whose action increases with the duration of contact with the blood.

The fact is that the breakdown of red blood cells increases when the spleen is distended. By acting on the energy, we have observed that a distended spleen is always accompanied by a barely perceptible spleen pulse, a common sign of serious insufficiency. After tonification of the spleen, the organ returns to its normal size, the red blood cells no longer decrease in number or amount of hemoglobin, and the signs of lassitude and lack of concentration disappear. The destruction of the cells does not represent the excess of a specific function of the spleen, but rather a mechanical filtration which increases when the filter increases in size. The psychological function of the spleen is a vital one and diminishes with the weakening of the organ.

The role of the spleen as a reservoir for holding blood is well known. Experimentation on this aspect of the spleen is not extensive enough to cite key issues and commentaries. We do know that the spleen empties of blood during exercise and digestion.

Since the quality of the blood has great influence on the energy, the role of the spleen is vitally important in its action on lassitude arising from energetic deficiency. The spleen also exhibits a strong effect on the evolved man (frontal lobes), which can restore energy.

Chapter IX
Occasional Stimulants of Energy

The Endocrines

I. Endocrines and Energy — II. Pituitary — III. Adrenals — IV. Thyroid — V. Parathyroid

I. Endocrines and Energy

We believe we have made an important discovery regarding the endocrine glands and energy: the pulses give a functional indication of each of the four main endocrine glands. Through the pulses, we can enhance our knowledge of the action and interaction of these endocrine glands and note changes occurring after clinical use of their related hormones.

Perhaps the most significant observation is that stimulation of the command point of a given endocrine gland normalizes production of the single hormone produced in abnormal quantities by this gland; the others do not respond to the stimulation. This has been especially noted of the pituitary gland, which produces more than thirteen hormones, several of which oppose each other in function. This is also true of the feedback interaction of one hormone to another. Among the other endocrines influenced, only the one needed will respond.

We know that the power of these hormones is extraordinary at incredibly minute levels. It is acknowledged (Dale, Hédon) that pituitary hormones induce the contraction of the uterus *in vitro* in Ringer's solution with only one hundred billionth of a dilution (equivalent to the fifth or sixth centesimal homeopathic solution).

We also know that the quantities produced by the endocrines are not constant in all circumstances. In cases of external or internal excitation, e.g., emotion, shock, cold or heat, discharges are produced which stimulate the functions under their action for short periods. They are intermittent stimulants of energy.

It is not believed that reserves are retained in the body. Rather, it appears that when the need passes, the quantities dispersed throughout the blood are eliminated.

Stimulation of the command point of a given endocrine gland will regulate hormonal production: in case of an overall insufficiency, this stimulation will return hormone production to normal, full levels; in the case of an external or internal excitation, this stimulation causes the gland to secrete one or more of its necessary hormones at the exact instant they are needed and in a quantity marvelously precise and infinitesimally small. This assures their effect without risk of either excess or insufficiency.

Finally, the importance of the endocrines is illustrated by the fact that extirpation of the pituitary gland (Hédon) or thyroid causes death. Main writes:

> [The hormone's] prolonged (chemical) administration generally causes the atrophy of the gland which produces the hormone. For example, androgen produces atrophy of the interstitial cells, probably by inhibition of the pituitary gonadotropin. Desoxycorticosterone, although not representing all the hormones of the adrenal cortex, causes its atrophy, however, perhaps through the inhibition of the pituitary corticotropin.

We know that the ingestion for only a few days of adrenalin causes sclerosis of the arterial walls and weakening of its endocrine gland. Such a danger is not to be feared when acupuncture is used to maintain normal levels by re-establishing the natural function of each endocrine gland.

The liver, here also, plays an important role in regulating the action of certain hormones. It detoxifies them through transformation into a less active form. Thus, testosterone is transformed by the liver into androsterone, and estrodiol is transformed into estrone (Main). The action on the energy must make use of this function of the liver, since it has been remarked that after tonifying the liver energetically, autointoxication seems to decrease or disappear.

The ability to measure the function of the endocrine glands through the pulse and to regulate hormone production through action on the energy should greatly enhance future studies in endocrinology. Indeed, this field is a difficult one, especially given the following facts regarding the endocrine glands:

1)   Each may secrete more than one hormone; the pituitary, for example, secretes more than thirteen.

2)   As previously stated, the use of chemical hormones atrophies the gland. The chemical hormone can have the same formula as the human hormone while not possessing all its elements.

3)   They stimulate or inhibit one another. The immediate modification of the pulses allows us to observe and determine this. For the hormones which are ingested or injected, however, only the results allow us to judge.

4)   Certain endocrine functions are dependent on prior action by another gland; e.g., adrenalin is released only after the parathyroids have first increased the calcium in the blood; the ovaries respond fully only after gonadotropin has been released from the pituitary.

Thus, it is often sufficient to tonify the pituitary for the ovaries to return to their full function, true also of the thyroid, corticoadrenals, kidneys and liver. At the same time there will be contraction of the vessels, of the smooth muscles, etc.

The word "endocrine" means internal secretion. Some authors, taking this literally, have put under this label any secretion which pours into the blood, be they secretions from the liver, pancreas or even parasympathetic and sympathetic systems, which are not really glands. Of course, the pituitary, adrenals, thyroid, parathyroid, ovaries and testicles are included under this label.

It is clear that one must study the ovaries and testicles as important sources of sexual energy — their insufficiency and excess act on procreation as well as on the male or female psychological characteristics.

Below we will discuss the energetic functions of the pituitary, adrenal, thyroid and parathyroid glands. The following research, however, is beyond the scope of this work and not included:

1)   The exact nature of the hormones secreted and the food which contains useful elements.

2)   The sensitive mechanisms which activate production of one hormone and not another; those which establish the proper infinitesimal proportion of hormones.

3)   The mechanisms which determine when the hormonal effects are sufficient and regulate hormonal output. The processes which destroy or transform hormones not broken down in use.

Here, instead, we will discuss the multiple effects produced by stimulation of a given acupoint on the endocrine system. We will also discuss the organ or the part of the body which requires this temporary stimulation. The receptivity of the peripheral tissues plays a primary role.

The effects of tonifying or dispersing a command point of a given endocrine gland correspond well with endocrine research in the West. We must keep in mind that stimulation of a command point produces only the needed effects of those listed below. Likewise, only those organs disordered in some manner will respond. The endocrines work similarly — the hormones whose effects are needed are produced while the others are not.

Some command points act immediately on the whole endocrine system. All abnormalities in hormone production are normalized for the given individual.

Gaohuangshu (BL-38, IS BL-43): numerous blood analyses have shown an equilibrated and harmonious production of all the hormones. In addition, there is a general increase of red blood cells and hemoglobin and afterwards the presence of an element in the blood conferring a general immunity. China and Japan attribute to this acupoint only a great tonifying power.

Inferior side of the spinous process of the sixth cervical vertebra (between C6 and C7): I have discovered this acupoint after extensive experimentation. It is not mentioned in the Far Eastern texts. It will either tonify or disperse the pituitary, and through the latter, all the endocrines. The only hormones and endocrines which respond to this stimulation are the ones needed.

Leg-*sanli* (ST-36): by acting on the general energy and thus nervous centers, it also acts on all the endocrines.

A specific command point exists for each endocrine gland. By modifying the gland's supply of energy, this point can activate or inhibit its hormone production.

II. The Pituitary Gland

The command point which I believe I have discovered is on the inferior edge of the sixth cervical vertebra, bilaterally at the lateral angle of the medial tendon.

The pulse discovered is on the right wrist, section V, deep level, both sides of the artery. The point acts only on the pituitary hormones which are malfunctioning. This is an isolated action, useful as some of the hormones work in opposite ways — antidiuretic and pancreatrophin (vasopressin), lactogenic and mammotropin (prolactin), etc.

The measurement and management of the pituitary hormones is very much complicated by the interactions with the other endocrines. The pituitary is tonified by the sympathetic system, the adrenals and ovaries. It is dispersed by the ovaries and testicles. The pituitary itself tonifies all the other endocrines, the kidneys and the pancreas. It can also be used to disperse the pancreas. Urine flow can be diminished by it.

The relative insufficiency-excess of the pituitary is as follows:

Insufficiency	Excess
Lack of attention, absent, distracted, mental immaturity, proud; supple moral sense, diplomacy; easy fears; slow, apathy, lassitude, heaviness, asthenia (adrenals -).	Strong character, energetic, even aggressive; masculine women; needs to act, needs little sleep (adrenals +).
Muffled voice, mostly medium range.	
Growth hormone: small, grows late; small head, jaws, mouth, hands and feet. Teeth too tight, late in coming in; with age, teeth displaced forward, loose, fall out.	Tall, nose and chin too large, hands and feet large to the point of acromegalia, gigantism.
Vasopressin: hypotension, Particularly systolic (adrenals -). Capillaries and vessels relaxed (adrenals -, parathyroids -).	Hypertension, particularly systolic (adrenals +). Vessels and capillaries contracted (adrenals +).
Gonadotropin: insufficient ovaries, weak menses, frigidity, sterility; testicles insufficient, sexual diminution; late puberty; adiposity (ovaries -, testicles -).	Genital hyperexcitation; precocious puberty (testicles +). Women: ovaries excessive, abundant, frequent menses, migraine from menses (ovaries +).
Mammotropin (prolactin, lactogen): breasts too large.	Small breasts.
Oxytocin: weak lactation, uterine muscles relaxed.	Heavy lactation, menstrual spasms, uterine muscles contracted, vaginismus.
Vasopressin (antidiuretic hormone): insufficient urine (vasopressin +).	Abundant urine (vasopressin -).
Diabetogenic hormone: diabetes insipidus (vasopressin -).	Diabetes mellitus (diabetogenic +).
Premature balding.	Thick, abundant hair.
Intermedin: skin retains water and fat; cellulitis, becomes fat from excess work and insufficient food, gets thin from rest and abundant food; fatty anemia; eunichoid obesity, damp skin (sympathetic -, parasympathetic +); pale skin (intermedin -).	Emaciation; dehydration; dry skin (sympathetic +, parasympathetic -). Brown, dark skin (intermedin +).
Insufficient basal metabolism (pituitary -).	Excessive basal metabolism (pituitary +, thyrotropin, corticotropin +, thyroid + or -).

III. Adrenals

The command point of the adrenals, which we believe to have discovered, is *fengfu* (GV-15, GV-16), located bilaterally at the angle of the inferior edge of the second cervical vertebra and the medial tendon. This point acts on both glands and on two hormones that we know of (corticotropin and adrenalin), according to need. We have discovered a pulse on the right wrist, section V, superficial level; each side of the artery reflects one gland.

They are tonified by the pituitary, sympathetic system, thyroid, parathyroid and calcium. They are dispersed by the pancreas, and potassium.

They tonify the pituitary and the sympathetic system, and retain salt; they disperse the pancreas, liver (sugar), thyroids and ovaries; they release potassium.

One adrenal gland can be in excess and the other insufficient.

There are two parts of each gland: 1) The cortex, which forms adrenocorticotropin (corticotropin), estrogen and androgen (in equal quantities up to puberty, then that particularly specific to the sex). Retains salt, excretes potassium. 2) The medulla, which produces adrenalin (which has a bad effect without calcium). Its artificial use for several days causes sclerosis of arterial tissues, and atheroma.

Insufficiency	Excess
Apathy (corticotropin -, Na -, K +, pituitary -) shock. Asthenia, non-resistance to force, to infections, to cold (adrenals -, pituitary -). Slow recuperation. Slowness, heaviness, fatigue (adrenals -, pituitary -). Coldness, cold extremities, damp (adrenals -, pituitary -). Work is difficult and slow (adrenals -, thyroid -). Needs sleep, poor sleep, tired in the morning (spleen -, pancreas -).	Active, energetic, (adrenals +, pituitary +, potassium -). Resistance to force, shock, infections, cold (adrenals +). Heat, irritability; works without stopping, needs to act (adrenals +, pituitary +). Needs little sleep, gets up early (adrenals +).
Thinness with weakness (pituitary -).	Fullness; hypertonic obesity.
Weak muscles, non-excitable (corticotropin -, pituitary -, parathyroid +).	Muscles strong, excitable to the point of pain or contractions (corticotropin +, pituitary +, parathyroid +).
Blood coagulation slow (liver -, large intestine -). Insufficient blood volume; hypotension (adrenals -, pituitary -). Heart slow, or rapid and small (adrenals -, thyroid -). Block or fibrillation (adrenals -, potassium +).	Blood coagulation rapid (liver +, large intestine +). High blood volume (sodium +, urea +). Strong and rapid heartbeat. Vessels have increased tone, hypertension to the point of sclerosis. Capillaries contracted.
AV node conduction insufficient. Lax vessels, hypotension. Contracted coronary vessels. Permeable capillaries. Edema (adrenals -, pituitary -). Cutaneous arterioles. Raynaud's syndrome (pituitary -).	Cutaneous arterioles contracted (pituitary +). Coronary arteries relaxed.
Increased urine quantity, diminished color; retains fewer salts and urea (adrenals -, pancreas -, testicles -).	Quantity of urine diminished, deeper color. Excess urea, retains salt (adrenals +, corticotropin +). Acute edema of the nose, blocked nose. Pulmonary edema.
Convulsions from excess insulin to the point of coma (corticotropin -).	Burning of stomach one hour after meals or after sweets to the point of adrenokinetic diabetes (pancreas -, corticotropin +).

Corticotropin decreases insulin and sugar production of the pancreas and augments sugar production of the liver.

Insufficiency	Excess
Androgen insufficiency (men) and estrogen insufficiency (women). Ovaries insufficient, large breasts, insufficient menses (pituitary -, ovary -).	Ovaries in excess, small breasts, abundant and frequent menses (pituitary +, ovary +).
Mydriasis, exophthalmia (pituitary +, thyroid +).	
Insufficient basal metabolism.	Excessive basal metabolism.

IV. Thyroid

There are several command points for the thyroid which we believe we have discovered: at the inferior edge of the fourth cervical vertebra, bilaterally along the medial tendon; also, *huagai* (CV-20).

I have also discovered its pulse, on the right wrist, section V, middle level, inferior part; each side of the artery reflects one lobe.

Its hormone, thyroxine, acts at about one six millionth in the blood. It is tonified by the pituitary (thyrotropin), parasympathetic system, and iodine; it is dispersed by the parathyroids, sympathetic system, adrenals, insufficiency of iodine and zinc; it is antagonized by paraxanthin.

It tonifies the sympathetic, pituitary and adrenals; it disperses the parathyroids (eliminates calcium and retains phosphorus).

The relative insufficiency-excess of the thyroid is as follows:

Insufficiency	Excess
Slow comprehension, weakened intelligence, memory slow and insufficient, apathy (parathyroid -).	Rapid understanding, quick but superficial intelligence; sensitive, passionate; quick but unreliable attachments; easy rage, egoistic; anxiety, insomnia.
Heart slow, hypotension.	Rapid heart rate, tachycardia, hypertension.
No appetite, gains weight, does not burn calories.	Continual appetite, emaciation, burns calories too quickly.
Insufficient menses (pituitary -). Sterility.	Abundant menses; sexual hyperexcitation.
Dull, sunken eyes (parasympathetic +, sympathetic -). Swelling under the eyes or even of the face.	Eyes too bright, bulging (sympathetic +).
Cellulitis.	Red skin.
Pale mucus membranes.	Red mucus membranes and lips.
Receding gums, late dentition.	Decalcified teeth, frequent caries, protruding upper teeth.
Nails dull, soft (parathyroid -).	Bright, hard nails (parathyroid +).
Insufficient basal metabolism.	Excessive basal metabolism.
Cold in the eyes or teeth. Cold skin.	Always hot, sensitive to heat, heat flushes (pituitary +, adrenals +).

Instability: sudden crises, congestions, secretions, asthma, migraines, urticaria, eczema.

V. Parathyroids

The command points for the parathyroids, which we believe we have discovered, are at the inferior edge of the fifth cervical vertebra: two points, each on the angle between the vertebra and the medial tendon. The pulse is on the right wrist, section V, middle level, superior part, each edge of the artery reflecting each lobe.

They are tonified by the pituitary, and dispersed by the thyroid.

The parathyroids tonify the pituitary, the ionized calcium of the blood and the liver. They disperse the thyroid, the soluble calcium of the bone, phosphorus and the adrenals (salt).

In fact, by their action on calcium, they assure an equilibrium 1) between calcium of the blood and of the bone; 2) between calcium of the blood and phosphorus (Ca 5mm: P 100); and 3) between calcium of the blood and salt (Ca 2: Na 100).

Vitamin D in small doses increases blood calcium and thus acts in the same manner as tonifying the parathyroids. In strong doses, vitamin D acts in the same manner as dispersing the parathyroids — calcium in the blood is diminished while more is deposited in the bone.

The relative insufficiency-excess of the parathyroids is as follows:

Insufficiency	Excess
Insufficiency of ionized calcium in the blood; excess of phosphorus in the blood.	Excess of ionized calcium in blood; insufficiency of phosphorus.
Anxiety, fear; nightmares, aversion to the night; agitation, mental instability.	Indifference, calm, sadness, depression.

Insufficiency

Hyperesthesia; strong and easy neuralgia; hypersensitivity of the arm on pressure.

Itching, pruritus.

Muscles tense, tics, trembling, blinking, convulsions, eclampsia, spasms, stiffness, contractures (adrenals +).

Heart and vessels contracted (adrenals +). Spasmodic hypertension, arterial spasms (adrenals +, pituitary +).

Insufficiency of the thyroid, liver, small intestine.

Large intestine, ureters contracted.

Always hot (thyroid +).

Excess

Diminished sensitivity to pain, less subject to pain.

Muscles weak, soft (adrenals -, pituitary -). Blackouts or epileptic falls, sudden weakness.

Hypotonic heart and vessels, capillaries lax and permeable (adrenals -, pituitary -). Cell permeability diminished. Less edema (adrenals -).

Thyroid, liver, small intestine in excess.

Large intestine, ureters relaxed.

Alternately hot and cold.

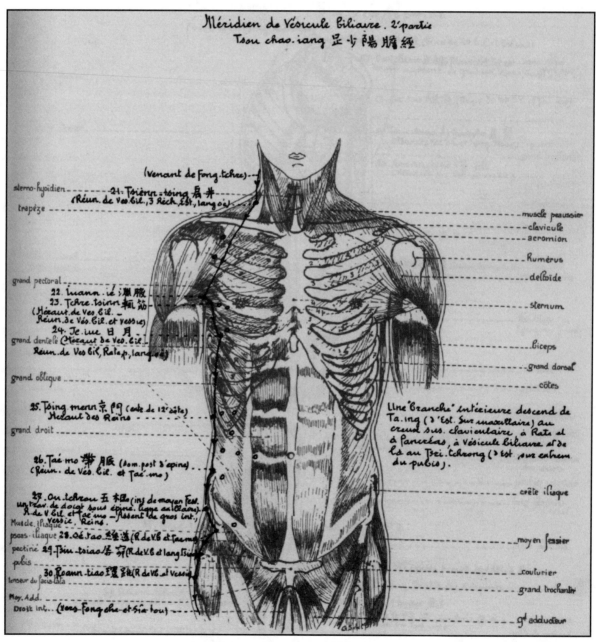

Meridian of the gallbladder (part 2) (GSDM)

Part III

Action on the Energy

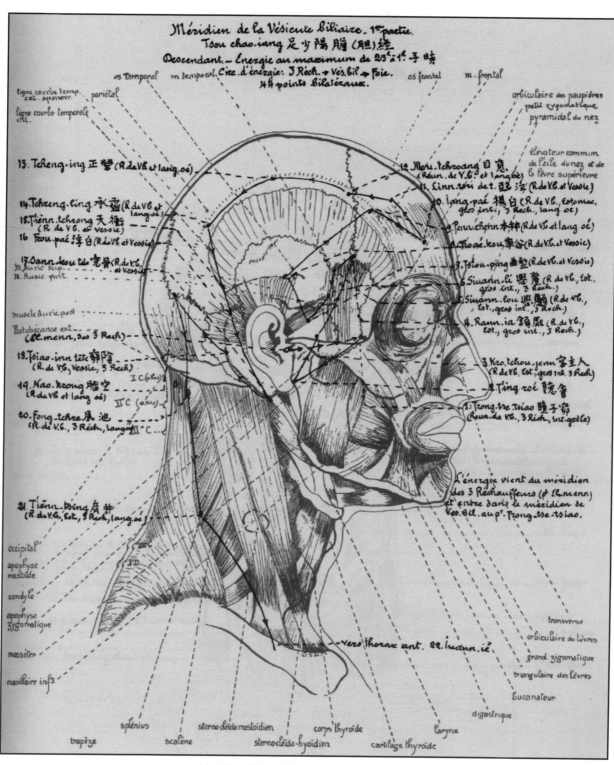

Meridian of the gallbladder (part 1) (GSDM)

Chapter I

Action on the Energy (I)

The Laws of Action on the Energy

The practical knowledge of vital energy has made apparent the importance of the universal law under which all things are subsumed — the law of yin-yang relativity. We can have knowledge of things only through their differences. If all were identical, we could know nothing; we perceive only relativities. This law also profoundly governs the science of energy, for the understanding of apparent relations as well as for the conception of what must be done to correct the relative dysfunction.

The first application to energy is that it exists for us by reason of its greater or lesser intensity, that is, of its excess-insufficiency relativity — the one or the other being relative to the individual and to circumstances. This is a notion of considerable importance, because from the beginning it determines the cause and the method to use.

This relativity of more and less, or yin-yang, demands considerable attention. A so-called illness can have one or the other of two opposite causes. Thus, there is a myopia with protruding eyes, which is an excess, and myopia with sunken eyes, which is an insufficiency. To act on both in the same manner would risk one being treated in reverse, either checking or aggravating it.

The result of this is the absolute necessity of perceiving clearly the possible measures of excess or insufficiency. The radial pulses are the most complete measure, the most detailed and the most sure. Their precise knowledge and careful use before, during and after all action is of the greatest importance for those who want to act without failure. Without the guidance of the pulses there is no science of energy; there are only ''tricks'' and some rote formulae which are used with risk.

It is for this reason that it is indispensable to absorb thoroughly the implications of the law of relativity on the notion of illness. ''The illness is not the invader; rather, it is the problem which invites the invader.'' Without the patient, there is no illness. If the whole body, or one of its parts, or some cells are deprived of their regular, constant and harmonious supply of indispensable energy, they wither and can resist neither disaggregation nor exterior forces. With a completeness of energy the being remains intact, adapting itself immediately. It is in this way that we remain alive. It is not a question of an exterior illness-entity having an independent existence of its own. The illness is only the expression and consequence of the disturbance of energy, more or less, in that part of the individual that does not have a harmonious supply of vitality and begins to disintegrate.

While the cause is always an insufficiency or an excess, we must know how and where ''to tonify'' and ''to disperse'' in order to correct it; i.e., we must know how to re-establish the harmonious supply of energy and the equlibrium of the yin-yang energies.

But this action is complex. We must know which command of the body is necessary to which meridian and to which point to address ourselves, and whether we must act on the mental or physical plane. We must also evaluate the reaction of the patient; action and reaction are relative.

The interactions of the organs cause any action upon a single organ to act on two others in the same way, and also on two others in the opposite way, with two local actions able to neutralize or add to the effect.

Finally, there are the points which command either the whole body, or all the energy of activity, or all the energy of inactivity, or which cause the excess of the producer organs to pass into the insufficiency of the distributor organs and vice versa. Also, there is the point which commands all the disturbed organs. To ignore them is to forego a great aid; to use them inappropriately will upset the entire system.

The means of action itself must be chosen according to the possible reaction of the subjects, their age, constitution, the season, etc.

The task is not easy. To learn is not enough; we must understand each case and each subject.

Chapter II

Action on the Energy (II)

The Illness Defined by the Battle Against It

I. Classification of the Battles — II. Homeopathy and the Science of Energy

I. Classification of the Battles

What is the "illness" we must combat to help the action of the energy? It is difficult, if not impossible, to glean from the innumerable and scholarly works on illness a description of this enemy itself; rather, we can find only some definitions of the word. Thus it comes to mind to study the problem in another way: by considering the many methods used to fight against this multifarious evil.

The battles themselves can be classified according to the goal they try to reach. Their strategy illustrates their conception of the enemy they combat. However, one should not forget, "Without patients, no illnesses."

1) *The enemy is immaterial.* Behind the different words used, the same idea is always found: there is an invasion, either by an imaginary being itself, or by its power, influence, obsessions, etc. Let us briefly note:

At the beginning of history and in primitive populations, the illness was either the devil himself or "a spell cast." We terrify the demon by incantations, war dances, the terrible cure of the drums, the screams of the sorcerers. For spells there are icy baths, passage through the flames, etc; results must have been obtained, because these methods have not been abandoned.

In the Middle Ages, there was the battle against the devil and the use of mysterious medicines transmitted from antiquity and considered to be magic. Among the means used was the *auto-da-fé* of the Inquisition: the illness-devil was burned with the patient.

These days, exorcisms, which are much more numerous than we might imagine, sometimes give excellent results against the compulsion to do evil, the persecuting wrath of paranoiacs — the "executioners of the family," as the great neurologist Gilbert Robin writes.

What once was called "spells" and what now is called possession, compulsions or obsessions, phobias, false ideas, etc., are treated successfully by the true methods of lay exorcism: psychoanalysis, psychiatry, Christian Science, etc. The causes of mental illnesses treated in this way are badly defined, but the problems are still considered as being outside the patient.

When the "illness" is characterized by monomania, phobia, madness, etc., and becomes extreme, the battle consists of confinement in a sanitarium with similar treatment as in the old days: cold baths and electric shocks, instead of the passage through flames (which might also be a great shock), etc.

We laugh at the books of the Middle Ages which minutely describe the names, the appearance, the customs, the subtle attacks of each of the demons. But in front of the pyre, there was no laughter.

There was always the old medicine, scientific and clear, from Hippocrates and Galen. Until the eighteenth century, however, it was quickly obscured by the qualifying ideas of magic. It became allopathy and, with the help of living plants which had effects known for millennia, it fought illnesses defined by their appearances. Each one had a summarizing name. "The magisterial prescription," which was carefully adapted to the patient and to the form of the illness, is not practiced any more. Already, allopathy does not show the illness as an exterior entity, but as a cluster of symptoms, of personal reactions of the subject to the exterior elements — cold, heat, food, drinks.

The illustrious Trousseau relates an experience which merits our consideration in the battle against disease. In his inaugural lecture from the Chair of Therapeutics he recounted how, after thirty years of directing the services of a clinic, he asked himself if the results he obtained were truly due to the value of the medications. The following year, in order to judge, he stopped all medication. Then, he said, he formally observed that without medicines, the cures were more rapid and more complete. He could explain this fact only by noting that the patients did not have to cure themselves of the medicines. We might suggest that the medicines create a new illness destined to combat the first. Would the medicine thus constitute an exterior ally, coming to chase away the occupant, but causing additional damage in the process?

2) *The enemy is material:* With modern "pasteurism" we clearly have the conception of a material, exterior enemy having its own life and "seeking something to devour": the microbe. But while the characteristics of the life and customs of the imaginary demons were based before on the declaration of the patient (sorcerers, etc.), and from the

confusion after torture, we now have numerous scholarly works describing appearances and behaviors of the microbes. Just as we always combated the demon, now microbes also are "tamed." We use them as allies and inject them into the blood to combat the occupants, the "untamed" microbes.

Our epoch has renounced the idea of elimination of the "peccant humours" of Molière, which is now a laughable idea. The Faculty does not preach bleeding and purgation anymore. By a natural mental process, this ridicule has moved French medicine away from the Latin (still used by all other countries) and has thrown it into the Greek, from which are formed almost all the new barbarisms of medicine and science. Let us recall that Washington, suffering from digestive trouble, was killed in twelve hours by a bleeding of 2.8 liters; Byron, having resisted eight days of diet and purgation, was killed on the eighth day by a bleeding of 2 litres.

To clarify the profound affective tendency of the battle against illness, the invading enemy, it is possible to do a close comparison between the idea of burning the possessed to destroy the demon and what now renders such services: remove the occupant by operating on the occupied organ, or by destroying it with X-rays.

Finally, in our Faculties, pathology and therapeutics are taught separately. The patient and the remedy are learned in a few months during seven years of study.

3) *There is no enemy.* Homeopathy, in its battle for health, reveals a totally new concept to the West. There is no exterior-illness entity which is the same for all. The individual is unique. Each one expresses his personal disequilibrium by a certain number of problems which are the signs of deep disequilibrium of the subject. There is fundamentally the observable similitude between the group of signs special to each person, and the signs of poisoning by a substance which has never been absorbed by the subject.

The battle consists of giving "dynamizations" of the substance for which the signs of poisoning are the same as those of the different troubles. These "dynamizations" fortify the energy of the patient; they do not combat anything.

Hahnemann bases his theories on the concept of the "terrain," the hereditary and ancestral constitution, with its "miasms," the actual value of which must evidently be re-examined. There is ancestral syphilis, vital weakness or psora, abnormal proliferations from hereditary gonorrhea or sycosis and a medical miasm from medicines. Each group of constitutions is more inclined to certain problems.

However, Hahnemann insists so strongly on the importance of mental symptoms that we are led to consider physical problems as the consequence of psychological reactions proper to each person faced with the difficulty of their existence.

Kollitch, an authorized commentator on Hahnemann, explains that the illness is a dynamic disequilibrium of the living being. It is a question of disturbances of the vital energy, translating themselves through the alterations of the physical and psychological functions.

It is exactly this idea which is at the basis of the science of energy. We shall see further some other relationships of great utility between these two concepts.

Conclusions

In the truest sense: "Without the patient, there is no illness."

In effect, very healthy people do not know what illness is and go through epidemics without being affected. Health is a natural immunity: the happy fullness of energy and of vitality.

The Far East has taught from great antiquity that all lesional problems are preceded by a more or less prolonged functional disturbance, and that the latter has been preceded by a derangement of the energy, either in excess or insufficiency. When intervention is undertaken in order to re-establish a harmonious and constant supply of energy, the functional troubles cease and the lesion heals and disappears (when possible).

The *Nei Jing* says:

> *The more than 445 illnesses are in reality only one — a derangement of energy; because they are all a consequence of this.*

A great treatise on energy, the *Da Cheng* of the sixteenth century A.D., says:

> *The hundreds of illnesses all start with the energy, then extend into the muscles, bones and organs through the meridians.*

Thus, there are no illnesses, but only disturbances of the energy.

Two important factors are thus apparent:

1) Many problems which replace or succeed each other have the same cause. Thus, migraines, eczema and asthma are caused by problems of the biliary passage (liver and gallbladder) which itself is caused by a sensitivity (instability of energy) to certain emotions acting on the psyche.

2) The same problem can come from different and sometimes opposite causes. Thus, myopia with enlarged eyes and myopia with sunken eyes; or obesity from excess food without activity, and that with excessive activity and insufficient food; or gout of the ''rich'' and gout of the ''poor.''

To utilize the same method of intervention for conditions that stem from opposite causes will in the one case obtain results by chance, and in the other case will aggravate the condition.

Microbes can live and proliferate only in a favorable terrain. The pasteurian diagnosis, which defines an exterior entity, a microbe to fight, does not exist in energy. It is replaced by the measure of the intensity of the energy, either total, multiple, or local, by the radial pulses — the potential of the vitality of the subject. Where the energy is in balanced fullness, the microbe dies.

In the science of energy, there is thus no battle against an ''illness,'' which does not exist in itself. There is only the material manifestation, proper to each person, of his energetic derangement. The whole art consists of knowing where the supply of energy is insufficient or excessive and of knowing how to equilibrate this supply, to put it back to the normal condition for each person. Thus, having known where the excess or the insufficiency is through the radial pulses, we stimulate or reduce the control of the area, which is deranged by stimulating in the appropriate way the special command point of the involved meridian.

II. Homeopathy and the Science of Energy

In the battle for health, homeopathy and the science of energy have some similarities that are useful to note. 1) Both recognize and study only the troubled subject who is himself different from any other. 2) The problem does not exist outside the unique patient since it can be produced from several causes and since each cause can produce several different problems. 3) Neither uses material substance which, according to Trousseau, creates an additional illness that the patient must cure along with the illness. This needs development:

In homeopathy, the substances given for the cure are not, properly speaking, medicines, but ''dynamizations of substances.'' Enemies of homeopathy, not wishing to understand its results, state that there is no material at all in these ''dynamizations.'' The instruments which have been perfected to register the strength of the dynamized substances and which distinguish them from dynamized water or alcohol under the same conditions prove that while there is no longer any matter, the energy remains. Is it not because we are ignorant of exactly what is energy, that we can deny effects that have been observed for more than 150 years?

This ''energy'' observed in the dynamizations is absolutely special to the substance from which it has been extracted. Likewise, each command point of the meridians has its special dynamic action which no material introduction of any substance can give.

Each dynamized product acts not upon a universal morbid entity, but upon the energy of the individual expressing its disequilibrium through numerous symptoms, syndromes or special problems affecting either the whole being, or its left or right half, or a group of organs, muscles, bones, or vessels, or one organ. In the science of energy, each command point acts in the same way.

Thus, homeopathy and the science of energy, by their insubstantial dynamization, cannot be thought of as destroying an enemy. They both must be seen and used to give to the ''form'' the local or multiple energy for correcting a malfunction of the vital strength, either total or partial; that is, they help the living being to give to each cell and group of cells the harmonious supply of energy without which all disintegrates and dies. Energetic disturbances cause the beginning of disaggregation, which is the functional trouble. If this disaggregation persists too long or too far, then a lesional problem is established, which is the death of a group of cells. The problem lies with the lack of resistance that allows the microbe to develop. It is not the microbe which causes the problem. This is the definition of ''illness'' for all action relating to the vital energy, which is special to each person.

Thus the ancient Chinese distinction is justified between: 1) Illnesses having a known duration that cure of themselves (five out of ten, even with microbes or functional disorders of one part of the body), which the energy of the form can correct by itself, mental and physical rest permitting the use of quantities of energy expended otherwise in work and worries. 2) Illnesses which do not cure themselves: deep and already lesional troubles of the form itself, too major for the patient's reserves alone.

The parallel action of both sciences is proven again by the identity of action of the dynamizations and of the command points. This is thanks to the discoveries made by Dr. Weihe, some fifty years ago. This scholar has shown, followed by Drs. Göhrum in Germany, Nebel in Switzerland, and Rouy, who has published in France, that when a certain syndrome is manifesting, a certain point of the body becomes painful on finger-pressure. So these "points of Weihe" are all exact Chinese points having an action almost identical to that of the dynamizations required by the syndrome.

A detailed comparison of the effects obtained by the points of Weihe and the command points has led me to discover that their lists complement one another. But the work must be done very scrupulously. It is too easy to affirm without verifying, to copy and copy badly.

One example is typical: a dynamization of *Raphanus sativus* is indicated for problems of the liver and spleen, gas and a curious aversion to children, particularly young girls; none of this is mentioned for *yutang* (CV-18) which is the Weihe point for *Raphanus sativus*. On the other hand, *yutang* has actions on the heart, respiratory passages and kidneys not mentioned for *Raphanus,* besides the common action of both on the stomach, etc. I examined some cases of swelling of the liver and spleen *(Raphanus)* accompanied by troubles of the heart, respiratory passages, stomach, intestines and kidneys *(yutang),* which I termed "syndrome of the eight organs." It is common in Asia and has been described in Germany for some years as "Roemheld's Syndrome." It was unknown in France (at least among the top specialists consulted) until the last edition (1952) of the *Dictionnaire Granier et Delamarre.* The idea came to me to stimulate the *yutang/Raphanus* concordant point. The result was immediate: the liver and spleen returned immediately to their normal size and their full function, ceasing to compress the stomach between them (gas, ptosis, sleeping after meals); above, the lungs (panting, false asthma), the heart (palpitations, embarrassment, false angina); below, the kidneys (prolapse, hypotension, pains) and the large intestine (constipation).

In many circumstances it has been possible for me to fill out each lists, from the other, and to obtain a more comprehensive effect.

There are some notable differences between homeopathy and the science of energy. Homeopathy studies the symptoms of the patient and searches for the same symptoms, the similimum in the effects of a substance; this similimum causes one to think of a syndrome that exists by itself as a reflection of the idea of an exterior illness entity, when in reality the remedy addresses itself to the constitutional tendency and the accidental failure of the energy.

The science of energy directly studies the disharmony of the flow of energy and corrects it. It teaches that each disharmony can manifest itself according to each individual (hereditary and infant constitution) through syndromes that are noticeably different from one another (temporary disturbances).

Homeopathy possesses its special symptoms, the *rubrics,* which indicate the remedy. The science of energy has pulses, which indicate the disturbed meridian and in what way to stimulate what point, when the patient and the therapist are not sufficiently sensitive to perceive the disturbance and the point by themselves.

Finally, let us mention that initially, for Hahnemann, the method of homeopathy was to look for the similimum in a single remedy, as the animist school still does today. One school, called "pluralist," tries to reach the similimum through several remedies, of which certain were "drainers." This clearly opposes the energetic action (which can be used without provoking reactions that cancel or multiply themselves) as it results in effects markedly different from the desired similimum effect.

There is still another difference: the knowledge of excess and insufficiency. However, many homeopaths teach that the low dilutions tonify and the high dilutions disperse. It would be enough, perhaps, if the homeopaths would be equal to acupuncturists in the method of distinguishing excess and insufficiency by the pulses, and to correct them by the proper dilutions.

On the other hand, it would seem that very sensitive people, by handling a homeopathic remedy, can tell on which organ and part of the body its principal action is, as we can say where the responses come by pressing on the pulses of the meridians.

In summary, the battles against illness can be classified into three groups:

1) Those addressed to the psyche, and through it to the physical organism.

2) Those designed to fight an exterior enemy, by addressing the physical body through shaking from shock, or through a new illness which forces it to fight (Trousseau) and which thus awakens the failing organism.

3) Those addressed directly to the vital force — total, multiple or local.

If we look closely, we will find that they all take their strength from the vital energy, and we are led to conclude that the so-called "illness" is in fact the proper manifestation for each individual of the disorder of their energy, of their vital force. This vital force no longer feeds, or feeds a region too much; the area begins to disaggregate and becomes suitable for the multiplication of the microbe.

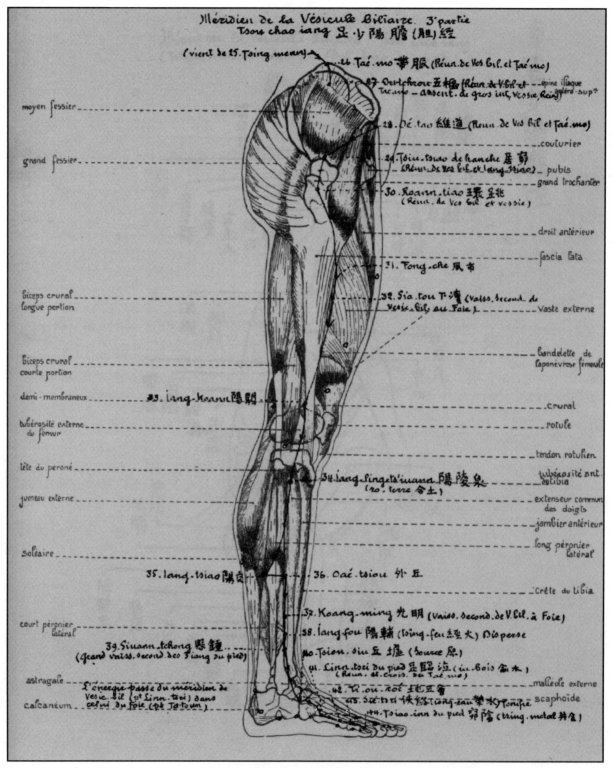

Meridian of the gallbladder (part 3) (GSDM)

Chapter III

Action on the Energy (III)

The Law of Relativity

I. The Law of Relativity — II. Insufficiency and Excess

I. The Law of Relativity

The law of relativity dominates all knowledge, all science. One can distinguish or discern things only through their differences, because it is on these differences that the action of energy is based. From high antiquity this law has been constantly studied and applied to all knowledge by the ancient Chinese under the name of *yin-yang;* these are the opposed and relative terms of all things.

In its relation with yang, yin is the negative pole: cold, humidity, heaviness, material, slowness, immobility, water, obscurity, night, low, the left, physical, the north face of the mountain, the shadow; decrease.

In its relation with yin, yang is the positive pole: warmth, dry, light, immaterial, quick, active, sunny, the day, the light, high, the right, mental, the south face of the mountain and the sun, increase.

One should not commit the error of attributing a separate existence to each of these opposite aspects. High exists only in relation to low and can be low for that which is higher; cold exists only in relation to warmth, etc. The whole universe obeys this dialectical yin-yang relativity, but alternating and opposed: day and activity for animals and plants, night and sleep for all that lives, temperature 0.5° C more at four in the afternoon than at four in the morning, etc.

II. Insufficiency and Excess

Applied to disturbances of energy, which are either general, multiple or local, and which manifest themselves through "illnesses," this law obliges us to observe that all illness, all disturbance of energy, can manifest itself through one of the two aspects of the excess-insufficiency relativity.

As soon as the intensity of the energy deviates from the equilibrium, from the normal fullness, it can only be insufficient or excessive.

Certain authors have spoken of "non-circulation," but by examining the question closely, one will notice that this non-circulation causes excess upstream and insufficiency downstream. If it is generalized, it is all the meridians which are in excess or insufficiency.

On the other hand, just as there is no yin or yang by itself, there is no insufficiency or excess by itself, but only in relation to the norm of each individual, a norm which is absolutely his own. Thus, a person can be in habitual perfect health with a blood pressure of 120/70, which would be accompanied by a great weakness and would be an insufficiency in a person having habitually 160/90. On the other hand, it would be an excess for someone in good health at 100/60. A temperature of 10° C. is cold for a Mediterranean person, but warm for an Eskimo; a weight of 5 kg. is heavy for an infant but light for a man; a heart beating at 60 can be properly full if that is its norm; it would be very slow for a person whose heart generally beats at 75.

Thus in order to act it is important to understand the insufficiency or excess for each person according to their norm. This knowledge, overall as well as in the detail of the moment, is given through the pulses. It remains relative to the lasting measure given by the physical and vital aspect of each person.

For example, large lymphatic types will have pulses that are soft and a little elevated, beating poorly; big vigorous types will have pulses that are supple, of average elevation and beating well; large, plethoric types who are in excess will have pulses that are hard, jerky and beating violently. These same distinctions can be seen in thin, exhausted people, or those who are normally vigorous, or hypernervous. Only what differs from these norms will be troubled, either for one pulse or for several.

Certain difficulties may be encountered; for example, if the totality of the pulses is without a beat, the first temptation is to think of insufficiency. But one should know that this total absence of perceptible beats can be caused by a contracture which is a serious excess (of the parasympathetic or adrenals). The pulses are then harder, the harder they are pressed. It can also come from complete exhaustion and continuing weakness (pulses are then not palpable even by pressing more and more), implying a serious insufficiency. The same difference can be found on the pulse of an organ, and this warrants attention.

For the whole organism, a table of the excess-insufficiency relative to perceptibly opposite troubles can be edifying.

Insufficiency	Excess
Empty, asthenic, apathetic, tired without cause, regains strength slowly; slow, heavy of mind.	Active, never tired or is able to regain strength very quickly; alive, light, quick of mind.
Sad, without gaiety, tired of everything.	Gay, enthusiastic, too happy, too agitated.
Slow, reactions slowed down or weak.	Lively, reactions too rapid, impulsive.
Dull, sad eyes.	Brilliant, alive eyes.
Pale, grey, tense face.	Alive complexion, warm, relaxed face.
Interior cold, cannot become warm; does not sweat; looks for sun and dryness.	Too hot, even in shadow, sweats easily, looks for shade and humidity.
Pale, cold extremities; difficult fever.	Extremities hot, easy and strong fever.
Annoyed, inattentive, distracted, cannot fix the attention and concentrate.	Interested in too many things, imagination always in movement.
Attenuated pains.	Intense, unbearable pains.

The pulse of the organ gives the measure for each organ, but this is relative to the other pulses and to the individual. A pulse of an organ can be elevated, a sign of excess, but will not be in excess if usually all the other pulses are elevated equally.

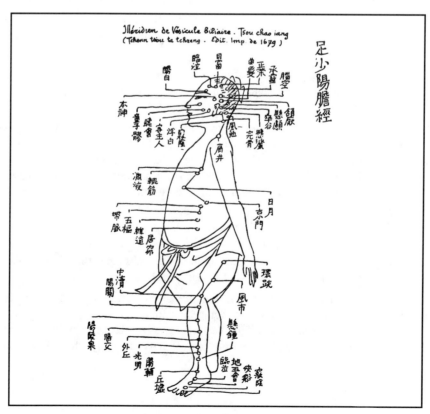

Meridian of the gallbladder (DACH)

Chapter IV

Action on the Energy (IV)

Measures of Insufficiency and Excess. Significance of the Radial Pulses

I. Multiple Aspects of the Pulses — II. Ensemble of the Two Wrists — III. Relativity of the Two Wrists — IV. Relativity of the Three Levels of Blood Pressure — V. Location, Aspects and Significance of Each Pulse of the Organ Meridians

The explanations of the pulses have been given in Chapter III, Part I, of this volume. Here, only their significances are explained.

Since all disturbances of energy — either total, multiple or local — can only manifest through insufficiency or excess, it is essential that we know how to differentiate one from the other, and how to recognize dysfunctional organ meridians. For that, we must know how to observe the constant and precise indications which the radial pulses can give and to how to interpret them well. Without this knowledge it is singularly audacious and even dangerous to dare, while in the dark, to modify any part of the mechanism which is so complex and intricate, and which regulates the production, distribution, etc., of the energy, consequently modifying all the functions of the body and mind.

I. Multiple Aspects of the Pulses

The radial pulses are linked to the higher centers and the organs through the autonomic nervous system. The pulses constantly reflect the functions of the autonomic nervous system and are instantly modified at the same time as the organs and higher centers. If there is an excess, it will be shown on the pulse and in the form that this excess can assume (congestion or inflammation, contracture, etc.). If, on the other hand, there is an insufficiency, the different forms (weakness, distention, etc.) which it can take will be represented at the pulse.

It is enough to have expertise in discriminating the different qualities that can be perceived in a pulse relative to other pulses, and to be able to judge the function of each organ. The interpretation of these qualities is complicated by the fact that one pulse cannot represent a simple quality: it represents always a combination of two, three or more qualities. This fact makes it difficult to construct an apparatus that registers so many different qualities at the same time, a task so easily performed by the fingers.

An apparatus may show the elevation of a pulse, but not its hardness, and if it registers the hardness, it will be inadequate for the width, etc. It seems that only with the fingertips can one discern each of the combined qualities, and study each simple quality that enters into combination. These important qualities and their significance are as follows:

1) *Height.* Elevated: abundance of energy, also great pain. Low: weakness.

2) *Resistance.* Soft (easily compressed): insufficiency of blood, atony of the organ. Hard: excess, contraction of the organ to the point of stopping.

3) *Width.* Narrow: contraction, nervousness, or weakness. Wide: distention, congestion.

4) *Movement.* Rapid: fever, or general or local recent agitation. Slow: general or local insufficiency, cold. Arythmic: irregular: hasty, excess thyroid; slow movements: insufficiency of thyroid; intermittent: general vital weakness; jerky: spasms, pain.

5) *Shape.* Irregularity of height: the arrival of energy is insufficient, weak or hindered. Short, sharp: retraction, pain. Without form: weakness, serious insufficiency.

6) *Force.* Good beat: good vital resistance, good function. In excess: hypertension. Violent beating: passing or habitual nervous hyperexcitation, excess blood or energy. Soft beating: vital weakness, emptiness of energy or blood.

7) *Location.* Beyond the location: healthy fullness of energy. Behind: exhaustion, emptiness of energy.

Various combinations of pulse qualities commonly occur. For example, a pulse is not thought to be simply elevated. At the same time it may be either soft or hard, narrow or large, intermittent or regular, etc. In these combinations each single quality carries its significance, and the particular combination of pulse qualities gives the most precise information about the function of each organ, or group of organs, or about the whole body.

Given the number of simple qualities, their possible combinations are endless. This is precisely what allows us to deduce the disturbance, which is absolutely unique to each individual, and the underlying cause of the dysfunction of energy. Often it is possible to deduce the material state of the organ from the indications of energy dysfunction. These indications can be disturbed by the nervous state, or through intoxication by food, drinks, tobacco, or medication.

Here we will offer only some general indications about pulse combinations for: 1) The two wrists together. 2) The one wrist relative to the other. 3) The relation and significance of the three tension levels of each wrist. 4) The location, aspects, and significance of each pulse of the organ meridians.

II. The Two Wrists Together

It is good for the left (blood, husband) to be a little stronger than the right (nervous energy, wife).

When the two wrists have the same qualities, it represents the general vitality, the total energy.

Elevated, wide, hard: fullness, excess volume of blood, and at the same time excess of energy and blood.

Elevated, soft: nervousness, weakness.

Nonexistent, soft: exhaustion, lack of strength, continual fatigue, insufficiency of energy and blood.

Hard, low, to the point of being without beats: excess of the parasympathetic, insufficiency of the sympathetic with diastolic and systolic hypertension and lack of blood.

III. The One Wrist Relative to the Other

The right wrist (yang, wife) represents the great producers of energy, so it has been called "mouth of energy" by the ancients; it reflects the mental activity. The psyche — emotions, feelings, thoughts — is the cause of all problems of excess or insufficiency. Moreover, it contains the pulse of the three nervous centers and of the triple warmer.

The left wrist (yin, husband) most represents the distributor organs and purifiers of blood; the physical life and exterior influences are the cause of problems of excess or insufficiency. It was thus called "human meetings."

The left wrist (physical, husband) must be a little stronger and beat harder than the right (mental, wife), which must not dominate.

Left strong, right weak: solid or exaggerated physical condition, but nervous and mental life tired, weak; follows sorrow, cold or heat, or habitual excess of eating. If pregnant, probably a boy.

Right strong, left weak: lives on nerves, by will, irritable; has suffered moral shocks or hyperstimulating worries, etc. If pregnant, probably a girl.

IV. The Relation and Significance of the Three Tension Levels

The superficial pulses (diastolic pressure, yang), which represent the producers of energy, describe the mental activity ("nervous life"), the energy of activity (yang).

The middle pulses (intermediate pressure) are nearer to the diastolic or systolic pressure according to the wrist. On the right (yang), the pancreas and lung, although viewed as yin organs, are also organs of blood and of the energy of activity (yang) — the pancreas through sugar and the lungs through air; they are linked to the superficial pulses. On the left (yin), the liver and kidney-filtration, purifiers of the blood, are linked to the deep pulses.

The deep pulses (systolic pressure, yin) represent the physical life, the blood and the circulation.

When all the superficial pulses (yang) are like a wire at both wrists, the deep pulses (yin) being weak, the energy of activity dominates the emptiness of the energy of physical rest; the nerves dominate. If the wire is narrow, it is from weakness or pain; if it is big and ample, it is from excess stimulants.

When all the deep pulses are strong with the superficial pulses weak, the physical life dominates, the blood is abundant; there is strength but no activity; there can be plethora.

All the deep pulses weak (except that of the vessels, which is strong), and all superficial pulses strong (except that of the triple warmer, which is weak): dominance of the parasympathetic over the sympathetic.

All the superficial pulses weak (except the triple warmer strong), with all the deep pulses strong (except the vessels): dominance of the sympathetic over the parasympathetic.

V. Location, Aspects and Significance of Each Pulse of the Organ Meridians

After the discovery of the radial pulses, the ancients counted three segments on the radial artery, but certain levels of each of these segments did not have any correspondence with an organ. Observations made since I began teaching acupuncture in France have allowed me to: 1) Specify the locations of the pulses. 2) Find the organ-pulse correspondences of the levels still without connections. 3) Describe the organ-pulse relation of new segments. 4) Specify the meaning of the qualities according to the described organ.

At the two wrists, starting from the palm, segment I is shown as having two neighboring groups: first, on the radial artery (which deviates and goes towards the thumb), and second, a branch which detaches from it at the radius at an angle towards the palm (radiopalmar artery). The latter has only two levels (superficial and deep on the left, superficial and middle on the right), while there are three levels of this segment at the radial artery itself and on all the others.

Right wrist (energy, nerves, producers of energy).

I. Radiopalmar, right superficial: large intestine. The part of the pulse near the palm corresponds to the rectum and anus; in the middle, the transverse colon; the part near the radius, to the ascending colon and cecum.

Supple, a little elevated: good function.

Narrow and hard: spasms, spasmodic constipation, or diarrhea due to irritation and pain.

Nonexistent: relaxed or atonic.

Elevated, wide: gas, aerocolia, swollen.

Rising to the palm, narrow and agitated: intestinal worms (particularly pinworms); if not agitated, hemorrhoids.

The middle like a wire and agitated: trichocephalus and other intestinal parasites.

Part near the radius swollen and hard: retention of matter, does not empty totally.

All the pulses swollen and hard: has not been to the toilet.

I. Radiopalmar deep: lungs. Medial edge of the artery: left respiratory passages. Radial edge: right respiratory passages. Part near the radius: upper passages, throat, trachea, bronchus. Part near the palm: lower lung. Middle: middle-lung.

Low and supple: good function.

Nonexistent: insufficient function to the point of paresis, cannot expand the chest, does not take enough energy of activity from the air.

Narrow and hard: spasms (of the bronchi when near the radius).

Elevated, wide, hard: inflammation (congestion or bronchitis, pneumonia, pleurisy or edema according to the part of the pulse).

I. Radial artery, right. Radial edge: right half of the body. Medial edge: left half of the body. Superficial: inferior third of the governor vessel (and sympathetic): genitourinary function.

I. Radial artery, right middle: middle third of the governor vessel (and sympathetic): digestive function.

I. Radial artery, right deep: superior third of the governor vessel (and sympathetic): respiratory and cerebral functions.

II. Right superficial: stomach.

Supple, moderately elevated: good function.

Swollen, elevated, wide: indigestion or recent large meal, aerogastria, sleepy after meals, stomach does not empty. If, in addition, the pulses of the spleen and liver are nonexistent: spleen and liver are distended.

Narrow and hard: cramps, pain.

Nonexistent or very weak: slow digestion.

Narrow, long and elevated: frequent dreams, nightmares, even to the point of mental hyperexcitation.

Large, strongly beating: recent big meal, alcohol, coffee.

II. Right middle: pancreas.

Elevated, firm without hardness, well formed: good function.

Elevated, large, long, soft: insufficiency, stomach burns one or two hours after ingestion of jams, pastries; probability of diabetes; does not digest chestnuts, beans, fats; this often happens after worries and sorrow.

Short, narrow, pointed, hard: inflammation of the head of the pancreas.

If soft with nonexisting pulse of the spleen: spleen and liver distended.

II. Right deep: spleen.

Well formed, a little elevated, quite firm: good function, reason (synthetic mind, moral consciousness).

Nonexistent: insufficiency and distention, accompanied also by distention of the liver also compressing surrounding organs, anemia.

Soft, low, slight insufficiency: tired in the morning, sleep has not given rest, better after 5 p.m. Or, if more serious: tired also in the evening, cannot concentrate easily or for a long time, attention wanders, lack of synthetic mind, of moral consciousness, moderate anemia; if serious, can reach the point of leukemia.

Short, pointed, hard: inflammation of spleen, pain.

III. Right superficial: triple warmer.

Well formed, moderately elevated: supple, good function.

By itself: represents the activity of the three great functions.

Same qualities on all the superficial pulses (yang producers): Weak: energy of activity, nerves below the individual average. Strong, hard tight: excess of nerves, of energy of activity. If a little narrow: lives on will, excess of nerves over weakness, pain aggravated during the night, irritability.

Hard with all the superficial pulses soft (and the deep hard except the vessels): Dominance of the sympathetic over the parasympathetic.

Alone soft and weak when all the other superficial pulses are hard and all the deep pulses soft except the vessels: Insufficiency of the sympathetic and relative excess of the parasympathetic.

III. Right middle: vessels.

Supple, quite ample: good function and good state of the vessels (lower half of the middle pulse) and of the veins (upper half).

Hard by itself, contracted: hypertension, arteries, veins without suppleness.

Very hard: arteriosclerosis which can be an excess of arterial contracture.

Soft by itself, without form: hypotension, arterial circulation insufficient, relaxed veins, swelling of ankles during walks, heat.

Hard, ample, with all the superficial pulses except the triple warmer, and softness of all the deep pulses (distributors): excess of the parasympathetic which can reach the point of the pulses being without beats and hard.

Soft or nonexistent with all the superficial pulses (producers) except the triple warmer, with hardness of the deep pulses: insufficiency of the parasympathetic and relative dominance of the sympathetic.

III. Right deep: sexual organs. The radial edge of the artery responds to the right organs, the medial edge to the left organs. The lower part of the pulse (near the eminence) responds to the lower part of the organs (women: uterus; men: glans); the middle part to the middle organs (women: fallopian tubes; men: penis); the upper part to the upper organs (women: ovaries and the upper pavillion; men: testicles, epididymis).

Well formed, moderate elevation and resistance: sexual organs in good function and state. Reflects the material condition as well as the activity of the hormones; less sure for erection and pleasure, which depend more on the mental state.

Hard and ample: inflammation, congestion, to the point of tumor.

Soft, ample: swelling.

Nonexistent: insufficiency.

Hard and pointed: pain (women: cyst, tumor).

For women, menses are announced seven days earlier by a clearly increased beat on the edge of the artery representing the ovary and fallopian tubes, this beat becoming stronger and stronger as the time of the period approaches; it stops on the arrival of the menses. If the beat continues, one should consider an ovarian or fallopian tube congestion. From nine to eleven days after the end of the menses, there is ovulation and the beat has the same intensity as for the seven days preceding the menses.

In pregnancy, the two edges of the artery are large and firm. A flattened dome: a boy (the left pulse is then stronger than the right). With the top edge sharp: a girl (the right pulse is then stronger). All intoxication (tobacco, alcohol, medicines) interferes with these qualities and their meanings.

Elevated, hard, beating vigorously: sexually hyperexcitable.

Soft, weak: without sexual desire, or tired.

In part, this pulse is linked to that of the vessels because of its action on the heart and circulation. Thus, the ancients grouped them under the name of "heart governor."

IV. Right. This segment (which I discovered and extensively experimented with prior to 1940) responds to the function of the three nervous centers.

IV. Right superficial: spinal cord, medulla. The radial edge responds to the left of the spinal cord, the medial edge to the right. The proximal part of the pulse responds to the upper part of the spinal cord; the distal part of the pulse responds to the lower part of the spinal cord. The medulla is represented at the upper extremity by two lateral points.

Supple, but not soft, well formed but neither narrow nor wide and beating softly: perfect function.

Hard, narrow, elevated, tight: rapid and violent reactions, before having reflected — more reflex than reflection; also, uncontrollable irritability.

Elevated, wide, hard: inflammation to the point of motor or sensory problems, upper or lower according to the part of the pulse.

Soft without form: slow reactions, weak.

Nonexistent: possibility of paralysis.

Lateral projections show displaced vertebra; the sacrum is close to III.

IV. Middle: cerebellum, pons. The distal part of the pulse responds to the cerebellum, the proximal lateral points to the pons. Radial edge of the artery: left half of the cerebellum and pons. Medial edge: right half. The equality between the two sides is essential to proper function — any differences indicate problems with coordination of movement.

Supple, well formed, quite elevated: good function.

Elevated, wide, hard: inflammation of one side of the organ. If there is a lesion, the head as well as the trunk turns to the side of the lesion.

Soft to nonexistent: bad coordination of movements, awkwardness.

IV. Right deep: brain. Radial edge: left side of the brain (the command points are on the right side of the body). Medial edge: right side. Proximal part of the pulse: posterior brain, occipital lobes. Proximal middle part: parietal and temporal lobes. Distal middle part: central brain. Distal part: anterior lobes, posterior and anterior frontal lobes (anterior lobes nearer to III).

Slightly elevated, slightly firm, beating well: good function.

In total, nonexistent: cerebral anemia, arterial spasm, weakness, vertigo, inability to hold attention or concentrate; seen in cerebral anemia or in hemiplegia (opposite limb).

Elevated, wide, hard: cerebral congestion, headache when bending forward, heaviness of the head. Each part has its separate significance (q.v. brain chapter: nervous centers).

V. Right superficial: adrenals.

Elevated: active.

Nonexistent: weak.

V. Right middle: thyroid (inferior part), parathyroids (superior part).

Parathyroid nil: insufficiency of calcium in the blood, excess of phosphorus, pains, tightness.

Strong parathyroid: excess blood calcium, muscles soft, insufficiency of phosphorus.

V. Right deep: pituitary.

Left wrist.

I. Left (as for I of the right wrist) two segments: one on the radiopalmar artery, one on the radial artery.

On the radiopalmar artery:

I. Radiopalmar left superficial: small intestine. The distal part, near the palm, responds to the jejunum and ileum; the proximal part, near the radius, to the duodenum.

Supple and formed, moderately elevated: good function.

Agitated and hard: tapeworm.

Hard, narrow, like a wire: spasm.

Elevated, wide, soft: fermentation, gas.

Flaccid to nonexistent: recuperates only slowly from physical or psychological fatigue; insufficiency of the "personal molecule."[1]

I. Radiopalmar left deep: heart. The radial side of the artery responds to the left side of the heart, the auricle of which receives the blood coming from the lungs and the ventricle of which expels it into the aorta. The medial side responds to the right side of the heart, which receives the venous blood and sends it to the lungs. The proximal half responds to the ventricles, the distal half to the auricles.

Quite elevated, of good form, beating well: good function.

Low, soft, hardly beating: insufficiency, heart can get tired, panting after climbing stairs, malaise from emotions, moments of depression, bad sleep at night, anxiety; at the extreme, anguish, insufficient circulation, cold. Perhaps following pulmonary troubles, asthma, prolonged discomfort from distended spleen, or following sorrow, etc.

Absent: tendency to weakness, grey fog at moments.

Arhythmic, intermittent, irregular strength: general exhaustion, excess work or worries, or bad nourishment, particularly with the first weakness of age.

On the radial artery:

I. Radial left superficial: conception vessel: lower genitourinary third (and parasympathetic, *tianzhu,* BL-10).

I. Radial left middle: conception vessel: middle digestive third (and parasympathetic).

I. Radial left deep: conception vessel: upper respiratory third (and parasympathetic).

II. Left superficial: gallbladder. Involves the entire biliary reflex with gallbladder, common bile duct, Oddi's sphincter, etc.

Slightly elevated, supple, quite short: good function.

Elevated, hard, narrow: gallbladder constricted, blocking the bile flow; migraines; skin eruptions; may be followed or replaced by constipation or asthma.

Elevated, wide, soft: biliary sediments from insufficiency; ill from atony.

Elevated, hard, spherical: stones.

Nonexistent: collapses when faced with an effort, finds everything beyond one's strength.

II. Left middle: liver. The radial side of the artery responds to the anterior lobes (particularly bile). The medial side responds to the posterior lobes (particularly antitoxic).

A little elevated, supple, well formed: good functions.

Low, soft, hardly perceptible: insufficiency, bad digestion of fresh cream, chocolate, fried foods, very often of eggs and omelettes; constipation, migraines, skin problems or problems of the respiratory passages, etc. Also observed when distended along with the spleen.

Elevated, wide, hard: blood congestion or even tumor.

A little elevated, narrow, tight: pains, parasites, trematodes?

II. Left deep: blood pressure. Very slightly perceptible when the pressure is normal for the individual. Nonexistent when the pressure is lower than normal. More and more elevated and hard as the pressure is higher than normal.

III. Left superficial: bladder. At the distal extremity of the pulse there is a small pointed pulse: the sphincter? Distal: (men) the prostate, when it is congested. When the body of the bladder is soft, the sphincter is contracted and vice versa.

A little elevated, a little wide, supple: good function.

Large and hard: retention.

Elevated, narrow, hard like a wire: frequent urgings, urgent but little urination, spasms, inflammation of the bladder, cystitis.

Soft, nonexistent: relaxation to the point of atony or flaccidity, need to urinate very great at the least emotion; in excess, cannot retain urine for a long time, to the point of incontinence.

III. Left middle: kidney-filtration (glomerules). The radial edge of the artery responds to the kidney-filtration on the left, the medial edge to that of the right.

Good elevation, quite wide, supple: good function.

Hard, narrow: insufficient filtration.

Nonexistent but hard at the bottom: exaggerated filtration, urine very abundant, kidney contracted (glomerules and capillaries).

Nonexistent, but soft and wide at the bottom: lets everything pass (albuminuria), abundant urine, kidney relaxed.

Nil: removed.

III. Left deep: kidney-excretion and secretion (tubules). Radial edge of the artery, tubules of the left kidney; medial edge, those of the right kidney.

Good elevation, quite large, resistant without hardness: good function.

Weak, soft: excretes and secretes little, urine with little color (pale yellow), often with relaxed filtration, then urine very abundant, tubules without vitality.

Nonexistent: removed or paralyzed; atrophy.

Nonexistent due to being hard and without beats: hypertension of the diastolic, contracted tubules absorbing too much but excreting well, urine colored or full.

Elevated, wide, soft: swollen.

Elevated, wide, hard: congestion.

IV. Left: mental. For twelve years, I have explored and experimented on this segment with constant success. The relativity of the three parts is most important.

IV. Left superficial: evolved consciousness. This pulse responds to the moral consciousness, to reason, comprehension, synthesis, judgment, common sense, nonsuggestability — the evolution which differentiates the human from the animal. Goes much beyond the sense of conscious perception of ''awareness'' in the West. Radial edge of the artery: right frontal lobes. Medial edge: left frontal lobes.

Elevated, beating well, supple but not soft: good observation, good deduction, moral consciousness, reason, synthesis (2 + 2 = 4), true intelligence.

Soft, without form, to nonexistent: sees and hears but neither concludes nor acts in conformity; suggestible, bad morals, easily discouraged, weak character.

Quite elevated, narrow, hard like a wire: fixed ideas, obsessions. The conscious is led by the unconscious, to the point of hallucinations.

IV. Left middle: automaton and parrot. The medial edge responds to the left parietal and temporal lobes, present memory and consciousness, particularly of words, or phrases — what appears before a thought which often does not come, much like a parrot. The radial edge responds to the opposed right parietal and temporal lobes, the hereditary memory, entirely unconscious, the talents and hereditary impulses good or bad which cause blind action before the person is even aware of the thought of action, like a dog that hunts in the chase without any training: the automaton. The parietal lobes respond to all the points that act on sensitivity, the sensations; the temporal lobes respond to the organs of sense.

Automaton (radial edge):

Elevated, well formed, quite resistant: intensity of the hereditary impulses (good or bad), blind activity (good or bad) to the point of fanaticism; traditionalist or revolutionary, conformist or innovator.

Low, soft to nonexistent: weakness of the hereditary impulses, succumbs to influences, victim of circumstances.

Parrot (medial edge):

Elevated, well-formed, beats well, resistant: good memory, can speak on any subject with conviction but without vision or personal invention; good talent, but no genius, succeeds at school and in examinations, deceives. Thinks only in known phrases, speaks and writes only by sentences already made, ideas and words are rarely his own, replaces reality with words which hide everything from him. Knows without understanding.

Low, soft, slightly perceptible: lack of memory, difficulty in memorizing. Words do not represent reality for him and he is always searching for them. He can have genius if he finds his way, but it takes a long time to acquire talent.

IV. Left Deep: primate. Responds to the deepest and least acknowledged primitive instincts in our nature: conquest, destruction, violence, breaking, burning, bestial sexual satisfaction; its love is only ''manual, anal, or vaginal masturbation,'' pride and persecution.

Elevated, large, hard: primitive instincts and pride dominant, need to humiliate and persecute to aggrandize oneself, lack of enthusiasm for the beautiful and good; egoist. A good executive, resilient to work. Strong sex appeal, seductive. Clever without intelligence.

Low, without form, to nonexistent: no taste for life, regards all with indifference, prefers to be restrained than to conquer, indifferent to money or to power, without sex appeal, without authority.

V. Left: organs of sense. I discovered these and have experimented with them since before the Second World War.

V. Left superficial: eyes, vision. Radial edge: left eye. Medial edge: right eye.

Elevated, well formed, beating well: eyes in good condition; good vision (according to age and health).

Elevated, hard, narrow: pain.

Elevated, hard, wide: congestion.

Low, soft, badly formed, beating weakly: tired vision, atony or insufficiency of energy.

V. Left Middle: ears, hearing. The radial edge of the artery responds to the left ear; the medial edge to the right ear.

Elevated, well formed, supple: good function according to age and health.

Hard, narrow, like a wire: pain.

Elevated, wide, soft: inflammation.

V. Left, Deep: smell, taste. Smell and taste seem inseparable and obedient to the same points.

Elevated, well formed, supple: good function.

Soft to nonexistent: weakness or loss of smell and taste.

Notes

[1] The protein molecule unique to each individual, which is manufactured in the small intestine.

Chapter V

Action On The Energy (V)

Tonification and Dispersal. Action and Reactions.

I. The Basic Principle — II. Tonification and Dispersal: 1. Significance of the Terms 2. Real Effect Obtained by Tonifying or Dispersing 3. Effects on the Equilibrium of the Functions — III. Action-Reaction Relativity: 1. Action-Reaction 2. Groups of Reactions 3. General Laws of Reaction

I. The Basic Principle

All so-called "illness" is only the personal expression and consequence of an energetic problem. Energetic problems can only manifest through an excess or insufficiency. The aim of action can only be to re-establish the equilibrium and fullness normal and habitual to the individual. Therefore, it is useful to tonify insufficiencies and to disperse excesses until normal fullness, partial or total, is re-established.

Before elaborating upon tonification and dispersal, however, we should clearly establish the principle of all action, and its opposition to Western concepts. Moreover, we should call attention to the individual and the circumstances. *There are no standard actions or standard effects, but only action-reaction relativities.*

To conceive and undertake an action which gives success without fail, always keep in mind one essential principle: *The action addresses itself only to the vital energy, the insufficiency or excess of which it aims to correct in order to re-establish a harmonious fullness in the whole body and in all the organs.*

From which it must follow: *There are no key points curing such and such an "illness," but rather "commands" of areas.* It is not a question of a fight against such and such a microbe: the energy masters them all. The action regulates the intensity of the energy, which maintains the life of the terrain and the defense of the vital command.

Thus, for the common cold, *hegu* (LI-4) does not act against the cold; it does not try to destroy the microbe. Its action is only to disperse the excess, the congestion of the nasal mucosa, by re-establishing the normal rhythm which does not allow the microbe to live. The cold thus disappears. To disperse the excess of a gallbladder supresses an excess of cholecystitis, and with this the various problems it causes also disappear.

However, the effects of proper actions do not only re-establish the equilibrium of the energy of a troubled organ which expresses its trouble through an "illness." They also include the correction of the general energy and the return to immunity, thanks to which we live and without which we would disintegrate bit by bit. This disintegration is "illness," and complete disintegration is death.

II. Tonification and Dispersal

The objective is thus to tonify the insufficiencies of energy and to disperse the excesses. The significance, the explanations and the implications of these words are many.

Significance of the terms.

Tonification is the word I have chosen to represent the ideogram which describes the idea of "help," "supplementation," "reinforcement," "to fill an emptiness." In a general way it means to increase the supply of energy, to give life, to stimulate the physical or mental strength, to revive the form, to re-establish the appearance and the usual function and to cause them to reach the highest level which the form permits. This goes much beyond the idea of stimulation.

All insufficiencies must be tonified. To tonify an excess generally has no effect, but occasionally may be dangerous.

The more one uses the ascendant rhythms of energy, the more one tonifies. Thus, the more the organ is insufficient, the more easily the organ is tonified — such are the meridians at their minimum or their rising: the energy of yang activity at the waxing of the moon and rising of the sun, and in clear, warm weather, and at the waning of the moon and the dwindling of summer.

A sick organ responds to a weak stimulation, while a strong organ remains insensitive (Arndt). Tonification of a convalescent provides great benefit.

Dispersion translates an ideogram which represents the concept of "spreading," "drainage," "making emptiness," "to remove over-fullness." In a general way it means to diminish the excess supply of energy, the hyperactivity of the form, to re-establish their functions at their lower habitual level. This goes much beyond the idea of inhibition.

All excess must be dispersed. To disperse an emptiness generally has no effect, but occasionally can be harmful.

The more marked the excess, the easier it is to disperse. Thus the meridians at their maximum and at their decrease: the energy of yang activity after its maximum at noon, and after the summer solstice, or the energy of yin inactivity after its maximum at midnight, or after the full moon and after the winter solstice.

The table of general insufficiency and excess (q.v., Illness chapter) as well as the comparison of insufficiency-excess of each organ meridian given in different chapters, allows us to have greater ability to determine when we must tonify and when we must disperse.

The best means of tonifying or dispersing are described in the chapter entitled "Methods of Action."

The real effect obtained by tonification or dispersion.

In a general way, tonifying an organ supplies it with energy which causes it to attain fullness if empty. To disperse an organ in excess thus empties the excess and returns it to normal fullness. But from where does the energy supplied by tonification come? Where does the energy go which is expelled by dispersion, since energy can neither be lost nor created?

With careful verification, measuring the pulses for all changes produced after each needle, I have observed that for tonfication or dispersion, the effects obtained may be classified into two groups — the one corroborated by a measurement and easily explicable; the other verifiable, but for which I have not yet found the explanation.

In most cases, it is easy to observe that either by tonifying or dispersing, two organs respond in the same way and two others respond in the opposite way when it is a question of a single stimulated organ. The energy is transferred from some to others.

For the commands of either all the yang or all the yin, we note that to tonify all the deep empty pulses when all the superficial pulses are in excess (and vice versa) causes the excess to pass into the emptiness and return everything to normal fullness. It is thus a question of the transfer of energy.

The ancient authors recommend that to tonify, make the needle penetrate, then wait for "the energy to come to the needle," which is discernible when it is pinched by the skin; then penetrate even deeper; then again a third time. This has the purpose and effect of causing the energy of yang activity of the exterior surface to pass into the energy of yin inactivity, which is deeper. To disperse, drive the needle in with one push to the deepest level and come back to the superficial level in three steps by waiting at each step for the energy to hold the needle. They were looking for an internal-external transfer.

To corroborate this idea we must indicate that effects of the same kind are always obtained for the organs whose pulses are at the same tension level; on the other hand, the opposite effects are obtained for the organs whose pulses are at a different tension level. To tonify a yang organ always tonifies other yang organs and disperses yin organs and vice versa — thus there is a yang-yin or yin-yang transfer (q.v. Chapter VIII of this volume, "The Hierarchy of Commands").

There is another particular case less easy to understand, though also completely verifiable, which concerns the effects of some command points on the total energy. For example, tonifying leg-*sanli* (ST-36) will affect all the yang and yin organs and pulses without exception. To disperse it disperses them all. From where comes this energy that floods all the organs? To where goes this energy that leaves all the organs? It does not seem to be a question here of a transfer between yin and yang. The only hypothesis of action would still seem to be that of a transfer between the form and the deep reserves of energy. But these reserves are not yet known; the brain is suggested as an accumulator. This explanation remains a hypothesis for the moment. However, two facts support it:

1) When the practitioner incorrectly estimates the intensity of the possible reaction of the patient and uses needles too strongly, stimulates too large a number of points, or puts sessions too close together, the patient becomes exhausted and without vitality for a more or less long time — a few days to several weeks.

2)   When a point has been stimulated, it is as if discharged and it returns to its usual effect only after several days, according to the recuperative abilities of the patient; this implies reserves.

On the other hand, without food and drink, life and even activity can be sustained for some time. Moreover, regular work can continue while food and drink are very irregular in quantity and quality, which implies reserves from which the organism draws according to its needs and reforms according to its potential. Are these reserves taken from the transformation of assimilated and stored products in the organism, in the cells? From the transformation of latent energy into active energy (of yin energy into yang energy)?

On the other hand, without air life is quickly extinguished. This is explained perfectly through chemistry, but we must juxtapose this with the fact that even with all the needed air, but without sun or light, plants and animals lack color, and are weakened and anemic. Is this lack of yang solar energy? Lack of reserves of yang energy?

Effect on the functional equilibrium.

When a meridian is tonified, the organ is invigorated and receives a greater intensity of energy; its functions are augmented. When dispersed, its activity is diminished along with its functions.

But the functions of an organ-meridian are not always simple. They often appear contradictory. Thus, a point on the meridian of the small intestine (*shaoze,* SI-1) acts on all secretions: sweat, saliva, milk, fluids of the eye, urine, etc. By tonifying this point, we observe that urine is increased while all the other secretions are diminished. By dispersing it, urine is diminished and all the other secretions are increased.

These opposing results surprise us until, upon reflection, we have understood that the urine and all the other secretions replace and balance each other; the more liquid goes out through the urine, the less is left for the other secretions. The less urine that goes out, the more the other secretions are fed. The two groups balance each other in order to maintain the equilibrium of fluid in the body.

On further reflection, it becomes evident that the bladder is the most normal pathway for the evacuation of liquid, the others being occasional pathways that may be used for replacement. The conclusion is that to tonify the small intestine augments the urine, to disperse it diminishes the urine. ''It divides solids and liquids,'' write the ancients, ''sending the solids to the large intestine and the liquids to the kidney and bladder.''

The large intestine produces antihemorrhagic vitamin K. By tonifying it, we increase this production and its antihemorrhagic action on the organism. But perhaps because of this the menses are sometimes diminished or stopped; there is a tonification of the blood which becomes less fluid, tonification of the tissues which become less permeable, more contracted — thus, there is an augmentation of their energy. Dispersing the large intestine diminishes the production of antihemorrhagic vitamin K; the menses are increased as well as all hemorrhages. The tissues become dispersed and relaxed. The blood is more fluid; the energy is diminished. It is the energy which we must thus consider, not the blood.

Several points also have some apparently contradictory effects but in reality have an equilibrating consequence.

III. Action-Reaction Relativity

Action-reaction.

Besides the tonification-dispersal relativity, there is an important action-reaction relativity. That is, theoretically, it is possible to say that a strong and prolonged action tonifies, while a weak and short action disperses. But we must add that a certain action which will tonify if the reaction is appropriate may neither disperse nor paralyze if the reaction is not appropriate.

What is a strong stimulation for one is a weak stimulation for another, and vice versa. In a weakened individual, a sick organ will respond more than a robust individual or a strong organ. An enumeration of some facts will clarify this issue.

1) *To transfer:* a person suffering from an excess of nerves and exhaustion of physical vitality: if his nerves (yang) are dispersed, he will have a crisis of tears and complete exhaustion. If the physical vitality (yin) is tonified, the nerves are relaxed, the excess passes into the insufficiency of the physical vitality and the benefit is immediate. The dispersal of nerves which are greatly in excess gives maximum relaxation. Tonification of a greatly insufficient physique provides maximum strength by taking from the nerves only the quantity of energy in excess.

2) *To tonify:* to tonify a weakened person's energy too strongly exhausts him for a relatively long time and never gives the full effect desired. One should only increase digestion and respiration, the taking in of energy. Tonifying the local insufficiency of a weakened person gives weak and less durable results; he should first be fortified.

To tonify by numerous points or at intervals which are too frequent diminishes the effect of each point and the response of the person in proportion to the number of points and sessions. A new session with the same points, if it is too soon, can have an opposite effect, and disperse instead of tonify.

To tonify an old person with weak needles gives weak and delayed results. To tonify a weakened person with strong needles is to risk fainting, and in all cases, exhausts him for a long time. The results are minimal.

3) *To disperse:* to disperse a local excess in a weakened person increases his exhaustion; one should tonify the opposite. To disperse a weakened person with strong needles or by action at too many points weakens seriously and for a long time.

To disperse even with appropriate needles, but every day, or every two days and with numerous sessions, exhausts the patient for a long time, and leaves the person without immunity, even if the excess aimed at has been cured.

To disperse any point is to discharge it for many days.

In conclusion, the effect of the action depends to a great extent on the possible reactions and is the result of three forces:

a)   The intensity of the action: strong (thick), medium or weak (thin) needles and the number of moxas; also the greater or lesser number of points stimulated; also the closeness of multiple sessions (when only one should be enough in cases of recent incidence).

b)   The rhythms of energy: increase of yang energy of activity from midnight to midday, from the full to the new moon and from the winter solstice to the summer soltice; with a decrease from midday and the waning moon and from the summer solstice. Increase of energy of yin inactivity from midday, the new moon and the summer solstice with a decrease from midnight, the full moon and the winter solstice.

c)   The intensity of the possible personal reaction: capacity varies greatly from young to aged, or from strong to weak people.

Groups of reactions.

The individual reaction is of great importance; one should take precautions in order to obtain the maximum immediate results as well as to avoid fainting or a slow and weak response. The palpation of the pulses *in toto* gives the information. The Loch apparatus gives a number, but it is useful to obtain some of the revealing signs.

Although each individual is unique in form and reactions, there are certain analogies (without identity) between individuals. These lead us to conceive of the relativity of some opposed groups, either physically or mentally.

The thin and the fat. The thin have thin skin and their subcutaneous fat is minimal. The needle thus reaches the subcutaneous tissue where the point is at a shallow depth. Insert the needle shallowly and use a small number of moxas.

But there is a relativity among thin people:

There are people who are thin from an excess of energy. They are active, always in movement, with bright eyes and sonorous voices. In the West, they are termed "nervous." Fine needles, or at the most, intermediate-sized ones should be used. Among the points with multiple effects choose what corresponds to all the troubled organs and verify the results immediately at the pulse; often one point is enough. Large needles or numerous points are very tiring and provide slow results (often taking two weeks) and even risk producing unintended results.

There are people who are thin from exhaustion, poor nourishment, sorrow or despair. They are immobile and slow, with dull eyes and a timberless voice. In the West, they are termed "pretubercular." They should never be dispersed. Use intermediate-sized needles at one or two points at the maximum, stimulating the production of energy by assimilation and respiration. If they have had a mental or physical shock as a cause, begin with the point that removes the shock. Wait at least a week for the regulation of any failing organs, and to see if the stimulated organism has not already responded.

Fat people have thick skin. To reach the subcutaneous tissue where the points and meridians are found, one must go through the subcutaneous fat, the thickness of which varies from some millimeters to centimeters. It is only by reaching the subcutaneous connective tissue that the full effect is obtained. The closer one approaches this level, the clearer and more durable are the effects.

But fat people also have their relativity:

There are those for whom the energy is asleep, who move slowly with heaviness and for whom thought is numbed, the voice without sonority, the eyes without expression. For these it is useful not only to puncture deeply, but also to use intermediate or large-sized needles. Many points are often necessary to obtain the desired effect. The points with multiple effects produce little result.

There are also fat people whose mental or physical power rises with their excess development. They are hyperactive, quick in thought and action, with bright eyes and powerful voices, and great strength. For these, although one must always traverse the subcutaneous fat, thin or intermediate-sized needles give excellent results. The points give all their effects and those with multiple effects act completely. It is not necessary to puncture several points to obtain the same effect.

Mental and physical. The opposition here is between those the Far East distinguished as either "esteemed" or "unesteemed."

The esteemed were those individuals hereditarily selected for generations for their elevated qualities. From the third century B.C., in fact, to be nominated for bureaucrat it was necessary to have parents and grandparents from both sides who passed examinations. Until modern times, there was only concern with the development of higher qualities of Confucian reason.

We also have our intellectuals, hereditary urbanites. This mental selection strongly induces physical refinement and greater sensitivity.

The unesteemed were the physical types: manual workers with hereditary development bearing on strength, thickness of tissue, lack of sensitivity and in consequence less cultivation of the mind. We would call these opposite groups: sensitives and manuals or mental and physical, or from the point of view of reason and of the moral consciousness of this relativity, the evolved and the primates.

When the mind dominates, in all cases sensitivity and reactions are greater and quicker. With them one should always be concerned that one might go beyond their equilibrium and disturb the energy. Thus, thin or intermediate needles inserted shallowly, and points with multiple effects, should be used.

When the physical dominates, sensitivity and reaction are reduced, response takes time, but is good. Use strong (thick) needles. Points with multiple effects do not work well; several points are easily supported at full depth.

Children and old people. Children have form and energy in the rhythm of growth; they are easy to stimulate. It is often sufficient to use one of the points which commands the general energy. At the beginning of the problem, massage is sufficient and moreover can be recommenced as soon as the improvement stops. The needles must be very fine, and one is often sufficient.

Old people, or those people for whom aging accompanies or preceeds their age, are both weak and have diminished reactions. They must have strong (thick) needles, but they bear many points poorly. Daily moxa is recommended for them. Do not disperse, but tonify the opposite aspect. Tonify the sexual energy.

Exhausted-plethoric. There is a group of exhausted people who faint with too strong a needle and for whom one should first stimulate the energy taken in air and food. There are also the congestive plethoric types, for whom one should relax the arteries and diminish the volume of blood.

Intoxicated people. There are people who become intoxicated from poisons, medicines, tobacco, alcohol, coffee, tea and even from water; also from food, unhygienic drinks, coffee with milk, quantities of drinks during and after meals, etc. They all have a dulled energy, which is difficult to stimulate; their responses are slow and diminished. One should use strong needles, starting with the point which detoxifies, that is, which suppresses the unconscious and irresistible need for poison, *shuaigu* (GB-8).

General laws of reaction.

In general, puncturing a patient who is standing up, using even the finest needles, will surely cause weakness, if not fainting, and will block the effect of the action. The patient should be lying down and relaxed; the energy is thus more easily moved or sent to the organ. All tightness blocks its flow. A patient with an empty stomach is a weak patient. After a heavy meal, the energy is busy with digestion. After great physical or mental fatigue, the available energy is less abundant.

A bad and even dangerous acupuncturist is known by the way in which he does not attend to the possibilities of reaction. He riddles the patient with innumerable needles whose strength he has not measured, having no concern for the precise location. He ignores the measure of the energy through the pulses, taking no thought to the effect of each meridian on other meridians, and requires the patient to come every day or every other day and anticipate numerous sessions. One session well done would be enough for those cases that do not go beyond the already very large framework of the science of energy. Only after improvement has ceased should a new session be required.

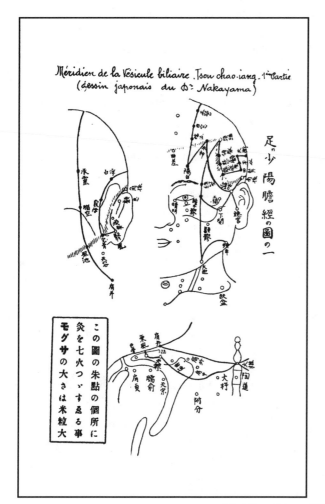
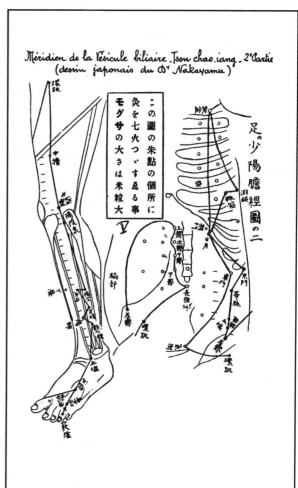

Meridian of the gallbladder (Nakayama)

Chapter VI

Action On the Energy (VI)

Interaction of the Organs and of the Parts of the Body

I. The Laws of Interaction 1. Laws of Similar Effects 2. Laws of Opposite Effects — II. Application to the Organs — III. Mechanical Interaction of Neighbors — IV. Interaction of Parts of the Body — V. Interaction of the Elements and the Planets — VI. Consequences of the Interaction: Multiple Effects of the Points

I. Laws of Interaction of the Organs

It is impossible to act on one organ without acting on many others. This law, already described in antiquity under some of its effects, has been developed and refined as a result of the scrupulous reading of the pulses after the insertion of each needle and also due to the availability of new instruments for measuring the energy. It is specified that:

It is impossible to modify the intensity of the energy of one organ without simultaneously affecting:
1)   *In the same way the energy of two other organs.*
2)   *In an opposite way the energy of two other organs.*

The effect in the same way and the effect in the opposite way obey certain laws.

We shall see further that certain points have in addition the possibility of modifying the intensity either of the whole body or of one part of the body, or of the totality of the yin or yang organs or of several organs, etc. From this comes, in addition to the regular interactions, the existence of a hierarchy of commands.

Laws of similar effects.

These laws exist only between organs at the same level, either between producers, or distributors. That is, either between superficial yang pulses (the producers), or between deep yin pulses (the distributors). It does not apply to parts of the organism.

Two sure laws: husband-wife and mother-child of the same level.

1) *Husband-wife: it is impossible to modify the intensity of energy of one organ-pulse without modifying in the same way the organ-pulse at the same level and segment of the opposite wrist.*

The ancients had adopted the image of the husband-wife because it is impossible to undermine the husband without the wife suffering equally; the husband likewise suffers from all undermining of the wife. This image recalls, moreover, that the solidity of the couple depends on the dominance of the husband — if the wife commands, everything goes wrong. So it is necessary that the left wrist (husband, the physical life) should be a little stronger than the right wrist (wife, nervous life) so the individual will be fully balanced and will not be at the mercy of his feelings and nerves.

The husband-wife groups are: (yang) small intestine-large intestine, gallbladder-stomach, bladder-triple warmer; (yin) heart-lungs, liver-spleen-pancreas, kidney filtration-vessels, kidney excretion-sexual organs.

2) *Mother-child at the same level: it is impossible to modify the intensity of one organ-meridian without modifying in the same way the organ-meridian that precedes it or follows it at the same level in the flow of energy.*

The old image refers to the upstream organ meridian as the mother. The downstream meridian is considered the child.

The mother nourishes the child: if the mother is in fullness, her child will be well-nourished. Tonifying the mother will tonify the child. If the mother is empty, her child will be malnourished. Dispersing the mother will disperse the child.

The child receives food from the mother and empties her. If the child is full to excess, he does not suck; the mother goes into excess. Tonifying the child will tonify the mother. A starved child empties the mother. Dispersing the child will disperse the mother.

Antiquity did not teach any exception to the mother-child rules. We have observed that it applies only to the succession at the same level of the pulses. Between different levels the law of contrary effect or that of the coupled meridian intervenes.

The mother-child couple at the same level are (yin) liver-lung, spleen-pancreas-heart, kidney-vessels and sexual organs; (yang) small intestine-bladder, triple warmer-gallbladder, large intestine-stomach.

Laws of opposite effects.

These laws exist only between couples of the different levels formed from one yang producer organ (superficial pulses) and one yin distributor organ (deep pulses). There are two laws: maximum-minimum (midday-midnight) and coupled meridians.

1) *Maximum-minimum (midday-midnight).* It is impossible to tonify one organ-meridian at the hour of its daily minimum without dispersing in proportion the organ meridian which has its maximum at the same hour. It is equally impossible to disperse an organ-meridian at the hour of its daily maximum without tonifying in proportion the organ-meridian which has its minimum at the same hour.

Let us recall that each meridian each day receives its maximum energy during two hours and its minimum twelve hours later, for two hours. In fact, the rise during these two hours reaches its highest in one hour and almost immediately goes down in the next hour.

As there are twelve meridians, it is absolutely necessary that the hour of maximum of one coincides with the hour of minimum of another, and always with a twelve-hour interval, always between one yang **and** another yin meridian.

These couples form at the pulse crossings between superficial and deep, which helps to find **them**:

Between pulses I and II left: heart (deep) and gallbladder (superficial), small intestine (superficial) and liver (deep).

Between pulses III left and I right: kidney (deep) and large intestine (superficial), bladder (superficial) and lung (deep).

Between pulses II and III right: stomach (superficial) and vessels-sexual organs, particularly sexual organs (deep), spleen-pancreas (deep) and triple warmer (superficial).

Regarding the understanding and utilization of these contrary effects, our observations have led us to the conclusion that it is a question of command points which balance yin and yang, energy and blood, solids and liquids, etc.

Thus: 1) Production of vital elements (small intestine) and their distribution (liver). 2) Absorption of yang energy from the air (lungs) and its reduction (bladder assent points). 3) Stimulation of the energy (gallbladder) and circulation of blood (heart). 4) Production of energy by sugar (pancreas) and its distribution (triple warmer). 5) Production of yin energy by sugar (stomach) and through it the vital stimulation (sexual organs). 6) Equilibration and excretion of solids (large intestine) or of liquids and solubles (kidney).

2) *Coupled Meridians.* These couples have two special peculiarities. In addition to terminal connections to each other, they are connected by a branch *(luo)* by which they flow into one another when the terminal connection is not sufficient for this passage. A special point on each meridian allows us to activate or slow down this movement (passage-point).

In addition, the couples are always formed from a superficial (yang) and a deep (yin) pulse. In one way they obey their special law of contrary action of coupled meridians and in another way that of the mother-child because they always follow each other in the flow. That is to say:

1)   *When the two meridians superimposed by the pulse are of equal intensity, it is the mother-child law which prevails: each acts in the same way on the other.*

2)   *When the intensities are clearly different, tonifying the weaker disperses the stronger, or dispersing the stronger tonifies the weaker: an action in the contrary way which is proper for the coupled meridians balancing yin and yang.*

These couples of the meridians are those at the same segment: Right I — large intestine (child) and lung (mother). Right II — stomach (mother) and spleen-pancreas (child). Right III — triple warmer (child) and vessels-sexual organs (mother). Left I — small intestine (child) and heart (mother). Left II — gallbladder (mother) and liver (child). Left III — bladder (mother) and kidney (child).

In summary:

1) Action in the same way: *Husband-wife:* symmetrical pulses, same level at the opposite wrist. *Mother-child:* following each other in the flow at the same pulse level. This applies also to the coupled meridians if they are of the same intensity, although at different levels.

2) Action in the opposite way: *maximum-minimum (midday-midnight):* crossed pulses, one superficial and one deep. Left I and II, Left III and Right I, Right II and III. *Coupled meridians* if different in intensity; for each segment, the superficial with the deep.

The application of these laws follows; it may be observed also with medicines acting specifically, in a tonifying or dispersing manner, on one organ.

II. Application to the Organs

Lung (yin, maximum 4 a.m., minimum 4 p.m.). To tonify, tonify the lung (direct), liver (mother), heart (husband), and disperse the large intestine (coupled meridian if in excess), bladder (maximum at 4 p.m.). To disperse, act in the opposite manner.

Large intestine (yang, maximum 6 a.m., minimum 6 p.m.). To tonify, tonify the large intestine (direct), stomach (child), small intestine (husband), and disperse the lung (coupled meridian if in excess), kidney (maximum at 6 p.m.). To disperse, act in the opposite manner.

Stomach (yang, maximum 8 a.m., minimum 8 p.m.). To tonify, tonify the stomach (direct), large intestine (mother), gallbladder (husband); disperse the spleen-pancreas (coupled meridian if in excess), heart governor (maximum 8 p.m.). To disperse, act in the opposite manner.

Spleen (yin, maximum 10 a.m., minimum 10 p.m.). To tonify, tonify the spleen-pancreas (direct), heart (child), liver (husband), and disperse the stomach (mother or coupled meridian if in excess), triple warmer (maximum at 10 p.m.). To disperse, act in the opposite manner.

Pancreas: same as the spleen.

Heart (yin, maximum at midday, minimum at midnight). To tonify, tonify the heart (direct), spleen-pancreas (mother), lung (wife); and disperse the small intestine (coupled meridian if in excess), gallbladder (maximum at midnight). To disperse, act in the opposite manner.

Small intestine (yang, maximum 2 p.m., minimum at 2 a.m.). To tonify, tonify the small intestine (direct), bladder (child), large intestine (wife), gallbladder and stomach (digestive system), and disperse the heart (coupled meridian if in excess), liver (maximum at 2 a.m.). To disperse, act in the opposite manner.

Bladder (yang, maximum 4 p.m., minimum 4 a.m.). To tonify, tonify the bladder (direct), small intestine (mother), triple warmer (wife); disperse the kidneys (child or coupled meridian if in excess), lungs (maximum 4 a.m.). To disperse, act in the opposite manner.

Kidney (yin, maximum 6 p.m., minimum 6 a.m.) To tonify, tonify the kidney (direct), heart governor (child and wife) and disperse the bladder (coupled meridian if in excess, and mother), large intestine (maximum 6 a.m.). Also, through the bladder, the respiratory passages. To disperse, act in the opposite manner.

Heart governor (yin, maximum 8 p.m., minimum 8 a.m.) To tonify, tonify the heart governor (direct), kidney (mother and husband); disperse the triple warmer (coupled meridian if in excess), stomach (maximum at 8 a.m.). To disperse, act in the opposite manner.

Triple warmer (yang, maximum 10 p.m., minimum 10 a.m.) To tonify, tonify either 1) Sympathetic: triple warmer and all the distributor yin organs, or 2) Energy of activity: triple warmer and all the yang producer organs, or 3) Triple warmer (direct), gallbladder (child), bladder (husband) and disperse the heart governor (mother or coupled meridian if in excess), spleen-pancreas (maximum at 10 a.m.). To disperse, act in the opposite manner.

Gallbladder (yang, maximum midnight, minimum midday). To tonify, tonify the gallbladder (direct), triple warmer (mother), stomach (wife), and disperse the liver (child or coupled meridian if in excess), heart (maximum at midday). To disperse, act in the opposite manner.

Liver (yin, maximum 2 a.m., minimum 2 p.m.) To tonify, tonify the liver (direct), lung (child), spleen-pancreas (wife), and disperse the gallbladder (coupled meridian if in excess), small intestine (maximum 2 p.m.) To disperse, act in the opposite manner.

III. Mechanical Interactions of Neighbors

Besides groups of organs all responding either in a similar or opposite manner to the action on the energy of one of the organs in the group, we must mention, with some interpretive reservations, the insufficiency or excess of energy mechanically caused by the distention or retraction of a neighboring organ.

Each organ in the body takes up only the space that is strictly indispensable to its normal size. Its distention squeezes its neighbors and irritates or blocks them. Its exaggerated retraction leaves a free space and causes ptosis and prolapse of its neighboring organs.

Thus, a spleen distended from insufficiency (also the liver, the husband) presses the heart (child) to the point of simulating angina pectoris. It presses the lungs (and causes panting, which can be mistaken for asthma), the stomach (mother) which is pushed down inferiorly and which is treated as aerophagia or ptosis, the pancreas (which can make digestion difficult and even simulate a false diabetes), the large intestine in two places (forbidding the passage of hard or half-hard stools and simulating a chronic constipation and even an intestinal obstruction), the small intestine (with oppressive fullness and difficult digestion of starches, meat and fat), the kidneys (with pains, blood pressure problems, sometimes emission of blood, ptosis of the right kidney in women, problems of the left kidney in men). The pulses of the spleen and liver in this case are almost nonexistent. That of the stomach is swollen, of the heart contracted and agitated, of the lungs contracted, and of the two intestines hard.

A retraction of the two intestines causes a ptosis of the stomach. Irritation of the rectum from pinworms (oxyures) is communicated to the bladder, irritation of which can bother the female organs. Ovaries and the cecum-appendix can irritate one another, etc.

In these groups of neighbors, the more marked pulse indicates the responsible organ and the organ which is the victim.

IV. Interactions of Parts of the Body: "The Great Puncture"

Instruments which measure the energy have permitted us to verify and to extend certain observations made by antiquity, observations which render the greatest services in the management of energy. The opposite polarization of whole parts of the body is involved here. We fall back on the yin-yang law of relativity; electrically, the positive and negative poles.

If one applies an electrode on a part which is a yang positive pole and the other electrode on a part which is a yin negative pole, the needle moves and gives a potential. But if one applies an electrode on two yang parts — the same side of an arm or hand, and particularly along the same meridian — the needle does not move. It gives no potential.

It seems thus that the designations "positive-negative," "yin-yang" of each part of the body correspond to an energetic-electric reality and not to some theoretical idea as some people have thought.

Thus, positive-yang are: the right lateral half of the body, the upper half from the waist, the cutaneous surface, the external side of the limbs, and the back. Likewise, negative-yin are: the left lateral half of the body, the lower half from the waist, the internal organs, the internal face of the limbs, and the anterior thorax and abdomen. But it is a matter of relativity: thus, the head is yang relative to the extremities, while the upper limbs are yang relative to the lower limbs.

Practically, for the management of energy, every stimulation causes a transfer of equal quantity on the opposite term. Thus, if there is excess in the right side, tonification of the left side at the symmetrical point will cause the excess of the right to pass into the insufficiency or even normality of the left. To tonify the external yang side of a limb will empty the internal yin side of its excess. The yang pains of the head are dispersed by tonifying the yin hands. The pains of the shoulder and arm are dispersed by tonifying the feet, the excess of the right part of the face by tonifying the left part. Insufficiencies of the right arm are tonified by dispersing the left arm.

For the action to be fully successful, one must choose the symmetrical point on the opposite branch of the same meridian for the opposite puncture, for the symmetrical part of the body. For different limbs or opposite sides of the body or limbs or different parts of the body, choose a point of the meridian opposite (by the midday-midnight law) to the meridian crossing the troubled part, that is, a yin meridian point for a yang meridian problem, and vice versa.

Thus, migraines of the right temple (yang, gallbladder in excess) will be helped by tonifying a point of the yin heart meridian, particularly on the left hand. An excess of the yang large intestine is dispersed by tonifying a yin kidney point on the foot; an excess of the yin kidneys by tonifying a yang large intestine point on the hand — particularly on the opposite side.

If the improvement is not complete, it is possible, since the energy is directed towards the opposite side, to directly treat the troubled area.

For the parts of the body as well as for the organs, through the transfer of the energy, *it is impossible to tonify one region without tonifying another of the same sign and to disperse another of the opposite sign, and vice versa.*

An old aphorism states: "When the tiger is in the house, it is wise to open the doors and windows before taking him by the tail."

V. Interaction of the Elements and the Planets

Liver: wood, Jupiter. Heart: fire, Mars. Kidneys: water, Mercury. Spleen-pancreas: earth, Earth. Lungs: metal, Venus.

Each element (and each astral influence) endangers one element and benefits another. Thus, fire (Mars, the heart) endangers wood (liver, Jupiter); we must protect the liver when the heart is sick. The fire (Mars, heart) is put in danger by the kidneys (water, Mercury). The spleen (earth) benefits the liver (wood, Jupiter), but destroys the lungs (metal, Venus), etc.

We know of the cardiorenal and hepatocardiac reflexes, etc.

This law of the five elements is very interesting, but it would be abusive to give it a predominance and quasi-preference in a process as complex as the management of energy.

VI. Consequences of the Interactions: Multiple Effects of the Points

In addition to all these interactions, each point of a meridian has in addition to its own action on a function of its organ: 1) An effect on one or several functions of two or more organs in the same way. 2) An effect on one or several functions of two or more organs in an opposite way. 3) An effect on the parts of the organism crossed by its meridian. 4) An effect on certain of the parts of the organism crossed by the meridians on which it acts, either in the same way or in an opposite way. 5) An effect according to its strength in the hierarchy of the organs (see further: Chapter VIII).

Moreover, there are still more varied effects, such as when a problem of one organ has caused problems in organs in relation to it, and these in their turn provoke dysfunctions in organs in relation to them. The problem eventually extends to the entire organism.

In a case which started with chronic cholecystitis, eleven different "illnesses" were observed, for which the patient took eleven different medicines each day. If one of them was stopped, the "illness" which it "cured" was hardly felt.

This shows the importance of always searching for the original problem, the "root," and to see after some days if all the other troubles, the "branches," fall away by themselves. It is thus possible with a single point or single needle to improve problems so numerous as to appear to have no connection with each other.

It is in this spirit that, having found the first problem and the point which commands it, we would be wise to check again in Part IV as to whether or not all the subsequent problems are listed for this point. This practice alone will allow us to understand the multiple effects of the points and the interactions of the organs.

Chapter VII

Action On The Energy (VII)

The Eight Vessels of the Marvellous Meridians: Qi Jing Ba Mai

I. Captors of External Yin or Yang Energy 1. Yin, Conception Vessel: Ren Mai 2. Yang, Governor Vessel: Du Mai — II. Regulators of the Intensity of Yin or Yang Energy 1. Yin, the Internal Submalleolar Vessel: Yinqiao Mai 2. Yang, External Submalleolar Vessel: Yangqiao Mai — III. Organic Producers of Yin or Yang Energy 1. Yin, Chain of Yin: Yinwei Mai 2. Chain of Yang: Yangwei Mai — IV. Yin and Yang Nervous and Motor Distributors 1. Yin, Vessel of Attacks: Chong Mai 2. Yang, Belt Vessel: Dai Mai

In antiquity it was noticed that certain points have analogous and very powerful effects on the energy itself, and its nervous and motor manifestations. These points, some of which are located on the two median lines and other of which are borrowed from other meridians, have been combined into groups which have been given the general name of the ''eight vessels of the marvellous meridians.'' The points have a mutual response in each group. Their command points (each vessel has one such point) have mutual responses in pairs, two times two yin and two times two yang. Their groupings are not theoretical, but the result of careful observations and experiments.

Among these eight vessels are included: 1) The two median lines (governor and conception vessels); 2) Six groups of points borrowed from different meridians.

The eight have in common a command point borrowed from a meridian (for the median lines also), which awakens a mutual response in a command point of another vessel. Thus *lieque* (LU-7), command point of the conception vessel and *zhaohai* (KI-3, IS KI-6), command point of the internal submalleolar vessel *yinqiao mai,* and so forth. (A captor of energy is coupled with a regulator of intensity, and an organic producer with a nervous and motor distributor.) Tradition describes them as each having special effects, for which a list is given.

Our observations and instrumental measurements have led us to recognize the great importance of capturing, balancing and alternating the two forms of the vital energy (of yang activity and of yin repose), either in the vital force itself or in the groups of meridians which produce it (yang) or distribute it (yin). This occurs in pairs in the same way and in pairs in the opposite way (tonifying and dispersing).

All disequilibrium between the two forms of energy, between the two opposed groups, is manifested through special, general disorders which are impossible to comprehend and cure without knowing clearly the opposing characteristics of these channels and especially their command points. We thus try to describe them by classifying them in pairs according to their major opposing roles.

Let us point out, first of all, the important fact that all tonifying action on one diminishes the energy of the opposite member of its group in exact correlation. All dispersing action on one increases the opposite energy of the other in exact correlation. They are thus passage points between opposite groups: 1) The captors of yin or yang energy linked to the regulators of intensity of yin or yang energy; 2) The organic producers of yin or yang energy linked to the nervous or motor distributors of yin or yang energy.

In order to manipulate them one should not forget that by the alternation of yin and yang energy of day and night, of the moral-cerebral and physical life, it is essential to determine the solar rhythm, so that the yang energy may be tonified during the rising of the sun and the yin energy tonified during its descent. On the other hand, as is said above, to tonify the yin, disperse the yang; to disperse the yin, tonify the yang.

I. Captors of External Yin or Yang Energy

''Captors'' implies summons and reception of energy of external origin: yin-sexual and yang-astral. Perhaps there is a transformation of this external energy by a process heretofore ignored. Tonifying one aspect disperses the other. Each is linked to a regulator of intensity.

Yin energy: conception vessel (ren mai).

Described in detail in Part IV: ''Meridians, median lines.'' The yin energy comes in large part from sexual stimulation. This is the center of the instinct for reproduction which makes the active power of the being. In addition to the genitourinary functions, it also supplies energy to the respiratory and digestive functions.

If in excess: illnesses of women; men: problems of the genital apparatus; pains of the head and nape; abdomen full, swollen, painful; abscesses of mouth and tongue. If insufficient: pruritis, heaviness of the lumbar region.

Command point: *lieque* (LU-7), mutual response with *zhaohai* (KI-3, IS KI-6), command point of the internal submalleolar vessel, *yinqiao mai,* regulator of yin energy intensity.

This vessel contains all the herald points of the triple warmer, through which its energy is distributed, and two herald points for the vessels and sexual organs. All these points have a mutual response with those of the lung. Its points are enumerated in Part IV, ''Meridians; median lines.''

Yang energy: governor vessel (du mai).

Described in detail in Part IV: ''Meridians; median lines.'' The yang energy is of astral origin captured by the back and particularly the vertebral column. In addition, its origin, like the conception vessel, is at the perineum (*huiyin,* CV-1), and participates in the sexual energy, the center of which is at the perineum.

It acts on physical strength, mainly of the back, but also on mental force, on the character. If insufficient: bent walk, the head falls forward, lack of strength, weakness of character. If in excess: stiff back, heat in the middle of the back; headache, hallucinations, pains of the eyes, hyperexcitation, epilepsy.

Its command point is *houxi* (SI-3). All the points of the small intestine and governor vessel have a mutual response. *Houxi* awakens a mutual response in *shenmai* (BL-62) of the external submalleolar vessel, *yangqiao mai,* regulator of the yang energy.

Its other points are enumerated in Part IV: ''Meridians, median lines.''

These two median lines, acting like captors of energy, are each linked to a vessel which allows the regulation of the intensity of the captured energy. Tradition suggests that they have their ''root'' at the point *qichong* (ST-30) in the lower abdomen (with the vessel of attacks, *chong mai*).

Let us recall that each one has an ascending current on the right and a descending current on the left and that the stimulation of a point on the right of one is perceived in the left current of the other and vice versa. The result is that there is an alternating continual current connecting the two lines, the capturing of the yin of night and the yang of the day.

Another final analogy is that their pulses give the measure of the parasympathetic and of the sympathetic (conception vessel: parasympathetic; governor vessel: sympathetic).

II. Regulators of the Intensity of Yin or Yang Energy

These two vessels, one yin and one yang, each have yin with yin, yang with yang mutual responses of their command points with the captors of energy described above.

Yin energy: internal submalleolar vessel (yinqiao mai).

Regulates the intensity of the yin energy of rest, the inactivity of nocturnal sleep.

If in excess, disperse (dominance of yin energy over the yang energy during the day). Aggravations marked at the middle of the day, improving at sunset and at night; or aggravation in the middle of the day, or increasing from sunrise. Migraines, congestive headaches, contractions, attacks of epilepsy during the day (remitting at night), but good sleep. If insufficient: tonify. Domination of yang energy at night: aggravations at night, headache at night, cramps or convulsions at night, poor sleep.

Command point: *zhaohai* (KI-3, IS KI-6); mutual response with *lieque* (LU-7), command point of the conception vessel, captor of yin energy.

This vessel also includes two points borrowed from the kidneys and bladder, *jiaoxin* (KI-8) and *jingming* (BL-1).

Yang energy: external submalleolar vessel (yangqiao mai).

Regulates the intensity of the yang energy of activity, of waking, daytime. If in excess, disperse. Aggravations at sunset and sunrise: crises, pain and nocturnal congestion, nighttime headaches, poor sleep. If insufficient, tonify. Dominance of yin energy: fatigue, lassitude, weakness in the day and, if the yin energy dominates, aggravations during the day with improvement at sunset.

(SI-3), command point of the governor vessel, captor of yang energy.

This vessel includes some other points borrowed from the stomach and bladder: *pucan* (BL-61), *fuyang* (BL-58), then on the face, cheek-*juliao* (ST-6, IS ST-3) and *chengqi* (ST-4, IS ST-1)

III. Organic Producers of Yin and Yang Energy

For these two groups it is impossible to tonify one without diminishing the other with equal intensity. To disperse one without increasing the energy of the other in the same way is also impossible. They are thus equalizers allowing the assurance of balance between production and distribution (thus the expenditure of energy) between the two internal and external regions of the body, between the superior and inferior crossing.

Yin: chain of yin (yinwei mai).[1]

Commands all the yin meridian organs (deep pulses), distributors of energy and blood: heart, lungs, spleen-pancreas, liver, kidney, vessels-sexual organs.

If in excess, all the deep pulses are clearly stronger than the superficial ones. The most apparent problems are internal excesses of the thoracic organs: heart pains, hypertension, tight chest, contraction of the lungs, respiratory disturbances. Also some external weaknesses: weakness of the shoulder and superior limb, hand and thumb, and of the opposite inferior limb.

If insufficient, all the deep pulses are clearly weaker than the superficial pulses. There are then thoracic internal weakness of the heart, hypotension and weak respiration. Also external excess: pain of the anterior side of the shoulder and superior limb, hand, thumb and of the opposite lower limb.

The command point is *neiguan* (PC-6), which is thus the passage point between all the yin and yang meridians, but it acts primarily on the abdominal organs: the spleen-pancreas, heart, stomach and intestines.

This vessel has other points acting in the same way, all yin, borrowed from the conception vessel, liver, spleen-pancreas, kidney. Conception vessel: *tiantu* (CV-22), *xuanji* (CV-21). Liver: thorax-*qimen* (LR-14). Spleen-pancreas: *fuai* (SP-16), *fuhe* (SP-13). Kidney: *zhubin* (KI-9).

Yang: chain of yang (yangwei mai).

Commands all the yang (superficial pulses), producers of energy: stomach, intestines, gallbladder, bladder.

Its excess (excess of all yang meridians) manifests through fever, headaches from heat, storms, or pains or problems of the skin from weather changes, pains or swellings of articulations particularly of the hand and heel, swellings of the parotid glands (mumps), diarrhea. Sometimes storms paralyze the life.[2] In brief, excess of yang (external) meridians and excess of the contralateral limbs. Its insufficiency (emptiness of the yang meridians) manifests as cold, lack of enthusiasm, loss of strength from weather changes, especially snow or rain. In brief, insufficiency of the yang (external) meridians, and excess of the contralateral limbs.

Its command point is *waiguan* (TW-5), which is also the passage point between the yin and yang meridians as well as the top and bottom of the body. It has a mutual response with foot-*linqi* (GB-41), command point of the belt vessel *dai mai,* a nervous and motor distributor which also commands the yang meridians.

The yangwei mai has other points, all yang, having similar effects, borrowed from the triple warmer, governor vessel, gallbladder, bladder and small intestine: *naohui* (TW-13), *naoshu* (SI-10), *tianliao* (TW-15). At the nape: *yamen* (GB-14, IS GV-15), *fengfu* (GV-15, IS GV-16), *fengchi* (GB-20); the skull: *naokong* (GB-19), *chengling* (GB-14, IS GB-18), *zhengying* (GB-13, IS GB-17), *muchuang* (GB-12, IS GB-16), head-*linqi* (GB-11, IS GB-15). On the shoulder: *jianjing* (GB-21). On the leg: *yangjiao* (GB-35). On the foot: *jinmen* (BL-63).

IV. Yin and Yang Nervous and Motor Distributors

The roles of these two vessels are complicated by the fact that one of them commands all the yin meridians, the other all the yang meridians. When tonified, they disperse the meridians of the opposite sign and when dispersed, they tonify them. They are thus equally used as passage points between the yang energy of the meridians and their yin energy. This is in addition to their role in nervous and motor external activity.

Yin: vessel of attacks (chong mai).

The word "attacks" or "assaults" must be understood as meaning a crisis of nerves or of pains or of circulation, of motor function, or even hyperexcitation.

In fact, the insufficiency of the vessel manifests through all spasms, contractions, pains and other excesses of the yang energy of activity, of internal organs or the external organism. By tonifying, all the yang organ meridians in excess are dispersed, particularly the abdominal organs, and all the yin organ meridians are tonified, particularly the contralateral thoracic meridians on the surface of the body. It is thus a distributor of the energy of yang activity of the abdomen and of the external surface.

Its insufficiency is manifested through an excess of the stomach and intestines: spasms and external contralateral contractures, and also by an excess of menses — it is called "sea of blood" for women having their menses. The insufficiency of the yang producer organs, particularly the stomach and intestines, can cause excess of the heart and spleen-pancreas. Its excess manifests through weakness of the abdominal organs, insufficiency of menses, nervous and motor atony, contralateral above and below.

Its passage point is *gongsun* (SP-4), which is the passage point between the spleen-pancreas and stomach. There are mutual responses with *neiguan* (PC-6) of the chain of yin, *yinwei mai,* all producers of yin energy; it commands all the yin meridians at the expense of all the yang meridians and has a deep action on the heart and lungs.

This vessel is said to start with the conception vessel and the governor vessel at the point *huiyin* (CV-1) at the perineum. From there it rises, borrowing all the kidney points on the abdomen up to and including *youmen* (KI-21). It rises (through the kidney meridian?) and surrounds the mouth borrowing the branches of the conception vessel and governor vessel.

Tradition says that in women this vessel does not surround the lips — thus the lack of a beard. For eunuchs, being cut at the root, the result would be the same regarding this lack. No experiments have been made in order to determine whether it diminishes superfluous hair if dispersed.

Its other points are: *henggu* (KI-11), *dahe* (KI-12), *qixue* (KI-13), *siman* (KI-14), *zhongzhu* (KI-15), *huangshu* (KI-16), *shangqu* (KI-17), *shiguan* (KI-18), *yindu* (KI-19), *tonggu* (KI-20) and *youmen* (KI-21)

All these points are important for their action on spasms, contractions, inflammation, congestion, contracting pain and also on nervous and motor atony.

Yang: belt vessel (dai mai).

The belt vessel acts on all the yang organ meridians, producers of energy, and in an opposite way, on all the yin distributor organ-meridians. It is said to surround all the meridians at the waist like a belt, hence its name. It acts by crossing the external body, muscles and ligaments as well as the nipples and even the ovaries and eyes, and "harmonizes top with bottom."

Its insufficiency manifests through the insufficiency of the yang meridians, as cold or slowness or weakness of the lumbar area and the inferior limbs, or as inflammation and paralyzing pains of the shoulder and of the opposite upper limb, the opposite eye, the opposite nipple or the opposite ovary. Its excess manifests through the excess of yang meridians, as pains of the lumbar area and lower limbs, or weakness of the shoulder and opposite limb, opposite eye and nipple or opposite ovary.

Its action is thus felt as crossed and opposite up to the waist on the same side, and at the top of the body on the opposite side. To tonify yang disperse yin and vice versa.

Its command point is foot-*linqi* (GB-41), which is said "to make flow easily" the conception vessel and vessel of attacks (both yin), and thus acts on all the troubles of menses and lactation.

There are mutual responses with *waiguan* (TW-5), command point of the chain of yang, *yangwei mai,* producer of yang energy which itself acts also in crossing. They are both said "to harmonize the top with the bottom."

There are other points having the same actions, all yang and of the gallbladder: *weidao* (GB-30, IS GB-28), *juliao* (GB-28, IS GB-29), hip-*wushu* (GB-27), *daimai* (GB-26).

Chapter VIII

Action On The Energy (VIII)

The Hierarchy of Commands

1. The Form. 2. Total Energy. 3. Energy of Activity: Yang. 4. Energy of Inactivity: Yin. 5. Passages between Energy of Yang Activity and Yin Inactivity. 6. The Parasympathetic System. 7. The Sympathetic System. 8. All the Yang Producer Organs. 9. All the Yin Distributor Organs. 10. Parts of the Body. 11. Parts of the Organism.

A ''form'' exists which always protects us and which regulates growth, harmonious development, the exact repairs within the plan of the individual, longevity perhaps, and surely immunity against all exterior physical or mental shock. There is a totality of energy, an intensity of life, which allows each person to use his faculties to the highest degree. It is impossible to act on a vital command of an organ without modifying at the same time in a similar or opposite way several other organs, and that according to precise laws which extend to the parts of the organism. Further, the pulses allow us to measure the intensity of the energy in the whole body or in one of its parts (see preceding chapters). Moreover, there are certain points which command more or less large groups or parts of organs. It is therefore shortsighted and sometimes even dangerous to limit oneself to the energetic equilibration of each organ.

On the other hand, the higher the plane of energy where problems are cured, the more complete will be the return of the whole individual to usual vitality, even to the point of achieving the maximum development of what comprises his particular body, mind and moral faculties. This is provided, of course, that an inappropriate intervention does not disturb the undamaged planes of command, which must not be upset.

When all the disharmonized commands have been re-established in their full intensity of energy, the organism makes all the problems (the so-called ''illnesses'') immediately disappear with the ease with which the organism normally prevents disease, because, as has been said in other chapters, an organic problem is always preceded by a more or less prolonged functional disturbance, and this by an unperceived derangement of energy. It is always possible to find a cause for this in some prolonged error of hygiene or in a mental shock.

We understand thus the chasm which separates this science of the vital energy from acupuncture as practiced by those who puncture anywhere, without caring for the exact locality of the command points, or for the measure of the energy in all places in the body, or for the flow of the energy, or for the interactions of the organs or of the hierarchy of commands. To act in this way is to debase the management of commands of life to the level of simple response points, to blind counterirritation.

The hierarchy of commands and the interaction of the organs must never be confused. The interaction of the organs as previously clarified is formed of associations of organs, each acting on the other members of its group, either similarly or in opposition. It seems that the members of each group are associated in order to maintain the equilibrium of energy by increasing or decreasing together or by taking or giving to one another.

On each of its levels, the hierarchy of commands rests on the strength of certain points of certain meridians, on a great number of organs and parts of the organism. The power of each point is observed concurrently with the action of the point on certain functions of the meridian and on the related organs.

Thus there is the action of a point of the stomach (leg-*sanli,* ST-36) on the total energy and the whole being and on the gallbladder (husband), large intestine (mother) and spleen-pancreas (child and coupled meridian). If we admit that the stomach is at the base of the production of energy, how can it make such a general and rapid distribution? Why do not all the points of the stomach meridian have the same effect? Is it a matter of a special function of the stomach?

The same questions can be posed for each of the command points governing one or the other of the different levels of the hierarchy. Studies and future observations, through compilation, will perhaps permit us to resolve most of these problems. At present, we are only able to give the name of the points and their effects on each of the groups and levels as they have been observed and measured.

The hierarchy of commands can thus be established in its general outlines and its most active points:

1) The individual, unique form.
2) The total energy.
3) The yang energy of activity.
4) The yin energy of inactivity.
5) Passages between yang energy and yin energy, commanders of all the yang meridians or all the yin meridians.
6) The parasympathetic system, commander of the yang meridians.
7) The sympathetic system, commander of the yin meridians.
8) All yang organs and yang energy.
9) All yin organs and yin energy.
10) Parts of the body.
11) Parts of the organism.

The individual, unique form.

The form, which assures growth, repair, etc., and which is strictly personal to the individual, is fed by the small intestine, spleen-pancreas, gallbladder and governor vessel:

Insufficiency: *houxi* (SI-3), *dadu* (SP-2), *xuanzhong* (GB-39), *bailao* (GV-13, IS GV-14 *dazhui*).

Total energy.

Measurable by the combination of all the pulses.

The best results are obtained by taking careful account of the rising of the sun, the moon and the year for tonifying, and their descent for dispersion.

Only one point acts on the total energy without any transfer: leg-*sanli* (ST-36).

It is also possible to act on the total energy without transfer by acting at the same time and in the same way on the energy captors: conception and governor vessels.

The yang energy of activity.

Seen in activity, vivacity, brilliant eyes, the timbre of the voice, etc. The command point of the external submalleolar vessel, *yangqiao mai* (*shenmai,* BL-62), is the most efficacious; the other points are less so.

The yin energy of inactivity.

Seen in heaviness, somnolent aspect, etc. The command point of the internal submalleolar vessel, *yinqiao mai* (*zhaohai,* KI-3, IS KI-6), is the most efficacious; its other points are less so.

Passages between all the yin and yang meridians.

These points transfer the excess of one to the insufficiency of the other to tonify the insufficiency or to disperse the excess.

Yang meridians (superficial pulses): *waiguan* (TW-5), command point of the chain of yang, *yangwei mai,* on which its other points act slightly. Yin meridians (deep pulses): *neiguan* (PC-6), command point of the chain of yin, *yinwei mai,* on which its other points act slightly, but the points of the heart governor have a marked action.

The parasympathetic system, commander of the yang meridians.

Measurable by its pulse and the totality of yang and vessel pulses: *tianzhu* (BL-10).

The sympathetic system, commander of the yin meridians.

Measurable by its pulse and the totality of the yin and triple warmer pulses: *fengchi* (GB-20).

All the yang producer organs and yang energy.

Hegu (LI-4), *zhongzhu* (TW-3).

All the yin distributor organs and yin energy.

Taichong (LR-3), *zhongchong* (PC-9).

Parts of the body.

All parts: either internal-external, or up and down, or right-left, etc. To tonify, disperse the opposite; to disperse, tonify the opposite. *Dabao* (SP-21), the great *luo* of the spleen, acts on all meridians, although especially on the yin.

Lateral half on the same side: in the reverse way on the opposite side: large intestine: *quchi* (LI-11), *jianyu* (LI-15); gallbladder: *huantiao* (GB-29, IS GB-30).

Upper limb: direct action (and opposite on the other upper limb): *yangchi* (TW-4), hand *wangu* (SI-4). See T1, T2, T3 of the same side. Opposite action and on the opposite lower limb: foot-*linqi* (GB-41).

Lower limb: direct action (and opposite on the other lower limb): Thigh-*futu* (ST-32), *yinchi* (ST-33), *yaoyang-guan* (GV-3). Opposite action and through the opposite upper limb: *houxi* (SI-3), *sanjian* (LI-3), *hegu* (LI-4), *waiguan* (TW-5).

Parts of the organism.

All the muscles: on the same side: *yanglingguan* (GB-34): external muscles; *chengjin* (BL-56): internal and external muscles; arm-*shanglian* (LI-9): upper limb same side, opposite lower limb, also *quyuan* (SI-13).

All bones: dazhu (BL-11); periostium: foot-*shangqiu* (SP-5).

Bone marrow: xuanzhong (GB-39) on the same side of the body.

Blood: gaohuangshu (BL-38, IS BL-43); to a lesser degree *pohu* (BL-37, IS BL-42). See: *geshu* (BL-17), assent point, but reunion of blood?

Arteries: can tonify or disperse, upper limb same side and lower limb opposite side: *taiyuan* (LU-9). Tonify only (also crossed): *zhongchong* (PC-9); disperse only (contralateral): *daling* (PC-7).

Veins: lower limb same side, opposite upper limb: thigh-*futu* (ST-32) can tonify or disperse. Equally crossed: above all disperse foot-*shangqiu* (SP-5).

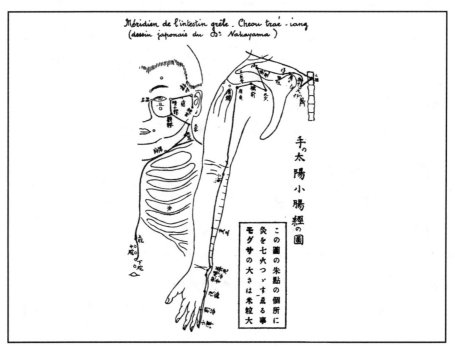

Meridian of the small intestine (Nakayama)

Chapter IX

Action On The Energy (IX)

The Means of Action

I. Needles — II. Moxa — III. Massage — IV. Sound — V. Electricity — VI. Magnetism

The exact effect produced by the action taken on the command points by different means, already extensively experimented upon, has not been clearly explained.

The word "excitation" is used when it is a question of dispersing or tonifying a point. In fact, certain instruments allow us to observe that by "excitation" there is always a discharge and never a charge. In effect, a point excited in one way or another (tonified or dispersed) is without power for several days. Its sensitivity diminishes or even disappears as soon as it has been touched; it appears to be discharged. Only rest recharges it.

On the other hand, the organism can be discharged (dispersed) or recharged (tonified) according to the action and according to the sort of instrument used.

Historically, the *Nei Jing* mentions the usage of stone needles and recommends the "new" needles of copper as being softer and more efficient. It again mentions the use of moxa made with still-glowing ambers. Some works cited since the Christian era mention steel or gold needles, "which are more elegant," until the time when the effects of the different metals were compared.

I. The Needle

The needles[3] could be more correctly called pins, because for a long time there has been no eye, but a head. The term has remained from the first needles of copper, which were really for sewing. However, a thread of copper was passed through the eye and wound to delimit the depth of insertion. The same system was used later for the needles of iron, and then steel.

The law of action-reaction relativity governs the effect of the needle: the effect depends both on the action of the needle and on the reactive capacity of the patient.

In other words, a strong needle will greatly tire a weakened person and even risk making him faint, or more, retard and even diminish the desired effect. The same strong needle on a physically strong person will obtain all the desired effects without fatigue. The reaction is conditioned by the hour, by the lunar cycle and by the astrological house. The energy is superficial in summer; it is deeper in winter. Hence a strong needle will be supporting and even useful in winter; it will tire the patient in summer. It is useful at the full moon for the yin and at the new moon for the yang, etc.

It is important to observe the mass of the metal, whether the needle is long and quite thin or more short and thick in body (although equally thin at the point). The shape of the head seems important; if the head is of precious stone, it clearly adds to the strength, one explanation being that the precious stones are impermeable to the waves which circulate in the body (which are negative or positive) or which escape from the body through the metal.

A handle shaped like a sphere gives effects which are more or less regular, whether the atmospheric electricity is positive or negative. This sphere has the value of an antenna, its length determined by the thinnest thread that can be extended from it.

A sharp handle, on the other hand, absorbs the maximum exterior waves and gives effects which vary completely with the weather. A pointed lightening rod attracts the thunderbolt which a sphere does not attract.

Experiments allow us to distinguish three degrees of strength:

1)   The strong needle, which one should use only in winter, in cold weather, on people with good resistance, and in very small numbers — only one if possible. In this group the strongest, and at the same time the most manageable (gold for tonifying, silver for dispersing) is 3 to 4 cm. in length, and in thickness from 1 to 2 mm., with a handle of precious stone and a fine point tapered with a long gradient.

2)   The intermediate needle, in summer, can be a little too strong for weak people — intellectual and nervous types — but in winter a little too weak on people who react well, although it can still give good average results. It should be (in gold or silver) 3 or 4 cm. in length, in thickness from .9 to 1 mm, with a small spherical head of the same metal.

3)   Thin needles, adapted for people with lively reactions, are for children and for old people in summer; they are insufficient in winter.

Two varieties are used (gold or silver): length of approximately 3.5 cm., with a small head of the same metal; thickness of .6 or .7 mm.

Some very fine needles are from .1 to .2 mm. thick, and from 6 to 7 cm. long, with a head 1 cm. long and .3 mm. thick. They are put in with the help of a tube. The needle is made to enter the point by tapping with the finger: this is used widely in Japan. In spite of their smoothness, they can still cause fainting if the patient is very tired and is punctured while standing.

In pharmacies in the north of China acupuncture needles of iron and steel are sold with a length from 10 to 25 cm. and a thickness from .9 to 1.2 mm. Their effect is too strong and often goes against the goal hoped for. The acupuncture masters in China use gold needles from 3 to 4 cm. in length and only a millimeter thick at the maximum.

The metal has a multiple importance:

1)   For dispersing: silver is best; to tonify, gold is best.[4]

2)   For disinfection: gold and silver quickly kill all microbes. When carefully wiped with cotton saturated in alcohol before and after use, they have never caused abscesses, as often happens with a hypodermic needle of steel, which is hollow. These solid needles, which must be kept highly polished, are not designed to promote the survival of a microbe. In all cases, gold and silver needles placed in a virulent culture have shown dead microbes after about thirty seconds.

3)   For oxidation: gold and silver do not oxidize, but they are dotted after a certain number of punctures as if the body eats into an infinitesimal part; one should then polish them.

Copper is very good for tonifying: it oxidizes black after the first puncture and must be rubbed with sandpaper. Steel is attacked relatively quickly when not highly polished.

For the natural action of the metal, which is added to that of the puncture: silver with zinc is strongest for dispersing, to calm pains, inflammation and fever. Gold with copper is strongest for tonifying, for giving life, to act against all weaknesses.

In antiquity it was observed that all yellow or red metals were the strongest for tonification and all white metals were strongest for dispersal, the grey being neutral. Our modern electricians recognize that yellow or red metals are positive, the white metals negative. A sensitive hand, placed a few centimeters from or above a gold needle feels a current, some waves rising towards the wrist, centripetally. Above a silver needle the waves go towards the fingers, centrifugally. Some perceive hot waves for the gold and cool for silver.

Iron, steel, platinum and nickel are less strong than gold for tonifying and less strong than silver for dispersing. However, steel with manganese strongly tonifies, but disperses with difficulty.

On the other hand, gold and silver are soft and puncture poorly when they are pure. An appropriate alloy is necessary to give hardness, but should permit bending in case of a false movement so the point does not break off under the skin. Mr. Souteyrand, an expert in metals, has had the patience and skill to study the alloys of different metals, according to the similar effects of each one. Thus, gold and red copper with 700 parts of gold, and silver and zinc with 665 parts of silver, give the best results for puncturing and do not break.

II. Moxa

The word "moxa" comes from Japanese *mogsa,* or *mogusa,* their term for the artemisia from which it is made. It was introduced in Europe, in the seventeenth century, by the first Dutch travellers returning from Japan.

The antique method in China is to use a small ball "the size of a small bird's dropping," made of a mixed powder from one kind of artemisia (*artemisia urens,* a variety of wormwood), which is then placed in the hole of a coin and burnt like tinder (the fire on the surface of the skin), thereby emitting a live heat. It seems that artemisia projects onto the point some more active elements than any other plant. Would we now say there are ions?

Some people burn it directly on the skin and create a blister. The Japanese use small stems of this tinder applied with small touches on the skin, or kept there, but placed over one or two thicknesses of paper to avoid burns.

The importance attached to artemisia emphasizes that in the moxa there may be two elements: almost burning heat and the ions of artemisia (absinthe being particularly stimulating in effect). It is the most tonifying, but cannot be used every day, as the skin is quickly attacked and the point emptied. From three to five times are common doses.

In France, some very good results have been obtained with heat alone, by means of rapid touches like the pecking of a chicken, made with a shaving brush, the hair of which has first been put in boiling water in order to be charged with heat, and then shaken hard in order to remove the excess water. Each touch must give the impression of a puncture (of heat), the brush being immersed again as soon as this sensation stops; a spoon is also used.

In this system only the element of heat remains. It can be renewed every two days without the point ceasing to be active, but not for more than one month. So it is wise to stop one week out of every two in order to allow the point the time to recharge.

A moxa apparatus giving heat puncture exactly controlled according to the skin has been invented by Mr. Leplus.

When the sun is shining, an extremely energetic method consists of concentrating the rays of the sun with a lens and heating without burning.

III. Massage

The tip of the finger is pressed on the command point and is passed over the skin in order to rub the subcutaneous tissue. It is equally possible to massage the meridian with the palm of the hand. Go against the flow for dispersal, with the flow for tonification.

Massage does not frighten children and sensitive people. It causes neither shock nor fatigue, but it can be rather painful and the results are not lasting except for children, very sensitive people and very recent cases. Physical people can be massaged every day according to need.

Specialists in magnetism estimate that the magnetic power of the masseur has a very great importance. In effect, while it is possible to massage oneself, the results are more clear and durable when done by someone else. It seems that the left hand takes energy (disperses) and the right hand gives energy and tonifies.

IV. Sound

The instrument invented by Mr. Leplus, the sonopuncturist, transmits to the desired point a vibration at audible frequency and both tonifies and disperses, better than massage and the same as moxa.

V. Electricity

Continuing experiments were made by the late Dr. Dimier with all varieties of electricity, either with electrodes on the point, or with a needle inserted and connected by a copper wire to the apparatus. At best, the results were not noticeably stronger than those obtained with the finger. In addition, they were erratic, according to the constantly changing polarity of atmospheric electricity. Also, beyond a few microamperes, the electricity did not seem to penetrate, but rather spread over the skin with a prickling or burning sensation.

VI. Magnetism

Human magnetism gives certain results but must be repeated. It is applied by the imposition of the hand either on the pulses, on the points, or by following a meridian. The instruments invented to measure human energy in the different parts of the body have allowed us to observe its existence in each person and to measure its effects.

The verification of magnetism by measuring the modification of different pulses, by imposing in one way or another one hand or the other on one of the points which commands the pulse examined, has permitted us to notice the following facts. They were observed on apparatus newly invented for measuring the energy and registering the pulses.

1)   The part of the body most active for receiving exterior energy is the center of the palm of the hand (point *lao-gong,* PC-8) and for giving energy, the pad of the finger tip. The fingers project the maximum measured intensity; the index finger is the most powerful.

2)   The two hands do not have the same action. For right-handed people, the right hand gives energy, tonifies; the left hand takes energy, disperses. For left-handed or ambidextrous people, the right hand takes energy, disperses; the left hand gives energy, tonifies.

3)   If the hand is kept above a point or an organ, soon a special heat is felt, and the pulse corresponding to the point or organ is modified.

4)   By keeping the hand palm side up (supinated) inhalation during the day elicits the senstation that some waves are clearly more alive than when the hand is turned palm side down (pronated) and the superficial pulses increase. If the hand is held palm down (pronated) during the day, the waves are weaker and the pulse even drops. At night they are clearly more alive, and the deep pulses are increased.

Does the upturned palm receive yang astral energy? Atmospheric positive electricity? Does the palm down receive yin terrestrial energy during the night, the terrestrial negative electricity? Individual disparities make these experiments difficult.

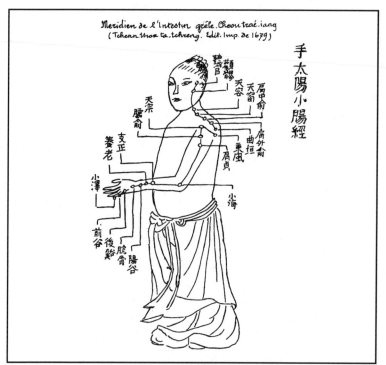

Meridian of the small intestine (DACH)

Notes

[1] The French term means "chain" but is used in the sense of "regulation." — Trans.

[2] The author's meaning is unclear. We suppose it to mean that the person cannot function during storms. — Trans.

[3] The best have been developed, after research and experiments, by Mr. Souteyrand, jeweler and expert in metals, 23 Rue Racine, Paris.

[4] The point *zhonglushu* (BL-29), punctured with a gold needle, redresses a displaced sacrum in a matter of minutes. Punctured with a silver needle, the sacrum does not move, but punctured again with gold in the hollow left by the silver (which has been removed), the sacrum goes back in place in a few minutes.

Chapter X
Action On The Energy (X)

The Causes of Failure

I. In the Subject — II. Temperature — III. In the Practitioner

When all the necessary conditions of experimentation are joined in the practitioner as well as in the subject, the desired results should be integral and almost immediate in a recent case. If this does not occur, one or several of the conditions are missing. One must then look for a cause of the failure.

I. In the Subject

All effect is either simply delayed for a few hours or diminished if there has been recent absorption of analgesics or anesthetics from the aspirin group, or from barbiturates. Morphine has a marked inhibiting action, as well as cocaine, which has no particularly opiate effect, except when taken in great quantities.

Regular food poisoning, coffee with milk, coffee in large quantities, tobacco, alcohol, excess liquid and particularly excess water (which are true intoxications) have the same effect of delay or diminution.

II. Temperature

Cold, even if not very great, always delays the full result, at times even for eight days, the effect being felt suddenly at the end of the delay. Storms, heavy wind, heavy rains, thunder, etc. also diminish the result or delay it until the end of the storm. Sometimes, without it being possible to specify why, the effects are reversed, and the pains increase.

III. In the Practitioner

To expect an action from energy which it cannot give:

The standard is recent functional disturbances, with no material organ physically affected. They give and must give complete results. The more recent the disturbance, the more complete is the response of the organism. This person has not yet accepted defeat, given up the battle and organized a new type of life. Thus, an acute case of shoulder neuralgia can be stopped with one needle and will not leave a trace. If it dates from more than three weeks, a secondary problem, ankylosis, occurs to block the painful movement; the pain then demands many needles. Those caused by ankylosis must be conquered through exercise.

On the other hand, lesions never stop immediately. At most, in certain cases, one can hope to revive the battle of the organism, of the form, which takes up again its work of reconstruction and succeeds, when it is materially possible, to remake the injured tissue entirely, sometimes without leaving even a trace or scar.

1)   To ignore the measure of the energy through the pulse to the point of not knowing if one should tonify or disperse, or which meridian causes the trouble, or which is the point of this meridian which commands the disturbed function.

2)   Not to consider the energy of the individual but the "illness-enemy;" to pay attention only to the apparent problem and not look for the true, deep cause, the dysfunction of energy from physical shock or hygienic mistakes. In other words, to try to sponge up the water without closing the open tap.

3)   Regarding the muscles, vessels or bones: to ignore that they depend first on the meridian which traverses them and gives them their energy.

4) Not to know or not take the trouble to find the precise location of the desired point. To be content with the sensation of bruising announced by the patient, a sensation which can also be well felt several centimeters away from the point, particularly on the meridian, and if the pressure of the finger is violent. We must pass the finger lightly to find the hollow of the point; to assure oneself that the pulse of the organ and the organ respond when one is on the point and do not respond when one is away from it, even by a few millimeters; to ask the patient if he perceives the "something" which passes in the meridians mainly at the hands and feet (not everyone feels this), and even less frequently noticed, if there is a response, a sensation in the related organs. The refined practitioner listens to his own body to perceive the dysfunction of the patient and the point which will correct it.

5) To thrust the needle in as for injections, instead of carefully placing the tip at the center of the point by using a guide which slides into the bottom of the small hollow, and then putting it in slowly. The pain is not felt by the epidermis if the point is carefully found at the center (where the pain is almost nil) and at the desired depth. Thrusting generally causes one to miss the center and in addition, by bruising the subcutaneous tissue where the point is found, causes useless pain.

6) To fail to use the hour of minimum of the meridian for tonifying and of maximum for dispersal. The hour and yin weather (afternoon and dark weather) for tonifying the yin, and the hour and yang weather (morning and clear weather) for tonifying the yang. To ignore the lunation cycle and the seasons; not to act according to the moment, on the yin by the yang and on the yang by the yin.

7) To fail to use the possibility of making the excess yin pass into yang and vice versa.

8) Not to know how to discern troubles from excess yang energy (in the evening and at night) from those of excess of yin energy (in the morning and at noon).

9) To ignore, above all, the opposition between insufficiency and excess, between tonifying and dispersing.

10) To ignore the interaction of the organs or parts of the organism and to make punctures which contradict each other.

11) To riddle the patient with punctures, which prevent any reaction and exhaust him even when they do not neutralize themselves, ignoring that most of his problems stem from one dysfunction and can be stopped with only one needle.

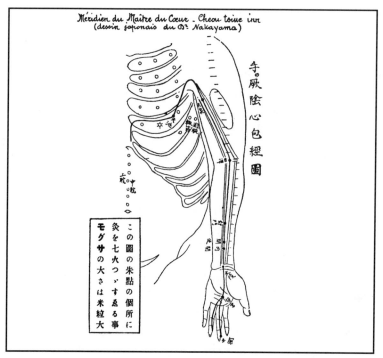

Meridian of the heart governor (Nakayama)

Volume IV

Meridians, Points,
and Their Symptoms

Meridian of the heart governor (GSDM)

Introduction

I. Using the Meridians and Points

Always remember that what we look for, measure and correct through the meridians and points is energy, either total, multiple or local. Without energy there is no existence. If the energy is excessive or insufficient, problems occur. If the energy is harmoniously full, there is health, strength and immunity.

Thus, by examining the pulses and the individual, we first gain an overview of the total energy and then look for how to correct the intake — by the median lines, with food and drink, the astral waves, by exercise and air, from human emanations and through the people around us.

This is the search for how to distribute the energy harmoniously through the meridians to the organs and to all the parts of the body.

To act: refined people and those who have learned to listen to themselves perceive the points for stimulation on themselves (there are very often only one or two); there is a clear feeling of prickly heat. All people are surrounded by waves which they emit with more or less intensity, waves which reflect their condition at the moment. If they are not closed through a dogmatic teaching which negates and paralyzes them, all people according to their refinement perceive the waves of others (sympathy, antipathy, love, repulsion) and can train themselves to measure and analyze these waves on their own body.

Finally, remember that the points command the energy of the affected area, and thus the area itself, according to the particular energetic dysfunction and type of problem. In order to do this, certain points have a special power for which the meridian connection is sometimes difficult to understand. Thus

1)   For the total energy: will to live, vegetative vitality; for the psychic, primitive instincts; primate: *baihui* (GV-19, IS GV-20). The capturing of energy, the recharge, is assured.

   a)   For the astral energy of activity, yang, the mental and physical strength, by *houxi* (SI-3), command point of the governor vessel.

   b)   For the sexual energy, yin, which animates the great physical, sexual, digestive and respiratory functions, through *lieque* (LU-7), command point of the conception vessel.

2)   The unique role for the body of leg-*sanli* (ST-36), which increases or diminishes all the energies of the whole body at once without any perceptible displacement of energy in any other part of the body, suggests that it is perhaps related to the energy of all the cells.

3)   For the intensity of the energy, either yin or yang: the intensity of the yin energy of inactivity, of rest, of sleep, of cold, in the whole body is regulated by *zhaohai* (KI-3, IS KI-6). The intensity of yang energy, of activity, of wakefulness, of cerebral activity, of heat, in the whole body is regulated by *shenmai* (BL-62).

4)   For the equilibrium of the yin and yang meridians. All the yin meridians of distribution and purification are commanded by *neiguan* (PC-6), but to tonify it disperses all the yang meridians and to disperse it tonifies all the yang meridians.

   Taichong (LR-3) acts also on all the yin meridians but with a very weak, opposite effect on the yang meridians.

   All the yang meridians (producers of energy) are commanded by *waiguan* (TW-5), but to tonify it disperses all the yin meridians and to disperse it tonifies all the yin meridians.

   Hegu (LI-4) also acts on all the yang meridians but with a very weak, opposite effect on the yin meridians.

5)   Energy of the skin: *sanli* of the leg (ST-36), *lieque* (LU-7).

6)   Energy of the skeleton.

   a)   Bones: all their troubles, *dazhu* (BL-11); their pains: foot *dadu* (SP-2), *taibai* (SP-3), *xuanzhong* (GB-39).

   b)   Bone marrow, bony sutures: *xuanzhong* (GB-39), of the flat bones, red and white cells, sternum.

   c)   Periosteum: *shangqiu* of foot (SP-5).

   d)   Joints: *xiguan* (LR-7) *yangfu* (GB-38).

7)   The energy of the muscles: lower limb same side, superior limb opposite, muscles of the yang side (external), *linqi* of foot (GB-41), muscles of the yin side (internal), *gongsun* (SP-4). Half of the body, same side: *yanglingquan* (GB-34).

8)   Blood, red cells; *gaohuangshu* (BL-38, IS BL-43).

White cells: polynuclear (streptococcus, pus, abscess): *xuanzhong* (GB-39). Mononuclear (staphylococcus, pemphigus, psoriasis, impetigo, etc.): *dadu* of foot (SP-2).

9)   Vessels.

a) Arteries: *taiyuan* (LU-9), tonifies and disperses, *daling* (PC-7), disperses.

b) Veins: Thigh, *futu* (ST-32): all troubles; foot: *shangqiu* (SP-5), pains, heaviness; *chengshan* (BL-57) and *chengjin* (BL-56), hemorrhoids, internal varicosities.

10)   Internal and external mucosa: *xuanzhong* (GB-39).

11)   Nerves: leg-*sanli* (ST-36); excess: *tianjing* (TW-10); pains: *kunlun* (BL-60), *qihai* (CV-6).

12)   Encephalon: from the pulse, part of the meridian of the governor vessel. Brain: anterior lobes: *dadu* of the foot (SP-2), *fenglong* (ST-40); parietal and temporal lobes: *qianding* (GV-20, IS GV-21), *xiajuxu* of leg (ST-39); occipital lobes: *baihui* (GV-19, IS GV-20), *shanglian* of leg (ST-37). The whole brain: *xinhiu* (GV-21, IS GV-22). Cerebellum: *yanglingquan* (GB-34); medulla: *qiangjian* (GV-17, IS GV-18).

13)   Spinal cord: part of the meridian of the governor vessel, the different points of the governor vessel, mostly *bailao* (GV-13, IS GV-14 *dazhui*).

14)   Endocrines: pulse — no meridian, although their points are on the cervical part of the governor vessel.

Pituitary: inferior edge of sixth cervical.

Parathyroids: inferior edge of fifth cervical.

Thyroid: inferior edge of fourth cervical.

Adrenals: inferior edge of third cervical.

15)   Top and bottom of the body.

a) Top of the body (head, thorax) direct action; limbs, extremities, opposite action (to disperse warms the hands and feet, to tonify calms them): *yuzhong* (KI-26).

b) Lower body (lower limbs) direct action: upper limb, opposite action: foot *linqi* (GB-41).

c) Upper body and organs, also abdomen: *tianshu* (ST-25).

d) Middle of the body and organs (liver, spleen-pancreas): *yinlingquan* (SP-9).

e) Lower body and genital organs: *diji* (SP-8).

II. Searching for the Cause through the Pulse

For every problem there is a deep, original, sometimes old mental or physical cause which has attacked our vital force. The apparent problems are only its consequences and manifestations. When this cause, this ''root'' is found and corrected, all its consequences, its branches, immediately fall. It is this for which the science of energy, true acupuncture, searches in order to return full strength to the vital force.

In effect, it is our vital force which makes us insensitive to all bad influences, to fatigue, to sorrow, to mental exhaustion, as well as to hyperexcitation such as anger, to the excesses of our vital functions. It is this which gives us the full enjoyment of our possibilities, the possibility of adapting ourselves instantly to a brusque cold, to sun or shade. If the vital force is wholly in excess or wholly insufficient, life stops. If it excessive or insufficient in a part of the body, any problem is possible.

Even the skeleton is displaced when the vital force weakens, and it is immediately put back in place when strength has been returned to the vital force. Some instruments (Dr. Brosse) have registered that when the mental and physical vital force is full and intact, the heart and the lungs can be stopped voluntarily (yogis) without signs of death.

Only the pulse can give us the clue to the attack on the vital force. An attentive reading and synthesis of its indications can lead us to the goal. They indicate the malfunctioning organ-meridian and even the points of the meridians necessary. It is enough to know the points that are active at the time and then act in the desired way on those points.

III. Recognizing and Choosing Meridian Lines and Median Lines

The meridian.

1) When only one pulse is excessive or insufficient, the choice of a meridian is obvious.

To recognize the course and to be sure of its identity, we must be absolutely certain that under the pressure of the finger it evokes certain sensations which vary in intensity according to the person and the circumstances. These sensations under pressure consist of "responses" **a)** along the course, **b)** in the organ of the meridian, **c)** in the pulse of the meridian, **d)** in sensitive people, in the organ related to the meridian.

Each meridian has its own responses which allow us to recognize it.

2) When several pulses (thus meridians and organs) are in disequilibrium, one in excess, some others insufficient, we must choose the meridian for which the reactions cover all the disorders. Recall the explanation in the chapter "Interaction," describing how each organ-meridian stimulated in one way acts in the same way on several organs, and in the opposite way on other organs. Thus it is enough to act on the one meridian which will produce all the effects we want. To act on all the meridians would risk neutralizing some actions and clouding the energy. Assessment of the pulses in light of the laws of interaction will allow us to determine which organ the meridians influence in the same way or in the opposite way.

3) When all the pulses without exception are in excess or insufficiency, there is only one point that corrects them all in the same way: leg-*sanli* (ST-36). This point is enough.

The two median lines.

Their courses allow us to commit almost no error, provided, however, that we do not forget that both are double — the flow of energy rising on the right and going down on the left of the thin median separation. Each double point is separated in the conception vessel by a very narrow ridge, in the governor vessel by the narrow, medial epispinal tendon.

The points on the narrow flow of the right act on the left half of the body; those on the left flow act on the right half.

Anterior line: yin. Distribution of energy in the internal organs: cold, depression.

Posterior line: yang. Physical and cerebral strength: fever, hyperexcitation.

IV. Recognizing the Point

Each meridian has an important point for the energy itself, among those which command the functions of its associated organ and the energy of its related regions.

1) *The exact location of the points:* They are not easy to find; we must learn to recognize them. As many true points as there are on the meridians, there are also points that give some, but never as many, analogous effects: those which are neither all the same nor of equal strength; and those which are the wrong points. And then again there are points of limited effect which are the points "off the meridians," or "new points;" and finally, there are purely local points of command, the "local points."

Antiquity gives only the distances from point to point; it is with care that I have corrected even the evident mistakes.

2) *The true points:* These are determined from several indications and must exhibit all of them.

a) A sensitivity to pressure, a kind of bruising, like a "black and blue mark"; a sensitivity which is stronger in nervous people when the point commands an organ that is in excess. This sensitivity is the same for all varieties of points. As the fingertip is passed slowly along the surface of the skin, the smooth skin becomes sticky at the point. When passing the finger one centimeter from the skin feel a flow of waves can be felt at the point; when the finger is moved up and down this flow seems solid and seems to strike the finger.

b) An awakening in the meridian of "something that passes," an "electric flow."

c) A response in the related organ, like a wave, which mostly comes by moving the finger on the point.

d) A response on the pulse of this organ.

e) A response of the same sort in the related nervous center and always on the opposite side (contralateral).

f) A (sense of) puncture in the true point upstream and downstream on the meridian.

g) A response in the organs in relation to the principal organ.

h) A response in the pulses of the related organs.

i) A response, finally, in the part of the body commanded by the point, and as well in all other regions of the body that are in disequilibrium.

j) On themselves, sensitive people perceive a warm pressure on the point which commands the cause of all their problems.

The three last manifestations often pass unperceived by the subject and the practitioner whose physical strength surpasses their mental strength or whose memory has been developed too much at the expense of the spirit of observation of others and of themselves.

Finally, the true points have something special that all sensitive people and those accustomed to "reading" and "listening" to the sensations of their organs and the parts of their bodies can perceive without error. By pressing on a true point a slight sensitivity awakens in the preceding and following point on the meridian; only the true points respond.

3) *The false points:* on each meridian there are some points other than the true ones. Inexperienced and inattentive people might mistake these for the true points.

Their effects are not comparable to those of the true points in intensity of reaction, in the duration of the desired effect, or in the number of effects produced.

Pain under pressure is their single trait in common with the true points. So we must never base ourselves on this single sign.

4) *The new points, or those outside the meridians.* In addition to the true points all located on meridians or the median lines, there are points on the body with fixed places having exact effects. Some of them are located on meridians and, in addition to their own strength, they have in part the strength of the whole line of the meridian. Others are clearly outside the meridians. A list of them is given following the meridians.

It is possible to recognize them by the sensation in the part of the body which they command and from the pain awakened under the pressure of the finger.

5) *Center of pain points:* Local neuralgias, contusions, weakness or contractures of muscles, etc. sometimes awaken at the center of the pain, a particularly painful point under the pressure of the finger which often has no relation with any of the points described above.

Only used in "reaction-acupuncture" (local) they give good results when the pains are recent, but in fact they do not remove the cause, the functional trouble or more deeply, the energetic problem which is the true cause.

V. Choosing the Point

Choice of the point.

The condition of the pulses indicates the troubled organ and consequently the meridian and pulse to correct. When there is only one, or if there are several, it indicates the one commanding all the others in the desired manner (see chapter "Interaction"). We must still choose which meridian point will best improve the particular problem of the organ.

For this there are two methods:

One is based on the indications of the pulse. By pressing on the pulse of the organ, a sensitive person who is sure of his faint sensations, will feel on himself the best indicated point of the meridian, and if he is sensitive, the subject will indicate this also to the practitioner.

The second method relies on the memory of all the effects of all the points on the meridian. This leaves a choice if there are several meridians troubled in different ways. One must choose what will tonify the insufficient ones and at the same time disperse those in excess, a heavy work for the memory, which allows many errors. Also, many acupuncturists are content to use some important points without noticing that very often one point is neutralized by others when they stimulate more than one.

The acupuncturist who cares for perfection and who wants success ten times out of ten will use the first method.

We summarize below the rules which are easy to remember through their connections with the pulses and which the examination of the pulses will immediately bring to mind.

Interaction of the organs.

These interactions can be said to exist, for all action, either through direct effects in the same way as given by the action, or in a contrary way (tonifying disperses, dispersing tonifies), or in accordance with the relation of the intensity of the pulses in one way or the other.

1)   Direct effects (in the same way).

  a) Husband-wife law.

On the wrist the pulses of the same segment at the same level on the two wrists react on one another in the same way. Tonifying one tonifies the other; dispersing one disperses the other. The couples (husband-wife) thus formed are:

Segment I.   Right to left — superficial: large intestine and small intestine; middle and deep: lungs (respiratory passages) and heart.

Segment II.   Superficial: stomach and gallbladder; middle and deep: vessels — sexual organs, kidney — filtration and reabsorption.

  b) Mother-son law.

In the flow of energy the upstream meridian is the mother; the downstream meridian is the son. Thus a meridian is the mother of the meridian which follows it and the son of the one which precedes it.

This law, however, is dominated by the law of the unequal coupled meridians (see below) for the pulses which are found superimposed on the same segment, one yin and one yang. The mother-son law acts only for the pulses at the same tension-level (two yang or two yin).

The succession in the flow of energy is as follows:

Lungs - large intestine - stomach - spleen-pancreas - heart - small intestine - bladder - kidneys - heart governor - triple warmer - gallbladder - liver - lungs, etc.

2)   Opposite effects (tonifying disperses, etc.)

  a) Midday-midnight law

Every two hours a pulse-organ-meridian receives its maximum energy for the day and at the same time another meridian is at its minimum energy. Twelve hours later the same pair have inversed charges: what had its maximum will have its minimum; what had its minimum will have its maximum. The pairs thus formed act in a contrary way on one another. It is impossible, for example, to tonify the large intestine without dispersing the kidneys and vice versa. It is impossible to disperse the large intestine without tonifying the kidneys.

These pairs are always formed with the superficial pulse of one segment and a deep pulse of the neighboring segment. There is thus a crossing between segments: Left I and II (small intestine-liver, gallbladder-heart), Right II and III (stomach-heart governor, triple warmer-spleen-pancreas)), between Left III and Right I (bladder-lungs, large intestine-kidneys).

  b) Unequal coupled meridians.

Between the superficial yang and middle-deep yin of each segment there is formed a coupling of meridians. *If they are unequal in intensity,* there is interaction in a contrary manner.

It is enough to tonify the weaker meridian for the stronger to be weakened in proportion. It is enough to disperse the stronger meridian for the weaker to be increased in proportion.

In summary: all action on the organ meridians, point and pulse acts:

1)   In the same way on two other organs according to the husband-wife law (symmetrical right-left pulses) and according to the mother-son law (upstream-downstream in the flow of the energy except for the unequal coupled meridians).

2)   In the opposite way on two other organs: according to the midnight-midday law (one meridian has its maximum and the other its minimum at the same hour), and according to the law of coupled meridians when they are unequal.

3)   Effects on the same side of the body (ipsolateral) or on the opposite side (contralateral).

   a) Most of the points produce their effects on the same side of the body as the stimulated point.

   b) Certain points produce their effects on the opposite side of the body.

   c) Some others, for example on the left foot, produce their effects on the upper right part of the body, etc. These crossed effects are exceptional but constant for certain points.

   d) All points, whatever they are, act in the opposite nervous centers (contralateral).

These are facts the laws and explanations of which have not yet been made precise, but it is essential to take notice where the two sides of the body are not troubled in the same way and where it is useful to correct only one side.

These differences can be detected in two ways:

First, the memory: easy for some points, but difficult on the whole.

Mostly, by "listening" to oneself if the subject is not able to feel on himself the responses awakened by the point under the pressure of the finger.

Let us cite, among the points with a contralateral effect: *houxi* (SI-3) and *hegu* (LI-4).

Among the points with crossed effects: foot *linqi* (GB-41) and *waiguan* (TW-5).

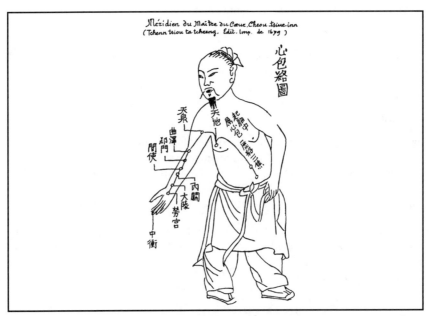

Meridian of the heart governor (DACH)

Editor's note: The author planned to include the **Points of Weihe** in Part IV. However, his premature demise did not allow him to achieve this arrangement in the original French edition. However, these notes have been moved to Part IV in this edition.

Part I

The Meridians

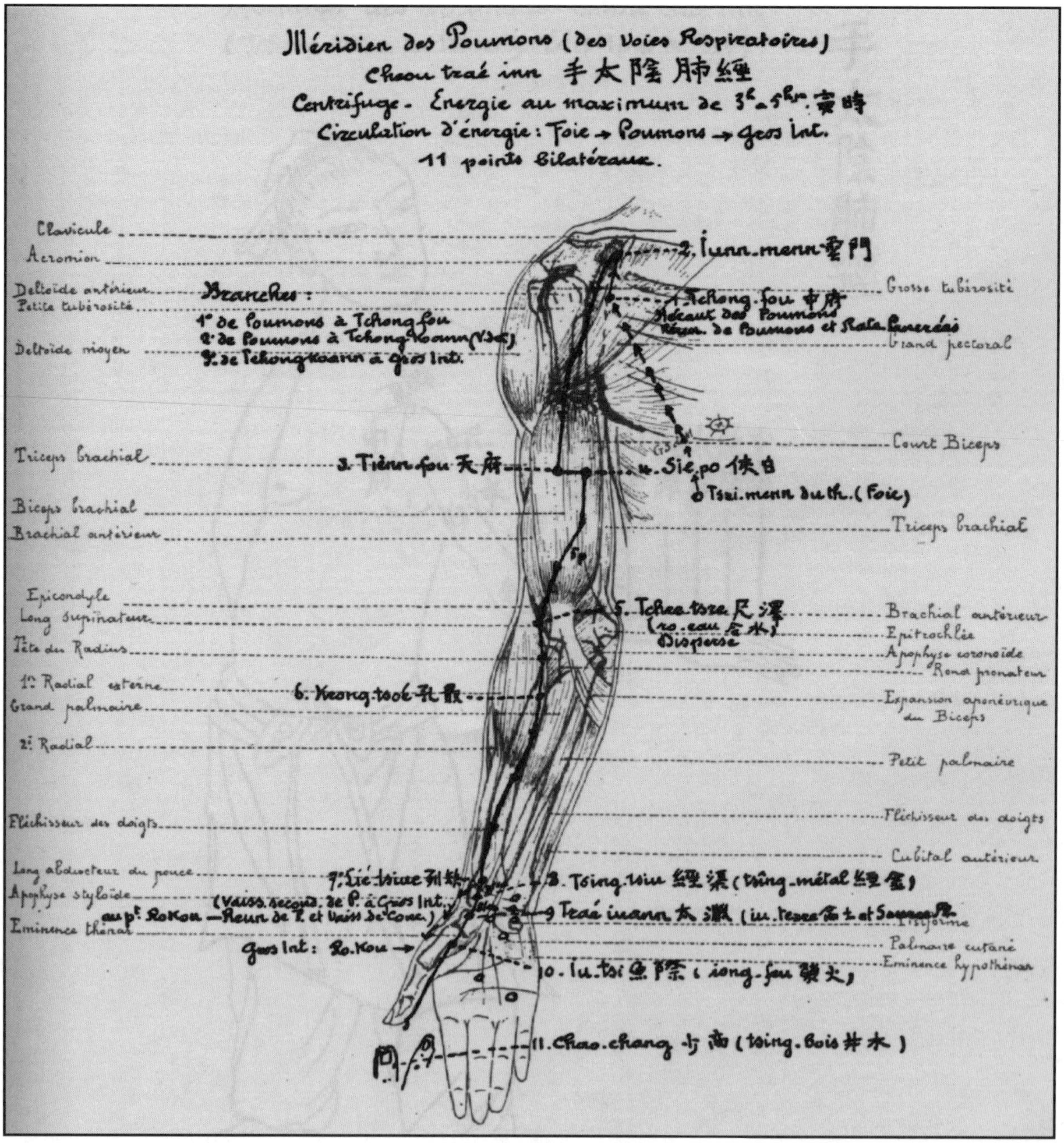

Meridian of the lungs (GSDM)

Chapter I

Lungs

Respiratory Passages

In reality the meridian called the lung meridian controls all the respiratory passages. It is among the distributor organs (''treasure,'' yin, deep pulse) although charged with taking in and assimilating the elements of the air and planets which are yang and bring us the energy of yang activity. (Controls H ions in the blood and oxygen).

All its points awaken a response in the mid-brain and the opposite side of the cerebellum.

These respiratory passages are contracted, congested and inflamed by the vagus (*tianzhu*, BL-10; *zhongwan*, CV-12). They are dilated, decongested, by the sympathetic system (*fengchi*, GB-20; *zhangmen*, LR-13).

Dryness activates them to the point of irritation; humidity blocks them (as well as the skin) to the point of engorgement and inflammation. Worries, regrets or sadness weaken them to the point of panting (excess of the vagus), and they are dissipated by joy or anxiety.

Tonifying the lungs necessarily tonifies the heart and disperses the bladder (increases urine).

They are tonified by dispersing the bladder and kidneys and by tonification of the heart.

They are tonified or dispersed by the large intestine according to its relative strength.

Insufficiency: weak respiration; chest not dilating; no breath; changing complexion; shoulder and back cold; dry skin; abundant and frequent urine; sudden depressions; weakness; fever from anxiety, from tears and sobbing.

Excess: fullness of the chest; shoulders and back hot; colored and feeble urine; perspiration; poor inhalation of breath; cough; sputum; loving and tender character; easily cries or laughs uproariously; subject to problems from excess of respiratory passages; dreams of flying (excess of the upper part of the body).

To tonify: *taiyuan* (LU-9), to disperse: (LU-5).

The energy comes from the liver (*qimen* of the thorax, LR-14) through a direct branch to *zhongfu* (LU-1). It passes into the large intestine from *shaoshang* (LU-11) to *shangyang* (LI-1).

LU-1   *zhongfu* — central workshop

The Chinese tradition places *yunmen* as the first point of the lung. But by pressing on *zhongfu* it is this which has a response in the branch coming from *qimen* (last point of the liver, LR-14), in the liver itself as well as in the meridian of the lungs and the lungs.

Anterior upper shoulder at the level of the medial crease; at the inferior point of the projection of the coracoid process; in the angle of the superior edge of the second rib (the first under the clavicle) and of the medial superior edge of the tendon of the pectoralis minor, inserted on the coracoid process; in a hollow.

Three finger-widths below and medial to *yunmen* (LU-2); linked by a direct branch to *qimen* (LR-14). Three FW[1] medial and inferior to *jianyu* (LI-15). Three lateral to *kufang* (ST-14).

When tonified:
   Tonifies respiratory passages, heart, spleen-pancreas, temporal-parietal lobe, medulla, automatic parrot, inferior spinal cord, three endocrines, liver.
   Disperses the bladder.
   Dispersing acts in the opposite way.
   Here the energy coming from the liver (*qimen*, LR-14) by a direct branch enters the meridian of the lungs.

Direct effects:
   Herald point of the lung (respiratory passages) (troubles with cold or depression). Painful in troubles of the posterior side of the lungs. It awakens around 3:00 a.m. (the lungs not being nourished by energy coming from insufficient liver); spasms of the voice muscles; stuttering cough; thick or liquid mucus; tonsillitis. Full, painful chest, lungs contracted; without respiration, cannot sleep; asthma, emphysema, pulmonary tuberculosis; pulmonary infections.
   Eyes: red, painful, eyelids swollen, conjunctivitis.
   Heart: troubles — recurrent fever.
   Vomiting crisis from gallbladder excess (food and drinks do not go down), swollen abdomen.

Opposite effects:

Bladder: irritation or urine with fetid odor; excess uric acid, tonify.

Lymph nodes: Tumors (superative adenitis).

Parts of the body:

Hair, skin of the cranium (scalp), all troubles, opposite.

Red cheeks, warm; congested capillaries; acne rosacea, opposite.

Face swollen, skin painful, opposite.

Wrist and back of the hand swollen. Inferior and superior limb swollen, opposite.

Point of Weihe: Right: Benzoic Acid. Red stains on the face, acne rosacea. Wrist swollen; swelling around the ears; ulcerated tongue; beating of the temporal arteries; asthma increased in the evening; heart pain; kidney pain; urine: changing color, repulsive odor, incontinence, excess uric acid.

Left: Euphrasia. Influenza, whooping cough during the day; hay fever; inflamed eyelids, red and hot cheeks; eyes tear without stopping; mucus lining of the nose inflamed; conjunctivitis; constipation or dysentery; bladder: irritation at night; prostatitis; short menses with ophthalmia; beginning of measles, eyes inflamed.

LU-2 *yunmen* — door of the clouds

Superior anterior arm: three FW under and exterior (lateral) to the projection between the humerus and thorax (coracoid process); in the angle of the superior edge of the three ''major'' muscles (pectoralis, latissimus dorsi, teres) and the lateral edge of the vertical tendon of the short head of the biceps (inserted on the coracoid process); in the hollow. On the medial edge of the tendon of the long head of the biceps; on the inferior edge of transverse insertion of the subscapularis muscle.

Three FW above *zhongfu* (LU-1); point following: *tianfu* (LU-3) in the middle of the biceps. Two FW lateral to *jiquan* (HT-1); four medial to *binao* (LI-14).

When tonified:

Tonifies: lungs, heart, liver, spleen-pancreas, three nervous centers, three psychologies, three endocrines, finger joints and sexual organs.

Disperses opposite kidney, vessels, bladder, triple warmer.

Dispersing acts in the opposite way.

To puncture too deeply causes vertigo or fainting?

Direct effects:

Insomnia around 3:00 a.m.

Energy up; coughing fits; cannot breathe; nervous cough, causes vomiting.

Tonsillitis; fullness and agitation of the chest; bronchitis; pulmonary congestion; pulmonary tuberculosis.

Heart: all troubles.

Liver and spleen: distended.

Urethra, penis.

Parts of the body:

Skin of the opposite side of the face and lips; acne; scruff; perleche.

Arm cannot be lifted (contracture of teres major and of caraco-brachialis).

Fingers; wrist, dorsal hand; tightness, pain.

Point of Weihe: Sepia.

LU-3 *tianfu* — celestial workshop

Biceps brachialis, mid-height, mid-width; four FW above the anterior elbow crease, in a hollow between the short and long heads of the biceps. On the superior edge of a transverse ligament.

Preceding point: *yunmen* (LU-2). Two FW approximately medial and slightly above *xiabai* (LU-4). Three lateral and above *qingling* (HT-2).

When tonified:

Tonifies the respiratory passages, heart, temporal and parietal lobes, parrot. Opposite eye, room-of-tears (under the eye) opposite, opposite cheek, anterior shoulder and upper limb.

Disperses the bladder, opposite side of large intestine.

Dispersing acts in the opposite way.

Direct effects:

Talks to himself, talks alone or does not talk much, loss of memory, or cerebral congestion, possibility of apoplexia, vertigo.

Poisoned by gas, carbon dioxide, etc.: tonify.

Bronchitis; crisis of asthma preventing eating; pulmonary plaque; vomiting blood through mouth and nose.

Eyes: all troubles; tears, dizziness; myopia.

Hard of hearing.

Malaria, tumors.

Parts of the body:

Neck: lateral, opposite, sternocleidomastoid muscle, opposite.

Anterior shoulder.

All the nerves of the anterior shoulder and upper limb: painful or weak.

Chronic rheumatism, mostly articular.

LU-4   *xiabai* — close to the whiteness

Anterior external arm, four FW above the elbow (epitrochlear). On the anterior edge of the humerus and the inferior edge of the transverse bulge (opposite insertion of the brachioradialis and deltoid). Between the lateral edge of the biceps and the medial edge of the brachialis anterior; in a hollow.

Two large FW lateral and a little under *tianfu* (LU-3), four above *chize* (LU-5). Three anterior (medial) to arm-*wuli* (LI-13).

When tonified:

Tonifies the respiratory passages, heart (upper valves), temporal and parietal lobes, automaton-parrot, opposite upper eyes, chest.

Disperses the bladder, large intestine, opposite.

Dispersing acts in the opposite way.

Direct effects:

Heart: valves, upper part, nervous palpitation; pain of the heart, short of breath, internal pains of the chest.

Coughing fits.

Fits of dry vomiting.

LU-5   *chize* — swamp of the foot, elbow crease

Front of the elbow, lateral third; in the angle of the superior edge of the large transverse bulge of the joint, of the medial edge of the large muscle (supinator longus) and of the inferior edge of the transverse tendon of the biceps; in a hollow; lateral to the deep radial artery.

Four FW under *xiabai* (LU-4); five above *kongzui* (LU-6), three medial to *quchi* (LU-11); three lateral to *quze* (PC-3).

When dispersed:

Disperses the respiratory passage, heart, cerebellum, primate, lateral opposite of the body, face, liver, spleen-pancreas.

Tonifies the large intestine, small intestine, bladder.

Tonifying acts in the opposite way.

Direct effects:

Sneezing: cold in the head and of the throat; thick mucus; bronchitis, pains on the side; asthma, pleurisy; congestive pulmonary tuberculosis; fever; without equal for spitting of blood.

Less energy; depression; chagrin, sobbing, melancholia, agitation; chronic meningitis of children; spasms of convulsions of children.

Dry mouth and tongue; swollen abdomen; incessant vomiting and diarrhea.

Heart: sharp pain, pain into the arm, short of breath (angina of chest), hypertension.

Opposite effects:

Frequent need to urinate; paralysis of bladder.

Parts of the body:

Lateral half of the body, muscles and bone, sharp pain; upper limb extensors; anterior and lateral lower limb, contractions or contracture, or flaccidity or swelling; nervous paralysis.

For the face.

Back: contracture or pain; lumbar, vertebrae, pain; lumbar vertebrae, pain.

Anterior shoulder and anterior, exterior upper limb: cold, pain or contracture.

Elbow: anterior, exterior — sharp pain or numbness and pain with the hand and forearm.

Lumbar, inguinal fold; anterior, lateral lower limb; upper and lateral part of instep.

LU-6 *kongzui* — deepest hollow

Anterior, external face of the forearm; six FW above the wrist; in the angle of the medial edge (towards the ulnar bone), with the supinator longus of the radius and the edge of the insertions of the angular muscles coming from the inner elbow (pronator muscles); between the bone and the radial artery, very close to the bone; in a hollow. On the flexor longus of the thumb and deep to the common superficial flexors (ungual phalangeal).

Five FW under *chize* (LU-5); five above *lieque* (LU-7).

When tonified:

Tonifies the respiratory passages (mostly larynx, opposite trachea), heart, temporal-parietal lobes, palmar articulations of the fingers, dorsal face of thumb, articulations of the opposite lower limbs, opposite face.

Disperses the opposite side of the large intestine, small intestine, bladder.

Dispersing acts in the opposite way.

Direct effects:

Larynx, opposite vocal cord, husky voice, hoarse, loss of voice; swollen throat; headache; coughing and spitting of blood?

Opposite effects:

Fever with perspiration: to disperse causes perspiration?

Parts of the body:

Arm and elbow: pain and weakness.

Palmar side of the fingers, dorsal side of thumb. Patient does not grasp very well, awkward, weak or stiff joints; arthritis mostly of thumb and index finger.

LU-7 *lieque* — aligned hollow

Anterior forearm (palm up, supinated); three FW above the wrist (one above the head of the radius); on the line of the index finger; in the angle of the lateral (radial) edge of the large tendon (large palmar) and the inferior edge of a transverse bulge; in a hollow; on the medial (ulnar) edge of the radial artery; on pulse V (right, endocrines; left, organs of sense.)

Five FW under *kongzui* (LU-6), a little above *jingqu* (LU-8); separated by the large palmar tendon from *neiguan* (PC-6).

When tonified:

Tonifies the respiratory passages, conception vessel, its pulse and *xinhui* (GV-21, IS GV-22), all yin; distributor organ-meridians (deep pulses), posterior part of frontal lobes, cerebellum, medulla oblongata, spinal cord, psychology, on the left: sense organs, on the right: endocrines. Skin, muscles, bones opposite, face opposite, anterior shoulder, lateral arm, posterior forearm, wrist, hand, fingers, mostly index and dorsal side of thumb (radial nerve) same side: *zhaohai* (KI-3, IS KI-6).

Disperses the bladder, large intestine.

Dispersing acts in the opposite way.

Acts on the opposite half of the body and of the nervous centers (except superior limb same side).

It is important to clearly discriminate excess (heat, congestion, inflammation, hard, deep pulses) from insufficiency (cold, weakness, deep pulses weak).

Point of command of the conception vessel (rising on the right and descending on the left), all the yin energies; furnishes energy to the triple warmer and through it to all the meridians.

Acts on the sexual problems of women and of men; the skin, swelling of abdomen, etc. responds to *zhaohai* (KI-3, IS KI-6), which commands the energy of yin inactivity.

Point of passage between the lung and large intestine: causes the excess to pass from one to the other. If excess in the lungs: heat in chest, back, palms of the hands and fingers; abundant perspiration, difficult and painful urination. If insufficiency: cold of the back, shivering, weak and rapid breath, yawning, frequent and abundant urination, weakness of the four limbs. To tonify disperses the large intestine, to disperse tonifies it.

Direct effects:

Loss of memory, yawning, nervous tremors, emotiveness, crisis of hopelessness (also hemiplegia); shivering from cold or nerves.

Laughs too easily. Or fantastic visions, hallucinations.

Internal organs, mostly yin distributors (deep pulses): sharp pain in the chest, heart and abdomen.

Respiratory passages: influenza, throat opposite, tonsils, larynx, cough, trachea; bronchioles; abundant mucus; fever from lungs; pulmonary congestion (contracted breath, less energy for breathing), rusty, red sputum.

Eyes: sties, abscesses, eyelids — opposite — do not close.

Teeth: sharp pain.

Mouth and tongue: abscess; saliva and sputum.

Opposite effects:

Troubled digestion (food does not descend), epigastric pain; painful abdomen, swollen, full, serious diarrhea. Swollen hemorrhoids.

Frequent and profuse urination (mostly at the beginning of the night).

Genital apparatus: breath abscess, inflammation. After pregnancy, stiffness, cannot speak, lumbar pain, cold in the naval. The dead fetus does not come out.

Men: pain in the penis during emission.

Parts of the body:

Skin: inflammation; burns from any source; chemical, fire, sunburn; itching, pain, shiny skin with much hair?

Blood: illness or troubles of blood.

Thorax opposite:

Body: flaccidity from shock; sudden swelling of limbs.

Opposite to (vertex) or side of head: sharp pain. If insufficiency, tonify; if excess, disperse.

Opposite side of face swollen; neuralgia; paralysis (orbicularis muscles) of lips relaxed, mouth awry, eyelids do not close; tics, spasms, trismus.

Wrist and hand without strength, flabby; hands awkward.

Lumbar: lassitude opposite.

LU-8 *jingqu* — passage for the meridian

Anterior wrist (palm up, supination); external third (towards the thumb).

On the superior edge of the internal extremity of the head of the radius; on the lateral edge of the large tendon of the palmaris longus; exactly at the angle of the bone and the medial edge of the radial artery; in a hollow.

One FW under *lieque* (LU-7); one above *taiyuan* (LU-9); separated from *daling* (PC-7) by the tendon of palmaris longus and at its level.

When tonified:

Tonifies the respiratory passages, cerebellum, mid spinal cord, heart, palm of the hand, palmar side of fingers, dorsal side of thumb.

Disperses the bladder, stomach.

Dispersing acts in the opposite way.

Direct effects:

Opposite side of throat: inflammation; tonsillitis; trachea; larynx, bronchioles; energy at the top; coughing fits; chest full, contracted panting, dyspnea; back and chest squeezed.

Fever without perspiration; heart pain, pericarditis.

Opposite effects:

Epigastrium; nausea, vomiting; spasms of the esophagus and cardiac sphincter.

Parts of the body:

Serious rheumatism.

Lateral part of neck; nape and opposite scapula contracted; pain.

Hand: palmar aponeurosis; dorsal side of fingers, dorso-lateral side of thumb: rheumatism, weakness, medial and radial nerves?

Knee and leg opposite.

LU-9   *taiyuan* — supreme abyss

Front of the wrist (palm up, supination): lateral third (lateral towards the thumb). In the large hollow between the carpal bone (bottom of thumb) and the radial bone; in the angle of the inferior edge of the carpal bone and the medial (ulnar) edge of the tendon of the palmaris longus and the radiopalmar artery, which detaches itself from the radial artery medial towards the palm; in a hollow; in the scaphoid-trapezoid joint.

One FW below *jingqu* (LU-8); one above *yuji* (LU-10); one large FW lateral to *daling* (PC-7) and one FW above its level.

When tonified:
Tonifies the respiratory passages, heart, vessels, aorta, mid-brain, spinal cord, external, opposite eye: *shanzhong* (CV-17).
Disperses the large intestine, kidney, stomach.
Dispersing acts in the opposite way.

Direct effects:
Tonification point (and source?) of the respiratory passages (from the nose to the lung). Atonic respiration; cannot breathe in the cold; cough from cold drinks; contracts the swollen respiratory passages; pains crossing the chest from breathing.
Throat, opposite: tonsils, cough, mucus, trachea. Bronchus: pains in the side. Or bleeding, spits blood, flabby respiratory muscles; emphysema; bleeding lungs?
Arteries, veins: reunion of the vessels (on the left: aorta, artero-sclerosis; hypotension, rough pulse, decline of sexual energy and blood. Aorta: pain in the sub-clavicular hollow. Heart: weakness, pain.
Counterflow energy (nerve crisis, anger) "hyperexcited speech, vicious speech," insomnia from internal agitation, malaise; sometimes hot, sometimes cold; shivering from cold.
Eyes: red, painful, congested, conjunctivitis, cataract, keratitis.
Dry throat: eructation and vomiting.
Bladder: incontinence "without measure" through contractions (sphincter of the bladder relaxed) — disperse; atonic bladder (contracted sphincter), tonify. Urine: color changed by acid.

Opposite effects:
Kidney — excess: tonify; insufficiency: disperse.
Stomach — large intestine; opposite parotid; opposite salivary glands.

Parts of the body:
The whole body on the same side.
Skin: "perverse" troubles of skin.
Nervous pains (from energy); energy piercing the two breasts, pain spreading into the sub-clavicular fossa.
Chest and shoulder: pain. Line of the thumb on the forearm; pain.
Wrist: arthritis; thumb and palmar side of the index, muscles of thenar area.

LU-10   *yuji* — an area of the fish

Palm; base of the thumb (thenar eminence); one FW above the wrist; about half-width. Between the two muscles (lateral side of the thumb, of the short flexor of the thumb; medial to the short abductor of the thumb); at the angle of the inferior edge of the bony prominence (tubercle of the scaphoid bone) and of the insertion on it of the short abductor; deep: on the opposing muscle; in a hollow.

One FW below *taiyuan* (LU-9); following point: *shaoshang* (LU-11) on the ungual phalanx of the thumb; two fingers lateral to *shenmen* (HT-7).

When tonified:
Tonifies the respiratory passages, auricle of the heart, cerebellum, upper spinal cord, opposite nose, opposite tip of the tongue, opposite side of the throat (tonsils, larynx), opposite breast.
Disperses the bladder, stomach, large intestine.
Dispersing acts in the opposite way.

Direct effects:
Less energy, malaise, fear, anguish; chagrin, insomnia.
Chattering of teeth, from shivering, nervousness, cold or from malaria.
Bleeding mouth (gums); teeth (mostly canines, superior and opposite), pain or loose.

Tongue, opposite side of tip; yellow tongue, fever, headache, vertigo.

Opposite side of throat, coldness, pain, inflammation; opposite tonsils; larynx, dryness or inflammation, pain; loss of voice (aphonia); cannot speak (aphasia); cough causing pain in the chest and back, causing discharge of urine, cannot breathe.

Perspires a lot.

Opposite auricle of heart, all trouble; rheumatic heart?

Alcoholism. Abdomen: painful even without food.

Opposite breast, inflammation to the point of abscess.

Parts of the body:

Paralyzing rheumatism; circulating rheumatism, or generalized; deviation of the vertebral column?

Thumb, index, middle fingers: pain, movements, weakness of flexion.

LU-11   *shaoshang* — lesser merchant

Thumb, angular phalanx, index finger side (medial interior edge) about mid-width: at the angle of the inferior edge of the prominence of the bone near the joint and the dorsal edge of the palmar tendon (flexors), in a hollow.

Preceding point: *yuji* (LU-10); symmetrical to *guiku* MP-29a) on the lateral edge.

The energy passes from the meridian of the lungs by a branch following the thumb-index finger joint to the meridian of the large intestine (*shangyang,* LI-1).

When tonified:

Tonifies all the yin distributor organ-meridians (deep pulses), cerebellum, spinal cord, lateral opposite side of eye, opposite side of nose, opposite side of throat (tonsils, larynx): chin, in front of the ears, posterior knee, calf, dorsal side of fingers.

Disperses all the yang producer organ-meridians (superficial pulses).

Dispersing acts in the opposite way.

Direct effects:

Point of passage between yin and yang meridians.

Insomnia; cerebral congestion (red face, suddenly falling); acute or chronic meningitis of children; tonic or clonic convulsions.

Chattering of the teeth; shivering.

Violent perspiration; perspires and is icy.

Opposite nose; coryza, obstructed or bleeding.

Opposite side of throat; opposite tonsillitis, inflammation; opposite larynx; cough causing acute pain of the shoulder and of the sub-clavicular fossa; fits of coughing.

Pulse slow, fever of a yin organ.

Eyes lateral and opposite.

Opposite effects:

Dry lips (excess of digestive tract); abundant saliva.

Tongue: inferior side, swollen, painful.

Parotid: inflammation; mumps: pain in front of the ears.

Esophagus: contracted (eructation, vomiting, troubled digestion, regurgitation of food.)

Gallbladder: obstruction; jaundice.

Abdomen: noise, gas.

Parts of the body:

Opposite side of chin: inflammation, swelling, itching.

Dorsal sides of fingers (extensors); pains, cannot open or close (contracted) or flabby hand.

Notes

[1] FW refers to finger-widths.

Chapter II

Large Intestine

The large intestine has close connections to the energy: relaxed, it saps the energy and great danger relaxes it. Contracted or irritated by worms, it makes people irritated and nervous to the point of convulsions or mental problems. It acts directly on the throat, nose and complexion.

It produces antihemorrhagic vitamin K (completed and stored in the liver); the different B vitamins, all antinervous (also in the liver), and perhaps other vitamins as well.

It cannot function without a healthy fullness of the liver, nor without a good function of the small intestine and pancreas.

In the flow of energy it is preceded by the lungs (mother) with which it forms a pair of linked meridians. It is followed by the stomach (son); the small intestine is its husband. Its maximum energy is at 6:00 a.m. and from 5:00 a.m. to 7:00 a.m., hour of minimum for the kidneys. Its minimum is at 6:00 p.m., the maximum of the kidneys. It is stimulated by the vagus system and calmed by the sympathetic system. It is impossible to tonify it, mostly in the afternoon, without dispersing the kidney-filtration and without tonifying the small intestine (husband). Dispersing disperses the small intestine and tonifies the kidney. The reaction of the lungs depends on the relation of energy of both pulses.

In Europe, its acknowledged function is that of storing and evacuating stools. The stools give useful information through their appearance. Hard and very dark: excess of liver, concentrated bile; very clear, pale yellow: little bile, relaxation of the liver; shining like fat: insufficiency of the pancreas and small intestine; grey: insufficiency of the small intestine.

For the signs of excess or insufficiency, see Part II, Chapter V.

LI-1 *shangyang* — yang of the merchants

Hand, index finger, angular phalanx, facing the thumb, mid-width; at the angle of the inferior edge of the swelling of the bone at the articulation and at the dorsal edge of the palmar tendon (flexor longus); in a hollow.

Following point: *erjian* (LI-2), on the phalanx.

When tonified:
Tonifies the large intestine, small intestine, stomach, gallbladder (superficial I and II), inferior occipital lobes, temporo-parietal lobes, pituitary and thyroid glands.
Disperses the kidneys.
Dispersing acts in the opposite way (superficial I and II), tonifying the kidneys.
The energy coming from the meridian of the lungs *(shaoshang)* enters here into the large intestine meridian by a branch which follows the palmar side of the articulation.

Direct effects:
Pituitary? Thyroid?
Opposite incisors: pain, loose; opposite side of the mouth: dryness or inflammation.
Achloropsia (cannot distinguish colors).

Opposite effects:
Ears: buzzing or deafness from shock: tonify opposite side.
Lungs: congestion (panting, fullness, fever): tonify opposite side.

Parts of the body:
Skin of the face: inflammation, pain, swelling or itching.
All the muscles of the opposite side of the mouth.
Pains like a collar, opposite side at the level of the first and second ribs.
Upper limb same side, lower limb opposite side.

LI-2 *erjian* — second interval

Hand, index finger facing the thumb (lateral, external); just in front of the metacarpophalangeal articulaion; in the palmar angle of the head of the phalanx; exactly on the head and dorsal edge of the flexors, in a hollow.

Preceding point: *shangyang* (LI-1), on the small phalanx; point following: *sanjian* (LI-3), at the mid-length of the metacarpal.

When dispersed:

Disperses the opposite large intestine, the small intestine; stomach, inferior occipital, inferior frontal lobes, opposite teeth mostly molars. Lateral side of eye, opposite; opposite ear; corner of lips and opposite cheek, pectoral muscles, anterior shoulder, lateral side of arm, nose, back of the throat.

Tonifies the opposite kidney, urethra and sphincter of bladder, prostatitis on the same side, lower thumb, opposite knee, dorsal lateral side of foot.

Tonifying seems to increase the dispersal of the organs, but tonifies the parts of the body.

Direct effects:

Disperses the excess of the large intestine (less than *sanjian,* LI-3). Colic, spasms, spasmodic constipation, diarrhea from inflammation; typhoid fever (with *sanjian,* LI-3 and *hegu,* LI-4).

Heart weak, contracted arteries.

Eyes: foggy vision, cannot see clearly?

Opposite buzzing?

Mouth or throat, tonsils: inflammation; tired tongue.

Opposite teeth, mostly molars; loose teeth, or pain.

Esophagus contracted.

Jaundice.

Nose: coryza, opposite.

Chills: excess cold; laryngitis, asthma, pleurisy.

Urine stopped from cold, sphincter, prostatitis, urethra.

Parts of the body:

Opposite orbicularis muscles of mouth.

Pectoral muscles.

Anterior, shoulder, posterior arm, same side (pains with shivering or flaccidity); upper thumb, anterior superior knee, opposite.

LI-3 *sanjian* — third interval

Dorsal hand (palm down, pronation); long bone of the index finger (second metacarpal) at mid-length; by the palmar head of the swollen head of the body of the long bone; on the index finger facing the thumb (second metacarpal), lateral edge, along the head a little under (before) the transverse insertion of the fist dorsal interosseous muscle; in a hollow.

Four FW above *erjian* (LI-2); two below *hegu* (LI-4); one large FW above and medial to hand-*zhongdu* (MP-17 IS M-UE-23a).

When dispersed:

Disperses the opposite large intestine, small intestine, bladder (expulsor muscles), stomach; opposite eye, ear, nose, teeth, throat, tonsils, nape and shoulder; articulations of the five dorsal fingers and the base of the thumb, opposite medial, upper knee, opposite dorsal large toe.

Tonifies the kidneys on the same side, heart.

Acts on lungs according to the relation with its coupled meridian.

Tonifying seems to increase its effects.

Direct effects:

Great emotional agitation, likes to lie down.

Disperses the energy of the large intestine (*erjian,* LI-2): spasmodic constipation, pains, contractions (pulse small, hard). Or diarrhea from inflammation, gas (pulse swollen), colic, great noise, violent diarrhea; typhoid fever (with *erjian* and *hegu,* LI-2 and LI-4).

Weak heart, contracted arteries.

Mouth and lips dry, swollen tongue, opposite incisors and canines (pain increased from cold drinks).

Stomach: inflammation, a lot of thready saliva, mouth and lips dry, food does not pass (retarded digestion).

Abdomen and chest full.

Throat: tonsillitis (thorn in throat); difficult respiration, obstructing mucus.

Nose: opposite back of throat; coryza or oozing blood.

Opposite eye, (pain); opposite ears: buzzings?

Bladder: expulsor muscles (of treasure).

Parts of the body:

Nape and posterior shoulder, opposite, scapula dispersed on opposite side; elbow; thumb and dorsal side of fingers, same side.

''When the energy is in the upper limbs, first of all *sanjian*.''

Opposite, upper, medial knee; opposite, medial large knee (painful gout), upper, medial opposite arch of the foot.

LI-4 *hegu* — bottom of the valley

Dorsal hand: between the superior (posterior) heads of the first and second metacarpals, just between the head of the metacarpal of the thumb and the dorsoradial artery; in a hollow; on the superior edge of a small ligament.

Two FW above *sanjian* (LI-3); two below yangxi (LI-5); two from hand-*zhongdu* (MP-17, IS M-UE-23a).

When tonified:

Tonifies the opposite large intestine and all yang meridians, the three nervous centers, three organs of sense; opposite pituitary; opposite side of face and head, nose, eye, ears, teeth; tonsils, throat, opposite trachea, lateral side of neck, upper shoulder, lateral face of arm, posterior forearm, opposite wrist and hand and dorsal side of fingers; lumbar region, anterior, medial lower limbs and opposite dorsum of foot; stops hemorrhages, menses: tonify.

Disperses the opposite kidney filtration; opposite vessels and sexual organs.

Dispersing acts in a contrary manner.

Direct effects:

Commands the energy (*sanyinjiao*, SP-6, commands the blood), all the yang organ meridians, producers of energy (*taichong*, LR-3, commands the six yin).

Weakness and emptiness; weakness of the nerves; great perspiration from weakness; insomnia from weakness.

Opposite large intestine: production of antihemorrhagic vitamin K by the large intestine and of the anti-neuralgic vitamin B complex. Atonic constipation, difficult and not very abundant stools: tonify; inflammation, diarrhea: disperse; typhoid fever (elevated, prolonged fever, diarrhea, sweats, vomiting, lumbar pain): disperse.

Fever: fever from chills (and violent cough); intermittent fever; measles, German measles, scarlet fever.

Heart opposite side: troubles of rhythm — tonify if weak, disperse if excess.

Opposite side of tongue: heavy, stiff.

Loose teeth: tonify; all teeth painful, caries: disperse.

Opposite side of throat: sore throat, opposite tonsillitis; laryngitis; false croup: disperse; obstructing mucus, tracheitis; blocked respiration, asthma.

Opposite eye: weakness, vision weak and foggy: tonify; beginning of cataract, keratitis.

Opposite ear: deafness? ''If the blood is thick, disperse; if it is fluid, tonify;'' buzzing from emptiness.

Taste-smell: anosmia: tonify. Congestive headaches opposite side: tonify; opposite cerebral congestion: tonify.

Acute meningitis (to the point of ''false death''): tonify; cerebral spasms: tonify; cerebral anemia: disperse.

Opposite side of nose — congestive coryza: tonify; fluid at the beginning: disperse; sinusitis: disperse; fissures.

Blood: fluid blood: tonify; hemorrhaging easily, prolonged: tonify; menses too abundant: tonify). Bleeding nose: tonify; spits blood: tonify; intestinal hemorrhages, retinal hemorrhages, glaucoma, congestion of eyes: tonify. Bleeds easily, too thick: disperse. Fear of blood-clots: disperse. Luminous zigzag before the eyes; thick insufficient menses, not coming: disperse.

Confinement: disperse (relaxes the energy of the tissues and detaches the placenta) and tonify *sanyinjiao* (SP-6).

Conception: too easy — tonify; too difficult — disperse.

Kidney-filtration: profuse urine (and dry skin): disperse.

Insufficient urine (sweats a lot): tonify.

Parts of the body:

Skin: dryness or with squamation: tonify; acne on the opposite side of the face: tonify.

Spasms of infants.

Opposite tetanus (contracted muscles, acute pain); disperse. Trismus, contracted jaw, opposite: disperse.

Swelling on opposite side of face: tonify; acne: disperse; paralysis of opposite facial nerve: tonify.
Lateral side of neck, upper shoulder, lateral face of arm, wrist, hand and opposite dorsum of fingers.
Lower scapula, opposite lower back.
Opposite lumbar area, lower opposite limb; opposite medial leg and knee; opposite dorsum of foot and large toe.

LI-5 *yangxi* — little valley of yang

Dorsal wrist (palm down, pronation), lateral side (base of the thumb); at the angle of the inferior edge of the radial apophysical prominence and of the dorsal edge of the tendons forming the anterior crest of the short extensor of the thumb and the abductor longus of the thumb; in a hollow.

Two large FW above *hegu* (LI-4); separated by the lateral head of the radius from *pianli* (LI-6); one FW lateral to *zhongquan* (MP-14, IS M-UE-33).

When tonified:

Tonifies all the yang meridians (superficial pulses, producers of energy), frontal lobes, spinal cord, opposite ear, opposite lateral edge of eye, scalp, lumbar area, opposite upper and lower limbs, abdominal muscles, genital apparatus.
Disperses all the yin meridians (deep pulses, distributors).
Dispersing acts in an opposite way.
Has a response with *weizhong* (BL-54, IS BL-40) and the kidney meridian. Has effects on the lumbar area analogous to those of *weizhong* (BL-54, IS BL-40).

Direct effects:

Insufficiency: gripped by emotions, sudden weakness, troubled, upset, cannot breathe.
Excess: hyperexcited speech, happy laughter, hallucinations.
Fever, agitated mind to the point of delirium; hemiplegia?
Opposite lateral side of eye painful; inflammation; keratitis; floating spots before the eyes; cataract.
Opposite ear, pain, buzzing, deafness?
Opposite upper teeth: pain, caries.
Nose: opposite coryza, tonsillitis; sore throat, saliva, cough, sputum, cannot breathe, malaise; tuberculosis of children?
Hyper- or hypotension.
Penis; perineum; impotence; acute or chronic orchitis on the opposite side.
Opposite side, skin: all problems — dry and squamous or wet with pus.

Parts of the body:

Internal or external headache.
Opposite scalp, back, lumbar area.
Opposite abdominal muscle.
Upper limb same side.
Thumb same side, base, dorsal lateral: joints and nail.
Opposite anterior medial face of the lower limb.

LI-6 *pianli* — lateral succession

Dorsal side of the forearm (palm up, supination; three FW above the wrist; at the angle of the medial (ulnar) edge of the radius and the inferior edge of the transverse prominence (inferior insertion of the flexor longus?) of the thumb; between the bone and the supinator longus; in a hollow.

Separated from *yangxi* (LI-5) by the head of the radius, three FW under *wenliu* (LI-7). A branch passes through *zhongquan* (MP-14, IS M-UE-33), *weilaogong* (MP-13, IS M-UE-23) and *changdu* (MP-16, IS M-UE-23b), up to *zhongchong* (PC-9).

When tonified:

Tonifies the large intestine, small intestine, opposite side of the heart, opposite lung, brain, cerebellum, medulla oblongata, spinal cord, eye and ear; opposite incisors, thumb and index finger, opposite knee.
Disperses the opposite kidney.
Dispersing acts in the opposite way.
Point of passage between large intestine and lungs (see *lieque,* LU-7). If excess: dental caries, deafness; mental troubles; if insufficiency: cold of the incisors; digestion stopped, weakness. Also, ''child'' of the lung; if the

lungs are stronger than the large intestine, tonify. If lungs are weaker, disperse.
Mental troubles, speaks a lot: disperse; or weakness: tonify.

Direct effects:

Opposite incisors cold: or loose, or painful, or caries.
Opposite side of throat: tonsillitis, dry throat.
Opposite side of stomach: digestion blocked: tonify.
Opposite eye: foggy or obscure vision.
Opposite ear: pains or buzzing? or deafness?

Opposite effects:

Opposite side of nose: congestive coryza; or bleeding: tonify.
Urine: abundant, frequent needs at night and at beginning of night: tonify; edema, urine insufficient: disperse.

Parts of the body:

Opposite scapula.
Lateral upper arm, same side; forearm (radial and supinator muscles).
Also thumb and index fingers.
Anterior face of knee and opposite leg.

LI-7 *wenliu* — tepid flow

Forearm, palm up, supination; six FW above the wrist (mid-length of the forearm); at the angle of the anterior edge of the bone and of the inferior edge of a transverse eminence; between the supinator and flexor longus of the thumb; in a hollow; on the posterior edge of the supinator longus; on the anterior edge of the posterior radial artery coming from the posterior side; palm down (pronation), on the ulnar edge of the radius.

Three FW proximal to *pianli* (LI-6): one FW under arm-*xialian* (LI-8), at the level of *sidu* (TW-9).

When tonified:

Tonifies the large intestine, small intestine, temporoparietal lobes, stomach; mouth, gums, teeth, opposite side of lips; knee, opposite leg, upper shoulder, arm of same side.
Disperses the heart, lungs, opposite kidney.
Dispersing acts in a contrary manner.

Direct effects:

Easy laughter, hyperexcited speech, hallucinations; insanity, hyperexcitation.
Violent shock, four limbs swollen, tongue protrudes (?), cerebral congestion; apoplexy, hemiplegia, mouth awry (?).
Mouth and opposite side of tongue: inflammation, pain.
Opposite gums, teeth: pain.
Diaphragm in excess: crisis of eructation or vomiting, or abundance of saliva; gas in the stomach, aerogastria, aerophagia; abdomen: pains and growling; pelvic basin: spasms.

Opposite effects:

Respiratory passages in excess: bronchitis; top of lung: catarrh; pleurisy, tuberculosis.

Parts of the body:

Local pains, neuralgia.
Headache, face swollen.
Shoulder without strength: abductor longus of thumb, upper limb same side.
Anterior side of the knee: opposite leg.

LI-8 *xialian* — inferior angle

Forearm, palm up, in supination: seven FW above the wrist (five large FW below the head of the radius). Just at the anterior edge of the radius with the supinator longus; at the angle of the inferior edge of a transverse eminence (the inferior insertion of the shorter supinator); in a hollow; on the inferior edge of the insertion of the pronator.

One FW above *wenliu* (LI-7); one FW under arm-*shanglian* (LI-9).

When tonified:

Tonifies the large intestine, opposite brain, opposite ear; dorsal and palmar muscles of hand and thumb; knee, opposite anterior leg.

Disperses the opposite kidney, opposite lung.

Dispersing acts in the opposite way.

Direct effects:

Extraordinary fits of hopelessness; hyperexcited speech; walks blindly without direction (escapades), congestion from heat to the point of apoplexy.

Large intestine: the point is very sensitive in cases of diarrhea and even more in cases of intestinal tuberculosis, diarrhea after meals, noisy discharge and wind.

Small intestine: insufficiency, face without complexion, bad digestion, (mostly carbohydrates, meat, fat), pain at navel, dry lips, flowing saliva.

Asthma, cannot walk; inflammation of bronchioles; pleurisy; tuberculosis.

Opposite breast, inflammation or abscess.

Pelvic basin: spasms, fullness.

Urine with blood, flaccidity of bladder.

Parts of the body:

Rheumatism from cold, humidity, wind; rheumatism of skin.

All joints of same side of upper limb. Tennis elbow: pain of forearm and elbow, particularly from pouring drinks or from holding a racquet, neuralgia of the radial and supinator muscles (of the musculocutaneus nerve); thumb, all anterior and posterior muscles.

Causes the hand to lift: back of the hand.

Dorsal toes, lower limb, opposite anterior knee.

Sacrum and opposite lumbar muscles.

LI-9   *shanglian* — superior angle

Forearm, thumb up: four FW from the head of the radius (under the epicondyle). Just at the edge of the anterior angle of the radius; on the radial edge of the internal radial muscle; deep to the superior edge of the insertion of the flexor longus of the thumb; in a hollow.

One FW above arm-*xialian* (LI-8); two FW below arm-*sanli* (LI-10).

When tonified:

Tonifies the large intestine, opposite and central inferior lateral side of brain.

Yang energy (heat, movement). Opposite spinal cord; strength of hand (flexors by the extensors). Lumbar, heat and articulations of the upper limb on the same side and opposite lower limb.

Disperses the opposite kidney.

Dispersing acts in the opposite way.

Direct effects:

Point is painful in cases of cerebral fatigue, excess work. Fatigue to exhaustion of the brain; encephalitis, diplopia, urine stopped; paralysis of the bladder.

Breathless (dyspnea) headache.

Cerebral headache: from excess work and emotions; from cerebral congestion, from encephalitis, from meningitis, from inflammation of the brain.

Hiccoughs from inflammation of the brain, from hemorrhage or cerebral anemia.

Diarrhea from excess energy of the large intestine (and typhoid): "can serve as a reunion point for the large intestine."

Cold into the bone marrow; cold of the upper limb side and inferior opposite limb.

Parts of the body:

Upper limb same side: joints. Hand: grips without strength (weakness of flexors). Thumb: sprain or rheumatism.

Opposite lower limb: joints; mid part of back between the scapula, opposite (rhomboids and dorsal intercostal muscles).

Opposite lumbar muscles and vertebrae.

LI-10   [arm-]*sanli* — third mile

Forearm, thumb up: two large FW under the round head of the radius (which is above the epicondyle). On the posterior edge of the sharp edge of the radius; just in the angle of a curve of the radius; between the two radial muscles, above a transverse bulge; deep to the short supinator. Palm down (pronation); ulnar edge of the radius.

Two FW above arm-*shanglian* (LI-9); one large FW under *quchi* (LI-11). Separated by the supinator longus from *chize* (LU-5).

When tonified:

Tonifies the large intestine, heart, vessels, lungs, liver, spleen-pancreas, posterior frontal lobes; radial muscles, supinator longus, supinator teres; warms the extremities; breasts; half of the body same side; face, lips, opposite gums.

Disperses the bladder sphincter.

Dispersing acts in the opposite way.

Direct effects:

Also called "the point which awakens" (in reality *xingxingxue,* TW-9a), because massaging it awakens one from a faint, from weakness, from indigestion malaise, from loss of ability to make sound, loss of awareness and energy in cholera or apoplexy; or tongue dancing from the right to left.

Heart, arteries, veins (see TW-9a), influenza, flu; circulation, cold at the extremities (see TW-9a).

Very painful in constipation; all digestive troubles.

Dental caries, opposite side; dental abscess, fluxion, opposite side; loose, displaced molars, opposite side.

Lips: swollen, opposite side.

Ears: buzzing, opposite side?

Parotid glands: inflammation, same side.

Breasts: inflammation of mammary glands.

Lymph nodes of the neck or axilla: inflammation (adenitis).

Carbuncle, serious abscesses.

Parts of the body:

External headache, stiff nape, visual dizziness.

Cheek, maxilla, opposite side of chin, inflammation of tissues; or facial paralyses, flaccidity of the opposite lower eyelid, ectropion of the opposite lower eyelid.

Elbow and forearm, same side: pain, radial nerve; extensors and supinators.

"A quick blow paralyzes the arm and hand for a moment."

Hand: can neither open nor close, or contracted.

Opposite lower back: acute pain.

Opposite knee, lower leg and instep.

LI-11   *quchi* — swamp of the curve

Elbow flexed, lateral side (extensors): in the radiohumeral articulation; in the angle of the superior edge of the round head of the radius, below the epicondyle and of the deep condyle of the humerus. When the elbow is extended, the point is covered by the supinator longus, which is on the anterior edge.

One FW above and in front of arm-*sanli* (LI-10), four below *zhouliao* (LI-12); three anterior to *chize* (LU-5).

When tonified:

Tonifies the large intestine, small intestine, liver, all nervous centers, the three endocrines and three levels of the psyche, half-body same side, face, eyes, ears, gums, teeth, all opposite; anterior radial muscles, supinators, extensors.

Disperses the stomach, gallbladder, kidney.

Direct effects:

Depression, fear, forgetfulness; dreams of uncultivated fields.

Tonification point of the large intestine. Atony of the peristaltic reflex, of secretion and absorption, of the battle against the micro-organisms; insufficiency of anti-hemorrhagic vitamin K and of anti-neuralgic vitamin B; skin in bad condition, menses too abundant or too frequent; atonic constipation (big stools coming with difficulty); or stool badly formed.

Parotitis, mumps.

Stomach.

Master of troubles of eyes, ears, throat, teeth, mouth, face.

Red and painful eyes.

Ears: pain, pain in front of the ears.

Opposite effects:

Throat: pain, cannot speak; squeezed larynx; tonsillitis, diphtheria (mortal occlusion of the throat), tonify.

Teeth: pain, loose.

Fever not stopping after typhoid, tonify.

Menses: insufficient or slightly arrested, disperse (if anemia, *gaohuangshu,* BL-38, IS BL-43).

Thirst: if one drinks, perspiration; if one does not drink, dry skin: tonify.

Prolonged low fever: tonify; prolonged fever at the end of typhoid; scarlet fever; eruptive illnesses.

Kidney (hard, elevated pulse): tonify; bladder (soft pulse): disperse.

Parts of the body:

Troubles of skin; dry skin: tonify. Troubles of dry skin or to the point of squamousness: tonify; itching (pruritis) like the gnawing of insects, itchy skin with sores: tonify; swelling and redness of the hand and arm.

Furuncles and pimples on the hands, anterior fatty abscesses (lipoma)? Tubercular abscesses on the arm.

Headache, neuralgia; swelling of the head?

Opposite side of face, facial neuralgia (cheek, temple, cheekbone, upper teeth); neck: inflammation, swollen lymph glands.

Intercostal neuralgia; upper dorsal spine; deviation of the spine from paralysis, opposite scapula.

Back pain; lumbar area: contraction, pain on rising.

Axilla: pain or weakness.

Radial nerve (extensors, supinators?).

Articulations of the lower and upper limb, same side.

Shoulder, lateral side of arm, wrist, entire upper limb: acute pain, cannot lift.

Arm and elbow: numbness, becoming thin, without strength, slow muscles, cannot lift, can neither groom nor dress oneself.

External elbow: pain, arthritis, contracture or flaccidity; elbow and forearm pain.

Hand weak (does not obey, cannot keep tight), flaccidity or contracture.

Skin of the hand red, swollen, irritated; furuncles and pimples on the back of the hand; dorsal side of thumb: pain.

Toes on same side contracted.

LI-12 *zhouliao* — hollow of the elbow

Lateral side of the arm: two FW above the lateral epicondyle of the elbow; at the angle of the anterior edge of the humerus and the posterior, inferior edge of the muscle at an angle (brachialis anterior); in a hollow.

Four FW above *quchi* (LI-11); two below *wuli* (LI-13); two in front of *qinglengyuan* (TW-11); three posterior to *xiabai* (LU-4).

When tonified:

Tonifies the large intestine, posterior frontal lobes, opposite ear, lateral side of opposite side of the neck, shoulder-arm articulation.

Disperses the opposite kidney (and lumbar region), lung, same side.

Dispersing acts in the opposite way.

Direct effects:

Likes to sleep?

Opposite effects:

Tuberculosis from shock? Congestion?

Opposite kidney (and lumbar area).

Parts of the body:

Opposite lateral side of the neck.

Glenohumeral articulation; pain, ankylosis or arthritis. Upper limb: flaccidity, or contracture, pain, or tightness; cannot flex the elbow (weak brachialis anterior).

LI-13   *wuli* — fifth mile

Lateral side of the arm; five FW above the lateral epicondyle of the elbow; on the humerus; on the anterior edge of the external posterior bony prominence of the humerus; on the inferior edge of the large opposite tendinous insertion of the brachialis and deltoid.

Two FW above *zhouliao* (LI-12); three under *binao* (LI-14); three posterior to *xiabai* (LU-4).

When tonified:
Tonifies the large intestine, bladder, endocrines, opposite eye; hand, wrist, dorsal forearm same side; opposite, lateral lower limb.
Disperses the lung and kidney on the same side.
Dispersing acts in the opposite way.

Direct effects:
Contractures of intestine and bladder. Large intestine or small intestine: spasms to the point of contracture, obstruction and occlusion.
Bladder: sphincter contracted to the point of retention and occlusion.
Emotional agitation, fear, deranged mind, restless; likes to lie down.
Opposite eye; darkened vision.
Endocrines: all troubles.

Opposite effects:
Lungs, kidney same side: energy in upper body; cough, spits blood; pneumonia, tuberculosis from shock? congestion?
Lymph glands (adenitis); lymphangitis.

Parts of the body:
Articular rheumatism (from wind and humidity) upper and lower limb or pain of articulations, shoulder, elbow, wrist, back of thumb, same side, hip, knee, opposite foot.

LI-14   *binao* — deltoid and arm

Lateral aspect of the arm: three FW below the lower part of the large head of the humerus; six FW below the acromion; on the angle of the anterior edge of the prominence at the mid-length of the humerus and the inferior edge of a transverse insertion (the extremity of the insertion of the pectoralis major, latissimus dorsi and teres major); between two bundles of the deltoid muscle; on the upper part of a hollow above the opposed insertions of the deltoid and brachialis anterior.

Three FW above arm-*wuli* (LI-13); two large FW below and posterior to *jianyu* (LI-15); three FW anterior and below *xiaoluo* (TW-12); four FW posterior and below *yunmen* (LU-2).

When tonified:
Tonifies the large intestine, all the yang producer meridians (superficial pulses, opposite side of the lower spinal cord, lumbar area).
Disperses the opposite kidney.
Dispersing acts in the opposite way.

Effects and parts of the body:
Lymph glands.
Opposite side of head: pain.
Muscles of the opposite side of the face and under the eyes.
Scapulo-humeral articulation: cannot lift arm (acts on pectoralis major, latissimus dorsi, teres major).

LI-15   *jianyu* — deltoid of the shoulder

Anterior shoulder; in the hollow between the anterior edge of the clavicle, on the upper medial edge of the humerus, lateral and superior to the prominence of the coracoid process; just in the angle of the apophysis of the humerus.

Two large FW above and anterior (medial) to *binao* (LI-14); point following: *jugu* (LI-16) in the angle of the acromion; three large FW medial and anterior to *naohui* (TW-13); four FW lateral to *zhongfu* (LU-1).

When tonified:

> Tonifies the large intestine, posterior frontal, temporal and parietal lobes; weakly tonifies all the meridians; lateral half of the body (from nape to hands and feet).
>
> Disperses kidneys, arteries, heart, bladder sphincter.
>
> Dispersing acts in the opposite way.

Direct effects:

> Weakness, loss of energy, cold.

Opposite effects:

> All troubles of fever; prolonged fever; fever from nerves or neuralgia; eruptive fevers; tonify.
>
> Hypertension: tonify; arteriosclerosis: tonify.
>
> Right or left hemiplegia — special preventive and curative: tonify.

Parts of the body:

> Skin: dry, burnt complexion. All eruptions with or without fever.
>
> Lymph nodes; tumors (suppurative adenitis?).
>
> Half-body, same side: muscles and bones, acute pain; contracture.
>
> Head and face on the opposite side: spasms.
>
> Spasms or pain from head to scapula.
>
> Shoulder and upper limb: all troubles (infraspinatus, brachialis anterior, extensors and supinators; cannot lift the hand to the head; rheumatic pains or contractures (all to disperse). Or swelling, weakness, thinness: tonify. However, "frequent moxa makes the upper arm thin."
>
> Anterior lateral lower limb; anterior thigh (anterior rectus m.) lateral anterior lower leg (tibialis anterior m. extensor).

LI-16   *jugu* — big bone

Upper extremity of the shoulder; angle of the acromion; just on the medial edge of the acromioclavicular articulation; on the acromial insertion of the trapezius muscle; deep on the infraspinatus; in a hollow.

Preceding point: *jianyu* (LI-15) inferior edge of infraspinatus; following point: *tianding* (LI-17); middle of the lateral side of the neck, three FW medial to *jianshugu* (MP-10); three FW anterior to *jianliao* (TW-14).

When tonified:

> Tonifies the large intestine, spleen-pancreas, liver; inferior posterior frontal lobes, shoulder, arms, lateral posterior side of neck, knee and anterior leg.
>
> Disperses the opposite kidney, lung.
>
> Dispersing acts in the opposite way.

Direct effects:

> "Broken heart, vomits blood; forcing blood back into the chest," violent anger, broken vessels.
>
> Convulsions of children; epilepsy from fear.

Parts of the body:

> Lateral, posterior side of neck.
>
> Arms cannot be lifted from the side (weakness of the trapezius, infraspinatus, deltoid).
>
> Shoulder and upper limb: rheumatic neuralgia, acute pain on movement, knee and anterior lower leg.

LI-17   *tianding* — celestial cauldron

Lateral side of neck; about three FW under the bony prominence behind the ear (mastoid process); on the anterior and superior edge of a small round deep prominence (the lateral point of the third cervical vertebra); between two muscles.

Preceding point: *jugu* (LI-16); four FW under and posterior to neck-*futu* (LI-18); two under and before *tianchuang* (SI-16); three under and a little more in front of *tianyou* (TW-16).

When tonified:
>   Tonifies the large intestine, throat, shoulder, lateral upper limb and external posterior lower limb.
>   Disperses the opposite kidney.
>   Dispersing acts in an opposite manner.

Direct effects:
>   Throat: inflammation, pain; tonsillitis.
>   Laryngitis: sudden muteness, loss of voice, paralysis of the hyoid muscles; internal ear.

Parts of the body:
>   Lateral side of neck, from ear, upper and posterior shoulder, lateral face of upper limb, wrist, hand, dorsal side of fingers.
>   Lower limb of the same side, posteromedial aspect.
>   Back: muscles of the opposite side.

Points of Weihe: Right: Stramonium. Indecent speech; hands constantly on the genital organs; sexual erethism; offends, insults, beats; delirium tremens; hallucinations; hears voices; expression of terror; wide-open eyes; paralysis (contracture) of the muscles of expression and locomotion; stumbling walk (Parkinsonism?); anuria, spasmodic asthma.

Left: Belladonna. Inflammation of throat, nose or eyes; hoarseness; congestive headaches; inflammation of the brain; sudden pains; fever with sweat; scarlet fever: preventive and curative; parasympathetic system (which contracts throat, bronchus, inflames the stomach, etc.)

LI-18 *futu* — suddenness tamed

Superior lateral side of the neck just under the inferoposterior angle of the lower jaw; in the angle of the anterior edge of the muscle on the slant (sternocleidomastoid), and on the superior edge of a narrow transverse muscle (belly of the digastric muscle).

Four FW above and anterior to *tianding* (LI-17); following point: *heliao* (LI-19), under the nostrils; two FW anterior and under *tianrong* (SI-17); three under *jiache* (ST-3, IS ST-6); two above and posterior to *renying* (ST-9); two in front of *tianchuang* (SI-16).

The large intestine meridian crosses *daying* (ST-8, IS ST-5) and *dicang* (ST-7, IS ST-4).

When tonified:
>   Tonifies the large intestine, small intestine, spleen-pancreas, articulation of hip and opposite hip, parotid glands, opposite lateral salivary glands, throat and opposite larynx, opposite orbit of the eye, opposite side of upper lip.
>   Disperses the opposite kidney, stomach.
>   Dispersing acts in a contrary manner.

Direct effects:
>   Salivates in excess (flowing in rivulets); parotid glands; opposite lateral salivary glands.
>   Opposite side of throat; chronic angina, cough with much saliva, suffocating, swollen throat, tonsillitis opposite; opposite tracheitis; coughing fits, energy at the top; hoarseness; sudden muteness; laryngeal spasms; acute paralysis of the opposite hyoid muscles; edema of the opposite side of the uvula.
>   Opposite orbital neuralgia; opposite facial paralysis.

Parts of the body:
>   Opposite upper lips: trembling.
>   Platysma muscle of neck.
>   Articulation of the opposite hip: arthritic pains; opposite gluteus minimus and medius muscles; adductors.

Points of Weihe: Right: Bartya Carbonica. Hypertrophy of all glands, ganglia or tumors on the neck, tonsils, prostate; hoarseness from too much talking; cough of old people with difficult respiration; paralysis of tongue; lack of appetite, quickly satisfied; fetid odor of the feet; trembling hands; physical and psychological weakness.

Left: Tonca, Cumaruma. All neuralgias; orbital pains; pains of articulation of hip; trembling upper lip.

LI-19 *heliao* — hollow of cereals

Upper lip; one half FW inferior and lateral to the inferior edge of the nostril; at the angle of the upper edge of the orbicularis muscle of the lips and the medial edge of the elevator of the upper lip; in a hollow.

Preceding point: neck-*futu* (LI-18) under the maxillary angle; two inferior and posterior to *yingxiang* (LI-20); at the same level and lateral to *shuikou* (GV-25, IS GV-26 *renzhong*); two FW anterior (medial) to *juliao* (ST-4, IS ST-3); three FW anterior and superior to *dicang* (ST-7, IS ST-4), which the large intestine meridian crosses.

When tonified:

Tonifies the large intestine, small intestine, ear, top of the throat, nose, parotid glands, stomach.

Disperses the opposite kidney.

Dispersing acts in an opposite manner.

"Sends energy to the large intestine. Massage calms, softens and warms the large intestine."

Nose: incessant, clear flowing (spasmodic colds?); or blocked nose, bad smell (ozena?); blood oozing from both nostrils.

Hardness of hearing.

Mumps. Contracted jaws, trismus.

Motor point of the upper lip.

LI-20 *yingxiang* — encountering perfumes

Beside the nose: one half FW lateral to the mid-height of the nostril; at the angle of the inferior edge of the bony horizontal edge and the anterior (medial) edge of the canine and elevator of the upper lip; in a hollow.

Two FW above *heliao* (LI-19); one branch causes the energy to pass from the large intestine to the stomach at *touwei* (ST-1, IS ST-8), by traversing the edge of the nose to *yintang* (GV-23a, IS M-HN-3) and *shangxing* (GV-22, IS GV-23), and then redescending to *touwei* (ST-1, IS ST-8).

When tonified:

Tonifies the large intestine, heart, bladder, stomach; nose, maxillary sinus, lung.

Disperses the opposite kidney, lung.

Dispersing acts in the opposite way.

Direct effects:

Weakened atonic sense of smell; abundant and clear coryza; maxillary sinusitis; blocked nose, bad odor (ozena?); abscess of the nose; fatty inflammation of the nose; growths.

Nasal asthma, panting, respiration without results.

Scarlet eyes, swelling (if serious add *taichong,* LR-3).

Parts of the body:

Face: inflammation of the tissues, swelling, scratching, pruritis like gnawing insects. Intermittent contractions of the mouth and face; closed eyes, closed mouth: contracture (excess of facial nerve).

Swollen lips, painful.

Facial paralysis: mouth awry: tonify flaccid side, disperse contracted side. Acts on elevator muscles of upper lip.

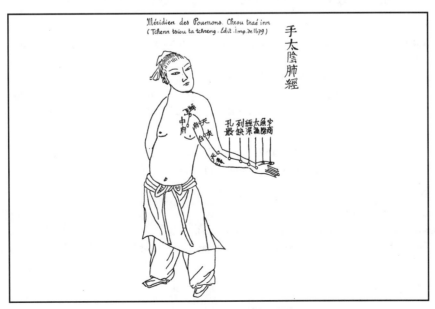

Meridian of the lungs (DACH)

Chapter III

Stomach

According to the physiology of energy, the stomach is "the origin of everything." Classified as a yang organ, producer of yang energy, it extracts food and drink coming from the earth, which is yin — thus the total yin and yang energy. One of its points, *qichong* (ST-30), is the reservoir of this energy whence the triple warmer, charged with its distribution to all the organ-meridians, draws it.

It is stimulated, tonified, nervously activated, by the parasympathetic system (*tianzhu,* BL-10), and inhibited, distended, dispersed, slowed down by the sympathetic (*fengchi,* GB-20).

The feelings have a great action on its function, and its function has a great action on the feelings.

1) Causing insufficiency (inhibits, disperses the stomach): chagrin or sorrow (which stimulates the heart governor), obsession, excess thoughts (which inflame the pancreas) cause insufficiency (inhibiting or dispersing the stomach); joy, heat and exercise cause excess.

2) Excess of the stomach can cause serious mental hyperexcitation comparable to the vapors of alcohol, which excite the stomach. It causes incessant dreams to the point of violent nightmares. Insufficiency of the stomach causes sadness, discouragement and a lack of taste for life as well as for food.

When tonified, it also tonifies the gallbladder (husband-wife), the large intestine (mother) and the spleen-pancreas (child) if they are equal (coupled meridian); and disperses the heart governor (midday-midnight) and spleen-pancreas (unequal coupled meridians); dispersing acts in the opposite way.

Its maximum energy is at 8:00 a.m. (minimum hour of the heart governor); its minimum is at 8:00 p.m. (maximum hour of the heart governor).

Tonification point: *jiexi* (ST-41); dispersal point: *lidui* (ST-45); source point: *chongyang* (ST-42); passage point: *fenglong* (ST-40) which connects to *gongsun* (SP-4).

ST-1 *touwei* (IS ST-8) — chain of the head

Upper temple, anterior part: at the angle of the lateral inferior edge of the frontal bulge, of the lateral edge of the vertical ridge of the frontal crest and of the inferior edge of the horizontal relief (superior temporal crest).

Following point: *xiaguan* (ST-2, IS ST-7), at the external corner of the eye; separated by the frontal crest from *yangbai* (GB-10, IS GB-14) by the frontal bulge from head-*linqi* (GB-11, IS GB-15); two FW anterior to *muchuang* (GB-12, IS GB-16); one large FW above and anterior to *sizhukong* (TW-21, IS TW-23).

When tonified:

Tonifies the stomach, gallbladder, occipital lobes, small intestine, eyes, eyelids, face same side.
Disperses heart, vessels.
Dispersing acts in the opposite way.
The energy comes from the large intestine meridian point *yingxiang* (LI-20), at the side of the nostrils, by a branch passing through *jingming* (BL-1) and *zanzhu* (BL-2) and turning above the eyebrow.

Direct effects:

Eyes: tired or very diminished vision (amblyopia, blindness).
Eyelids: clinging; purulent conjunctivitis; abundant tears.

Parts of the body:

Acute pain above the eyebrows.
Face: pain on one side, facial neuralgia, facial paralysis.
Internal headaches (congestive), "head as if broken and eyes as if torn out." If dizziness with fainting, tonify.

ST-2   *xiaguan* (IS ST-7) — lower barrier

Cheek: in the angle of the lateral inferior edge of the cheekbone and of the inferior edge of the large muscles (masseter); in a hollow.

Three FW below *chengqi* (ST-4, IS ST-1); three narrow FW above *dicang* (ST-7, IS ST-4).

When tonified:
Tonifies the stomach, large intestine, heart, gallbladder, anterior temporal lobe; ears, jaw, cheek; spleen-pancreas (equal coupled meridians).
Disperses vessels, spleen-pancreas (unequal coupled meridian).
Dispersing acts in the opposite way.

Direct effects:
Vertigo on turning, fainting (Meniere's syndrome).
Ears: buzzing, deafness, pain, otitis.
Teeth: pain, dental abscess, congestion.

Parts of the body:
Face: facial nerve, trigeminal nerve; yawning; spasms of the face; jaw dislocated; facial paralysis; eyes do not close; facial neuralgia.

ST-3   *jiache* (IS ST-6) — maxillary

Inferior, posterior cheek: just in the anterior angle of the posterior rise of the rising branch of the protrusion of the inferior posterior point of the maxillary bone. Between the two insertions of the large muscle which hardens by clenching the teeth (masseter muscle); in a hollow.

Three FW lateral to *dicang* (ST-7, IS ST-4); two FW lateral and a little above *daying* (ST-8, IS ST-5); two FW under *tinghui* (GB-2).

When tonified:
Tonifies: stomach, large intestine, small intestine, anterior temporal lobes, eyes, forehead, throat, larynx, trachea, nape and upper back.
Disperses: vessels.
Dispersing acts in the opposite way.

Direct effects:
Hoarse voice, loss of voice.
Dental cavities: pain; teeth: acute pain.
Hemiplegia? Total paralysis?

Parts of the body:
Skin: facial acne.
Upper part of the face: forehead, swelling, inflammation.
Facial paralysis (of the facial nerve), mouth awry and drooping, saliva, inferior eyelids do not close.
Facial neuralgia (of the trigeminal nerve).
Contracted jaw, cannot open the mouth, cannot chew (trismus); cheek and jaw and chin: acute pain or swollen.
Neck: all the muscles: pain or atrophy, cannot look to the rear.
Stiff nape; pain in nape and posterior shoulder.

ST-4   *chengqi* (IS ST-1) — receiver of tears

Lateral to the lateral corner of the eye; a little lateral to the angle of the lateral edge of the orbital arch and the superior edge of the zygomatic arch. Just at the superior edge of the suture of the zygomatic arch and the cheekbone; in a hollow.

Three FW just under *touwei* (ST-1, IS ST-8); one FW lateral and a little above *sibai* (ST-5, IS ST-2); separated from *quanliao* (SI-18) by the zygomatic arch; two FW anterior and below *tongziliao* (GB-1).

When tonified:
Tonifies the stomach, small intestine, inferior occipital lobe, eyes, skin of the face: *yangqiao mai* (yang energy).

Disperses: vessels; conception vessel.

Dispersing acts in the opposite way.

Direct effects: dispersion:

Eyes: distant vision foggy (pupil contracted, ciliary muscles relaxed). While looking, "the pupils itch." Sees badly in shadow and even worse at night: disperse (pupils contracted). Eyes winking and moving (spasms of the facial nerve); red eyes, painful, tears coming out; keratitis.

Ears: buzzing? Deafness?

Face: facial nerve spasms ("face moving," tightness, eyes winking and moving, mouth agitated, impeded speech, tics of nape and neck).

Parts of the body:

Spasms of all the muscles of the face and of the corner of the mouth and eye.

ST-5 *sibai* (IS ST-2) — four whitenesses

Face: under the middle of the eye; on the superior edge of the cheekbone at the point where it turns forward; on the bone of the orbital arch; under a notch on its superior edge.

One FW in front of and below *chengqi* (ST-4, IS ST-1); one large FW lateral and above *juliao* (ST-6, IS ST-3); one in front and above *quanliao* (SI-18).

When tonified:

Tonifies stomach, inferior occipital lobe, facial nerve.

Disperses vessels, conception vessel.

Dispersing acts in the opposite way.

Direct effects:

Eyes: itching, painful, streaming tears; pain of the eyeball; keratitis eyes red, painful, headache; dizziness; streaming tears, bad vision.

Eyelids blinking without stopping.

Face: spasms.

Sinusitis? "Illnesses in which one cannot speak."

ST-6 *juliao* (IS ST-3) — great hollow

Cheek: in the angle of the anterior (medial) edge of the cheek bone and of the inferior edge of the large prominence of the orbital arch; in a hollow.

One large FW above and in front of *sibai* (ST-5, IS ST-2); three a little above and anterior (medial) to *yingxiang* (LI-20); one large FW under and lateral to *jingming* (BL-1).

When tonified:

Tonifies stomach, large intestine, small intestine, heart, eyes, tip of the nose, corner of the mouth, face, jaw; *yangqiao mai.*

Disperses vessels, conception vessel.

Dispersing acts in the opposite way.

Direct effects:

Eyes: myopia, sees badly at a distance (pupils contracted, ciliary muscles relaxed); disperse. Brown floating spots before the eyes; blind even in light? (internal veiling of the retina?); cataract covering the lens?

Eyes: red, painful, tears coming out; keratitis, trouble of the cornea; eyes itching; veil of flesh on the eye (pterygion); eyes blink without stopping (nystagmus); inferior eyelid.

Nose: acute or chronic coryza; maxillary sinusitis; swelling, pain on the tip of the nose.

Parts of the body:

Face: facial paralysis (of the facial nerve) "from cold or wind on the lips or cheek," "attack of warmth on the lips or cheeks"; pain on the jaw, swollen, from wind or cold on the face.

Canine muscle, elevator of the upper lip zygomaticus minor muscle, corner of the lips falling: flaccidity of the above muscles.

Facial nerve: spasms or contracture.

Facial neuralgia (trigeminal neuralgia), cheekbone, eye.

ST-7   *dicang* (IS ST-4) — silo, grainary of earth

Cheek: two FW (IS: one FW) lateral to the corner of the mouth; in the angle of the anterior and inferior edge of the large muscle (masseter), and of the lateral edge of the vertical artery (facial artery).

Three FW below *juliao* (ST-6, IS ST-3); two FW above and a little medial to *daying* (ST-8, IS ST-5). The meridian of the large intestine passes through *dicang*.

When tonified:

Tonifies the stomach, medulla oblongata, spinal cord, large intestine, liver, spleen-pancreas (equal coupled meridian).

Yangqiao mai (yang energy of face and skin): orbicularis muscles of eye and mouth; tongue and lips, cheek, cutaneous muscles of cheek and neck. Disperses vessels, spleen-pancreas (unequal coupled meridians).

Dispersing acts in the opposite way.

Direct effects:

Muscles of eye, eyelids, mouth, tongue, cheek and neck.

Eyes: convergent strabismus; spasms or atrophy of all the eye muscles; eyes moving without stopping stagmus); incessant eye pain.

Eye: myopia, attacks of foggy vision; hemeralopia (does not see in shadow).

Eyelids: cannot close (lagothalmia); blinking.

Worms in the distributor organs (Distoma hepaticum?), easy production of pus?

Parts of the body:

Mouth and eye: spasms of all the muscles.

Tongue: contracture, cannot speak, loss of voice.

Face: facial paralysis (of the facial nerve), slow mouth, does not obey, flowing saliva.

Facial neuralgia, eye and forehead (superior trigeminal nerve?)

Cutaneous muscles of cheek and neck.

ST-8   *daying* (IS ST-5) — great meeting

Jaw: two FW in front of the inferior, posterior angle; at the angle of the inferior edge of the jaw and anterior edge of the vertical artery (facial artery); deep, on the myohyoidius muscle.

About two FW below and lateral to *dicang* (ST-7, IS ST-4) under the corner of the mouth; following point: *renying* (ST-9); four FW superior and medial to neck-*futu* (LI-18). The meridian of the large intestine passes through *daying*.

When tonified:

Tonifies the stomach, teeth, lateral neck and anterior face; cerebellum, large intestine, nostrils.

Disperses the vessels.

Dispersing acts in the opposite way.

Direct effects:

Teeth (particularly molars) opposite side: pain, caries.

Opposite salivary glands, opposite parotid (swelling of opposite jaw and neck; mumps).

Eye: spasms of the eyeball; external muscles same side, internal muscles opposite side; lymph nodes and pain of the front of the neck.

Parts of the body.

Facial nerve.

Face: facial paralysis (mouth awry, disturbed, does not obey, impeded speech, stiff tongue, eyelids do not close, painful eyes).

Face: contractions, spasms (of facial nerve). Spasms of the lips, mouth, lateral neck and nape; contracted jaw, trismus.

Facial pain (linked to trigeminal nerve?).

ST-9   *renying* — human meetings or external sensations

Front of the neck; two FW on either side of the medial line, at the level of the upper point of the thyroid cartilage (larynx); at the angle of the anterior edge (medial) of the large muscle (sternocleidomastoid); deep, the strong artery (carotid artery) and on the superior lateral edge of the thyroid cartilage; in a hollow.

Four FW below *daying* (ST-8, IS ST-5); two above *shuitu* (ST-10); two on either side of *lianquan* (CV-23).

When tonified:

Tonifies the stomach, gallbladder, posterior part of inferior frontal lobe, anterior temporal lobe, tongue, throat, larynx, esophagus.
Disperses the vessels.
Dispersing acts in the opposite way.

Direct effects:

Vocal cords hoarse; voice which cracks on high notes (vocal cords on the two sides at different tension).
Tongue: hypoglossal nerve (tongue, motor function, vasoconstriction of the mucosa).
Throat: swelling or abscess.
Cough: panting at expiration, cannot breathe out (emphysema), fullness of chest.
Lymph nodes.

Parts of the body:

Goiter; Basedow's disease.
Cutaneous muscles of neck.

ST-10   *shuitu* — sudden water

Front of the neck: about two FW from the medial line, at the level of the joints of the thyroid cartilage (larynx) and cricoid cartilage (sublaryngeal); at the angle of the anterior edge of the muscle (sternocleidomastoid muscle); deep, with the carotid artery and at the superior edge of the transverse bulge; in a hollow.

Two FW below *renying* (ST-9); four FW above and anterior (medial) to *quepen* (ST-12).

When tonified:

Tonifies the stomach, heart, large intestine, posterior part of inferior frontal lobes, shoulders, arm, wrist, opposite dorsal and palmar muscles of hand, perineum, anus; teeth same side; throat.
Disperses the vessels.
Dispersing acts in the opposite way.

Direct effects:

Throat: excess energy (energy in the upper body), spasms, cough, spasmodic cough; whooping cough; painful, swollen, or abscessed throat.
Particularly the left point: breasts hard before menses; impotence or excess from continence; asthma, bronchitis, cannot breathe, little energy for inhalation and exhalation.
Particularly the right point: skin, pruritis, fissures, cracked; urticaria.
Opposite posterior shoulder, posterior arm, opposite radial side of forearm, opposite wrist and hand, dorsal and palmar sides.
Perineum, anus.
Hypertrophied lymph nodes?
Paralysis; same ascending?

Point of Weihe: Right: Petroleum. Hands and feet smell; eczema, fissures, rough fingers, cracked; chilblains; ulcerated nostrils; herpes of the perineum; itching of urethra; prostatitis, hoarseness, cough.

Left: Conium Maculatum. Weakness from moving the head, mostly to the left; hard breasts before menses; impotence from excess or continence; fetid local sweats; urticaria; urinates often at night; scrofular troubles or paralytic or cancerous; ascending paralysis; aphonia; dyspnea; hypertrophy of the lymph nodes.

ST-11 *qishe* — home of energy

Lower neck: just at the lateral superior edge of the point (horn) of the sternum (manubrium); in the angle of the superior medial edge of the insertion of the sternocleidomastoid muscle and at the point of the bone; deep, on the sternohyoideus; in a hollow.

Two FW below *shuitu* (ST-10); on either side of *tiantu* (CV-22).

When tonified:
  Tonifies the stomach, cerebellum, pons; back of the throat, upper respiratory passages, tongue, uvula, genital organs.
  Disperses the vessels.
  Dispersing acts in the opposite way.

Direct effects:
  Suffocating sobs.
  Throat: coughing fits, "energy in the upper body"; chokes on sputum; amygdalitis; unending pain in the throat; tracheitis; tongue (right point right side, left point tip), thrush, inflammation.
  Eyes: paralysis of the muscles?
  Bad digestion.
  Diaphragm: spasms.
  Tumors? Ulcers? Furuncles? Wounds? Acne, eczema; thrush, freckles?

Parts of the body:
  Lateral neck: pain or stiffness.
  Posterior shoulder and scapula: contracted muscles, painful into posterior arm (cubital neuralgia).
  Sternoclavicular joint.

  Point of Weihe: Right: Muriatic acid. Blood; itching, freckles; acne; eczema on the back of hand; ulcers on the lower extremities; scarlet fever; ulcerated tongue; thrush; hoarse throat; swollen uvula; tonsillitis, false membrane; abhorrence of meat; hemorrhoids during pregnancy; rapid, small, weak pulse, one stop every three beats; extremities heavy and weak.

  Left: Lachesis. Extreme loquacity; speaks quickly, stutters, stammers, hypersensitive, susceptible, distrustful; headache at menopause; deep intoxication, better from discharges, worse from sleep; cannot bear a tight collar; coughs from speaking or from tight neck; tonsils purple and also the pharynx; neck of the bladder contracted; epigastric pain; flaccidity of the penis; nymphomania; leukorrhea; muscles of the eye paralyzed; facial neuralgia; furuncles, ulcers; scabs; whistling in ears; appendicitis.

ST-12 *quepen* — basin of the point

Anterior lateral neck; three large FW lateral to the swelling of the clavicle (horn of the sternum); just above (behind) the clavicle; in the angle of the deep, superior edge of the first rib and of the lateral edge of the hard muscle (anterior scalenus) with the strong artery (carotid); in a hollow.

Four FW lateral to *qishe* (ST-11); two FW medial above *qihu* (ST-13).

When tonified:
  Tonifies the stomach and other yang organ meridians, producers (superficial pulses); all elevator muscles of the arm, supinators and extensors.
  Disperses the vessels (carotid sinus?).
  Dispersing acts in the opposite way.

Opposite effects:
  Weakness and irritability of the nerves: tonify; loquacity, grimaces, cannot support neck and waist: tonify; insomnia from nervousness, from hyperexcitation or anxiety: tonify; trembling or agitation of the limbs: tonify (Parkinsonism, sclerosis in patches?).
  Arteries: carotid beats strongly: tonify; hypertension: tonify (acts on the carotid sinus); paroxysmal tachycardia, tonify.
  Coughs incessantly, nervously, dryly: tonify; asthma ameliorated after expectoration (chronic bronchitis) particularly in the morning: tonify; acute bronchitis; pleurisy; after a chill, prolonged warmth of the chest, fever, cough, panting; lung abscess.
  Lymph nodes?
  Acne unresponsive [to treatment].

Parts of the body:
  Neck, shoulder and upper limb, elevator muscles (deltoid, trapezius); extensors of arm (triceps); supinators,

radial muscles; extensors of the fingers; flaccidity, paralysis of Erb (or contracture or inflammation). Shoulder, subclavicular fossa: inflammation, ulcers, abscess, suppurating lymph nodes.

Point of Weihe: Right: Zincum Met. ''Zinc is to the nerves what iron is to the blood.'' Thyroid; trembling, agitation in the legs, must move; melancholia; intolerance of wine; chronic headaches; thin and weak; incessant cough; spitting of blood; panting after expectoration; pain in the neck; burning along the spinal column.

Left: Hyosciamus Niger. Loquacity; grimaces, antics; cerebral troubles of children; sensitivity; hyperexcitation or anxiety; trembling or contraction of the legs or agitation; delirium tremens.

ST-13   *qihu* — sidegate of the energy

Lateral superior thorax just under the clavicle: three FW lateral to the sternoclavicular angle; at the angle of the inferior edge of the clavicle and the lateral edge of the clavicular insertion of the pectoralis major; in a hollow.

Two FW inferior and lateral to *quepen* (ST-12); two superior and medial to *kufang* (ST-14); three lateral to *shufu* (KI-27); three medial to *zhongfu* (LU-1).

When tonified:

Tonifies the stomach, respiratory passages, heart; larynx, lower eyelids, diaphragm, armpit, thumb, heel and sole of foot; temporal and parietal lobes.
Disperses the vessels, genital organs.
Dispersing acts in the opposite way.

Direct effects:

Inferior eyelids, same side.
Loss of taste; nausea, spasms of the diaphragm; desires earth and plaster, etc. [geophagia?]; suffocating cough, cough coming from diaphragm, nausea, whooping cough; asthma, difficulty in breathing; chronic bronchitis, phlegm in the morning; pleurisy; pneumonia; pulmonary tuberculosis?

Parts of the body:

Skin: acne, warts, eczema.
Fetid perspiration of the feet, armpits, hands or occiput and forehead.

Point of Weihe: Right: Calcarea Carbon. Soft, weak, angry character; upper lip swollen; big head; hoarseness, short respiration, cough, emphysema; desire to eat earth, paper, plaster; early menses, profuse; slight urine; obesity; distended glands, lymph nodes; sweating of occiput and forehead, cataract.

Left: Nitricum Acidum. Chronic headaches of the occiput; desire to eat earth, paper, plaster; difficult vomiting; coughing in sleep; dyspnea; diplopia; paralysis of the lower eyelids; little urine; vulvar pruritis; prolapsed uterus; ulcerations of the cervix; acne, eczema; warts; abundant fetid perspiration of the hands, feet or armpits; chronic liver troubles.

ST-14   *kufang* — house of the treasure

Lateral superior thorax: two FW lateral to the angle of the sternum and the second rib; in the angle of the edge under the extremity of the first rib and of the inferior edge of the oblique muscle (clavicular fascia of the pectoralis major). A little above the superior edge of the second rib; between the oblique muscles (sternal and clavicular fascia of the pectoralis major); one large FW under the clavicle; in a hollow.

Two FW below *qihu* (ST-13); two FW above *wuyi* (ST-15); two FW lateral to *yuzhong* (KI-26); two FW medial to *zhongfu* (LU-1).

When tonified:

Tonifies the stomach and all yang producer organ-meridians (superficial pulses), anterior frontal lobes, superior occipital lobes, medulla oblongata, spinal cord, half of body, same side.
The point is crossed by the gallbladder meridian coming from *jianjing* (GB-21) and going to *yuanye* (GB-22) through *tianquan* (PC-2) and *jiquan* (HT-1).
Disperses vessels and all the yin distributor organ-meridians (deep pulses).
Dispersing acts in the opposite way.

Direct effects:

Distinguish clearly from the stomach pulse whether to disperse or tonify. The right point is always necessary and sometimes sufficient for the psyche; the left point acts more on the skin.
All physical or psychological consequences of shock, moral or physical: think of shock in the face of all physical or psychological troubles following an accident, emotional or recurring, even if it is a matter of vertebral

displacements, of skin troubles, eruptions, sore throat and loss of voice, after operations, etc.

Worries, preoccupations, obsessions: afraid to be touched or even looked at; alternates between gaiety and wickedness; moral or physical hypersensitivity; brain fatigue from excess work or worries.

Following accidents or operation; following contusions of breasts, swellings to the point of tumors; falling, bumps, bumps on the skull.

Throat contracted from emotion.

Hoarseness from too much speaking; inactivity of the lungs; breathes in and out with difficulty; coughing fits, energy on top; bronchitis; pleurisy; lung congestion (congestion of the chest); salivary troubles; spits pus and blood in clots.

Skin: troubles, mostly on the face, infantile eczema, impetigo, beginning of eruptive fevers (measles, German measles and scarlet fever).

Parts of the body:
Half of the body, same side.

Point of Weihe: Right: Arnica. All physical or psychological shock, bruises, bumps, blows, breast tumors from contusion, falling, contusion of the brain. Psychological shock, mourning, strong emotions, contraction of the throat and organs; hoarse throat from too much speaking; does not want to be looked at or touched; alternates between gaiety and wickedness; vertigo from moving the head; red cheeks; taste and gas of rotten eggs; spasmodic retention; short and difficult respiration; cough with coagulated blood.

Left: Viola Tricolor (and Calendula?). Eruptions and growths of the skin of the face and head; infantile eczema on the head, crust of milk; impetigo, pruritis with lymph nodes; sycosis; warm face and sweating after meals.

ST-15 *wuyi* — draft-screen of the bedroom

Anterior superior thorax: two large FW lateral to the angle of the sternum and the second rib; in the angle of the inferior edge of the second rib (first under the clavicle) and of the superior edge of the sternal fascia of the pectoralis major; under the clavicular fascia; in a hollow.

Two FW below and slightly medial to *kufang* (ST-14); three tightened fingers above *yingchuang* (ST-16); three FW lateral to *shencang* (KI-25); three FW medial to *jiquan* (HT-1).

When tonified:
Tonifies the stomach, large intestine, cerebellum, inferior spinal cord.
Disperses the vessels.
Dispersing acts in the opposite way.

Direct effects:
Repressed worries; malcontentment, melancholia.
Salivating (elderly people); inflammation of the esophagus; thready saliva.
Coughing fits; energy in the upper body; cough, panting; bronchitis, pleurisy; tuberculosis of children; coughs blood and pus.
Difficult orgasm; breast cancer.
Sensitive to humidity and cold.

Parts of the body:
Skin: urticaria, painful skin, cannot tolerate clothes.
Superficial swelling of the whole body (same side from hemiplegia? hydrogenoids?)
Hemiplegia of the upper and lower limbs of the same side; flaccidity or contracture.
Tonic convulsions? cramps in extension from hemiplegia?
Pectoralis major.

Point of Weihe: Aranea Diadema. Hydrogenoid; extreme sensitivity to cold and humidity, which causes swellings; swollen liver; facial neuralgias, intercostal and lumbar neuralgia, abdominal neuralgia; pains in the long bones; feels parts of the body as too large; clots in the last drops of urine.

ST-16 *yingchuang* — window of the chest

Chest: two large FW lateral to the sternum; two FW just above the nipple (men); at the angle of the inferior edge of the third rib (second under the clavicle in this place) and of the lateral (external) edge of the intercostal ligament; in a hollow; on the pectoralis major.

Three FW under *wuyi* (ST-15); two FW above *ruzhong* (ST-17); three FW lateral to *lingxu* (KI-24); two FW medial to *tianchi* (PC-1).

When tonified:

Tonifies the stomach, large intestine, medulla, cervical vertebrae, trachea, throat, lips, articulation of the hip, back of elbow.

Disperses the sexual organs, breasts.

Dispersing acts in the opposite way.

Direct effects:

Spasmodic, unceasing cough at night; whooping cough (nausea?); cough, cannot sleep, short respiration, suffocates, full chest; tracheitis; bronchitis; lung congestion (congestion of chest); pleurisy?

Swollen lips; swollen tonsils.

Esophagus: inflammation; stomach: bitterness, bitter burps; intestine: diarrhea, noises.

Lungs thickened?

Opposite effects:

Breasts: mammary glands; breasts too big; breast abscess; abscess on chest and on side; breast cancer.

Swollen prostate.

Parts of the body:

Articulation of hip: pain.

Dorsum of hand: swelling.

Point of Weihe: Right: Drosera Rotundif. Spasmodic cough; whooping cough; night cough; sore throat from too much speaking; tickling in the larynx; asthma during dentition; laryngitis, tuberculosis of larynx; vertigo, falling to left; cold of left cheek; pain of hip joint; stiff feet; aversion to sourness.

Left: Spongia Tosta. Suffocates at night; awake after midnight with pain and anxiety of the heart, violent and quick palpitations. All glands hypertrophied: thyroid, testicles, breasts, prostate, lymph, neck and nape, submaxillary, mesenteric, and thoracic; frequent and abundant urine; hands insensitive and swollen.

ST-17   *ruzhong* — middle of the breast

Just in the middle of the nipple. Tradition forbids needles and moxa at this point, and I have not wanted to try any experiments. Thus, it is only mentioned.

ST-18   *rugen* — base of the breast

Under the breast (men), two FW under the nipple; at the angle between the inferior edge of the fifth rib (the nipple is on the bottom of the fourth) and the lateral edge of an intercostal ligament; in a hollow.

Two FW just below *ruzhong* (ST-17); two FW above and slightly lateral to *burong* (ST-19); three FW lateral to *bulang* (KI-22); two FW medial to *qimen* (LR-14).

When tonified:

Tonifies the stomach, large intestine, lower and middle ribs.

Disperses the liver, bottom of the lung; sexual organs.

Dispersing acts in the opposite way.

Direct effects:

Chagrin, mental pain, (emphysema?).

Food causes severe choking; chest fullness and suffocation, chest pain; energy in the upper body that does not descend; coughing fits from looking up.

Cholera: cramps and weakness.

Opposite effects:

Swollen breasts; heat and pain in the breasts rising to above clavicle; menses continuing after the sixth day.

Parts of the body:

Ribs (particularly middle and lower): neuralgia; flaccidity or contracture; pain in the cold, cannot touch.

Forearm: pain, swelling (radial line).

ST-19   *burong* — not at ease

Lower lateral thorax (men), four FW directly below the nipple; three tightened FW lateral to the sternum; in the angle between the superior edge of the sixth rib (the seventh being the last joint on the sternum) and the lateral edge of a vertical intercostal ligament; in a hollow.

Two FW below *rugen* (ST-18); two FW above *chengman* (ST-20); two large FW lateral to *youmen* (KI-21); three FW medial to *shidou* (SP-17).

When tonified:

Tonifies the stomach, upper respiratory passages, superior and posterior shoulder, small intestine.

Dispersing acts in the opposite way.

Direct effects:

Stomach: pain; hypersecretion; stomach cancer.

Intestines: noise when empty; intestinal cancer; intestinal worms.

Respiratory passages: cough, panting, pain in chest and back; obstruction from mucus; asthma; nervous spasms; spits blood?

Heart: pain, endocarditis; angina of the chest.

Parts of the body:

Superior and posterior shoulder. Shoulder and chest: all the muscles?

ST-20 *chengman* — receive fullness

Mid-thorax: vertical from the nipple; at the level of the inferior extremity of the sternum; in the angle between the inferior edge of the sixth rib (the seventh being joined to the sternum) and the lateral edge of one tendon (insertion of the rectus abdominus).

Two FW below *burong* (ST-19); two above *liangmen* (ST-21); three lateral to *jiuwei* (CV-15).

When tonified:

Tonifies the stomach, heart, epigastrium, cerebellum, spleen-pancreas, vessels, lung.

Disperses the triple warmer.

Dispersing acts in the opposite way.

Direct effects:

Intermittent heartbeats, from emotional agitation or age. Or rapid and weak: hard and contracted arteries. Aortitis (pain under the clavicle); dyspnea, insomnia.

Stomach: thready saliva, mucus; difficulty swallowing; illnesses of the stomach; lack of appetite (cold in stomach); swollen abdomen (tympanism); noisy intestine; diarrhea; peritonitis; jaundice; infantile diabetes?

Attacks of dyspnea, does not eat; breathes with the shoulder; respiratory mucus; saliva with blood and pus; spits blood (hemoptysis). Convulsions with orgasms (nervous crises).

Parts of the body:

Painful skin?

Epigastrium: muscles hard and painful.

Swollen extremities.

Lower limbs hard and painful.

Point of Weihe: Right: Crataegus. Sympathetic system; heart irregular, intermittent, weak, rapid; skin, hands and feet cold and blue; dyspnea on the least effort with pain of the heart and under the left clavicle; insomnia from aortic troubles; infantile diabetes; edema; dissolves the arterial deposits from arteriosclerosis.

Left: Strophanthus. Heart weak, rapid, irregular; cardiac muscles weak; increases systolic beat and diminishes rapidity; irritable heart in smokers; arteriosclerosis of the aged; swollen extremities; urine increased; dyspnea on effort; dipsomania.

ST-21 *liangmen* — door with beam

Thorax: approximately vertical from the nipple; on the inferior edge of the seventh rib (the last joint on the sternum); on the lateral edge of one intercostal ligament; in a hollow.

Two FW below *chengman* (ST-20); two FW above *guanmen* (ST-22).

When tonified:

Tonifies the stomach, large intestine, small intestine, lumbar vertebrae, hypothalamus (anterior), parasympathetic.

Disperses the spleen-pancreas.

Dispersing acts in the opposite way.

Effects:

Weakness and tightness or agitation; insomnia after midnight?

Stomach: all troubles, mostly from excess; acute gastritis; gastroenteritis; cramps of the stomach; no appetite; bad and difficult digestion; irritable stomach.

Does not digest starches (insufficiency of the small intestine), pain or burning of the stomach one hour after lunch (starches, sweets, pastries).

Shining, slippery stools (insufficiency of the small intestine and pancreas); grey stools (insufficiency of pancreas); ulcer of duodenum?

Point of Weihe: Right: Gummi Gutti. Stomach painful and irritable after eating, gastroenteritis; diarrhea with bile.

Left: Arsenicum Album. Loss of memory; exhaustion with anxiety and agitation; insomnia; worse after midnight; pulse slow, irregular; hemorrhages easily; neuralgia; all illnesses of the skin: urticaria, etc.; ulcers; cancer; stomach troubles from fruit, ice cream; distended liver and spleen; stool small and slow; incontinence or ascites; hay fever.

ST-22   *guanmen* — door of the barrier

Lower lateral thorax: one large FW lateral to the angle of the eighth and ninth ribs; approximately vertical from the nipple; in the angle between the inferior edge of the eighth rib and the anterior (medial) edge of an intercostal ligament; in a hollow.

Two FW below *liangmen* (ST-21); two FW above and lateral to *taiyi* (ST-23); about at the level of *tonggu* (KI-20).

When tonified:

Tonifies the stomach, liver, kidney, medulla oblongata, spinal cord, eyelids, extremities.

Disperses the gallbladder.

Dispersing acts in the opposite way.

Effects:

Stomach: troubles mostly from excess; retention, cramps of the stomach, bad breath, frequent fullness of the stomach; bile in the stomach, burns; eructations; no appetite.

Intestine: inflammations, spasms, violent pains, pain around the umbilicus; small intestine and pancreas in excess; constipation or diarrhea.

Jaundice from obstruction of the gallbladder, cannot empty itself.

Eyelids: blinking (facial nerve: orbicularis muscle closes?)

Insufficient urine: edema, swelling of the body, or incontinence.

Point of Weihe: Right: Chelidonium Majus (*hunmen*, BL-42, IS BL-47). Liver distended, insufficient; jaundice (from obstruction of the biliary canal); constipation or crisis of diarrhea; frequent need to urinate; trembling, tics, pain under the right scapula; spasms of the eyelids.

Left: Carbo Vegetabilis. Flatulence and eructation; fetid breath; burning in stomach a half hour after eating; burning diarrhea; cold; violent; chilblains; fear of dark.

ST-23   *taiyi* — great curvature

Epigastrium: on the edge of the ribs; just at the medial (anterior) edge of the union of the tenth on the ninth rib (the eleventh being a floating rib with a free end); on the rectus abdominus; in a hollow.

Two FW below and medial to *guanmen* (ST-22); approximately two FW below and lateral to *huaroumen* (ST-24); two FW medial to *fuai* (SP-16); four FW medial to *zhangmen* (LR-13); one FW lateral and superior to *shiguan* (KI-18); about at the level of *xiawan* (CV-10).

When tonified:

Tonifies the stomach, gallbladder, posterior part of the mid-brain (sympathetic).

Disperses the heart.

Dispersing acts in the opposite way.

Effects:

Mental troubles: demented hyperexcitation; tongue out; escapades [walks crazily].

Troubles of the stomach from excess; inflammation; acute gastritis, cramps of the stomach.

Intestines: pains, spasms, all troubles; beriberi, heart distended; agitation of the heart; coronaries? veins.

Parts of the body:

Extremities very cold.

Point of Weihe: Right: Carduus Marianus. Melancholy; vertigo, falls forward; liver jaundice, stones, portal system; varicose veins, hemorrhoids, ulcers; diarrhea, vomiting, pains in the large curvature of the stomach, asthma.

Left: Squilla Maritama. Mucus lining of stomach and respiratory passages; bronchitis of old people with diminished hearing; tonifies heart, mostly coronary and peripheral vessels; kidneys; red points on the body; icy extremities.

ST-24   *huarou[men]* — sliding flesh [gate]

Abdomen: at the level of one large FW above the navel, at the inferior edge of the tenth rib and at the point of the eleventh rib; approximately vertical to the nipple; two FW under the anterior angle of the union of the tenth on the ninth rib; at the lateral edge of the rectus abdominus; in a hollow.

Two FW below *taiyi* (ST-23); one large FW above *tianshu* (ST-25); about two FW lateral to *shangqiu* (KI-17); four FW from *shuifen* (CV-9).

When tonified:

Tonifies the stomach, salivary glands, anterior opposite frontal lobes.
Dispersing acts in the opposite way.

Effects:

Hyperexcitation, vomiting fits; epilepsy, tongue out.
Salivary glands (sublingual and parotid), pain under the tongue and at the inferior angle of the jaw and towards the ear.
Tongue: inflammation, aphthae, lesion, swelling.
Stomach: chronic or acute inflammatory troubles, vomiting, pain, vomiting of blood (hematemesis), ulceration of stomach.
Intestines: chronic inflammation.
Uterus: endometritis, abnormal menses, leukorrhea.
Kidneys: inflammation, edema.

ST-25   *tianshu* — celestial axis

Abdomen: at the level of and about three FW lateral to the umbilicus; at the lateral edge of the vertical muscle (rectus abdominus); on the aponeurosis of the union with the external oblique muscle; in a hollow.

One large FW below *huaroumen* (ST-24); one FW above *wailing* (ST-26); two FW lateral to *huangshu* (KI-16); one large FW medial to *daheng* (SP-15).

When tonified:

Tonifies the stomach, large intestine, small intestine, temporal parietal lobes, automaton-parrot, superior occipital lobes, primate, ureters.
Disperses the kidney, spleen-pancreas.
Dispersing acts in the opposite way.

Effects:

The three memories (hereditary, subconscious and conscious); the primitive instincts, the primate; home of the automaton-parrot and of the primate; delirium of typhoid fever; malaria with hyperecited speech or depression; irritable, susceptible, passionate, pains aggravated by movement and in the daytime.
Stomach: chronic troubles; gastritis, chronic or acute; drinks too much, eats without assimilating, becoming thin; vomiting (cholera); vomiting of blood.
Stomach and intestine: cutting pains.
Assent point of the large intestine: (troubles from feelings, with coldness and depression; prolonged diarrhea from atony or from emptiness or inflammation, or from cold stopping the digestion, or liquids; does not finish.
Dysentery with blood; sharp intestinal pain from cold or humidity, with excess of food; chronic troubles; swelling of intestines; worms in duodenum or large intestine.
Pancreas insufficient (left point), from misfortune, emotion, or emptiness, or with pain.
Heart: intermittent beats from indignation or malaria.

Kidney: inflammation; little urine; edema; face swollen.

Menses: irregular or difficult, painful; metrorrhagia: tonify; metritis.

Middle of the body: all troubles.

Point of Weihe: Left: Staphysagria. Aggravated by being touched, at night, the new moon, from indignation; susceptible, capricious; sees things that are lower; gnarled fingers; eyelids inflamed, right side; colic, flatulence; constipation or diarrhea with tenesmus; ulcerations of the mouth; frequent urine; heart irregular from indignation or chagrin; irregular menses; sexual hyperexcitation.

Right: Bryonia. Pain aggravated by movement and in the daytime; ear pain; eliminates mucus through the intestine and kidney. Constipation or diarrhea of nondigestion; colic with swelling; vomiting, excessive thirst; congestion of the lungs; menses early or suppressed; ovary pains; little urine, very irritable, easy anger.

ST-26 *wailing* — exterior hill

Abdomen: at the level of one FW under the umbilicus; approximately three large FW from the median line; on the lateral edge of the rectus abdominus; a little medial to the vertical rise of the external oblique muscle; in a hollow.

One large FW under *tianshu* (ST-25); two FW above *daju* (ST-27); two FW lateral to *zhongzhu* (KI-15); approximately three large FW from abdomen-*yinjiao* (CV-7).

When tonified:

Tonifies the stomach, small intestine, genital organs, rectus abdominus.
Dispersing acts in a contrary way.

Effects:

Intestines (particularly small intestine): spasms (exhausting pains, heart as if suspended).
Uterus: painful contractions; neuralgia of the lower pelvic area; rectus abdominus: contractions, contracture or flaccidity.

ST-27 *daju* — large eminence

Abdomen: at the level of half the distance from the umbilicus to the pelvis; approximately three large FW from the midline; on the lateral edge of the rectus abdominus; a little medial to the vertical rise of the external oblique muscle, in a hollow.

Two FW below *wailing* (ST-26); one large FW above *shuidao* (ST-28); about two FW lateral to *siman* (KI-14); three or four large FW from *shimen* (CV-5)

When tonified:

Tonifies the stomach, large intestine, bladder, genital organs, superior occipital lobes, primate, posterior frontal lobes, half of body on same side.
Dispersing acts in the opposite way.

Effects:

Insomnia (particularly from worries, boredom); great emotional agitation, deranged mind, emotional sensitivity, fear of touch and of the air.
Great thirst? Constipation?
Urine difficult or stopped?
Testicles relaxed or falling; scrotal hernia?

Parts of the body:

Half of the body without strength, lateral weakness, laziness.
Rectus abdominus.
Plantar part of heel.
Skin?

Point of Weihe: Right: Ignatia. Sensitivity to fear, surprise; insomnia from worries, malcontentment; focused, sad, changeable; lump in the throat; urine abundant and like water; inflammation of the mouth; digests heavy foods better; hard stools; pain in the bones; burning pain in the heel; jerking in the arms or legs.

Left: Ranunculus Bulbosus. Irritable; sensitive to air or touch; fog before the eyes; pain in the eyeball and forehead; burning and itching skin; illnesses of skin: herpes, shingles, painful corns, spasmodic hiccough.

ST-28   *shuidao* — ureter, way of water

Abdomen: at the level of three FW above the pelvis (one below the pelvic-umbilical midpoint); about three FW from the medial line on the lateral edge of the rectus abdominus; a little medial to the rise of the external oblique muscle.

One large FW below *daju* (ST-27); one large FW above *guilai* (ST-29); two FW lateral from *qixue* (KI-13); three FW lateral from *guanyuan* (CV-4).

When tonified:

Tonifies the stomach, gallbladder, large intestine, opposite eye, opposite ear, posterior frontal lobes.
Disperses the genital organs, spleen-pancreas, kidneys.
Dispersing acts in the opposite way.

Effects:

Depression, exhaustion.
Atrophy of the opposite optic nerve; convulsive movements of the eyes; buzzing.
Opposite gums retracted.
Prolapsed rectum? Constipation?
Triple warmer (genitourinary functions) "warm and knotted."
Painful menses; inflammation of the ovaries; spasms of the uterus or insensitivity of the vulva, vagina.
Men: orchitis; or insufficient erection.
Insufficient or stopped urine; bladder inflammation (cystitis); or frequent urination at night?

Parts of the body:

Inflammation of the spinal cord.
Back and lumbar tight and painful.
Contractures or cramps of hands, feet, calf.

Point of Weihe: Right: Phosphoricum Acidum. Prostration; indifference; emptiness; physical or mental overwork; profuse and frequent urine at night; night sweats; atony of the optic nerve; eyes pressed into the head; buzzing, growling; does not hear well; retracted gums; liver distended; diarrhea; prepuce: herpes, edema, pimples of blood.

Left: Cuprum Met. Contractions; cramps in the hands, feet and calves; cramps of the stomach, hiccough; contraction of the chest, dyspnea; convulsive movements of the eye; nocturnal incontinence; prolonged and retarded menses.

ST-29   *guilai* — recurrence, periodicity

Abdomen: at the level of one FW above the pelvis; about three FW from the medial line; on the lateral edge of the rectus abdominus; a little medial to the vertical rise of the external oblique muscle; in a hollow.

One FW under *shuidao* (ST-28); one FW above *qichong* (ST-30); about two FW lateral from *dahe* (KI-12); about three FW lateral to *zhongji* (CV-3).

When tonified:

Tonifies the stomach, large intestine, superior occipital lobes, primate, eyes, ears, same side.
Disperses the genital organs.
Dispersing acts in the opposite way.

Effects:

All spasms; lump in the throat from emotion.
Women: accumulations, tumors in organs or clots in the blood.
Swollen tonsils (cryptic?), swollen lymph nodes in the throat.
Stomach and intestines: gas, spasms of energy of the small intestine.
All trouble of the male or female genital system.
Women: sterility; arrested menses; ovaries: inflammation; uterus: atony.
All trouble, displacement, prolapses; metritis, leukorrhea in excess; vagina: inflammation; clitoris: pain?
Men: Penis: non-erection; or painful erections; undescended testicles (cryptorchidia); inflammation (orchitis).

Point of Weihe: Right: Palladium. Ovaries; uterus displaced or descended; leukorrhea with mucus; twinges from the pubis to navel and breasts; arrogance, flamboyant in social settings, likes to be approved of, susceptible, violent; pains at the top of the head, from ear to ear.

Left: Mercurius Iodatus Flavus. Inguinal nodes swollen; pain in the throat with ganglia; tumors or cancer of the breast; lump in the throat; swallows without stopping; tongue yellow at the base, worse on the right; secreting tonsils (cryptic).

ST-30   *qichong* — assaults of energy

Abdomen, lower lateral: in the angle of the superior edge of the apparent extremity of the transverse bone (pubis) and the medial edge of the muscle passing above the pubis (psoas); in a hollow. The medial branch of an artery.

One FW below *guilai* (ST-29); the meridian goes towards the exterior and at two FW crosses *chongmen* (SP-12) in order to go four finger widths on the lateral edge of the sartorius muscle, at *biguan* (ST-31). One small FW lateral to *zigong* (MP-35, IS M-CA-18); two FW from *henggu* (KI-11); about four FW from *qugu* (CV-2).

When tonified:

Tonifies the stomach, triple warmer, temporal-parietal lobes, superior part of the occipital lobes; automaton-parrot; primate.
Disperses the genital organs.
Dispersing acts in the opposite way; responds with *taibai* (SP-3).

Effects:

"Important point for the general vitality." "The source activating the transformation of food and drink into energy through the stomach and the distribution of this energy to the twelve meridians through the triple warmer, the stomach being the source of all." "All the energy-producing organs are linked to *qichong*."
"First point on the vessel of attacks (abdominal line of the kidney; spasms, contractions)." "Root of the conception and governor vessels." "Commands the triple warmer, of which it is the reservoir of energy."
All troubles of the genital organs, men and women; swelling. Coldness at orgasm, etc.
Women: sterility; troubles and desperations at not having children; troubles of pregnancy, "child assails the heart," delivery pains; difficulties of delivery; commands the contractions of the uterus when the time of delivery approaches; placenta not coming by itself.
Ovaries; inflammation; insufficient or delayed menses; uterus: all troubles; displacement, particularly lateral.
Men: insufficient erections; painful erections when sleeping on the back; pain of the penis and of the two testicles; neuralgia of the spermatic canal. Testicles: inflammation, swelling, pain, orchitis.
Stomach and intestines: heat, fermentation, gas.
Kidney or bladder stones: "urinates stones, eased by passing of red sand." Retention (abdomen full, hot, cannot urinate); ureter: inflammation.

Parts of the body:

Lumbar area: pains.
Thigh: pains (crural neuralgia) on the medial face of the lower limb.

Point of Weihe: Right and Left: Juniperus Com. Inflammation of the kidney; feeble urination of the aged with bad digestion; cough with feeble, cloudy urine; urine with the odor of violets, changeable; stoppage of urination; hydropsy; retention; prostatic discharge; pain of the lumbar region.

ST-31   *biguan* — barrier to articulation

Anterior face of the thigh: about four FW below the inguinal crease; about at the mid-width of the thigh; on the medial edge of the large lateral muscle (tensor facia lata muscle); on the lateral edge of the oblique muscle (sartorius); in a hollow.

The meridian comes from *qichong* (ST-30) by crossing *chongmen* (SP-12); four FW above thigh-*futu* (ST-32).

When tonified:

Tonifies the stomach, large intestine, small intestine, spinal cord; articulation of the hips, knees, insteps, lumbar region.
Disperses the genital organs.
Dispersing acts in the opposite way.

Effects and parts of the body.

Throat and lower pelvis.
Lumbar area, contracture or pain and flaccidity.
Lower limb: weakness to the point of paralysis; cannot extend or flex.

Hip joint: arthritis, pain.

Anterior thigh: weakness or contracture (femoral-cutaneous nerve, obturator and crural nerve?) vastus lateralis and medialis; rectus anterior.

Knee: weakness, cold.

Arch: flaccidity.

ST-32   *futu* — lying hare

Thigh: anterior, external face, eight FW above the patella; on the lateral face of the femur; in the angle between the lateral edge of the rectus anterior and the superior edge of a transverse bulge; on the vastus lateralis; in a hollow.

Four FW below *biguan* (ST-31); four FW above *yinshi* (ST-33); four FW anterior to *xiadu* (GB-32).

When tonified:

Tonifies the stomach, superior part of the posterior and frontal lobes and middle part same side, medulla oblongata, spinal cord; opposite face of the upper limb, anterior opposite face of the lower limb (force, heat) and heel on the same side.

Disperses the veins, heart, auricles, genital organs, kidneys, lung, skin.

Dispersing acts in the opposite way.

Opposite effects:

Veins: "reunion of the veins," all trouble.

Varicosity (if the tissue has not lost its elasticity); phlebitis; periphlebitis; venous return; heart: auricles.

Eyes: Phosphenes (moving lights).

Skin: chicken pox: inflammation with pustules; eruptions.

Asthma in the middle of the night; edema of the lungs.

Kidney: edema, legs swollen. "It is the way of water."

Women: all trouble of the genital organs, mostly uterus.

Parts of the body:

Lower limb: opposite face, same side. All trouble; cold; weakness; flaccidity or pain, agitation, cramps; contractures; acts particularly on the rectus anterior and vastus lateralis muscles.

Upper limb anterior and opposite face; hand contorted by maleficent excitation.

ST-33   *yinshi* — market in shadow

Anterior lateral face of the thigh: four FW above the patella. Anterior lateral face of the femur: in the angle between the external edge of the large anterior tendon (triceps) and the inferior edge of a transverse bulge; on the vastus lateralis; in a hollow.

Four FW below thigh-*futu* (ST-32); three large FW above *liangqiu* (ST-34); four FW anterior and above knee-*yangguan* (GB-33).

When tonified:

Tonifies the stomach, heart, cerebellum, opposite side of superior part of the posterior and frontal lobes, middle part same side, medulla oblongata, opposite spinal cord, opposite upper limb, lower limb same side.

Disperses the genital organs.

Dispersing acts in the opposite way.

Direct effects:

Lack of strength, relaxing of force, little energy.

Slow heart, stops every twenty or thirty beats; "removes the root of heart pain accompanied by trembling hands treated by *shaohai* (HT-3)."

Diabetes; beriberi?

Opposite effects:

Genital organs: pains in the lower pelvis; spasms of the uterus.

Contracted vagina (vaginismus).

Parts of the body:

Opposite upper limb: shoulder, arm, posterior forearm, dorsum of hand, thumb.

Lumbar area same side: cold like ice; pain "which prevents looking at anything."

Lower limb same side: cold like ice; lateral thigh and lumbar area; pain, or cold, or weakness, flaccidity or contracture; knee: cold as ice, or pain, arthritis, or paralysis; can neither extend nor flex; feet: arthritis.

ST-34   *liangqiu* — hill of the roof-beams

Knee: in the angle between the upper lateral edge of the patella and the lateral edge of the large anterior tendon (triceps) and deep on the top edge of the femur; on the lower edge of a transverse bulge; in a hollow.

Three large FW below *yinshi* (ST-33); following point: *dubi* (ST-35).

When tonified:

Tonifies the stomach, gallbladder, large intestine, small intestine, lumbar area, anterior face of lower limb, great toe, medial plantar heel.

Disperses the genital organs, breast, opposite nipple, heart; posterior muscles of thigh and knee.

Dispersing acts in the opposite way.

Great emotional agitation.

Opposite effects:

Opposite breast, nipple: all trouble; pain, swelling, abscess.

Parts of the body:

Lumbar area, ischium, knee (and posterior muscles of knee and thigh); foot: pain, or lassitude, cannot extend the leg, makes the knee and tip of the foot lift.

Anterior knee: weakness, swelling, arthritis, pain, contraction.

Anterior leg, tibia: cold; foot: big toe.

Medial, plantar heel: pain.

ST-35   *dubi* — calf's nose

Anterior lateral knee: in the angle between the lateral edge of the anterior patellar-tibial tendon and the superior edge of the head of the tibia; one FW below and lateral to the inferior edge of the patella; in a hollow.

Five FW below *liangqiu* (ST-34); three FW above leg-*sanli* (ST-36); this is the lateral *xiyan* (MP-38a).

When tonified:

Tonifies knee problems arising from insufficiency.

Dispersing relieves knee problems arising from excess.

Effects:

Knee: weakness, flaccidity, or pain; arthritis; acute pain from cold or wind.

Patella: swelling, abscess, pain.

ST-36   [leg-]*sanli* — third mile

Inferior lateral knee; one FW anterior to the round head of the fibula; in the angle between the deep inferior edge of the head of the fibula and the tendinous edge of the large muscle along the tibia (anterior tibialis); on the anterior edge of a narrow muscle along the head of the fibula (extensor longus); in a hollow.

One branch of the meridian of the stomach separates here, goes towards the head of the tibia, then descends along the lateral edge of the tibia and rejoins the meridian at *fenglong* (ST-40). Some false points are also found there at the level of the true ones.

Three FW below *dubi* (ST-35); three FW above leg-*shanglian* (ST-37, IS *shangjuxu*); one anterior to *yanglingquan* (GB-34).

The right point acts on the radial edge of the two wrists and the left on the ulnar edge.

When tonified:

Tonifies all the meridians and pulses on the same side, yin and yang, blood, vessels, muscles, nerves, skin, bone; conception and governor vessels.

Dispersing acts in the opposite way.

Effects:

Tonifying in the morning tonifies particularly the yang energy of activity; the yang meridians, all yang parts of the body, brain, skin, and nerves.

Tonifying in the evening tonifies particularly the yin energy of rest; the yin meridians, all yin parts of the body, blood, muscles and bone. But to tonify too much, and to tonify the digestion in the evening or too often after the age of thirty, causes the blood pressure to rise, and can cause nausea, insomnia and congestions.

Distinguish clearly between excess or insufficiency of total energy on the same side.

Alternation of yang and yin energy during the day and night, activity and rest, high and low, when it does not alternate harmoniously.

All physical or vital troubles caused by emotions (joy, sorrow, anger, worries, fear), nervous centers, nerves, the psyche, eyes, ears, smell, taste, internal organs, blood, vessels, muscles, bone, skin.

All the varieties of yin or yang emptiness of energy (not alternating): yin does not nourish the yang; yang remains without nourishing the yin.

Emptiness of yin (in the lower body), excess of yang (in the upper body): insomnia, headache at night, frenetic agitation, frenetic speech or laughter, uncontrolled behavior or fury, great insults or nerve crises.

Emptiness of yang (in the upper body), excess of yin (in the lower body): frequent sighing, discouraged, lack of liveliness, prolonged melancholy, sadness, ''terrorized by ghosts,'' aversion to cold, chattering of the teeth, apprehension, vertigo, weakness, lack of memory.

Eyes: preventive and curative: for excess of yang (in the upper body) tonify in the evening. Twice a week with moxa from eight to sixteen years can prevent and diminish myopia, astigmatism and hyperopia. For insufficiency of yang (in the upper body): weakened vision from age or weakness, the effect is doubled with moxa after needles; foggy vision, lower eyelids falling (extropia), add arm-*sanli* (LI-10).

Ears: songs of cicada aggravated in the evening, tonify in the evening; aggravated in the morning, tonify in the morning.

Heart: all troubles; fullness, swellings; sudden pain (angina of the chest), tonify in the evening.

Vessels: All troubles; arteries hard, contracted; hypertension: disperse; hypotension: tonify.

Blood: all troubles; thick blood.

Thinness: from emptiness, cold, fatigue, exhaustion, tuberculosis, following typhoid. Moxa two times per week.

Mouth: all troubles; bitter, fetid breath.

Vomits easily, on boats, cars or airplanes.

Poisoning from food or toxins.

Stomach: no appetite, aversion to the smell of food; atony; does not empty, indigestion. (Tonifying this point, along with *jiexi* (ST-41), in front of a fluoroscope, shows the stomach to empty in ten minutes instead of the normal three-quarters of an hour); weakness of the stomach with a red face and cold feet during meals and in the daytime.

Chronic or acute gastritis, acidity, hypersecretion, pain; stomach troubled by emotion.

Abdomen: ''without equal for all abdominal troubles;'' swollen abdomen (tympanism); pain; peritonitis; heat in the abdomen even without food.

Swollen small intestine.

Large intestine: atony, constipation from emptiness; all diarrhea, prolonged diarrhea, from undigested food, etc.; dysentery; cholera, fever; beriberi; diarrhea from malaria.

Throat: all problems; respiratory passages: all mucus, cough with abundant mucus; hemoptysis; rising energy attacking the upper body; dyspnea; breathlessness from emptiness.

Breasts: swelling, abscess.

Menses: insufficient or delayed.

Difficult delivery: tonify; after delivery, hemorrhage, fainting: disperse.

Urine insufficient or not coming; fullness and hardness of the lower pelvis; stone in the bladder, or frequent urination at night from excess: disperse; from atony: tonify. Incontinence from excess of the bladder: disperse; from insufficiency of the sphincter of the bladder: tonify; inflammation of the bladder (cystitis).

Swelling: all varieties of swelling from energy; from edema or wind (cold?, neuralgia?); swelling of the breasts; swelling of knee, anterior leg or feet.

Pain from rheumatism (wind and humidity).

Parts of the body:

Facial paralysis, contracted jaw (trismus).

Stiff nape.

Four limbs: weakness, flaccidity; or pain, fullness.

Upper limb: pain or bad cold in the elbow; pain or weakness in the hand or fingers (particularly the thumb and index finger).

Perineum, lumbar area: cannot bend or straighten, pain. If extended to the feet, tonify; if extended to the hip, disperse.

Lower limb: weakness, pain, cannot remain standing for a long time; knee: weakness, flaccidity, swelling or pain; knee and lower leg, anterior, tibia: swelling, numbness or pain; foot: great curer of all troubles: weakness, flaccidity, swelling or pain, heat; big toe, medial; sole of foot: medial half.

ST-37   *shanglian* (IS *shangjuxu*) — upper edge [of leg]

Anterior lateral lower leg: three FW below the head of the fibula; in the angle between the inferior edge of a transverse membrane (aponeurosis of the leg) and the anterior edge of the extensor longus, which runs along the fibula; posterior edge of a large muscle running along the fibula (tibialis anterior); in a hollow.

Three FW below leg-*sanli* (ST-36); three above *tiaokou* (ST-38).

When tonified:

Tonifies the stomach, large intestine, small intestine, all yin meridians (distributors, deep pulses), opposite superior occipital lobes, primate, spinal cord same side, anterior lower leg, arch of foot; posterior (frontal lobe, half of the body).
Dispersing acts in the opposite way.

Effects:

Primitive instincts and vitality, primate; cerebral anemia.
Intestines: atony, diarrhea after eating, intestinal tuberculosis, colic, cutting pain, loud rumblings.
Stomach: lack of appetite; stomach inflammation (gastritis), stomach heat; difficult digestion, beriberi, swelling of the upper part of body, dyspnea, energy in the chest.
Insufficiency of yin distributor organs.
Difficult release of urine.

Parts of the body:

Bone marrow: cold and pain.
Spinal cord same side.
Half body same side: flaccidity or contractures.
Lumbar area: pain: lower limb: pain; knee: rheumatism, swelling from water or wind; tibialis anterior cramps; lower leg and foot: numbness; feet: swelling; difficulty lying down and getting up.

ST-38   *tiaokou* — mouth in pieces

Anterior, lateral face of the lower leg: six FW under the heads of the tibia and the fibula; in the angle between the inferior edge of a transverse bulge in a hollow, and the anterior edge of the extensor longus, which runs along the fibula; on the posterior edge of the large muscle running along the tibia (tibialis anterior).

Three FW under leg-*shanglian* (ST-37 IS *shangjuxu*); three FW above leg-*xialian* (ST-39, IS *xiajuxu*); one large FW above and anterior to *yangjiao* (GB-35).

When tonified:

Tonifies the stomach, superior posterior frontal lobes, large intestine, radial line of the upper limb, lower limb.
Disperses the vessels.
Dispersing acts in the opposite way.

Effects:

Large intestine: all trouble; edematous beriberi.
Rheumatism, particularly from humidity.
Radial line of the upper limb.
Lower limb: all trouble; weakness, flaccidity, cannot remain standing for a long time; cold; swelling (edema of the feet?); or pain, cramps; thigh: mostly medial; knee: cold, numbness, weakness, slowness, or pain; feet: cold, numbness, weakness, slowness to the point of flaccidity, does not obey; or rheumatism, pains, gout, swelling; sole: cold or heat.

ST-39 *xialian* (IS *xiajuxu*) — lower angle [of the leg]

Anterior, lateral face of the leg: six FW above the external malleolus; on the posterior edge of the large muscle running along the tibia (tibialis anterior); in the angle of the upper edge of the transverse bulge; in a hollow; on the anterior edge of the muscle running along the fibula (extensor longus).

When tonified:

Tonifies the stomach, temporal parietal lobes, automaton-parrot, skin muscles, half of body of the same side.
Disperses the arteries, opposite breast, ureters.
Responds to *qianding* (GV-20, IS GV-21).
Dispersing acts in the opposite way.

Direct effects:

The three memories: automaton-parrot; opposite temporoparietal lobes. For violent or sudden emotions, or serious depression; or hyperexcitation; frenetic speech; congestion or cerebral anemia.
Stomach: lack of appetite, stomach heat, does not eat, dry lips, saliva comes out without being felt; amygdalitis; beriberi: without strength, "sinks into heaviness."
Insufficiency of the small intestine; face without hue.
Large intestine: dysentery with pus and blood.

Opposite effects:

Arteries weak: disperse; hard, strong: tonify.
Opposite breast: abscess.
Urine difficult, painful.

Parts of the body:

Same half of the body: flaccidity or contracture.
Hair too dry, falling, dry seborrhea.
Skin: cannot sweat, "rheumatisms of the skin," chilblains: disperse.
Corns on the feet: tonify; soft corns (between the toes) dropping off after three weeks; skin becoming detached between the toes, wetness, odor.
Muscles of the same side: all trouble; muscular rheumatism; rheumatism from cold, wind, humidity, cannot move.
Knee: acute pain; pain mostly from going down steps; anterior swelling of lower leg: pain; foot: flaccid, does not lift; rheumatism at the base of the toes (metatarso-phalangeal), pain from putting the foot down; posterior heel: pain.

ST-40 *fenglong* — abundance and prosperity

Lateral, anterior face of the lower leg: five FW above the external malleolus; in the lower angle of two muscles which narrow (the posterior edge of the tibialis anterior, which runs along the tibia, and the anterior edge of the extensor longus, which runs along the fibula); in a hollow.

When tonified:

Tonifies the stomach, gallbladder, knee, foot on the same side, wrist, hand on the same side, opposite mid-brain, opposite frontal lobes; evolved man.
Disperses the spleen-pancreas, opposite lung.
Dispersing acts in the opposite way; responds to *xinhui* (GV-21, IS GV-22).

Direct effects:

Stomach: pain, burning, or swelling.
Heart and chest: boring pain.
Abdomen: cutting pain.

Opposite effects:

Point of passage between stomach and spleen-pancreas.

When tonified, it tonifies the stomach and disperses the spleen (right point) and pancreas (left point). Dispersing produces the opposite effect. Excess (hyperexcitation, insanity): disperse; weakness and flaccidity: tonify.

Evolved man: laziness, indolence, lassitude: disperse. Nervous crises, sudden bluish complexion, cannot speak, body wet and cold, hands like ice: tonify. Or, hyperexcitation, hallucinations: disperse.
Attacks of hyperexcitation, sings, gets up on tables, takes off his clothes: disperse.

Coldness, mucus, headaches, congestion of face and nose, sore throat, cannot speak: tonify; pleurisy?
Liver insufficiency; stool and urine difficult.

Parts of the body:
Knee: numb, difficult extension or flexion.
Lower leg becoming thin, flaccid foot.

ST-41   *jiexi* — enlarging valley

Anterior and superior arch, midway between the internal and external malleolus; in the angle between the upper edge of the deep transverse bone (astragalus) and the lateral edge of the large middle tendon (of the tibialis anterior); in a hollow; on the medial edge of the extensor longus.

When tonified:
Tonifies the stomach, gallbladder, posterior central lobes, sympathetic system, superior occipital lobes, primate, sense organs, tibialis anterior.
Disperses the spleen-pancreas, vessels, heart.
Dispersing acts in the opposite way.

Effects:
No appetite for life or food, boredom, tired mind; emotional agitation, deranged mind, anxiety, sorrow; depression from shock; convulsion, indigestion.
Mouth painful, bites his tongue (cheeks: *jinggu,* BL-64), swollen or painful tongue; teeth: pain.
Stomach: tonifies emptiness and insufficiency, atony of the muscles or secretions.
Tonifying causes an atonic stomach to empty; slow digestion; lazy stomach, still full and sensitive five hours after a meal.
Red face and cold feet, either from general weakness or from meals.
Swollen, distended abdomen, same for lower abdomen (tympanism).
Headache like a bar above the eyebrows and even in the eyes.

Parts of the body:
Rheumatism.
Face: inflammation of the skin of the face (and acne?) from weakness of the stomach, or from shock stopping the stomach.
Body: swollen from shock?
Lower limb: inflammation of the muscles; swelling of the thigh, knee, lower leg with numbness; cramps of cholera; particularly cramps of the anterior lower leg.
Arches: arthritis.

ST-42   *chongyang* — yang assault

Dorsal aspect of foot. In the angle of the anterior edge of the transverse bone (scaphoid) and the medial edge of the extensors. In a hollow behind the articulation of the second and third cuneiforms.

Three tight FW in front of *jiexi* (ST-41). Two FW behind *xiangu* (ST-43). The energy passes from this point to the spleen-pancreas meridian (to *yinbai,* SP-1).

When tonified:
Tonifies the stomach, large intestine, temporoparietals, opposite eye, opposite gums, medulla, spinal cord.
Disperses the vessels, heart.
Dispersing acts in the opposite manner.

Direct effects:
Jumps at sudden noises, at the slightest thing. Episodes of malaria; continually excited, sings, climbs on tables, marches around aimlessly. Epilepsy?
Aversion to cold, always cold, searches for heat.
Yawning; shivering from cold. Nervous fevers without temperature.
Source point of the stomach: can rectify its excess or insufficiency. Lack of appetite, does not eat. Vomiting.

Stomach fever (cold, cannot eat without distention). Epigastric pain.

Gums: inflammation. Teeth: caries, pain.

Intestines: abdominal distention, or hard and distended (typany).

Parts of the body:

Face: facial paralysis.

Opposite hand and foot.

Lower limb: pain, or flaccidity. Foot dropped, cannot be lifted; or inflammation, pain, arthritis. Instep inflamed.

ST-43 *xiangu* — hollowed valley

Dorsum of foot. Two FW behind the articulation of the base of the second and third toes. In the angle of the posterior (superior) head and the body of the long bone of the third toe (third metatarsal). In a hollow. Between the bone and the interdigital artery, vein and nerve.

Two FW in front of *chongyang* (ST-42). Approximately two FW behind *neiting* (ST-44). One FW medial to *diwuhui* (GB-42). Two FW lateral to *taichong* (LR-3).

When tonified:

Tonifies the stomach, opposite midbrain, opposite inferior eye and lachrymal duct.

Disperses vessels, heart, kidneys.

Dispersing acts in the opposite manner.

Direct effects:

Fever from all causes, malaria or nervousness without sweating. Shivering of malaria and sighing. Excessive nightsweats.

Eyes: swollen, hardened (glaucoma?); congestion.

Intestines: pains, spasms, noises; abdomen: pain.

Opposite effects:

Edema; edema of the abdomen (ascites).

Parts of the body:

Face: superficial swelling.

Feet: pain, tibialis anterior.

ST-44 *neiting* — interior pavillion

Dorsum of foot: at the articulation of the second and third toes; in the angle between the anterior head and body of the third metatarsal (of the third toe), towards the second toe; in a hollow; between the bone and vessel and nerve.

Two FW approximately in front of *xiangu* (ST-43); point following: *lidui* (ST-45), on the terminal phalanx of the third toe; one FW medial to *xiaxi* (GB-43); one large FW lateral to *xingjian* (LR-2).

When tonified:

Tonifies the stomach, temporoparietal lobes, medulla oblongata, spinal cord, automaton-parrot, face, gums, upper teeth, throat, scalp.

Disperses the vessels, heart.

Dispersing acts in a contrary way.

Effects:

Sequelae of malarial fever, nightmares, difficult dreams, swelling of hand and foot, yawning, nervous jerking of the extremities at night.

Detests human noises, looks for silence. Dispersing eases reception of bad news. Attacks of weakness, vertigo; shivering from cold.

Throat: spasms, choking, strangles from drinking or eating.

Stomach: total lack of appetite (anorexia), cannot eat, no taste for food, acidity, stomach does not empty, vomiting; women: food poisoning?

Abdomen: all trouble; swollen to the point of not being able to breathe; noises; fainting during menses.

Gums: inflammation.

Teeth: caries of the teeth and upper incisors, acute pain.
Eruptive illness?
Nose: bleeding?

Parts of the body:
Face: facial paralysis (of the facial nerve), swelling of the face.
Scalp: pain.
Upper and lower limbs: cold pains with white or red skin.
Foot: arthritis of the base of the toes (metatarso-phalangeal).
Sole: pain.

ST-45   *lidui* — cruel payment

Foot: third toe, ungual phalanx, about mid-width from the medial face (towards the second toe); in the angle between the swelling and the body of the bone, on the dorsal edge of the palmar tendon (flexor); in a hollow.

When dispersed:
Disperses the stomach, gallbladder, temporoparietal lobes, automaton-parrot, gums, tonsils, superior occipital lobes, primate.
Tonifies the sexual organs.
Tonifying acts in the opposite way.

Direct effects:
Nightmares and incessant dreams: exaggerated nervous reactions; jerks at sudden noises; excessive emotional agitation; heat, agitation; hyperexcitation to the point of insanity, tongue out.
Detests the houses of others; loss of vitality, neurasthenia, cerebral anemia.
Coma: ''like a cadaver, pulses abolished, perceives nothing.''
Malarial fever with hyperexcitation or freezing (algid).
Disperses the excess energy of the stomach. Stomach inflammation; stomach fever, (continuous cold, looks for fire, cannot eat without swelling up, bad digestion); aerogastria and epigastric swelling after meals; stomach pains; small cracks on the lips or mouth.
Loss of appetite; or excessive hunger (bulimia), digestion too rapid.
Teeth: cold of the teeth; caries of incisors or molars.
Throat: inflammation, pain.
Nose: cold, acute rhinitis, sinusitis.

Opposite effects:
Heart: pain, edema.
Kidney: edema, ascites.
No longer knows sexual pleasure?

Parts of the body:
Skin: humid or purulent illnesses.
Bony tuberculosis?
Face: risorius and obicular muscles of the lips weakened, flaccid, atrophied, mouth awry; or contracture; or superficial swelling.
Nape: swollen, pain.
Groin: pain, inflammation of tissues.
Knee: swelling, pain; lower leg: cold.
Feet: pain; or cold.

Chapter IV

Spleen-Pancreas

Energetically, the only link between the spleen and pancreas is that they each respond to one branch — right or left — of the same meridian. Physiologically, or nervously, they react with one another. They both have their maximum at 10 a.m. and their minimum at 10 p.m., the opposite of the triple warmer.

Logically, the effects of each point on this double meridian should be separated into those belonging to the spleen and those belonging to the pancreas. This separation, however, is potentially arbitrary, given the present state of insufficient knowledge in the West regarding these two organs. Thus it is wise to interpret prudently the recorded and proven effects of these points. Nevertheless, the separate functions, pulses and branches of the two organs can be described.

The West and Far East agree on the spleen's action on the purity of the blood. It was known in antiquity that ''the spleen takes the blood and sends it purified to the organs.'' Today, we ascribe to it the destruction of used red blood cells, elimination of foreign particles and bacteria and the temporary storage of blood during rest and digestion (it returns the blood during exercise and digestion — low blood pressure). The more distended the spleen, the more it destroys even unused red blood cells, thus causing increased anemia of red cells, hemoglobin or platelets.

It forms large and medium mononuclear white cells, which are seen abundantly in skin illnesses such as psoriasis, eczema, impetigo, etc.

The Far East has added the spleen's proven powerful action on the anterior lobes (anterior frontal) of the brain, the harmonious force of which gives reason, moral consciousness, a synthetic mind which resolves problems (supports what one knows and hears), concentration without the attention wandering; briefly, the true intelligence separated from the cleverness of the primate: the evolved human.

The meridian of the pancreas is on the left — that of the spleen on the right.

The pulse is Right II Deep.

Maximum: 10 a.m. (minimum hour of the triple warmer); minimum at 10 p.m. (maximum hour of the triple warmer). Tonifying the spleen disperses the triple warmer (mostly at 10 p.m.). Dispersing the spleen at 10 a.m. tonifies the triple warmer.

Husband-wife: liver; no action on the spleen can be undertaken without acting in the same way on the liver and vice versa.

Linked meridian and mother: stomach; they act on one another in the opposite way in spite of the position for the stomach.

Weakening to the spleen: obsessions, humidity, summer heat, excess sugar.

Strengthening to the spleen: beef, rye, yellow color.

Contracting and emptying to the spleen: adrenals.

Insufficiency: poor intellectual work, cannot concentrate, cannot easily resolve problems of mathematics or life; lazy, without gaiety or enthusiasm; distracted; dreams of rocks, of houses in ruins in the rain, of stretches of water, lakes or the sea; tired in the morning; sleep does not removed fatigue, body heavy, better from the end of the afternoon, a night person; always tired; heart weak.

Tonification points: foot-*dadu* (SP-2), tonification point, *taibai* (SP-3), source point. Toward 10-11 a.m., *zhongzhu* (TW-3). *Fengfu* (GV-15, IS GV-16) for the adrenals.

Excess: mental depression, exaggerated worrying, always preoccupied, neurasthenic, sad and discouraged about everything, loss of memory. Dreams of songs, music, of heaviness of the body, of not being able to run or get up. For the physique: heavy body, feels swollen and hot; heavy and swollen legs; pains in the articulations or bones, the periosteum. Women: excessive menses; varicosity, varicose ulcers; cholesterinemia.

Dispersing points: foot-*shanqiu* (SP-5), dispersal point; *taibai* (SP-3), source point; *fenglong* (ST-40), passage point.

Troubles: If the pulse of the spleen is soft or non-existent, it is worthwhile verifying whether the liver pulse has the same qualities. One can then be sure that the spleen and liver have greatly increased in volume (three finger-widths all round), compressing the stomach between them and forcing it down, squeezing the large intestine and the kidneys, pressing the heart and lungs upward, causing great fatigue in the morning or all day; swelling of the stomach after meals; swelling of the waist; panting to the point of palpitations.

SP-1   *yinbai* — hidden whiteness

Foot, medial side (facing the other foot), great toe, ungual phalanx; mid-width; in the angle between the swelling and the body of the bone; on the dorsal edge of the palmar tendon (flexor); in a hollow.

Following point *dadu* (SP-2); symmetrical to *dadun* (LR-1), lateral side of the big toe.

When tonified:

Tonifies (on the left) pancreas, (on the right) spleen, liver, vessels and sexual organs, anterior frontal lobes.
Disperses stomach, intestines.
Dispersing acts in the opposite way.
Here, the energy coming from the meridian of the stomach (*chongyang,* ST-42) enters the spleen-pancreas meridian.

Direct effects:

Contrary children, fears visitors, timid, attacks of fear; acute meningitis of children, or clonic convulsions, agitated; loss of awareness (evolved person), recognizes nothing, coma, but with normal pulses: "the yin energy is up," tonify.
In the chest: heat, pain, panting, cannot lie down in peace.
Menses too abundant, too prolonged; disperse; uterus: spasms.
Spleen-pancreas and heart: pain.

Contrary effects:

Thirst, vomiting.
Stomach: food does not descend; acidity one hour after meals; fullness, swelling, hyperchlorhydria (tonify, particularly the left point).
Intestines: acute enteritis; violent diarrhea; peritonitis; cold in the abdomen.

SP-2   *dadu* — great capital

Medial edge of the foot (facing the other foot); just behind the large joint of the base of the big toe; in the palmar angle between the anterior head and the body of the long bone (first metatarsal of big toe); needle along the metatarsal; in a hollow.

Preceding point *yinbai* (SP-1); two FW anterior to *taibai* (SP-3); one large FW medial (internal) to *xingjian* (LR-2).

When tonified:

Tonifies spleen (right point and pancreas left point), liver, heart, vessels, anterior frontal lobes, inferior occipital lobes, bladder (expulsor muscles), rectus abdominus, lumbar area, sacrum, knee.
Disperses stomach, kidney, bladder (sphincter), gallbladder.
Dispersing acts in the opposite way.

Direct effects:

Acts on the anterior cerebral lobes (anterior frontal).
Lack of moral awareness (sees his desires and not their consequences); lack of inner discipline; lack of emotional control; obstinate, contrary children.
Mental fatigue: cannot fix attention for long; cannot concentrate on one subject for long duration.
Lack of synthetic mind, does not compare facts with previous knowledge; accepts gossip, everything which is said; cannot resolve mathematical problems, nor those of life (cannot superimpose data immediately), two plus two do not immediately equal four.
Euphoric, friendly, but egoistic, without tact, without distinction of social differences. Superficial mind, without individuality; no interior life, lack of foresight.
If excess: exaggeration of worries, insomnia, anguish, agitation and anxious depression; dreams of stony pass, of ruins in the rain.
Physically, from insufficiency: does not recuperate easily from fatigue (see *houxi,* SI-3) of overwork; body heavy, lassitude, fatigue of the whole body, mostly on waking; better in the evening, a "night person"; weakness of the hands and feet.
Blood: tonifying greatly increases the number of white cells (leukocytes), which abound in most skin illnesses

— psoriasis, eczema, pemphigus, impetigo, etc — and which defend against staphylococcus and protect mucus membranes; acts also against abscesses.

Abundant mucus; fullness of the chest.

Pancreas (left point — insufficient): does not digest or like starches, fat, meat. Sugar and pastries cause acidity in the stomach about one hour after eating; diabetes.

Heart: pain from worms, mostly ascaris.

Opposite effects:

Stomach: pain in the hollow of the stomach; stomach cramps; vomiting from pregnancy, vomits easily, fits of vomiting.

Cholera: vomiting and diarrhea.

Abdomen: fullness.

Skin: bad abscesses.

Parts of the body:

Whole body: lassitude, laziness.

All joints painful.

Bone: pains.

Anterior shoulder: pain in the joint.

Hands and feet: weak, cold.

Rectus abdominus: spasms, contracture.

Lumbar area: pain, can neither bend nor straighten; old pains.

Lower limb: pains, particularly medial face.

Medial face of the knee: pain.

Ankle and foot: swelling, particularly on the right and without edema; feet and hands weak, cold.

SP-3   *taibai* — supreme whiteness

Foot, medial edge (medially facing the other foot): about mid-length; in the angle between the dorsal edge of the body and the posterior head of the long bone (first metatarsal of the great toe); on the dorsal edge of the plantar muscle (adductor of the great toe); in a hollow.

Two FW behind *dadu* (SP-2); two FW ahead and medial to *gongsun* (SP-4); two medial to *taichong* (LR-3).

When tonified:

Tonifies spleen (right point) pancreas (left point), liver, anterior frontal lobe, evolved man, heart, small intestine, large intestine, all bones, joints, lumbar area.

Disperses the triple warmer.

Dispersing acts in the opposite way.

Direct effects:

Source point of the spleen-pancreas, acts on insufficiency or excess.

Heaviness, laziness, lassitude, mostly when walking; numbness of the limbs, difficulty walking; or fever, agitation, malaise; heavy, congestive headache; fits of energy (nervous crises); cramps.

Stomach: gas, nausea, spasms, pain of the epigastrium; acidity, hyperchlorhydria; stomach and heart: pain from ascariasis (roundworms); bad digestion; lack of appetite.

Abdomen: cutting pain; swelling of abdomen and fullness of the chest.

Intestines: difficult stools, or stopped stools; spasms of pain; intestinal hemorrhages; diarrhea with pus and blood; vomiting, cholera.

Heart: pains, slow pulse.

Parts of the body:

Bone: pains; joints: pains.

Nape: pain.

Lumbar area: pain; lower limbs: heaviness or numbness, flaccidity or pain or contracture.

SP-4   *gongsun* — son of the prince

Foot: medial edge (medially facing the other foot), mid-length; in the inferior angle between the joint of the first metatarsal and the first cuneiform bone; between the posterior edge of the proximal head of the metatarsal of the big toe and the anterior edge of the cuneiform bone; in a hollow.

Two FW posterior and lateral to *taibai* (SP-3); two large FW ahead of foot-*shangqiu* (SP-5); two large FW medial to *chongyang* (ST-42).

When tonified:

Tonifies spleen (right point, pancreas left point), liver, heart, sexual organs, kidneys, frontal lobe, lower spinal cord, great toe same side, thumb same side.

Disperses stomach opposite, small intestine opposite, large intestine opposite; gives a response in *neiguan* (PC-6, opposite).

Dispersing acts in the opposite way.

Direct effects:

Excess yang energy — internal or external contracting pains; excess of stomach, intestines, sexual organs.

Opposite effects:

Command point of vessel of attacks (yin: frenetic attacks, nervous crises, external or internal violent or sudden pains, contractions, fits of energy, mostly of the abdomen and heart; women: pains from menses or lactation; yin insufficient, does not counterbalance the yang). Tonifying disperses excess yang, responding in *neiguan* (PC-6) opposite, which acts on all yin energies and is a passage between yin and yang (cf. *waiguan,* TW-5).

Passage point between the spleen-pancreas and stomach. If excess yang, there are cutting pains of intestines or stomach: tonify. If insufficiency of yang, the stomach is swollen, causing the abdomen to become swollen, tympanism: disperse. To tonify, transfer the excess of the stomach and intestine into the insufficiency of the spleen-pancreas, heart, kidney.

Dispersing acts in the opposite way.

Stomach, opposite: all illness from insufficiency, cannot eat; swollen, spasms of the pyloris, disturbed heart: disperse.

Stomach opposite: all illness from excess pain, inflammation, vomiting; tonify.

Cancer of the stomach.

Spleen (right point) and pancreas (left point): pains, acute pain of the heart: disperse; fever from spleen-pancreas (vomits and is depressed); disperse.

Opposite intestines: all trouble from excess, tonify; from insufficiency: disperse. "Diarrhea from inflammation is immediately cured": tonify. Intestinal hemorrhages, all pain of the abdomen from excess: tonify.

Heart: all varieties of pain, from excess: disperse; from insufficiency: tonify. Heart pain with swelling of face or head; acute pain of the heart and spleen-pancreas: disperse; malaria, heart pain; heart inflammation.

Hypertension from aerogastria compressing the heart: tonify.

Cough, attacks of suffocation: tonify.

Kidney: edema; disperse.

Genital organs: women: menses coming too often or irregularly: disperse. Spasms of lower pelvic region: men: blow to the testicles (massage).

Parts of the body:

External or internal contracting pains, same side.

Head or face: swelling with pain of the heart.

Limbs: thumb same side, great toe same side.

Start with it for: aerogastria, gas in stomach or intestines, bad digestion, hiccoughs, incessant diarrhea, jaundice, heart pain, fever of the different organs, pain in the limbs; finish with *neiguan* (PC-6).

SP-5 [foot-]*shangqiu* — mound of the merchant

Foot, medial edge (medial side of the great toe): one small FW in front of the medial malleolus; in the angle between the posterior edge of one transverse bone (scaphoid) and of the bone under the malleolus of the talus; in a hollow; under the tendon of the tibialis anterior.

Two large FW above and behind *gongsun* (SP-4); five FW under *sanyinjiao* (SP-6); one large FW medial to *jiexi* (ST-41); separated by the tibia and malleolus from *dazhong* (KI-6, IS KI-4).

To disperse:

Disperses spleen (right point), pancreas (left point), liver, evolved man, frontal lobes, kidney, periosteum.

Tonifies stomach, large intestine, small intestine, all opposite.

Tonifying sometimes augments the dispersion.

Direct effects:

Dispersal point of the spleen (right point) and pancreas (left point): all their excess; fever of spleen-pancreas (abdominal swelling, vomiting, depression); congestion, heat or pain of the spleen-pancreas; convulsions from excess insulin.

From excess of the spleen: excessive destruction of red cells, excess of white cells.

Pessimism, anxiety about the future, exaggeration of the importance of worries, agitated depression, no joy, deep sighs, chagrin, obsessions; overscrupulous; excessive religiosity, excessive altruism to the point of masochism or nightmares; nervous crises; convulsions from excess insulin, hysteria? acute or chronic epilepsy?

Stomach: lack of appetite from excess of the spleen-pancreas: disperse. Stomach: laziness, disperse; or inflammation: tonify. Base of the tongue stiff.

Swollen abdomen, noises in the intestines; disperse. Large intestine: disperse. Large intestine: spasmodic constipation, or inflammatory diarrhea: tonify; hernia, outside or inside.

Whooping cough.

Parts of the body:

Veins: varicose veins painful particularly at night; phlebitis; periphlebitis, hemorrhoids, fissures, fistulas.

Periostitis: pains of the bone; abscess of the bones; decalcification; bony rheumatism.

Joint pains; wrist, cubital side.

Lower limb: anterior hip and medial thigh (hip joint).

Knee: dry arthritis; pain on effort (mostly medial face).

Arch of foot: pain.

SP-6 *sanyinjiao* — reunion of three yin

Medial surface of the lower leg; four FW below the bone of the ankle (medial malleolus); on the tibia, just on the lateral edge of the narrow relief of the posterior side; in a hollow; on the inferior edge of a bulge; at the level of the top of the relief, mid-width.

Five FW above foot-*shangqiu* (SP-5); two large FW below *lougu* (SP-7); one FW ahead and above *jiaoxin* (KI-8); three FW above and a little posterior to *ligou* (LR-5).

When tonified:

Tonifies spleen (right), pancreas (left), liver, kidney, frontal lobes, cerebellum, pons, spinal cord, sexual organs, raises the blood pressure, warms the extremities.

Disperses stomach and intestines.

Dispersing acts in the opposite way.

Direct effects:

Laziness, lassitude, heaviness; insomnia from fatigue; weakness of nerves and brain; contrariness (children), fear of visitors, timid; aged people, empty of energy.

Cold of the whole body, or the limbs, or of the extremities.

Yawning until the jaw dislocates.

Blood and circulation: (compare energy of *hegu*, LI-4, and vitamin K — antihemorrhage), angina of the chest; arteriosclerosis; hypotension; tonify. Hypertension: disperse; bleeding hemorrhoids: disperse; hemorrhages: disperse.

Genital system: women: all troubles of blood, insufficient menses, difficult conception, easy miscarriage: tonify (insufficient blood, excess energy). Profuse menses, easy conception, no miscarriages: disperse (excess blood, insufficient energy). Menses: delayed — if from weakness, anemia: tonify; if with fullness, pains, spasms, disperse. Menses too abundant, too prolonged, red discharge; metrorrhagia, mostly after confinement: disperse.

Menopause: all troubles, hot flashes, night sweats; tonify (and disperse *hegu*, LI-4). After menopause: if obese, tonify; if rheumatic, disperse.

Leukorrhea: tonify.

Conception difficult, miscarriages easy: tonify. Paralysis of uterus, sterility: tonify (and disperse *hegu*, LI-4).

Conceives too easily: disperse (and tonify *hegu*, LI-4).

Confinement prolonged, difficult: disperse. After delivery, metrorrhagia: disperse; fainting: tonify.

Pains of the clitoris or vagina: disperse.

Men: testicles, all trouble; penis pain, seminal losses: tonify; gonorrhea in the morning; urethritis.

Stomach: inflammation, thready saliva; bad digestion, painful, or weak, insufficient.

Stomach and intestines: chronic troubles.

Vomits water after meals, vomits mucus after drinking and with pain.

Intestines: abdomen swollen, full; pain, spasms, constipation; or dysentery; thick diarrhea from undigested food; bleeding hemorrhoids; cholera, cold of the extremities; beriberi; insufficient, empty gallbladder.

Spleen (right point) and pancreas (left point): insufficiency, waist swollen.

Liver insufficient and swollen.

Kidney: "way of the kidney": disperse, five times in succession; urine insufficient, to the point of anuria; or incontinence: tonify; incontinence of children.

Hernia, intolerable pain under the umbilicus, urine stopped.

Parts of the body:

Cold of the extremities same side.

Back at the level of the scapula same side.

Lower limb mostly medial: cold flaccidity; or pain, contracture; anterior and inferior knee, pains; anterior lower leg, cramps: tonify; feet: cold, flaccidity, cannot walk.

SP-7 *lougu* — valley of the outflow

Medial lower leg; seven FW above the medial malleolus; on the tibia; just on the lateral edge of the narrow relief of the posterior side; on the inferior edge of a bulge.

Two large FW above *sanyinjiao* (SP-6), two FW under *diji* (SP-8), one FW posterior and a little above leg-*zhongdu* (LR-6); two FW above and anterior to *zhubin* (KI-9).

When tonified:

Tonifies spleen (right point) and pancreas (left point), liver, kidneys, genital organs, cerebellum, posterior nape, along the vertebrae to the bottom of the scapula, same side.

Disperses stomach, large intestine.

Dispersing acts in the opposite way.

Direct effects:

Loss of vitality, neurasthenia (weakness of the nerves); yawning; sorrow; nervous crises from weakness; hysteria? stiffness? Spleen (right point) and pancreas (left point) insufficient, distended along with the liver; swollen abdomen, gas; beriberi.

Heart: angina of the chest, cold.

Extraordinary leakage. Men: seminal losses.

Kidneys, bladder: profuse urine, day and night: tonify; or insufficient: disperse; ureters: inflammation.

Augmentation of volume and weight from water retention: disperse. Thinness from too abundant urine: tonify.

Parts of the body:

Rheumatism and pain from humidity.

Nape, along the dorsal spine to the level of the base of the scapula, all the muscles.

Posterior interior thigh to the knee, all muscles.

Four last toes: flexor commonalis (without the great toe).

SP-8 *diji* — celestial elasticity

Medial face of the lower leg: three FW under the head of the tibia; on the tibia at the posterior edge; in the angle between the inferior posterior edge of the tibia and the inferior edge of the transverse bulge; at the level of a notch in the bone; in a hollow.

Two FW above *lougu* (SP-7); following point: *yinlingquan* (SP-9), in the joint of the knee.

When tonified:

Tonifies spleen (right point), pancreas (left point), sexual organs, kidneys, hip joint, posterior knee, anterior arch, plantar side of big toe.

Disperses the stomach.

Dispersing acts in the opposite way.

Direct effects:

Sexual organs: Men: testicles insufficient; sperm insufficient, without active spermatozoa. Women: vaginal secretions too abundant: tonify; or insufficient: disperse; menses too abundant: tonify. Leukorrhea: tonify; congestion of uterus: tonify.

Kidney: insufficiency of urine to the point of anuria and abdominal edema (ascites).

Opposite effects:

Stomach: cramps, no appetite; pasty diarrhea.

Parts of the body:

Hip joint, mostly posterior.

Posterior knee, anterior arch (extensors of the toe) flabby: tonify; and flexor longus of the great toe flabby: tonify (great toe up and the other four down).

SP-9 *yinlingquan* — source of the internal plateau

Medial face of the knee: just at the edge of the angle between the head and body of the tibia; in a hollow, at the inferior edge of a transverse bulge.

Preceding point: *diji* (SP-8); seven FW below *xuehai* (SP-10); separated by a medial ligament from *ququan* (LR-8).

When tonified:

Tonifies opposite internal organs: spleen (right point), pancreas (left point), cerebellum, pons, pericardium, urethra, gallbladder sphincter, prostate, opposite body same side, sacrum, medial thigh, central knee, sole.

Disperses stomach, intestines, bladder.

Dispersing acts in the opposite way.

Direct effects:

Spleen (right point), pancreas (left point).

Contrary effects:

All trouble of the abdominal and genitourinary organs (''of the middle and bottom'').

Stomach: eructation, yawning, does not like food, vomiting, swelling of the epigastrium, cold of epigastrium and weakness in the cold; intestines in opposite side of abdomen; diarrhea after eating, explosive diarrhea with all the symptoms of cholera (bilious or sporadic cholera). Cholera: spasms, attacks of panting; peritonitis; intestinal pains, opposite; swollen abdomen in the cold with fullness of the sides.

Liver: jaundice from excess wine; beriberi.

Bladder sphincter: insufficiency, flaccidity, incontinence, loss of control of urine which is not felt to flow, urine coming out in torrents: tonify. Excess: opposite sphincter contracted — retention, hard abdomen, less urine: disperse; sand or stones in the bladder; urethral inflammation, blenorrhagia.

Opposite kidney and ureter: tonify.

Opposite sexual organs: pains; women: spasms and all tumors; vagina: inflammation; men: prostatitis, seminal loss.

Heat in the chest?

Parts of the body:

Body: external half, same side; medial upper limb and dorsal hand; inferior lumbar area sacrum; posterior hip joint; lower limb: medial thigh, rotator and adductor muscles; foot: sole.

SP-10 *xuehai* — sea of blood

Medial face of the superior part of the knee; slightly above the angle between the posterior edge of the femur and the large inferior head (medial condyle); in the superior part of the hollow; in the angle of the femur and the lower edge of an oblique muscle (vastus medialis).

Seven large FW above *yinlingquan* (SP-9); two large FW below thigh-*jimen* (SP-11).

When tonified:

Tonifies the blood, spleen (right point) pancreas (left point), heart, vessels, sexual organs, kidneys (opposite), opposite bladder sphincter.

Disperses urine, large intestine, small intestine, lateral calf, hip joint, lateral knee, lateral dorsum of foot.

Dispersing acts in the opposite way.

Gives a response at abdomen-*yinjiao* (CV-7) and in *chengjin* (BL-56).

Alarm point of the lower warmer (compare abdomen-*yinjiao*, CV-7, genitourinary functions). ''The more the triple warmer functions, the more blood there is, the less urine.''

Called also ''the house of blood, where the yang and yin are stopped, the meridian comes back and flows. In men (erection?) it flows again; in women it remains for a long time'' (menses?).

''It is the way of the blood of the uterus'': insufficient menses, pain; or delayed, with malaise: tonify. Blood of the menses with clots: disperse; red discharge: disperse; ovaries: inflammation; uterus: endometritis, leukorrhea: tonify. Men: prostatitis; urethra: blenorrhagia; testicles: orchitis.

Blood: all trouble; bad blood from excess food or excess effort and work.

Skin: all purulent inflammations; all abscesses, abscess of genital area, hot abscess of calf recurring over the years (osteomyelitis).

All fevers.

Urine: ''the flow of urine depends on the lower warmer (the more it functions, the less urine there is), and of the small intestine (the more it functions, the more urine there is)''; acts on a relaxed bladder sphincter: abundant urine during the day and at the beginning of the night to the point of incontinence: tonify; or contracted, urine rare to the point of retention: disperse.

Opposite effects:

Stomach: contracted, spasms: tonify; atonia, does not empty: disperse.

Intestines, abdomen: acute or chronic peritonitis; abdomen: swelling and fullness from counterflow of energy (spasms).

Parts of the body:

Lateral hip joint.

Posterior, lateral thigh: pain.

Knee and posterior, lateral calf.

Lateral dorsum of foot.

SP-11   *jimen* — portal of the winnowing machine

Medial thigh, about mid-width: three FW above the protuberance of the lower head of the femur (medial condyle); in the angle between the posterior edge of the tibia and the lower edge of the transverse mass; in a hollow; between the bone and semimembranosus muscle.

Two large FW above *xuehai* (SP-10); following point: *chongmen* (SP-12) of the groin; one FW above and posterior to *yinbao* (LR-9).

When tonified:

Tonifies the spleen (right point), pancreas (left point), posterior frontal lobes, lower spinal cord, groin, bladder, prostate gland, urethra, genito-abdominal nerve. Lateral calf, lateral dorsum of foot.

Disperses stomach, small intestine, large intestine.

Dispersing acts in the opposite way.

Direct effects:

Groin: pain, swelling; painful, swollen ganglia of the groin, to the point of abscess.

Sphincter of the bladder: either relaxed to the point of incontinence or contracted to the point of retention; prostate, urethra: all trouble; either relaxed or contracted, or inflamed, blenorrhagia (urethritis).

Lower part of the lateral abdomen: pain.

Parts of the body:

Groin: lateral calf (lateral gastrocnemius); dorsum of foot, lateral.

SP-12   *chongmen* — door of assaults

Groin: mid-distance from the apparent extremity of the pubis to the inferior point of the crest of the hip (anterior superior iliac spine); on the lower edge of the deep oblique rise (iliac bone); in a hollow in the triangle between the medial edge of the iliac muscle on an angle towards the hip (causes the leg to lift and cross) and the lateral edge of the muscle (greater psoas) passing above the iliac bone (and inserted on the lumbar vertebrae); deep is the pectineus muscle; in the angle between the psoas and the iliac bone.

Preceding point: thigh-*jimen* (SP-11); three large FW under *fushe* (SP-13); two large FW lateral to *qichong* (ST-30).

When tonified:

Tonifies spleen (right point), pancreas (left point), sexual organs, opposite breast, anterior thigh, medial.

Disperses stomach, large intestine, small intestine.

Dispersing acts in the opposite way.

Crossing point of spleen-pancreas, stomach and liver meridians.

Direct effects:

Sexual organs: spasms or inflammation. *1)* Men: spermatic canal? pain; epididymitis: inflammation; testicles: inflammation (orchitis). Tonifying can help erections. *2)* Women: ''the fetus rises, worries the heart, inhibits breathing,'' difficulties of lactation in opposite breast; inflammation of the mammary glands; white discharge (endometritis); metrorrhagia.

Contrary effects:

Stomach: spasms, cramps, or inflammation; epigastrium: swollen, blocked; large intestine: spasms, colic, acute pain; abdominal swelling (tympanism); prolapse, urine and stool stopped (stoppage of functions).

Parts of the body:

Anteromedial thigh.

SP-13 *fushe* — house of workshops

Inferior lateral abdomen: one half FW in front of the lower point of the crest of the hip (anterior superior iliac spine) and from the insertion onto it of the sartorius muscle; on the external oblique muscle; above the deep prominence of the iliac bone; in a hollow; on the iliac muscle.

Three large FW above *chongmen* (SP-12); three large FW under *fujie* (SP-14); one small FW lateral to *guilai* (ST-29).

When tonified:

Tonifies spleen (right point), pancreas (left point), liver, kidneys, oblique muscles of abdomen, iliac muscle, superior occipital lobe.

Disperses stomach, large intestine.

Dispersing acts in the opposite way.

Direct effects:

Fits of energy with spasms and fullness.

Spleen (right point) or pancreas (left point): pains, inflammation.

Abdomen: fullness, contractions and pains; intestines, cecum: inflammation; appendicitis; intestinal spasms and fainting from cholera; poisoning from lead (severe headache and intestinal troubles); paralysis of the intestines, constipation.

Parts of the body:

Abdominal muscles (particularly the oblique muscles).

Iliac muscles; anterior face of lower limb.

Point of Weihe: Right: Antimonium Crudum.

Left: Cannabis Indica.

SP-14 *fujie* — knot of the abdomen

Lateral abdomen; a little anterior and under the anterior and superior angle of the crest of the hip; about mid-distance from the iliac bone and the free end of the eleventh rib. In a hollow of the oblique muscles; about at the level of two FW under the umbilicus.

Three large FW above *fushe* (SP-13); two FW under *daheng* (SP-15); about three large FW in front of *daimai* (GB-26); one large FW lateral to *wailing* (ST-26).

When tonified:

Tonifies spleen (right point), pancreas (left point), kidneys, opposite sexual organs.

Disperses stomach, large intestine.

Dispersing acts in the opposite way.

Direct effects:

Loss of vitality; weak, annoyed, distracted; proud, contemptuous.

Cough, fits, dyspnea.

Paralysis of the penis, non-erection.

Contrary effects:

Large intestine: boring pain up to the heart, colic, peritonitis, diarrhea and spasms of the intestine; beriberi; abdominal cold.

SP-15　*daheng* — great transverse

Lateral abdomen, at the waist, mid-distance between the iliac crest and the free end of the eleventh rib; at the level of the umbilicus; about at the vertical of the point of the hip; on the oblique and transversus muscles; one large FW lateral to the rectus abdominus muscle; in a hollow.

Two FW above *fujie* (SP-14); four FW under *fuai* (SP-16); about two FW lateral to *tianshu* (ST-25).

When tonified:

Tonifies spleen (right point), pancreas (left point), anterior frontal lobes, evolved man, opposite half of the body. Dispersing acts in the opposite way.

Direct effects:

Easy sorrow, overwhelming tears, deep sighing, deep shock, nervous crises, great cold.
Epidemic flu; great perspiration.
Spleen very enlarged, leukemia; diminishes coagulation?

Contrary effects:

Intestines: serious diarrhea; chronic inflammation of the intestines; chronic dysentery (with blood); heat in the abdomen — often needs to move the bowels; or stoppage of stool; intestinal worms.

Parts of the body:

Opposite upper and lower limb; difficulty in lifting or moving them.

Point of Weihe: Ceanothus.

SP-16　*fuai* — mourning of the abdomen

Inferior lateral thorax between the ninth and tenth ribs; in the lateral angle of the anterior meeting of the ribs; on the inferior edge of the ninth rib; on anterior edge of a vertical tendon; in a hollow.

Four FW above *daheng* (SP-15); five FW under *shidou* (SP-17); four FW lateral to *taiyi* (ST-23); two FW lateral to *zhangmen* (LR-13).

When tonified:

Tonifies spleen (right point), pancreas (left point), and all yin meridians (chain of the yin).
Disperses stomach, large intestine, small intestine.
Dispersing acts in the opposite way.

Direct effects:

Cold, sensitive to cold.

Contrary effects:

Stomach: pains, burning, acidity, does not empty; undigested food; ulceration, ulcer of the stomach.
Intestines: pains, intestinal hemorrhages, stools with blood and pus.

SP-17　*shidou* — cave of nourishment

Lateral thorax: upper edge of the seventh rib (between the sixth and seventh ribs); about two FW lateral from the line of the nipple; in a hollow.

Five FW above *fuai* (SP-16); two FW under *tianxi* (SP-18); one FW anterior to *qimen* (LR-14); three FW lateral to *burong* (ST-19).

When tonified:

Tonifies stomach (right point), pancreas (left point), liver; ends of fingers, eyes, ears.

Disperses stomach, intestines.

Dispersing acts in the opposite way.

Direct effects:

Aggravated between 2 and 4 a.m. (solar time); great weakness.
Liver: pain; pain under the right scapula.

Contrary effects:

Diaphragm, stomach: always a noise of water in the area of the diaphragm and stomach; pain in the diaphragm. Pleurisy, and with purulence; noise of water in the pleura. Eyes: flying spots.

Ears: buzzing?

Point of Weihe: Kali Carbonicum. Great weakness; aggravated between 2 and 4 a.m. solar time; from rest, from pressure; extreme dryness of the scalp; ends of the fingers; medial arm swollen; floating spots before the eyes; buzzing; pain in the region of the right scapula, bottom of right lung, back; asthma; pointed pain in the region of the liver; liquid in the pleura or stomach.

SP-18 *tianxi* — celestial flow

Lateral chest: about mid-distance from the vertical of the nipple and the armpit; on the inferior edge of the fifth rib (the third being just under the armpit); in a hollow.

Two FW above *shidou* (SP-17); two FW under *xiongxiang* (SP-19); one FW lateral and under *tianchi* (PC-1); two FW lateral to *ruzhong* (ST-17); two FW anterior (medial) to *zhejin* (GB-23).

When tonified:

Tonifies spleen (right point), pancreas (left point), breast same side, lungs.

Disperses stomach.

Dispersing acts in the opposite way.

Direct effects:

Cough: violent fits; acute or chronic bronchitis, dyspnea, pulmonary congestion, pain and fullness of the chest; chronic pneumonia.

Contrary effects.

Nausea; stomach ulcer.

Parts of the body:

Breast same side: swelling, ulceration to the point of deep abscess.

Point of Weihe: Kali Chlor.

SP-19 *xiongxiang* — region of the chest

Lateral thorax: mid-distance from the vertical of the nipple to the vertical of the armpit; on the inferior edge of the fourth rib (the third being just under the armpit); in a hollow.

Two FW above *tianxi* (SP-18); two FW under *zhourong* (SP-20); two FW lateral and slightly under *yingchuan* (ST-16); two FW medial to *zhejin* (GB-23).

When tonified:

Tonifies spleen (right point), pancreas (left point), liver, opposite lumbar muscles.

Disperses stomach, diaphragm, lower esophagus, large intestine.

Dispersing acts in the opposite way.

Contrary effects:

Contracted esophagus (particularly lower), cannot swallow or make the food go down, regurgitation of food, excess saliva. Stomach and diaphragm: spasms.

Parts of the body:

Back and opposite lumbar muscles: difficulty in turning or bending to the side; lumbar muscles opposite: contracture or flaccidity.

Point of Weihe: Right: Creosotum.

Left: Sabadilla.

SP-20 *zhourong* — circulating blood

Lateral chest; mid-distance from the vertical of the nipple to the vertical of the armpit; on the inferior edge of the third rib (which is just under the armpit); in a hollow.

Two FW above *xiongxiang* (SP-19); one large FW medial to *dabao* (SP-21 and behind); two FW medial to *yuanye* (GB-22); two FW lateral to *wuyi* (ST-15); two FW inferior and medial to *jiquan* (HT-1); two FW inferior and lateral to *kufang* (ST-14).

When tonified:
>   Tonifies spleen (right point), pancreas (left point), opposite throat, sexual organs, opposite eye.
>   Disperses the stomach.
>   Dispersing acts in the opposite way.

Direct effects:
>   Hypersensitivity to touch, pain, cold, air; aggressiveness, very irritable; coughing fits, energy in the upper body; coughs and spits pus, pulmonary congestion; bronchitis; pleurisy.
>   Sexual hyperexcitation?

Contrary effects:
>   Swollen upper lip?
>   Contracted esophagus: cannot swallow or make the food go down, regurgitation.
>   Large intestine, hemorrhoids; troubles of rectum and anus; prolapse of rectum?
>   Swollen eyelids.

Parts of the body:
>   Tendency to suppuration (particularly the left point).
>   Chest and back pain; intercostal pain.

>   **Point of Weihe:** Right: Hepar Sulfur.
>   Left: Ratanhia.

SP-21 *dabao* — large envelope

Lateral chest: slightly in front of the vertical of the armpit; under the third rib (which is just under the armpit), in the angle of the anterior edge of an intercostal ligament; under the inferior edge of the pectoralis major; in a hollow.

One large FW lateral to *zhourong* (SP-20); two FW under *jiquan* (HT-1); one large FW inferior and medial to *yuanye* (GB-22).

When tonified:
>   Tonifies spleen (right point), pancreas (left point), all the yin distributor organ meridians, posterior frontal lobes, cerebellum, medulla oblongata, sense organs, half of the body internal and external, same side and upper part.
>   Disperses all the yang producer organs and the lower half of the body on the same side; responds to *yanglingquan* (GB-34).
>   Dispersing acts in the opposite way.
>   Here the energy leaves the meridian of the spleen-pancreas to enter through a branch into that of the heart, *jiquan* (HT-1).

Direct effects:
>   Acts on the lateral and medial side of the body on the same side, except the eye, the upper and medial in the direct way and the lower and lateral in the opposite way.
>   Unites and harmonizes upper and lower body, right and left, interior and exterior, chest and back.
>   ''The great secondary vessel of the spleen-pancreas'' commands all the secondary vessels, yin and yang, one in addition to the twelve meridians and the two of the medial lines.
>   ''Irrigates, through the spleen-pancreas, all the yin distributor organs.''
>   If excess: the whole body is painful. If insufficient: all the articulations are relaxed (see insufficient pituitary).

Parts of the body:
>   Eye: right, external opposite muscular asthenopia?
>   Larynx same side; vocal cords; respiratory passages: little energy, dyspnea; pleurisy; pneumonia.
>   Heart on same side: endocarditis.
>   Kidneys same side: eliminates salt poorly, swollen: tonify (see adrenals); urine diminished; bladder: paralysis?
>   Half of the body, same side, medial and lateral aspects; direct action on the upper half, opposite action on the lower half; direct action on the entire medial aspect, opposite action on the entire lateral aspect; opposite action on the opposite side of the body.

>   **Point of Weihe:** Right: Allium Cepa.
>   Left: Senega.

Chapter V

Heart

Deep pulse I, left wrist: maximum hour: noon (minimum hour of the gallbladder), minimum: midnight (maximum hour of the gallbladder). Husband-wife: lungs; mother: spleen-pancreas.

Child and linked meridian: small intestine.

It is therefore impossible to act on the heart meridian without acting:

1)   In the same way on: heart, lungs, spleen-pancreas, brain, particularly anterior frontal lobes and on the small intestine when the pulses are equal.

2)   In the opposite way on: gallbladder (particularly according to the rhythm of the energy), small intestine (according to the inequality of the pulses).

Besides its action on the circulation (thus the yin energy of inactivity, of calm) and the distribution of material vitality, the heart is closely linked to the psyche (through the intermediary of the autonomic nervous system and the endocrines). The emotions act strongly on it; its more or less energetic functioning causes the personality to more or less influence other people.

For action on the mind as well as the heart, it is the most important of the meridians, and commands: moral depression (*jiquan*, HT-1 and *shaofu*, HT-8); moral hyperexcitation (*lingdao*, HT-4); mental depression (*shaohai*, HT-3); excess or insufficiency from emotional agitation (*tongli*, HT-5); mental or physical excess or insufficiency (*shenmen*, HT-7); mental and physical weakness (*shaochong*, HT-9); physical excess or insufficiency (*yinxi*, HT-6).

HT-1 *jiquan* — source of the axis

Lateral upper thorax: at the bottom of the fold of the shoulder, and towards the arm; in the angle between the upper edge of the inferior bulge of the pectoralis major, the sternal fascia and the medial edge of the deep vertical muscle (the coracobrachialis, which passes between the pectoralis major and latissimus dorsi); in a hollow of the groove between the sternal fascia and the clavicular fascia of the pectoralis major.

Following point: *qingling* (HT-2). The energy comes from a direct branch of the spleen-pancreas (*dabao*, SP-21). One large FW under *tianquan* (PC-2), two FW medial and inferior to *yunmen* (LU-2).

The point is crossed by the meridian of the gallbladder coming from *tianjing* (GB-21) through *kufang* (ST-14) and *tianquan* (PC-2) to go to *yuanye* (GB-22).

When tonified:
Tonifies the heart, spleen-pancreas, lungs, opposite frontal lobes, pericardium, pectoralis major, internal upper limb, anterior distal limb, throat, extremity of the tongue.

Disperses the gallbladder, bladder, small intestine in excess.
Dispersing acts in the opposite way.

Direct effects:
Joylessness, sorrow, moral depression, regrets; heart: all troubles.
Respiratory passages, bronchi (asthma); lungs: pleurisy.

Contrary effects:
Bladder.
Tongue: extremity.
Dry throat, violent thirst; dry retching.

Parts of the body:
Shoulder and upper limb: cold.
Pectoralis major: contracture (hand pulled towards the other shoulder).
Or flaccidity (hand cannot reach the other shoulder).
Hemiplegia? Flaccidity?

HT-2 *qingling* — the immateriality of sky

Anteromedial elbow: one FW lateral to the bone of the elbow (epitrochlea); in the angle between the upper edge of the large transverse prominence of the articulation and the anterior edge of the insertion on an angle on the epitrochlea (pronator teres muscles); in a hollow.

Preceding point *jiquan* (HT-1, on the pectoralis major); two FW above *shaohai* (HT-3).

When tonified:

Tonifies the heart, lungs, opposite frontal lobes, throat same side, extremity of the anterior shoulder, posterior upper limb, dorsal hand.

Disperses the gallbladder, bladder.

Dispersing acts in the opposite way.

Direct effects:

Heart. Lung same side: inflammation, intercostal pains, shivering, fever.

Parts of the body:

Anterior extremity of the shoulder, posterior arm, posterior forearm, dorsal hand; cannot put on clothes, cannot fully extend the arm, cannot flex the elbow.
Motor point of the cubital nerve?

HT-3 *shaohai* — smaller sea

Medial, anterior elbow: two FW inferior and lateral to the internal prominence of the bone (epitrochlea); in the angle between the inferior edge of the large transverse rise of the articulation and the upper edge of a large muscle on an angle (pronator teres); in a hollow; medial to the deep brachial artery.

Two FW under *qingling* (HT-2); following point: *lingdao* (HT-4); one FW medial to *quze* (PC-3).

When tonified:

Tonifies the heart, all yin organs (distributors, deep pulses), three nervous centers, three endocrines, three levels of the psyche, opposite eye, opposite half of the body on the same side, armpit, wrist and palmar side of fingers.

Disperses the gallbladder, bladder.

Dispersing acts in the opposite way.

Direct effects:

Mental depression, forgetfulness, stupidity, loss of vitality, cerebral anemia.
Acute encephalitis (diplopia, visual troubles, headaches) opposite; opposite meningitis; epilepsy (tongue out, vertigo, falling, salivation, moaning), occasional frenetic attacks.
Heart: acute pain, shivering hands, pericordial pain.
Teeth: pain, cold.
Pulmonary tuberculosis, depression, weakness.

Contrary effects:

Children: trembling, swellings, scratching: tonify.
Breasts: pain, swelling: tonify.
Ganglia in the armpit (adenitis, suppurating), pain in the armpit, side, elbow and nape: tonify.

Parts of the body:

Face: opposite facial neuralgia.
Lateral neck and opposite nape: pain; side: pain.
Half of body same side: flaccidity, weakness or contracture, pain.
Anterior shoulder: arm, medial elbow, anterior wrist, hand and palmar side of fingers.
Lateral, anterior lower limb.

HT-4   *lingdao* — way of immateriality

Anterior wrist (palm up, in supination); on the line of the little finger; four FW above the palm, two FW above the head of the ulna; in the angle between the radial (lateral) edge of the ulna and the tendon of the flexor carpi ulnaris muscle, and of the inferior edge of a transverse bulge; on the ulnar edge of the ulnar artery; in a hollow.

Preceding point: *shaohai* (HT-3); two FW above *tongli* (HT-5); separated from *jianshi* (PC-5) by the artery and the tendon of the palmaris longus and flexors; separated by the flexor carpi radialis from *zhizheng* (SI-7); at the level of *lieque* (LU-7).

When tonified:

Tonifies (contracts) all the yin meridians, particularly the opposite heart, governor vessel, three nervous centers, three levels of the psyche, three endocrines, three sense organs; heats the opposite half of the body.
Disperses (diminishes) the aorta, opposite vessels, all the yang meridians, conception vessel.
Dispersing acts in the opposite way.

Direct effects:

Sorrow and frenetic fear: tonify; convulsions, hysteria: tonify.
Moral hyperexcitation.
Icy to the bone from cold, warms himself at the fire, opposite half: tonify.
Opposite larynx, cannot speak, suddenly mute; if weak, swellings: tonify. If pain, inflammation or contracture: disperse.

Contrary effects:

Opposite heart: weak, tonify; contracted, disperse. Opposite aorta, carotid, opposite arteries ample and hard: tonify (contracts them); soft, a little elevated: disperse; hypertension: tonify; hypotension: disperse.
Stomach: dry vomiting, tonify.

Parts of the body:

Opposite half of the body: tonifying warms.
Hand, thumb, fingers, dorsal and palmar sides; medial elbow.

HT-5   *tongli* — village of passage

Wrist, anterior face (palm up, in supination): on the line of the little finger; in the angle between the superior (posterior) edge of the transverse head of the ulna, and the lateral head of the tendon of the flexor carpi ulnaris muscle, between it and the ulnar artery; in a hollow.

Two FW under *lingdao* (HT-4); one FW above *yinxi* (HT-6); separated from *yanglao* (SI-6) by the flexor carpi ulnaris muscle, and from *daling* (PC-7) by the ulnar artery and the palmaris longus secondus muscle.

When tonified:

Tonifies the heart, lung, same side; anterior frontal lobes, evolved man, small intestine if equal, posterior articulation of the shoulder, posterior arm, anterior knee, anterior lower leg, dorsum of foot.
Disperses the gallbladder, small intestine if stronger, large intestine, bladder, opposite eye.
Dispersing acts in the opposite way.

Direct effects:

Psychological agitation, cardiac, gallbladder.
Psychological agitation (stage fright of artists, etc.) can cause contraction and cold or enervation and heat.
Or little energy, cold, shock, cannot speak (acute contraction of the hyoglossal muscle), face without expression, vertigo-fainting, anxiety, heart tight.
Or face hot, agitation, headache, heavy limbs, palpitations, speaks precipitously, agitated apprehension.
If the shock has been serious: fever, heat, initial euphoria, then after several days frequent yawning and sorrow, facial heat without sweat, headache, sudden muteness, no longer speaks, eye pain, palpitations.
Cardiac agitation: from emotion; or tight heart, circulation as if stopped, intermittent beats, or palpitations, precipitous or irregular beats.
Bladder agitation: from emotion: urgent and frequent need to urinate, abundance of clear urine, to the point of incontinence, or stoppage.
Eyes: bloodshot eyeballs, pain.
Sore throat, tonsillitis; long and dirty teeth? black face?
Overly abundant menses; metrorrhagia, miscarriages.
Swollen abdomen, constipation.

Parts of the body.
   Upper limb pain and numbness with pain of the heart and chest.
   Posterior shoulder joint, posterior arm.
   Anterior knee, anterior lower leg and dorsal foot.

HT-6   *yinxi* — valley of yin

Anterior wrist (palm in supination): on the line of the little finger; in the angle between the inferior edge (towards the palm) of the head of the ulna and of the lateral edge (towards the lateral thumb) of the large tendon of the flexor carpi ulnaris (inserted on the pisiform bone); on the medial (ulnar) edge of the ulnar artery; in a hollow.

One FW below *tongli* (HT-5); one large FW above *shenmen* (HT-7); separated by the flexor carpi ulnaris from *yanggu* (SI-5).

When tonified:
   Tonifies the heart, cerebellum and pons, medulla oblongata and spinal cord, small intestine, opposite eye and cheek bone, opposite throat, face same side, anterior shoulder, anteromedial upper limb, anterior lower leg, dorsum of foot.
   Disperses the gallbladder, stomach.
   Dispersing acts in the opposite way.

Direct effects:
   Emotional agitation of the physical energy causing excess or insufficiency; weak heart.
   Through terror of energy: insufficiency. Emptiness in revolt, attacks of weakness, vertigo and fainting, slack tongue, loss of voice, cannot speak (flaccidity of the hyoglossal muscle?) fear of cold, shivering in the bath; stomach cannot empty; leukorrhea.
   Excess: fits of energy, nervous crises, tight throat, heart and chest pains, nervous palpitations, lack of breath, fullness of chest, congested nose, blocked nose, nosebleeds; contracted stomach, violent nausea, hematemesis; violent diarrhea; night sweats.
   Fever from a bad cold.
   Children: tuberculosis of the bone?

Parts of the body:
   Anterior shoulder and anterior medial upper limb; anterior lower leg, dorsum of foot.

HT-7   *shenmen* — door of the evolved

Palm, near the wrist, on the line of the little finger: on the hypothenar eminence; on the inferior and lateral edge (towards the fingers and thumb) of the round bony head (pisiform bone); on the medial edge of the ulnar artery; on the upper edge of the transverse mass (palmar aponeurosis); in the angle between the bone and the lateral edge (towards the thumb) of the insertion of the adductor of the little finger; in a hollow.

One large FW below *yinxi* (HT-6), three above *shaofu* (HT-8), separated by the adductor from hand-*wangu* (SI-4).

When tonified:
   Tonifies the heart, opposite brain, spinal cord, all the yin meridians, shoulder and anterior upper limb; hand and thumb, palmar and dorsal muscles (pancreas with the left point, spleen with the right point).
   Disperses all the yang meridians.
   Dispersing acts in the opposite way.

Effects: "important point for illnesses of the personality and of the heart, great master point of all the internal organs, home of the evolved man and of the sexual energy"; source point of the heart.
   Psychological troubles with excess or with physical insufficiency.
   With excess: excessive sorrow, frenetic sobbing, or frenetic laughter and sighing; mad anger; absurd false ideas, violent hallucinations; frenetic epilepsy ("the five epilepsies of adults and children"); insomnia from hyperexcitation.
   With insufficiency: little energy; numerous sighs; stubborn forgetfulness, forgets names; fear; stupidity of nature and spirit; depression to the point of cerebral anemia; anguish; shivering from cold, aversion to cold, prefers a warm climate; arms and hands cold; impeded tongue, speaks poorly (flaccidity of the hypoglossal muscle).
   Heart: source point of the heart, corrects excess or insufficiency.
   Excess: heart and arteries contracted; nervous palpitations; rapid heart (tachycardia); great agitation of the heart; desire to drink cold water; sad at heart; pain in the heart, bar on the chest; "when there is an excess of energy in

the heart, this point unifies the sexual energy and guides the energy''; intermittent fever with agitation.

Insufficiency: weakness of the heart; tiring heart; weak beats without energy, unequal in amplitude.

Arteries: hypertension, or hypotension.

Nose blocked, congested to the point of nosebleeds: disperse.

Stomach: energy troubled, vomiting of blood (hematemesis): tonify, or lack of appetite (mental anorexia?): disperse.

Sexual organs; hemorrhages after delivery: disperse.

Flaccid urethra; does not feel the urine pass, up to the point of incontinence: tonify.

Tonsillitis; asthmatic attacks; hot palms.

Ganglia.

Parts of the body:

Anterior shoulder; anteromedial upper limb.

Hand, thumb fingers, palmar and dorsal muscles; hand contracted.

Forearm and hand: cold.

Anterior lower leg; arch.

HT-8   *shaofu* — lesser workshop

Palm, line of the joint of the ring and little fingers: one FW above the joint; just at the superior lateral edge of the prominent angle of the bone at the bottom of the little finger (head of the fifth metacarpal bone). Towards the angle of the head of the fourth metacarpal. Between the bone and the insertion of the small muscle (fourth lumbricalis muscle); in a hollow. On the medial edge of the interosseous artery; on the ''heart line.''

Three FW below *shenmen* (HT-7); following point: *shaochong* (HT-9); one FW medial from *laogong* (PC-8), in the angle of the head of the ring finger.

When tonified:

Tonifies the heart, cerebellum, pons, all yin meridians (particularly sexual organs, kidney excretion), side, posterior extremity of the shoulder, posterior arm, radial forearm, dorsal muscles of thumb and index fingers.

Disperses all the yang meridians (mostly bladder).

Dispersing acts in the opposite way.

Direct effects:

Little energy, fear of people, deranged mind, fearful, deep sighs; or agitation, fullness.

Shivering from cold.

Throat: as from adenoid growths, irritation, burning interior, heat of the palms.

Sexual organs, either pains, itching (pruritis) or weakness: women: menses too abundant, vulvary pruritis, pains of the vagina, or prolapsed uterus; men: swelling of the testicles (orchitis); disturbing erections, or insufficient erections.

Contrary effects:

Bladder retention: tonify; or incontinency: disperse.

Parts of the body:

Side: intercostal pain; axilla.

Shoulder: posterior extremity; lateral posterior arm; elbow: contraction, pain.

Radial forearm (supinators); contracted hand, does not extend; retraction of the palmar aponeurosis (Dupuytren?) thumb and index finger; dorsal muscles.

HT-9   *shaochong* — lesser attack

Hand: little finger; terminal phalanx, ring finger side (lateral); mid-width of the finger; in the angle between the inferior edge of the prominent angle of the prominence of the bone and the dorsal edge of the palmar tendon (flexor); in a hollow; slightly ahead of the bulge; between the body and the flexor; on the posterior edge of a ligamentous mass.

Preceding point: *shaofu* (HT-8) on the palm; symmetrical to *shaoze* (SI-1) through a short dorsal branch.

When tonified:

Tonifies the heart (ventricles), frontal lobes, all yin meridians, governor vessel, opposite eye and ear, throat and tongue same side, extremities.

Disperses all the yang meridians, particularly gallbladder and stomach.

Dispersing acts in the opposite way.

Direct effects:

Psychological, physical and cardiac weakness.

Moments of weakness and discouragement; eyes dull, voice without timbre, exhausted face, drawn; grey fog, sensations of momentary weakness to the point of fear of fainting; weakness after fever.

Sadness, sorrow, without zest; fear, apprehension, anxiety; Emotional agitation with trembling; children; emotivity with agitation.

Mind weak; dreams of smoke, fire, flames.

Heart: tonification point, particularly the ventricles; weak heart, insufficient, easily tired; either slow (bradycardia), or nervous palpitations from weakness.

Opposite eye, opposite ear.

Tongue and throat on the same side; dry throat, thirst; swollen and painful larynx; abundance of mucus, weak lungs, pleurisy, coldness.

Sexual organs: offensive odor, white or red discharges with weakness of the heart or fever.

Parts of the body:

Intercostal neuralgia.

Anterior shoulder and internal anterior upper limb, pain or contracture; palmar side of index finger and thumb; painful elbow, cannot be extended.

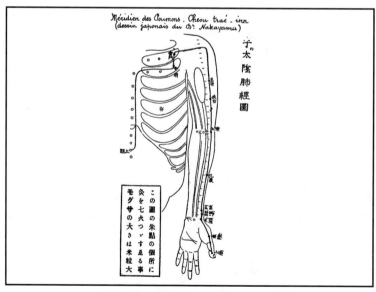

Meridian of the lungs (Nakayama)

Chapter VI

Small Intestine

In the West, the importance of the small intestine lies in the production of the completely separate albumin molecules; in the action of the duodenum on the pancreas; in the digestion of meat, fat and starches; and the reciprocal action on the gallbladder.

The Chinese add to this its value as a producer of energy — ''life given to dead food''; its action on the heart, of which it is the child and the coupled meridian; its interaction with the liver — it is tonified by dispersing the liver, and dispersed by tonifying the liver (midday-midnight); its relation with the governor vessel, each of their points acting on one another; and its action on the organs of sense: eyes, ears, smell-taste.

Its maximum is 2 p.m. (minimum hour of the liver); its minimum is 2 a.m. (maximum hour of the liver). Upstream is the heart meridian (mother); downstream is the bladder meridian (son). The large intestine is its wife.

It thus acts always in the same way on the large intestine and bladder, and in a contrary way on the liver. When equal to the heart, it acts in the same way. When different, it gives the heart its excess or brings the heart's excess to itself.

Its tonification point, *houxi* (SI-3), causes rapid recuperation from fatigue and weakness, and commands the entire governor vessel (physical, mental and moral strength); it diminishes the waste from food through better assimilation, and from this acts against rheumatism. It also acts on the muscles, and increases urine and decreases stools and other secretions.

Its dispersing point, *xiaohai* (SI-8), acts against swelling of the flesh and skin from wastes; diminishes the excesses and fevers of the governor vessel and its excesses of physical strength such as Saint Vitus Dance, tics, perhaps epilepsy and also the stiffness of nape and back.

SI-1 *shaoze* — smaller marsh

Dorsal hand (palm down, pronation); little finger, terminal phalanx; slightly behind the medial angle of the nail; in the angle between the inferior edge (towards the nail) of the bony mass of the terminal phalanx at the articulation and the dorsal edge of a short insertion (of the internal lateral ligament); in a hollow.

When tonified:
　　Tonifies (augments) urine, small intestine, large intestine when smooth, tonifies heart, bladder, upper opposite nape.
　　Disperses kidneys, liver; diminishes all secretions — saliva, sweat, milk, etc.
　　Dispersing acts in the opposite way.

Direct effects:
　　Secretions: tonifying increases urine and decreases secretions; dispersing does the contrary. Milk insufficient or not coming after delivery: disperse. Or too abundant, breasts swollen, painful: tonify. Saliva like paste, with warm and dry mouth: disperse; no sweat, dry skin from insufficiency of small intestine: tonify. Or from excess: disperse. Algid malaria without sweat: disperse. Abundant urine (and insufficient secretions): disperse; insufficient urine (and abundant secretions): tonify.
　　Eyes: do not release fluids, stay swollen and hard; pterygium; cataract.
　　Throat: pain, tonsillitis, laryngitis.
　　Nose: incessant bleeding.
　　Enlarged heart; cold pains, cold under the heart.
　　Internal headaches; convulsions.

Parts of the body:
　　Inferior chin: swelling.
　　Opposite medial nape: all troubles.
　　Little finger contracted or flaccid; anterior cubital edge of the forearm.

SI-2   *qiangu* — anterior valley

Hand: medial edge of the little finger; phalanx, in the palmar angle between the inferior (anterior) head and the body of the bone; on the dorsal edge of the palmar tendon (flexors); in a hollow.

Preceding point: *shaoze* (SI-1), near the ungual angle; two FW distal to *houxi* (SI-3).

When tonified:

Tonifies the small intestine, vessels, large intestine, kidneys, posterior frontal lobes, heart (according to its relation with the opposite inner ear), lateral neck and nape, breast, thumb, forearm, stomach, gallbladder.
Disperses the heart, lungs, sexual organs and kidneys.
Dispersing acts in the opposite way.

Direct effects:

Weakened sight or myopia from age or weakness, opposite eye.
Opposite inner ear, surrounding pain, buzzings?

Contrary effects:

Opposite nose: colds, congestion between nose and throat, blocked nose, nosebleeds: tonify.
Coughs; coughing fits: tonify.
Heart enlarged and fatty: tonify.
Opposite breast: milk insufficient after delivery: disperse; inflammation of mammary glands: tonify.

Parts of the body:

Opposite jaw: swollen to the back of the ear, swollen chin.
Lateral nape and neck, mid-height same side; pain, either swelling or contracture; cervical vertebrae.
Radial forearm: medial thumb and index finger; flexor of the little finger; medial surface of the thigh.
Medial (internal) arch, same side.

SI-3   *houxi* — posterior vale

Hand: medial edge; on the lateral line of the little finger (palm up, in supination); just above (behind) the articulation of the base (metocarpophalangeal) of the little finger; in the angle towards the palm between the head and the deep muscle opposing under the superficial muscle (adductor); in the angle of the head and palmar muscle.

Two FW above (behind) *qiangu* (SI-2); two FW under (distal to) hand-*wangu* (SI-4): at the level of hand-*zhongzhu* (TW-3).

When tonified:

Tonifies the small intestine, large intestine, gallbladder; raises the pulse of the governor vessel, dorsal spinal cord same side, opposite brain, *xinhui* (GV-21, IS GV-22), inferior posterior frontal lobes, cerebellum, spinal cord, lateral eye, opposite temple, muscles of the upper limb and hand extensors, triceps of the same side, opposite anterior and inferior limb, anterior opposite external arch, *shenmai* (BL-62).
Disperses the liver.
Dispersing acts in the opposite way.

Direct effects:

Command point of the governor vessel on the dorsal spine: yang energy (physical and psychological weakness); does not recuperate rapidly from fatigue, from a shock; tired or unduly depressed and for too long a time; cries easily; dreams of narrow passages.
Or psychological or physical hyperexcitation, unduly hyperexcited for too long a time.
Heart: all troubles of rhythm.
Tonification point of the small intestine (see functions of small intestine); does not like meat; bad digestion; borborygmus after fats or starches; abdominal swelling; grey or fatty stools; pancreatic diabetes.
Fever, chills and heat; seasonal, epidemic fevers; shivering and stiff nape (flu?).
Eye (medial side, same side, and external lateral, same side): farsighted; congested, red eyes; acute headache; cold tears; eye forming a veil; cataract; keratitis; opposite external upper eyebrow; pain.
Opposite ear buzzing? Deafness?

Direct effects on urine; inverse effects on secretion.

Pulmonary edema (congestion, suffocation in the middle of the night): tonify. (Increases urine, diminishes secretion). Bronchitis: tonify; tonsillitis.
Kidneys and bladder: insufficient urine (abundance of saliva, sweat, mucus, etc.): tonify; abundant urine (weak secretions): disperse.
Tooth congestion, swollen cheek or throat: tonify opposite side; opposite teeth.

Parts of the body:

Opposite neck and nape.

Opposite body or face: all external trouble; facial neuralgia or paralysis (ear and maxillary angle).

All the muscles of half the body; same side upper limb (posterior wrist, fingers, triceps, extensors). And (through T3) opposite side inferior limb, lower leg, external anterior arch; motor function of the extremities.

Opposite foot: external, anterior arch; toes (extensors); tetanus.

Through the governor vessel: weakened back, head tilted: tonify; stiff back: disperse. Heat in the middle of the back.

Head, vertex, medial nape: pain, stiff nape, cannot look behind; torticollis; eyebrows: neuralgia.

Begin with it for equilibrating top and bottom, motor function of the extremities. Equalizes urine and secretions (insufficient urine with abundant sweat, mucus, etc.); red eyes, throat, cough. Pain in the eyebrows, teeth. Finish with *shenmai* (BL-62).

SI-4   *wangu* — wrist bone

Hand, palm up, in supination; on the medial edge (internal line of the little finger); one large FW below (distal to) the bony prominence of the ulna; in the angle between the inferior and dorsal edge of the small, round bone towards the palm (pisiform) and the dorsal edge of the muscle inserted on its inferior face (adductor muscle of the little finger); between it and the unciform bone of the fifth metacarpal, in a hollow.

Two FW proximal to *houxi* (SI-3); two FW distal and palmar to *yanggu* (SI-5); one proximal and dorsal to *shenmen* (HT-7).

When tonified:

Tonifies the small intestine, all the producer organs (yang, superficial), spinal cord, dorsal vertebrae same side, opposite cervical vertebrae, governor vessel, particularly stomach and gallbladder. All articulations of the vertebrae, the upper limbs, same side and lower limbs, base of the nape same side, opposite hip; sense organs.

Disperses all distributor yin organs (deep), conception vessel, occipital lobes, mid-brain.

Dispersing acts in the opposite way.

Direct effects:

Source point of small intestine: tonifies insufficiencies; or disperses excess (vomiting, irritated stomach, gallbladder, jaundice): disperse.

Hyperexcited apprehension, agitated melancholy, hyperexcited speech; convulsions; meningitis, contracted fingers.

Attacks of perspiration, cold then hot, intermittent fever, headache.

Eyes: cold in the eyes, tears flowing in the cold, or flowing; congestion of cornea; veil of the cornea, beginning of cataract; all eye troubles on the opposite side.

Opposite ears: buzzing, tonify?

Touch: diminished sensations.

Pleurisy, pain at the bottom of the ribs; tuberculosis of children.

Parts of the body:

All troubles of the face, posterior shoulder and upper limb same side. Opposite face, from the ear to the chin; cheek, jaw, chin (swelling, pain or flaccidity); opposite lateral neck; articulations of the cervical vertebrae.

All articulations of the upper limb same side and lower limb opposite side.

Crackling cervical vertebrae.

Poliomyelitis: gluteus medius and minimus (lateral atrophia).

Upper limb same side; joints, tight pain; opposite elbow: contracture or arthritis, cannot be extended or flexed; swelling of the opposite wrist; opposite hand: without force, cannot hold anything, writer's cramp, pain; fingers: sense of touch, tight pains, stiffness or contraction.

Opposite hip: gluteus medius and minimus (poliomyelitis); opposite lower limb, opposite joints.

SI-5 *yanggu* — yang external valley

Wrist, ulnar edge (on the lateral line of the little finger): in the angle between the inferior edge (towards the fingers) of the dorsal prominence of the ulna and the posterior dorsal edge of the large anterior tendon (flexor carpi ulnaris muscle); in a hollow.

Separated from *yanglao* (SI-6) by the ulnar prominence; two FW above and dorsal to hand-*wangu* (SI-4). Separated by the tendon of the flexor carpi ulnaris from *yangchi* (TW-4).

When tonified:

Tonifies opposite side of abdomen (small and large intestines), liver, spleen-pancreas, opposite brain; sexual organs, opposite lateral neck, external side of thumb and of the great toe, eyes, ears, knee and great toe on the same side.
Disperses the kidney.
Dispersing acts in the opposite way.

Direct effects:

Extravagant speech or laughter; escapades (walks blindly without direction); or head bent, looks to right and left; giddiness, vertigo, fainting.
Scarlet eyes, inflamed from pain or wind.
Ears: buzzing? deafness?
Mouth: chews the cheeks; inflammation; babies cannot suck; gums: inflammation.
Teeth: upper opposite caries and pain.
Painful hemorrhoids.
Impotence?

Parts of the body:

Lower opposite jaw and chin: inflammation of the tissues; pain on the chin; lateral neck opposite.
Hand: external side of thumb. Forearm: flexor and pronator muscles (cubital nerves). Wrist: cubital.
Knee: great toe, same side.

SI-6 *yanglao* — help for the aged

Lower forearm: palm up (in supination); ulnar edge; two FW above the wrist. A little above the head of the ulna; between the anterior edge of the ulna and the flexor carpi ulnaris muscle. In the angle between the flexor carpi ulnaris and the inferior edge of a transverse mass; in a hollow.

Separated by the ulnar prominence from *yanggu* (SI-5); two large FW below *zhizheng* (SI-7); one FW superior and medial to *zhigou* (TW-6).

When tonified:

Tonifies opposite small intestines and large intestine, opposite eye, eyelid, opposite ear, opposite inferior occipital lobe, upper limb, cubital nerve, opposite joint of the lower limb.
Disperses liver, kidney.
Dispersing acts in the opposite way.

Direct effects:

Opposite eye: vision easily tired, vision darkened; congestion of the eyeball; opposite eyelids, inflammation; opposite ear.

Contrary effects:

Opposite kidney (reabsorption and excretion), reabsorption in excess: tonify; too relaxed: disperse.

Parts of the body:

Upper limb: cubital and posterior internal side, cubital nerve; pain, contracture or flaccidity; hand cannot be lifted up, flexed; contracture or flaccidity; flexors, pronators; acts on the extensor carpi ulnaris muscle; thumb, same side.
Articulations of the opposite lower limb, great toe same side.

SI-7   *zhizheng* — correct limb

Forearm: palm up, in supination; on the ulnar edge; four FW above the wrist. Between the anterior edge of the ulna and the flexor carpi ulnaris; in the angle between the flexor carpi ulnaris and the upper edge of a transverse mass; in a hollow.

Two large FW proximal to *yanglao* (SI-6); two FW distal to *xiaohai* (SI-8); separated by the flat surface of the ulna from *sanyangluo* (TW-8).

When tonified:
> Tonifies the small intestine, opposite mid-brain, opposite mid-height of the spinal cord; half-body, same side; hand, fingers.
> Disperses the heart.
> Dispersing acts in the opposite way.

Direct effects:
> Passage point between small intestine and heart (*tongli,* HT-5, to the small intestine). If excess: painful or contracted articulations; if insufficient: sties or warts.
> Recoil of [energy from intense] feelings. From shock: emptiness, fear, emotional agitation, depression, sorrow, regrets. Debilitating decline of the nerves and brain. Hyperexcited apprehension, hyperexcited speech.
> Florid diabetes (likes to eat, gets fat, thirsty): tonify.
> Sties (on the eyelid), opposite: tonify. Face: miliary, little white pimples, opposite: tonify; warts: tonify.
> Face easily congested: becomes red easily.

Parts of the body:
> Jaw and under the chin, opposite, (swelling, pains).
> All stiff or contracted articulations, pain or spasms: disperse.
> Posterior shoulder and upper limb (weakness).
> Hand does not tighten, pain or contracture: disperse. Fingers: articulations (swelling, acute pain, either contracture or flaccidity): disperse.

SI-8   *xiaohai* — small sea

Mid-length of the forearm: ulnar edge; palm up, in supination. Between the anterior edge of the ulna and the flexor carpi ulnaris and the superior edge of a transverse mass; in a hollow.

Two FW above *zhizheng* (SI-7); following point: *jianzhen* (SI-9); separated from *sidu* (TW-9) by the dorsal width of the bone.

When tonified:
> Tonifies the small intestine, medulla oblongata, spinal cord; opposite lateral eye; dorsal hand and finger-muscles.
> Disperses the liver.
> Dispersing acts in the opposite way.

Direct effects:
> Disperses the small intestine (pains, spasms of the central abdomen opposite); stomach painful from one to two hours after eating, excess of the governor vessel, excess nervous commands, force, etc.
> Agitated insanity.
> Chorea (agitating neuritis, tics, trembling).
> Epilepsy (bleating, tongue out)?
> Eyes: opposite internal corner; opposite ear: lobes.
> Mouth and tongue opposite side: inflammation; opposite gums: swelling.
> Opposite teeth: caries, inflammation, loose teeth; jaw and under the chin: swelling (dental fluxion); upper and lower jaw: pain.
> Heart: all troubles; algid malaria.
> Pulmonary edema.
> Retention of water in the tissues?
> Swelling: itching, shivering.
> Swollen cervical lymph nodes; armpit: swollen nodes.

Parts of the body:
> Opposite lateral side of the neck; swelling or inflammation of the tissues; torticollis, spasms or contracture.
> Posterior shoulder and posterior arm; all posterior muscles; extensors of the arm.

SI-9 *jianzhen* — true shoulder

Posterior shoulder: just under the inferior edge of the scapulohumeral articulation (glenoid fossa); in a hollow; on the superior edge of the teres minor.

On the inferior edge of the infraspinatus muscle; arm towards the other side of the body.

Preceding point: *xiaohai* (SI-8); four FW lateral and under *naoshu* (SI-10); four FW below and posterior to *jianliao* (TW-14); at the level of and medial to *xiaoluo* (TW-12).

When tonified:
> Tonifies the small intestine on the same side, gallbladder, posterior frontal lobes, longissimus dorsi to the lumbar area, posterior arm, glenoid articulation.
> Disperses the liver, heart.
> Dispersing acts in the opposite way.

Direct effects:
> Headache and pain of the chin?
> Opposite ear: buzzings? deafness?

Parts of the body:
> Arm cannot be put behind the back or lifted from the side. Teres minor: contracture or flaccidity. Scapulohumeral articulation: inflamed, rheumatism, ankylosis, pain.

SI-10 *naoshu* — ascent of the deltoid

Posterior shoulder: just at the upper edge of the articulation of the scapula and humerus (glenoid). On the upper edge of a muscle on an angle (infraspinatus); about one FW under the spine of the scapula.

Four FW posterior and above *jianzhen* (SI-9); two FW lateral to *tianzong* (SI-11); two FW below and lateral to *tianliao* (TW-15); three FW medial to *jianliao* (TW-14).

When tonified:
> Tonifies the small intestine same side, scapulohumeral articulation, deltoid, infraspinatus, posterior arm, gallbladder.
> Disperses the liver.

Parts of the body:
> Ear same side.
> Lateral opposite side of neck: swelling, pain.
> Scapula: swelling, inflammation (from cold?) pain.
> Scapulohumeral articulation inflamed, pain of the scapula and the posterior arm; arm without strength, numb.

SI-11 *tianzong* — heavenly ancestors

On the scapula: one FW under the inferior medial prominence of the transverse angle of the spine (of the scapula); in a hollow; on the infraspinatus. Two FW medial and under *naoshu* (SI-10); two FW lateral to *bingfeng* (SI-12); two large FW under *tianliao* (TW-15).

When tonified:
> Tonifies the small intestine, large intestine, stomach, lateral neck, upper shoulder extremity (circumflex?); jaw, same side.
> Disperses the liver.
> Dispersing acts in the opposite way.

Parts of the body:
> Jaw and chin: swelling, same side.
> Lateral side of neck and superior shoulder and extremity of the shoulder (circumflex nerve?) all the muscles, (trapezius, deltoid); cannot lift the arm or turn it backward: disperse. Disperses infraspinatus, teres major (which pull the arm down) with the latissimus dorsi.

SI-12   *chengfeng* (IS *bingfeng*) — to ride the wind

Scapula about mid-height: one FW lateral to the medial edge; one FW medial and inferior to the inferior medial prominence of a transverse rise (spine of the scapula); on the trapezius and infraspinatus; in a hollow.

Two FW medial to *tianzong* (SI-11); two FW below *quyuan* (SI-13); at the external level of *gaohuangshu* (BL-38, IS BL-43).

When tonified:

Tonifies the small intestine, posterior shoulder, scapulohumeral articulation, posterior, superior arm.

Disperses the liver.

Dispersing acts in the opposite way.

Effects and parts of the body:

Lateral nape, posterior shoulder, muscles of the scapula, scapulohumeral articulation, posterior shoulder: contracture or flaccidity, or pain, neuralgia, rheumatism.

SI-13   *quyuan* — curve of the wall

Posterior shoulder: on the superior edge of the scapula; about one-third medial. On the lateral edge of a penetrating angle of the bone (coracoid notch); in the angle of the posterior edge of the muscular insertion; on the trapezius and serratus anterior; on the inferior edge of the infraspinatus; in a hollow.

Two FW above *bingfeng* (SI-12); about four FW inferior and lateral to *jianwai* (SI-14); two FW medial to *tianliao* (TW-15); two FW lateral to *pohu* (BL-37, IS BL-42).

When tonified:

Tonifies the small intestine, large intestine, stomach, nape and posterior shoulder, upper arm, lateral part of back.

Disperses spleen-pancreas.

Dispersing acts in the opposite way.

Effects and parts of the body:

All muscles, nape, posterior shoulder, back on the same side, attachments of the posterior upper arm, radial forearm, thumb; lower limb, meridian of stomach and spleen-pancreas; pains; flaccidity or contracture; muscular rheumatism, general rheumatism.

SI-14   *jianwai* — outside the shoulder

Lateral base of the nape: one FW under the crest of the shoulder; in the angle between the inferior edge of the first rib and the lateral edge of the vertical muscles (iliocostal and levator scapulae muscles); in a hollow.

Four FW inferior and medial to *quyuan* (SI-13); two FW posterior to *jianzhong* (SI-15); one large FW superior and lateral to *fufen* (BL-36, IS BL-41); two FW lateral to *bailao* (GV-13, IS GV-14, *dazhui*) and slightly above *dazhu* (BL-11).

When tonified:

Tonifies the small intestine, bladder (lateral line of the back), lung, temporoparietal lobes, nape and posterior-superior shoulder, posterior arm.

Disperses the heart, liver.

Dispersing acts in the opposite way.

Effects and parts of the body:

Neck and nape: torticollis; pain or cold.

Cold from nape to posterior elbow.

All the muscles of the nape, posterior shoulder, posterior arm, scapula, back: pain, general muscular rheumatism (trapezius, latissimus dorsi, rhomboids, deltoids, triceps, extensors of the forearm on the arm, muscles of the scapula).

Eye: external corner? pleurisy?

SI-15   *jianzhong* — middle of the shoulder

Neck: posterolateral base; between the anterior edge of the trapezius and the posterior edge of the hard vertical muscle (scalenus posterior). At the level of the sixth cervical vertebra; towards the trapezius and the muscles which it covers (iliocostal and levator scapulae muscles); in a hollow.

Two FW ahead of *jianwai* (SI-14); mid-height from *tianchuang* (SI-16); one large FW medial to *jianjing* (GB-21).

When tonified:

Tonifies the small intestine, large intestine, lung, eyes, lateral neck, temporoparietal lobes, occipital lobes.
Disperses the heart, gallbladder, spleen-pancreas.
Dispersing acts in the opposite way.

Direct effects:

Eyes: weakened vision, tired, amblyopia, beginning of amaurosis; obscured vision; insufficient coordination of the two eyes (asynergy).
Ears: buzzing, throbbing and hissing.
Heart: respiratory passages, bronchitis, cough until spitting blood; dyspnea.

Parts of the body:

From the lateral neck to the scapula: contractions, pain or flaccidity (acts on the iliocostal and levator scapulae muscles).

SI-16   *tianchuang* — celestial window

Lateral side of neck: three FW under the prominence behind the ear (mastoid process); in the angle between the posterior edge of the large muscle on an angle towards the front (sternocleidomastoid), and deep, the splenius of the neck, and the inferior and posterior edge of a small round prominence of a deep transverse relief (lateral transverse process of the second cervical vertebra, the axis); in a hollow.

Two FW inferior and posterior to *tianrong* (SI-17); about four FW superior to *jianzhong* (SI-15); one FW inferior and anterior to *tianyou* (TW-16); two FW above *tianding* (LI-17); three FW below *yifeng* (TW-17).

When tonified:

Tonifies the small intestine, inferior frontal lobes, temporoparietal lobes, lateral eye and ear same side; posterior shoulder; upper scapula; anus.
Disperses the liver.
Dispersing acts in the opposite way.

Direct effects:

Lateral eye (external).
Ear: buzzing, pain or deafness.
Throat: cannot speak; difficult respiration.
Anus: oozing fistulas.

Parts of the body:

Face and head: swelling or pain from cold or wind; painful jaw.
Nape, posterior shoulder and upper scapula: torticollis, painful contracture.

SI-17   *tianrong* — celestial face

Upper lateral neck, a little behind the posterior, inferior angle of the maxilla; in the angle between the anterior edge of the prominence of the mastoid and the insertion on it of the sternocleidomastoideus; in a hollow.

Two FW superior and anterior to *tianchuang* (SI-16); one FW under *yifeng* (TW-17); following point: *quanliao* (SI-18); two FW behind neck-*futu* (LI-18).

When tonified:

Tonifies the small intestine, respiratory passages, inferior occipital lobes, opposite lateral side of eye on same side, throat, larynx.
Dispersing acts in the opposite way.

Direct effects:

Throat irritated ''like brambles,'' cannot speak without panting and cough; coldness, fever, chest full, cannot breathe.

Teeth: loose incisors, caries and pain of the incisors, swollen gums.

Swollen tongue (abscess of the lower face?).

Saliva, attacks of vomiting.

Ears: buzzing? deafness?

Awakens a response in the points commanding the blood: *gaohuangshu* (BL-38, IS BL-43) and *geshu* (BL-17).

Tumors? (adenitis?). Lateral neck swollen, pain, itching, abscess, tumors of the tongue, lower face.

Parts of the body:

Chest and back: contraction at the level of the scapula.

Spinal nerves.

SI-18   *quanliao* — palace of hearing

Cheek: on the anterior edge of the lobe, at the point where it is attached to the cheek; a bit under the lower bulge of the ear.

About two FW above *tianrong* (SI-17); point following: *tinggong* (SI-19); about one FW under *ermen* (TW-23, IS TW-21); one FW in front of *tinghui* (GB-2).

When tonified:

Tonifies the small intestine, bladder, separate, inferior frontal and temporoparietal lobes, inferior occipital lobes, ear, lateral eye, upper canines, masseter muscle, radial side of arm, arch, great toe, opposite throat (larynx).

Disperses the liver.

Dispersing acts in the opposite way.

Direct effects:

Ear: buzzings; continuous whistling or songs of cicada; wax, inflammation of the external canal; deafness.

Lateral side of eye: weakness, trachoma.

Throat (larynx): loss of voice, aphonia, hoarseness, noise in the larynx.

Upper teeth (canine): pain; maxilla; contracture, trismus.

Epigastrium: fullness, pain.

Parts of the body:

Posterior shoulder and radial arm (extensor and radial muscles); lateral side of the thumb: pain; dorsum of hand.

Arch, great toe (liver meridian).

♦ SI-19   *tinggong* — hollow of the cheek

Cheek; in the angle between the anterior edge of the vertical branch of the lower jaw and the superior edge of the large oblique muscle (masseter muscle); about three FW above the inferior edge of the maxilla.

Preceding point: *quanliao* (SI-18), on the lobe; one FW behind *ermen* (TW-23, IS TW-21).

The energy leaves the small intestine meridian here in order to pass into the bladder meridian at *jingming* (BL-1) at the internal corner of the eye through a branch which follows the lower eyelid.

When tonified:

Tonifies the small intestine, bladder, medulla and spinal cord, triple warmer, lower surface of the eyelid on the same side, canines, corner of the mouth.

Disperses the liver.

Dispersing acts in the opposite way.

Direct effects:

Eyes: unceasing blinking, lower eyelid.

Face: facial neuralgia (facial nerve), sensitivity of the upper canines and of the cheek bones and jaw, with swelling.

Face: facial paralysis (trigeminal nerve), mouth to the side, eyes shut badly, corners of the mouth falling from age or fatigue, curvature of the spine? opposite.

Chapter VII
Bladder

The bladder meridian commands the bladder, the sphincter of the bladder and the urethra, as well as the prostate in men.

It is unique in that its pathway follows along the back in two parallel lines which concern all the organs, including the bladder, indicating that the bladder has an action on all the organs. The lateral line branches at *tianzhu* (BL-10) and includes points which are almost all tonification points (*pohu*, BL-37, IS BL-42; *gaohuangshu* BL-38, IS BL-43; *yixi* BL-40, IS BL-45, etc.). The medial line, on the other hand, which branches at *dazhu* (BL-11), contains only dispersal points: all the names end with the word *shu,* which means ''assent.'' Each one corrects the excess of a particular organ, accompanied by fever or hyperexcitation, and provoked by external elements: wind, heat, cold, etc.

Thus we may consider the meridian of the bladder as having power over all the organs. In addition, it acts on the blood (*gaohuangshu* BL-38, IS BL-43), the parasympathetic (*tianzhu* BL-10), pains (*kunlun* BL-60), the eyes (*jingming* BL-1; *zanzhu* BL-2; *yuzhen* BL-9), the internal and external automatic smooth muscles (*chengshan* BL-57), intestinal worms (*zhiyin* BL-67) and the energy of yang daytime activity (*shenmai* BL-62), and thus sleep.

Finally, the bladder, aside from its role as a reservoir, seems to act by stimulating the production of urine by the kidneys and by stimulating the erection of the penis and clitoris.

For the two lines of the back, tradition follows the enumeration first through the medial line (the assent points), and then through the lateral line.

The meridian (supreme yang of the foot) is a yang producer of energy. Its maximum is at 4 p.m. solar time (minimum hour of the lungs). Its minimum is at 4 a.m. (maximum hour of the lungs). The upstream meridian (mother) is the small intestine; that downstream (child) is the kidney; the wife is the triple warmer.

The tonification point is *zhiyin* (BL-67 and last); the source point is *jinggu* (BL-64); the dispersal point: *shugu* (BL-65); the assent point is *pangguangshu* (BL-28); the herald point on the abdomen is *zhongji* (CV-3).

Tonifying the small intestine increases the urine; dispersing it decreases the urine.

Tonifying the bladder fortifies and contracts the expulsor muscles and relaxes the sphincter. Dispersing the bladder relaxes the expulsor muscles and tightens the bladder sphincter.

BL-1   *jingming* — clarity of the pupils

Anterior cheek: one small FW under the medial corner of the eye; on the inferior edge of the flat bulge of the orbital arch; in the angle of the medial edge of the insertion of the elevator of the upper lip; in a hollow. Lateral and superior to the levator communalis of the upper lip and the wings of the nose.

Three FW under *zanzhu* (BL-2); one FW medial to *chengqi* (ST-4, IS ST-1); four FW medial to *tinggong* (SI-19); one large FW above *yingxiang* (LI-20). The point receives a branch coming from the small intestine (*tinggong,* SI-19). Another, coming from the large intestine (*yingxiang,* LI-20), crosses it in order to go to *touwei* (ST-1, IS ST-8) through *zanzhu* (BL-2) and *yuyao* (MP-4, IS M-HN-6).

Tradition describes it as the reunion of the bladder, stomach, small intestine, *yangqiao* (chain of the yang) and *yinqiao* (chain of the yin).

When tonified:
   Tonifies the bladder, opposite eye (mostly the retina), small intestine, large intestine, inferior occipital lobe and also all yang meridians.
   Disperses all yin meridians, particularly the lungs.
   Dispersing acts in the opposite way.

Direct effects:
   Opposite eye: all troubles of vision, eyeball, eyelid, mostly from excess or insufficiency of blood, ''the bladder meridian has much blood and little energy''; disperses the bladder and stomach and the eyes.
   Vision becoming unclear: cannot see in darkness (contracted iris?) does not see anymore: disperse. Distance vision not clear (contracted iris?): disperse. Inflammation of the retina: disperse; cataract, pupils covered with a veil.
   Redness and pain of the medial corner of the eyeball, red eye, with veil; photophobia; inflammation of the cornea (keratitis). Children: eyes with growths, a veil of flesh from medial area to corner (pterygium).
   Inflammation of the eyelids (conjunctivitis), tears, itching; conjunctivitis in babies (blenorrhagic?).
   Hates the cold; congestive headaches, fainting.

BL-2   *zanzhu* — tight bamboo

Eyebrows: one half FW on either side of the median line; in the angle between the lower edge of the crest of the arch of the eyebrow and the lateral edge of the suture of the nasal bone and frontal bone; in a hollow.

One half FW on either side and a bit under *yintang* (GV-23a, IS M-HN-3).

Three FW above *jingming* (BL-1); following point: *meichong* (BL-3) above the forehead; two large FW medial to *yuyao* (MP-4, IS M-HN-6).

When tonified:

Tonifies the bladder, all yang meridians, eye, ear, teeth and tongue on the same side; lateral knee; opposite inferior occipital lobes; anus.

Disperses the lungs; all yin meridians.

Dispersing acts in the opposite way.

Direct effects:

Hyperexcited mind, nightmares, hallucinations; or serious depression to the point of loss of consciousness.

Sneezing when in light or wind.

Acidity of all the secretions (particularly the right point), sour body odor, loose teeth, gums: inflammation.

Eye: the vision clears after three sessions; weak vision (amblyopia), sees everything unclearly (weakness of the iris, which stays open); obscured vision, does not see without strong light (contracted iris); cataract.

Lateral muscles on the same side; medial on the opposite side; convergent strabismus; coordination (synergy) of the eyes, red and painful eyes, inflammation of the cornea; nystagmus.

Eyelids: inflammation, conjunctivitis, excess tears, blinking, cannot sleep; blepharitis, trachoma; ophthalmia of the newborn.

Ear: diminished hearing or buzzing from acidity of the secretions.

Kidneys: albumin during pregnancy; Bright's disease?

Intestines: colic with fetid wind; contracted anus?

Rapidly spreading ulcer?

Parts of the body:

Headaches in the area of the eyebrows; between the eyebrows.

Face: pain, tongue, teeth, jaw.

Point of Weihe: Right: Magnesia Carb.

Left: Mercurius Corr.

BL-3   *meichong* — attack on the eyebrows

Top of the forehead: one FW on either side of the medial line; at the posterior edge of the protuberance of the frontal bone at the average hairline (superior edge of the insertion of the frontal muscle).

On the lateral edge of the median vertical rise.

One FW on either side of *shenting* (GV-23, IS GV-24); preceding point: *zanzhu* (BL-2, on the eyebrow); two FW in front of *qucha* (BL-4); two tightened FW above and medial to head-*linqi* (GB-11, IS GB-15); three FW medial to *muchuang* (GB-12, IS GB-16).

When tonified:

Tonifies the bladder, large intestine, back of the eye, maxillary sinus, ear.

Disperses the lungs.

Dispersing acts in the opposite way.

Direct effects:

Internal headaches, blocked nose, particularly maxillary sinusitis.

All varieties of epilepsy?

Frontal muscles.

BL-4   *qucha* — minister of the curve

Anterior skull: about one FW on either side of the medial line; two tightened FW in front of the posterior (superior) edge of the frontal bone. About mid-distance between the posterior edge of the frontal bone and the transverse rise of the upper insertion of the frontal muscle; in the angle of the lateral edge of the longitudinal rise; in a hollow; on the posterior edge of a slight flat (transverse) rise.

Two FW posterior to *meichong* (BL-3); two FW anterior to *wuchu* (BL-5); two large FW medial and anterior to *muchuang* (GB-12, IS GB-16); one large FW lateral to *shangxing* (GV-22, IS GV-23).

When tonified:
> Tonifies the bladder, large intestine, inferior spinal cord and lumbar area, temporal-parietal lobes, same side, eye same side, ear, frontal sinuses, half of head and body, limbs same side.
> Disperses the kidneys.

Direct effects:
> Eye: weak vision (amblyopia); foggy vision.
> Nose: coryza; greasy inflammation of the nose, blocked nose? bleeding of the nose, abscess of the nose.
> Enlarged and fat heart?

Parts of the body:
> Body: heat, agitation; burning heat attacking the top of the head, pain and swelling at the top of the head; congestive headache.
> Face: paralysis, particularly of the frontal muscle, facial neuralgia.
> Head and nape: pain.

BL-5   *wuchu* — five places

Head: in the angle between the posterior edge of the parietal-frontal suture and the longitudinal rise at about one large FW on either side of the medial line; in a hollow.

Two FW posterior to *qucha* (BL-4); one large FW anterior to *chengguang* (BL-6); one large FW on each side of *xinhui* (GV-21, IS GV-22); one large FW medial to *muchuang* (GB-12, IS GB-16).

When tonified:
> Tonifies the bladder, superior posterior frontal lobes, eye and cheekbone, incisors same side, opposite inferior limb, mostly the knee, liver.
> Disperses the lungs, gallbladder.
> Dispersing acts in the opposite way.

Direct effects:
> Epilepsy, eyes lifted; loss of consciousness, does not recognize anybody.
> Eye: diminished vision, not clear; eyes lifted?
> Upper teeth, mostly incisors, canines.
> Stomach: burning, fullness. When tonified, disperses the gallbladder and tonifies the liver.

Parts of the body:
> Posterior shoulder at the superior medial angle of the scapula.
> Cervical vertebrae and upper thoracics: stiffness or pain on the same side.

BL-6   *chengguang* — receives light

Head: top (vertex); one large FW on either side of the medial line; one large FW posterior to the frontal-parietal suture; about two FW in front of the occipital-parietal suture; in a hollow.

One large FW posterior to *wuchu* (BL-5); one FW in front of *tongtian* (BL-7); two FW medial to *zhengying* (GB-13, IS GB-17); one FW lateral and anterior to *qianding* (GV-20, IS GV-21).

When tonified:
> Tonifies the bladder, lateral eye same side, posterior cheek, nostrils, anterior deltoid, upper shoulder, inferior occipital lobe.
> Disperses the small intestine and large intestine.
> Dispersing acts in the opposite way.

Direct effects:
> Dizziness, vertigo after shock; internal headaches.
> Eye: darkened vision; cataract; keratitis.
> Nose: clear, abundant discharge; or loss of smell, blocked nose.

Parts of the body:
> Mouth awry; lateral cheek bone.
> Anterior deltoid, upper shoulder.

BL-7 *tongtian* — communicates with the sky

Head: top (vertex); one FW on either side of the median line; one large FW anterior to the occipital-parietal suture; two large FW posterior to the frontal-parietal suture; in a hollow.

One FW posterior to *chengguang* (BL-6); one large FW anterior to *luoque* (BL-8); one FW lateral and posterior to *qianding* (GV-20, IS GV-21); two FW medial to *chengling* (GB-14, IS GB-18).

When tonified:

Tonifies the bladder, opposite inferior occipital lobe, anterior lower limb same side, anterior deltoid, nostrils, trachea, upper bronchus, lateral side of eye.
Disperses the large intestine.
Dispersing acts in the opposite way.

Direct effects:

Darkened and weak vision.
Hearing weak?
Nose: coryza with clear and abundant discharge, blocked nose, loss of smell, fissure of the nose, abscess of the nose.
Bronchus: chronic bronchitis; panting but breathes without exertion?
Hypertension, headache from bending forwards or standing up suddenly, to the point of vertigo and loss of consciousness.

Parts of the body:

Face: facial paralysis, contracture of all the muscles of the mouth, flaccidity of the same; facial neuralgia, pain at the cheekbone.
Tumors?

BL-8 *luoque* — track of the veins

Head, summit, posterior and a little lateral; one large FW to each side of the median line. Just anterior to the occipital-parietal suture, on the parietal bone, on the medial edge of a small bony protuberance; in a hollow.

One large FW posterior to *tongtian* (BL-7); following point: *yuzhen* (BL-9) at the lateral, posterior tuberosity; one large FW on each side of *baihui* (GV-19, IS GV-20); two large FW medial to *chengling* (GB-14, IS GB-18).

When tonified:

Tonifies the bladder, temporal-parietal and posterior frontal lobes, muscles of the lateral neck and the nape to the scapula, posterior shoulder, posterior upper limb, knee, ear, eye, same side.
Disperses the lungs.
Dispersing acts in the opposite way.
Repression of worries; delusions, lack of animation; depression, dizzy head; or hyperexcitation, escapades, mad walking; illness of the vitality.
Blind pupil? internal veil; sees nothing; everything seems badly lit.
Buzzing? deafness?
Swollen abdomen, fullness, cannot breathe.

Parts of the body:

Lateral neck and nape to the scapula: all muscles.
Posterior shoulder, upper limb, posterior side.
Anterior knee, inferior thigh, upper part of lower leg.

BL-9 *yuzhen* — pillow of jade

Lower occiput: two FW above the inferior edge of the skull; two FW from the median line; in the angle between the inferior edge of a flat, transverse rise and the posterior (medial) edge of a flat rise; in a hollow.

Preceding point: *luoque* (BL-8) at the occipital-parietal suture; point following: *tianzhu* (BL-10); two large FW medial to *naokong* (GB-19).

When tonified:

Tonifies the bladder, inferior occipital lobes, eye, canines, same side; nose, posterior shoulder, posterior upper limb.

Disperses the lungs.

Dispersing acts in the opposite way.

Direct effects:

All pain of the eye, ocular neuralgia; eyes as if torn out, sharp pain in the eye if one suddenly stands, bends, or extends; cannot bear the cold or the wind? (in the eyes). Headaches from contraction of the ocular vessels, going to the interior of the head with unbearable pain.

Myopia?

Heavy head from lack of sleep; pain from cold in half of the head, pain at the top of the head; pain at the back of the head (occipital neuralgia).

Facial neuralgia; cheek, middle branch of the trigeminal nerve.

Nose: blocked, or smells nothing.

Abundant perspiration: disperse; not coming: tonify.

Writer's cramp?

Parts of the body:

Muscles of the nape: trapezius, trachelomastoid, splenius of the head, posterior scalenius.

BL-10   *tianzhu* — celestial column

Nape: two FW from the median line; one FW above the inferior edge of the cranium; in the angle between the posterior (medial) edge of the superimposed insertions of the trapezius and the trachelomastoid muscle and of the deep lower edge of a bony rise; in a hollow.

Two FW under *yuzhen* (BL-9); five FW above *dazhu* (BL-11); separated by the trapezius from *fengchi* (GB-20); about six FW superior and slightly medial to *fengmen* (BL-12); six FW superior and medial to *fufen* (BL-36, IS BL-41).

From this point, the lateral line of the bladder meridian separates and descends through *fufen* (BL-36, IS BL-41) on the vertical of the medial edge of the scapula, until *chengfu* (BL-50, IS BL-36); it laterally parallels the direct line of the assent points, which rejoins it at *chengfu* (BL-50, IS BL-36). The medial line descends from *dazhu* (BL-11).

When tonified:

Tonifies the parasympathetic system (cold, perspiration, pupils contracted, arteries) all the yang producer organs (superficial pulses); anterior mid-brain, radial nerve, conception vessel, opposite half of the body and abdominal organs.

Disperses the heart, governor vessel and half body same side.

Dispersing acts in the opposite way.

Direct effects:

Cold: sweat, at the palms, etc.: disperse; heat, dryness: tonify.

Parasympathetic system (vagus nerve, glossopharyngeal nerve, connective nerves), pulse of the vessels and all the yang pulses: excess: disperse; insufficiency: tonify.

Glossopharyngeal nerve: tongue, sensitivity and vasodilation; larynx, motor function; saliva in excess: disperse.

Parasympathetic: vessels and all yang producer organs (stomach, two intestines, bladder, gallbladder).

Tongue: motor function and vasoconstriction (parasympathetic), sensitivity and vasodilation (glossopharyngeal nerve).

Glosso-labio-pharyngeal paralysis.

Throat, larynx and pharynx: sensitivity and motor function. Contractions or inflammations: disperse; weakness: tonify; blocked nose, mouth open: disperse; weak nerves, chilled from the emotions: disperse; insomnia: disperse; vertigo from heights (legs soft, foggy, sudden weakness): disperse; perspiring palms from emotions: disperse.

Eyes: contracted pupils (miosis): disperse.

Ears: weakened hearing from inflamed eustachian tubes: disperse. Contracted arteries (coronary arteries relaxed): disperse. Coronaries contracted, arteries supple; aorta too strong: disperse; hypertension: disperse.

Heart slow, contracted, arrhythmic, unequal: disperse.

Blood too fluid, slow coagulation, slow healing: tonify.

Contracted bronchus, spasms, asthma: disperse.

Contracted esophagus and cardiac sphincter, food does not descend: disperse.

Contracted stomach (cramps, spasms, pain, dreams, nightmares): disperse.

Liver, spleen-pancreas, kidney, lung: insufficiently dilated; disperse.

Bladder: expulsor muscles contracted, sphincter relaxed: disperse; expulsor muscles relaxed, sphincter contracted: tonify.

Large intestine contracted, anal sphincter relaxed: disperse (spasmodic constipation).

Large intestine relaxed, sphincter contracted: tonify (atonic constipation).

Small intestine in excess: disperse; insufficient: tonify.

Genital system in excess, sexual hyperexcitation: disperse. Women: ovaries in excess, menses too abundant, too long or frequent, neck of the uterus stays open: disperse; ulvary pruritis. Men: from hyperexcitation, non-erection, inhibited testicles: disperse.

Parts of the body:

Skin: wet from emotions, palms soaked: disperse.

Nape: stiffness, pain, cannot turn the head, spasms; writer's cramps?

Arch of the foot: motor problems.

BL-11 *dazhu* — great shuttle

Upper back: one small FW from the angle of the inferior lateral edge of the first thoracic vertebra (the seventh cervical being the most prominent), on the lower edge of the first rib; in a hollow; between two vertical muscles. The flow descends along the medial line (of the assent points) towards *fengmen* (BL-12).

Five FW below *tianzhu* (BL-10); two FW medial and superior to *fengmen* (BL-12); three large FW medial to *fufen* (BL-36, IS BL-41); one FW lateral and below *bailao* (GV-13, IS GV-14, *dazhui*); one large FW medial and above *taodao* (GV-12, IS GV-13); two tightened FW below *jianwai* (SI-14).

When tonified:

Tonifies the yin distributor organs (deep pulses), medulla oblongata, spinal cord, thoracic spine, all the bones; governor vessel, eye same side, opposite breast, eyebrow, opposite; responds to *qubin* (GB-7) opposite.

Disperses the bladder, triple warmer, gallbladder, governor vessel.

Dispersing acts in the opposite way.

Passage point between the governor and conception vessels. When tonified, tonifies conception vessel and disperses governor vessel; dispersing does the opposite.

Reunion of the bones: all their troubles. Vertebrae: pains, abscess, Pott's disease, vertebral rheumatism, bony tuberculosis.

Direct effects:

All opposite articulations: pain, inflammation, rheumatism — hip, knee, shoulder, arm, etc.

Weakness to the point of paralysis, bruised, cannot remain standing for long; malaise, feels badly treated, nervous spasms, nervous agitation, contractions, shivering, headache; or insanity with contracted muscles; body twisted, dizziness, massive contractures.

Prolonged fever from shock or suppression; tertiary fever, vertigo. Eye same side; ciliary muscles (affecting shape of lens for visual accommodation of distant objects); ciliary neuralgia.

Acts on the yin organs.

Cough, bronchitis, pulmonary tuberculosis.

Parts of the body:

Nape, lateral neck, posterior shoulder, arm; can neither bend nor lift the head; spasms from the nape to scapula; sensation of cold in the shoulder and back; lumbar muscles: contracture opposite side; can neither bend nor straighten?

Point of Weihe: Phellandrium Aquaticum. Bronchitis, emphysema, walking causes fatigue; eyes: ciliary neuralgia, pain and burns at the temples and above the eyes; photophobia; breasts: pain at the nipple, at the lacteal vessels spreading to the back.

BL-12 *fengmen* — door of wind (neuralgia)

Upper back: about two FW on each side of the first cervical vertebra; in the angle between the inferior edge of the second rib and the medial edge of a vertical muscle (iliocostalis); on the edge of the rhomboids; in a hollow.

Two FW lateral and inferior to *dazhu* (BL-11); two FW medial and superior to *feishu* (BL-13); two FW inferior and lateral to *jianwai* (SI-14).

The flow comes from *dazhu* (BL-11).

When tonified:

Tonifies the bladder, large intestine, anterior mid-brain (parasympathetic), eye same side, back.

Disperses the lungs.
Dispersing acts in the opposite way.

Direct effects:

Likes to sleep.

All heat of the yang (upper body, skin, lung, etc.): puncture often.

Easily troubled by cold; preventive for influenza; trouble of the respiratory passages. Nose: colds, sneezing often: disperse deeply; cough: cough from cold to the point of stomach troubles, short breath, whooping-cough, hay fever (heat of chest, cannot expand), bronchitis, pleurisy, pneumonia, pulmonary tuberculosis.

Eye: congestion or hemorrhage of the retina of the vitreous body.

Parts of the body:

Head and brain: heat, headache after drinking.

Head (top) and nape: stiffness.

Acne, particularly on shoulder and back; abscess on the back: puncture frequently.

Point of Weihe: Millefolium. Hemophilia; all external or internal hemorrhage; troubles from arrested menses; varicose pain during pregnancy.

BL-13   *feishu* — assent of the lungs

Upper back: mid-distance from the upper medial point of the scapula to the spinal cord (third thoracic); between two vertical muscles (iliocostalis, longissimus dorsi); on the inferior edge of the third rib; on the upper edge of the rhomboid; in a hollow.

Two FW under *fengmen* (BL-12); two FW above *jueyinshu* (BL-14); two FW lateral to *shenzhu* (GV-11, IS GV-12); two FW medial to *pohu* (BL-37, IS BL-42).

When tonified:

Tonifies the bladder, stomach, skin, mouth.

Disperses the respiratory passages, liver.

Dispersing acts in the opposite way.

Direct effects:

Blinding boredom; desires to kill himself.

Assent point of the lungs (troubles from external action with fever or hyperexcitation). All inflammation of respiratory passages: cough, mucus, whooping cough, bronchitis, pleurisy, pneumonia, pulmonary congestion, abscess of the lungs, tuberculosis: panting, spits, blood, fever, perspiration; asthma, spasm paralyzing the lungs. Heart: endocarditis; pericarditis?

Vomiting, vomits water after meals; reactions to poisons; gastritis of drinkers or gout sufferers? Babies: nutritional problems. Thrush.

Mouth: inflammation, dry mouth and tongue, no appetite.

Jaundice?

Parts of the body:

Skin: pain, itching (pruritis), tumors.

Lumbar area: pain?

Point of Weihe: Antimonium Tartaricum. All problems of the respiratory passages; gastritis in cases of gout or alcohol intoxication; white tongue with red sides and center; worms; urinary problems; debility; violent pain of the lumbar and sacral areas.

BL-14   *jueyinshu* — assent of the least yin

Back: mid-distance from the thoracic spine to the scapula at the level of the inferior edge of its crest; between two vertical muscles (iliocostalis and longissimus dorsi); on the inferior edge of the fourth rib; on the trapezius and rhomboid; in a hollow.

Two FW under *feishu* (BL-13); two FW above *xinshu* (BL-15); two FW medial to *gaohuangshu* (BL-38, IS BL-43).

When tonified:

Tonifies the bladder, lungs, vessels.

Dispersing acts in the opposite way.

Assent point of the vessels (troubles from external action with fever or hyperexcitation).

Direct effects:

Malaise from the sun, from heat; nosebleeds.

Heart: troubles or pains; stays contracted with agitation and malaise; heart enlarged and fat? pericarditis; internal agitation on the seventh day of typhoid?

Altitude sickness; fits of vomiting.

Teeth: molars, acute pain.

Respiratory passages: all troubles; coughing fits with fullness of the chest; emphysema, pneumonia.

Herpes of the vulva or prepuce?

Point of Weihe: Right: Agaricus (Amanita). Loquacity and indifference; chorea; trembling and agitation; incessant movement of the head; nosebleeds of old people; vertigo from the sun; oppressed intermittent heart with red face; violent cough; beginning of phthisis; stomach and intestinal gas; frequent, urgent needs to urinate; sexual excitation.

Left: Robinia (yellow locust). Acidity of fluids; acidity of the stomach with frontal headache; acid vomiting; too rapid digestion of the albuminoids; acid discharge and blood between menses; herpes of the vagina or vulva; nymphomania.

BL-15   *xinshu* — assent of the heart

Back: at the level of the upper third from the spine of the scapula to its lower point; mid-distance from the scapula to the thoracic spine; between two vertical muscles (iliocostalis, longissimus dorsi); just at the inferior edge of the fifth rib; in a hollow; on the trapezius and rhomboid.

Two FW under *jueyinshu* (BL-14); two FW above *dushu* (BL-16); at about the level of *shendao* (GV-10, IS GV-11), about two FW medial to *shentang* (BL-39, IS BL-44).

When tonified:

Tonifies the bladder.

Disperses the heart, lungs, brain, skin.

Dispersing acts in the opposite way.

Direct effects:

Loss of memory; fear; cries when talking of his unhappiness; dreams of dead people; overwhelmed by melancholy; delusions; convulsion (or epileptic fit?), scarlet lips, walks rapidly; muteness. Children not talking until several years old; all emptiness of yin or yang from youth; cold panics at interviews or examinations.

Assent point of the heart. Troubles from external excitation with fever or hyperexcitation; master point of heart troubles (from excess contraction with mental troubles); heart pain extending to the chest and back; congestion of the heart? When one lies down, he can not get up, sweats; heart distended; endocarditis; apoplexy; contracted heart: one hundred moxas.

Eyes: one pupil dilated, the other contracted; blinking, troubled vision.

Jaundice: yellow face, cannot taste food; vomiting.

Incisors: pains. Esophagus: spasms, contractions, hematemesis.

Nosebleeds; coughs and spits blood, beginning of tuberculosis, old tuberculosis: one moxa per year of age.

Skin: acne, abscess; eruptions of measles and scarlet fever.

All troubles with trembling, contractions of fingers and toes, of throat.

Point of Weihe: Gelsemium. Troubles with trembling; trembling of the four limbs, spasms, convulsions, contraction of fingers or toes; one pupil dilated, the other contracted; troubles of vision and vertigo; buzzing; troubles from sudden emotion or at examinations; or, when appearing in public, loss of means of expression; insomnia; frequent and abundant urine; spasms of throat, uvula, hoarseness; lassitude, heart on the point of stopping, fatigue with trembling; develops eruptions in measles; acute pains of the muscles; catalepsy; pains of muscles of nape and back; scarlet fever.

BL-16   *dushu* — general assent point

Back: three FW above the inferior point of the scapula; mid-distance from the scapula to the thoracic spine; between two vertical muscles (iliocostalis, longissimus dorsi); on the inferior edge of the sixth rib; in a hollow.

Two FW under *xinshu* (BL-15); two FW above *geshu* (BL-17); about two FW on either side of *lingtai* (GV-9, IS GV-10); two FW medial to *yixi* (BL-40, IS BL-45).

When tonified:

Tonifies the bladder, ribs and sides, stomach, abdomen.

Disperses the heart, sexual organs.

Dispersing acts in the contrary way.

Direct effects:
    General vitality; troubles of energy, counterflow of energy (nervous fits).
    Heart: pain; cold and warmth going and coming? endocarditis, pericarditis.
    Stomach: all trouble; cramps of the stomach.
    Abdomen: loud noises (aerocolia), pain.
    Ribs and side: pain.

BL-17   *geshu* — assent of the diaphragm

Back: about two FW from each side of the thoracic spine (sixth and seventh ribs); at the level of one FW above the inferior point of the scapula; mid-distance from the scapula to the vertebral column; between two vertical muscles (iliocostalis and longissimus dorsi); at the lower edge of the seventh rib; in a hollow.

Two FW under *dushu* (BL-16); four FW above *ganshu* (BL-18); about two FW on either side of *zhiyang* (GV-8, IS GV-9); two FW medial to *geguan* (BL-41, IS BL-46).

When tonified:
    Tonifies the bladder, heart, sternum, temporal-parietal lobes, stomach.
    Disperses the triple warmer, lungs.
    Responds to *xuanzhong* (GB-39), *gaohuangshu* (BL-38, IS BL-43) and thigh-*futu* (ST-32).
    Dispersing acts in the opposite way.

Direct effects:
    Desire to rest and not talk.
    Reunion of blood. All trouble of blood; syphilitic troubles: tabes, bubo, excrescences?
    Heart: all trouble; endocarditis, pain, heart enlarged and fat, angina of chest; digestion blocked, rising pain, weak heart; prevents paralysis of the heart.
    Vomits and sweats: contracted esophagus; stomach: pain and swelling, inflammation of the stomach; does not assimilate; blocked digestion; cold and mucus in the stomach; nutritional troubles; ulcers; stomach fevers, cannot eat; stomach cancer.
    Intestines: inflammation, intestinal hemorrhages.
    Swollen throat: loss of voice.
    Cough and panting after meals; asthma, bronchitis, pleurisy.

Parts of the body:
    The whole body constantly wet, sweats without reason, sweats at night; weakness of the four limbs.
    Bone: cold and heat; bony tuberculosis.
    Generalized rheumatism; shoulder and back stiff, can neither bend or straighten; heaviness and fullness of the limbs; stiffness or spasms of the head and nape?
    Painful swellings of the body; swelling from emptiness; swelling of the ankle and foot.

Point of Weihe: Phytolacca. Blood diseases; syphilitic eruptions, bubos, birthmarks, warts, pains of tabes; painful induration of testicles, pain of the penis, swollen glands; fibroid tissues; bleeding mouth, swollen throat, loss of voice without a sound; diphtheria; stabbing pains in the eyes from swallowing; mumps; sand under the eyelids; weak heart from age; feeble urination; two frequent and too abundant menses; chronic rheumatism, back stiff; pain at the heel; feet or ankles swollen; obesity.

BL-18   *ganshu* — assent of the liver

Back: one large FW under the inferior angle of the scapula; about mid-distance from the scapula to the thoracic spine; between two vertical muscles (iliocostalis and longissimus dorsi); at the lower edge of the ninth rib; in a hollow.

Four FW below *geshu* (BL-17); two FW above *danshu* (BL-19), about two FW lateral to *jinsuo* (GV-7, IS GV-8) on the tenth thoracic vertebra; two FW medial to *hunmen* (BL-42, IS BL-47).

When tonified:
    Tonifies the bladder, eyebrows, shoulder, sides, temporal-parietal lobes.
    Disperses the liver.
    Dispersing acts in the opposite way.

Direct effects:
    A lot of discontent and sadness, ''ruminates on his misfortunes,'' vertigo, little energy. Or hyperexcitation from emotion; hysteria, bends backwards; weakness, vertigo after illnesses from fever.

Assent point of the liver (troubles from external excitation with fever or hyperexcitation). Black around the eyes and even to the forehead; congestion of the liver, jaundice.

Stomach: chronic illnesses; eats without digesting; cramps of the stomach; distention; hematemesis?

Duodenum: troubles, or worms; intestinal hemorrhage.

Eyes: obscured vision as if at dusk; cold tears flowing.

Preventive for flu.

Sexual organs: puerperal fever; vagina: contracture, also of the muscles of the leg with pain in the lower pelvis and cold or hot convulsions?

In the nose: acidity, irritation; bronchitis: cough, pain on the side, contractions to the point of not breathing; hemoptysis.

Pain at the eyebrow.

Shoulder: acute pain; sides: acute pain extending to the vertebrae; turned, cannot return to the front.

Point of Weihe: Chenopodium.

BL-19   *danshu* — assent of the gallbladder

Back: four FW under the lower angle of the scapula; between two vertical muscles (iliocostalis and longissimus dorsi); at the lower edge of the tenth rib; in a hollow; on the latissimus dorsi.

Two FW under *ganshu* (BL-18); two FW above *pishu* (BL-20); two FW medial to *yanggang* (BL-43, IS BL-48); two large FW on either side of *zhongshu* (GV-6a, IS GV-7).

When tonified:

Tonifies the bladder, liver, temporal-parietal lobes, axilla.

Disperses the gallbladder, small intestine.

Dispersing acts in the opposite way.

Direct effects:

Assent point of the gallbladder (problems from external excitation with fever or hyperexcitation). Excess vesicules, dry or bitter mouth and nausea in the morning, migraine, outbreaks on the skin, or asthma, particularly in the morning; jaundice, yellow eyes, jaundice from alcohol; pains at the pharynx; contracted esophagus, food not descending, not digested.

Heart: fullness, swelling; hypertension.

Respiratory passages: bad cold, fever, headache, sore throat, mucus, little energy and breath; fear of stretching, cannot rest; internal chest painful, mostly the sides; pleurisy, tuberculosis, fever.

Bone: tuberculosis.

Axilla: swelling and inflammation of the lymph nodes (adenitis).

Face becoming red and blotched.

BL-20   *pishu* — assent of the spleen-pancreas

Back: approximately two FW on each side of the eleventh thoracic vertebra; between two vertical muscles (iliocostalis and longissimus dorsi); at the lower edge of the eleventh rib; in a hollow; on the latissimus dorsi.

Two FW below *danshu* (BL-19); two FW superior and slightly lateral to *weishu* (BL-21). In the angle of and under the last rib; two FW on each side of *jizhong* (GV-6); two FW medial to *yishe* (BL-44, IS BL-49).

When tonified:

Tonifies the bladder, spleen-pancreas, stomach, eyes, lumbar areas.

Disperses the lung, heart.

Dispersing acts in the opposite way.

Direct effects:

Assent point of the spleen-pancreas (problems from external excitation with fever or hyperexcitation; all problems from excess of spleen or pancreas or stomach).

Stomach: all trouble and excess energy and inflammation; hematemesis; cramps; can eat, but becomes thin; contracted esophagus; vomiting.

Intestines: swollen and painful abdomen with chest and back pain, serious diarrhea with fever, mucus, vomiting, thinness, diarrhea of bile; eats a lot; bad body odor.

Diabetes.

Eyes: children not seeing at dusk.

Opposite effects:

Heart: angina of the chest, breathlessness, contraction and pain of the side; heavy body.

Contracted kidneys, not functioning, cold and heat; pain of lumbar area; edema, stiffness and tightness of the lumbar vertebrae.

Bone: pains, twisted from pain.

BL-21 *weishu* — assent of the stomach

Back: one large FW on each side of the twelfth thoracic vertebra; on the inferior edge of the last rib; between the muscle along the thoracic spine (longissimus dorsi) and the edge of the twelfth rib, in an angle; on the latissimus dorsi; deep, on the lateral superior edge of the transverse process of the first lumbar vertebra; in a hollow.

Two FW below *pishu* (BL-20); two FW above *sanjiaoshu* (BL-22); one large FW medial to *weicang* (BL-45, IS BL-50).

When tonified:

Tonifies the bladder, stomach, intestines, skin, back, lumbar area.

Disperses the lung.

Dispersing acts in the opposite way.

Direct effects:

Assent point of the stomach (problems from external excitation with fever or hyperexcitation). All problems of the stomach from excess: very hungry, cannot eat, upset stomach, vomiting; children vomiting their milk, vomiting without eating; bad digestion, vertigo after eating, stomach cramps, burning in the stomach, hyperchlorhydria, distended stomach, eats a lot; fetid body odor; thinness of children, cannot produce flesh; cancer of the stomach.

Intestines: pain of the abdomen, swelling, noises; constipation or diarrhea; worms in the duodenum; cancer of the intestines.

Distended liver, jaundice.

Urination stopped; blue-black urine? Kidneys: inflammation.

Eyes: diminished vision, tired; cannot see at dusk.

Humidity entering?

Bad abscess.

Parts of the body:

Back: contractures; tightened muscles; back, lumbar and vertebral pain.

BL-22 *sanjiaoshu* — assent of the triple warmer

Lumbar area: one large FW on either side of the inferior edge of the first lumbar vertebra; two FW under the last rib; between two vertical muscles (iliocostalis, longissimus dorsi); on the superior edge of the transverse process of the second lumbar vertebra; on the latissimus dorsi, in a hollow.

Two FW below *weishu* (BL-21); two FW above *shenshu* (BL-23); two FW medial and slightly above *huangmen* (BL-46, IS BL-51); two FW on either side of *xuanshu* (GV-5).

When tonified:

Tonifies the bladder, triple warmer, stomach, intestines, dorsal muscles.

Disperses the kidney, lung.

Dispersing acts in the opposite way.

Direct effects:

Assent point of the triple warmer (problems from external excitation with fever or hyperexcitation). Tight and weakened nerves; all internal organs: old troubles, chronic contractions, pain.

Stomach: food not passing, headache; thinness, can neither eat nor drink; fits of vomiting; stomach cramps; eats but does not digest.

Stomach and intestines: chronic, old trouble; swollen, painful abdomen; gushing diarrhea.

Gallbladder: spasms, tightness.

Genital organs: men — seminal emissions.

Kidney: inflammation; the point is painful in cases of renal troubles; incontinence?

Parts of the body:

Shoulder, back, lumbar area: contracted muscles, stiffness, pain.

BL-23   *shenshu* — assent of the kidney

Lumbar area: approximately one large FW on either side of the lower edge of the second lumbar vertebra, between the second and third; between two vertical muscles; on the lower edge of the point of the transverse process of the second lumbar; on the medial edge of the insertion of the greater psoas; in a hollow.

Two FW below *sanjiaoshu* (BL-22); two FW above *qihaishu* (BL-24); two FW medial and slightly inferior to *huangmen* (BL-46, IS BL-51); two FW on either side of *mingmen* (GV-4).

When tonified:

Tonifies the bladder, large intestine, spleen-pancreas, liver, bone, lumbar muscles, knees, feet, superior occipital lobe, primate.

Disperses the kidney, lung, adrenals.

Dispersing acts in the opposite way.

Direct effects:

All emptiness: shivering under the sun, cold at the lumbars, heavy body.

Assent point of the kidneys (problems from external excitation with fever, or hyperexcitation). Inflammation of the kidney (nephritis). Either slow, feeble urine, edema of the face in the morning, edema of the lung, pain of the kidneys relieved by walking (epithelial nephritis, enlarged kidney); or abundant urine, acute pain of the kidney from waiting too long to urinate; spasms of the bladder, incontinence of the urethra; edema under the eyes (''room of tears'') (interstitial nephritis); or Bright's disease (illness of the adrenals). Albumin in the urine, blood with the first drops of urine, enlarged and fat kidney, or emptiness of the kidney, urine abundant, frequent need to urinate from weakness of the kidney; visual dizziness, dim vision.

Adrenals: excess or insufficiency.

Male sexual organs: impotency (non-erection); desire to sleep alone.

Sperm lacking.

Seminal losses from weakness; dreams of demonic spirits; women: difficult, painful menses; knees and feet feel as if broken after orgasm.

Hemorrhoids; liver enlarged and fat, distended; yellow face; jaundice of tuberculosis in women; diarrhea, undigested food, particularly when cold; burning of stomach; intestinal hemorrhages.

Diabetes from excess adrenals.

Heart: pain, as if suspended?

Thinness even when eating abundantly, aggravated in the cold, from emptiness of tuberculosis, or from coitus during menses? Tuberculosis: all troubles: spits blood, blood in the intestines.

Bones: tuberculosis.

Parts of the body:

Heavy head, warm body, red warm face.

Intercostal neuralgia.

Lumbar area: pains when sitting down or getting up; lumbar muscle contractures.

Buttocks, posterior thigh, posterior knee: pain; contracted knees.

Feet cold like ice; or contracted, or weak, lacking.

Point of Weihe: Berberis (see abdomen-*zhongzhu*, KI-15). Kidneys: pain, sand; urinary troubles; frequent urination; liver trouble; headache from bile with dirty tongue and vertigo; indigestion from bile; gallbladder stones; burning of the stomach; troubles at menses; hemorrhoids.

BL-24   *qihaishu* — assent of the sea of energy

Lumbar area: one large FW on either side of the interval between the third and fourth lumbar vertebrae (the upper edge of the fourth lumbar extends to the iliac crest); on the lateral edge of a vertical muscle; on the inferior edge of the transverse process of the third lumbar vertebra; in a hollow.

Two FW under *shenshu* (BL-23); two FW above *dachangshu* (BL-25); one FW medial to *zhishi* (BL-47, IS BL-52). There is no point between the third and fourth lumbar vertebrae.

When tonified:

    Tonifies the bladder, intestines, anus.

    Disperses the sexual organs.

    Dispersing acts in the opposite way.

Direct effects:

    Intestines: spasms, pains; anus: hemorrhoids, fistulae.

    Hypertension.

    Blenorrhagia.

Parts of the body:

    Posterior knee; posterior lower leg and foot.

BL-25 *dachangshu* — assent of the large intestine

Lumbar area: one large FW on either side of the mid-height of the fourth lumbar vertebra. On the upper edge and medial to the prominent angle of the iliac crest; between the muscles (common mass) and the transverse muscles; in a hollow.

Two FW under *qihaishu* (BL-24); two FW above *guanyuanshu* (BL-26); two FW medial and slightly under *zhishi* (BL-47, IS BL-52). There is no point between the fourth and fifth lumbar vertebrae.

When tonified:

    Tonifies the bladder, large intestine, small intestine, lumbar muscles.

    Disperses the lungs.

    Dispersing acts in the opposite way.

Direct effects:

    Assent point of the large intestine (problems from external excitation with fever, or hyperexcitation). Intestine: inflammation, noises, old constipation or serious diarrhea, swollen abdomen, appendicitis, inflammation of the cecum, intestinal hemorrhage, beriberi.

    Thinness, does not assimilate; eats a lot, stays thin. Or assimilates too much, does not burn it; obesity.

    Kidneys: inflammation, or contraction; urine slow, difficult; or incontinence, urethritis, blenorrhagia.

    Dryness has entered the body?

Parts of the body:

    Lumbar area: pain, lumbar or vertebral muscles contracted; lumbar vertebrae: stiffness, pain.

    Lumbar area; medial posterior lower limb.

BL-26 *guanyuanshu* — assent of the origin of the barrier

Lumbar area: in the deep angle of the upper edge of the sacrum and of the medial edge of the hip bone, at the upper opening of the sacroiliac articulation; on the lower edge of the transverse process of the fifth lumbar vertebra. One FW on either side of the lumbosacral articulation; in a hollow; on the common mass of the lumbar and vertebral muscles.

Two FW under *dachangshu* (BL-25); two FW superior and medial to *xiaochangshu* (BL-27); above *shangliao* (BL-31); one FW on either side of back-*yangguan* (GV-3).

One branch proceeds to the sacral foramen, the other one along the edge of the sacrum.

When tonified:

    Tonifies the bladder, sexual organs, heart, lower pelvis, large intestine.

    Dispersing acts in the opposite way.

Direct effects:

    Weakness and emptiness after flu.

    All female troubles with pains and spasms: "way of the blood of the uterus," painful menses.

    Large intestine: serious diarrhea, swelling, emptiness.

    Contracted bladder, difficulty in urination.

Parts of the body:

Lumbar area: pain, contracted lumbar muscles; sacroiliac arthritis.

Upper extremity of the sacroiliac articulation.

Articulation of the hip, posterior face and posterior side of calf.

BL-27   *xiaochangshu* — assent of the small intestine

Bottom of the back: in the angle between the lateral edge of the sacrum and the inferior edge of the iliac crest. In the angle of the insertions of the gluteus medius and maximus; in a hollow.

Two FW inferior and lateral to *guanyuanshu* (BL-26); one FW lateral to *shangliao* (BL-31); two FW medial to *baohuang* (BL-48, IS BL-53).

When tonified:

Tonifies the bladder, small intestine, large intestine, knee, lower leg, anterior lateral foot.

Disperses the lungs.

Dispersing acts in the opposite way.

Direct effects:

Assent point of the small intestine (problems from external excitation with fever or hyperexcitation). "Dispersing relaxes the small intestine with noises of water flowing."

Intestines: cold of the two intestines? Stools difficult, or blocked; or diarrhea, dysentery with pus and blood (infectious dysentery); or with blood and heaviness of the rectum; painful spasms of the intestines; hemorrhoids, congestive headaches.

Diabetes; unbearable, dry mouth; fatigue, emptiness.

Bladder: red, insufficient urine; swelling and fullness of the lower abdomen, strangling pains; "little secretion of the bladder and triple warmer"; or incontinence.

Heat has entered the body?

Painful swellings: swollen feet.

Parts of the body:

Lumbar vertebrae: stiffness and pain; ischium: pain.

Knee, lower leg and foot: lateral anterior face.

BL-28   *pangguangshu* — assent of the bladder

Bottom of the back: on the lateral edge of the sacrum; about two FW under the iliac crest. At the bottom of a marked notch of the bone; at the inferior opening of the sacroiliac articulation; on the insertion of the gluteus maximus on the sacrum; in a hollow.

Two FW under *xiaochangshu* (BL-27); two FW above *zhonglushu* (BL-29); at the level of the second sacral foramen, *ciliao* (BL-32).

When tonified:

Tonifies the bladder, sexual organs, large intestine, lumbar muscles, sacrum and posterolateral knee, feet.

Disperses the lungs, kidneys.

Dispersing acts in the opposite way.

Direct effects:

Assent point of the bladder (problems from external excitation with fever or hyperexcitation). Inflammation of the bladder (cystitis), frequent pressing need, with little urine, dark urine, pain or spasms of the lower abdomen, or incontinence; urethra: inflammation.

Large intestine: constipation, or serious diarrhea; pain in the abdomen; beriberi.

Female sexual organs: all problems; metritis; genital abscess.

Bone: pain, fever, aches (dengue fever).

Parts of the body:

Sacroiliac articulation: arthritis, contracted lumbar muscles, lumbar pains, pains of thigh and posteromedial face of the knee.

Posteromedial knee and foot without strength, or contracted; can neither extend nor flex.

BL-29   *zhonglushu* — assent of the central vertebrae

Bottom of the back: on the lateral edge of the sacrum; about four FW under the iliac crest. In a large notch of the bone, at about the level of the third sacral foramen. On the gluteus maximus; deep, the inferior edge of a transverse muscle (piriformis muscle); in a hollow.

Two FW under *pangguangshu* (BL-28); two FW above *baihuanshu* (BL-30); one large FW lateral to *zhongliao* (BL-33); three FW medial to *zhibian* (BL-49, IS BL-54).

When tonified:

> Tonifies the bladder, large intestine, lumbar area, buttocks, anterior lateral thigh.
> Disperses the kidneys.
> Dispersing acts in the opposite way.

Direct effects:

> Spasms of the intestines, kidneys, tonic convulsions, stiffness.
> Intestines: painful spasms, or inflammation, dysentery, swelling of abdomen, pains at the side, peritonitis: or cold of the intestines? Beriberi.
> Kidneys: spasm, contraction, bladder (restrains); insufficient urine; sweats, thirst, emptiness.
> Diabetes: renal?

Parts of the body:

> Lateral lumbar muscles: contracted, painful.

BL-30   *baihuanshu* — assent of the sphincter

Bottom of the back: just at the edge of the lower prominent angle and lateral to the sacrum; in the angle of the inferior edge of the insertion of the gluteus maximus; in a hollow.

Two FW below *zhonglushu* (BL-29); two FW above and lateral to *huiyang* (BL-35); at the level of the fourth sacral foramen.

When tonified:

> Tonifies the bladder, vitality, heat, cerebellum, lower posterior leg (Achilles tendon), large intestine, anus, perineum, hypogastric plexus.
> Dispersing acts in the opposite way.

Direct effects:

> Nervousness, emotional agitation, fear, apprehension, fatigue, exhaustion, emptiness; or hallucinations, heat.
> Large intestine: constipation from general emptiness.
> Kidney: insufficiency of urination, from emptiness; bladder (sphincter).

Parts of the body:

> Half body: flaccidity (mostly of the extensor muscles).
> Anus, perineal muscles: pains, contracture, or flaccidity; muscles of the sacrum.
> Displaced sacrum (tonify the soft hollow side; disperse the hard, contracted side).
> Lumbar area, ischium: pains; Achilles tendon.
> Jiujitsu: knock out point; kuatsu: revival point.

BL-31   *shangliao* — superior hole [first sacral foramen]

In each first sacral foramen; upper part of the sacrum; one large FW under the superior edge of the sacrum; one FW medial to the angle between the sacrum and the iliac crest; in an elongated hollow.

One large FW below *guanyuanshu* (BL-26) from where the line of the edge of the sacrum and that of the sacral foramen branches; one large FW medial to *xiaochangshu* (BL-27); one FW above *ciliao* (BL-32).

When tonified:

> Tonifies the bladder, large intestine, sexual organs, spleen-pancreas, anterior knee, heel, dorsum of toes, bone.
> Disperses the gallbladder.
> Dispersing acts in the opposite way.

Direct effects:

> Point of passage between gallbladder and spleen-pancreas: fits of vomiting, nose bleeds, constipation, urine insufficient or stopped.
> Sexual organs: women — sterility, metritis, painful menses, prolapsed uterus with discharge. Men — orchitis,

inflammation of the epididymis.

Bone: all trouble.

Parts of the body:

Anterior knee: cold and pain in the area of the patella to the point of paralysis of the knee; if kneeling, cannot get up.

Lumbar area and ischium: pain. Posterolateral aspect of the thigh.

Heel pain.

BL-32   *ciliao* — second hole (second sacral foramen)

Sacrum: in the second sacral foramen; two large FW under the superior edge of the sacrum. Three large FW below the inferior edge; one large FW medial to the upper notch of the edge of the bone; in a hollow.

One large FW below *shangliao* (BL-31); one large FW above *zhongliao* (BL-33); one large FW medial to *pang-guangshu* (BL-28).

When tonified:

Tonifies the bladder, sexual organs, large intestine, lumbar area, anterolateral side of the knee.

Disperses the lungs, kidney.

Dispersing acts in the opposite way.

Direct effects:

Loss of energy and strength, falls down easily, weakness from hemiplegia; paraplegia from lumbar area to foot, without strength to the point of flaccidity.

Cold in the pores of the back; cold and weakness of the area of the front of the knee.

Intestine: constipation, intestinal noises.

Vomiting, nosebleeds.

Kidneys: insufficiency; urine red, or urine not arriving.

Genital organs, women: insufficiency of ovaries and uterus, sterility; painful, insufficient menses, white discharge: tonify; red discharge: disperse; prolapsed uterus. Men: orchitis. Both sexes: blenorrhagia; urethral inflammation.

Parts of the body:

Lumbar area and genital organs: pain.

Paraplegia, hemiplegia, lower limb weakness; or pain from the sacrum to the heel.

Thigh, posterior inferior side.

Knee: weakness and pain when going up and down stairs.

Posterior side of the knee and lower leg: pain; calf and big toe: pain.

Feet: purely nervous pains.

BL-33   *zhongliao* — central hole (third sacral foramen)

Sacrum: in the third sacral foramen; two FW above the inferior edge; three FW below the upper edge; one large FW medial to the lateral edge, in a notch; in a marked hollow, near the spinal eminence.

One large FW below *ciliao* (BL-32, second sacral foramen); one above *xialiao* (BL-34, fourth sacral foramen); one large FW medial to *zhonglushu* (BL-29).

When tonified:

Tonifies the bladder (detrusor?), gallbladder, liver, sexual organs, lateral side of the lower limb, perineum.

Disperses the lungs, triple warmer.

Dispersing acts in the opposite way.

Direct effects:

Intestines: spasms, difficult or stopped stool. Or diarrhea after eating (intestinal tuberculosis?), swollen abdomen, vomiting.

Bladder (detrusor): urine insufficient or stopped (weakness of the extensor muscles?); urethra: inflammation.

Tuberculosis: all the troubles of the different forms.

Genital organs: spasms; women — insufficient menses; difficult, painful, metritis, white discharges; at orgasm: weakness, loss of strength; men: orchitis.

Parts of the body:
Lumbar area, sacrum: pain; posterior part of knee: pain; external side of heel.

BL-34   *xialiao* — lower hole (fourth sacral foramen)

Bottom of sacrum: one FW above the lower edge; close to the spinal eminences. One large FW medial from the lateral edge; in a hollow.

One FW under *zhongliao* (BL-33, third sacral foramen); two large FW above *huiyang* (BL-35); one large FW medial to *baihuanshu* (BL-30).

When tonified:
Tonifies the bladder, heart, sexual organs, kidney, lumbar area, heat, dryness.
Dispersing acts in the opposite way.

Direct effects:
Humidity causing spasms or heat or cold or disturbances of the skin or breath.
Large intestine: constipation, or blood coming with the stool, or gas forcing one to evacuate stool.
Urethra, sphincter of bladder, prostate; urine insufficient or stopped (vesical spasm, prostatitis?); urethra: serious inflammation with bleeding; blenorrhagia.
Sexual organs: greenish discharge that cannot be checked; pain. Blenorrhagia, metritis, pain and itching in the organs, syphilis of women, chancre, bad discharge, sweats; insufficient, difficult, painful menses. S4 (nervi splanchnici pelvini).

Parts of the body:
Lumbar area: painful, cannot twist, pain spreading to ovary or testicles.
Lower limb — knee and calf: pain; external face of heel.

BL-35   *huiyang* — reunion of the yang

Coccygeal region: at the level and one large FW on either side of the interval between the first and second coccygeal vertebrae; one large FW under the lower edge of the sacrum; in a hollow.

About two FW inferior and medial to *baihuanshu* (BL-30); two FW under *xialiao* (BL-34); four FW above *chengfu* (BL-50, IS BL-36).

From this comes the name "reunion of the yang." From this point, the numbering ascends to the lateral paravertebral line.

When tonified:
Tonifies the bladder, triple warmer, sexual organs, urethra, anus, external malleolus.
Dispersing acts in the opposite way.

Direct effects:
Lassitude, lack of energy of yang activity; either energy of cold or of heat.
Sexual organs: men — non-erection, impotence, seminal losses; women — inflammation of the vulva, hardness of the perineum (preparing for delivery). Both sexes — sweating of the sexual organs, cold dampness of the organs, itching (pruritis) of the genital regions; blenorrhagia.
Bladder: incontinence?
Large intestine: constipation or diarrhea; anus: pain, old hemorrhoids; intestinal hemorrhages, inflammation of the intestines; abdominal cold?

Parts of the body:
Displaced coccygeal vertebrae; coccyx pain.

BL-36   *fufen* (IS BL-41) — adjoining division

Upper back: one FW above the medial superior angle of the scapula; on the superior edge of the second rib; on the lateral edge of the superimposed vertical muscles (iliocostalis under the levator scapulae); in a hollow.

One very large FW lateral to *dazhu* (BL-11); one very large FW above *pohu* (BL-37, IS BL-42). One large FW under and a bit lateral to *jianwaishu* (SI-14). Its current comes from *tianzhu* (BL-10) via a lateral branch.

When tonified:

Tonifies the bladder, triple warmer, small intestine, chin, posterior shoulder and nape. Disperses the lungs. Responds to *fengchi* (GB-20).

Dispersing acts in the opposite manner.

Direct effects:

Sympathetic?

Wind and cold entering the pores.

Lungs: catarrh of the apex of the lungs. Tuberculosis from shock?

Parts of the body:

Contractions of the posterior shoulder and nape, preventing the head from turning; painful spasms; muscular rheumatism.

BL-37 *pohu* (IS BL-42) — portal of the primate

Upper back: On the medial edge of the scapula, at the angle between its superior and medial thirds, and the inferior edge of the second rib. On the medial inferior edge of the insertion of the levator scapulae. On the lateral edge of the iliocostalis muscle. In a hollow; on the rhomboid.

One very large FW below *fufen* (BL-36, IS BL-41); one very large FW above *gaohuangshu* (BL-38, IS BL-43); two FW lateral to *feishu* (BL-13); two FW medial to *quyuan* (SI-13).

When tonified:

Tonifies the bladder, large intestine, primate, eyes, upper back.

Disperses the lung.

Dispersing acts in the opposite way.

Direct effects:

Primate: weakness, exhaustion, paresis; or agitation, fullness.

Lungs: ''discharge from all orifices'' (inflammation of all mucous membranes?); panting; cannot rest, coughing attacks, asthma, bronchitis; ''cold and heat'' of the lung, pneumonia, atrophy of the lung, emptiness, exhaustion of the lung, tuberculosis from emptiness, exhaustion.

Parts of the body:

Increases red blood cells, in small quantities.

Course of the ulnar nerve:

Upper back: posterior shoulder, nape, posterior arm, forearm and ulnar side of hand; without strength; pain or contracture. Nape and shoulder: pain and contracture after having carried too heavy a weight; contracture of the rhomboids and serratus anterior.

BL-38 *gaohuangshu* (IS BL-43) — vital centers

Upper back: elbows held in front in order to separate the scapulae, which cover the point when they are in normal position. By following the inferior edge, towards the back, of the relief on an angle to the spine of the scapula, the finger falls between the third and fourth ribs, in a triangular hollow. The point is in the lateral inferior angle of the hollow, on the superior edge of the fourth rib and of a tendon on an angle (serratus anterior), in a groove on an angle between rhomboids major and minor; on the trapezius.

One very large FW below *pohu* (BL-37, IS BL-42); one very large FW above *shentang* (BL-39, IS BL-44); two FW lateral to *jueyinshu* (BL-14); two FW lateral and slightly above *bingfeng* (SI-12).

When tonified:

Tonifies the bladder, vessels, heart, red cells, the three nervous centers, the three endocrine glands, lower sternum (*jiuwei*, CV-15), shoulder, back.

Disperses the lungs.

Dispersing acts in the opposite way.

Direct effects:

In cases of anemia, instantaneous production of red blood cells, for approximately the quantity which is lacking, which mature in 15 to 18 hours. Often there is momentary fatigue and the back is a little stiff. It is good to reduce the swelling of the spleen first, if distended, because it destroys more red blood cells than the body can make (in the marrow of the flat bones, sternum and ribs): tonify *yutang* (CV-18).

Exhaustion, weakness, cold; moments of exhaustion; all recent or old problems from weakness (except congestive tuberculosis with spitting of blood).

Weakness and decline of the yang energy of activity; loss of memory; weakness of the nerves (neurasthenia). All troubles of ''frenetic doubts, wild errors''; frenetic attacks from weakness, hysteria?

All varieties of tuberculosis.

Pulmonary tuberculosis, atonic and noncongestive; constellated lungs, troubles from weakness of the respiratory passages, susceptibility to cold, sensitivity of the respiratory passages, mucus, coughing fits; energy in the upper body; bronchitis, pleurisy.

Tuberculosis of the bones; decalcified, softened bone, Pott's disease.

Tuberculosis of the spinal cord; weakness of the limb; painful back with fatigue from cold or during coitus; shoulder and back pains.

Stomach: the stomach does not empty because of anemia and slowed digestion; swelling of the stomach disappearing at 600 m. altitude; hiccoughs, diaphragm, vomiting, nausea.

Sexual organs: men — wet dreams; women — menses not coming because of anemia, weakness.

BL-39   *shentang* (IS BL-44) — room of the evolved

Back: at the level of one third from the spine of the scapula to the lower angle; in the angle between the medial edge of the scapula and the inferior edge of the fifth rib; in a hollow; between the bone and the iliocostalis muscle; on the rhomboid.

One very large FW below *gaohuangshu* (BL-38, IS BL-43); one very large FW above *yixi* (BL-40, IS BL-45); two FW lateral to *xinshu* (BL-15); at the level of *shendao* (GV-10, IS GV-11).

When tonified:

Tonifies the bladder, temporal-parietal and frontal lobes, heart, back and posterior arm.

Dispersing acts in the opposite way.

Direct effects:

Shivering when bathing, hot and cold.

Respiratory passages: fullness of the chest, energy rising and suffocating; bronchitis; panting.

Heart: all problems?

Parts of the body:

Iliocostal muscle: contracture, pricking pains.

Thoracic and lumbar vertebrae: stiffness.

Shoulder, lateral arm, posterior forearm: acute pain.

BL-40   *yixi* (IS BL-45) — cries of pain

Back: at the level of two thirds from the spine of the scapula to its lower angle at the medial edge of the scapula, and at the lower edge of the sixth rib; in a hollow; on the rhomboid.

One very large FW below *shentang* (BL-39, IS BL-44). One very large FW above *geguan* (BL-41, IS BL-46); two FW lateral to *dushu* (BL-16); four FW on either side of *lingtai* (GV-9, IS GV-10).

When tonified:

Tonifies the bladder, midbrain (?), elbow, hand.

Dispersing acts in the opposite way.

Direct effects:

Insomnia from fatigue, exhaustion; great shock, sweat.

All fevers: prolonged fever of one of the five yin distributor organs, fever from cold or heat, fever from energy. Fever from melancholy, all troubles with fever, intermittent fever.

Violent sweat at night, or from shock.

Heart: all fever from the heart; pericarditis.

Eyes: pain; obscured vision, vertigo.

Stomach: counterflow of food, vomiting, nausea; children: headache while eating.

Parts of the body:

Tonic convulsions, stiff, from cold.

Chest: pain spreading to the four sides, to the armpit, to the back of the arm.

Back, shoulder and lumbar area: pain; scapula, medial edge: pain.

BL-41   *geguan* (IS BL-46) — barrier of the diaphragm

Back: at the level of one FW above the inferior angle of the scapula; in the angle between the scapula and the lower edge of the seventh rib; in a hollow on the latissimus dorsi, rhomboid.

One very large FW below *yixi* (BL-40, IS BL-45); four FW above *hunmen* (BL-42, IS BL-47); two FW lateral to *geshu* (BL-17); four FW on either side of *zhiyang* (GV-8, IS GV-9, superior edge of T7).

When tonified:
> Tonifies the bladder, esophagus, large intestine, back.
> Disperses the kidney.
> Dispersing acts in the opposite way.

Direct effects:
> Esophagus: spasms, contractions; eructations; much saliva, nauseous, belches and vomits, neither drink nor food descends.
> Large intestine: abundant and frequent stools.
> Kidney: colored urine.

Parts of the body:
> Back: pain and contracture (of the latissimus dorsi).
> Stiff vertebrae.

BL-42   *hunmen* (IS BL-47) — door of the automaton-parrot

Back: at the level of three FW below the lower angle of the scapula; four FW on either side of the upper edge of the tenth thoracic vertebra; on the inferior edge of the ninth rib; on the vertical of the medial edge of the scapula; in a hollow.

Four FW below *geguan* (BL-41, IS BL-46); two FW above *yanggang* (BL-43, IS BL-48); two FW lateral to *ganshu* (BL-18). There is no governor point at T9; at T10: *jinsuo* (GV-7, IS GV-8).

When tonified:
> Tonifies the bladder, liver, parrot-automaton, heart, muscles.
> Dispersing acts in the opposite way.

Direct effects:
> Parrot-automaton (the three memories).
> Liver: all problems.
> Large intestine: diarrhea, spasms, colic, noises, aerocolia.
> Esophagus: contraction, salivation, vomiting; food and drink do not descend.
> Stomach: cramps, bad digestion.
> Heart: pain spreading to chest and back.

Parts of the body:
> Muscular rheumatism; contracted muscles, bone pain.

> **Point of Weihe:** Right: Chelidonium Majus (see *guanmen*, ST-22). Pain under the scapula; trembling, shaking; spasms of the eyelids; distended liver, jaundice, obstruction of the biliary canal; constipation or attacks of diarrhea; frequent need to urinate.
>
> Left: Terebenthina. Liver, kidneys.

BL-43   *yanggang* (IS BL-48) — firmness of yang

Lower, lateral back: approximately four FW under the inferior edge of the last rib; approximately four FW on either side of the superior edge of the eleventh thoracic vertebra; in a hollow on the inferior edge of the tenth rib.

Two FW below *hunmen* (BL-42, IS BL-47); one large FW above *yishe* (BL-44, IS BL-49); two FW lateral to *danshu* (BL-19); four FW on either side of *jizhong* (GV-6).

When tonified:
> Tonifies the bladder, liver, stomach, pancreas, heart.
> Dispersing acts in the opposite way.

Direct effects:
> Liver: all trouble; jaundice: face, eyes and body yellow, urine brown-red, rough.
> Stomach: pains, cramps, food does not descend, no appetite.
> Large intestine: stools upset, noise and pain; pain from worms (tapeworm).

Diabetes, hot body, swollen abdomen.

Heart: endocarditis, rib pains (pleurisy?).

Muscular rheumatism.

Point of Weihe: Capsicum. Vital heat lowered; cold face with burning ears, mental exhaustion or wasting, in old people; when coughing, fetid odor from the lung; hiccough; pain from the hip to the foot.

BL-44　*yishe* (IS BL-49) — home of the imagination

Inferior lateral back: about four FW on either side of the upper edge of the twelfth thoracic vertebra; approximately two FW above the lower edge of the twelfth rib; on the lower edge of the eleventh rib; nearly above the end of the twelfth rib; in a hollow.

One very large FW below *yanggang* (BL-43, IS BL-48); two FW above *weicang* (BL-45, IS BL-50), lateral to *pishu* (BL-20); four FW on either side of *xuanshu* (GV-5).

When tonified:

Tonifies the bladder, liver, kidney, stomach, back.

Disperses the lung.

Dispersing acts in the opposite way.

Direct effects:

Contracted esophagus, atonic stomach, bad digestion, lack of appetite.

Liver: all troubles, jaundice, red-brown urine.

Diabetes: fever, thirst.

Contrary effects:

Lungs: fits of sneezing; pleurisy.

Parts of the body.

Rectus abdominus: weakness or contracture.

Point of Weihe: Solidago Virga. Congestion and pain of the kidneys; urine feeble or difficult; albuminuria; Bright's disease; frequent chills; sneezing attacks, cough; dyspnea; bronchitis; fibroids, distended uterus, lower limbs, dermatitis.

BL-45　*weicang* (IS BL-50) — storehouse of the stomach

Lumbar area: on the lower edge of the last rib (twelfth); about three FW on either side of the twelfth thoracic vertebra; in a hollow; on the lateral edge of the mass of the lumbar muscles.

Two FW below and slightly medial to *yishe* (BL-44, IS BL-49); slightly above *huangmen* (BL-46, IS BL-51); three FW on either side of *jizhong* (GV-6); one large FW lateral to *weishu* (BL-32).

When tonified:

Tonifies the bladder, stomach, cerebellum, kidney, abdomen, lumbar.

Dispersing acts in the opposite way.

Direct effects:

Abdominal organs: atony (stomach, small intestine, liver, kidneys).

Local edema.

Parts of the body:

Lumbar, back, thoracic vertebra: pain.

BL-46　*huangmen* (IS BL-51) — door of the vital centers

Lumbar area, about one FW below the last rib; about three FW on either side of the thoracic spine (second lumbar vertebra); on the lateral edge of the lumbar muscles; deep, at the level of the lower edge of the extremity of the transverse process of the first lumbar vertebra; in a hollow.

One FW below *weicang* (BL-45, IS BL-50); two FW above *zhishi* (BL-47, IS BL-52); one large FW lateral to *sanjiaoshu* (BL-22); three FW lateral to *xuanshu* (GV-5).

When tonified:

Tonifies the bladder, stomach, large intestine, sexual organs, opposite breast, medulla oblongata, spinal cord, lumbar and thoracic muscles.

Dispersing acts in the opposite way.

Direct effects:

Abdominal organs: troubles from spasms.

Stomach: cramps, contractions.

Large intestine: habitual constipation; hard stools.

Gallbladder: spasms.

Opposite breast: all types of problems, inflammation of the mammary glands (nodules).

Parts of the body:

Lumbar area and back: muscles contracted, painful.

BL-47 *zhishi* (IS BL-52) — home of the decision-will

Lumbar area: a little above the iliac crest; about three large FW on either side of the upper edge of the fourth lumbar vertebra; on the latissimus dorsi and lumbar muscles; in a hollow.

Two FW below *huangmen* (BL-46, IS BL-51); three FW above and medial to *baohuang* (BL-48, IS BL-53); two FW lateral to *dachangshu* (BL-25); about two FW medial to *daimai* (GB-26).

When tonified:

Tonifies the bladder, medulla oblongata, spinal cord, stomach, large intestine, genital organs, prostate, articulation of hip.

Dispersing acts in the opposite way.

Direct effects:

"Nature blocked and tied from the emotions"?

Stomach: bad digestion, food and drink not digested.

Large intestine: cholera, vomiting and diarrhea attacks, abdomen full and swollen; the two sides contracted and painful.

Genital organs: all problems — swelling, pain; blenorrhagia; men: penis painful; special point for seminal discharge during dreams; military gout [poor man's gout]; prostate; women: swollen vulva.

Kidneys: inflammation; urethra: inflammation.

Parts of the body:

Lumbar muscles contracted; pain and stiffness of the lumbar area.

Jiujitsu: knock-out point, and even of death?

Point of Weihe: Coccus Cacti. Upper eyelids inflamed; sensation of foreign body under the upper eyelid; spasmodic cough; kidney stones, anuria, general dropsy, ascites.

BL-48 *baohuang* (IS BL-53) — vital center of the uterus

Upper buttock: two FW lateral to the top of the sacrum; in the angle of the inferior edge, very deep to the edge of the iliac crest; on the medial edge of a muscular bundle (gluteus medius); deep, the insertion of the gluteus minimus; in a hollow.

Three FW inferior and lateral to *zhishi* (BL-47, IS BL-52); four FW above *zhibian* (BL-49, IS BL-54); two FW lateral to *xiaochangshu* (BL-27); about four FW medial to hip-*wushu* (GB-27).

When tonified:

Tonifies the bladder, sexual organs, stomach, large intestine, lumbar area, sacrum, lower limb, gluteus muscles.

Dispersing acts in the opposite way.

Direct effects:

Abdomen, anus, sexual organs: inflammation.

Stomach: bad digestion.

Abdomen swollen, hard, painful; constipation; intestinal noises; anus: hemorrhoids.

Bladder: inflammation (cystitis); urine stopped (retention, lower abdomen swollen); urethra: inflammation.

Sexual organs — women: all troubles; uterus; men: testicles; orchitis; prostatitis.

Parts of the body:

Infantile paralysis (poliomyelitis): flaccidity of the gluteus medius and minimus.

Lumbar area: pain; stiffness and pain of the lumbar vertebra; sacrum and lower limb to the heel: pain (sacroiliac arthritis).

BL-49 *zhibian* (IS BL-54) — beside the row

Buttocks: mid-width and mid-height; deep, the superior edge of the neck of the femur, articulating in the hip, also a transverse muscle (piriformis muscle); on the inferior edge of the gluteus medius; on the gluteus maximus; in a hollow.

Four FW below *baohuang* (BL-48, IS BL-53); six FW below *chengfu* (BL-50, IS BL-36); three large FW lateral to *zhonglushu* (BL-29); four FW medial to *huantiao* (GB-29, IS GB-30).

When tonified:
Tonifies the bladder, small intestine, urethra, bladder sphincter, prostate, posterior face of the thigh, calf, central brain, medulla oblongata, lower warmer.
Disperses the lungs.
Dispersing acts in the opposite way.

Direct effects:
Illnesses of women.
Cystitis, urine very much colored.
Hemorrhoids swelling from time to time.
Heaviness of the coccyx, cannot get up.

Parts of the body.
Lumbar area, lumbar vertebrae, external part of the posterior side of the lower limb: pain mostly of the lateral posterior area of the knee.

BL-50 *chengfu* (IS BL-36) — receives support

Upper and posterior thigh: under the buttocks; on the gluteal crease; on the lower edge of the gluteus maximus; between two vertical muscles (lateral: quadratus femoris muscle; medial: semitendinosis muscle). Deep, one FW below and lateral to the point of the ischium; in a hollow.

Six FW below *zhibian* (BL-49, IS BL-54); five FW above *yinmen* (BL-51, IS BL-37); about five FW medial to *huantiao* (GB-29, IS GB-30).

Here, the lateral line coming from *tianzhu* (BL-10) and the medial line coming from *dazhu* (BL-11) rejoin with that of the sacral foramina branching at *guanyuanshu* (BL-26) and rejoining the medial branch at *huiyang* (BL-35).

When tonified:
Tonifies the bladder, large intestine, anus, sexual organs, back, lumbar area, buttocks, ischium, posterior thigh.
Dispersing acts in the opposite way.

Direct effects:
Large intestine: constipation, insufficient stool, difficult stool; anus: hemorrhoids old or like wounds.
Kidney, bladder: urine insufficient or stopped.
Sexual organs: insufficiency; men: seminal losses: women: sterility, insensitive uterus.

Parts of the body:
Back and lumbar area: pain and cold; buttocks: pain or cold or swelling; ischium: pain; posterior thigh: pain.

BL-51 *yinmen* (IS BL-37) — door of prosperity

Posterior thigh: around the median line, a little lateral; five FW under the point of the ischium. In the angle between two large muscles (lateral: biceps femoris; medial: semitendinosis); in a hollow.

Five FW below *chengfu* (BL-50, IS BL-36); the point following is *fuxi* (BL-52, IS BL-38) on the lateral condyle.

When tonified:
Tonifies the bladder, blood, back, lumbar area, posterior thigh.
Dispersing acts in the opposite way.

Direct effects:
Blood thickened, circulation slow; ''bad blood from having lifted too heavy a weight.''

Parts of the body:
> Back and lumbar area: contracture, stiffness, pain.
>
> Lower limb, mostly posterior side: all trouble, sudden weakness, falling down from sudden bending of the thigh or the lower leg (poliomyelitis).
>
> External part of posterior thigh weak, swollen or contracted, inflamed.

BL-52   *fuxi* (IS BL-38)   —   superficial vale

Lateral posterior knee: in the angle between the superior edge of the large projection (lateral condyle of the femur) and the medial edge of the tendons on an angle (plantaris muscle, lateral gastrocnemius muscle); in a hollow on the edge of the plantaris.

Preceding point: *yinmen* (BL-51, IS BL-37), at five FW below the ischium; three FW above *weiyang* (BL-53, IS BL-39).

When tonified:
> Tonifies the bladder, large intestine, small intestine, gallbladder, hip joint, posterolateral knee.
>
> Dispersing acts in the opposite way.

Direct effects:
> Heat in the lower abdomen.
>
> Small intestine: heat; large intestine: heat, spasms, constipation, urination stopped.

Parts of the body:
> Hip: joint without action, immobilized.
>
> Posterior, lateral face of the lower limb: pain or flaccidity.
>
> Posterior lateral thigh and knee: cramps after walking, exertion, cramps or cholera. Flaccidity.

BL-53   *weiyang* (IS BL-39)   —   exterior of the delegate [popliteal crease]

Posterolateral knee. At the lateral extremity of the crease of flexion: between the medial edge of the great tendon of the biceps femoris and the lateral edge of the lateral gastrocnemius; in a hollow.

Three FW below *fuxi* (BL-52, IS BL-38); three FW superior and lateral to *heyang* (BL-55); one FW lateral to *weizhong* (BL-54, IS BL-40).

When tonified:
> Tonifies the triple warmer and all the yang (thus yang energy); bladder meridian, urethra, prostate, back of the ear, nape, shoulder and scapula, thoracic longissimus muscles, lateral buttock muscles, popliteal crease, calf, dorsal side of the great toe.
>
> Disperses vessels, lung.
>
> Dispersing acts in the opposite way.
>
> Acts on all the yang (and yang energy) and kidney filtration. Tradition says: additional assent point of the triple warmer and special point of passage between the bladder and kidney. In general, excess yang in external and internal muscles; spasms, pains.

Direct effects:
> Urethra, sphincter, prostate: contractions, spasmodic incontinence, spasmodic retention (urine stopped, hardness and pain of the abdomen spreading to the sexual organs); prostatitis; urethritis, pain in the lumbar area.
>
> Genital organs: spasms, tremors.

Contrary effects:
> Congestive headache; fever.
>
> Lung; chest swollen, full; pulmonary plaque.

Parts of the body:
> Back of the ear: pain.
>
> Nape, posterior shoulder and scapula; lateral gluteus muscles, waist, longissimus thoracis, scapula; posterior knee, lateral gastrocnemius: contractions, cramps.
>
> Axilla: swelling, pain.
>
> Dorsum of great toe.

BL-54 *weizhong* (IS BL-40) — middle of the delegate

Knee, posterior face (popliteal crease); lateral third of the crease of flexion; one FW medial to the lateral ropy tendon (biceps femoris); in the angle between the lower edge of the crease of flexion and the medial edge of lateral gastrocnemius; in a hollow.

One FW medial to *weiyang* (BL-53, IS BL-39); two FW above *heyang* (BL-55); responds with *houxi* (SI-3).

When tonified:

Tonifies kidney (excretion-secretion) sexual organs, governor vessel, anterior and posterior frontal lobes of the liver, evolved man, superior occipital lobes, primate; along the sacrum and half-width of the back (iliocostal area), scalp same side.
Disperses opposite large intestine, bladder.
Dispersing acts in the opposite way.

Direct effects:

Cerebral congestion, apoplexy; nosebleeds.
Blood: old troubles, chronic, intractable, "great tonic for the blood."
Skin: old problems, intractable; pruritis; leprosy: puncture and bleed three times in a row.
Scalp, same side: great shock, hair and eyebrows fall out, grow again with white hair. Tonifying returns the white or grey hair to its original color.
Kidney: reabsorption; abundant urine, without color: tonify. Urine slow, feeble: disperse.
Abundant sweat: disperse; or fever without sweat: tonify.
Bladder: retention, scarlet urine, abdominal pain. If from spasm, pain on pressure: disperse; if from atony, swollen abdomen, contraction in cold, less pain: tonify.
Influenza, flu.
Genital organs: orgasm radiating into the spinal cord.

Contrary effects:

Large intestine: spasms: tonify; cholera, strangling pains of the abdomen: tonify. Bleeding hemorrhoids: tonify.

Parts of the body:

Nervous paralysis of all kinds, all troubles; paralysis of the whole body, nervous paralysis returning periodically.
Head always bent, falling; tonifying makes the head and body erect.
Lateral gluteus muscles, thoracic muscles (iliocostal), muscles of the nape and head, same side: weakness. When the sacrum is displaced to one side, tonifying the other side helps to straighten it. Also true for vertebrae; tonifies the lumbar muscles. Dispersing acts in the opposite way.
Hip joint: arthritis or pain.
Lumbar area: all trouble, or pain; cannot, without pain, bend, lift up a heavy object or straighten: disperse. Or weakness, cannot stand from sitting position: tonify.
Posterior thigh: muscles, weak or contractures.

BL-55 *heyang* — reunites the yang

Calf: about two FW under the transverse fold of the back of the knee, about mid-width; in the superior angle between the two bellies of the gastrocnemius; exactly at the angle of the lateral gastrocnemius and the lower edge of a transverse mass; in a hollow.

Two FW below *weizhong* (BL-54, IS BL-40); three FW inferior and medial to *weiyang* (BL-53, IS BL-39); two FW above *chengjin* (BL-56).

When tonified:

Tonifies the bladder, mid-brain, large intestine, sexual organs, back, lumbar area, posterior lower limb, dorsum of foot.
Dispersing acts in the opposite way.

Direct effects:

Large intestine, sexual organs, lower limbs: excess.
Large intestine: obstruction, or intestinal hemorrhage.
Genital organs: pain, inflammation, metritis; uterus; metrorrhagia, metrorrhagia and miscarriage; ovaries, vagina: spasms; lower abdomen: spasms, discharges.
Men: testicles, orchitis.

Parts of the body:
   Lumbar area: pain; thigh and posterior knee: heat, inflammation; difficulty walking with shoes; leg, lateral heel, anterior arch.

BL-56   *chengjin* — receives the muscles

Calf: mid-height, mid-width; between the two sides of the gastrocnemius; in the angle between the lateral gastro.I (BL-55) Two FW below *heyang* (BL-55); two FW above *chengshan* (BL-57).

When tonified:
   Tonifies the bladder, large intestine, anus, hemorrhoids, veins, medial and lateral muscles; cerebellum; from the occiput to the heel; thoracic arch.
   Dispersing acts in the opposite way.
   Responds to *xuehai* (SP-10).

Direct effects:
   Large intestine: constipation or diarrhea; anus: hemorrhoids.
   Veins: internal varicosity, calf and feet numb and heavy.

Parts of the body:
   Axilla: swollen.
   Half of the back of the body: from the occiput to the heel or hand (nape, back, lumbar area, upper limb and posterior lower limb): contracture, pain or weakness; flaccidity.
   Posterior face of upper and lower limb: swelling or numbness, or cramps; cramps of cholera.
   Posterior heel (and Achilles tendon?): contracture, hardness, pain.

BL-57   *chengshan* — receives the mountain

Bottom of the calf, mid-width: in the angle of separation of the two gastrocnemius muscles, at a tendinous point which separates them (beginning of the Achilles tendon); in the angle between the point and the lateral gastrocnemius; in a hollow; on the lower edge of a transverse mass.

Two FW below *chengjin* (BL-56); two FW superior and posterior to *feiyang* (BL-58), which is posterior and slightly inferior to *waiqiu* (GB-36).

When tonified:
   Tonifies the bladder, cerebellum, anus, medial and lateral muscles, anterior lower leg mid-height.
   Dispersing acts in the opposite way.

Direct effects:
   Contractions of the medial or lateral muscles; distended veins; contusions.
   Stomach: the food does not descend; vomiting.
   Large intestine: pain of abdomen, colic and diarrhea; constipation from energy or heat.
   Bladder: neck of the bladder contracted, urine difficult; or urine stopped from cold. Urethra: inflammation, blenorrhagia.
   Hemorrhoids: special for all hemorrhoids, fissures or fistulas: tonify. Anus: itching, or pain during stool; contractions.

Parts of the body:
   Special for all contractions of lateral and medial muscles. Special for cramps; cramps of cholera; contracture or cramps of the thigh, calf, Achilles tendon, feet or sole; tetanus: contracted, painful muscles.
   Contusions: first needle *chengshan* (BL-57), then the site of the injury.
   Swelling of the fingers, of the feet: beriberi: swelling of knee and foot.
   Vertebra, lumbar area: acute pain from twisting.
   Lower and upper limb: sudden shooting pain of poliomyelitis.
   Lower leg: weak, cannot stand for a long time, old rheumatism of the lower leg.
   Foot: great toe bent up; four other toes clenched.
   Sole: heat under foot.

BL-58 *feiyang* — gliding flight

Posterolateral lower leg, about mid-height: seven FW above the lateral malleolus. One large FW posterior to the peroneus muscle; one small FW under the lateral union of the lateral gastrocnemius muscle on the Achilles tendon; on the lateral edge of the tendon, in a transverse groove; on the soleus muscle.

Two FW below and lateral to *chengshan* (BL-57); three FW above and posterior to *fuyang* (BL-59); one small FW lateral and slightly below *waiqiu* (GB-36).

When tonified:
> Tonifies the bladder (urethra and sphincter), kidney filtration and excretion; posterior and frontal lobes, upper and lower warmer, heart, vessels, organs, anus, nose, all joints same side, four toes (extensors), great toe (flexor muscle), nape and opposite upper back.
> Disperses bladder (sphincter), large intestine, lung, small intestine.
> Dispersing acts in the opposite way.
> Responds in *taixi* (KI-5, IS KI-3).

Direct effects:
> Counterflow energy, convulsions, depression, tongue out; hysteria, epilepsy, vertigo-fainting; bladder; sequela of left-side hemiplegia, trembling, weakness; cannot stay standing or sitting for a long time. If sitting, cannot get up.
> Bladder (body) and kidney (filtration, excretion): if excess; nose blocked, posterior headache and pain of the upper back; if insufficient, nose flowing and even bleeding.
> Nose blocked: disperse; nose flowing and even bleeding: tonify.

Parts of the body:
> Nape and opposite upper back: acute pain; headache, opposite side.
> All joints; rheumatism: pain same side.
> Lumbar, hip, buttocks: acute pain, or weak: cannot stand up from sitting; hemiplegia: walks without lifting the foot, as if gliding.
> Lower leg and foot: numbness, swelling.
> Calf: acute pain, or cramps.
> Flaccid foot, four toes immobile or contracted (acts on extensor muscles), great toes bent up (acts on flexor muscles).

BL-59 *fuyang* — additional yang

Lateral leg: four FW above the lateral malleolus, just at the posterior edge of the peroneus; on the upper edge of a transverse mass; on the anterior edge of the soleus muscle, in a hollow.

Three FW below and slightly anterior to *feiyang* (BL-58); four FW above *kunlun* (BL-60); one very large FW posterior to *guangming* (GB-37).

When tonified:
> Tonifies the bladder, prostate (pericardium), opposite superior occipital lobes, axilla, four limbs, liver; face, same side; lumbar area; lower limb, same side; upper limb, opposite side.
> Dispersing acts in the opposite way.
> Responds in *dazhong* (KI-6, IS KI-4).

Parts of the body:
> Face: neuralgia (of the trigeminal nerve), or paralysis (of the facial nerve), lower jaw.
> Face, under and in front of the ear, same side.
> Posterior shoulder, opposite.
> Lumbar area, hip joint: pain turning in the groin, same side.
> Anterior and posterior lower limb, anterior thigh and knee: pain or numbness, heaviness, weakness to the point of flaccidity, pain when getting up from sitting position.
> Foot: turned inward: tonify; turned outward: disperse; sprain of lateral malleolus; great toe: flexor hallucis longus.

BL-60 *kunlun* — Mount Kunlun

Posterolateral ankle; in the angle between the posterolateral edge of the lateral malleolus and the upper edge of the calcaneus and the anterior edge of the posterior peroneal tendons. Anterior to the posterior peroneal artery, external saphenus nerve and vein; in a hollow.

Four FW below *fuyang* (BL-59); two tightened FW above *pucan* (BL-61).

When tonified:
> Tonifies the bladder, all yang meridians, parathyroid glands; half-body, same side: pain, spasms.
> Disperses all the yin meridians, all the nervous centers (response mainly in the mid-brain): endocrines (except parathyroids), levels of the psyche, organs of sense.
> Dispersing acts in the opposite way, acts on all pain.

Direct effects:
> Insufficiency of thalamus, which inhibits sensations.
> Special for all pains, internal or external, all cramps and contractions, all swellings, all forms of pruritis. In general, half-body same side, recent or slight pain: disperse; serious or old pain: tonify.
> Insomnia from moral pain, or discontent, irritation or physical pain. Babies: insomnia, pains and all teeth problems.
> Head: congestive headache, with vertigo, bleeding nose; tics of the head.
> Eye (medial part, opposite; lateral part, same side): acute pain, congested or swollen.
> Ear, same side: pain.
> Gums, teeth, same side: acute pain, all troubles of teeth of babies (pains, diarrhea, etc.)
> Stomach: pains, cramps, acidity.
> Intestines: pains, colic, spasms; beriberi: diarrhea and swelling of the lower limb; bleeding hemorrhoids.

Opposite effects:
> Hypertension (congestive headache, nosebleeds, bleeding hemorrhoids); apoplexy, coma; hemiplegia: weak and painful limbs; heart: pain radiating into the back.
> Sexual organs: pains, swelling; men: testicles, orchitis; women: pain during menses; vagina: pain or swelling; vulva: pain or swelling or pruritis; difficulty and malaise of pregnancy (can cause miscarriage). Confinement, lessens and reduces the number of the pains, makes the child come more quickly, makes the placenta descend.
> Cough: fits with expectoration and suffocation; cough with response in the back and vertebral column, lumbar area. Asthma: stops the suffocation and the pain; lungs paralyzed from spasms, suffocation; or congestion.

Parts of the body:
> Skin: all pruritis, all swelling, abscess or acne of the back, pain from abscess, wounds, bruises.
> Swollen lymph nodes, painful, poisoned.
> All pain from spasms, from convulsions of children.
> Vertebral column: pains, fatigue, deviation; lumbar and sacral vertebrae: pains of displacement.
> Shoulder and back: contractures, hardness, pain.
> Upper limb, same side: all pain or swelling.
> Lumbar area, sacrum, coccyx, ischium: pains, swelling, contracture.
> Lower limb, same side: all pain or swelling; beriberi: red swelling of the leg and foot. Posterior knee: contracture, or swelling, arthritis; ankle: pain, sprain or rheumatism.
> Foot: old pain, cramps, cannot be put on the ground, as if bursting, or weakness, cannot lift the foot, walks without strength, to the point of flaccidity.
> Arch: pain, arthritis.
> Sole: acute pain.

BL-61 *pucan* — help of the servant

Lateral heel: on the bone; below the angle between the anterior edge of the vertical long tendon and the posterior edge of the ankle (lateral malleolus) and the eminence of the bone; in a hollow.

One FW below *kunlun* (BL-60); about two FW above *shenmai* (BL-62).

When tonified:
> Tonifies the bladder, mid-brain (thalamus), large intestine, half-body opposite, lateral heel.
> Dispersing acts in the opposite way.

Direct effects:

    Opposite side of the body, all pain (less effective than *kunlun,* BL-60).

    Hyperexcited speech, delusions, hallucinations, talks all the time (?), tongue out, then coma (epilepsy?).

    Large intestine: cholera (cramps, agitation, pain, vomiting, diarrhea); beriberi.

Parts of the body:

    Half-body, opposite side.

    Upper limb, opposite; hand: pain.

    Lumbar area, opposite sacrum: pain; opposite lower limb; opposite lateral knee; opposite lateral leg; peroneus longus muscle.

    Opposite foot: flaccidity; extensors of the toes; lateral heel and sole.

BL-62   *shenmai* — perforating vessel

Lateral foot: just under the lateral malleolus, below the lower edge of the last transverse bone (calcaneus); in the angle between the posterior edge of the tendons turning towards the front (peroneus longus muscle, and under it, the posterior peroneus brevis), and the superior edge of a horizontal muscle (abductor digiti minimi muscle); in a hollow.

    About two FW below *pucan* (BL-61); one large FW posterior to *jinmen* (BL-63).

When tonified:

    Tonifies the bladder, all the energy of yang activity, all that is yang (brain, heat, spasms, skin, body and limbs same side, particularly the right side).

    Disperses cold, energy of yin inactivity, swelling.

    Dispersing acts in the opposite way.

    All energy of yang activity, wakefulness, cerebrum, heat. Command point of the *yangqiao mai,* "vessel of the external hollow," which commands all the yang energy; responds with *houxi* (SI-3), the command point of the governor vessel (cerebral energy and physical strength). If excess: aggravation at night, better in the middle of the day, with insomnia, hyperexcitation, irritability, heat.

Direct effects:

    Obsessions, repression of feelings and ideas, helps to speak and unbosom oneself: disperse; hyperexcitation, delirium from fever or emotion, convulsion or epilepsy at night: disperse. Can cause convulsions in the day. If during the day, disperse *zhaohai* (KI-3, IS KI-6), which can provoke convulsion at night; apoplexy: disperse.

    If insufficient: slowness and lassitude of mind, somnolence, vertigo, cannot open one's heart, heavy sleep at night, chills. (Tonifying acts like a cup of coffee.)

    Without cause, head foggy, empty, vertigo, feels as if on a boat: tonify; sleeps too deeply: tonify.

    Insomnia: disperse.

    Heat: extraordinary heat, even in shadow and cold: disperse; head sweats: disperse, or internal cold, cold from extreme fatigue, chills: tonify.

    Hot flushes and violent sweats of menopause: disperse.

    Skin: acne, furuncles, boils: disperse. Prevents their repetition (furunculosis).

    Eye same side: pain, dizziness, dizziness from shock (or nerves): disperse.

    Ear same side: pain, bleeding: disperse; buzzing: tonify.

    Teeth: same side, pain (particularly molars).

    Stomach: cramps, spasms.

    Bladder: incontinency during very heavy sleep (often due to spina bifida); disperse every evening until the sleep becomes lighter and the need to urinate awakens; prostate and sphincter.

Parts of the body:

    Articulations: pain, hardness, contractures, ankylosis; or relaxed.

    Head: acute pain, mostly above the eyebrows like a bar, congestive headache, migraine, external pains of the head.

    Body: swelling, back bent, stiff.

    Extremities: troubles with mechanical or involuntary motions, awkwardness, cold, pain, or weakness.

    Lumbar area: pain, rheumatism of the lumbar vertebrae from cold, muscles contracted or weak.

    Upper limb: joint pains.

    Lower limb: pain; or swelling: tonify.

Lower leg (region of the tibialis anterior muscle): numbness, cannot stand for a long time, weakness, swelling or pain; contracture.

Foot sprain, pain and swelling: disperse.

Begin with it for: abscess, joint pain, nape and back pain with contracture or flaccidity; does not speak; or agitation; finish with *houxi* (SI-3) if necessary.

BL-63 *jinmen* — gate of gold

Lateral edge of the foot: about two FW below and a little in front of the lateral malleolus. In the angle between the upper edge of a horizontal muscle at the edge of the sole (abductor digiti minimi muscle), and the posterior edge of the inferior point of the cuboid bone; in front of the calcaneus; in a hollow.

One large FW in front of *shenmai* (BL-62); two FW posterior to *jinggu* (BL-64).

When tonified:

Tonifies the bladder, anterior frontal lobe, heart, stomach, eye and ear same side; lower abdomen, knee, lower forehead.

Disperses mid-brain (striopallidum).

Dispersing acts in the opposite way.

Direct effects:

Eye: same side, "home of the tears."

Ear, same side: buzzing or pain; otitis: bleeding.

Stomach: vomiting, nausea, peritonitis.

Bladder: fevers (red face, hyperexcitation, abundant sweat, pain in the lumbar area, vertigo).

Malaria: several attacks per day without interruption.

Opposite effects:

Epileptoid troubles, dependent on the striopallidum, which inhibits the involuntary movements and thoughts.

Excess of the striopallidum: disperse. Absence, distraction without apparent cause, fog and vertigo to the point of falling, body trembling, cannot stand for a long time.

Insufficiency of the striopallidum, uncontrolled movement, children beating their head against the furniture or on the ground, infants with shaking head, throwing it back, mouth open; epilepsy, whinnying, falls, loss of consciousness; convulsions or spasms of children.

Parts of the body:

Forehead: pain above the eyebrow; head: tics, movement.

Sudden cramps; cramps from cholera.

Knee: paralysis of the patellar area.

Knee: anterior lower leg: arch, numbness.

BL-64 *jinggu* — bone of the capital

Lateral edge of the foot: one half FW in front of the big bony eminence at mid-length (tubercle of the fifth metatarsal); in the angle between the upper edge of the metatarsal and the anterior edge of the insertion of the peroneus brevis; on the upper edge of the muscle forming the edge of the sole (abductor digiti minimi muscle), in a hollow.

Two FW anterior to *jinmen* (BL-63); two FW posterior to *shugu* (BL-65).

When tonified:

Tonifies the bladder, posterior inferior frontal lobes, liver, gallbladder.

Disperses lung, heart, kidney.

Dispersing acts in the opposite way.

Direct effects:

Emotional agitation: neither drinks nor eats; insanity, hyperexcitation; meningitis; cerebral congestion, congestive headaches, heat in the head, cerebral anemia, vertigo.

Source point of the bladder: can tonify or disperse. Directly: prostate, sphincter, urethra; opposite way: expulsor muscles (detrusor muscle).

Eye same side: medial corner congested; cataract starting at the medial corner of the pupil.

Opposite effects:

Heart: all trouble with pain and visual dizziness; malaria with convulsions.

Parts of the body:
    Vertebral column: all troubles — displacements, deviation.
    Chews the cheek.
    Muscles: contractures?
    Lateral neck: nape, back and lumbar area same side: stiffness, pain.
    Hip joint, hip, lower limb and foot: pain.
    Foot: contracture, turns inside, lateral edge low, difficulty extending and raising foot.

BL-65 *shugu* — linking bones

Foot, lateral edge: in the angle between the lower edge of the head and body of the fifth metatarsal; on the upper edge of a longitudinal muscle (abductor digiti minimi); in a hollow.

Two FW in front of *jinggu* (BL-64); two FW posterior to *tonggu* (BL-66); two FW lateral to foot-*linqi* (GB-41).

When dispersed:
    Disperses the bladder, cerebellum, spinal cord, large intestine, lacrimal canal, head, skin, back, lumbar area, posterior hip joint, posterior knee and calf.
    Tonifies the lung.
    Tonifying acts in the opposite way.

Direct effects:
    Dispersal point of the bladder (pulse of the bladder narrow, hard). Bladder: irritation to the point of inflammation (cystitis), spasms; need to urinate frequent and urgent.
    Stones in the bladder.
    Large intestine: occlusion with pain in the lumbar area; or diarrhea; anus: hemorrhoids.
    Teeth: pain of the incisors.

Opposite effects:
    Lung: congestion, or edema with diminished urine.

Parts of the body:
    Head: acute pain at the top, headaches during defecation.
    Lacrimal canal (medial canthus) contracted, swollen, obstructed; tears flow without stopping; ear: deafness?
    Skin: ache, abscess (particularly on the back).
    Movement inside the skin (fibrillations).
    Opposite head, cheeks, nape: pain; stiff nape; opposite nape: atrophied muscles.
    Back, lumbar area; pain as if broken; from the back of the head to the opposite foot: pain.
    Hip and lower limb: stiff joints, hip stiff, cannot bend (ankylosis?).
    Posterior knee: tied up; calf: cramps, as if torn.
    Cannot bend the foot.

BL-66 [foot-]*tonggu* — communicating valley

Foot; lateral edge: just in front of the articulation of the base of the fifth toe; in the lower angle between the inferior, anterior (plantar) edge of the head of the phalange and the upper edge of the abductor; in a hollow.

Two FW in front of *shugu* (BL-65); one FW behind *zhiyin* (BL-67 and last); two FW lateral to *xiaxi* (GB-43).

When tonified:
    Tonifies the bladder, medulla oblongata, frontal lobes, upper spinal cord, stomach, ear, throat, lateral neck, eye, lumbar area, buttock and posterior opposite thigh.
    Disperses the heart.
    Dispersing acts in the opposite way.
    Deranged mind, emotional agitation; cerebral anemia or cerebral congestion, vertigo, nosebleeds, pain of the nape, headache, visual dizziness. Frequent yawning.
    Eyes: obscured vision.
    Stomach: old inflammation, mucus of the stomach (thready); liquids remain, food non-digested.
    Nose: chronic coryza — clear flow from attacks.
    Uterus: congestion?

Point of Weihe: Spigelia?

BL-67 *zhiyin* — extreme yin

Foot, fifth toe, lateral face, ungual phalanx; in the angle between the inferior, anterior edge of the swelling of the bone and the superior edge of the flexor; in a hollow.

One FW distal to *tonggu* (BL-66).

When tonified:

Tonifies the bladder, all the yin distributor meridians (deep pulses); posterior frontal lobes, posterior hypothalamus (sympathetic system), upper half of the face and body (particularly the thorax).

Disperses the kidneys, all yang producer meridians (superficial pulses).

Dispersing acts in the opposite way.

Direct effects:

The energy coming from the meridian of the kidney (*yongquan,* KI-1) enters the bladder meridian here.[2]

Contracted thoracic and pelvis organs; parasitic worms.

Tonification point of the bladder. All weakness, atony, atonic retention, urination insufficient or stopped (tonifies the expulsor muscles and relaxes the vesical sphincter): tonify; incontinence (expulsor muscles too strong and sphincter relaxed): disperse.

All varieties of parasitic worms (intestines or stomach: threadworms, lamblia and even tapeworms, etc.); makes them come out the next day and gives immunity against them if the treatment is redone three new moons following; all trouble caused by worms (nervousness to the point of convulsions, hyperexcitation to the point of insanity, pain in the abdomen or stomach, vertigo, etc.).

Opposite side of nose blocked, head heavy, headache: tonify; chronic coryza, flowing clearly from a crisis: disperse.

Eyes: pain, congestion; cataract?

Ears: buzzing? deafness?

Arteries and veins: hypotension: tonify. Hypertension, hardness: disperse. "Rheumatism paralyzing the vessels"?

Ice cold malaria (without sweat, with palpitation, nervous form).

Genital organs: weak uterus: tonify; contracted: disperse. Accelerates birth delivery; delivery with infant's hand presenting first; menstrual periods not coming because of atonic ovaries: tonify; or from spasms with pain: disperse.

Parts of the body:

Opposite face and half-body, particularly the thorax.

Face, all problems.

Lateral neck, nape and entire shoulder.

Thorax and sides: pain like a belt, having no fixed location.

Back, from lumbar area to coccyx: pain.

Opposite lower limb, foot: arthritis; sole: heat.

Notes

[1] The last works of the author seem to indicate that the points 31, 32, 33, 34, 35 of the bladder meridian could be linked with the governor vessel between points 2 and 3 of the governor vessel. — ed.

[2] This seems to be a mistake in the text, for the energy of the bladder meridian goes into the kidney meridian, not the other way around as stated here. — ed.

Chapter VIII

Kidney

Although having only a single meridian, each kidney has two pulses — left III middle radial: left kidney, glomerules, filtration; middle ulnar: left kidney glomerules, filtration; left III deep radial: right kidney (reabsorption-excretion-secretion tubules); deep ulnar: right kidney (reabsorption-excretion-secretion tubules).

Their maximum hours are 5:00 p.m. to 7:00 p.m. (minimum hours of the large intestine). The bladder is the upstream meridian (mother) and also the linked meridian; the heart-governor is the downstream meridian (son) and also the wife. Tonifying the kidney-filtration tonifies the vessels and disperses the large intestine and the bladder. Tonifying the kidney excretion-secretion tonifies the sexual organs and disperses the large intestine. Dispersing acts in the opposite way.

The parasympathetic system inhibits it, contracts it; the sympathetic system tonifies it, dilates it. Dispersing the glomeruli (*jiaoxin,* KI-8, and *rangu,* KI-2) augments the filtration (quantity of urine). Tonifying the tubules (*fuliu,* KI-7, and *yongquan,* KI-1) augments the excretion-secretion (color of the urine, the solids). Tonifying the glomeruli diminishes the filtration; dispersing the tubules diminishes the color.

Tonifying the tubules, if it is necessary, can cause renin secretion (vasopressin, which forms angiotensin) which raises the blood pressure if it is too low for filtration.

In the Far East, it is said, "Kidneys receive their life from the hair of the head and from the skin (which receives it from the lungs) and give it to the bone."

They command, for the mind: decision-will, seductiveness, (*fuliu,* KI-7), inferiority or failure complexes, with their opposite, that of authority (*dazhong,* KI-6, IS KI-4), "abhorrence of living" and despair (epigastrium-*shangqiu,* KI-17, and *shencang,* KI-25).

For the physical: the most important is the rectification of faulty heredity: *zhubin* (KI-9). Most kidney points affect the sense organs, particularly *yongquan* (KI-1). The sexual organs are affected by *dahe* (KI-12), *qixue* (KI-13) and *siman* (KI-14). For vomiting from all causes: *youmen* (KI-21) and *tonggu* (KI-20). Kidney points also are used for spasms and sudden pain through all the points of the abdomen (which form the "attack vessel," *chong mai,* the command point of which is *gongsun,* SP-4). They also affect head and body hair, with *weizhong* (BL-54, IS BL-40).

They are greatly affected by emotions, cold and heat.

KI-1   *yongquan* — bubbling source

Sole of the foot: about one-third lateral, approximately mid-length: at the level of and at two FW medial to the anterior edge of the lateral eminence of the foot (tubercle of the fifth metatarsal); in the angle between the medial edge of the lateral muscle (abductor digiti minimi) and the anterior edge of a transverse mass; in a hollow. Slightly lateral to the flexor digitorum brevis muscle.

Two FW lateral and in front of *rangu* (KI-2). A branch goes along the abductor digiti minimi muscle and curves around this on the lower face up to the lateral face of the distal phalange [of the fifth toe] at *zhiyin* (BL-67), causing the energy to pass from the meridian of the kidney to that of the bladder.

When tonified:
>   Tonifies the kidney excretion-secretion (tubules), medulla oblongata, spinal cord, superior occipital lobes, primate, organs of sense, heart, arteries, pancreas, sexual organs, mouth, throat, larynx, lung, posterior shoulder, upper and lower limb same side.
>   Disperses the large intestine, stomach, small intestine, bladder.
>   Dispersing acts in the opposite way; responds with *fuliu* (KI-7).

Direct effects:
>   Little energy, voice husky, without timbre, to speak is an effort; timidity, apprehension, easy sadness, easily upset, memory confused, forgets easily; yawning, likes to stretch, does not want to speak; but as soon as sitting, wants to stand up; hot fainting, hot feet; weakness, "face black like carbon"?
>   Or fits of hyperexcitation. Children: convulsions; acute or chronic meningitis? Epilepsy with pain at the heart? The whole body: prickling numbness; pain, neuralgia; cramps of all limbs; cramps from cholera; articular rheumatism.
>   Kidney: deep pulse (reabsorption-excretion-secretion; tubules).

Insufficiency: tonify (insufficiency of tubules, of excretion): colorless urine; frequent need to urinate night or day; pain in the kidneys from waiting too long to urinate; skin dry, little perspiration; edema below the eyes (home of the tears); cramps at night.

Excess: disperse (tubules in excess). Insufficient urine, colored, difficult; contracted kidneys: lumbar pain; abundant sweat; hypertension (of minima); headache from bending; edema, ascites; cramps from excess of kidney; excess urea in the blood; deep pulse sinking, hard.

Bladder: spasms, retention, lower abdomen contracted.

Arteries: hypertension of the minima: disperse; incessant nosebleeds.

Heart: agitation, palpitations, tachycardia, sudden unbearable hot pains; interior of chest as if bound.

Eruptive fevers: measles, German measles, scarlet fever; fever from all inflammation, starting from numbness of the lumbar area.

Liver, gallbladder, jaundice, body yellow, chest bound, stool stopped.

Sexual organs: men — sexual weakness, non-erection; women — sterility, without children, uterus displaced or in spasm, prolapsed uterus. Both sexes: blenorrhagia.

Sense organs: Eyes darkened, bad sight, eyelids falling (ptosis). Ears: buzzing, deafness (from excess of kidney): disperse. Smell-taste diminished or lost.

Mouth, tongue and throat dry, opposite; drinks a lot: tonify.

Throat: pain and swelling, can neither swallow nor speak; fever, cough, closed throat (acute tonsillitis), disperse opposite.

Larynx: mute, aphonia, weakness to the point of flaccidity of the hyoid and glosseus muscles, dyspnea, suffocation from laughing, coughs and spits blood.

Opposite effects:

Large intestine: excess — stool difficult, or diarrhea, pain of the abdomen and sides; heaviness in the anus and lower abdomen. Spasms of small intestine, painful. Cholera: cramps, pain of the abdomen, cold, fainting.

Stomach: inflammation. Even fasting, no desire to eat. Drinks a lot.

Parts of the body:

Half body, same side: pain or cramps; or rheumatism of joints or numbness.

Shoulder, upper limb, same side: all trouble. Lumbar area; pain.

Lower limb: pain, contracture or weakness; medial posterior thigh: pain; feet: cold to the knee, or pain, cannot touch the ground; five toes: pain; sole: cold or hot, contracture.

𝔦 KI-2 *rangu* — valley of approbation

Sole of the foot; one-fourth of the width; one large FW in front of the heel bone (calcaneus); in the angle between the anterior edge of a transverse mass and the lateral edge of the muscle forming the medial edge (abductor, and deeper, the flexor of the great toe); in a hollow; on the medial edge of the flexor digitorum brevis muscle.

Three FW in front of and lateral to *zhaohai* (KI-3, IS KI-6); two posterior and medial to *yongquan* (KI-1). At the level of and lateral to (separated by the adductor) foot-*shangqiu* (SP-5) and the scaphoid eminence.

When dispersed:

Disperses kidney filtration, glomeruli (increases urine), medulla oblongata, spinal cord, lower conception vessel, all the yin distributor organ meridians, sexual organs, ear and throat same side, feet, contusions.

Tonifies the bladder, lower part of the governor vessel, large intestine and all the yang producer meridians. Responds in *jiaoxin* (KI-8).

Tonifying acts in the opposite way.

Direct effects:

Psychological: Excess: excess decision-will and personality. Insufficiency: apprehension, anxiety as if afraid of being arrested, melancholy and fullness, tongue relaxed, weakness, cold in the chest.

Dispersal point of the kidney filtration (glomeruli). Excess kidney-filtration: disperse (pulse of kidney-filtration narrow, hard); feeble urination, edema, abundant nights sweats with no apparent cause, abundant saliva (epithelial nephritis, glomerulonephritis?); maxima hypertension. Excess urine from diabetes: tonify; abundant urine, particularly at the end of the night; incontinence in the morning, dry mouth, little sweat.

Bladder, urethra: inflammation (cystitis, urethritis); difficult urination.

Heart: inflammation, pain as if pierced, weakened; pulse: rapid with a pause every ten or twenty beats (decline of energy), or normal speed with a pause every third beat: disperse; tonifying increases the irregularity.

Arteries: maxima hypertension from kidney excess (glomerulonephritis, causing production of renin, which forms in the liver angiotensin), or from distention of the liver and kidney.

Blood: furunculosis, succession of furuncles: disperse; septicemia: disperse; blood poisoning: disperse.

Sexual organs: men and women: blenorrhagia, inguinal nodes; women: sterility; ovaries inflamed; uterus: congestion or prolapse, insufficient or difficult menses; leukorrhea, contracted vagina, spasm (vaginismus), pain piercing chest and side, lower abdomen swollen; vulva: swelling, congestion, pruritis; numbness of legs during orgasm; delivery: first child — eclampsia, convulsions, jaw contracted (trismus). Men: flaccidity of the penis, impotence (diabetes), insufficient sperm, tired, seminal losses.

Ear same side: inflammation.

Throat same side: inflammation, acute tonsillitis; can neither swallow nor spit; swelling under the tongue; abundant saliva, even with blood.

Cough, little energy, dyspnea, fullness of the chest and sides.

Pancreas: diabetes, glycosuria, violent sweats, impotence, dry mouth: disperse.

Opposite effects:

Large intestine: diarrhea to the point of never leaving the bathroom.

Parts of the body:

Falls: internal contusions, "bad blood remaining in the abdomen."

Knee: pain as if pierced or separated; lower leg: numbness, cannot stand up for a long time. Feet: one hot, one cold, cramps in the feet, mostly at night, arch swollen, cannot walk, hot soles.

KI-3   *zhaohai* (IS KI-6) — mirroring ocean

Foot, medial face: just under the medial malleolus; in the angle between the inferior edge of the last bone (calcaneus) and the posterior edge of the vertical tendons (flexor digitorum and flexor pollicis longus muscle; in a hollow; slightly above the plantar cushion.

Three FW posterior and above *rangu* (KI-2); one FW below *shuiquan* (KI-4, IS KI-5).

When tonified:

Tonifies yin energy of inactivity, kidneys, cerebellum, pons, lower spinal cord, diaphragm, lumbar area, halfbody same side.

Disperses the bladder, throat and sexual organs.

To tonify, act in the opposite way.

Direct effects:

Commands the yin energy of inactivity, of sleep, of lassitude. Point of command of the *yinqiao mai* (vessel of the the lateral hollow), which acts on all troubles from insufficiency or excess of yin energy; responds with *lieque* (LU-7), which commands the conception vessel; reunion of all the yin meridians.

Exhaustion, lassitude, weakness either of women or old people, insomnia from insufficiency of yin energy, thus dominance of yang energy; great nervous troubles with hyperexcitation and pain, great malaise without knowing where the evil is; constant sorrow without joy: disperse.

Aggravation of all troubles in the middle of the day: disperse. Cramps or epileptic fits in the middle of the day: disperse. (Retards them at night or abolishes them.) All troubles increased in the middle of the day: of the heart, lung, chest, lower abdomen, throat and diaphragm.

Eye: sees stars or is in shadow (ophthalmic migraine).

Diaphragm: strange energy, sudden spasms, hiccoughs, vomiting: disperse.

Opposite effects:

Throat: pain, tonsillitis, larynx strangled with mucus, saliva or dry throat, unappeasable thirst (diabetes or dipsomania): tonify.

Upset stomach: tonify.

Abdomen: enlargement or inflammation from alcohol; colic, gas, constipation or urgent diarrhea; intestinal spasms: tonify. Frequent or constant intestinal hemorrhages: tonify; constipation of women: tonify.

Lower pelvis and throat: linked troubles: disperse; lower abdomen: spasms, pains; heat and pain of the sides of the lower abdomen.

Sexual organs: sudden jumps and hardening (spasms), blenorrhagia. Men: non-erection (diabetes); or erections without cause; pruritis; testicles: orchitis. Women: during menses, pain of the vagina, cannot retain the fetus: tonify. Pains of virgins during menses: tonify. Menses difficult, frantic malaise, excess vaginal secretions, "fluids clearly flowing": disperse. After delivery, the placenta does not descend: disperse.

Bladder: nervous pain: tonify; urethra: inflammation, burning urination.

Parts of the body:
    Limbs and lumbar area without strength; cannot sit with confidence.
    Lateral atrophy from great nervous trouble (polio?).
    Sprain of the internal malleolus.

KI-4   *shuiquan* (IS KI-5) — water source

Heel, medial face: one large FW below and slightly behind the medial malleolus; in the angle between the inferior edge of the transverse superior edge of the calcaneus and the posterior edge of the vertical tendons (flexor communis, then flexor pollicis longus, then tibialis posterior); in a hollow.

One FW posterior to *zhaohai* (KI-3, IS KI-6); two FW under *taixi* (KI-5, IS KI-3).

When tonified:
    Tonifies the kidney, sexual organs, superior occipital lobes, cerebellum, uterus, urethra, opposite eye (muscles), medial heel.
    Dispersing acts in the opposite way.

Direct effects:
    For several days before menses: depression, sadness, easy tears: tonify; or irritability, nervousness, aggressiveness: disperse.
    Menses insufficient or impeded, due to spasms: disperse; from weakness: tonify; prolapsed uterus?
    Men: non-erection? urethritis?
    Opposite eye: myopia; problems of distant vision: tonify.

Parts of the body:
    Medial plantar heel.
    Flexor communis digitorum pedis muscle.

KI-5   *taixi* (IS KI-3) — supreme vale

Top of the medial side of the heel, in the angle between the posterior edge of the medial malleolus and the tendons running along it (flexor communis, then in front of the flexor proper, then the tibialis posterior); in a hollow. In front of the anterior peroneal arteries, veins and nerves.

Two FW above *shuiquan* (KI-4, IS KI-5); two small FW below *dazhong* (KI-6, IS KI-4).

When tonified:
    Tonifies the kidney excretion-secretion (tubules) and all the yin distributor meridians (except vessels), spleen-pancreas, eye same side, ear same side, tip of the tongue, bottom of the palate, tonsils, opposite throat, opposite parotid gland.
    Disperses kidney filtration (glomeruli), vessels, large intestine, stomach, bladder (urethra, sphincter).
    Dispersing acts in the opposite way; responds with *feiyang* (BL-58).
    ''If the patient has this pulse (interior peroneal artery) he will live; if not, he will die.'' (?)

Direct effects:
    Point of passage between kidney and bladder (*feiyang*, BL-58). If excess: urine and stool are diminished or stopped; if insufficient: pain in lumbar area and vertebra. Tonifying makes the excess of the bladder pass into the insufficiency of the kidney and diminishes the frequent needs and irritation of the bladder. Dispersing causes the excess of the kidney to pass into the insufficiency of the bladder; increases urine and stool; calms the irritation of the kidneys.
    Point of passage between kidney excretion-secretion and kidney filtration; acts on the glomeruli; dispersing the tubules contracts the glomeruli. Kidney insufficiency: abundant urine, little sweat, saliva and secretion: disperse (tubules in excess, hypertension, glomeruli insufficient, relaxed). Excess: scant urine, abundant sweat, saliva and secretion: tonify (hypotension, tubules insufficient, glomeruli in excess, contracted).
    Tonifying gives humidity and heat, ''prevents the humidity of the earth from stopping the kidneys'' (?) Fever of kidneys: (a lot of sweat, thirst, vomit, desire for solitude, pain of lumbar area and legs).
    Heart: pain as if pierced; feet and hands cold and ''if there is dyspnea, he will not live'' (true angina of the chest): disperse; endocarditis.
    Arteries: hypertension. If excess of tubules: disperse; if excess of glomeruli: tonify. Tonifying tonifies the sexual organs and disperses the arteries (point of passage).

Cough: fullness of mucus, breathlessness: disperse; coughing fits with prolonged fever; rusty saliva, wet pleurisy, dry pleurisy.

Pancreas: diabetes, impotency, thirst, abundant urine, pain in right abdomen, emaciation, bad breath (nephritis?).

Sexual organs: women — opposite breast: inflammation; uterus: spasms and pain, deposits; paresis of hands and feet; contracted vagina. Men — impotency from sexual excess or from diabetes.

Ear same side: buzzing from emptiness of kidney: tonify.

Eye same side: swelling, pain.

Mouth, opposite side; heat, saliva like paste, inflammation of the mouth; yawning; back of the opposite palate; opposite throat; tonsillitis: pain, swelling, chronic angina; teeth: pain same side.

Opposite effects:

Diaphragm spasms, hiccough: tonify.

Large intestine: constipation from atony: disperse; dysentery: pain in abdomen and side: tonify.

Stomach: "causes the energy of the stomach to go out and circulate with the yang." Melting thinness, no appetite, regurgitation of food, vomiting: tonify; all trouble with vomiting: tonify.

Parts of the body:

Four limbs weak and cold, extremities cold after fever, extremities weak; leg, knee, calf numb, weak or swollen.

Medial malleolus: all troubles and sprains.

Babies: swelling of the umbilicus.

KI-6   *dazhong* (IS KI-4) — big bell

Medial side of the ankle; in the angle between the upper edge of the medial malleolus and the tibia; in the angle between the edge of the tendon that runs along the malleolus (tibialis posterior muscle) and the superior edge of a ligament at an angle (achillo-malleolar); on the flexor communis and the edge of the flexor pollicis longus between the tibialis posterior and the Achilles tendon; in a hollow.

Two small FW above *taixi* (KI-5, IS KI-3); two large FW below *fuliu* (KI-7).

When tonified:

Tonifies the kidney, superior occipital lobe, primate, spinal cord, lower lumbar area, medial malleolus, authority, respiratory passages.

Disperses the bladder, prostate, large intestine, digestive passages.

Responds with *fuyang* (BL-59).

Dispersing acts in the opposite way.

Direct effects:

Inferiority and failure complex, lack of authority; apprehension, emotional agitation; misanthropy, desire to exclude oneself from the world and close one's door; melancholy without joy; little energy, desire to lie down; stupidity, easily or constantly cold; little warmth.

Respiratory passages; energy in the throat, spasms of throat, noise in the larynx; cough, mucus; breathlessness; "swelling of chest."

Heart: nervous palpitation from emotion, from timidity.

Opposite effects:

Mouth, opposite: heat, inflammation; tongue opposite; dryness, inflammation, aphtha; gums opposite, pain, weakness, teeth loose.

Contracted esophagus, nausea, vomiting, food does not descend, stays in throat.

Large intestine: constipation, stool difficult or stopped.

Prostate: has a response in *fuyang* (BL-59).

Parts of the body:

Vertebrae and abdomen: stiffness with shivering in the bath.

Lumbar vertebrae: pain, little energy.

Medial ankle: sprain and pulls; flexor pollicis longus.

KI-7 *fuliu* — flows again

Medial lower leg; two FW above the medial malleolus; one half FW posterior to the posterior edge of the tibia, between two muscles; on the posterior edge of the tibialis posterior muscle; on the anterior edge of the flexor communis; on the lower edge of a transverse mass; in a hollow.

Two FW above *dazhong* (KI-6, IS KI-4); one FW inferior and posterior to *jiaoxin* (KI-8).

When tonified:
Greatly increases urine and stool; tonifies kidney excretion-secretion (tubules), superior part of occipital lobes, primate, medulla oblongata, spinal cord, vessels, eyes, ears, back of the throat, last molars, all on the same side.
Same side: upper limb, lower limb (medial gastrocnemius, medial thigh, hip, lumbar area).
Disperses the large intestine, stomach, bladder.
Dispersing acts in the opposite way.
Responds with *yongquan* (KI-1), *zhigou* (TW-6), and *xuehai* (SP-10).

Direct effects:
Decision-will insufficient, lack of character, dreams of being in water, in a flood, on the edge of the precipice; or unhappy, speaks a lot, peremptory, easily angered.
Cold to the marrow; cold of the lower legs and feet; cannot get warm; intensely cold after catching a chill.
Kidney excretion-secretion (tubules): right III pulse deep, sunken, soft; urine without color, or scant to the point of anuria; sweats without cause, or incessantly, in streams, hot, at night; saliva in excess.
All varieties of edema: swelling, mostly ankles, feet. Tonifying increases the excretion of salt, urinary solids and water (tubules) without changing the middle pulse (filtration, glomeruli); verifies the permeability of the adrenal capillaries.
Heart, arteries: Insufficiency: minima hypotension. Excess: minima hypertension (excess of renin and of blood volume); nosebleeds, bleeding hemorrhoids.
Sexual organs: men — tonifying causes nocturnal erections; prostatitis, orchitis, testicles.
Bladder, urethra: inflammation, blenorrhagia; cystitis, urethritis, urine burns like fire, pain at the level of the kidney.
Eye same side: troubled vision, glaucoma; ear and back of mouth same side, teeth: inflammation.

Opposite effects:
Large intestine: tonifying greatly increases the stool and disperses inflammation. Stool insufficient, difficult, gas, spasms, pain of the lumbar area, to the point of occlusion, peritonitis, spasms from intestinal worms, diarrhea burning to the anus, bleeding hemorrhoids after stool.
Stomach: tonifying causes acidity, burning.

Parts of the body:
Spinal cord: inflammation causing paralysis, mainly of the lower limb; lateral neck, under and behind the ear, same side.
Upper limb, same side, anterior face of the biceps — pronators, flexors.
Lower limb: flaccidity.
Arch: weakness, flaccidity; contracture or pain.
Flexor digitorum longus muscle, contracted, toes tightened; heel: pain.
Medial gastrocnemius: cramps or weakness.
Medial thigh: weakness or contracture of the adductors and rotators.
Hip-joint: pain, arthritis.
Lumbar area, lumbar muscles flaccid: can neither stand up nor stretch.
Contractures: cannot bend forward.

KI-8 *jiaoxin* — mutual confidence

Medial lower leg: three FW above the medial malleolus. Just on the posterior edge of the tibia; in the upper part of a hollow; between bone and muscle (flexor communis muscle). Slightly above the upper transverse edge of the muscle which disappears under the tibia (tibialis posterior muscle); on the lower edge of a transverse mass (fibers of the flexor communis).

One FW above and in front of *fuliu* (KI-7); one FW under *sanyinjiao* (SP-6); four FW inferior and anterior to *zhubin* (KI-9).

When tonified:

Tonifies the kidney-filtration (glomeruli), sexual organs, posterior frontal lobes, spinal cord, hip joint, lumbar area, thigh, anterior and lateral lower leg and knee; opposite teeth.

Disperses the large intestine, stomach.

Dispersing acts in the opposite way; strongly increases urine, stool and menses.

Direct effects:

Kidney filtration glomeruli: glomeruli contracted (pulses of kidney filtration hard and narrow, or hard and sinking); urine insufficient or stopped. Dispersing strongly increases the quantity of urine without increasing the color (urinary solids): ''urine stopped by heat or energy''; minima hypertension.

Sexual organs: women: if spasms, pain in the lower pelvis, difficult menses, coming badly: disperse; four limbs numb during orgasm: disperse; prolapsis of uterus: tonify; sweat of genitals: disperse. Men: scrotal hernia?

Opposite effects:

Sexual organs: women: menses insufficient, or impeded due to excess vitamin K (antihemorrhagic) produced by the large intestine: disperse; blood flowing without stopping to the point of metrorrhagia: disperse; miscarriage: disperse.

Large intestine: dispersing increases and facilitates the insufficient stool from the atonic large intestine. Tonifying diminishes inflammation or spasms of the large intestine, provoking constipation to the point of occlusion, or violent diarrhea from inflammation; peritonitis; all irritation from intestinal worms.

Stomach: dispersing causes excess and burning; tonifying calms it.

Opposite teeth: pain; caries?

Parts of the body:

Opposite spinal cord: inflammation.

Opposite nape, shoulder, back, lumbar area.

Hip joint, pain going into inguinal area, same side.

Lower limb: flaccidity or contracture, thigh and knee, anterolateral lower leg; toes contracted.

KI-9   *zhubin* — built riverbank (levy)

Medial lower leg: about mid-height, mid-width; seven FW above the medial malleolus. In the anterior angle between the large posterior tendon (Achilles) and the lower edge of the medial gastrocnemius, at its union with the Achilles tendon; in a hollow; on the soleus muscle.

Preceding point: *jiaoxin* (KI-8); two FW anterior and behind *sanyinjiao* (SP-6), where the meridian passes; seven FW below *yingu* (KI-10).

When tonified:

Tonifies the kidney, sexual organs, superior part of the occipital lobes, primate, lower conception vessel, lower governor vessel, gums, penis, uterus; four flexors of the toes, great toe: extensors.

Disperses the large intestine.

Dispersing acts in the opposite way.

Direct effects:

Rectification of faulty heredity or ancestral defects. Tonifying during pregnancy, preferably twice, once at three months and once at six months (once is already enough) gives the child an especially luminous complexion; sleeps at night, laughs during the day, does not get sick or if he does, the cure is within a few hours or days, according to the case. The child will have none of the bad characteristics of the parents, but rather a healthy mind, morale and body.

Prevents miscarriage (must be done as soon as possible, even before conception; prevents the spasms of pregnancy).

Adults and children: unstable temperament and character, capricious, unhappy; frenetic and insulting speech, hyperexcitation, fury, changing moods, appearances of insanity (paranoia); tongue cut [cracked?], flowing saliva, nausea, hysteria. Babies: spasms, pains, cannot suck; spasms of energy.

Lead poisoning (saturnism): headache, teeth loose, nausea, etc.

Teeth loosening, displaced forward in the mouth, gums inflamed.

Lower abdomen, bladder, sphincter of bladder: spasms.

Scrotal hernia? Hernia of baby from birth.

Parts of the body:
   Lower back herpes; lumbar pain.
   Calf (gastrocnemius, soleus), medial foot: cramps; flexor longus digitus: contracture or spasms.

KI-10   *yingu* — valley of yin

Posteromedial face of the knee: on the medial extremity of the transverse crease; on the lateral edge of the tendon (semitendinosis); on the lateral edge of the medial gastrocnemius; in a hollow.

Around eleven FW above *jiaoxin* (KI-8); seven FW above *zhubin* (KI-9); three large FW under *yinlingquan* (SP-9).

When tonified:
   Tonifies the kidney, sexual organs, medial part of the lower limb and posterior knee, cerebellum, pons, spinal cord, sacrum, vertebra same side, lateral part of eye same side, medial part of eye opposite.
   Disperses the large intestine.
   Dispersing acts in the opposite way.

Direct effects:
   Kidneys: edema, dark urine, pain in the abdomen and umbilicus; ''men as if attacked by ascites; women as if pregnant''; distention of the lower abdomen.
   Bladder: difficult urination, contraction, pain in the genital organs, spasmodic retention; urethral inflammation.
   Abundant, flowing saliva; tongue relaxed; swelling under the tongue.
   Sexual organs: women — large lipped vulva, inflammation, vulvar pruritis; vagina: inflammation, constant white discharge: tonify; metrorrhagia: disperse. Men: non-erection; penis: glands: pain or insensitivity.

Parts of the body:
   Sacrum and vertebrae, same side; readjusts them.
   Lower limb, medial: posteromedial knee pain as if pierced through; arthritis.
   Posterior knee: pain; or contracture or arthritis.
   Lower leg: medial gastrocnemius.
   Foot: particularly the great toe — gout, swollen, painful, red, weak, heavy.

KI-11   *henggu* — transverse bone (pubis)

Lower abdomen: just at the upper edge of the transverse bone (pubis); one large FW on either side of the median line. In a hollow; mid-width on a large vertical muscle (rectus abdominus muscle); on the lateral edge of a vertical artery (superficial abdominal).[1]

One FW below *dahe* (KI-12); one large FW on either side of *qugu* (CV-2); three FW medial to *qichong* (ST-30).

When tonified:
   Tonifies the kidney, heart, sexual organs, superior occipital lobes, lower spinal cord, primate, medial part of opposite eye, ear same side, eyelids, under the eye (''home of the tears''), tongue opposite side; inferior face of penis.
   Disperses the large intestine, stomach.
   Dispersing acts in the opposite way; a point of the attack vessel *(chong mai)*.

Direct effects:
   General weakness, exhaustion, becomes red at the least emotion; trembling? cramps?
   Insufficiency, exhaustion of the internal organs.
   Medial side of opposite eye, eyeball congested, red, painful, ''home of tears,'' swollen, eyelids red.
   Mouth: opposite side of tongue: cryptic tonsillitis?
   Kidneys contracted, spasms, feeble urine
   Sexual organs: pain. Women — uterus laterally displaced, sensitivity or pain of the vagina, fibrous uterus? Men — seminal losses.
   Heart: easily tired, anemia.

Opposite effects:
   Large intestine: spasms, spasmodic constipation; colic.
   Bladder: spasm, retention, difficult micturition, pain, to the point of urine not coming, lower abdomen swollen, bladder inflammation (cystitis), bladder flaccidity, nocturnal incontinence? urethra: blenorrhagia.

Parts of the body:
Opposite lateral calf and foot.

Point of Weihe: Ferrum Metallicum. Lips red, swollen, burning tongue, general weakness, anemia, trembling, cramps: follicular tonsillitis; bladder: pain, incontinence in the aged; vomits after eating or after midnight; sensitive vagina, uterine fibroids; seminal losses.

KI-12   *dahe* — great respectability

Lower abdomen: about one FW above the pubis and two FW on either side of the median line [see footnote for *henggu,* KI-11]; mid-width on the large vertical muscle (rectus abdominus); in a hollow; on the lateral edge of the vertical artery (superficial abdominal artery).

One FW above *henggu* (KI-11); one FW below *qixue* (KI-13); one large FW on either side of *zhongji* (CV-3); two FW medial to *guilai* (ST-29); one FW medial to *zigong* (MP-35, IS M-CA-18).

When tonified:
Tonifies the kidney, sexual organs, superior occipital lobes, primate. Opposite lateral side of eye, base of the penis.
Disperses the large intestine.
Dispersing acts in the opposite way.
One of the points of the vessel of attack *(chong mai).*

Direct effects:
Sexual organs: special for the fallopian tubes — congested, sensitive; disperses the uterus. Chronic metritis, constant discharge: tonify; red discharge: disperse.
Men: insufficiency of sexual organ, sperm diminished, no erection, seminal loss from emptiness or exhaustion, testicle not descending (cryptorchidism) or re-ascending, gonorrhea, old blenorrhagia, urethritis; penis: pain at the base.
Lateral side of eye opposite: congestion, redness, keratitis.

KI-13   *qixue* — point of energy

Abdomen: about two FW above the pubis (three FW below the level of the navel). Two FW on either side of the median line [see footnote for *henggu,* KI-11]. Mid-width on the large vertical muscle (rectus abdominus); in a hollow; on the medial edge of the vertical artery (superficial abdominal artery).

One FW above *dahe* (KI-12); one FW below *siman* (KI-14); two FW on either side of *guanyuan* (CV-4); two FW medial to *shuidao* (ST-28).

When tonified:
Tonifies the kidney, sexual organs, brain, cerebellum, spinal cord, lateral side of eye, same side.
Disperses the large intestine.
Dispersing acts in the opposite way; a point of the attack vessel *(chong mai).*

Direct effects:
Sensitive to the cold, hands blue? Reddens easily?
Kidney: inflammation (nephritis) with paralysis of the bladder.
Sexual organs: women — special for the ovaries and the ends of the fallopian tubes (salpingitis).
All troubles: ovaries swollen, painful — congestion from cold or microbial inflammation, menses difficult, painful: disperse; or ovaries insufficient, menses insufficient or not coming or irregular; tonify; end of fallopian tube: inflammation, salpingitis, discharge. Men — testicles: orchitis; prostatitis? gonorrhea.
Lateral side of eye, opposite: congestion, redness, keratitis, muscular asthenopia?
Ear same side: whistling or ringing?
Measles: prevents or cures?

Opposite effects:
Stomach swollen with pain in the lumbar vertebrae, lumbar area contracted.
Large intestine: incessant diarrhea.

Parts of the body:
Articular rheumatism with swelling; great toe, gout; hands, articular pain.

Point of Weihe: Right: Rhododendron. Sleeps with legs crossed; eyes: muscular asthenopia, pain in the eye and in the temple, buzzing, deafness, fears thunder, aggravation before storms; rheumatism, gout, particularly during hot weather; swollen articulations, gout of great toe; pain in the hands.

Left: Pulsatilla. Soft, easily overridden, fears the opposite sex. Difficulty sleeping; sleeps with the hands over the top of the head. Men: sexual excitation, prostatitis, blenorrhagia. Women: swollen vulva. Menses stopped from shock, abundant sweat. Hands blue, lower lip cracked, veins dilated, visible, sensitive to cold. Preventive and curative of measles, styes, ophthalmia of newborn, stomach swollen after eating, knee pain.

KI-14   *siman* — four plenitudes

Abdomen: two FW below the level of the umbilicus (three FW above the pubis). About two FW on either side of the median line [see footnote for KI-11]; at the mid-width of a large vertical muscle (rectus abdominus muscle); in a hollow.

One FW above *qixue* (KI-13); one FW below *zhongzhu* (LI-15); two FW medial to *daju* (ST-27); two FW on either side of *shimen* (CV-5).

When tonified:
Tonifies the kidney, sexual organs, mid-brain opposite, spinal cord, eye same side.
Disperses the large intestine.
Dispersing acts in the opposite way.
A point of the attack vessel *(chong mai)*.

Direct effects:
Proud, contemptuous.
Kidney: acute nephritis, pyelitis?
Sexual organs: women — sensual desire, particularly in virgins.
Sensitive sexual organs; during menses, spasms in the uterus, painful "bad blood"; strangling pain, menses insufficient or stopped, contraction, pain, "accumulations," sterility.
Eye same side: atrophy of the pupils and optic nerve? cataract.

Opposite effects:
Large intestine: spasms, pain, intestinal occlusion, "water in the large intestine," pain below the umbilicus.

Point of Weihe: Right: Platina. Pride. Impulse to kill. Atrophy of the retina and optic nerve. Spasms of the pharynx. Obstinate constipation while travelling. Pain during menses; early and prolonged menses; sterility; hot flashes; sensitive sexual organs; sexual desire, mainly in virgins.

Left: Kali Bichromicum. Swollen eyelids, conjunctivitis; ophthalmia. Diphtheria. Swelling after meals, round ulcers, constipation or diarrhea. Vulvar pruritis, early menses, prolapsed uterus. Acute inflammation of the kidney; pyelonephritis; chronic, thick coryza. Dyspnea. Contractions, spasms. Inflammation of the mucosa with mucus. Sensitive heels. Acne.

KI-15   *zhongzhu* — central flow

Abdomen: at the level of one FW below the umbilicus; two large FW on either side of the median line [see footnote for KI-11]; mid-width on the large vertical muscle (rectus abdominus); in a hollow. One FW above *siman* (KI-14); one FW below *huangshu* (KI-16); two large FW on either side of *qihai* (CV-6); two large FW medial to *wailing* (ST-26).

When tonified:
Tonifies the kidney, anterior frontal lobes, sexual organs, base of the penis, inferior lateral side of the eye, same side; articulation of the fingers, heel.
Disperses the large intestine.
Dispersing acts in the opposite way; a point of the attack vessel *(chong mai)*.

Direct effects:
Sexual organs: women — lower pelvis: swelling, inflammation, heat. Ovaries: inflammation, swelling. Fallopian tubes: inflammation, swelling. Menses: insufficient, difficult, painful. Burning vagina, cutting pain during coitus. Men — testicles, inflammation, orchitis; spermatic canal: pain.
Lateral side of the lower part of the eye same side: congestion, redness, pain, keratitis, cataract.

Opposite effects:
Large intestine: inflammation, pain, constipation, particularly spasmodic; dry, hard or insufficient stool; or diarrhea with energy rising or descending with pain radiating into the lumbar area.

Parts of the body:
Head tight like in a helmet.

Hand: eczema? pain; finger joints: swelling, pain.
Heel: pain.

Point of Weihe: Right: Berberis (see *shenshu*, BL-23). Troubles of the liver, rheumatism with urinary trouble, hemorrhoids, abnormal menses; during urination, pain from the lumbar area to the sides; pain in the kidneys, gravel stones, frequent urination; pain in the testicles and in the spermatic canal. In the vagina, burns, cutting pain during sexual relations; shooting pain in the bladder and stomach; head tight as if in a helmet; eczema at the anus or hand; swelling of the finger joints; pain in the heel.

Left: Sepia. Nervous system, liver, uterus; asthma during the night, worse after first sleep, cough dry in the evening, mucus in the morning with back pain; hand, cold sweats, fetid sweat in the armpit and feet; palpitations in the evening, after meals with intermittence and anguish; attacks of heat during movement; generalized pruritis; illnesses of skin, bumps, skin eruptions, warts; headache during menses; heaviness of genital organs; crosses the legs; greenish discharges; incontinence during first sleep; frequent need (to defecate or urinate); nausea in the morning from sight or smell of food; anxiety, depression, all boredom and irritation, apathy; yellow stains around the nose and mouth; articulations of the fingers and toes.

KI-16   *huangshu* — assent of the vital centers

Abdomen: two large FW on either side and at the level of the umbilicus [see footnote for KI-11]; mid-width of the large vertical muscle (rectus abdominus); in a hollow.

One FW above *zhongzhu* (KI-15); two FW below *shangqiu* (KI-17); two large FW on either side of *shenguan* (CV-8, IS *shenque*); two large FW medial to *tianshu* (ST-25).

When tonified:
Tonifies the kidney, sexual organs, posterior frontal lobes, spinal cord, opposite eye, orbit, opposite ear, eustachian tube, heart.
Disperses the bladder (neck), large intestine.
Dispersing acts in the opposite way.
One of the points of the attack vessel *(chong mai)*.
Malaise, trembling, weakness, muscular atrophy, spasms.

Direct effects:
Heart: pain, inflammation, pericarditis.
Sexual organs: sterility, heat of the lower pelvis and abdomen; vagina contracted.
Opposite eye: back of the orbit, congestion, cataract, keratitis.
Opposite ear: tympanum thickened, eustachian tubes closed.

Opposite effects:
Stomach: spasms, pain.
Abdomen: contraction of the whole abdomen, cutting pain; omentum: spasms.
Large intestine: spasms, constant constipation, dried stools or constant diarrhea, jaundice, cirrhosis, hypertrophy of the liver?
Bladder: spasms of the neck.

Point of Weihe: Right: Mercurius Vivus (calomel). Mouth: inflammation, blackish tongue, eustachian tubes obstructed, tympanum thickened; diarrhea, anus painful; colic and vomiting of children; cirrhosis of hypertrophy of the liver; heart and kidney; troubles; prostatitis.

Left: Plumbum Metallicum. Weakness, trembling, flaccidity of the extensor muscles; muscular atrophy, pain in the eyes, as if too big; abdomen contracted, hard; colic, spasm of the anus, obstinate constipation, vagina contracted; spasm of the neck of the bladder, retention.

KI-17   *shangqiu* — turning of the merchants

Epigastrium: about one and one half FW above the level of the umbilicus. About one FW on either side of the median line [see footnote for KI-11]; mid-width on the large vertical muscle (rectus abdominus); in a hollow; at a level of the mid-height of the tenth rib.

Two FW above *huangshu* (KI-16); one FW below *shiguan* (KI-18); about one FW above and on either side of *xiawan* (CV-10); about one FW above and medial to *huaroumen* (ST-24); one FW under and medial to *taiyi* (ST-23).

When tonified:
Tonifies the kidney, sexual organs, cerebellum, pons, eye same side, opposite ear.
Disperses the large intestine.
Dispersing acts in the opposite way.
One of the points of the attack vessel *(chong mai)*.

Direct effects:

    Detests life, deep sadness, impatient.

    Eye same side: congestion or inflammation, keratitis, one pupil dilated?

    Opposite ear: itching. One ear red?

    Sexual organs: uterine spasms or congestion; vagina: acidity?

Opposite effects:

    Hiccough at meals, spasms of diaphragm or abdomen; stomach spasms; acidity.

    Small intestine: old inflammation, occasional pain; large intestine: constant constipation; interintestinal nerves: spasms.

Parts of the body:

    Bones: caries and syphilitic afflictions (nose, ear, mastoid process); knee or wrist: prolonged arthritis; swollen lymph nodes.

    Inflammation of the corners of the lips, of the cheek.

Point of Weihe: Right: Aurum Metallicum. Deep melancholy, abhorrence of living, impatience. Sees only the lower half of objects. Weakness of the extremities. Excess blood, diverse congestions. Caries of the bones of the ear, of the mastoid, of the nose. Bone problems from syphilis.

Left: Natrum Phosphoricum. One pupil dilated, one red ear. Troubles and chancre of the lips and cheeks. Arthritis of the knee or wrist. Swollen lymph nodes. Stomach or vaginal acidity.

KI-18   *shiguan* — stone barrier

    Epigastrium: about three small FW above the umbilicus; at the mid-distance from the medial edge of mid-height of the ninth rib and of the median line [see footnote for KI-11]; in a hollow; mid-width of the rectus abdominus muscle.

    One FW above *shangqiu* (KI-17); one FW below *yindu* (KI-19). About one FW below and on either side of *zhongwan* (CV-12); one FW medial and above *taiyi* (ST-23); one FW medial and below *guanmen* (ST-22).

When tonified:

    Tonifies the kidney, sexual organs, temporal-parietal lobes, spinal cord, upper back, lumbar area, eye, same side.

    Dispersing acts in the opposite way.

    A point of the attack vessel *(chong mai)*.

Direct effects:

    Weeps when listening to music; photophobia, dreams of flowing water; aggravated by humidity, sea, river, changes of weather, heat of bed.

    Eye same side: congestion.

    Genital organs: women — uterus congestion, "bad blood in the uterus," spasms or pain. Men — prostatitis, blenorrhagia, non-erection?

Opposite effects:

    Saliva in excess, spits up copious excretions; regurgitation of food; stomach spasms.

    Large intestine: constipation, pain in the abdomen and heart.

Parts of the body:

    Hot head and cold feet; periodic migraine.

    Skin: unpleasant odor, acne, furuncles, eczema.

    Upper back: pain as from a burning needle.

    Lumbar area and vertebrae: pain, stiffness.

Point of Weihe: Right: Natrum Sulfuricum. Tongue like a geographical map; photophobia, cold as ice, tears from hearing music, dreams of running water, aggravated by humidity, sea, rivers; pain in the hair; infantile asthma; itching nose; liver distended, cannot bear a tight belt, diarrhea after fruit; abundant urination with red sediment, pain in the vertebral column and burning needles in the upper back; inflammation around the nails (whitlow); burning soles; red excrescence on the body.

Left: Sulfur. Tongue red on edges and tip, white in the middle, all orifices red, eyelids, lips, ears; expels toxins through the skin, looks for a cool corner in the bed, hot head, cold feet; opens the windows and door at night; vertigo on rising, or on a bridge; aggravated by changes in the weather, or by remaining standing up, or from rest; sleeps on right side; acne, furuncles, eczema, fetid odor of the skin; dry, hard, frequent stools; urination mostly at night; periodic migraines; men: non-erection, sensitive liver.

KI-19 *yindu* — yin capital

Epigastrium: about three FW below the lower extremity of the sternum; at the level of the mid-height of the eighth rib, and at mid-distance from the rib to the median line; about mid-width of the vertical muscle (rectus abdominus); in a hollow.

One FW above *shiguan* (KI-18); two FW below *tonggu* (KI-20); about one FW on either side and above *zhongwan* (CV-12); one FW medial and above *guanmen* (ST-22); one FW medial and below *liangmen* (ST-21).

When tonified:
   Tonifies the kidney, sexual organs, heart, lung, cerebellum, pons, spinal cord, eye same side.
   Disperses the large intestine, stomach.
   Dispersing acts in the opposite way. A point of the attack vessel *(chong mai)*.

Direct effects:
   Sexual organs: women without children — congestion of uterus, strangling, unbearable pain.
   Heart: spasms of energy, fullness and agitation in the heart, pain in the heart during digestion.
   Lungs: swelling, dyspnea, pain in the lower ribs (emphysema).
   Eye same side: congestion, keratitis, cataract.

Opposite effects:
   Stomach: inflammation to the point of ulceration — copious thready saliva, chronic dyspepsia, nausea, vomiting.
   Large intestine: constipation with intestinal noise and pain.
   Jaundice.
   Hot fever, painful heat: disperse.

KI-20 *tonggu* — communicating valley

Epigastrium: one large FW below the lower edge of the sternum (without the xyphoid process). One FW medial and above the union between the seventh and eighth ribs; one FW on either side of the median line; mid-width of the rectus abdominus; in a hollow.

Two FW above *yindu* (KI-19); one FW below *youmen* (KI-21); one FW above and on either side of *juguan* (CV-14, IS *juque*); one FW medial and above *liangmen* (ST-21). Two FW medial to *chengman* (ST-20).

When tonified:
   Tonifies the kidney, lung, muscles of throat and tongue (hyoid muscle), nose, risorius muscle, cerebellum, pons, spinal cord, heart, eye same side.
   Disperses the stomach, diaphragm, large intestine, nose.
   Dispersing acts in the opposite way. A point of the attack vessel *(chong mai)*.

Direct effects:
   Emotional agitation, deranged mind, repression, delusions.
   Heart: fullness of chest, angina of chest?
   Eye same side: vision blurred, headache, congestion of the eyeball.

Opposite effects:
   Stomach: vomiting easily — in cars, at sea, in airplanes. Vomiting in pregnancy; stomach distended, liquids remain. Undigested food, chronic gastritis. Yawning.
   Clear and abundant coryza, chronic?

Parts of the body:
   Hyoid muscles: paralysis, muteness, cannot speak.
   Risorius muscle: flaccidity, mouth awry.
   Nape: stiffness.

KI-21 *youmen* — obscure door, cardiac sphincter

Epigastrium, base of the sternum: about one FW on either side of the median line. Just at the lower opening of the joint of the seventh rib on the lower extremity of the sternum; in a hollow; on the rectus abdominus muscle.

One FW above *tonggu* (KI-20); two FW under *bulang* (KI-22); three FW medial to *burong* (ST-19); one FW lateral to *jiuwei* (CV-15).

When tonified:

Tonifies the kidney, sexual organs, temporo-parietal lobe, medulla oblongata, spinal cord, breast, liver, tonsils. Disperses the stomach, esophagus, large intestine.

Dispersing acts in the opposite way. A point of the attack vessel *(chong mai).*

Direct effects:

Loss of memory, melancholy, aggravated by heat, by anger, bad humor, improved with rhythm and rhythmic movements, sleepy, but cannot sleep; children: one red cheek, cries in order to get an object, immediately throws it down, likes to be carried.

Sexual organs: hard, sensitive, swollen breasts.

Liver: all trouble with irregularity.

Lung: opposite tonsils: pain, incessant cough; bronchitis, intercostal pain.

Heart: pain in the chest.

Opposite effects:

All vomiting: car-, air-, or sea-sickness; morning sickness of pregnancy; vomiting of saliva, flowing saliva. Contracted esophagus, contracted cardiac sphincter, contracted stomach; from nervous upset or shock. Stomach does not empty, swollen epigastrium, no appetite.

Large intestine: dysentery with pus and blood.

Parts of the body:

Lumbar area, buttocks, posterior thigh.

Point of Weihe: Left: Cocculus. Motion sickness at sea, in cars, on airplanes, on trains; weakness and trembling of lower limbs, aggravated from tobacco; early, abundant menses, abundant and frequent urine, without color.

Right: Chamomilla. Nausea with weakness, somnolent but cannot sleep; one red cheek, ameliorated by rhythm (carried or rolled); capricious, bad humor; children who cry for an object and immediately throw it away, aggravated by heat, by anger, children who like to be carried, green diarrhea of children during dentition; early menses with unbearable mood and with colic, dry cough at night and during sleep, hard and sensitive breasts.

KI-22   *bulang* — veranda of the steps

Lower thorax: on the edge of the sternum. In the angle between the fifth and sixth ribs; on the lower edge of the fifth rib; in a hollow.

Two FW above *youmen* (KI-21); two FW below *shenfeng* (KI-23). At the level and on either side of *zhonging* (CV-16); two FW medial and a little above *burong* (ST-19).

When tonified:

Tonifies the kidney, cerebellum, lower part of the eye, nose, throat, lung, sexual organs.

Disperses the large intestine, stomach.

Dispersing acts in the opposite way.

Direct effects:

Indignation from injustice?

Lungs: little energy for breathing (inhaling or exhaling), asthma, cannot lift the arms, pain in the chest from coughing or breathing, intercostal neuralgia, bronchitis, pleurisy.

Nose same side blocked: fetid odor (ozena).

Opposite breast: pain, inflammation.

Eye same side: lower part.

Skin: all suppurating wounds: disperse.

Opposite effects:

Vomiting, without appetite. Esophagus, cardiac sphincter: inflammation, contraction.

Large intestine: spasms: tonify; weakness, atony: disperse.

Parts of the body:

Rectus abdominus.

Point of Weihe: Graphites. All suppurating wounds, skin eruptions, indignant from injustice, chest tight.

KI-23   *shenfeng* — mark of the evolved man

Chest: on the edge of the sternum; between the fourth and fifth rib; in the angle between the sternum and the lower edge of the fourth rib; in a hollow; at the level of the nipple; between the sternum and the mammary artery.

Two FW above *bulang* (KI-22); two FW below *lingxu* (KI-24). At the level of and three FW medial to *ruzhong* (ST-17); about one FW on either side of *shanzhong* (CV-17).

When tonified:

Tonifies the kidney, anterior mid-brain (vagus, anterior hypothalamus), vessels, sexual organs, lungs, ears.
Disperses the large intestine, nose.

Direct effects:

All congestive eruptions, coronaries; jiujitsu knock-out point.
Congestive eruptions; danger of congestion: at menopause; from excess of heat; from sunburn.
Heart: coronaries, angina of chest.
Lung: congestions, fullness of chest, difficulty in breathing, cannot breathe, fits of suffocating coughs, bronchitis, pleurisy, intercostal neuralgia.
Sexual organs: breast abscess.
Ears: congestive buzzing.

Opposite effects:

Nose congested, blocked; if inflammation, fetid odor (ozena).
Stomach: fits of vomiting, no appetite.

Parts of the body:

Face: half same side.

Point of Weihe: Glonoin. Congestive headache with beating; angina of chest, painful attacks while walking; congested from the sun, sunburn; congestive buzzing; changes related to aging.

KI-24   *lingxu* — emptiness of the immaterial

Chest: on the edge of the sternum: two FW above the level of the nipples (men); in the angle between the third and fourth ribs; in the angle between the sternum and the lower edge of the third rib; in a hollow; between the bone and the mammary artery.

Two FW above *shenfeng* (KI-23); two FW below *shencang* (KI-25); about two FW on either side of *yutang* (CV-18); about three FW medial to *yingchuang* (ST-16).

When tonified:

Tonifies the kidney, anterior frontal lobes, heart, sexual organs, cubital line of the upper limb, lung.
Disperses the large intestine, stomach.
Dispersing acts in the opposite way.

Direct effects:

Anxious, suspicious, feels the need to swear, sensation of having two opposed wills. Conscious memory weakened.
Heart contracted and painful with fatigue from walking; in angina of chest.
Respiratory passages, nose blocked, fetid odor (ozena), bronchitis, dyspnea, pleurisy, intercostal pain.

Opposite effects:

Vomiting without having eaten.

Parts of the body:

Upper limb, particularly the ulnar side of the forearm.

Point of Weihe: Anacardium. Heart: amnesia, anxious, suspicious, needs to swear, feeling oneself between two opposite wills, feeling of a blunt point penetrating a part of the body, pain in the stomach if empty.

KI-25   *shencang* — treasure of the evolved man

Chest: on the edge of the sternum; in the angle between the second and third ribs; in the angle between the sternum and the lower edge of the second rib; in a hollow; between the bone and the mammary artery.

Two FW above *lingxu* (KI-24); two FW below *yuzhong* (KI-26); about three FW medial to *wuyi* (ST-15); one FW on either side of *zigong* (CV-19).

When tonified:

Tonifies the kidney, anterior frontal lobe, medulla oblongata, spinal cord, lung, heart, radial line of the forearm, the two jaws, cheeks, temple, nape, back, knee, dorsum of hand, ears.

Disperses the stomach, large intestine.
Dispersing acts in the opposite way.

Direct effects:

Respiratory passages: excess; coughing fits, dyspnea, cannot breathe, fullness of the chest, bronchitis, pleurisy, pulmonary congestion, intercostal pain, cough preceded by tickling in the throat.

Weakness with age or overwork, insomnia from worries, stays on the unpleasant side of things, does not like life.

Ear: hearing diminished.

Opposite effects:

No appetite, esophagus contracted, or irritated (very hot drinks), stomach distended, mostly in the middle of the night, regurgitation of food, vomiting.

Parts of the body;

Two jaws: cheek, temple.
Nape, muscles of cervical vertebrae, back.
Radial side of forearm, dorsum of hand; cramps?
Knee.

Point of Weihe: Right: Ambra Grisea. Weakness from age or overwork, insomnia from worries. Remains on the unpleasant side of everything, does not like life; diminished hearing; cramps in the hands and fingers; swelling in the stomach and intestines after midnight; nervous cough preceded by tickling in the throat; atonic dyspnea.

Left: Angostura. Needs coffee, colic, burns at anus, atonic dyspnea, paralyzing rheumatism, difficulty walking, pain in the cheek, cheek-bone, temple, back, knee, caries of the long bones.

KI-26 *yuzhong* — in doubt

Chest: on the edge of the sternum; between the second and first ribs; in the angle between the first rib and the sternum; in a hollow; between the bone and the mammary artery.

Two FW above *shencang* (KI-25); two FW under *shufu* (KI-27 and last). Two large FW medial to *kufang* (ST-14); about one FW on either side of *huagai* (CV-20).

When tonified:

Tonifies the kidney, cerebellum, lower spinal cord, spleen-pancreas, liver, lung, vessels (all the yin organs), radial line of the upper limb, dorsum of the thumb and index finger, vocal cords.
Disperses the large intestine, stomach.
Dispersing acts in the opposite way.

Direct effects:

Bad humor upon waking, sensitive, easily angered but calms quickly (''flies off the handle''); thinks that nobody likes him; aggravated around 11 a.m. and from 4 to 6 p.m. Shaky mind, weak memory? reflection difficult?

All congestion, inflammation, spasms in the cerebrum, in all organs, from sun stroke, from suppression of menses, from arterial spasm.

Ears: itching.

Frequent urine.

Breasts: swelling, nodules? men: non-erection, rapid ejaculation?

Respiratory passages: congestion, inflammation, spasms; bronchus: asthma, cannot eat without an attack, bronchitis, pulmonary congestion, wet and dry pleurisy, pneumonia; vocal cords: ulcerations, or weakness.

Liver: small, insufficient.

Heart: palpitations (auricular fibrillations?), spasm of arteries, false arteriosclerosis.

Opposite effects:

Nose blocked, back of throat irritated; coughing fits.
Esophagus, stomach: spasms, contracture; excess of saliva, vomiting.

Parts of the body:

Hot head, cold extremities.
Upper shoulder, radial line of the upper limb; dorsum of thumb and index finger.

Below the left ribs: pain (splenic angle of the large intestine).
Cold hands or feet.

Point of Weihe: Right: Lycopodium. Weak memory, difficult reflection, bad humor upon waking (''flies off the handle''), easily angered and quickly calmed, sensitive, ''people don't like me.'' Worse on the right side and from 4 to 6 p.m.; eczema around the ears; one foot cold, the other hot; nodules in the breasts, non-erection, quick ejaculation; frequent urine; ulceration of the vocal cords; coughs while sleeping, pain in lower left throat, liver insufficient or small, atrophied.

Left: Veratrum Viride. All congestion or spasms, cerebral congestion from suppression of menses, sunstroke, pulmonary congestion, bronchial spasms, asthma, spasms of the esophagus; auricular fibrillations, palpitations; scant, cloudy urine; rheumatic fever; appendicitis; warts, bunions.

KI-27 *shufu* — workshop of the assent points

Upper chest: on the edge of the sternum; between the clavicle and the first rib; in the angle between the lower edge of the clavicle and the sternum, in their articulation; in a hollow.

Two FW above *yuzhong* (KI-26); one large FW on either side of *xuanji* (CV-21); one FW on either side and below *tiantu* (CV-22); two FW medial to *qihu* (ST-13).

When tonified:
    Tonifies the kidney, vessels, three nervous centers, three endocrines, three levels of the psyche.
    Disperses the large intestine, stomach.
    Dispersing acts in the opposite way.
    The energy leaves the kidney here and descends through a branch at an angle to enter the meridian of the heart governor at *tianchi* (PC-1).

Direct effects:
    Apprehension, attends misfortune, jumps at sudden noises, nervous irritability, agitation, unconquerable insomnia.
    Headache: from excess mental effort or from rheumatism, or from suppressed menses.
    Opposite eye: weakness of the ciliary muscle and of the sphincter of the iris, scotoma; heart, arteries, veins.
    Sexual organs: menses — pain and spasms before menstruation, all mental trouble or headache from stoppage of menses, arrested menstruation either from cold or moral shock.
    Lung: continual cough, energy in the upper body, violent cough, hoarseness, old asthma, pulmonary congestion, pleuritis, pleurisy, pain in the chest, intercostal pain.

Opposite effects:
    Digestive tract: thrush, painful tongue, lack of appetite, nausea, saliva, contracted esophagus, spasms; vomiting, food not descending.

Parts of the body:
    External nose: tip of nose red or inflamed.
    Muscular, rheumatic or nervous troubles, tics, trembling, cramps.
    Upper limb: course of the medial nerve, palm.

Point of Weihe: Right: Borax. Tip of the nose red, jumps at noises; violent cough, difficult breathing; tugging in the intercostal muscles; thrush; tongue and mouth cracked; vomiting mucus; headache at 2 a.m.; pain, heat, redness of fingers or toes.

Left: Cimicifuga.

Notes

[1] The current references give the kidney meridian as 1/2 cun from the medial line on its course up the front of the body to the level of *bulang* (KI-22) — ed.

Chapter IX

Heart Governor

Vessels, Sexual Organs

Under the name ''heart governor'' (because of its action on the circulation), the ancients describe a single meridian and a single pulse. Our research has enabled us to observe the existence of:

1) Two pulses — middle III right, vessels (lower half arteries, upper half, veins).

2) The almost exclusive action on the sexual organs of three points on the two branches and their exclusive action on the sense organs: *laogong* (PC-8) (sexual organs, tactility, smell and taste, and their effects on this pulse); *quze* (PC-3) (veins and hearing and their effect on this pulse); *tianquan* (PC-2) (sight and its effect on this pulse). All the other points have an almost exclusive action on the arteries.

The interactions are as follows: 1) In the same way: vessel points on kidney filtration (glomeruli); sexual organ points on kidney reabsorption-excretion (tubules); heart, with an equal intensity on the triple warmer. 2) In the opposite way on the stomach, with a very different intensity on the triple warmer.

The heart governor is modified: 1) In the same way by the kidney (level for level); 2) In the opposite way by the triple warmer, stomach.

The links between the heart, vessels, sexual organs and sense organs are such that we will see each of these points acting directly or indirectly on all these organs.

This double meridian is yin. Its general tonifying point is *daheng* (PC-9) (the tonification point of the sexual organs is instead *laogong,* PC-8). Its general dispersal point is *daling* (PC-7) (the dispersal point of the sexual organs being instead *laogong,* PC-8, which is thus the source). Its maximum of energy is at 8 p.m. (minimum hour of the stomach); its minimum is at 8 a.m. (maximum hour of the stomach). Its energy comes from the kidney meridian; it passes into that of the triple warmer.

Concerning the proper action of this meridian, heart problems from excess appear in all its points. For the most part, emotional agitation: *ximen* (PC-4), *neiguan* (PC-6) and *zhongchong* (PC-9) for loss of memory; *jianshi* (PC-5) for insecurity and apprehension; for timidity, fear of people: *ximen* (PC-4) and *laogong* (PC-8); fear with weeping at night: *zhongchong* (PC-9) and *jianshi* (PC-5); insomnia from fatigue and fever: *neiguan* (PC-6), and from excess blood, *daling* (PC-7); violent hallucinations, delusions of persecution: *jianshi* (PC-5). On the physical level, trembling of the extremities are specific to *quze* (PC-3); all congestive eruptions at *daling* (PC-7); weakness of the vessels, arteries or small veins with bleeding of the nose, stomach, in the stools or urine, or under the skin are specific to *ximen* (PC-4) and *laogong* (PC-8).

PC-1 *tianchi* — celestial pool

Thorax: men: one large FW lateral to the nipple.

Following point: *tianquan* (PC-2) at the shoulder-fold; one large FW lateral to *ruzhong* (ST-17); one medial to *tianxi* (SP-18).

When tonified:
Tonifies the heart governor (sexual organs, vessels), kidneys, anterior face of lower limb, cerebellum, pons, opposite eye.
Disperses the stomach, triple warmer, opposite side of the throat.
Dispersing acts in the opposite way.
Here, the energy coming from the kidney meridian (*shufu,* KI-27, at the angle between the clavicle and sternum) comes into the heart governor after going through *yingchuan* (ST-16).
The branch between the liver (*qimen,* LV-14) and lung (*zhongfu,* LU-1) borrows from the ascending meridian of the heart governor.

Direct effects:
    Energy in the upper body, congestion of the head or brain.
    Heart: troubles, pericarditis.
    Opposite eye: darkened vision, not clear.
    Breast: mammitis? Insufficient lactation?

Opposite effects:
    Opposite larynx and chest: respiratory noises.
    Stomach, diaphragm: fullness, agitation.

Parts of the body:
    Armpit: inflamed nodes (adenitis).
    Anterior face of the lower limb (stomach meridian).

PC-2 *tianquan* — celestial source

Anterior shoulder: one FW medial to the axillary fold; at the angle between the lower edge of the second rib (under the clavicle) and the lateral edge of the pectoralis major and, deeper, the pectoralis minor; in a hollow; on the lateral edge of a vertical muscle (coracobrachialis).[1]

Preceding point: *tianchi* (PC-1); following point: *quze* (PC-3) on the anterior part of the elbow; two FW below *zhongfu* (LU-1).

The point is traversed by the gallbladder meridian coming from *jianjing* (GB-21) through *kufang* (ST-14) and going to *yuanye* (GB-22) through *jiquan* (HT-1).

When tonified:
    Tonifies the sexual organs, all yin meridians, spleen-pancreas, mid-brain, cerebellum, medulla oblongata, spinal cord, heart, kidney, opposite eye, opposite lumbar area.
    Disperses the stomach, triple warmer.
    Dispersing acts in the opposite way.
    Response in the pulse of the eye.
    One of the three points of the sexual organs.

Direct effects:
    Opposite eye: weak vision, tired (amaurosis, amblyopia), obscured vision, foggy vision, not clear; special point for sight.
    Heart: palpitations, troubles, endocarditis.
    Throat: lung same side: cough, pain in the back, coughing fits, fullness of chest, back, sides, limbs.

Opposite effects:
    Stomach: nausea, epigastrium, upper abdomen: swelling.

Parts of the body:
    Chest, scapula, back, upper limb: pain particularly when coughing, chest disturbed, rheumatism.
    Upper limb cannot be lifted up or put behind the back, muscular rheumatism, acts on the pectoralis major, latissimus dorsi, teres major, pectoralis minor, coracobrachialis.

PC-3 *quze* — pool of the curve

Anterior and medial elbow: on the flexion fold; at the angle between the medial edge of the medial tendon of the biceps and the upper edge of the transverse mass of the joint; in a hollow; on the lateral side (towards the biceps) of the deep artery (humeral) and the deep muscle (brachialis anterior).

Preceding point: *tianquan* (PC-2); six FW above arm-*ximen* (PC-4); one large FW lateral to *qingling* (HT-2); separated by the biceps from *chize* (LU-5); one of the three points of the sexual organs.

When tonified:
    Tonifies the heart governor (particularly sexual organs), lung (superior lobes), opposite sacral nerves, anterior shoulder, anteromedial arm, medial elbow, anterior forearm, palm, thumb, index finger, terminal phalanx of the middle finger (median nerve), internal ear.
    Disperses the stomach, bladder, triple warmer.
    Dispersing acts in the opposite way.

Direct effects:
> Indecision and trouble, emotional agitation, or nervous crisis.
> Chronic bronchitis; pulmonary tuberculosis?
> Heart: pain, heat, agitation, myocarditis.
> Measles, German measles; scarlet fever?

Opposite effects:
> Vomiting, vomiting in pregnancy; vomiting of blood, intense thirst, dry mouth, cold in the abdomen.
> Parkinsonism: tonify. Multiple sclerosis: disperse. Elbow, forearm and hands agitated without stopping: if stopped by grasping the object, tonify; if increased by grasping the object, disperse. Also, head agitated with upper limb.
> Median nerve (anterior medial arm, anterior forearm, thumb, index finger, terminal phalanx of middle finger, anterior shoulder).
> Lower leg, opposite posterior foot.

PC-4   *ximen* — door of the vale

Anterior part of the forearm (palm up, in supination): six FW above the wrist; about mid-width; at the angle between the lower edge of a transverse mass and the radial (lateral) edge of a large tendon of the flexor; ulnar edge of the flexor carpi radialis; in a hollow.

Six FW below *quze* (PC-3); two above *jianshi* (PC-5); one medial to *kongzui* (LU-6); three lateral to *xiaohai* (SI-8).

When tonified:
> Tonifies the vessels, kidney filtration, temporal-parietal lobes, large intestine, heart, automaton-parrot, anterior part of forearm, palmar side of hand, thumb, index finger, terminal phalanx of the middle finger (median nerve).
> Disperses the stomach (right: great curve; left: pylorus), triple warmer, bladder, gallbladder.
> Dispersing acts in the opposite way. It has a response in leg-*xialian* (ST-39, IS *xiajuxu*).
> Memory, bleeding of nose, anus or stomach; median nerve.

Direct effects:
> Lack of memory; helps during psychoanalysis; fears people; fear, emotional agitation; hysteria?
> Vessels: hypertension (disperse); weakness of the tissues, bleeding.
> Heart: pain, myocarditis.
> Large intestine: bleeding hemorrhoids, also intestinal hemorrhage.
> Nose: bleeding.

Opposite effects:
> Stomach: bleeding. Vomiting of blood (hematemesis): tonify; belching, vomiting.

Parts of the body:
> Arm and anterior forearm, palmar side of hand, thumb, index finger and terminal phalanx of the middle finger (median nerve): pain, contracture, rheumatism: disperse; loss of touch, weakness, flaccidity: tonify.

PC-5   *jianshi* — intercalary messenger

Anterior forearm (palm up, in supination). Four FW above the palm, about mid-width; at the angle between the lower edge of a transverse mass and the radial (lateral) edge of a large medial tendon (flexor); in a hollow; on the ulnar (medial) edge of the tendon of the flexor carpi radialis; deep, the flexor pollicis longus.

Two FW below *ximen* (PC-4). One large FW above *neiguan* (PC-6); between the two *erbai* (MP-12, IS M-UE-20) points; separated by the flexor carpi radialis from *lieque* (LU-7), and by the flexor and ulnar artery from *lingdao* (HT-4).

When tonified:
> Tonifies the sexual organs, superior occipital lobes, primate, opposite sacral nerves, heart, kidney excretion, anterior face of the upper limb, axilla, tibia.
> Disperses the triple warmer, stomach.
> Dispersing acts in the opposite way.

Direct effects:
> Apprehension, insecurity, childhood timidity, always withdrawn, weakness of the nerves and brain; much

emotional agitation; moral sensitivity; has a need to move, violent hyperexcitation; nocturnal terror, hallucination (tormented by ghosts); delusions of persecution, strangeness, insanity.

Apoplectic attacks (flowing saliva, cannot pronounce words, foggy, falls); infantile convulsions.

Heart: all pain, rapid pulse, inflammation of the heart.

Fever, heart agitated, thirst; intermittent fever; a little cold, then intense heat.

Sexual organs (left point: ovaries, testicles; right point: penis, clitoris). Women: insufficient menses: tonify; uterus congestion or inflammation; metritis.

Respiratory passages: chills, sore throat, difficulty breathing in cold, chest tight.

Opposite effects:

Stomach: frequent belching; vomiting: from cold, from nerves, from cholera.

Parts of the body:

Axilla: swelling (adenitis).

Biceps and medial elbow: pain or contracture.

Thumb and index finger, the one near the other, median nerve.

PC-6 *neiguan* — internal barrier

Anterior forearm (palm up, in supination): three FW above the wrist, about midwidth; at the angle between the superior edge of a transverse mass and the radial (external) edge of the large median tendon (of the flexors); in a hollow; on the ulnar (medial) side of the strong tendon of the flexor carpi radialis; deep, the median nerve.

One large FW below *jianshi* (PC-5); one large FW above *daling* (PC-7).

When tonified:

Tonifies all the yin meridians, cerebellum, spinal cord; anterior elbow.

Disperses all the yang meridians.

Dispersing acts in the opposite way. Responds with *gongsun* (SP-4).

In general, mainly insufficiency of the yin or yang organs; also, excess of the heart, vessels, lungs.

Direct effects:

Passage point between all the yin meridians and all the yang meridians. Tonifying causes the excess yang to pass into the yin (and vice-versa).

Command point of the "chain of yin," *yinwei mai.* If excess: circulatory trouble, pain in the heart, chest contracted; if insufficient: emptiness, vertigo; responds with *gongsun* (SP-4, command point of the attack vessel, *chong mai:* nervous contractions, passage between the stomach-intestines and the spleen-pancreas).

Loss of memory for words, loss of decision-will, anxiety, emptiness, weakness, vertigo, grey fog in front of the eyes, lassitude, laziness, cold that does not stop.

Insomnia from fever caused by fatigue or emptiness.

Heart: insufficiency (troubles from emptiness, weakness, vertigo, grey fog, malaise), or myocarditis, endocarditis, pericarditis, pain in the heart and sides, circulatory troubles.

Hypertension (hard wrist pulse).

Intermittent fever, "can cure it by itself," fever of atonic tuberculosis.

Red eyes, congestion to the point of hemorrhage, troubled vision.

Sexual organs: placenta not descending.

Lungs: internal fullness of the chest, congestion, pain; all trouble from emptiness, with mucus and fever: tonify.

Opposite effects:

Stomach: insufficient, slow digestion: disperse; stomach swollen, painful: tonify; vomiting from emptiness: disperse; from gallbladder excess: tonify.

Intestines: all trouble from emptiness; to tonify "cures forever."

Acute pain: tonify.

Diarrhea: from weakness: disperse; from inflammation: tonify. Constipation from atony: disperse; from spasms: tonify. Rectal prolapse: disperse; hemorrhoids: tonify.

Bladder: irritating, painful urination: tonify.

Parts of the body:

Head: stiff.

Anterior elbow: painful, contracture or arthritis.

Wrist pulse hard, full; or arthritis.

Hand: palm hot; congested hand or pain; thumb: flexor pollicis longus; palmar and dorsal sides of fingers, median nerve.

Begin with *neiguan* (PC-6) for loss of memory, loss of words, mental troubles, anxiety or irrelevant laughter, epilepsy, stomach insufficiency causing indigestion or vomiting, atonic constipation, hemorrhoids, internal fullness — and finish with *gongsun* (SP-4).

PC-7 *daling* — great plateau

Anterior wrist (palm up, in supination): about mid-width; one FW above the wrist, at the angle between the upper edge of the transverse head of the radius and the lateral (radial) edge of the large tendon of the flexor; in a hollow; medial side of the strong tendon of the flexor carpi radialis.

When tonified:
Tonifies the vessels, sexual organs, kidney, lungs, throat, tonsils, cerebellum, opposite sacral nerves, armpit, anterior elbow and forearm, palm.
Disperses the stomach.
Dispersing acts in the opposite way.

Direct effects:
Excess indignation or feeling, frenetic discontent, chagrin, tears, apprehension, fear, insomnia from excess.
Disperses the vessels and sexual organs (heart governor); all congestion (cerebral, pulmonary, renal, local eye, etc.).
Arteries hard, ample; hypertension (anger, red or yellow eyes, body hot, hot palms, headache mainly when leaning over, wrist pulse hard; temporal artery visible); arterial spasms.
Heart agitated, pain, myocarditis, endocarditis, or intermittent (one stop every three pulsations).
Kidneys congested, painful; red urine.
Lung: chest painful, short breath, cough, angina, tonsillitis (headache, fever); tooth pain, and in the cheek.

Opposite effects:
Stomach: acute gastritis, vomiting, intestines: stool like blood.

Parts of the body:
Skin: inflammation with pus, abscess.
Armpit: swollen lymph nodes, adenitis.
Anterior elbow and forearm: pain or contracture.
Hand: contracture, spasms, writer's cramp, abscess in the whole hand, bubbles in the palm (dishydrosis), nutgall.
Thumb and index finger, palmar side: flexors.

PC-8 *laogong* — palace of fatigue

Center of the palm: on the line of the medius-annular joint; on the transverse line (the "head line" of palmistry); at the medial angle near the head and body of the third metacarpal; on the lateral edge of a tendon running along the metacarpal (annular flexor); in a hollow.

Five FW below *daling* (PC-7). *Zhongchong* (PC-9) is on the terminal phalanx of the middle finger; one lateral to *shaofu* (HT-8).

When tonified:
Tonifies all the yin meridians, particularly the sexual organs, sympathetic system, endocrine system, superior occipital lobes, inferior frontal lobes, spinal cord, tactility, smell-taste, between the nose and throat, tips of the fingers.
Disperses all the yang meridians, parasympathetic system.
Dispersing acts in the opposite way. Responds with *fengchi* (GB-20) opposite and *baihui* (GV-19, IS GV-20).
Third point of the heart governor acting particularly on the sexual organs.
The energy leaves the heart governor to enter the triple warmer by a branch to *guanchong* (TW-1).

Direct effects:
Fatigue, physical exhaustion, counterflow of energy from fatigue, timid, withdrawn, restless, anxious, easily discontented, or cannot stop laughing, primate; blood in the nose, stools or urine; hypertension; cerebral congestion.
Mouth: bad breath (adults or infants); opposite side of mouth: inflammation, difficulty in swallowing; opposite gums: inflammation (adults and children), abscess.

Throat opposite side: angina; sense of taste.
Lungs: cough, asthma, pain and fullness of the chest and sides.
Burning mucus, sense of smell.

Opposite effects:
Stomach: belching, vomiting, intense thirst, pain in the heart.

Parts of the body:
Skin: pain, inflammation, abscess, scabies.
Hand: modified sense of touch, writer's cramp, retraction of the palmar aponeurosis, rheumatism, pain, thumb, index finger, middle finger: pain, rheumatism, or weakness, flaccidity.
The palm and this point have a great importance for the taking of energy (left) or the giving of energy (right).

PC-9   *zhongchong* — central assault

Hand, middle finger, ungual phalanx; on the face of the index finger, at mid-width; at the angle between the lower edge (towards the tip of the finger) of the swelling of the bone at the joint and the dorsal edge of the palmar tendon (flexors); in a hollow.

Preceding point: *laogong* (PC-8); on the dorsal side of the middle of the terminal phalanx, one point of *shixuan* (MP-25-29, IS M-UE-1).

When tonified:
Tonifies the vessels, kidney filtration, heart, conception vessel (lower third, superficial pulse), opposite side of tongue, opposite inner cheek, opposite eye, temporal-parietal lobes, automaton-parrot, axilla.
Disperses the stomach, gallbladder.
Dispersing acts in the opposite way.

Direct effects:
Memory tired, inadequate; anxiety, irrational fears; malaise at night or in darkness; children: fear or weeping in the night or darkness.
Vessels: hypertension, or hypotension.
Heart: pain or agitation, fullness, inflammation, myocarditis, endocarditis, sudden pains with pain in the upper limb (angina of the chest), fullness of chest, red face.
Fever without sweat, body burning like fire, hot palms, agitation.
Kidney filtration: abundant urine: tonify; insufficient: disperse.
Opposite eye. Children cannot see at dusk.

Opposite effects:
Stomach, bladder.

Parts of the body:
Stiff tongue; inner cheek: rapidly spreading ulcers (with *guanchong,* TW-1).
Axilla: swelling, pain (lymph nodes, adenitis).
Upper limb: pain, can neither extend nor flex it, hand contracted; anterior elbow: contracture.

Note

[1] The location of this point is normally given as "two cun above the extremity of the auxiliary fold between the two heads of the biceps" (*Precis d'acuponcture Chinoise,* Beijing, p. 188, 1975 edition). — ed.

Chapter X

Triple Warmer

This meridian, although existing materially, does not correspond to any material organ. This makes it difficult to understand unless we consider that it acts entirely and completely on the yang energy of activity (like the heart governor, on the yin energy of inactivity). It is called the "father of energy and of yang."

In Japan, Dr. Sawada has written a large work about it, demonstrating that the triple warmer can correct almost all troubles.

All its points act on the opposite side of the brain and body and on the same side locally.

Each of its three branches commands one of the three great functions — the first or upper warmer: respiration and the energy of the external sheath; the second or middle warmer: the distribution of the energy coming from food and drink to the other meridians; the third or lower warmer: the distribution of the sexual energy and that of the genitourinary organs. It is thus said to command the circulation of energy and blood.

When the three are in excess together, the nerves are tight, with irritability and nervousness. When the three are insufficient, the whole body is without buoyancy, without vitality. Upper warmer empty: head tilted, brain empty, breathing causes fatigue, buzzings, obscured vision. Middle warmer empty; digestion and defecation troubled. Lower warmer empty: genitourinary organs function badly, the heartbeat is sometimes intermittent.

The conception vessel (yin) brings the energy to the triple warmer and is directly connected with it through the herald points: *shanzhong* (CV-17), which has a mutual response particularly with *guanchong* (TW-1) and which is the herald point of the upper warmer, *zhongwan* (CV-12), which has a mutual response with *sidu* (TW-9); abdomen-*yinjiao* (CV-7), which has a mutual response with *yangchi* (TW-4). There is also a herald point of the three warmers together, *shimen* (CV-5). On the other hand, the tonification point, hand-*zhongzhu* (TW-3) has a mutual response with all the herald points.

The pulse of the triple warmer is right III superficial. It is easy to distinguish three parts along its length: lower for the third warmer, middle for the second warmer, upper for the first, upper warmer. Each of these parts changes independently according to the vitality of the corresponding warmer.

When this pulse is full or insufficient along with all the superficial pulses, it represents the vitality of the yang energy.

On this meridian, the tonification point is hand-*zhongzhu* (TW-3). The dispersal point is *tianjing* (TW-10). The source point is *yangchi* (TW-4).

The assent point is *sanjiaoshu* (BL-22); the general herald point is *shimen* (CV-5). But each warmer has its herald point: the upper warmer point is *shanzhong* (CV-17), which responds in the lungs. The second, middle warmer point is *zhongwan* (CV-12), which responds in the stomach and parasympathetic. The third, or lower warmer point is abdomen-*yinjiao* (CV-7), which responds in the sexual organs and bladder.

Stimulating the meridian acts in the same way on the bladder and gallbladder, and in the opposite way on the sexual organs, spleen-pancreas and lung.

It has a strong action on the sense organs, ears, eyes and tongue-throat-nose, on the nervous vitality and nervousness; mentally, on sadness, regrets, nervous insomnia, irritability, etc., with *tianjing* (TW-10); on sensitivity to storms and weather changes through *waiguan* (TW-5); trembling, St. Vitus Dance, through *huizong* (TW-7); on the veins through *guanchong* (TW-1).

TW-1 *guanchong* — assault on the barrier

Hand, ring-finger: terminal phalanx, side towards the little finger (medial), mid-width; at the angle between the lower edge of the bulge of the bone and the dorsal edge of the palmar tendon (flexors); in a hollow.

Following point: *yemen* (TW-2).

When tonified:
　Tonifies the opposite side of the body, triple warmer (upper third), temporal-parietal lobes, opposite veins, heart, mid-height of the spinal cord; around the ear and the lateral part of the opposite neck, elbow, forearm and dorsal muscles of the hand; opposite knee, lower leg, front of opposite foot.
　Disperses the opposite side of the head, opposite eye and ear, throat, lungs, tongue same side, mouth.
　Dispersing acts in the opposite way.

Responds with *shanzhong* (CV-17).

Here, the energy coming from the heart governor point *laogong* (PC-8) follows a branch through the joint of the ring finger and enters the triple warmer.

It is a passage point between the top (head, eye, ear, throat) and the mid-lower area (heart, veins, forearm and lower leg).

Direct effects:

Opposite veins; heart: pain, agitation, numbness of the opposite upper limb.

Sexual organs: urination disturbed by the position of the fetus.

Opposite effects:

Excess energy in the upper warmer, counterflow of energy, cannot sleep, nervous fever, body burning, agitation, malaise: tonify.

Throat, larynx: nervous suffocation, pain, food not passing: tonify; opposite tonsillitis: tonify; dry mouth, tongue heavy, does not obey, dry vomiting, lack of appetite.

Opposite eye: acute pain, keratitis, cataract: tonify.

Opposite ear: pain, deafness, buzzing: tonify.

Parts of the body:

Opposite side of head: congestive pain, vertigo, fainting: tonify; around the ear and the lateral part of the opposite neck.

Opposite spinal cord, mid-height.

Elbow, forearm, wrist, dorsal muscles of opposite hand; or pain, weakness.

Opposite knee, lower leg, anterior foot.

TW-2 *yemen* — door of the humors

Dorsum of hand: head of the fourth metacarpal of the ring finger, at the joint of the phalanx; at the angle between the medial edge of the transverse ligament between the two heads; between the bone and the interosseous artery, interdigital veins and nerves; in a hollow.

Preceding point: *guanchong* (TW-1); three FW below hand-*zhongzhu* (TW-3); between *houxi* (SI-3) and *xiatu* (MP-18).

When tonified:

Tonifies the opposite body and brain, triple warmer (lower third), bladder, small intestine, lower spinal cord, temporal-parietal lobes; forearm, dorsum of hand, also same side.

Disperses the spleen-pancreas (right point), liver (left point), opposite eye, ear, gums, teeth, parotid glands, submaxillary glands, all opposite side.

Dispersing acts in the opposite way.

Responds with *shimen* (CV-5).

Passage point between the head and hand, liver, spleen-pancreas.

Direct effects (at the expense of the upper body):

Spleen (right point), pancreas (left point).

Hand: chilblains; back of the hand with red swelling up to the forearm; same side: disperse; opposite side: tonify; or weakness (can neither lift nor lower the hand).

Lateral side of elbow and posterolateral forearm, back of wrist; dorsum of hand: contracture, pain or weakness.

Opposite effects:

Congestion of opposite face and head; frenetic speech, hyperexcitation to the point of insanity: disperse; hot or cold from shock or emotional agitation, deranged mind, headache from cerebral anemia, vertigo, fainting: tonify.

Opposite eye painful, troubled, scarlet: tonify; cataract, keratitis.

Opposite ear pain, buzzing, violent or sudden deafness: tonify.

Mouth: opposite gum inflammation: tonify; opposite tooth pain, inflammation, caries (in the lower teeth, pain in the upper teeth): tonify.

Nose blocked: tonify; short breaths on inhalation and exhalation, parotid glands, opposite sub-maxillary glands, inflammation: tonify; insufficiency: disperse.

TW-3   *zhongzhu* — central islet

Dorsum of hand: line of the ring finger, on the lower angle and towards the little finger (medial), between the upper (posterior) head and the body of the long bone of the ring finger (fourth metacarpal). Just above a transverse mass; between the bone and the interdigital artery; in a hollow.

Three FW above *yemen* (TW-2); one above *yangchi* (TW-4); one medial to *wailaogong* (MP-13, IS M-UE-23).

When tonified:

    Tonifies the opposite side of body, triple warmer, all yang meridians, brain, spinal cord, opposite ear, opposite back, dorsum of hand same side, opposite lower leg and front of foot, opposite back of throat and larynx.
    Disperses the spleen (right point), pancreas (left point), vessels.
    Dispersing acts in the opposite way.
    Responds with the three herald points of the triple warmer and in *shimen* (CV-5), herald point of the entire triple warmer.

Direct effects:

    Tonification point of the triple warmer; all the yang meridians without buoyancy, react slowly and only slightly.
    Spinal cord: all trouble, particularly mid-height opposite.
    Opposite eye: foggy vision, cataract, keratitis.
    Opposite ear pain: disperse; hears badly: tonify.
    Throat: back of throat and opposite larynx; irritation, pain or itching.

Opposite effects:

    Arteries (particularly maximal and middle blood pressures); hypertension: tonify (congestive headaches, heavy head, giddiness, heat without sweat); hypotension: disperse (maxima weak).
    Spleen (right point); pancreas (left point).

Parts of the body:

    Opposite half of body, opposite part of head, cranium, temples, cheek, opposite jaw: pain or heat, red face.
    Nape, posterior shoulder, opposite back, opposite lumbar muscles: all problems.
    Opposite upper limb: all problems.
    Dorsum of hand, same side: redness, swelling (chilblains), blisters, furuncles, contracture, or flaccidity (can neither extend nor flex); fingers: pain, stiffness, contracture, flaccidity.

TW-4   *yangchi* — pool of yang

Dorsum of wrist: lower opening of the radio-ulnar articulation; lateral inferior edge of the prominence of the ulna (ulnar process); on the angle projecting from the radius, on the inferior edge; in a hollow.

One FW above *zhongzhu* (TW-3); two under *waiguan* (TW-5).

When tonified:

    Tonifies the triple warmer (particularly the lower warmer), heart opposite side (particularly the auricles), sexual organs, bladder (sphincter, prostate, urethra), spleen-pancreas, shoulder, pectoralis major, medial face of the arm, radial side of the forearm, palmar side of the hand, anterior part of lower limb.
    Disperses the bladder (body), vessels, kidney.
    Dispersing acts in the opposite way; responds with abdomen-*yinjiao* (CV-7).
    Herald of the lower warmer. Also responds with *shimen* (CV-5), herald of the entire triple warmer.

Direct effects:

    Source of the triple warmer (excess or insufficiency). Weak potential: tonify; nerves excited or tight: disperse; cold or heat.
    Heart (auricles): tonifying can agitate nervously, causing some missed beats (corrected by dispersing the sympathetic system at *fengchi* (GB-20).
    Malaise and agitation; heat of the body without fever, fever without sweats, intermittent fever, flu.
    Lymphatic vessels?
    Sexual organs: blenorrhagia; men: epididymitis, prostatitis; women: displaced uterus?
    Spleen (right point); pancreas (left point): diabetes, dry mouth.
    Bladder: sphincter, prostate, urethra.

Opposite effects:

    Bladder: expulsor muscles, detrusor muscle.

Kidney filtration and excretion.

Shoulder, pectoralis, medial arm, radial side of forearm, palmar side of hand.

Wrist: pain, rheumatism; hand: flaccidity or contracture.

Anteromedial face of the lower limb, medial half of the arch of the foot.

TW-5 *waiguan* — barrier of the yang

Dorsum of the wrist: in the upper (posterior) opening of the radius and ulna, (behind) the angle between the head and body of the ulna (lateral upper edge of the bulge of the ulnar apophysis) and the tendon of the anterior ulna; in the protruding angle of the radius: in a hollow.

Two FW above *yangchi* (TW-4); one below *zhigou* (TW-6); one below and medial to *huizong* (TW-7), in the anterior angle between the edge and process of the ulna.

When tonified:

Tonifies all the yang producers of energy, the three levels of the psyche, the three organs of sense, midbrain, spinal cord, sympathetic system, ear same side.

Disperses all the yin distributors of energy (makes the yin pass into the yang).

Dispersing acts in the opposite way.

Reponds with opposite *fengchi* (GB-20) (sympathetic system).

"To know only *waiguan* is important."

Direct effects:

Command point of all the yang energy, of the chain of yang *(yangwei mai),* which links all the meridians with yang weakness. If excess: elbow contracted. If insufficient; weakness to the point of flaccidity of the upper limb.

Passage point between the yin and yang meridians. Causes the excess of one to pass into the insufficiency of the other; acts on the yang.

All trouble from external temperature, or from changes of weather. Heat: headache, congestive eruptions, swelling: disperse. Cold: weakness, skin trouble, pruritis: tonify. Storm: neuralgic or congestive headache: disperse; loss of vitality: disperse. Wind or dryness: pain, neuralgia, asthma: disperse. Snow or humidity: rheumatism, loss of strength: tonify.

Sweats without reason, at night, body burns.

Eye same side: lateral muscles (medial opposite); all troubles of the eye: swelling, red pupils (glaucoma?).

Ear opposite: great buzzing, hears nothing due to deafness from rheumatism.

Nose: chronic coryza.

Opposite parotid: inflammation, mumps.

Opposite teeth and tongue.

Parts of the body:

Lateral neck and mastoid area: swelling.

Nape and back, same side: bones and muscles painful, stiff.

Upper limb same side, joints, elbow contracture, elbow and wrist: pain; wrist and dorsum of hand: flaccidity or contracture; five fingers: painful points.

Start with this point for these troubles; if the result is inadequate, end with foot-*linqi* (GB-41).

TW-6 *zhigou* — ditch like a fork

Posterior forearm (palm down, pronation): three FW above the wrist, about mid-width; between the radial edge of the medial tendon (extensor muscles of the middle finger and thumb) and the ulnar edge of the posterior radial artery, along the radius. On the inferior edge of the transverse muscle (abductor pollicis longus); on the upper edge of a point of a bony bulge of the radius; in a hollow.

One FW radial and above *waiguan* (TW-5); one radial and slightly below *huizong* (TW-7).

When tonified:

Tonifies the triple warmer and all the yang meridians, posterior frontal lobes, mid-brain, cerebellum, spinal cord, thumb and index finger and palmar side of the fingers same side; opposite knee, lower leg and anterior foot; opposite ear and eye.

Disperses the liver.

Dispersing acts in the opposite way.

Direct effects:

Yang energy of activity.

All nervous trembling: tics, chorea, agitation of the fingers same side and of the opposite feet; useful in Parkinson's disease (disperse), or multiple sclerosis (tonify).

Opposite eye: tics, movements (rectus lateralis).

Opposite ear: great buzzing? Deafness?

Opposite effects:

Liver.

Parts of the body:

Skin: pruritis.

Lateral elbow and radial side of forearm, thumb and index finger, continual agitation.

Palmar side of fingers: agitation, involuntary movements of the upper limb same side.

Knee, anterior lower leg, dorsum of opposite foot: agitation, involuntary movements.

TW-7   *huizong* — reunion of the ancestors

Posterior forearm: three FW above the wrist; two tight FW above the prominence of the ulnar process; at the angle between the lateral (radial) edge of the ulna and the tendon of the posterior ulnar bone and the lower edge of a tendon, in an angle (insertion of the extensor pollicis longus); in a hollow; between the posterior ulnar artery and the ulnar edge of the extensor of the little finger.

The meridian comes at a right angle from *zhigou* (TW-6).

One FW above *waiguan* (TW-5); one ulnar FW from *zhigou* (TW-6); one below *sanyangluo* (TW-8).

When tonified:

Tonifies the triple warmer, temporal-parietal lobes, automaton-parrot, spinal cord, opposite thyroid gland; upper limb, same side; lower limb same side.

Disperses the heart (auricles, coronary arteries), opposite side of spleen-pancreas, lung, lower third of the conception vessel, opposite sexual organs.

Dispersing acts in the opposite way.

Painful spasm of the heart (coronary arteries), opposite side of internal organs, or upper limb same side, or lower limb opposite.

Direct effects:

Large intestine same side: habitual spasmodic constipation; cholera: vomiting, diarrhea, cramps.

Opposite effects:

Chills; opposite sore throat, cough, red face, fever, chronic inflammation of the opposite respiratory passages: tonify.

Acute paralysis of the hyoidian muscles, total muteness, tongue paralyzed, cannot swallow (glosso-labio-pharyngeal paralysis?)

Sexual organs opposite side, "women for whom the conception vessel does not function" (superficial pulse and lower third of the conception vessel); from spasms? after delivery, fainting from loss of blood.

Parts of the body:

Skin: inflammation with pus or bubbles, scabies.

Axilla same side: superative adenitis, abscess, pain in the side and arm, muscles same side painful, tied up, contracted.

Lumbar area same side, contracted; women: "contracted vertebrae."

Upper limb, same side, mainly knee and lateral face of the lower leg.

TW-8   *sanyangluo* — secondary vessel of the three yang

Posterior side of the forearm, palm down (in pronation): four large FW above the wrist; at the angle between the medial (ulnar) edge of the median tendons (extensor of the extensor digiti minimi muscle) and of the lower edge of the tendon on an angle of the extensor pollicis longus muscle; in a hollow; on the radial edge of the posterior ulnar artery and ulna.

One FW above *huizong* (TW-7); one below *sidu* (TW-9).

When tonified:

Tonifies the opposite side of the throat, posterior frontal and temporal lobes same hemisphere, but opposite side of it, muscles of the opposite larynx, large intestine, temporal-parietal lobes, opposite half of body.

Dispersing acts in the opposite way.

Direct effects:

Opposite larynx: aphonia and violent aphasia, cannot speak.

Opposite incisors: pain. Intestinal worms.

Parts of the body:

Lateral neck, opposite side.

Opposite half of the body: can neither move nor desires to move.

TW-9 *sidu* — four trenches

Posterior forearm: about mid-width; palm down (in pronation); six FW above the wrist; at the angle between the medial (ulnar) edge of the median tendons (extensors: extensor digiti minimi) and of the lower edge of one tendon at an angle of the extensor pollicis brevis; on the radial edge of the posterior ulnar artery and ulna; in a hollow.

One FW above *sanyangluo* (TW-8); eight FW below *tianjing* (TW-10). At the level of *wenliu* (LI-7), *kongzui* (LU-6), arm-*ximen* (PC-4) and *zhizheng* (SI-7).

When tonified:

Tonifies all yang producer meridians, temporal-parietal lobes, opposite ear, throat opposite side, lower teeth and opposite lower jaw, opposite knee, (with *zhongwan,* CV-12).

Dispersing acts in the opposite way.

Direct effects:

Ears: deafness from sudden energy, buzzings.

Pain in the lower teeth and from the mandible to the opposite ear.

Back of the opposite throat: pain as if there were growths; difficulty inhaling and exhaling.

Parts of the body:

Thorax same side.

Upper part of the shoulder and lateral side of the base of the neck.

Extensor muscles of the fingers cannot be extended, extensor pollicis brevis (phalanx).

Opposite knee, medial side.

TW-9a[1] *xingxingxue* — point which awakens

Posterior forearm: two FW below the olecranon; at the angle between the anterior edge of the ulna and the lower edge of the olecranon.

When tonified:

Tonifies all the opposite nervous centers, triple warmer, opposite veins, lateral half of the opposite body; heat, circulation.

Disperses the vessels.

TW-10 *tianjing* — celestial well

Flexed elbow: upper posterior surface; in the lower and lateral part of the olecranon fossa, above the point of the elbow (olecranon); at the angle between the lateral edge of the median tendon of the triceps and the upper edge of the lower bony edge of the olecranon fossa; in a hollow.

Eight FW above *sidu* (TW-9); three below *qinglengyuan* (TW-11).

When dispersed:

Disperses the triple warmer, cerebellum, medulla oblongata, spinal cord, midbrain (thalamus), spleen-pancreas, all the yang producers, bladder sphincter, ear same side, external side of the eye same side, between the scapulae, lumbar and pelvis same side, nerves opposite half of the body, opposite edge of the artery (pulse III superficial).

Tonifying this point seems to disperse even more.

Direct effects:

Disperses the excess energy of the triple warmer (all superficial pulses tight and hard).

Relaxes nervous excess, psychological or physical reflexes too strong, chattering of teeth, nervous crises, convulsions, hyperexcitation to the point of insanity. In women who are very nervous, the sudden relaxation can cause a crying fit.

Nervous insomnia at the beginning of the night.

Emotional agitation, deranged mind, irritability, cannot bear people, exhausted and acts through will alone, repression of worries.

Great sadness, cannot sleep, great shock, all trouble, stupefied to the point of deafness, blindness, paralysis.

Shivering, trembling from nerves or cold.

Nervous hypertension only of the maxima.

Stomach contracted; no pleasure from food, abdomen painful.

Throat tight, cough, cannot speak without coughing, bronchitis with pus, pain in the chest and heart.

Intermittent fever: attacks during meals; beriberi attacking the upper parts.

Heart: troubles with rhythm (from nervous excess).

Eyes: lateral side of opposite eye, and medial side same side.

Eyelids: inflammation, conjunctivitis.

Lymph nodes: if fever: disperse; if not: tonify.

Skin: troubles increase from emotion, thoughts.

Parts of the body:

Lateral part of the head: pain from shock.

Jaw: inflammation, pain, swelling.

Lateral part of the neck: torticollis, pain into the posterior shoulder.

Scapula: pain, also medial muscles of the scapula (rhomboids).

Opposite lumbar area: pain.

Upper limb: pains from tightness.

Contusions, blows, trauma, pain in the lumbar area.

TW-11 *qinglengyuan* — abyss of limpid cold

Posterior arm: five FW above the olecranon process; posterior edge of the humerus and anterior edge of the triceps; on the lower edge of a transverse mass; in a hollow.

Three FW above *tianjing* (TW-10); six FW below *xiaoluo* (TW-12); about three posterior to *wuli* (LI-13).

When tonified:

Tonifies the triple warmer, large intestine, lower conception vessel; opposite eyes, ears, and cheek; shoulder, posterior part of upper limb, extensors, also bladder.

Disperses the pericardium, also kidneys.

Dispersing acts in the opposite way.

Direct effects:

Eyes: acute pain, opposite eye; opposite ears: buzzing.

Pain in the sides, shivering (also in pleurisy).

Parts of the body:

Posterior shoulder, muscles of the scapula, posterior muscles of the arm, forearm, hand (extensor muscles and deltoid muscle).

Motor point of the radial nerve (extensors, triceps).

TW-12 *xiaoluo* — the river during the thaw

Lateral, posterior arm; five FW below the acromion; on the posterior edge of the humerus; on the lower edge of the insertion of the deltoid; in a hollow.

Six FW above *qinglengyuan* (TW-11); three below *naohui* (TW-13).

When tonified:

Tonifies the triple warmer, bladder; posterior frontal lobes, spinal cord, all the articulations of the body, muscles of scapula, rhomboids.

Disperses the kidneys, vessels, lateral side of the opposite eye.

Dispersing acts in the opposite way.

Direct effects:

Malaise, headache from heat (disperse) or cold (tonify).

All articulations of the body, same side: periarthritis, rheumatism, pain; inflammation of the tissue and ligaments.

Parts of the body:

Nape, posterior shoulder: rhomboids, muscles of the scapula, joint between shoulder and arm (glenoid) (scapula moves on lifting the arm).

TW-13   *naohui* — reunion of the deltoid

Posterolateral side of the arm: three FW below the acromion; on the posterior edge of the humerus; at the angle of the lower edge of the transverse insertion (infraspinatus); in a hollow; just above the insertion of the teres minor.

Three FW above *xiaoluo* (TW-12); four below and a little before *jianliao* (TW-14); two below *jianzhugu* (MP-10); three behind *jianyu* (LI-15).

When tonified:

Tonifies the triple warmer, large intestine, infraspinatus, all finger and toe articulations same side, particularly dorsum; arch; throat.

Disperses the kidney same side, spleen-pancreas, vessels.

Dispersing acts in the opposite way.

Parts of the body:

Throat, same side: swelling.

Lateral side of neck and nape: lymph nodes hot or cold, tumors of all kinds, swellings.

Posterior shoulder: swelling.

Infraspinatus, deltoid: all troubles, cannot touch the opposite shoulder.

All articulations of the fingers and toes same side.

TW-14   *jianliao* — hollow of the shoulder

Posterior point of the shoulder: just in the angle between the lower edge of the lateral, posterior bulging angle of the acromion and the posterior edge of the muscle that passes under it (infraspinatus); in a hollow.

Four FW above and lateral to *naohui* (TW-13); five lateral to *tianliao* (TW-15); separated from *jianzhugu* (MP-10) by the supraspinatus muscle, and from *jugu* (LI-16) by the bone; four FW above and anterior to *jianzhen* (SI-9).

When tonified:

Tonifies the triple warmer, superior part of the scapula and lateral arm; bladder, lateral opposite eye; upper part of the nape same side.

Disperses the spleen-pancreas.

Dispersing acts in the opposite way.

Parts of the body:

Supraspinatus (which causes the arm to lift anteriorly and keeps it from being taken behind the back).

Humero-scapular articulation.

Nervous spasm, tics, involuntary movement of the posterior, lateral part of the head.

Posterolateral intercostal neuralgia.

Emergence of the radial nerve?

TW-15   *tianliao* — celestial hollow

About mid-width of the posterior part of the shoulder: just on the upper edge of the swelling of the transverse spine of the scapula; between the bone and the supraspinatus; in a hollow.

Five FW medial to *jianliao* (TW-14); following point: *tianyou* (TW-16), under and behind the ear; two FW lateral to *quyuan* (SI-13), behind *jianjing* (GB-21).

When tonified:

Tonifies the triple warmer, cerebellum, trapezius, supraspinatus, triceps, bladder.

Disperses the spleen-pancreas.

Dispersing acts in the opposite way.

Direct effects:

    Agitation, malaise, fullness of chest from heat or cold.

Parts of the body:

    Nape: extreme coldness or nervous contraction.

    Nape, posterior shoulder and arm: all trouble (trapezius, supraspinatus and triceps muscles).

    Wrist, thumb, index finger: rheumatic pain.

TW-16   *tianyou* — celestial opening

    Lateral side of neck: one large FW below and behind the bulge behind the ear (mastoid); at the angle between the posterior edge of a large muscle, on an angle towards the front (sternocleidomastoid muscle) and the lower edge of a deep, transverse prominence (transverse process of the first cervical vertebra — atlas). In front of a muscle on a posterior angle (splenius of the head).

    Preceding point: *tianliao* (TW-15); two FW below and behind *yifeng* (TW-17); one FW behind *tianrong* (SI-17).

When tonified:

    Tonifies the triple warmer, heart, stomach; superior, lateral side of eye same side, lateral superior side of ear same side, medial part of nape, cheek.

    Disperses the spleen-pancreas, liver.

    Dispersing acts in the opposite way.

Direct effects:

    Tonifying too much can swell the face and close the eyes?

    Spasms of the upper lateral side of the eye; or contracture (from energy, murky vision or pain); or red, congested eyes; or cataract.

    Ears, auditory spasm (from energy, hearing not very distinct, sudden deafness from energy), buzzing.

    Dreams of standing on the head.

    Congestive headache, internal; face hollow without complexion, or swollen.

Parts of the body:

    Lateral part of the neck: sternocleidomastoid muscle.

    Nape: splenius capitus, medial nape stiff or painful.

TW-17   *yifeng* — wind screen

    Head: behind the lobe of the ear; at the posterior angle between the lower point of the bony protrusion (mastoid) and the upper edge of the insertion on it of a large muscle (sternocleidomastoid muscle); in a hollow.

    Two FW above and in front of *tianyou* (TW-16); two FW below *qimai* (TW-18). One FW behind *tianrong* (SI-17); two FW below and in front of head-*wangu* (GB-17, IS GB-12).

When tonified:

    Tonifies the triple warmer, face same side, ears, lower gums.

    Disperses the opposite large intestine.

    Dispersing acts in the opposite way.

Direct effects:

    Internal and middle ear: buzzings? deafness: either with pain or with difficulty speaking or from blocked energy; acute pain of the ear, itching in the ear, cerumen.

    Lower teeth: pain.

    Parts of the body:

    Face: risorius muscle in contracture or flaccid; facial paralysis: mouth to one side, pain of the cheek.

    Jaw: frequent yawning; dislocation of the jaw; jaw contracted; trismus, teeth contracted when eating.

    Lower jaw and under the chin: inflammation.

    Neck and nape: lymph nodes, tonify (particularly the chain on the lateral part of the neck).

    Point of Weihe: Left: Tabacum. Nervous deafness. Increased secretions of ears, nose, eyes, mouth. Nausea. Murky vision. Congestion of the veins. Atrophy of the optic nerve; blindness. Floating spots before the eyes; central scotoma; vertigo when opening the eyes. Very easy vomiting: sea, car, plane, pregnancy. Cold skin, icy extremities. Trembling. Insomnia, anxiety, extreme depresssion, discontent.

Right: Sabina. Music is unbearable. Abundant menses; red discharge between menses, headache when menses come; sexual excitation; risk of miscarriage; after miscarriage, inflammation of the ovaries and uterus, placenta not expelled, intense pain afterward; blenorrhagia. Bladder and urethra: inflammation. Bleeding hemorrhoids. Pain in the anterior surface of the thigh, in the metatarsal bone, in the heel. gGut, gouty nodules of the fingers. Comedo (blackhead).

TW-18   *qimai* — vessel of stupidity

Head: behind the mid-height of the ear; at the angle between the upper edge of a transverse bulge and the anterior edge of the mastoid process; on the posterior edge of a vertical artery.

Two FW above *yifeng* (TW-17); one below *luxi* (TW-19); two in front of head-*qiaoyin* (GB-18, IS GB-11).

When tonified:

Tonifies the triple warmer, heart, inner ear and eustachian tube, anterior part of the eye same side.
Disperses the opposite large intestine.
Dispersing acts in the opposite way.

Direct effects:

Middle branch of the trigeminal nerve.
Emotional agitation, fear. Children: convulsions or epilepsy? from fear or spasms.
Vomiting or diarrhea without fixed time.
Eye: pupil, hollow of pupil abnormal (iritis).
Ear: eustachian tube.
Buzzing or deafness with congestive headache.

TW-19   *luxi* — breath of the cheeks

Head: between the posterosuperior attachment of the ear and the anterior edge of the upper point of the mastoid process. In the anterior upper angle of two flat reliefs; on the anterior edge of an artery. The ears vary considerably in their attachments.

One FW above *qimai* (TW-18); two under and behind *jiaosun* (TW-20).

When tonified:

Tonifies the triple warmer, posterior and inferior frontal lobes, medulla oblongata, opposite spinal cord.
Anterior eye same side, ear, gum and upper teeth.
Disperses the opposite large intestine and spleen-pancreas.
Dispersing acts in the opposite way.

Direct effects:

Acts on the upper branch of the trigeminal nerve.
Illnesses with trembling, convulsion, epileptic fit, chest and side responding.
Meningitis, internal headache, body hot, cannot sleep.
Murky vision, heavy head.
Ear: beginning of otitis (blocked and painful or swollen, progressing to the point of flowing and pus), buzzing, deafness from shock.
Smell and taste.
Children: vomiting of saliva; chest and side painful.
Teeth and upper gums.

TW-20   *jiaosun* — descendants of the horns

Above the ears: one FW posterior to the vertical anterior to the lobe (about mid-width of the ear). At the level of three FW above the transverse prominence of the zygomatic arch; on the superior, posterior edge of a bulge on an angle; on the upper edge of an artery (auricular artery).

Two FW in front of *luxi* (TW-19); one half FW above ear-*heliao* (TW-22) and *sizhukong* (TW-21, IS TW-23), on the extremity of the eyebrow. One FW below and posterior to *shuaigu* (GB-8).

When tonified:

Tonifies the triple warmer, thyroid, eye, corners of the lips, mouth, teeth and upper gums, anterior part of the opposite neck, opposite occipital lobes.
Disperses the opposite large intestine.

Dispersing acts in the opposite way.

Parts of the body:
    Trunk of the trigeminal nerve.
    Excess of thyroid: prominent eyes, goiter (swelling of the anterior opposite neck); inflammation of the cornea.
    Lips: corners stiff and hard.
    Mouth inflamed.
    Gums: all trouble, swelling from caries.
    Upper teeth: molars and incisors cannot chew.
    Jaw contracted, trismus.

TW-21   *sizhukong* (IS TW-23) — bamboo thread

Above and in front of the ear: two FW above a transverse relief of the zygomatic arch; on the extremity of the eyebrow; in a hollow.

One FW above *tongziliao* (GB-1); two FW anterior and slightly above *qubin* (GB-7).

When tonified:
    Tonifies all the yang producers (superficial pulses), lower opposite frontal lobes; face, opposite earlobes; eyelids, molars same side; wrist, hand, same side.
    Disperses the spleen-pancreas, liver, pericardium.
    Dispersing acts in the opposite way.

Direct effect:
    All headaches which are difficult to bear, opposite facial neuralgia, aversion to cold and wind (skin of cheek, corners of the lips, upper teeth).
    Eyelashes turned inward (entropion); red eyes, congested; keratitis, cataract?
    Convulsions; epilepsy (eyes raised, recognizes no one, salivation, hyperexcitation, attacks coming irregularly).

TW-22   [ear-]*heliao* — silo, hollow of the cereals

Cheek: at the level of the upper edge of the hollow of the ear. At the angle between the upper edge of the transverse relief of the zygomatic arch and the deep cartilaginous anterior edge of the ear; on the lower edge of a transverse artery (auricularis anterior); in a hollow.

One FW above *ermen* (TW-23, IS TW-21); one below *jiaosun* (TW-20).

When tonified:
    Tonifies the triple warmer, small intestine, large intestine, eye, ear, lower jaw.
    Disperses the gallbladder.
    Dispersing acts in the opposite way.

Direct effects:
    Sends some energy to the triple warmer? Tonifies it?

Parts of the body:
    Vision: contraction and agitation.
    Ear: great buzzing, or pain, also below the ear.
    Nose: clear discharge, maxillary sinusitis, swelling of the tip of the nose, pain from abscess.
    Thyroid?
    Head: pain and heaviness.
    Face: facial paralysis from cold (with rigor).
    Jaw: contracted (trismus); jaw, below the chin and neck: swelling.

TW-23 *ermen* (IS TW-21) — door of the ear

Cheek: just anterior to the tragus and at the level of the ear hollow, between the tragus and the vertical artery (auricular artery and nerve). Between two small deep bones; one half FW posterior to the rising portion of the maxilla; in a hollow.

The energy passes from here into the meridian of the gallbladder (at *tongziliao,* GB-1), in the posterior angle between the head and body of the mandible.

Two FW under *heliao* (TW-22); two above and anterior to *tinggong* (SI-19).

When tonified:

Tonifies the triple warmer, gallbladder, anterior temporal-parietal lobes, middle ear, eye and upper lids, below the eye, mouth, palate, upper teeth, gums, tongue, lips, cheek, perineum, prepuce, vulva, solar plexus.
Disperses the genital organs, breast same side.
Dispersing acts in the opposite way.

Parts of the body:

Ear, particularly middle: all troubles; pain, inflammation, otitis, pus, wax, deafness: disperse; buzzing.
Eye, orbit same side; nocturnal pain; lateral muscles? Iritis? Upper eyelids, same side.
Nose: bone painful, caries, ulceration, pereostitis.
Mouth: mucus, posterior palate, inflammation, aphthae; tongue, gum, uvula, opposite tonsils.
Lip: swelling.
Throat: globus hystericus, beating in the solar plexus.
Pharynx, esophagus, opposite stomach: spasms.
Perineum; vulva: swelling; breast: inflammation same side; prepuce.
Facial paralysis from cold (to the point of freezing).
Itching pain, or burning or pricking; insect bites.
Nervous spasms (particularly at night).
Local edema (uvula), prepuce, vulva, below the eye (home of tears).

Point of Weihe: Right: Apis Mel.

Left: Asa Foetida.

Note

[1] This point is not included in the international system. — ed.

Chapter XI

Gallbladder

The gallbladder meridian is a yang meridian (lesser yang of the foot). It starts in front of the ear,[1] zigzags down the head to the neck, descending from the shoulder to the side of the body and the lower limb. It consists of forty-four points. It is preceded in the flow by the triple warmer (mother), and followed by the liver (child). The stomach is the wife. It has its maximum at midnight (minimum hour of the heart) and its minimum at midday (maximum hour of the heart). Its coupled meridian is the liver.

The parasympathetic system contracts it, relaxes its Oddi's sphincter, and thus empties it. The sympathetic system acts in the opposite way. The parathyroid gland disperses it, relaxes and empties it; emotions trouble it to the point of anguish.

The meridian acts on the whole duodenal-vesicular biliary reflex, which is stimulated and tonified by a small quantity of fat (causing a flow of bile); but contracted and blocked by a large quantity of fat (stopping the bile and congesting the liver).

Its pulse is the left II superficial. If narrow and hard, disperse; if swollen and soft, tonify. If there are stones, the pulse will be large, round and hard. Do not treat without an X-ray to show the size of the stone. Treatment will cause only the small ones to be evacuated.

A healthy fullness governs its effects: ''All the organs receive their *elan* from the gallbladder. It nourishes the heart, which nourishes it.''

Troubled, it fills the stomach with bile. The large intestine is disturbed by its insufficiency with regard to its stimulation as well as its function. Dispersing the small intestine relaxes the gallbladder.

A gallbladder in prolonged excess (thus excess of stomach, insufficiency of heart and the evolved man) produces combativeness, aggressiveness, nervous irritability, strong character, stubbornness, decisiveness, explosiveness and discontent with everything. In excess it causes either migraine, neuralgia, rheumatic pain or eruption on the skin, pruritis, etc.; or asthma.

Insufficiency: lack of character, of daring, or confidence in oneself; apprehension, depression, cold, vain agitation, trembling, insomnia, dull eyes, gloominess; perspiration at night, particularly under the chin, dreams of brawls, insults and humiliations, of being naked, without shoes, of burning oneself.

Tonify: *xiaxi* (GB-43), passage point *guangming* (GB-37); or disperse *ligou* (LR-5). Herald point: *jingmen* (GB-25). To tonify the parasympathetic system: *tianzhu* (BL-10) (see mother-child, husband-wife and midday-midnight rules).

Excess: on waking, nausea, or bad taste in the mouth or dry mouth; dusty complexion, migraines, pains like suspenders; contracted calves; swelling in the popliteal crease; cannot look to the right or left; likes silence; unhappy, irritable; envious, jealous; impelled to do evil through speech or acts, quarrels.

Disperse: *yangfu* (GB-38), passage point *guangming* (GB-37); or tonify: *ligou* (LR-5) from gallbladder to spleen-pancreas *shangliao* (BL-31). To tonify the sympathetic system: *fengchi* (GB-20). See T6, T7, T8, assent point: *danshu* (BL-19).

GB-1   *tongziliao* — hole of the pupil

Cheek: lower temple; two FW lateral to the lateral corner of the eye. One FW above the angle of the posterior edge of the vertical suture (temporosphenoid) and the upper edge of the transverse prominence of the zygomatic arch.

Three FW in front of *kezhuren* (GB-3, IS *shangwan*); separated from *hanyan* (GB-4) by a horizontal suture; two FW above and lateral to *chengqi* (ST-4, IS ST-1).

When tonified:
  Tonifies the gallbladder, small intestine, triple warmer, spinal cord same side, opposite occipital lobes, opposite retina, opposite eyelids, opposite ear, cheek, index finger, anterior lower limb, arch of the foot.
  Disperses the heart.
  Dispersing acts in the opposite way.

Direct effects:

> Eye: all troubles of the eye from energy (excess), distant vision troubled (contracted pupil). Retina: does not distinguish colors (achloropsia); weakened vision; inflammation of retina, congestion of retina or hemorrhage; cataract?
>
> Eyes: acute pain, itching of the eyes, congestion of the eyeball (glaucoma), keratitis.
>
> Eyelids: orbicular muscles of eye (of the facial nerve, eyelids shut) ptosis, blepharoptosis; or eyes not closing (lagophthalmia); conjunctivitis (tears flowing, itching, photophobia, headache).

Parts of the body:

> Face: spasms or paralysis (facial nerve), neuralgia (trigeminal).

GB-2   *tinghui* — reunion of hearing

Cheek: one half FW in front of the hole of the ear. A little under the posterior angle of the head and body of the maxilla; on the superior edge of an insertion on the bone (risorius); between the bone and the vessels (superficial temporal artery and vein); in a hollow.

Two tightened FW above and posterior to *ermen* (TW-23, IS TW-21 by name, SI-19 *tinggong* by location) to which it is connected through a branch; one small FW under ear-*heliao* (TW-22, IS TW-21 *ermen* by location); two FW posterior to *kezhuren* (GB-3).

The energy coming from the triple warmer (*ermen,* TW-23, see above) passes here into the gallbladder meridian.

When tonified:

> Tonifies the gallbladder, triple warmer, superior occipital lobes, bladder, middle and inner ear, posterior molars, lower jaw, upper lip, upper eyelids.
>
> Disperses the heart.
>
> Dispersing acts in the opposite way.

Direct effects:

> Delusions, joyless; escapades (walks blindly without direction), stupidity.
>
> Insomnia after 3 a.m. (solar time) from cerebral hyperactivity; eats, drinks quickly.
>
> Middle and inner ear: eustachian tubes, buzzing, song of cicada, deafness from energy, wax, inflammation of the middle ear (otitis), acute pain, itching (pruritis) in the ear.
>
> Eyelids: conjunctivitis?
>
> Teeth, particularly the posterior upper and lower molars (pain, abhorrence of cold food and drinks).
>
> Bladder: difficult urination, cancer of the bladder? Prostatis, urethra; perspiration at night?

Parts of the body:

> Jaws: dislocation, trismus, cannot open the mouth.

> **Point of Weihe:** Right: Coffea.
>
> Left: Taraxacum.

GB-3   *kezhuren* (IS *shangguan*) — host and guest

Face: about mid-distance from the ear to the edge of the orbit (orbital arch); at the angle between the transverse edge of the zygomatic arch and the posterior edge of the upper prominence of the arch; above the anterior edge of the condyle of the maxilla.

Three FW under and behind *tongziliao* (GB-1); two tightened FW lateral to *tinggong* (SI-19); two FW under and anterior to ear-*heliao* (TW-22, IS TW-21 *ermen* by location); three FW under *qubin* (GB-7).

When tonified:

> Tonifies the gallbladder, triple warmer, occipital lobes, lateral side of the opposite posterior part of the eye, ear, teeth, canines, edge of the nose.
>
> Disperses the lungs.
>
> Dispersing acts in the opposite way.

Direct effects:

> Troubles of the eyes from energy (excess): pain, particularly lateral, darkened sight, foggy, inner veil of the retina (weakness of optic nerve), achloropsia (does not distinguish colors), sees through only half of one eye (hemianopia).

Ear: pain, buzzing, deafness.

Children: epilepsy? (or convulsions?) contractions, flowing saliva.

Nose: swelling of the mucus membranes.

Teeth: pain, pain and noise on chewing.

Parts of the body:

Face: facial paralysis (facial nerve), eye and mouth screwed to one side; corner of the mouth (commissure): contracture or flaccidity.

Cheek: muscles of skin.

Face: neuralgia (middle and lower branches of the trigeminal nerve).

GB-4 *hanyan* — heavy chin

Temple: approximately two FW lateral to the extremity of the eyebrow. A little above the lateral edge of the vertical prominence (between the parietal-sphenoid suture and the upper edge of the horizontal prominence (the temporoparietal suture); on the point of the parietal bone.

Separated from *tongziliao* (GB-1) by a horizontal mass. One medial (anterior) FW to *xuanlu* (GB-5). Two FW under *muchuang* (GB-12, IS GB-16); three tightened FW under and lateral to *touwei* (ST-1, IS ST-8).

When tonified:

Tonifies the gallbladder, upper posterior frontal lobes same side, opposite side of the lower stomach, medulla oblongata; rectus externus of the eye same side; inner opposite thumb; articulations of the upper molars, upper limb same side, lower limb opposite.

Disperses the heart.

Dispersing acts in the opposite way.

Direct effects:

Children: convulsions? Epilepsy from fear?

Eye: muscles — rectus externus same side, rectus internus opposite (external ocular motor nerve).

Ear: pain? buzzing? deafness?

Nose: sneezing without stopping — inflammation of the mucus membrane.

Parts of the body:

Face: facial paralysis, flaccidity of the eyebrow muscle, tic or spasms.

Migraines, pain in half the head, corner of the eye, impression of tightening, pains of the head, giddiness, sees nothing.

Rheumatism of the joints, upper limbs same side and lower limbs opposite.

Upper limbs same side: arthritis, pains of all the joints, particularly thumb, opposite dorsal side of index finger: tonify.

Opposite lower limb: hip, medial knee and big toe.

GB-5 *xuanlu* — suspended skull

Temple: three FW lateral (posterior) to the extremity of the eyebrow, two FW above the horizontal prominence of the zygomatic arch; at the angle between the anterior edge of the vertical mass (temporal-parietal suture) and the upper edge of the horizontal suture of the same bones; on the point of the parietal bone.

One FW lateral to (behind) *hanyan* (GB-4); one FW medial (anterior) to *xuanli* (GB-6); one under and a bit medial (anterior) to *benshen* (GB-9, IS GB-13); two above and lateral to *kezhuren* (GB-3, IS *shangwan*). One above and lateral to *tongziliao* (GB-1).

When tonified:

Tonifies the gallbladder, opposite side of medulla oblongata, both eyes, all muscles except the rectus interior; ear lobes, cheek, nostrils, canines, thumb.

Disperses the heart.

Dispersing acts in the opposite way.

Direct effects:

Weakness of brain and nerves.

Eye: all muscles (except external rectus); upper lids, ciliary muscles, sphincter of the iris (common ocular motor nerve).

Eyelids: upper: eyes do not close (lagophthalmia): disperse; dropping of the eyelids (ptosis): tonify.
Ear: lobes.
Excessive thirst; teeth, particularly canines: pain.
Nose: thick, incessant discharge.

Parts of the body:
Facial congestion.
Cerebral congestion. Pain at the vertex; occipital pain.
Migraine [with pain at] the external canthus.
Hand: medial dorsal surface. Anterior thigh and knee.

GB-6 *xuanli* — suspended hundredth

Temple: one FW anterior to the vertical line from the anterior edge of the ear. Two FW above the transverse relief of the zygomatic arch. At the angle of the superior edge of a slight transverse relief (on the inferior curve) and the posterior edge of a vertical relief. In a notch of the temporal-parietal suture.

One FW lateral (posterior) to *xuanlu* (GB-5). One-half FW anterior to *qubin* (GB-7). Two large FW under *zhengying* (GB-13, IS GB-17).

When tonified:
Tonifies the gallbladder, stomach, triple warmer; eye (oblique muscles), premolars, face.
Disperses the heart (and liver, according to their interrelationship).
Dispersing acts in the opposite way.

Direct effects:
Weakening of the nerves and brain.
Eye: grand oblique muscle (superior) same side; minor oblique (inferior) opposite side. Eyelids: acts on the obicularis oculis. Closed eyelids: disperse; eyelids that do not open (lagophthalmia): tonify.
Internal nose: inflammation.
Teeth: premolars.
Heat and burning in the digestive tract (no appetite, palpitations, fever without perspiration).

Parts of the body:
Headache; migraines.
Face: scarlet skin, inflamed, painful.
Lateral side of opposite little finger; metacarpophalangeal articulation, at the insertion of the short abductor and its antagonist.
Anterior thigh.

GB-7 *qubin* — twisted bun

On the lateral side of the head: three FW above the transverse relief of the zygomatic arch; one FW anterior to the vertical from the anterior edge of the ear. At the angle of the superior edge of a slight horizontal relief (inferior curve) and the anterior edge of a vertical relief. Between two horizontal reliefs.

One half FW posterior to *xuanli* (GB-6); one in front of and a bit under *shuaigu* (GB-8). Two large FW under and posterior to *zhengying* (GB-13, IS GB-17). Two large FW under and anterior to *chengling* (GB-14, IS GB-18); one above and a bit anterior to *sizhukong* (TW-21, IS TW-23); one above and very much anterior to *jiaosun* (TW-20).

When tonified:
Tonifies the gallbladder, liver (according to its interrelationship), small intestine, occipital lobes, spinal cord, eye, cheek, molars, maxilla, chin, opposite side of throat (tonsils), anterior upper neck, lateral base of thumb.
Disperses the heart.
Dispersing acts in the opposite way.

Direct effects:
Shock, depression?
Eyes, weakness of vision.
Molars: caries, loose.
Throat: opposite tonsils.

Parts of the body:
> Migraine, temple and top of the head.
> Upper jaw (vertical branch), cheek bone, bone of the nose; frontal prominences: pain.
> Facial neuralgia.
> Ring finger, little finger, opposite palmar side.
> Lateral side of dorsum of thumb: long abductor and short extensor (responds at *yangxi,* LI-5).

GB-8   *shuaigu* — valley of the assembly

Lateral side of the head: three FW above the level of the zygomatic arch at the vertical of the anterior of the ear; at the angle between the upper edge of the transverse mass (inferior curve) and the anterior edge of the vertical prominence; one FW posterior to *qubin* (GB-7); three large FW lateral to *benshen* (GB-9, IS GB-13); one half FW under *chengling* (GB-14, IS GB-18); two above and anterior to *tianchong* (GB-15, IS GB-9); one above and anterior to *jiaosun* (TW-20).

When tonified:
> Tonifies the gallbladder, stomach, liver, large intestine, spinal cord, opposite parietal-temporal lobes, cheek, lateral side of the neck, palate.
> Disperses the heart.
> Dispersing acts in the opposite way.

Direct effects:
> All problems from any kind of intoxication (alcohol, poisons), drug addiction (alcohol, tobacco, coffee, water, toxins, opium, etc.)
> Malaise after intoxication: headache, nausea, vertigo, pain of the eye.
> Mouth: palate.
> Upper teeth and gums.
> Eyes: rectus internus of both eyes. Upper lids of both eyes.
> Middle and internal ear; vertigo (of Meniere?).
> Cough: mucus.

Parts of the body:
> Headache due to drunkenness: frontal prominences to nape.
> Lateral part of neck (scalenius and sternocleidomastoid muscles).

GB-9   *benshen* (IS GB-13) — fundamental evolved man

Upper temple: four FW above the transverse mass of the zygomatic arch. At the angle between the posterior edge of the frontal parietal suture and the lower edge of the prominence of the superior curve.

Three FW anterior and above *shuaigu* (GB-8); two FW posterior to *yangbai* (GB-10, GB-14); one small FW under *muchuang* (GB-12, IS GB-16); one above *hanyan* (GB-4).

When tonified:
> Tonifies the gallbladder, posterior frontal lobes opposite and inferior, wrist, hand same side and opposite, opposite spinal cord.
> Disperses the heart.
> Dispersing acts in the opposite way.

Direct effects:
> Epilepsy: with saliva, from fear.
> Children: cerebral congestion, hemiplegia.

Parts of the body:
> Nape and neck: spasms same side.
> Shoulder: posterior and opposite extremity.
> Tightened chest: can neither twist nor bend.

GB-10   *yangbai* (IS GB-14) — extended whiteness

Forehead: in the angle between the inferior and lateral edge of the frontal prominence and the medial edge of the vertical ridge (frontal crest).

Two FW anterior to *benshen* (GB-9, IS GB-13); two under and lateral to head-*linqi* (GB-11, IS GB-15); one above and medial to *touwei* (ST-1, IS ST-8).

When tonified:
> Tonifies the gallbladder, inferior opposite occipital lobes; eye: opposite rectus externus.
> Disperses the heart.
> Dispersing acts in the opposite way.

Direct effects:
> Master point for troubles of the eyes: myopia, hemeralopia, spasmodic contractions of the eyes, foggy; bright dancing circles; pains in the eyes and head, acute pain of the eyeball, pain and itching of the eyes; rectus superior and great oblique?
> Cold in the back, cannot get warm. Massaging warms the lower limb, same side.

Parts of the body:
> Face: paralysis (facial nerve), facial neuralgia (trigeminal): pain of forehead; facial spasms (facial nerve); forehead tics.

GB-11   [head]-*linqi* (IS GB-15) — near to tears

Forehead: upper edge and a bit medial on the frontal prominence, in a notch on the prominence; lateral edge of a vertical flat relief.

Two tightened FW above and medial to *yangbai* (GB-10, IS GB-14); three large FW medial to *muchuang* (GB-12, IS GB-16); about four FW under *qucha* (BL-4); about two FW inferior and lateral to *shenting* (GV-23, IS GV-24).

When tonified:
> Tonifies the gallbladder, all superficial (yang) organs, bladder, posterior eye, inferior occipital lobes, frontal sinus, lateral side of neck.
> Disperses the heart.
> Dispersing acts in the opposite way.

Direct effects:
> Weakened vision, coordination of the eyes (synergy), beginning of cataract, eye pain, congestion of the lateral corner of the cornea, excess tears, inflammation of the cornea, great oblique muscle?
> Eyelids: conjunctivitis (cloudiness of the eyes), tears, fear of light.
> Nose: frontal sinusitis (nose blocked, bad cold).
> Cerebral congestion, cerebral hemorrhage, sudden stroke (eyes reversed, great shock), epilepsy from fear, grinding the teeth.
> Malaria: two attacks per day.

Opposite effects:
> Heart: pain, and pain in the side.

Parts of the body:
> Temple, occiput, nape, torticollis, pain.
> Axilla: swollen (adenitis).

GB-12   *muchuang* (IS GB-16) — window of the eye

Head, top lateral side: four FW on either side of the medial line; in an angle between the posterior edge of the frontal-parietal suture and the upper edge of the horizontal mass (superior curve); just posterior to the vertical artery and vein.

Two FW lateral to head-*linqi* (GB-11, IS GB-15); one large FW anterior to *zhengying* (GB-13, IS GB-17), one half FW above *benshen* (GB-9, IS GB-13); two under *wuchu* (BL-5).

When tonified:

> Tonifies the gallbladder, eye (particularly lateral), molars and canines same side, opposite pectoralis major muscle, opposite upper arm, opposite lumbar area, lateral arch of the foot.
> Disperses the heart.
> Dispersing acts in the opposite way.

Direct effects:

> Eyes: tired vision, particularly from too much reading, eyes troubled. Tonification during three sessions gives a great clarity of vision; does not see far clearly, red and painful eyes, particularly in the lateral part.
> Teeth, particularly molars and canines: neuralgia of the alveoli, pain in the teeth, swelling of gums and cheek from dental caries, teeth loose and out of place, corner of the lips.
> Sinusitis.
> Attacks of fever from bad cold, acute pain of the head, sudden vertigo.

Parts of the body:

> Pectoralis major muscle: opposite sternal fascia, opposite breast.

GB-13 *zhengying* (IS GB-17) — correct stage

Head, lateral side of top: four FW on either side of the medial line; one FW lateral to the vertical frontal-parietal suture; upper edge of the horizontal mass (superior curve).

One FW lateral to *muchuang* (GB-12, IS GB-16); about two FW anterior to *chengling* (GB-14, IS GB-18); one above *shuaigu* (GB-8); two under *chengguang* (BL-6).

When tonified:

> Tonifies the gallbladder, orbicularis muscle of the lips, particularly upper, cheek, temple, dental alveoli, top of the head, pectoralis major muscle, opposite clavicular fascia, opposite deltoid, under the opposite scapula.
> Disperses the heart.
> Dispersing acts in the opposite way.

Direct effects:

> All fevers from chills or nerves.
> Eyes: darkened vision, visual dizziness, atrophy of the optic nerve.
> Mouth: palate.
> Dental alveoli: pain in the gums, particularly upper jaw.
> Teeth: particularly upper pain, caries.
> Lips: orbicularis muscle, particularly upper same side.

Parts of the body:

> Head: lateral side of top, posterior lateral part of neck, same side.
> Pectoralis major, clavicular fascia and opposite deltoid.
> Dorsum of wrist and hand same side.
> Under the scapula to the opposite lumbar area.
> Lateral opposite arch of the foot.

GB-14 *chengling* (IS GB-18) — receives the immaterial

Lateral top of the head: four FW on either side of the medial line; two tightened FW anterior to the vertical occipital-parietal suture; upper edge of the horizontal prominence (superior curve).

Two FW posterior to *zhengying* (GB-13, IS GB-17); one anterior and a little above *tianchong* (GB-15, IS GB-9); two under *tongtian* (BL-7); two above *shuaigu* (GB-8).

When tonified:

> Tonifies the gallbladder and all the yang, opposite inferior frontal lobes, nape, posterior and extremity of shoulder (trapezius and deltoid muscle), nose.
> Disperses the heart.
> Dispersing acts in the opposite way.

Direct effects:

> Encephalitis: internal opposite headaches.
> Nose: coryza, blocked nose, nosebleeds.
> Asthma (nasal), contracted respiration.

Parts of the body:
Posterior shoulder, deltoid muscle, lateral upper arm.

GB-15   *tianchong* (IS GB-9) — sky assault

Head: posterior and upper edge of the superior point of the mastoid, four FW above and posterior to the top of the ear, under the prominence of the curved line which ends on the anterior edge of the vertical of the occipital-temporal suture; at the angle of the mastoid suture.

One FW posterior to *chengling* (GB-14, IS GB-18); two above *fubai* (GB-16, IS GB-10); two FW posterior to *shuaigu* (GB-8); two below *luoque* (BL-8).

When tonified:
Tonifies the gallbladder, bladder, opposite inferior occipital lobes, last molar.
Disperses the heart, lung, nose.
Dispersing acts in the opposite way.

Direct effects:
Inferior branch of the trigeminal nerve.
Easy fear, great emotiveness, violent sobbing, from shock; trembling, stiffness, painful stretching (particularly at night).
Depression, convulsions, epilepsy.

Parts of the body:
Dental congestion: last molars, lower jaw.
Head and face: pain, internal headache.

GB-16   *fubai* (IS GB-10) — superficial whiteness

Head: behind the upper edge of the ear; at the angle between the posterior edge of the upper point of the mastoid and the anterior edge of the vertical occipital-temporal suture.

Two FW below *tianchong* (GB-15, IS GB-9); two above head-*wangu* (GB-17, IS GB-12); two above and slightly in front of head-*qiaoyin* (GB-18, IS GB-11); one large FW posterior to *luxi* (TW-19).

When tonified:
Tonifies the gallbladder, inferior occipital lobes, bladder, eye same side, inner ear opposite, lateral side of the neck and upper shoulder same side, thumb, lower jaw (lower branch of the trigeminal nerve).
Disperses the heart, lung.
Dispersing acts in the opposite way.

Direct effects:
Inner ear, opposite: buzzing like a hammer, deafness, upper last molar, same side; upper jaw: pain same side.
Tonsils, opposite: coughing fits; mucus; saliva; cannot speak nor breathe; dyspnea; exhalation difficult, tiring; asthma, internal fullness, attacks of heat and cold without a temperature.

Parts of the body:
Lateral part of the neck and upper shoulder same side: swelling, abscess, tumor or all inflammation, flaccidity or contracture of the same area, also of the posterior shoulder and upper arm, or arthritis.
Hand, thumb same side: arthritis.
Arch, same side: slowness, weakness, walks badly.

GB-17   *wangu* (IS GB-12) — mastoid (final bone)

Head: behind the ear: one small FW above the lower edge of the skull; at the lower angle between the posterior edge of the mastoid and the anterior edge of the insertion of the splenius muscle, in a hollow.

One FW below *fubai* (GB-16, IS GB-10); one lateral (anterior) to head-*qiaoyin* (GB-18, IS GB-11).

When tonified:
Tonifies the gallbladder, opposite superior posterior frontal lobes, bladder (expulsor muscles), eye, eyelids, "home of tears" same side, lower surface of the opposite side of the maxilla, opposite middle ear, upper and lower limbs same side.

Disperses the heart, bladder sphincter.

Dispersing acts in the opposite way.

Direct effects:

Ear: disequilibrium, falls (labyrinthine vertigo); middle ear: inflammation, pain behind the ear.

Eyelids: home of tears?

Eyes: coordination (synergy) of the two eyes.

Mouth: opposite lower gum — inflammation; opposite tonsils, opposite orbicularis muscle.

Opposite side of tongue: hypoglossal nerve (motor activity and vasoconstriction of the tongue).

Opposite effects: Tonify:

Heart: agitation, insomnia.

Arteriosclerosis (arteries contracted?).

Malaria: hyperexcitation.

Parts of the body:

Face opposite side, opposite lower jaw.

Opposite lower face: swelling, itching, pain, trigeminal neuralgia, facial nerve paralysis, opposite corner of the mouth paralyzed.

Opposite lower jaw: contracted, trismus.

Occiput, nape, splenius capitis: spasms, contracture, pain or swelling.

Upper limb (particularly the lateral part of the elbow and the dorsum of the wrist) same side.

Lower limb, same side (particularly knee, arch): falling arches.

GB-18   [head]-*qiaoyin* (IS GB-11) — yin of the opening

Posterior lower part of the head: about mid-distance from the ear to the posterior median line. One FW above the lower edge of the skull; at the angle between the lower edge of a transverse relief (line of the lower curve) and the posterior edge of the insertion of the splenius capitis muscle.

One FW posterior to head-*wangu* (GB-17, IS GB-12); one FW lateral to *naokong* (GB-19).

When tonified:

Tonifies the gallbladder, opposite lower brain, triple warmer, bladder sphincter?, eye same side, ear opposite, tongue opposite side, upper jaw and cheekbone opposite, back (medial line of the scapula).

Disperses the heart, lung.

Dispersing acts in the opposite way.

Direct effects:

Headache like a hammer blow, cerebral congestion, meningitis.

Eye same side: pain.

Opposite ear: buzzings, deafness, motor point of the posterior auricular nerve?

Mouth: bitter or disagreeable taste, or dry (particularly on waking).

Tongue, opposite side: cold, stiff, root of the tongue bleeding.

Opposite effects:

Coughing fits: tonify. Abscess of the bronchus and nosebleeds: tonify.

Parts of the body:

Bone: serious attacks of abscesses from tuberculosis.

Opposite surface of the nose, cheekbone to ear (and with buzzing?); trigeminal neuralgia of the middle branch (nose to ear).

Upper limb, same side: joints of posterior shoulder, posterior medial elbow, dorsum of wrist. Temporary paralysis? of the arm, cannot reach head or nose; agitation or cramps.

Lower limb, particularly posterior side of the thigh and calf: cramps or agitation.

GB-19   *naokong* — hollow of the brain

Posterior base of the skull: one FW above the lower edge; two large FW from the posterior medial line; in the angle between the lower edge of a transverse relief (line of the lower curve) and the lateral edge of large muscles (superimposed insertions of the trapezius on the semispinalis capitis muscle, in a marked hollow.

One FW medial to head-*qiaoyin* (GB-18, IS GB-11); one large FW above *fengchi* (GB-20); two lateral and below *yuzhen* (BL-9).

When tonified:

Tonifies the gallbladder, all yang superficial pulses (chain of yang) half brain opposite (meninges), medial part of the eye same side, corner of opposite lips and cheek, opposite teeth, occiput, nape, trapezius muscle.
Disperses the heart, lung.
Dispersing acts in the opposite way.

Direct effects:

Meningitis, encephalitis (heaviness with unbearable pain of the head, deranged mind, depression, trauma causing diplopia, pain in the eyes, foggy vision, vertigo).
Opposite ear: buzzing, deafness.
Unhealthy thinness.

Opposite effects:

Palpitations, attacks of fever.
Opposite side of nose: pain, pain of sinusitis, deep abscess of nose, nosebleeds, opposite nostril.
Asthma (nasal?), bad cold, pulmonary tuberculosis.

Parts of the body:

Occiput, nape, trapezius, posterior shoulder; nape stiff from cold; nape and shoulder: pain.

GB-20 *fengchi* — marsh of winds

Nape: one half FW below the angle between the lower edge of the skull and the lower edge of the large vertical muscle. Exactly at the angle between the medial edge of the lateral muscle (splenius capitis) and the upper edge of the lateral process of the second cervical vertebra, in a hollow.

One large FW below *naokong* (GB-19). About six FW above and medial to *jianjing* (GB-21); three tightened FW lateral and slightly above *tianzhu* (BL-10); one inferior and medial to head-*qiaoyin* (GB-18, IS GB-11).

When tonified:

Tonifies the sympathetic system (all the pulses of the yin distributor organs except the vessels — heat, dryness); triple warmer, all the yin, governor vessel, gallbladder, posterior midbrain (posterior hypothalamus) pons, medulla oblongata, spinal cord, three endocrines, opposite eye, ear and nose, mastoid, penis or clitoris, half-body same side.
Disperses (makes supple and relaxed) the vessels.
Dispersing acts in the opposite way.
Evokes a response in *yangchi* (TW-4) and *shanzhong* (CV-17).

Direct effects:

All effects of the sympathetic system (heat, dryness, dilation of pupils and arteries, etc.); insufficiency: tonify; excess: disperse.
Heat in excess, dryness: disperse; cold, sweating: tonify.
All nervous troubles: weakening of the brain and nerves, serious headache with acute pain in the brain, laborious dizziness.
Eyes: pupils too open (mydriasis): disperse; troubled vision, lack of clarity (luminosity): tonify; or pupils too open: disperse; glaucoma: tonify.
Ear: hearing trouble from excess energy; disperse.
Nose: all trouble, coryza.
Throat: pain.
Fever: does not sweat: disperse.
Loose teeth, displaced.

Opposite effects:

Heart: rapid and small, contracted, tight: tonify; warm feet and hands, shivers in bath, cold and hot: tonify.
Men: non-erection?

Parts of the body:

Vertebral column (governor vessel).
Neck and nape: pain, stiffness, cannot turn the neck, weakness of the muscles.

Shoulder and back: weakness of muscles — vertebral and thoracic — to the point of the displacement or deviation of the vertebra; shoulder, back, lumbar area, pain.

Posteromedial part of lower limb, particularly the lower leg.

GB-21   *jianjing* — well of the shoulder

Upper shoulder: five FW medial to the bony extremity (acromion). Just in front of the trapezius muscle, at the angle between the lower edge of a deep transverse mass (first rib) and the posterior edge of a hard vertical muscle (posterior scalenius); in a hollow.

Preceding point: *fengchi* (GB-20); following point: *yuanye* (GB-22).

Four FW medial to *jugu* (LI-16); one large FW lateral to *jianzhongshu* (SI-15); two FW posterior to *quepen* (ST-12); three anterior to *tianliao* (TW-15).

When tonified:

Tonifies the gallbladder, opposite side of brain, three psychological pulses, the three endocrines, half-body, kidneys.

Disperses the large intestine, liver; left point: pancreas; right point: spleen, heart, triple warmer.

Dispersing acts in the opposite way.

The large intestine and triple warmer meridians go through this point in order to continue their flow. The gallbladder meridian turns at a right angle towards the front, going through *kufang* (ST-14), *tianquan* (PC-2), *jiquan* (HT-1).

Direct effects:

Awakening of the nerves and brain, neurasthenia (chest twisted from melancholy), cerebral anemia, insufficiency of the sympathetic system.

Counterflow of energy (nervous crisis), cerebral congestion, apoplexy (blocked energy, saliva, cannot speak), hemiplegia; children: acute or chronic meningitis.

Contrary effects:

Commands the energy of the five yin distributor organs? and acts on all?

Heart: beriberi attacking the heart: tonify.

Left point: pancreas; right point: spleen; acute pain of the spleen or pancreas: tonify.

Respiratory passages: violent cough, cold and heat, cannot extend, bronchitis, catarrh in upper lung; tuberculosis.

Breast abscess: tonify; fibroma, cysts: tonify.

Difficult delivery; after delivery, attack of weakness, hands and feet icy; after premature delivery, lower limbs ice cold, post-partum metrorrhagia: tonify.

Parts of the body:

Contusions: pain in the abdomen, lower belly and lumbar area, same side.

Nape: pain, stiffness, cannot turn neck.

Shoulder and back as if tied, side and lumbar area: pain, scapula: acute pain, rheumatism of the scapula muscles, particularly subscapularis (inserted on the anterior head of the humerus), shoulder and arm as if pulled, tied, hand cannot reach the head.

Thumb and index finger.

Jiujitsu: knockout point; kuatsu: reinvigorating point.

GB-22   *yuanye* — abyss of the axilla

Axilla, midlength: lower edge of the fourth rib (the third being deep on the axilla); in a hollow.

Preceding point: *jianjing* (GB-21), passing through *kufang* (ST-14), *tianquan* (PC-2), *jiquan* (HT-1). Following point: *zhejin* (GB-23), having passed through *dabao* (SP-21) below the fifth rib and following the lower edge of the fifth rib; three FW lateral to *tianchi* (PC-1).

When tonified:

Tonifies the gallbladder, longissimus dorsi, lower posterior frontal lobes, axilla.

Disperses the heart.

Dispersing acts in the opposite way.

Direct effects:
Intercostal neuralgia from bronchitis or pleurisy, weakness, fullness of the chest.
Inflamed lymph nodes (superative adenitis), swelling and itching of the axilla.
Malaria, particularly left point (Ledum pal).

Parts of the body:
Latissimus dorsi: contracture, cannot raise arm.

Point of Weihe: Left: Ledum Pal.

GB-23 *zhejin* — brusque muscles

Lateral part of thorax: three FW lateral to the vertical of the nipple; inferior edge of the fifth rib; in a hollow; three lateral to and under the nipple (men).

Five FW under and anterior to *yuanye* (GB-22), passing through *dabao* (SP-21); one large FW under *tianchi* (PC-1); two above and medial to *riyue* (GB-24); one large FW above and lateral to *qimen* (LR-14).

When tonified:
Tonifies the gallbladder, opposite side of the brain, spinal cord, and back, eye and ear same side, bladder.
Disperses the heart.
Dispersing acts in the opposite way.
Herald point of the gallbladder (troubled by negative feelings, with feeling cold, or depression); see *riyue* (GB-24).

Direct effects:
Saliva in excess: stomach, liquid vomiting at night, acidity, hyperchlorhydria, retracted gums?
Nerve degeneration and weakness. Excess work, heavy sighs, sadness, worried and difficult speech. Children as if seized with horror, convulsed mouth. Fears at night; does not like to greet people? amnesia.
Asthma, cannot lie down, severe fullness of the chest.
Weakening vision.
Ear: whistling, ringing.
Heat in the lower pelvis.

Parts of the body:
Weakness particularly of the back, flaccid or contracted extremities.

Point of Weihe: Kali Phosphoricum.

GB-24 *riyue* — sun and moon

Lower lateral part of the thorax: four large FW lateral to the vertical of the nipple (and two below its level — men), inferior edge of the sixth rib (the nipple being on the superior edge of the fifth rib); in a hollow.

Two FW lateral and below *zhejin* (GB-23); six above and anterior to *jingmen* (GB-25).

When tonified:
Tonifies the gallbladder, cerebellum, opposite side of the lumbar area.
Disperses the heart, large intestine, stomach.
Dispersing acts in the opposite way.

Direct effects:
Happiness and unhappiness from moment to moment, heavy sighs, easily saddened, talkative with brash speech. Hysteria?
Herald point of the gallbladder: emotional problems, depression and feeling cold (see *zhejin,* GB-23).
Stomach (distention), acid vomiting at night, constant salivation, spasms of the diaphragm.
Heat in the lower pelvis.
Kidneys: inflammation.
Heaviness of the limbs.

GB-25 *jingmen* — door of the capital

Bottom of the lateral part of the thorax; at the angle between the inferior point of the twelfth and last rib and the anterior edge of the large vertical muscle (latissimus dorsi); in a hollow.

Preceding point *riyue* (GB-24); about three FW above *daimai* (GB-26). Two large FW under and posterior to *zhangmen* (LR-13); two above and anterior to *huangmen* (BL-46, IS BL-51, lateral to BL-21).

When tonified:

Tonifies the gallbladder, stomach, intestines, kidneys, medulla, spinal cord, eyes, ears, nose, throat, front of scapula, trapezius muscle and latissimus dorsi muscle.

Disperses the opposite breast, heart.

Dispersing acts in the opposite way.

Direct effects:

Herald point of the kidneys (emotional troubles, depression, feeling cold): insufficiency (clear, abundant urine), or inflammation (nephritis) with hypertension, pain of lumbar area, slow, feeble urine, pain radiating into the back, cannot breathe, acute nephritis (with large, white kidneys and insufficiency of urine).

Urine-stool balance, or abundant urine and scant stools, or scant (slow, feeble) urine and abundant stools.

Intestines: acute diarrhea, noises in the abdomen, swollen abdomen, tympanism, pain.

Contrary effects:

Opposite breast.

Parts of the body:

Shoulder and back, contractions from cold.

Scapula: pain, contracted muscles.

Lumbar area: pain, contracted muscles, and pain in lumbar area, abdomen and articulation of the hip, and intercostal area.

Intercostal pain?

Point of Weihe: Cantharis.

GB-26 *daimai* — belt vessel

At mid-distance of the superior edge of the iliac crest (top of the hip) to the last rib, about vertical to the axilla; three FW posterior to the anterior angle (of the ilium); on the anterior edge of the insertion on the hip of the large dorsal muscle (latissimus dorsi); in a large hollow (triangle of Petit).

About three FW under *jingmen* (GB-25); three above *wushu* (GB-27); about three large FW anterior to *dachangshu* (BL-25); four posterior to *fujie* (SP-14).

When tonified:

Tonifies the gallbladder, all yang meridians, brain, medulla, spinal cord, opposite upper part of eyelid, hip, all articulations.

Disperses all yin meridians, sexual organs, penis.

Dispersing acts in the opposite way.

''Point of the belt vessel which connects all the meridians at the level of the waist.''

Direct effects:

Abdomen relaxed, ''noise like water in a bag.''

Opposite effects:

Genitourinary system: contraction, pain: tonify.

Sexual organs: abdomen — contractions, pains, spasms. Women: insufficient or blocked menses, red or white discharge, ovaries — all trouble; uterus — spasms, endometritis; all women's troubles with spasms. Men: troubles of the testicles, orchitis, penis.

Kidneys: painful point when problems are present.

Parts of the body:

All articulations problems.

Latissimus dorsi muscles.

Lumbar area: acute pain.
Articulation of the hip, medial anterior part of the thigh.

Point of Weihe: Calcarea Phosphoricum.

GB-27 *wushu* — the five pivots

Lateral part of the hip: two FW posterior to the vertical anterior part of the hip (iliac crest); two FW under the upper part; at the angle between the inferior edge of the large prominence of the crest and the anterior edge of the insertion of the muscle (gluteus medius); above the insertion of the gluteus minimus; in a hollow.

Three FW under *daimai* (GB-26); two above *juliao* (GB-28, IS GB-29); two anterior to *baohuang* (BL-48, IS BL-53).

When tonified:
Tonifies the gallbladder, posterior frontal lobes, sexual organs, hypogastric plexus, large intestine, bladder; scapula, back, lumbar area, stomach, axilla, anterior thigh and knee.
Dispersing acts in the opposite way.
''Reunion of the gallbladder and belt vessel.''

Direct effects:
Hypogastric plexus: assent point of the large intestine, bladder, kidney, sexual organs, excess from external troubles, point of passage between kidney filtration and kidney reabsorption?
The whole interior of body contracted, particularly abdomen.
Stomach: cramps, large intestine: spasms.
Sexual organs — women: ovaries, inflammation; uterus, spasms; white discharge, metritis; red discharge. Men — spermatic tube: pain; epididymitis; opposite testicle: orchitis; testicles do not descend (cryptorchidia). Urethra: inflammation.

Parts of the body:
Hip, pelvis.
Helps to rise from sitting; pain and weakness in scapula, back, lumbar area; axilla; anterior thigh and knee.

GB-28 *juliao* (IS GB-29) — stays in the hole

Lateral part of hip: one small FW above the large bulge of the femur (greater trochanter); upper part of a large hollow; inferior angle between two muscles in front of the gluteus minimus (behind the gluteus medius).

Two FW under *wuchu* (GB-27); three above *weidao* (GB-30, IS GB-28).

When tonified:
Tonifies the gallbladder, large intestine, bladder, midbrain, articulations, ligaments, lower pelvis, lumbar area, gluteus medius.
Dispersing acts in the opposite way.

Direct effects:
Large intestine: inflammation of the caecum, enteritis.
Bladder: inflammation (cystitis).
Difficult menses; uterus: difficulties; white discharge; ovaries.
Caecum.

Parts of the body:
Gluteus medius and minimus: weakness and pain; poliomyelitis.
Articulations: stiffness, ankylosis, hard ligaments.
Scapula and chest, upper limb and hand: contracted muscles.
Lumbar area: pains radiating to the lower abdomen; hip: pain.
Knee stiff, can neither fold nor extend.

Point of Weihe: Colocynthis.

GB-29   *huantiao* (IS GB-30) — to jump into a hoop

Superior lateral part of the thigh: superior and anterior to the large bulge of the femur (greater trochanter); deep, the superior edge of the lower spine; between the anterior edge of the bone and the posterior edge of the large muscle (tensor fascia lata muscle) and of the insertion of gluteus medius.

One FW above *weidao* (GB-30, IS GB-28); eight FW above *fengshi* (GB-31).

When tonified:
>Tonifies the gallbladder, triple warmer, small intestine, posterior frontal lobes, spinal cord, lateral half of the body same side.
>Disperses the heart, arteries, skin.
>Dispersing acts in the opposite way.

Contrary effects:
>Arteries: tonification makes the arteries supple, can prevent arterial spasms, cerebral hemorrhages. Apoplexy, sudden stroke: tonify; arteriosclerosis, tonify.
>Pruritis of the whole body: tonify.
>Eruptive fever of whole body: measles, German measles, scarlet fever, chicken pox? smallpox?

Parts of the body:
>Rheumatic pain from cold, wind or humidity: tonify.
>Lateral half of the body same side: contracture or flaccidity, hemiplegia of right or left: tonify.
>Back: painful, swollen muscles; lumbar area: muscles contracted, cannot turn.
>Chest, axilla and side: pain in a specific spot.
>Posterior shoulder, dorsum of wrist and hand: joints, pain, rheumatism or weakness to the point of flaccidity.
>Lower limbs: hip joint.
>Medial side of gastrocnemius, plantar flexors of the big toe, extensors of the four toes: contractions, pain, weakness or flaccidity.

GB-30   *weidao* (IS GB-28) — path of the parallels

Lateral, superior part of the thigh, hip: anterior edge of the large bulge of the thigh (greater trochanter), angle of the deep anterior edge of the femur; posterior edge of the large muscle (tensor fascia lata); in a hollow.

Three FW below *huantiao* (GB-29, IS GB-30); five above *fengshi* (GB-31).

When tonified:
>Tonifies the gallbladder, stomach, triple warmer, small intestine, lung, genitourinary system, bladder, sexual organs, mid-brain, anterior part of the thigh and medial part of knee, hip joint.
>Three FW below *huantiao* (GB-29, IS GB-30); five above *fengshi* (GB-31).
>Disperses the heart.
>Dispersing acts in the opposite way.

Direct effects:
>Discouraged, weak, drops everything, awkward.
>Triple warmer (the three great functions) in excess.
>Coughing fits, mucus expelled by forced coughing.
>Constant vomiting attacks; nausea; intestines: inflammation.
>Cecum: inflammation; diarrhea; spasms; presses the abdomen inward.
>Edema: kidney and bladder contracted.

Parts of the body:
>Hip joint, gluteus maximus.
>Lateral side of the thigh, lateral part of knee.

>**Point of Weihe:** Stannum Metalicum.

GB-31   *fengshi* — market in the wind

Lateral part of thigh, about mid-height; five FW below the large, upper protrusion of the femur (greater trochanter). Ten FW above the lateral protrusion of the knee (lateral condyle); the angle between the posterior edge of a large flat tendon (band of the fascia lata) and the lower edge of a transverse mass; on the biceps femoris muscle.

Eight FW above the lateral bone of the knee (lateral condyle), *xiyangguan* (GB-33).

Two FW above *xiadu* (GB-32, IS *zhongdu*); eight FW below the greater trochanter, *huantiao* (GB-29, IS GB-30).

When tonified:

Tonifies the gallbladder, genital system, penis, lower limbs, lumbar area, middle of the back, shoulder, upper limb.

Dispersing acts in the opposite way.

Direct effects:

Sexual organs, penis.

Parts of the body:

Lateral half-body same side: all trouble, flaccidity, contracture.

Middle of back at the level of the scapula.

Posterior part of the upper limb and hand.

Lower limb: weakness, contracted muscles, buttocks, sacral nerves, posterolateral part of thigh, vastus intermedius muscle; knee: medial anterior; foot: serious swelling from rheumatism; plantar part of heel, medial sole, plantar part of big toe.

GB-32   *xiadu* (IS *zhongdu*) — lower torrent (IS middle of the canal)

Lateral thigh, about at the lower third; six FW above the lateral protruding bone of the knee (lateral condyle of the femur); at the angle between the posterior edge of a flat ligament (band of tensor fascia lata) and the lower edge of a transverse mass, on the vastus intermedius muscle; in a hollow.

Two FW below *fengshi* (GB-31); four above *xiyangguan* (GB-33); at the level and lateral to thigh-*futu* (ST-32).

When tonified:

Tonifies the gallbladder, cerebellum, lower spinal cord, lateral and anterior lower limb, perineum, anus, sexual organs, dorsum of hand.

Dispersing acts in the opposite way.

Direct effects:

Passage point between the gallbladder, anus and sexual organs.

Parts of the body:

Muscles cold?

Dorsum of hand.

Anterolateral lower limb: without strength to the point of flaccidity, contracture, pain; thigh: painful rheumatism; knee: cramps and pain after long effort; plantar heel.

GB-33   *xiyangguan* — external barrier of the knee

Upper, lateral part of the knee: two FW above the round head of the fibula; anterior to the posterior opening of the tibial-femoral articulation; at the angle between the upper edge of the head of the femur and the body of the bone; on the anterior edge of a large tendon (biceps femoris); in a hollow.

Four FW below *xiadu* (GB-32, IS *zhongdu*); three above *yanglingquan* (GB-34). At the level of and lateral to *liangqiu* (ST-34); three anterior to *weiyang* (BL-53, IS BL-39).

When tonified:

Tonifies the gallbladder, temporal-parietal lobes, knee, opposite sacral nerves, opposite side of the perineum, shoulder, elbow, wrist.

Disperses the heart.

Dispersing acts in the opposite way.

Direct effects:

Paralysis from shock, without action? lower limb paralysis?

Parts of the body:

Knee; mainly lateral, all trouble; pain, arthritis, can neither extend nor flex, cramps of the lateral part of the knee particularly after long effort.

Anterior part of lower leg and arch.

Upper limb, shoulder joint, elbow, wrist.
Perineum, sacral nerves opposite side.

GB-34 *yanglingquan* — source of the external plateau

Lateral, upper part of the lower leg, just at the anterior edge of the round head of the fibula. In the angle between the lower edge of the head of the tibia and the posterior edge of the insertion of the extensor digitorum longus muscle, in a hollow.

Three FW below *xiyangguan* (GB-33); six FW above *yangjiao* (GB-35); one large FW posterior and slightly below leg-*sanli* (ST-36).

When tonified:
Tonifies the gallbladder, posterior frontal lobes, cerebellum, medulla oblongata, all muscles of half the body same side, large intestine, bladder (body), eyes, ears, mouth (taste-smell).
Disperses the heart, liver, sphincter of anus and gallbladder.
Dispersing acts in the opposite way.
Responds in *dabao* (SP-21).

Direct effects:
Anguish, "fear of being arrested," heart, arteries, or throat contracted: disperse.
All trouble of the organism, external and internal, opposite side; gives strength, coordination, equilibrium. Tradition says "reunion of the spinal cord."
Reunion point for muscles: weakness of the muscles, cannot stand from a sitting position. Or cold of the muscles, atrophy, myelitis, poliomyelitis (makes the muscle grow, even the atrophied muscle if recent). Lack of resistance to fatigue, muscles flaccid from hemiplegia (if recent), or pains, cramps, contractures, St. Vitus Dance: muscles of the lower and upper limb, radial nerve, lateral side of neck.
False arteriosclerosis (muscles of the arteries contracted, spasmodic, hard).
Face swollen, itching? opposite.
Teeth: incisors, caries opposite.
Large intestine: anal sphincter contracted: disperse; or relaxed: tonify; constant constipation, either spasmodic (disperse) or atonic (tonify); abdomen swollen, tympanism.
Bladder: direct effect; sphincter of the bladder: opposite effect; relaxed: disperse; or contracted: tonify.

Parts of the body:
Half-body same side.
Upper limb: weakness or pain, or contracture. Hand, thumb: weakness or rheumatism, pain.
Lower ribs: pain. Lumbar area: shooting pain when sitting, or sharp pain. Coccygeal nerves, coccyx, sacrum: pain.
Hip, iliac crest: joint of the hip: pain or arthritis.
Lower limb: all trouble, walks heavily, weakness to the point of flaccidity, or spasms, cramps, cramps of cholera. Knee: weakness or swelling to the point of inability to flex it; pain, rheumatism, inflammation of the ligaments (periarthritis) particularly anterior and inferior. Foot: cannot be lifted, muscles lacking strength, to the point of flaccidity; or cold, colorless. Heel: lateral, posterior. Sole: except big toe.

GB-35 *yangjiao* — crossing of the yang

Lateral part of lower leg: six large FW below the round head of the fibula; angle between the anterior edge of the fibula (with peroneus longus muscle) and the upper edge of a transverse mass, posterior edge of the extensor digitorum longus; in a hollow.

Six FW below *yanglingquan* (GB-34); two above and posterior to *waiqiu* (GB-36); two posterior (lateral) to *tiaokou* (ST-38); at the level of *chengshan* (BL-57), between the gastrocnemius muscle.

When tonified:
Tonifies the gallbladder, medulla oblongata, throat, lung, coccyx, ischium, arch.
Disperses the heart, anterior frontal lobes.
Dispersing acts in the opposite way.

Direct effects:
Throat: pain, diphtheria, tonsillitis.
Chest full, swollen, painful, dyspnea.

Opposite effects:

Anguish, deranged mind, regrets, remorse, weakness and cold, or emotional agitation, hyperexcitation; hysteria?

Parts of the body:

Lower limb: pain, contracture or weakness; coccyx and ischium: pain; knee: weakness, peroneal nerve; arch: weakness; big toe: extensor pollicis longus muscle lifted: disperse; falling: tonify.

GB-36 *waiqiu* — curve towards the exterior

Lateral lower leg: six FW above the bone of the ankle (external malleolus), at the angle between the anterior edge of the fibula and the upper edge of a bulge curving backwards (groove of the peroneus muscle), on the inferior and anterior edge of peroneus longus muscle, in a hollow.

Two FW below and posterior to *yangjiao* (GB-35); one large FW posterior to and above *guangming* (GB-37); two in front of *feiyang* (BL-58); three posterior and slightly above leg-*xialian* (ST-39, IS *xiajuxu*).

When tonified:

Tonifies the gallbladder, posterior frontal lobes, midbrain, large intestine, opposite governor vessel, skin, flesh. Disperses the heart, kidney, lung, larynx.
Dispersing acts in the opposite way.

Direct effects:

Depression? weakness to the point of flaccidity? or epilepsy?
Skin: pain, wounds from animals, poison not being expelled, fever: moxa around the wound, bleed the site; wounds infected or healing badly.
Large intestine opposite side: atony? Beriberi.

Opposite effects:

Opposite heart: pain in the area, in the left thorax, fever from cold.
Larynx opposite side: inflammation; pleurisy: fullness and inflammation of the chest, pain in the side.

Parts of the body:

Lateral side of the neck and nape same side: pain.
Cervical, dorsal, lumbar vertebrae, sacrum opposite side (opposite governor vessel).
Lower leg: lateral part of calf: cramps; peroneal nerve.
Anteromedial part of the sole and dorsal edge of the short extensor of the four toes; flexor pollicis longus muscle.

GB-37 *guangming* — brilliant light

Lateral lower leg: five FW above the ankle bone (lateral malleolus); in the angle between the anterior edge of the fibula (with peroneus longus muscle), just at a small bony eminence, and the upper edge of a transverse mass (insertion of the peroneus anterior muscle); on the posterior edge of the extensor digitorum longus muscle.

One large FW under and anterior to *waiqiu* (GB-36): one FW above *yangfu* (GB-38); two posterior to *fenglong* (ST-40); one large FW anterior to *fuyang* (BL-59).

When tonified:

Tonifies the liver, heart, medulla oblongata same side, eyes opposite, anterior lateral part of lower leg, anterior part of sole.
Disperses the gallbladder, kidney.
Dispersing acts in the opposite way.

Direct effects:

Mostly insufficiency of the gallbladder and thus of the stomach with excess of the heart; evolved man, liver.
Loss of vitality, weakness, constitution not responding any more (without stimulus); cannot remain standing for a long time, cannot stand up from a sitting position. Illness or tuberculosis of the spinal cord?
Fever without sweat, with delirium?
Eye opposite side: acute pain or itching.
Feet and hands especially small.

Parts of the body:

Knee: pain; anterior, lateral lower leg: all trouble between the peroneus muscle and the tibia.
Lower leg and feet sluggish, weak, limping, cannot remain standing for a long time; hot and painful when

walking, or painful and numb during orgasm. Peroneus anterior (which lifts the lateral part of the foot), flaccidity or contracture. Foot: anterior part of sole, short extensor of the toes and long extensor of the big toe.

GB-38   *yangfu* — help for the yang

Lateral part of lower leg: four FW above the ankle bone (external malleolus); just at the anterior edge of the fibula; in the angle between the anterior edge of the upper prominence of a notch in the bone (the groove of the peroneus muscle) and the upper edge of a transverse mass; in a hollow. Posterior to the extensor digitorum longus and the peroneus anterior.

One FW below *guangming* (GB-37); two above *xuanzhong* (GB-39).

When dispersed:
>   Disperses the gallbladder, stomach, large intestine, small intestine, lung, skin, superior occipital lobes, primate, opposite upper limb, opposite joints, opposite axilla, lower limb same side, eye same side.
>   Tonifies the heart, liver, evolved man.
>   Tonifying acts in the opposite way.

Direct effects:
>   Dispersal point of the gallbladder: ashen complexion, eyes circled with black, nausea and bitterness or dryness in mouth on waking; cholecystitis; biliary mud or sand or even small stones in the gallbladder (the large ones are dangerous to try to evacuate).
>   Irritable, unhappy, finds all things bad, unyielding personality, decisive, stubborn, passionate, upset, susceptible, needs to act and attacks of weakness. Emotions, shock, are paralyzing, at the same time there is great courage and even audacity; bears a lot and suddenly explodes; sighs often; very worried about cleanliness to the point of exaggeration.
>   Migraines of the left temple, sometimes of the right, particularly after fatty food, chocolate, coffee with milk.
>   Eye same side: lateral corner and medial corner: pain.
>   Large intestine: obstinate constipation.
>   Insufficient liver.
>   Asthmatic fits. Throat inflamed or contracted.

Parts of the body:
>   Half of the body, opposite side: general pains without fixed location.
>   Opposite joints: pains, weakness.
>   Head pain of the opposite frontal prominences; inferior part of the chin, temples and occiput: pain.
>   Opposite armpit: swelling, pain, adenitis, suppurative adenitis.
>   Lumbar area: pain or "cold as if in water."
>   Lower limbs same side: pain or flaccidity or contracture, numbness of knee and leg same side. Opposite posterior knee: swelling of the popliteal crease or arthritis. Opposite arch of the foot: arthritis, pain.

GB-39   *xuanzhong* — suspended bell

Lateral part of the leg: two FW above the ankle bone (external malleolus); in the angle between the anterior edge of the peroneus muscle and the inferior edge of a transverse mass. Between the bone and the peroneus brevis muscle, which is just posterior to the extensor digitorum longus; in a hollow.

Two FW under *yangfu* (GB-38); three large FW above *qiuxu* (GB-40).

When tonified:
>   Tonifies the gallbladder, stomach, bladder, kidneys, posterior frontal lobes, bone marrow opposite side, polynuclear leukocytes.
>   Disperses the heart, liver, lungs.
>   Dispersing acts in the opposite way.

Direct effects:
>   Hyperexcited indignation sufficient to cause apoplexy; or exhaustion, cold.
>   Blood: tonifying puts a large number of polynuclear leukocytes into the blood (always numerous in inflammation, particularly streptococcal, of the blood, mucus, tissues). In cases of infection, causes high fever coming just at nightfall with a decrease and convalescence the next day. Septicemia. Abscess: if the white spot has not yet appeared, it will be reabsorbed within twenty-four hours. If the pus is already formed, causes evacuation and begins the rapid cicatrization from the root. Abscesses (furunculosis) will not recur. Abscess in the

brain; thick blood; arteriosclerosis; influenza; prolonged fever.

Indignation, rage sufficient to cause apoplexy; anxiety, hyperexcited worries.

Slow cicatrization, or emptiness, exhaustion, cold (acts on the conjunctive tissue, which cicatrizes?).

Reunion point of the bone marrow. All trouble of the bones: pain in the bones. Fracture: the suture is obtained in half or one third of the usual time and pain or inflammation stops (add *shangqiu*, SP-5, against periostitis). Inflammation of all the mucosa.

Inflammation of the digestive tract; heat of stomach, cannot eat; babies without appetite, not eating, abdominal fullness, distention of the stomach; aerogastria; intestines: inflammation, liquid diarrhea; anus: fistulas; beriberi.

Inflammation of the respiratory passages: nose: inflammation of the mucosa; nose congested, blocked, acute coryza, nosebleeds, dry nose, cough causing pain in the back or above the eyebrows; tonsillitis, prolonged bronchitis, bronchopneumonia, pleurisy, noncongestive tuberculosis.

Kidneys: inflammation, pyuria, profuse urine, painful urination.

Parts of the body:

Skin: itching (pruritis) of the lateral part of half of the body opposite side (excess urea). Lateral part of the half-body opposite: flaccidity or contracture. The four limbs cannot be lifted, difficulty in moving the feet, flaccid. Contraction of the muscles and pain in the bones.

Lateral part of neck, opposite: pain.

Upper part of the back opposite side: pain (levator scapulae of the scapula, iliocostal muscle). Hand: dorsum of wrist and radial side: pain.

Knee, lower leg, opposite foot: rheumatism from humidity; five toes: acute pain; medial side of great toe.

GB-40   *qiuxu* — fair of the hill

Lateral part of ankle: a bit under the anterior angle of the lateral malleolus; in the angle between the upper edge of the transverse bone (scaphoid) and the insertion of the extensor digitorum brevis muscle; in a hollow; in the upper part of the hollow.

Three large FW under *xuanzhong* (GB-39); four posterior to foot-*linqi* (GB-41); one large FW lateral to *jiexi* (ST-41); at the lateral angle of the malleolus and of the calcaneum.

When tonified:

Tonifies the gallbladder, superior occipital lobes, primate, stomach, spinal cord, face, lateral part of opposite neck, hip joint same side.

Disperses the heart, liver.

Dispersing acts in the opposite way.

Responds to and in *baihui* (GV-19, IS GV-20).

Direct effects:

Deep sighs, lassitude, weakness, emptiness; sitting, cannot stand.

Usually spasms, contractions, tightness.

Source point of the gallbladder: excess or insufficiency.

Opposite side of intestines: spasms, violent pain, nervous spasms; hardness of the abdomen, opposite side.

Contracted chest, difficult inspiration and exhalation; fullness, cannot breathe; pulmonary congestion, pleurisy.

Malaria, prolonged shivering.

Eyes: beginning of cataract; keratitis.

Parts of the body:

Opposite side of the face: swelling; lateral part of neck, opposite: swelling.

Axilla same side: painful swelling, suppurative adenitis.

Crotch: pain, pruritis?

Hip same side: arthritis, pain of the hip, groin, lumbar area, crotch, sacrum.

Lower limbs: numbness, cramps; calf same side: cramps, lateral and anterior leg and foot: cramps, foot turned to the interior and flexed: disperse; or turned laterally: tonify.

GB-41   [foot]-*linqi* — ready to cry

Dorsum of foot, between the fourth and fifth metatarsal bones (long bones of the fourth and fifth toes); at the mid-length of the bones; on the lateral edge of the tendon coming obliquely from the fifth toe (extensor digitorum longus muscle); on the medial edge (towards the toe) of the fourth metatarsal with the dorsal tendon (extensor digi-torum brevis); in a hollow; on the edge of a transverse mass.

Four FW under *qiuxu* (GB-40); one FW posterior to *diwuhui* (GB-42); one lateral to *chongyang* (ST-42); three medial to *jinmen* (BL-63).

When tonified:
   Tonifies the gallbladder, stomach, inferior occipital lobes, spinal cord, thyroid, mastoid, lower limb same side, upper limb, eye, opposite ear, opposite breast.

Disperses the heart, liver.
   Dispersing acts in the opposite way.

Direct effects:
   ''Harmonizes above and below.'' Tonifying disperses the upper body; dispersing tonifies the upper body.
   Troubles of insufficiency of the energy of yang activity; lymphatism, etc.
   Fits of weakness, rolling head; fears cold; non-resistance to external cold, shivers in cold water, internal cold, icy lumbar area, cold of lower leg and foot.
   Lymphatism; slowness, functions slow, repeated caries, coldness, swelling.
   Lymph nodes, lymphadenitis, adenitis: at the neck or nape or the subclavicular hollow, at the axilla; suppurative adenitis, tumors.
   All trouble with swelling.
   Mastoid: pain, swelling — swelling extending to the nape, cheek, eye.
   Throat opposite side: swelling, tonsillitis.
   Teeth same side: frequent caries, pain in all the teeth.
   Intestines, abdomen: all trouble; regulates the fat of the lower abdomen.
   Eyes lateral, opposite side: all troubles; acute pain, swelling, conjunctivitis, muscles of the eye: coordination, synergy.
   Opposite ear: pain, inflammation? sudden deafness?
   Lungs: cannot breathe, panting, cannot walk; difficulty inhaling and exhaling.
   Sexual organs: opposite breasts: problems of lactation; swelling, pain (mammitis); abscess; menses: difficult or insufficient; at orgasm, numbness of the leg.

Opposite effects:
   Heart: pain, endocarditis. Malaria: daily attacks at sunset.

Parts of the body:
   Half-body same side.
   Pains without fixed location; circulating rheumatism, pains throughout the body; pains in the joints; attacks of fever.
   Head: pain at the top (vertex); temple, opposite occiput: pain.
   Opposite mastoid, shoulder, back: pain.
   Shoulder and upper limb, hand, radial side: pain or contracture or flaccidity.
   Hip joint same side: pain.
   Lower limb same side: acute pain; ankle, foot: lateral side and base of the toe: pain, edema of the feet; heel: rheu-matism.

GB-42   *diwuhui* — fifth reunion of the earth

Dorsal and lateral part of the foot: one FW posterior to the joint of the fourth toe (metatarsophalangeal joint); in the angle between the lateral edge of the body of the fourth metatarsal and the anterior edge of the oblique tendon (extensor of the fifth toe); in a hollow.

One FW in front of foot-*linqi* (GB-41); one posterior to *xiaxi* (GB-43); two medial to foot-*tonggu* (BL-66); two lateral to *neiting* (ST-44).

When tonified:
   Tonifies gallbladder, temporoparietal lobes, eye, breast, tips of fingers and toes.
   Disperses the heart, lungs.
   Dispersing acts in the opposite way.

Direct effects:

>   Eye same side: itching, or acute pain.
>
>   Opposite breast: inflammation, mammitis, or abscess.

Opposite effects:

>   Lungs: pulmonary tuberculosis; exhaustion, spits blood?

Parts of the body:

>   Fingers or toes: problems of touch and sensitivity.
>
>   Dorsum of foot: pain, rheumatism; lateral side emaciated, dry?
>
>   Axilla: pain.

GB-43   *xiaxi* — narrowed valley

Dorsum of foot, just behind the joint at the base of the fourth and fifth toes; at the lateral angle of the head and body of the fourth metatarsal bone of the fourth toe; between the bone and artery, vein and nerve; in a hollow.

One FW in front of *diwuhui* (GB-42); following (and last) point: foot-*qiaoyin* (GB-44); on the terminal phalanx.

When tonified:

>   Tonifies the gallbladder, superior occipital lobes, primate, chest and opposite sides, ankle, toes, stomach, opposite maxilla, opposite eye.
>
>   Disperses the heart, sexual organs.
>
>   Dispersing acts in the opposite way.

Direct effects:

>   Insomnia from apprehension, worries, insecurity. All effort, all work seems too difficult, always procrastinates until enough courage is built up (the Chinese call audacious people ''large gallbladders'').
>
>   No audacity, detests meeting strangers, dreams of discomfort, of embarrassing situations, of being inadequately clothed in public, of humiliations, of rudeness.
>
>   Tonification point of the gallbladder: gallbladder not functioning, either swollen and not emptying or contracted and hardly perceptible from weakness (often from excess of the small intestine) to the point of fever from the gallbladder.
>
>   Opposite eye: unclear vision, cannot adjust focus; inflammation of the lateral corner; spasms of the ocular artery.
>
>   Opposite ear: itching, buzzing?
>
>   Bladder: spasmodic retention, lower abdomen hard, swollen.

Opposite effects:

>   Sexual organs: women: opposite breast: swelling, inflammation of the mammary glands, hardness, ulceration of the breast; men: orchitis.

Parts of the body:

>   Whole body: pain without fixed location.
>
>   Maxilla and below the chin, opposite side: pain or perspiration.
>
>   Chest and opposite sides: pain; intercostal neuralgia or cold or pain in the anterior chest and heart, cannot twist.
>
>   Posterior shoulder same side: sharp pain.
>
>   Lower limb: pain, or flaccidity or contracture.
>
>   Fourth and fifth toes: rheumatism (metatarsophalangeal arthritis).

GB-44 [foot]-*qiaoyin* — yin of the opening

Foot: fourth toe, terminal phalanx, facing the fifth toe (lateral side); in the angle between the anterior edge of the swelling and body of the bone near the joint and the dorsal edge of the palmar tendon (flexors); in a hollow.

Preceding point: *xiaxi* (GB-43).

When tonified:

Tonifies the gallbladder, stomach, temporoparietal lobes, opposite eye, ear. Lateral part of neck, lumbar area, diaphragm.
Disperses the heart, lungs, opposite breast; vessels.
Dispersing acts in the opposite way.

Direct effects:

Dreams of incubus or devils; cerebral anemia.
Opposite eye: pain of the medial corner; eyeball: pain.
Opposite ear: violent deafness?
Dry mouth, nausea, stiff tongue.
Veins: varicosity.

Opposite effects:

Respiratory passages: sore throat, laryngitis, coughing fits, pain, perspiration, impossible to breathe, pleurisy.
Weak heart, heart fat and enlarged?

Parts of the body:

Head pain, head and eye pain, tense face.
Lateral part of the neck: stiffness, pain.
Axilla and subclavicular hollow: swelling, abscess.
Opposite breast: tumors, cancer.
Upper and lower limbs opposite: agitation, cramps, agitation of the feet; cannot lift the elbow.

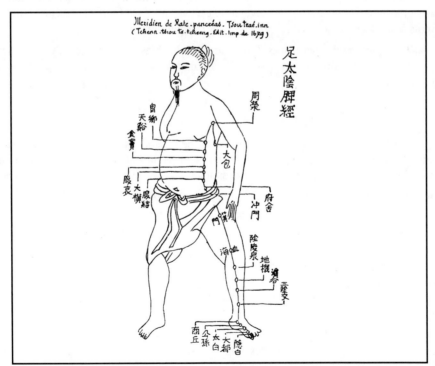

Meridian of the spleen-pancreas (DACH)

Notes

[1] In the International System the gallbladder meridian begins just lateral to the outer canthus of the eye. — ed.

Chapter XII

Liver

In the flow of energy, the liver meridian is preceded by the gallbladder meridian (its mother and coupled meridian), followed by the lung meridian (child). Its maximum energy is at 2 a.m. (local solar time), hour of the minimum activity of its opposite, the small intestine. It is symmetrical: the right branch from the spleen, the left branch from the pancreas (husband-wife); tonification point: *ququan* (LR-8); dispersal point: *xingjian* (LR-2); source point: *taichong* (LR-3).

The liver organ is tonified through the sympathetic system (*fengchi*, GB-20; *zhongzhu*, TW-3; *zhangmen*, LR-13); and the parathyroids (*yinxi*, HT-6). It is dispersed or inhibited through the parasympathetic system (*tianzhu*, BL-10; *yangchi*, TW-4; *zhongwan*, CV-12).

It is tonified by tonifying the spleen-pancreas and heart, or by dispersing the small intestine; it is tonified or dispersed by the gallbladder, according to the relative strength.

It is dispersed by the small intestine when this latter is tonified, and through the lung and spleen when they are dispersed.

It is weakened through unhappiness, worries and shocks (which cure obsessions); from cold (which contracts it); or from wind (which contracts the gallbladder). It is stimulated by heat, mainly humid.

A distributor organ (treasure, yin), it stores and distributes vitamins, blood and energy. According to Western thought, it has thirty-five functions, including the following (see Volume I). 1. Bile (particularly the left branch); blood, sugar, urea, acetone, antitoxic (particularly the right branch). 2. Skin, swellings, irritation, eruptions. 3. The nails. 4. Temperature of the body. 5. Spasms. 6. Digestion of fat. 7. Emotional imbalances: malcontentment-indifference, envy, jealousy, oppressiveness, worries, or combinations of these.

Insufficient: cold, waxy complexion, blue under the eyes, weakness, sees badly at twilight, subject to migraines or skin troubles or asthma, rheumatism, urea level low, gets worms easily, fits of hostility, envy. Dreams of trees, of forests, insomnia around 2 a.m. solar time, stool more or less yellow color.

Excess: dark complexion, brown marks, brown around the eyes, corner of the eyes swollen, hot breath, dark-colored urine, abundant and frequent to the point of incontinence, drowsiness, black or dark stool; dreams of unhappiness or humiliation.

LR-1 *dadun* — great abundance

Foot: big toe, terminal phalanx, lateral side (towards the second toe) about mid-width; behind the angle of the nail; in the angle between the anterior edge of a bony bulge of the last phalanx at the joint and the dorsal edge of the short insertion of the lateral articular ligament, between it and the dorsal tendon (extensor); in a hollow.

Following point: *xingjian* (LR-2) at the base of the joint; symmetrical to *yinbai* (SP-1) on the medial side.

When tonified:
Tonifies the liver, spleen-pancreas, genital organs, triple warmer, bladder (expulsor muscles), large intestine, small intestine, kidney.
Disperses the heart, bladder, sphincter, lower spinal cord.
Dispersing acts in the opposite way. To disperse energy:
Here, the energy coming from the gallbladder meridian (foot-*linqi*, GB-41) enters the liver meridian.

Direct effects:
Spasms of the arteries (including cerebral), of the abdominal organs, of the genitourinary organs.
Without joy, sighs, likes to lie down, attacks of heat or cold, headache, or nosebleeds. Children: acute or chronic meningitis? Sudden death: moxa. Coma?
Abdomen: eructation, vomiting, swelling and pain; contraction above and below and around the umbilicus, stool stopped from heat or excess energy, spasms of the small intestine, painful intestinal spasms, heat in the intestines, violent intestinal pain, urinary incontinence, pain in the heart.
Arterial spasms, excess energy in the heart.
Women: lower pelvis: spasms, pain in the uterus or vagina, prolapsed uterus, excessive menstrual flow.
Men: cryptorchidism; genital organs reascending into the pelvis; blenorrhagia, orchitis; glans, pain in head of the penis; prostatitis.

Swelling in perineum.

Bladder: spasms of the neck, frequent need to urinate, to the point of incontinence. Urethra: all problems.

Parts of the body:

Swelling: problems with swelling; all spasms; often the point is opposite to the trouble; tetanus.

Lumbar area and posterior lower limb.

LR-2 *xingjian* — acting interval

Dorsum of foot: at the metatarsophalangeal joint at the base of the big toe, facing the second toe; in the angle between the body and the head of the first metatarsal (great toe) and the posterior edge of a transverse ligament; in a hollow.

Preceding point: *dadun* (LR-1), on the terminal phalanx; following point: *taichong* (LR-3), between the posterior heads of the metatarsals.

When dispersed:

Disperses the liver, the six yin meridians (deep pulses), cerebellum, medulla oblongata, lower spinal cord, opposite eye, opposite gums and teeth, opposite palm and finger joints. Lower and anterior knee spasms; edema.

Tonifies the large intestine, small intestine, gallbladder.

Tonifying this point seems to increase the dispersion.

Direct effects:

Dispersal point of the liver; relieves the following: active congestion of the liver, pain in the liver spreading through to the heart, back side, vomiting of bile or of cold and acid liquid, bile in the stomach, stool (and urine) stopped, or pasty incessant diarrhea, with nausea.

Dusty complexion, blackish, or without color, grey skin; depression; cerebral anemia; psychological troubles, tears; deep sighs, suicidal tendencies.

Eyes: cannot see at dusk or in darkness, pupils contracted, miosis; failing vision, retinal insufficiency.

Ears: deafness?

Gums: inflammation; teeth: pain.

Heart: unbearable sudden pain; nervous palpitations.

Women: blood poisoning?

Large intestine or small intestine: spasms. Peritonitis.

Diabetes: exhausting thirst, dry throat.

Takes pleasure in drinking; violent sweats.

Genital system: women: cold, shivering, insufficiency, contracted vagina, pain in the lumbar area, menses too abundant or too prolonged, hemorrhage, metrorrhagia, miscarriage, white discharge. Men: erections from liver excess, pain in the penis.

Edema of the whole body (anasarca), edema of the feet and ankles, knee swollen, stopped urine (and stool), urination difficult with white foam; or incontinence?

Cramps, nervous pain from spasms, convulsions of children.

Parts of the body:

Nape, occiput. Pain in limbs and joints, arthritis, especially in big and second toes.

LR-3 *taichong* — supreme assault

Dorsum of foot: between the first and second metatarsals (big and second toes). A little in front of the deep angle between the posterior head and body of the first metatarsal; on the lateral edge of the extensor hallucis longus, between the bone and the lateral edge of the dorsalis pedis artery with the anterior tibial nerve and vein; in a hollow; in the angle between the bone and the anterior edge of the transverse ligament.

Three FW above *xingjian* (LR-2); three FW anterior to *zhongfeng* (LR-4).

When tonified:

Tonifies the liver and the other yin organs (distributor organs, deep pulses), temporoparietal lobes, automaton-parrot, opposite ear, opposite throat, and shoulder joint on opposite side, anterior lower leg.

Relieves spasms, swelling, excess energy in bladder.

Dispersing acts in the opposite way.

''If this artery beats, the patient will survive.''

''If a young girl of fourteen has this artery strongly beating, she can bear children.''

Direct effects:

   Source point of the liver (excess or insufficiency)

   Excess: fever from the liver (fullness of the lower pelvis, diminished urination, swollen bones of the knee); pain in the liver and heart; epidemic jaundice with fever; dusty face, blue-black; incessant sighs; vision of a black fog; pasty diarrhea finishing as liquid, bloody stools.

   Insufficiency: liver distended and insufficient; colorless or difficult stools.

   Swollen throat, noise in the larynx, dry throat, thirst.

   Nose: clear or thick discharge, coryza; fissures; swelling.

   Opposite eye: foggy vision, black fog; eye illnesses.

   Opposite ear: inflammation of the lobe; buzzing? deafness?

   Fits of vomiting, hematemesis.

Opposite effects.

   Veins: varicose ulcers, varicosities, arteries.

   Heart: pain, coronary spasms, angina of the chest.

   Genital system: pain, swelling, lower legs numb during orgasm; metrorrhagia, miscarriage; incessant discharges; blenorrhagia; men: orchitis (tonify); deficient or reduced testicles.

   Contractions of energy, internal and external spasms: tonify; cramps of cholera, feet and hands; spasms of the coronaries, of the arteries, of the lower pelvis, in the feet.

   Swellings of all sorts (except edema): tonify; caused by fatigue, emptiness, exhaustion (and tuberculosis?); throat, lips, axilla, thighs, knee, ankle, foot, bones of the foot (particularly the first cuneiform), shoulder, elbow, hand, fingers, etc.

Parts of the body:

   Lips: all trouble of the corners of the lips (dartre, perleche, etc.), swelling on side of mouth.

   Opposite shoulder: swollen articulation: tonify.

   Swollen axilla, suppurative adenitis: tonify.

   Swollen elbow: tonify. Opposite hand, fingers swollen; joint pain to the shoulder.

   Lumbar area and lower pelvis: pain, swelling.

   Lower limb: difficulty in moving, walking; swelling, numbness.

   Swelling of thigh, knee, lower leg (from attack of cold).

   Foot: pain in front of the medial malleolus, swelling, cold accompanied by blue facial color, cramps (from cholera), swelling of first cuneiform bone: tonify. Paralysis of the anterior tibial nerve, toes paralyzed, metatarsophalangeal arthritis (base of the toes).

LR-4   *zhongfeng* — central seal

   Arch, medial side (facing the big toe): about three FW anterior and lateral to the medial malleolus; in the angle between the anterior edge of a transverse bone (scaphoid) and the medial edge of the tendon of the extensor hallucis longus muscle; lateral to the flat tendon of the tibialis anterior; in a hollow.

   About three FW posterior to *taichong* (LR-3); about six FW in front of *ligou* (LR-5). Separated by the extensor hallucis longus muscle from *chongyang* (ST-42), by the tibialis anterior from *gongsun* (SP-4).

When tonified:

   Tonifies all yin organs, liver, genital organs, spleen-pancreas, kidneys, heart, brain, medulla oblongata, spinal cord, three endocrines; half the body, cold, weakness, flaccidity.

   Disperses all yang organs (superficial pulses, producer organs); spasms of the genitourinary system.

   Dispersing acts in the opposite way.

Direct effects:

   Liver: fever of the liver (excess of the lower pelvis region, insufficient urine, swelling of the knee): disperse.

   Shivering from cold; malaria, shivering from cold, bluish complexion: tonify.

   Walks with great difficulty; weakness, flaccidity, body and constitution without action, flaccidity of whole or part of the body: tonify.

Secondary effects:

   Nervousness, agitation, rapid speech: tonify. Spasms of the whole body, particularly the genitourinary area; tonic convulsions, stiffness: tonify.

   Stomach: no appetite, no pleasure from eating: disperse. Desire to drink, dry throat; pain in the hollow of the stomach.

Bladder: spasms of the neck; inflammation of the bladder; incontinence, urination difficult, painful or impeded; or white cloudy urine: tonify.

Lower pelvis region: spasms: tonify. Or pain; swelling: tonify.

Vagina: spasms, contractions, vaginismus, pain in the lumbar: tonify. Vaginal fluids too abundant: tonify. Blenorrhagia. Men: seminal loss: disperse; orchitis: tonify; prostatis: tonify.

Scrotal hernia?

Parts of the body:

    Occipital pain.

    Weakness of lower limb: weakness (walks with great difficulty); swollen knee.

    Feet cold as ice: tonify.

LR-5 *ligou* — furrow of the wood worms

Anterior side of the lower limb; lateral edge of the tibia. Three FW above the lower edge of the tibia; at the edge of an anterior notch of the bone. In the angle of the upper edge of a transverse mass; in a hollow.

Approximately six FW above *zhongfeng* (LR-4). Five FW inferior to *zhongdu* (LR-6). One and a half FW in front of and a little below *sanyinjiao* (SP-6); four FW below and in front of *guangming* (GB-37); three anterior and above *dazhong* (KI-6, IS KI-4).

When tonified:

    Tonifies the liver and the other yin organs (deep pulses, distributor organs), cerebellum, pons, posterior frontal lobes.

    Disperses the gallbladder and the other yang organs (superficial pulses), dorsal iliocostal muscles.

    Dispersing acts in the opposite way.

    Opposite cerebellum: if insufficient, spasms: tonify; if excess, weakness: disperse.

    Little energy, no joy, melancholy, deranged mind, fear, preoccupation, numerous sighs. If ''talkative without wisdom,'' puncture three times: tonify.

Direct effects:

    Heat, prolonged erection: disperse.

Opposite effects:

    Passage point between the liver and gallbladder. (Tonifying transfers the excess from the gallbladder meridian into the emptiness of the liver; dispersing does the opposite). If excess: prolonged erections; disperse. If insufficient: violent pruritis in some part of the body; tonify.

    Internal and external spasms: tonify

    Spasmodic cough, in the larynx, as if with growths: tonify.

    Heart, nervous palpitations: tonify.

    Intestines: spasms, abdominal pain: tonify. Spasms in abdomen, lumbar area, and back.

    Spasms during menses, menses difficult and painful: tonify.

    Bladder: spasmodic retention, urine difficult or stopped, violent pain from contractions: tonify.

Parts of the body:

    Itching, pruritis on some part of the body: tonify.

    Back, iliocostal, lumbar, dorsal and cervical muscles: contracted, painful, burning: tonify. Back seized, contracted, ''lumbar muscles tightened like the string of the cross-bow'': tonify.

    Lower limb: weakness and flaccidity: disperse.

    Lower leg and foot cold, numb; difficult to extend and flex: disperse.

    Arch: contracted, tonify; weak, disperse.

LR-6 *zhongdu* — central capital

Anterior lower leg just on the anterior edge of the tibia; between it and a large muscle (tibialis anterior muscle); in a hollow; in the angle on the upper edge of a transverse mass.

Five FW above *ligou* (LR-5); seven large FW below *xiguan* (LR-7); a little below the level of *lougu* (SP-7) and anterior to it.

When tonified:

    Tonifies the liver, posterior frontal lobes, temporoparietal lobes, opposite side of the face, opposite eye, ear and

throat, posterior palate, lower limb, medial side of the knee, genital organs.
Disperses the large intestine, gallbladder.
Dispersing acts in the opposite way.

Opposite effects:
Intestines: obstruction or occlusion; cancer; abscess or ulcer of the intestine, dysentery with blood; cholera; peritonitis: tonify.
Throat: inflammation, pain: tonify. Posterior palate.
Metrorrhagia after delivery or miscarriage: tonify. Metritis, discharge very heavy: tonify. Pain in the lower pelvis.
Scrotal hernia?

Parts of the body:
Lower limb: pain, weakness, flaccidity, can neither stand nor walk (astasia-abasia?); pain.
Knee: inflammation of the joint.
Sole: hot.
Big toe: base painful, rheumatism: tonify.

LR-7 *xiguan* — barrier of the knee

Upper medial side of the lower leg. On the tibia, just at the lower and medial edge of the anterior bulge of the anterior tibial tuberosity, on the lower edge of a transverse mass; in a hollow.

Four FW inferior and anterior to *ququan* (LR-8); seven large FW above *zhongdu* (LR-6).

When tonified:
Tonifies the liver, posterior frontal upper lobes opposite, lower part same side. Also: heart, spleen-pancreas, lungs, kidneys, pericardium, genital organs, knee, toes, articulations of the opposite lower and upper limbs, opposite throat, opposite ear lobe, opposite maxilla.
Disperses the large intestine and small intestine.
Dispersing acts in the opposite way.

Parts of the body:
Opposite ear lobes.
Opposite maxilla.
Painful articulations, articular rheumatism, opposite upper limb (particularly the wrist and fingers), opposite lower limb (particularly hip, medial part of knee, toes).

LR-8 *ququan* — source of the curve

Knee: medial side and lower part; in the posterior angle between the heads of the femur and tibia; in the angle between the head of the tibia and the posterior edge of the tibiofemoral ligament; in a hollow.

Four FW above and medial to *xiguan* (LR-7); eight FW below *yinbao* (LR-9); two FW above *yinlingquan* (SP-9); four above *diji* (SP-8).

When tonified:
Tonifies the liver, spleen-pancreas, heart, cerebellum, bladder (expulsor muscles); increases urine, genital organs, yang.
Disperses the skin, large intestine, swellings of the face, migraine, respiratory passages.
Dispersing acts in the opposite way.
The left point acts mainly on the bile, etc. The right point acts mainly on the antitoxic function. Their respective sensitivity is a differentiating sign.
The liver stores and distributes all vitamins; it transforms glycogen into sugar, etc.

Direct effects:
Tonification point of the liver. All its insufficiencies (yellow stools, constipation or migraine; or asthma, skin troubles, eczema, Quinke's edema, etc.)
Large intestine: colorless stool, yellow, badly formed; diarrhea finishing as liquid, intestinal ulceration; diarrhea with pus and blood, or constipation from liver insufficiency, lack of energy for evacuation; intestinal pain, troubles of the abdomen and umbilicus.
Eyes: confused vision or visual dizziness.

Blood: insufficient coagulation, oozing of blood (delayed, yet prolonged) at the least scratch, easily "black and blue," bruised.

Opposite effects:

Respiratory passages: asthma: tonify (cannot inhale, chokes at the least effort, after food), throat troubles, nosebleeds: tonify (for vitamin K). Colds or asthma from hay fever: tonify. All chronic trouble of the respiratory passages.

Genital system: menses are irregular, impeded: disperse. Swelling of the genital organs, of the vulva; itching, vulvar pruritis; prolapsed uterus: tonify. Pain in the clitoris. Men: premature ejaculation; seminal discharge from sexual fatigue; scrotal hernia?

Difficulty expelling urine, or impeded urination (spasm of the bladder sphincter): tonify. Constipation and retention from emptiness: tonify.

Urine uncolored, lemon or red, thick: tonify.

Skin: all trouble; itching, pruritis, uticaria, eczema, psoriasis: tonify.

Does not sweat.

Parts of the body:

Whole organism: extreme pain, same side.

Head: migraines (pain from one side of the head to the temple); face: sudden swelling (Quinke's edema); tonify.

Chest and abdomen: spasms, contracting pain.

Lower limb and thigh, particularly the medial side: pain, cramps.

Posterior part of the knee: contracture or pain or swelling (*yangfu*, GB-38): tonify.

Opposite upper limb: posterior muscles (triceps, carpal extensors).

LR-9   *yinbao* — envelope of the yin [organs]

Thigh, inferior third, medial surface: three FW above the condyle (lower head) of the femur, mid-width on the medial face of the femur; in the angle between the posterior (medial) edge of a longitudinal tendon and the lower edge (towards the patella) of a transverse mass; in a hollow.

Three FW above *ququan* (LR-8); three below thigh-*wuli* (LR-10); three anterior and below *jimen* (SP-11); three medial to *yinshi* (ST-33).

When tonified:

Tonifies the liver, heart, spleen-pancreas, cerebellum, spinal cord, kidney, opposite sacral nerves, perineum, testicles, ovaries, anus, posterolateral thigh, lateral part of the lower leg, lateral dorsum of the foot.

Disperses the small intestine and large intestine.

Opposite effects:

Urine too abundant, or cannot be retained for a long time: tonify. Urination difficult, stopped, with pain in the kidney while urinating: disperse (acts on kidney filtration).

Menses difficult, painful, with internal fullness, pain in lumbar area, lower pelvis, coccyx: tonify (excess of large intestine, antihemorrhagic vitamin).

Parts of the body:

Perineum: contraction or flaccidity, disperse before delivery.

Sacrum opposite: pains, contracture (sacral nerves).

Posterolateral part of thigh; lateral face of lower leg, lateral dorsum of the foot.

LR-10   [thigh-]*wuli* — fifth mile

Thigh, anteromedial surface: five large FW above a large protrusion of the femur at the knee (the medial condyle). About mid-width of the femur; in the angle between the posterior (medial) edge of a longitudinal tendon and the lower edge of a transverse mass; in a hollow.

Three FW above *yinbao* (LR-9); three below *yinlian* (LR-11); two FW above and anterior to *jimen* (SP-11).

When tonified:

Tonifies the liver, heart, mid-brain, cerebellum, lower spinal cord, thorax and anterolateral part of the opposite side of neck, opposite lower and upper limbs.

Disperses the opposite side of the large and small intestines, opposite side of bladder, opposite lung.

Dispersing acts in the opposite way.

Direct effects:
    Especially (?) for insomnia (causes sleep), or dry skin, lack of sweat: tonify.
    Weakness and decline after flu, fever from fatigue, likes to stretch.

Opposite effects:
    Intestines: great swelling, fullness, anal sphincter contracted.
    Pleurisy? tuberculosis from shock?
    Bladder: cannot urinate, retention, bladder sphincter contracted.

Parts of the body:
    Opposite upper limb: weakness.
    Muscles of the thorax and anterolateral side of the neck.
    Anterior, lateral opposite lower limb: moves slowly.
    Hip joint, anterolateral side opposite: weak, pain on movement.

LR-11 *yinlian* — yin angle

Thigh, medial face; eight large FW above the protrusion of the lower head of the femur (medial condyle); at the mid-width of the femur; on the anterior edge of the gracilis and posterior edge of the rectus femoris; in a marked hollow.

Three FW above thigh-*wuli* (LR-10); four below *yangshi* (LR-12, IS *jimai*).

When tonified:
    Tonifies the liver, spleen-pancreas, genital system, perineum, coccyx, anterior frontal lobes, posterior lower limb.
    Disperses the large intestine.
    Dispersing acts in the opposite way.

Effects:
    Genital organs: women who have not borne children: discontentment and rage? sterility? displaced uterus? abundant discharge, vulvar pruritis. Men: glans.
    Posterior lower limb: dragging pain, particularly at night; thigh: muscles of the medial surface.

LR-12 *yangshi* (IS *jimai*) — arrows for sheep (IS "quick pulse")

Upper medial surface of the thigh: just at the lower edge of the apparent extremity of the pubis. In a large hollow; in the angle between the bone and the lateral edge of the muscle passing over the pubis (psoas major muscle); just medial to the artery.

Four FW above *yinlian* (LR-11); following point: *zhangmen* (LR-13), between the ninth and tenth ribs.

When tonified:
    Tonifies the liver, genital system, psoas major muscle.
    Disperses the large intestine, small intestine.
    Dispersing acts in the opposite way.

Effects:
    Prolapse of the rectum?
    Ovaries.
    Testicles: epididymitis, inflammation, swelling; ovaries.

Parts of the body;
    Lumbar area hollowed (curved), lordosis, contracture of the psoas major muscle (needle inserted on the lumbar vertebrae): disperse.

LR-13 *zhangmen* — great door

Lateral part of the lower thorax: above the floating point of the eleventh rib, between the ninth and tenth rib; in the angle between the lower edge of the ninth rib and the anterior edge of a vertical ligament (intercostal). About two FW lateral to the lateral angle between the ninth and tenth ribs; in a hollow.

Preceding point: *yangshi* (LR-12, IS *jimai*), on the upper thigh. Four FW below *qimen* (LR-14 and last); two anterior (medial) to *fuai* (SP-16); two posterolateral to *taiyi* (ST-23).

When tonified:

Tonifies the liver and the five yin organs (deep pulses, distributor organs), brain opposite side, cerebellum, medulla oblongata, spinal opposite cord.

Disperses (slightly) all the yang organs (producer organs, superficial pulses).

Dispersing acts in the opposite way.

Direct effects:

Fear, little energy; attacks of weakness in the limbs on the same side; weakness from loss of organic liquids?

All the yin distributor organs (deep pulses): all trouble. Their "reunion point."

Herald point of the spleen and pancreas. Troubles from mental causes with cold and depression. Insufficiency of the spleen, either from excess food or growth, or from malaria; body hot and yellow, swelling of the spleen. Insufficiency of the pancreas, either from excess food, sugar or carbohydrates. Fullness, does not digest, regurgitation of food, eructation, vomiting, thinness, yellow body; gas in the stomach and intestines. Children: abdomen distended and thinness; overeating during hot season; during cold season, acute diarrhea. Also, dry and hot mouth, intestinal worms.

Violent cough, mucus, panting, pain in the heart, pain and fullness in chest and side; pulmonary tuberculosis?

Urine white, cloudy (phosphaturia?), or with red sediment (uric acid?); stones in the kidney and bladder.

Parts of the body:

Head: frontal and carotid arteries: intense beats?

Chest and abdomen: spasms of the muscles, cramps or contracture.

Side: pain, cannot sleep.

Dorsal vertebrae: pain. Lumbar vertebrae: acute pain from cold.

One hand hot, one hand cold?

Point of Weihe: Right: Nux Vomica. Vertigo with momentary loss of consciousness; irritable, criticizes everything, cannot bear noises or smells, hypersensitive, hyper-impressionable; insomnia after 3 a.m. solar time. Troubles from excess food, drugs, stimulants, from intellectual overwork, life in cities; nausea after eating, in the morning; swollen abdomen, swollen liver; dry cough, bleeding saliva; congestion of uterus, sexual excitation; spasm and pain of the neck of the bladder, frequent need to urinate with little result; lumbago.

Left: China. Apathetic, anxious, hypersensitive to touch; nervous erethism. Periodicity of the problems. Weakness from loss of organic liquids. Insomnia with somnolence during the day. One hand hot, one cold; dryness of the mouth and throat, great hunger, vomiting of undigested food; diarrhea; excess cholesterol; hypertrophy of the liver and spleen; very abundant gas, swollen abdomen, colic, regurgitation of bitter liquids; sexual excitation, congestion of the uterus, headache during menses; intense beating of the arteries of the head and carotid; neuralgia, rheumatic headache; intermittent fever.

LR-14 *qimen* — door of the epoch

Anterolateral thorax: five FW above the tip of the eleventh rib. Between the sixth and seventh ribs; two FW lateral to and below the nipple (men). In the angle between the lower edge of the sixth rib and the lateral edge of a vertical ligament (interosseous); in a hollow.

Four FW above and slightly lateral to *zhangmen* (LR-13). Four lateral to *burong* (ST-19); two below and lateral to *tianxi* (SP-18); two anterior to *riyue* (GB-24).

When tonified:

Tonifies the liver, spleen-pancreas, anterior and posterior frontal lobes, inside of the nose and upper part of the throat; accommodation and coordination.

Disperses the gallbladder, lungs.

Dispersing acts in the opposite way.

Direct effects:

Herald point of the liver (troubles of psychic origin with cold or depression); dark eyes, nausea, vomiting, after eating, vomiting water; pain under the right scapula.

Eyes: weakness of accommodation of each eye to light and to distance, also of coordination (synergy) of the two eyes.

Stomach: weakness.

Diabetes: thirst.

Chill which does not stop within the normal time, fullness of the chest after chills; chest contracted, cannot lie down without suffocation; pain in the chest, heat, agitation, mucus discharging incompletely, with difficulty; pleurisy; pneumonia.

Menses retarded, coming after their date, or difficult, painful; menopause: hot flashes, contracted chest, agitation; all problems after delivery; all problems from insufficiency of energy.

Part II

The Median Lines

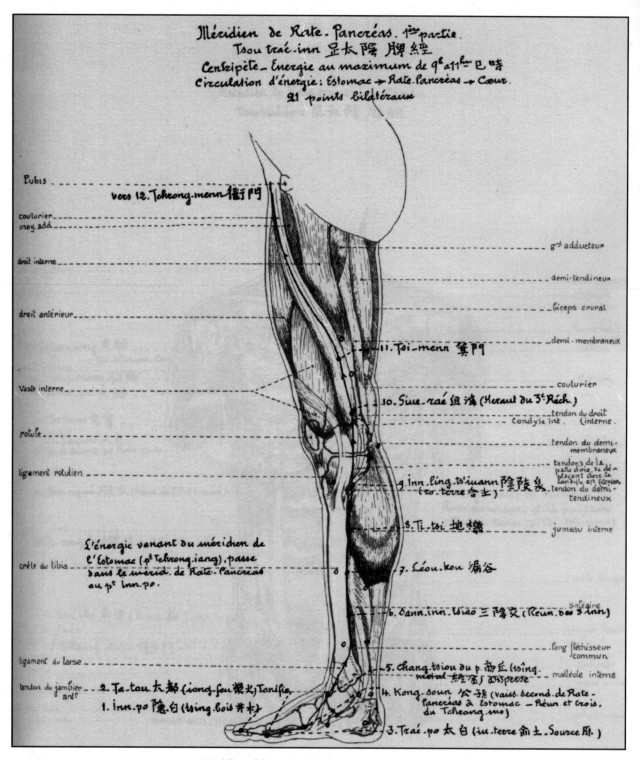

Meridian of the spleen-pancreas (part 1) (GSDM)

Chapter I

Anterior Median Line

Conception Vessel

(Ren Mai)

The two median lines are completely outside the double circle of the flow of energy. Together, they constitute a distinct circle of energy. Indeed, although their points have only one line, they are double, because each line is double, being composed of an ascending flow (right side of the body) and a descending flow (left side of the body). High antiquity counted them each as two, but this notion had been totally abandoned until we rediscovered their duality in our work. In addition, we have discovered something for which I have searched in vain through the collections of ancient and modern books: the two medial lines, which join at their extremities, form only one circle of energy. The ascending (right) flow of each is followed by the descending (left) flow of the other to rise again in the right flow, while the left descending flow rises through the climbing right flow of the other one. The crossing of the currents is made at the extremities.

The conception vessel has a point called ''meeting and crossing,'' which is *lieque* (LU-7). The right point acts on the ascending right flow of the conception vessel and continues in the left descending flow of the governor vessel (posterior line). Left *lieque* (LU-7) acts on the left descending flow of the conception vessel and rises in the right climbing current of the governor vessel.

The conception vessel carries all the herald points of the triple warmer, those of the small intestine and bladder and those of the sexual organs, vessels and heart.

The inferior third acts on the sexual life. The middle third, from umbilicus to sternum, acts on the digestive life. The upper third acts on the respiratory functions.

Right *fengchi* (GB-20) acts on the descending left flow of the conception vessel and the right ascending flow of the governor vessel. The left point acts on the right ascending flow of the conception vessel and the left descending flow of the governor vessel.

In fact, the conception vessel has:

1) An action on the total vital energy in the sexual, alimentary and respiratory manifestations.

2) A special link with the lungs, since the command point of the conception vessel is a point of the lungs, *lieque* (LU-7). All the points of the lungs awaken a response in the conception vessel. All the points of the conception vessel awaken a response on the pulse of the lungs.

3) A special link with the triple warmer, the herald points of which, all located on the conception vessel, distribute the general energy to all the meridians. The conception vessel would be the center, as it is recommended to treat it when the meridians no longer respond to stimulation, and in cases of disturbances coming from the interior and accompanied by cold or depression.

   These problems can manifest either from excess (the skin of the abdomen will be painful) or from insufficiency (there will be pruritis). There have also been noticed in cases of excess: spasms of men, abscess in the mouth, aphtha, head and nape pain. In cases of insufficiency: diseases of women, swelling and fullness of the abdomen, lassitude in the lumbar area. It is also said that when blood is in the conception vessel, the skin is smooth and the hair is abundant.

4) A close connection with the yin energy, since its command point is a point of the lungs (yin), and it awakens a mutual response in *zhaohai* (KI-3, IS KI-6), command point of yin energy and of the medial submalleolar vessel of yin energy, and from there, also with the kidneys (yin) through *zhaohai* (KI-3, IS KI-6).

CV-1   *huiyin* — reunion of the yin

Perineum, median line: in front of the anus and the anal sphincter. Between the bulbocavernosus muscles; in a hollow; two points one millimeter from each other laterally.

One branch passes on both sides of the anus and links the conception to the governor vessel at *changqiang* (GV-1); following point: *qugu* (CV-2).

When tonified:

Tonifies all the yin distributor meridians (deep pulses) and the conception vessel, governor vessel, anal and genital area, skin.

Disperses the bladder.

Dispersing acts in the opposite way.

Direct effects:

Passage points between the two medial lines. If insufficient: pruritis, either of the sexual organs or on all the skin. If excess: acute pain of the skin, either of the abdomen or of the body.

Anal pruritis, anal fistula; large intestine: constipation.

Sexual organs: all problems, pain extending in front and behind, abundant perspiration of the genital area, pain of the head and sexual organs. Women: intense vulvar pruritis: tonify; acute pain of the vulva and vagina: disperse; pain and inflammation of the vagina: disperse; cold in the genital system, insensitivity, menses stopped.

Bladder: urine stopped (retention); urinary meatus: heat or pain.

Drowning victims: legs up, head down and tonify: ''if urine comes out, will revive.''

Sudden death: tonify?

Parts of the body:

Skin: acute pain: disperse; or pruritis: tonify. Skin of the abdomen.

CV-2   *qugu* — bone-curve, pubis

Lower abdomen, medial line: just on the upper edge of the pubis (pubic symphysis). In a hollow; between the two rectus abdominus muscles. The two points are separated by a slight prominence (the linea alba).

Preceding point: *huiyin* (CV-1) in front of the anus; one FW under *zhongji* (CV-3); at one FW on either side is *henggu* (KI-11).

When tonified:

Right point: all right yin organs and all left yang organs (conception vessel ascending on the right and governor vessel descending on the left). Left point: the opposite. Inferior left occipital lobe; genital and urinary organs; lateral part of the neck; anterior upper shoulder, radial side of upper limb, thumb, medial surface of the lower limb.

Disperses the bladder.

Dispersing acts in the opposite way.

Direct effects:

Extreme cold from emptiness (anemia?); reddens at the least emotion.

Internal organs weak and empty (right point: right yin, left yang; left point: left yin, right yang).

Genital organs: spasms, pain or swelling. Blennorrhagia. Massages the whole organism. Women: uterus: inflammation, endometritis, itching pruritis; or displacement (particularly frontwards or backwards); ulceration of the neck of the uterus; prolapse; or metrorrhagia; or after delivery, does not contract sufficiently. After delivery, prolonged discharges, discharges of an extraordinary type. Men: seminal losses, prostatitis.

Opposite effects:

Bladder: inflammation (cystitis), blood, swollen lower pelvis, difficult urine, frequent need to urinate, incontinence of those with anemia; urethra.

Kidneys: nephritis after eruptions which have been driven into the interior?

Skin: acne; impetigo of the cheeks? ganglions? scrofula?

Parts of the body:

Lateral part of the middle of the neck; upper anterior shoulder, upper limb (radial line), thumb.

Medial surface of the lower limb: cold or numbness, weakness (acts on the obturator nerve and the rotator muscles of the thigh).

Point of Weihe: Ferrum Iodatum. Anemia, incontinence from anemia, inflammation of the kidneys after eruptions driven into the interior; acne, impetigo of the cheeks and lymph nodes; tumors; scrofula; sensation of insects in the urethra or scrotum; exophthalmic goiter from suppressed menses, white discharge, retroversion or prolapse of the uterus; when sitting, sensation of pressure ascending in the vagina.

CV-3 *zhongji* — central pole

Lower abdomen, medial line: one FW above the transverse bone (pubis). In a hollow; between the two rectus abdominus muscles; two points separated by the linea alba.

One FW above *qugu* (CV-2); one under *guanyuan* (CV-4); one FW on either side is *dahe* (KI-12).

When tonified:

The left point tonifies the descending flow of the conception vessel (left yin) and the ascending flow of the governor vessel (right yang); the right point tonifies the ascending flow of the conception vessel (right yin) and the descending flow of the governor vessel (left yang); three nervous centers, three levels of the psyche, three endocrines (except parathyroids), particularly the sexual organs, bladder; scapula, upper limb, hand, ulnar line; lower limb, lateral posterior.

Dispersing acts in the opposite way.

Direct effects:

''Numerous moxas suppress numerous troubles.''

Empty, cold, exhaustion; empty, decline of yang energy; delusions; loss of consciousness (coma?); cannot sleep, aggravated at night, in bed.

Herald point of the bladder (problems from emotions, with cold or depression): urine feeble, red, difficult, cannot urinate, urinates drop by drop, flaccid expulsor muscles, contracted sphincter; urethra: spasms, kidney pain when waiting for a long time. Or inflammation (cystitis), frequent need to urinate, passes little; urethra: pain or inflammation, blennorrhagic urethritis.

Sexual organs: women: breasts: all problems, problems from breast feeding; sterility: no male child? ''Puncturing four times can give a child.'' Sterility not depending on displacement of the uterus. After delivery: placenta not descending or uterine pain, or uterus not contracting, or bad, prolonged discharge. Menses: not coming or painful; vulva: swollen, painful, edema; or excess fluids, or heat and pain, or pruritis; perspiration of the genital area. Men: excess prostatic fluid, sterility, non-erection, seminal losses, prostatitis.

Heart: spasms of the coronaries? panting, knotted energy, pain.

Stomach: even having eaten nothing, cannot eat.

Large intestine: excess, swelling of abdomen, or heat, or colic (spasms).

Parts of the body:

Skin: redness, swelling, itching, erysipelas, cellulitis, smallpox, herpes; ligaments? fibrous tissues?

Swellings: of the eyelids? of fingers? of feet at night?

Red nose.

Scapula, upper limb and hand (ulnar line).

Posterolateral lower limb.

Point of Weihe: Rhus Tox (same as Rhus Radicans, cf. *naohu,* GV-16, IS GV-17). Aggravated at night, when resting, in bed; neuroarthritic conditions; rheumatic pain in the tendons, ligaments and fibrous tissues; afflictions of the mucous membranes, of the mouth; swelling of the skin, eyelids, fingers, feet at night, nipples, vulva; pruritis of the stomach; red skin, swollen, pruritis, erysipelas, herpes, chicken pox; cellulitis, cellulitis of the orbit; colored urine; teeth seemingly long and loose, painful gums; rheumatic iritis, the same suppurating; red nose; facial neuralgia worse in the evening; extreme agitation, insomnia before midnight.

CV-4 *guanyuan* — origin of the barrier

Abdomen, medial line: two FW above the pubis (three under the umbilicus), in a hollow in the groove between the rectus abdominus muscles; two points separated by a small prominence of the linea alba.

One FW above *zhongji* (CV-3); one under *shimen* (CV-5); on either side, at two tight FW, *qixue* (KI-13).

When tonified:

Tonifies the conception vessel: right point, the ascending flow of the conception vessel and the descending (left flow) of the governor vessel; left point: descending flow of the conception vessel and the ascending flow of the governor vessel. Anterior frontal lobe, opposite eye, evolved man, all yang organs (except the bladder), particularly the small intestine and kidneys; upper medial limbs and lower limbs, anteromedial same side.

Disperses all yin organs (except kidneys), particularly sexual organs, vessels, bladder.

Dispersing acts in the opposite way.

Direct effects:

Loss of strength, exhaustion, cold. All emptiness, from overwork, cold, weakness particularly from age; aging; internal cold; suffers from external cold.

Herald point of the small intestine (problems from emotions, with cold or depression). Diarrhea from atony and emptiness or from age, diarrhea not stopping; dysentery; intestinal hemorrhage; chronic inflammation of the intestine from weakness.

Opposite effects:

Bladder: retention, urine difficult, not coming, spasms of the neck of the bladder, cystitis, frequent minor urges to urinate with little result, urine escaping; urethra: inflammation.

Vessels: pulses sunken, without beats, or too full with blood in urine and stool (hypertension from weakness).

Kidney: decline of the kidneys, headache from decline of the kidneys, anuria, albuminuria, edema, renal stones.

Sexual organs: men: prostatitis, "wet dreams," loss of sexual energy; testicles: orchitis. Blennorrhagia. Women: "Point forbidden after the fourth month of pregnancy"? Dispersing can cause spasms of the lower pelvis region, or sterility from interruption "of the passages of conception" (blocked fallopian tubes, etc.). Cervix dilated: disperse; contracted: tonify. Ulceration or cancer of the cervix: tonify; yellow discharge, old problems.

After delivery, continual discharge, or the uterus does not contract; menses not coming: disperse; or menses not coming on schedule: disperse.

To revive victims of drowning: many moxas.

Parts of the body:

Lateral part of neck, same side.

Upper limb same side, medial part; palm.

Lower limb, same side, anteromedial part.

Point of Weihe: Hydrastis Canad. Mucosities, mucus thick, yellow or green, thick discharge flowing from the ears, inflammation of the eustachian tubes, rumbling; thick mucus in the urine; pain in the kidneys, yellow discharge, ulceration or cancer of the cervix, thick mucus in the back of the throat; sluggish liver; hemorrhoids; deep depression, irritable, miserable, aggravated at night, heat from movement.

✎ CV-5 *shimen* — stone door

Abdomen: medial line; about three FW above the pubic bone; about two FW below the umbilicus. In a hollow in the groove between the two rectus abdominus muscles. Under a deep transverse rise; two points separated by a slight rise of the linea alba.

One FW above *guanyuan* (CV-4); one below *qihai* (CV-6); on either side, at two close FW, *siman* (KI-14).

When tonified:

The right point tonifies the ascending flow of the conception vessel and the descending flow of the governor vessel; the left point tonifies the descending flow of the conception vessel and ascending flow of the governor vessel. All the yang organ meridians, distributors of energy. Opposite mid-brain (striopallidum); right point: penis (glans), clitoris; left point: testicles, ovaries; half body same side; shoulder and posterior upper limb, dorsum of hand, anterior lower limb same side.

Disperses the yin meridians.

Dispersing acts in the opposite way.

Direct effects:

Herald point of the triple warmer. Gathering point of all the energy distributed by the triple warmer to all the meridians; beginning and end of the ancestral energy; passes energy to the conception vessel.

Contracting energy of all the internal organs (excess or insufficiency).

Sexual organs: women: feminine pleasure. If insufficient, tonify (particularly the right point); if excessive, disperse. This prevents conception if totally deficient or excessive. Uterus: spasms, strangling pain in the lower abdomen; miscarriage, metrorrhagia.

Men: prostatitis. Both sexes: blennorrhagia? urethritis?

Stomach: bad digestion, nausea, vomiting, does not desire to eat, fullness of energy.

Intestine: constipation or diarrhea, chronic troubles; sudden spasms, pain, sudden swelling of the abdomen, intense pain; noisy small intestine? pain around the umbilicus spreading to the genital organs; omentitis; appendicitis; acute or chronic inflammation of the cecum.

Opposite effects:

Tuberculosis of the spleen or pancreas?

Kidneys: anuria, edema, abundant sweat.

Parts of the body:
>   Skin: retains water.
>   Perineum: retracted skin?
>   Half-body same side: tonification in excess can cause cramps or tightening.

CV-6   *qihai* — ocean of energy

Abdomen, medial line; two FW below the umbilicus. About one quarter of the distance to the pubic bone. In a hollow of the groove between the two rectus abdominus muscles; on the upper edge of a transverse bulge; two points separated by a small rise of the linea alba.

One FW above *shimen* (CV-5); one small FW below abdomen-*yinjiao* (CV-7). On either side, at the two FW, *zhongzhu* (KI-15).

When tonified:
>   The right point tonifies the mounting right flow of the conception vessel and the left descending flow of the governor vessel; the left point tonifies the left descending flow of the conception vessel and the right ascending flow of the governor vessel. All the yin organ meridians (deep and middle pulses), particularly vessels and sexual organs; nervous centers, three endocrines, three levels of the psyche, three sense organs; cheek, nostrils, same side; radial side of the upper limbs and medial part of the lower limb same side.
>   Disperses all the yang meridians.
>   Dispersing acts in the opposite way.

Direct effects:
>   Herald point of the vessels, of the yin energy, of the physical life.
>   General energy insufficient, all emptiness, insufficiency or exhaustion of the general energy; yin energy empty, yang energy abolished, as if after an illness. Lack of boldness, depression, desires death; weakness of the nerves (neurasthenia); loss of consciousness, eyes turned up, falls backward. Three pulses of the psyche weak; brain and cerebellum; three endocrines weak.
>   Insomnia from emotional agitation to the point of anxiety.
>   Muscular strength diminished.
>   Cold to the point of troubling the heart, with red face; if cold enters: warm the extremities and have the person eat onion tart; cold during digestion; cold under the umbilicus; trouble from cold or humidity, or from cold humidity or hot humidity; from cold, wind or heat.
>   Dries the sweat which streams (from weakness).
>   All mucus and discharges from weakness.
>   Sudden pain, special point; removes excessive suffering. All internal or external spasms, particularly from weakness.
>   Three organs of sense weak.
>   Heart: sudden and violent pain.
>   Asthma: contracted, cannot sleep, in anguish and panting day and night; congested by mucus.
>   Sexual organs: intractable cold or chronic problems. Men: "ocean of energy" for men? seminal discharges, testicles contracted, four limbs cold and weak. Women: "can produce a son," "thinness of women from having sex during menses"; ovaries: contracted; pain, spasms or swelling of the lower abdomen; menses: pain at the beginning, or insufficient or stopped, or red discharge to the point of metrorrhagia; white discharge, metritis after delivery; special for pains of women.

Opposite effects:
>   Alcoholism: "passion for alcohol"; emptiness of the gallbladder, elevated pulses, heat, energy in the upper body.
>   Abdomen: sudden tympanism, pain at the sides.
>   Intestines: cutting pain radiating to all the internal organs; acute pain under the umbilicus; chronic peritonitis or acute or chronic appendicitis.
>   Large intestine: constipation or diarrhea, inflammation of the cecum; intestinal hemorrhages.
>   Small intestine: spasms; or accumulations?
>   Bladder: special for insufficient urine. If kidney insufficient: tonify; if kidney in excess: disperse. Paralysis of the bladder, incontinence of children? Tonifying disperses the sphincter and body of the bladder. Inflammation (cystitis), frequent needs to urinate with little result, urine red and passes with difficulty. Urethral inflammation: tonify. Kidney and bladder: accumulations?

Parts of the body:

    Loss of physical strength.

    Babies: fontanelles not closing; children not developing.

    Lumbar area: sudden, acute pain.

CV-7 *yinjiao* — crossing of the yin

Abdomen, medial line: just under the umbilicus (at its cartilaginous edge). In a hollow; between the two rectus abdominus muscles; two points separated by the rise of the linea alba.

One small FW above *qihai* (CV-6); one FW below *shenguan* (CV-8, IS *shenque,* in the umbilicus).

When tonified:

    Tonifies the conception vessel: the left point tonifies the left descending flow of the conception vessel and the right ascending flow of the governor vessel; the right point tonifies the right ascending flow of the conception vessel and the left descending flow of the governor vessel; triple warmer, bladder, kidney, heart, genital organs, lumbar area, medial part of the upper knee.

    Dispersing acts in the opposite way.

Direct effects:

    Herald point of the triple warmer (genitourinary functions).

    Sexual organs: perspiration or pruritis of the organs. Women: sterility, miscarriage, vertigo from hemorrhage after delivery, discharges after delivery, menses difficult or insufficient or not stopping, strangling or cutting pain in the lower abdomen, vulvar pruritis of menopause, vagina contracted, strangling pain. Men: testicles: spasms, or pains from double orchitis.

    Kidneys: contracted or congested, cutting pain in the abdomen spreading to the genital organs, difficult urination, urethritis.

Parts of the body:

    Babies: fontanelles not closing.

    Lumbar area: pain or muscle contractures.

    Medial face of the upper part of the knee: pain, contracture, weakness.

CV-8 *shenguan* (IS *shenque*) — barrier for the evolved man

Umbilicus, center: two points; needles are forbidden, use moxa or massage.

One FW above abdomen-*yinjiao* (CV-7); one FW below *shuifen* (CV-9). On either side, at two FW, *huangshu* (KI-16).

When tonified:

    Tonifies the conception vessel: the right point tonifies the right, ascending flow of the conception vessel and the left, descending flow of the governor vessel; the left point tonifies the left, descending flow of the conception vessel and the right, ascending flow of the governor vessel. All the yin organ meridians (deep pulses) and all the yang meridians, opposite brain, three levels of the psyche, three endocrines, three sense organs.

    Dispersing acts in the opposite way.

Direct effects:

    All acute illnesses. An important tonic point, particularly for the organs and abdominal muscles; emptiness, decline; sudden death; dozes, but cannot sleep; dreams of black shapes?

    Cerebral anemia, or cerebral hemorrhage; hemiplegia that no longer improves: one hundred moxas.

    Bad circulation; prolonged cold and troubles of the yin and yang; arteriosclerosis?

    During sleep, noisy breath or snoring?

    Sexual organs: women: after delivery, swollen abdomen. Men: impotence?

    Large intestine: all diarrhea. Babies: incessant diarrhea, diarrhea from emptiness or great age; dysentery; chronic inflammation of the intestine, intestinal tuberculosis, emptiness and cold in the intestine, intestinal noise as if there were water flowing; tympanism.

    Edema?

Point of Weihe: Opium. Desires nothing; very sleepy but cannot sleep; dreams of black shapes; noisy breathing, snoring; face hot, red; vomiting; obstinate constipation; menses suppressed from fear.

CV-9   *shuifen* — division of the waters

Abdomen: medial line: just above the cartilaginous edge of the umbilicus. In a hollow; two points separated by the slight rise of the linea alba; on the lower edge of a transverse bulge.

One FW above *shenguan* (CV-8, IS *shenque,* in the umbilicus); one below *xiawan* (CV-10).

When tonified:

Tonifies the conception vessel; the right point tonifies the right, ascending flow of the conception vessel and the left, descending flow of the governor vessel; the left point tonifies the left, descending flow of the conception vessel and the right, ascending flow of the governor vessel; medulla oblongata, bladder, kidneys, lung, stomach, dorsal spine, lumbar area.

Dispersing acts in the opposite way.

Direct effects:

"Important point for promoting urination; master point of the kidneys." Edema, ascites, swelling of the face. Too frequent moxa can cause dehydration.

Stomach: atony, no appetite.

Intestines: atony, diarrhea, tympanism, intestinal noises "spreading up to the heart," pain around the umbilicus.

Parts of the body:

Cramps, spasms.

Baby: fontanelles not closing.

Vertebrae and lumbar area: contracture, pain going up to the heart.

Lower lateral thorax under the breasts.

Point of Weihe: Mezereum.

CV-10   *xiawan* — lower stomach

Epigastrium, medial line: about one FW above the umbilicus. About five FW below the sternum. In a hollow between the two rectus abdominus muscles. Two points separated by a small rise of the linea alba; on the lower edge of a transverse bulge.

One FW above *shuifen* (CV-9); one below *jianli* (CV-11); about two FW on either side is *shangqu* (KI-17).

When tonified:

Tonifies the conception vessel: the right point tonifies the right, ascending flow of the conception vessel and the left, descending flow of the governor vessel; the left point tonifies the left, descending flow of the conception vessel and the right, ascending flow of the governor vessel; stomach, large intestine, bladder.

Dispersing acts in the opposite way.

Direct effects:

Arteries: pulses abolished, or abolished and agitated.

Stomach: "master point," increasing thinness which does not stop, no food digested, stomach upset, cannot eat, vomits, dilation of the stomach, stomach cramps, chronic gastritis, constipation or diarrhea.

Abdomen hard and agitated; enteritis; blood in the stools.

Bladder: blood in the urine.

Vision: letters dance in front of the eyes.

Nails: white spots?

Point of Weihe: Silicea.

CV-11   *jianli* — established village

Epigastrium, medial line: two FW above the umbilicus (about five FW below the sternum). In the groove between the rectus abdominus muscles. In a hollow; at the level of the union of the ninth rib with the tenth; two points separated by a rise on the linea alba.

One FW above *xiawan* (CV-10); one FW below *zhongwan* (CV-12); three FW medial to *taiyi* (ST-23); two FW medial and above *shangqu* (KI-17); two FW medial and below *shiguan* (KI-18).

When tonified:

Tonifies the conception vessel: the right point tonifies the right, ascending flow of the conception vessel and the left, descending flow of the governor vessel; the left point tonifies the left, descending flow of the conception vessel and the right, ascending flow of the governor vessel; gallbladder, stomach, small intestine, large intestine, diaphragm, bladder (all yang).

Disperses the heart.
Dispersing acts in the opposite way.

Direct effects:

Gallbladder: spasms, pain; troubles from gallbladder excess; vomiting crises; migraine.
Stomach: no appetite, pain; diaphragm: spasms.
Abdomen: peritoneum, pains. Intestines: acute pain, energy in the upper body, swelling of the abdomen.
Lower pelvis, bladder, acute pain.
Edema: swelling of the body?

CV-12 *zhongwan* — central stomach

Epigastrium, medial line: mid-distance from the umbilicus to the lower point of the xyphoid process (three FW above the umbilicus, four large FW below the lower extremity of the sternum). In the groove between the two rectus abdominus muscles; two points separated by a slight rise of the linea alba. In a hollow; at the level of the mid-height of the medial edge of the ninth rib.

One FW above *jianli* (CV-11); one large FW below *shangwan* (CV-13). One and a half FW medial to *shiguan* (KI-18); four FW medial and above *taiyi* (ST-23); four FW medial and below *guanmen* (ST-22).

When tonified:

Tonifies the conception vessel: the right point tonifies the right, ascending flow of the conception vessel and the left, descending flow of the governor vessel; the left point tonifies the left, descending flow of the conception vessel and the right, ascending flow of the governor vessel. All the yang producer organ-meridians, except the triple warmer; occipital lobes; skin; parasympathetic system; vessels; sexual organs; responds in *tianzhu* (BL-10).

Direct effects:

All abnormal formations: tumors, fatty growths, lipoma and even cancer; all problems from vaccinations, intravenous injections, etc.
Parasympathetic system: excess or insufficiency.
Reunion point of all the organs which produce energy (superficial pulses, yang) commanded by the parasympathetic system (stomach, two intestines, bladder, gallbladder).
Worries, obsessions, sadness.
Herald point of the second warmer (digestive function); troubles from emotions, with cold or depression.
Herald point of the stomach: troubles from emotions, with cold or depression. All problems involving stomach pain; food and drinks are no longer digested. All types of vomiting: car, boat, pregnancy, etc.; lots of thready saliva. Stomach troubles from cold getting in: tonify; or from external heat: disperse; lassitude, insufficiency from excess food; stomach cramps; dilation of the stomach; spasms of the chest and gas in the stomach after drinking; or gastritis with fever: disperse. Cancer of stomach: disperse.
Diaphragm: spasms, pain.
Large intestine: colic, painful spasms, hard stools, diarrhea, feces released unknowingly, dysentery, cholera: vomiting and diarrhea; cancer of intestine: disperse.
Abdomen: sudden swelling, or heat in the abdomen, wants to drink.
Worms: ascaris (in the stomach): flukeworm (in the liver, also hydatid cysts?); thready saliva from worms.
Troubles of the uterus.

Opposite effects and on the opposite side of the body:

All the yin distributor organs (lung, heart, spleen-pancreas, liver, kidney): trouble or pain.
Respiratory passages: coryza, incessant asthma, suffocating mucus.
Spleen-pancreas: acute pain or congestion.
Heart: acute pain causing cold and stiffness of the whole body; heart swollen and dilated, yellow complexion.
Kidney: inflammation, urine stopped, swelling, panting, pain and hardness under the side.
Sexual organs: troubles of the uterus; vomiting from pregnancy: disperse; polyps, fibromas.
Cold having entered, stoppage of functions from cold, fever not stopping because of cold.
Heat causing troubles, head hot.

Parts of the body:

Receding gums?
Skin: involuntary movements (fibrillation); all abnormal growths: warts, corns, troubles of the skin and internal troubles after vaccination; can act against cancer, particularly of the stomach; polyps of the vocal cords? aphtha.

Point of Weihe: Thuja. Troubles from vaccination. All abnormal proliferations: warts, corns, polyps, tumors, cancers, fibroma, etc. Aphtha; polyps of the vocal cords; polyps of the uterus; prostatitis; teeth: caries of the roots, receding gums; profuse saliva, nausea. Stomach: swelling, cramps, constipation with frequent urge [to defecate]; frequent need to urinate, [but passing] with interruptions; vision: spots during the day and sparks at night; mental problems, exhaustion, rapid emaciation.

CV-13   *shangwan* — upper stomach

Epigastrium, medial line: two close FW below the point of the xyphoid process (three FW below the lower extremity of the sternum). Four FW above the umbilicus; in the groove between the two rectus abdominus muscles; in a hollow; two points separated by the linea alba.

One large FW above *zhongwan* (CV-12); one large FW below *juguan* (CV-14, IS *juque*); about two FW on either side is *liangmen* (ST-21); one large FW medial and below *yindu* (KI-19).

When tonified:
   Tonifies the conception vessel: the right point tonifies the right, ascending flow of the conception vessel and the left, descending flow of the governor vessel. The left point tonifies the left, descending flow of the conception vessel and the right, ascending flow of the governor vessel. Temporal parietal lobes, stomach, large intestine, upper limb (large intestine meridian), lower limb (stomach meridian).
   Disperses the heart.
   Dispersing acts in the opposite way.

Direct effects:
   Agitation and weakness of the mind, acts with haste and precipitation, sadness.
   All types of vomiting: from worms, from pregnancy, from cholera; of blood from ulcers or tuberculosis, etc.
   Diaphragm: spasms.
   Headache with nausea; menses with nausea.
   Worms (particularly stomach); nausea, saliva, vomiting, mucus, or dry cough, or pain in the heart, or pain in the spleen or pancreas.
   Tonic convulsions, stiff, from worms or from any type of poison; epilepsy from shock? or from spleen-pancreas problems?
   Stomach: dilated: painful gas in the entire epigastrium (aerogastria).
   Intestines: spasms, chronic inflammation; peritonitis.
   Heart: pain from food, agitation and heat in the heart? Cannot eat without trouble; illnesses with fever: disperse then tonify?

   Point of Weihe: Ipeca.

CV-14   *juguan* (IS *juque*) — great barrier

Epigastrium, medial line: two close FW under the lower extremity of the sternum (six FW above the umbilicus); just under the lower point (if there is one) of the xyphoid process. In a hollow of the groove between the two rectus abdominus muscles; two points separated by a small rise of the linea alba; at the level of the union of the eighth with the seventh rib.

One large FW above *shangwan* (CV-13); two tightened FW under *jiuwei* (CV-15). On either side, at the union of the eighth with the seventh rib, is *liangmen* (ST-21). One and a half FW medial and inferior to *tonggu* (KI-20); one and a half FW superior and medial to *yindu* (KI-19).

When tonified:
   Tonifies the conception vessel: the right point tonifies the right, ascending flow of the conception vessel and the left, descending flow of the conception vessel; heart, stomach, large intestine, upper limb (large intestine meridian), lower limb (stomach meridian), lungs.
   Dispersing acts in the opposite way.

Direct effects:
   Without strength, suffers from cold, does not eat, ready to faint with perspiration or cold sweat.
   Obsessions, false ideas coming incessantly, "phantom-cats" (oppression) fear, apprehension, attacks of hyperexcitation from emotions, tears; hysteria? epilepsy with cries, falling, loss of consciousness; children: violent convulsions.
   Herald point of the heart (problems from emotions, with cold or depression): all varieties of pain of the heart, particularly from weakness, insufficiency; agitation, malaise of the heart; pregnant women: heart troubles; pain of the heart, chest, back; short respiration (angina of the chest).

Stomach: attacks of vomiting without having eaten, easily vomits, vomits from coughing, or from hyperexcitation, vomits mucus, saliva, water, with acute pain of the heart; stomach: cramps or dilation, or thready saliva, or water; spasms of the diaphragm, hiccoughs.

Worms: intoxication, poisoning, causing anger, various pains or convulsions in children.

Abdomen: swelling or painful swelling. Cholera: vomiting or diarrhea, or first pain of the heart, or first vomiting, peritonitis.

Diabetes: jaundice, distended spleen-pancreas.

Cough: fits of coughing, energy in the upper body, urinates or vomits from coughing, respiratory mucus, bronchitis, abscess of the lungs, spits blood; chest and back pain; short respiration, fullness of the chest.

Lower abdomen swollen, sighs, heat, agitation.

Hernia protruding from cough.

Parts of the body:

Jiujitsu: point of knockout (and death?); kuatsu: revival point.

Pains from cold, tightening pains.

Sides and abdomen, pain from heart trouble, cannot lift the hand or arm.

Point of Weihe: Veratrum Album. Weakness, fainting with cold sweats and icy extremities; fear, tears; headaches from menses; hiccoughs; violent nausea; urinates from coughing, vomiting and diarrhea of cholera.

Jiujitsu, judo? point of knockout and even death.

Kuatsu: revival point.

CV-15 *jiuwei* — pigeon's tail

Epigastrium, medial line: one FW under the lower point of the sternum; mid-height and mid-width on the xyphoid process; in the hole of the xyphoid; two points separated by a slight rise.

Two tightened FW above *juque* (CV-14); one large FW under *zhongting* (CV-16). At one small FW on either side is *youmen* (KI-21).

When tonified:

Tonifies the conception vessel: the right point tonifies the right, ascending flow of the conception vessel and the left, descending flow of the governor vessel; the left point tonifies the left, descending flow of the conception vessel and the right, ascending flow of the governor vessel; sexual organs, corpus callosum, opposite lateral part of the eye, gums, throat, parotid glands, all same side; extensors, dorsum of wrist same side; lungs.

Disperses the anterior frontal lobes, temporoparietal lobes, evolved man, automaton-parrot, stomach, right half of the body.

Dispersing acts in the opposite way.

Responds in *gaohuangshu* (BL-38, IS BL-43).

Direct effects:

Source point of the vital centers. Little energy, dispersed vitality; ennui; does not like to hear human voices; weakening of the nerves and brain, nervous weakness, mental weakening, cannot find words, loss of memory; expects immediate misfortune; distracted; difficulty in falling asleep or total insomnia? diminished strength.

All varieties of epilepsy and convulsions in children or adults (epileptiform?); tightening.

Massage or moxa by bringing a match or lighted cigarette close.

Herald point of the sexual organs. Sexual troubles from prolonged abstinence. Or sexual hyperexcitation; hypotension, all pulses hard, without beats; headache at night radiating to the lateral corner of the eye.

Heart: pain or inflammation; myocarditis.

Opposite side of the throat: swelling, obstruction, pain, inflammation, swollen parotid glands; tonsillitis; cough, fullness of the chest, bronchitis, asthma, emphysema, pneumonia, spits blood.

Opposite eye: lateral commissure: pain, inflammation or weakness.

Opposite effects:

Mouth: ulcerations of the corners, skin eruptions, extreme thirst.

Swollen gums, same side; teeth moving towards the front, loose; vomiting; stomach: inflammation, pain.

Parts of the body:

Skin: hands hardening and peeling from place to place, particularly in spring and summer: tonify; herpes at the bottom of the back; bubbles on the soles of the feet; herpetic pruritis: tonify; bad body odor?

Drowning victims: keep head down, moxa with a lighted cigarette close or touching very quickly, causes the water to be thrown out of the lungs and stomach.

Point of Weihe: Mercurius Vivus and Solubis. Sleep retarded or total insomnia, aggravated at night and by heat of the bed, headaches at night, nightly yellow and viscous perspiration; red and painful throat; swollen tonsils; swollen gums, tongue keeping the imprint of the teeth; dartre, ulcerations of the corners of the mouth, extreme thirst; herpes at the bottom of the back; skin peeling in various places on the fingers, particularly in the spring; bad body odor; iritis; insufficient and hard liver; sexual hyperexcitation; numbness, stingings, trembling, cramps; tendency to hemorrhages; vertigo when extending oneself or standing up; forgetful, distractions, mental weakening; fears next misfortune; quarrelsome, peevish.

CV-16   *zhongting* — central pavillion

Sternum, midline: one FW above the lower extremity; just under the transverse rise connecting the two fifth ribs (upper part of the supra-xyphoidian fossa). In a narrow vertical groove; two points, one on either side of the groove.

One large FW above *jiuwei* (CV-15); one under *shanzhong* (CV-17). On either side, in the angle between the sternum and the lower edge of the fifth rib, is *bulang* (KI-22).

When tonified:
> Tonifies the conception vessel: the right point tonifies the right, ascending flow of the conception vessel and the left, descending flow of the governor vessel; the left point tonifies the left, descending flow of the conception vessel and the right, ascending flow of the governor vessel; cerebellum, spinal cord, heart, stomach, cardiac sphincter, esophagus.
> Dispersing acts in the opposite way.

Direct effects:
> Agitated, authoritarian, but fears dark places and storms, depressed; sleep curtailed; migraines of several days? vertigo on waking?
> Babies who regurgitate, or who vomit their milk as soon as they have taken it and it is not digested; spasms of the cardiac sphincter or of the esophagus; or contracture; adults: vomiting (sea, airplane, automobile).
> Opposite eye, tired vision, grey veil, black spots; atrophy of the optic nerve? paresis of the lateral muscles of the eye (external ocular motor nerve)? congestion of the retina?
> Teeth: alveodental periostitis, loose teeth.
> Stomach: burning pain, appeased by cold drinks.
> Throat: inflammation, tonsillitis, tracheitis; lungs: congestion, fullness of the chest and sides.
> Heart: arteries.

Parts of the body:
> Burning pains, sensations of burning on the skin.
> Upper back, between the shoulders: burning, stinging pain.

Point of Weihe: Phosphorus. Authoritarian, agitated, depressed, sleep interrupted, dreams of fire, fears dark places, storms; all burning pain; skin, stomach, excretions, discharges; burning pain between the shoulders; shivering, trembling when lying down, night sweats; chilblains; petechia, bruising; convulsions; scurvy; tired vision; foggy, greenish halo, black floating spots before the eyes; cataract; atrophy of the optic nerve; paresis of the common ocular nerve; edema surrounding the eyes, congestion of the retina; hears voices badly; vertigo on waking; migraines of several days; alveodental periostitis, loose teeth; weight on the chest; coughs particularly at night; profuse urine, pain in the urethra; hiccoughs, regurgitates, vomits bile; burning pain, particularly in the stomach, ameliorated by cold drinks.

CV-17   *shanzhong* — middle of the chest

Chest, medial line. Men: mid-distance between the two nipples; two FW above the lower edge of the lower extremity of the sternum; on the lower edge of the rise between the fourth ribs. At the top of a triangular hollow; in a narrow vertical groove; two points, each one on the edge of the rise of the groove.

One FW above *zhongting* (CV-16), one under *yutang* (CV-18); on either side, in the angle between the fourth rib and the sternum, is *shenfeng* (KI-23).

When tonified:
> Tonifies the yang energy. Tonifies the conception vessel: the right point tonifies the right, ascending flow of the conception vessel and the left, descending flow of the governing vessel; the left point tonifies the left, descending flow of the conception vessel and the right, ascending flow of the governing vessel; triple warmer (first warmer), stomach, breasts, cerebellum, medulla oblongata, lungs, liver and spleen-pancreas; forearm, hand, ring finger and little finger; lower leg, foot, all these same side.
> Disperses the yin energy.
> Dispersing acts in the opposite way.

Direct effects:

    Is always in a hurry, ahead of time; head seems empty?

    Reunion of the yang energy taken from the air. Tonification increases the force of inhalation and allows better retention of the breath (respiratory muscles); assimilation of air, oxygen and expulsion of the carbon dioxide; decreases the yin energy (increases the right hand, decreases the left).

    Herald point of the first warmer (respiratory functions). Problems from emotions with cold or depression; all troubles of the respiratory functions; energy in the upper body, hoarseness, clearing of the throat, cough, coughing fits, short respiration, spits mucus, bronchitis, dyspnea, cannot eat, lungs oppressed, energy compressed in the chest, gasping for air, abscess of the lungs.

    Breasts: insufficient lactation: tonify on right and left; or inflammation of the mammary glands, tumors: disperse.

    Esophagus and cardiac sphincter contracted, spasms; food does not descend, spits or vomits saliva; babies regurgitate their undigested milk; spasms of the diaphragm, hiccough.

    Stomach does not digest, acidity; thinness.

    Liver and spleen-pancreas distended (stomach compressed, swelling after meals, short respiration, palpitations from effort).

    Capillaries narrowed; ulcers?

Parts of the body:

    Ligaments, cartilage, articulations (periarthritis?)

    Painful rheumatism of the region of the heart; intercostal neuralgia, middle and low.

    Hand and foot same side, cold.

    Point of Weihe: Argentum Metallicum or Foliatum. Is always in a hurry; head seems empty; articulations, ligaments, cartilage; swollen ankles; rheumatism of the elbow or knee; serious back pain; walks bent over; writer's cramp, withered or blocked capillaries, ulcers; larynx; aphonia; coughs when laughing; scrapes in order to clear the voice; dyspnea, asthma, needs cool air; frequent abundant urine; prolapsed uterus; thinness.

CV-18   *yutang* — room of jade

    Chest, medial line: three FW above the lower extremity of the sternum; on the lower edge of the rise connecting the third ribs; in the hollow of a vertical groove.

    One FW above *shanzhong* (CV-17); one under *zigong* (CV-19). On either side, in the angle between the third rib and the sternum, is *lingxu* (KI-24).

When tonified:

    Tonifies the conception vessel: the right point tonifies the right, ascending flow of the conception vessel and the left, descending flow of the governor vessel; the left point tonifies the left, descending flow of the conception vessel and the right, ascending flow of the governor vessel; spleen-pancreas, liver, heart, lungs, kidneys, pituitary gland, palmar side of thumb and index fingers.

    Disperses the esophagus, stomach, large intestine.

    Dispersing acts in the opposite way.

Direct effects:

    Syndrome of the eight organs: spleen-pancreas and liver distended, crushing the stomach between them; above, the lungs and heart; below, the large intestine and kidneys. Prostration on waking or for the whole day; stomach swollen after meals with sleepiness. Short breath; palpitations from effort or at night. Slow defecation and attacks of diarrhea; hyper- or hypotension. Aggravates all problems of the eight organs.

    Aversion to little children, particularly little girls.

Parts of the body:

    Palmar side of the thumb and index fingers.

    Point of Weihe: Raphanus Sativus. Pain of the liver and spleen, gas above and below, difficult to expel; gas after operations; sore throat, pain from uterus to throat; nymphomania; sexual insomnia; edema of or under the lower eyelid; aversion to children, particularly little girls.

CV-19   *zigong* — purple palace

    Chest, medial line of the sternum: at the lower edge of the rise connecting the second ribs. In the hollow of a vertical groove; two points, each on the edge of the groove.

One FW above *yutang* (CV-18); one under *huagai* (CV-20); on either side, in the angle between the second rib and the sternum, is *shencang* (KI-25).

When tonified:
> Tonifies the conception vessel: the right point tonifies the right, ascending flow of the conception vessel and the left, descending flow of the governor vessel; the left point tonifies the left, descending flow of the conception vessel and the right, ascending flow of the governor vessel; lungs, heart, stomach, throat, esophagus, mastoid to the cervical vertebrae.
> Dispersing acts in the opposite way.

Direct effects:
> Powerful bactericide? old syphilis (bubos, skin easily fissured, ulcers?); throat: angina, diphtheria, back of the throat, eustachian tubes, coughing fits, agitation of the heart.
> Tracheitis, bronchitis, pleurisy, pulmonary congestion, pulmonary tuberculosis; heart and vessels contracted: disperse.
> Mouth: aphtha, saliva like paste, food and drink not descending (spasms of the esophagus); attacks of vomiting.
> Stomach: vomiting of blood (hematemesis).

Parts of the body:
> Nape: mastoid to cervical vertebrae (splenius capitis).
> Chest and sternum extending to the sides: acute pain.
> Thumb and fingers: stiff or painful or swollen joints.

Point of Weihe: Mercurius Iodatus Ruber. Powerful bactericide; throat: pain, ulceration, dark red pillars, scrapes the throat; diphtheria; coryza; bad hearing; aphtha; old syphilis; bubos, skin with small fissures and ulcers.

CV-20 *huagai* — flowered cover

Upper chest, midline: two FW under the upper edge of the sternum. At the lower edge of the rise connecting the two first ribs; in the hollow of a vertical groove; two points, each on the edge of the groove.

One FW above *zigong* (CV-19); one under *xuanji* (CV-21); on either side, in the angle between the first rib and the sternum, is *yuzhong* (KI-26).

When tonified:
> Tonifies the conception vessel: the right point tonifies the right, ascending flow of the conception vessel and the left, descending flow of the governor vessel; the left point tonifies the left, descending flow of the conception vessel and the right, ascending flow of the governor vessel; lungs, mid-brain (anterior hypothalamus, vagus), large intestine, palmar side of the thumb and index finger, sexual organs, thyroid gland, tonsils, larynx, skin, nose, eustachian tubes.
> Dispersing acts in the opposite way.

Direct effects:
> Thyroid: swelling at puberty; swollen glands.
> Larynx: stuttering; spasms of voice muscles; loss of ability to make sound, aphonia, tonsillitis.
> Throat contracted, nothing passes, asthma, spasms of the bronchus, panting, cannot speak, contracted, energy in the upper body, coughing fits; pleurisy, painful fullness of the chest, sides, limbs; uterine fibromas?

Parts of the body:
> Polyps in the nose and eustachian tubes?
> Skin: eruptions (yellowish), favus, scab like milk? ulcers with varicose veins?

Point of Weihe: Calcarea Iodata. Profuse and yellow secretions, yellow eruptions; favus; milky scabs; greenish mucus of old cough; polyps in the nose and ears; varicosities and painless ulcers; tonsils with puzzling secretions; distention of the glands; goiter at puberty; fibrous uterus; pain in the chest after anti-syphilitic treatment.

CV-21 *xuanji* — armillary sphere

Upper sternum, midline: on the lower edge of the ligamentous rise connecting the two clavicle bones. In the hollow of a vertical groove; two points, each on the edge of the groove.

One FW above *huagai* (CV-20); one under *tiantu* (CV-22). On either side, in the angle between the clavicle and the sternum, is *shufu* (KI-27).

When tonified:

    Tonifies the conception vessel: the right point tonifies the right, ascending flow of the conception vessel and the left, descending flow of the governor vessel; the left point tonifies the left, descending flow of the conception vessel and the right, ascending flow of the governor vessel; stomach, lungs, cerebellum, nose, back of the tongue, palate, opposite eye, ear same side, sense organs.

    Dispersing acts in the opposite way.

Direct effects:

    Sense organs: taste-smell, tactility, vision, hearing (eustachian tubes).

    Mouth: palate; tongue: upper and back part; sublingual salivary glands.

    Throat: sore throat, tonsillitis, abscess of the throat, coughing fits, energy in the upper body; asthma, panting, cannot speak, cannot sleep, malaise day and night, becoming thin; pulmonary congestion.

    Contracted esophagus; stomach: burning, cramps or pains, does not empty.

Parts of the body:

    Skin of face, of chest: painful.

    Sternoclavicular articulation: neuralgia or arthritis.

    Lateral palmar part of the thumb.

    Point of Weihe: Bromium. Throat: hoarseness, swelling, redness, inflamed tonsils; all kinds of cough, whooping cough, diphtheria, asthma, swollen and indurated glands, goiter, parotitis (mumps); orchitis, ovaritis; breast tumors, prostatitis; acne, scabs, particularly on the face and arms; tickling of the nose; burning of the stomach from the tongue to the stomach.

CV-22 *tiantu* — celestial spring

    Front of the neck, bottom, midline: on the posterior edge of the upper edge of the sternum; two points, each in the angle between the sternum and the posterior edge of the head of the clavicle.

    One FW above *xuanji* (CV-21); three FW under *lianquan* (CV-23); one large FW medial and inferior to *qishe* (ST-11).

When tonified:

    The right point tonifies the right, ascending flow of the conception vessel and the left, descending flow of the governor vessel; the left point tonifies the left, descending flow of the conception vessel and the right, ascending flow of the governor vessel; opposite side of the body; larynx same side; vocal cords same side; throat same side, tonsils same side, lung opposite side, stomach opposite side, face opposite side, veins opposite side; thyroid same side; cerebellum.

    Dispersing acts in the opposite way.

Direct effects:

    Throat: larynx, all kinds of cough and hoarseness: laryngitis, tonsillitis, whooping cough, spasms of the larynx, pain, inflammation, swelling of the throat, abscess of the throat, cold or dryness of the throat, tightness under the tongue; acute spasms of the hyoidian muscles, cannot speak.

    Ear: opposite, inflammation of eustachian tubes.

    Asthma: panting, cannot sleep: moxa; mucus; energy compressed into the lung; abscess of lungs.

    Thyroid: goiter, painful swelling of the front of the neck.

    Vomiting, spasms of the esophagus.

    Stomach: acidity, burning after pastries and sweets, profuse saliva from worms (ascariasis).

    Jaundice?

    Veins: varicosities; breast: tumors.

Parts of the body:

    Glands, swelling: thyroid, parotitis (mumps), testicles? ovaries? prostatitis?

    Skin of the face easily congested, acne.

    Hammering pain in the heart and back.

    Tumors (particularly throat, front of neck).

CV-23 *lianquan* — source of the angle

    Front of neck, midline: mid-height above the prominence and the two horns of the thyroid cartilage, larynx, Adam's apple. At mid-height of the transverse cartilage (hyoid bone); in the hollow of a vertical groove between the insertions of the sternocleidohyoidian muscles; two points, on the edge of each insertion.

Three FW above *tiantu* (CV-22); following point on the chin: *chengjiang* (CV-24). Two FW on either side and lower down is *renying* (ST-9). Three FW on either side and above is neck-*futu* (LI-18).

When tonified:
> Tonifies the conception vessel: the right point tonifies the right, ascending flow of the conception vessel and the left, descending flow of the governor vessel; the left point tonifies the left, descending flow of the conception vessel and the right, ascending flow of the governor vessel; salivary glands, lower part of the tongue, mouth, throat, bronchus, lungs; chain of the yin *(yinwei mai)*.
> Dispersing acts in the opposite way.

Direct effects:
> Excess saliva, vomiting of saliva.
> Tongue: lower part swollen, painful, contracture or atrophy of all glossal muscles; difficulty in speaking.
> Mouth: abscess; throat: inflammation.
> Cough, bronchitis, asthma.
> Dispersing too much can cause a spinal deviation?

CV-24   *chengjiang* — receives the noodles

Chin, midline: upper edge of the prominence (tuft of hair). In the lower curve of the vertical groove of the suture of the two parts of the lower jaw; on the inferior edge of the orbicular muscles of the lips; two points on either side of the groove.

The right rising flow of the conception vessel goes around the mouth and joins the governor vessel at *shuigou* (GV-25, IS GV-26, *renzhong*). The left, descending flow receives a branch encircling the mouth and coming from *shuigou* (GV-25, IS GV-26, *renzhong*).

Preceding point: *lianquan* (CV-23). On either side, under the corners of the mouth, is *dicang* (ST-7, IS ST-4).

When tonified:
> Tonifies the conception vessel: the right point tonifies the right, ascending flow of the conception vessel and the left, descending flow of the governing vessel; the left point tonifies the left, descending flow of the conception vessel and the right, ascending flow of the governing vessel; posterior frontal lobes; half-body same side; spleen-pancreas, heart; orbicular muscles of lips, opposite side of face.
> Dispersing acts in the opposite way.

Direct effects:
> Apoplexy, hemiplegia? epilepsy? can awaken from a loss of consciousness.
> Nose: growths.
> Mouth: children: abscess, phagedenic chancre?
> Teeth: pain in the molars and incisors.
> Diabetes, thirst, obscured vision.
> Incontinence? edema?

Parts of the body:
> Face: paralyzed, eye and mouth awry, difficult speech, cannot speak, or swelling.
> Neck and nape stiff, contracted, spasms, closed eyes.

Chapter II

Posterior Median Line

Governor Vessel
(Du Mai)

The governor vessel starts from the bottom of the coccyx (being connected to the conception vessel through a branch from *huiyin,* CV-1). It follows the spine, ascends to the skull, descends over the forehead and nose and terminates on the upper gum.

Each of its points is double. On the spine, they are on the inferior, lateral edges of the vertebrae, in the angle of the lateral edge of the median tendon; on the skull they are on either side of a slight rise. They form two currents, a rising flow on the right side, and a descending flow on the left side. At their extremities they pass into the conception vessel, changing side and direction of flow.

Using the governor vessel is recommended when the meridians no longer respond, and also in cases when the problem is accompanied by fever, physical agitation or mental hyperexcitation.

Systemically, it governs the strength of physical and mental activity, particularly for men. The small intestine points that command it act on the thoracic spinal cord on the same side, and on the cervical spinal cord, medulla, cerebrum and cerebellum on the opposite side.

The lower third, from the coccyx to the last thoracic vertebrae, acts on the sexual force and the strength of the lower limbs. The middle third, from the twelfth to the fifth thoracic, acts on the digestive organs, stomach, liver, gallbladder and spleen-pancreas. The upper third, up to the skull, acts on the thoracic organs, lungs, heart and the spinal reflexes. The cervical spine acts on the endocrine glands. On the skull the points act on different parts of the brain.

The command point of the governor vessel is *houxi* (SI-3); moreover, all the points of the small intestine and the governor vessel act on the two lines. *Fengchi* (GB-20) also strongly acts on the governor vessel.

The pulse, ignored by the Far East, is right IV on the radial artery. Superficial: sexual and urinary functions; middle: digestive functions; deep: respiratory and circulatory functions, as well as cerebral functions.

Most of its points act on the spinal cord.

It constitutes a reserve of energy for strength and male activity under its different forms.

In fact, it can be seen in three distinct ways, or groups of actions:

1)   The effects of its points on the nervous centers: brain, cerebellum, medulla oblongata, spinal cord.

2)   The effects of its points on the energy of yang activity, or insufficiency (the meridians which do not respond to the action of the needles), or excess (problems accompanied by fever or hyperexcitation and coming from excesses of the surrounding yang energy, from heat, cold or wind).

3)   The interlinking of its flow with that of the conception vessel. Tonifying the governor vessel on the right tonifies its descending flow and the ascending flow of the conception vessel and vice versa.

Its two currents pass with a change of direction into the conception vessel at the perineum at *huiyin* (CV-1), and under the nose at *shuigou* (GV-25, IS *renzhong, GV-26)* through two branches, right and left, encircling the mouth via the external edge of the obicularis muscle of the lips.

4)   Its connections with the vessel of the yang energy, the lateral submalleolar vessel *(yangqiao mai),* and with the small intestine (the duodenum, which makes the albumin molecule, specific to each individual and the source of life). In fact, the general command point of the governor vessel is the tonification point of the small intestine, *houxi* (SI-3). When this point is pressed, there is an awakening of a response in the lateral submalleolar vessel point *shenmai* (BL-62), and reciprocally. Thus there is a link through *shenmai* with the bladder meridian, which covers the back with its two lines, and which acts on the strength of the back and the yang energy.

Tradition has recognized the governor vessel as controlling the strength of the body and mind. If there is excess, the back is stiff and painful. If insufficient, the head is bent forward, falling. Its troubles would be, if insufficient: lack of vigor and of mental strength and of personality. If in excess: physical or mental hyperexcitation, hallucinations, neuralgia of the head, propensity to fevers, epilepsy, stiffness or heat of the back, pain in the eyes.

GV-1 *changqiang* — prolonged stiffness

Between the anus and coccyx, midline, on the levator ani muscle, a little under the last coccygeal vertebra, in a hollow.

Following point: *yaoshu* (GV-2) at the base of the sacrum; separated from *huiyin* (CV-1) by the anus; two points separated by a small medial rise.

When tonified:
> Tonifies the governor vessel, spinal cord, medulla oblongata, superior occipital lobe, primate, sexual organs, eyes, heart, lumbar area.
> Disperses the conception vessel, large intestine, anus.
> Dispersing acts in the opposite way.

Direct effects:
> Passage point between the governor and conception vessels (to *huiyin*, CV-1). If excess: back, lumbar area and vertebral column stiff, heavy, sensitive. If insufficient: the head falls, the body is arched, the top of the head is sensitive.
> Insufficiency: emotional agitation, fear, depression. Excess: hyperexcitation, meningitis; epilepsy? convulsions from cold?
> Eyes: problems, bad vision, "does not look to the right," fault of accommodation?
> Heart: pain?
> Genital organs: men: non-erection, dreads sexual fatigue and cold food, seminal discharge, phagedenic chancre of the genital area, chronic blennorrhagia.

Opposite effects:
> Anus: hemorrhoids, fissures, flowing fistulas, pain, itching, "master point."
> Large intestine: prolapsed rectum, serious diarrhea, diarrhea of bile, intestinal hemorrhages, or stool and urine difficult.

Parts of the body:
> Pain at the top of the skull.
> Children: fontanelle not closing.
> Vertebral column and lumbar area: heaviness, stiffness.

GV-2 *yaoshu* — assent point of the lumbar area

Bottom of the back: between the coccyx and sacrum, midline, in the sacro-coccygeal hiatus; deep, the cauda equina (end of the spinal cord). Two points separated by a small medial rise.

Separated from *changqiang* (GV-1) by the coccyx and from *yaoyangguan* (CV-3) by the sacrum. One large FW above and medial to *huiyang* (BL-35); two medial to *biahuanshu* (BL-30).

When tonified:
> Tonifies the governor vessel, sexual organs, back, lumbar area, lower limbs, particularly on the anteroteral side.
> Disperses the large intestine, anus, bladder, urethra.
> Dispersing acts in the opposite way.

Direct effects:
> Sexual organs: blennorrhagia. Women: menses blocked, uterine problems.

Opposite effects:
> Anus: hemorrhoids.
> Bladder: quantity of urine insufficient; red color; urethra: inflammation (blennorrhagia).

Parts of the body:
> Back and lumbar area: pain, lumbar area stiff, troubles of the lumbar vertebra.
> Lower limb, particularly the anterolateral surface: extreme coldness or weakness to the point of flaccidity; foot weak to the point of flaccidity "without action."[1]

GV-3 *yaoyangguan* — barrier of the yang

Lower back, midline: between the fifth (last) lumbar vertebra and the upper edge of the sacrum. [This point is usually located between the fourth and fifth lumbar vertebrae. — Trans.] Two points separated by the median tendon; in the angle between the tendon and the sacrum; in a hollow.

Separated from *yaoshu* (GV-2) by the sacrum; following point: *mingmen* (GV-4), between the second and third lumbar vertebrae; two FW medial to *guanyuanshu* (BL-26).

When tonified:

Tonifies the governor vessel, mid-brain opposite, lower limbs, knee, foot, all the nerves.
Disperses the large intestine, anus, sphincter of the bladder.
Dispersing acts in the opposite way.

Direct effects:

Nerves injured, fingers crushed, shingles, pains after operations etc. Trouble and lesions of the spinal cord or coccyx.
Feeling of insects on the face, hands etc.
Large intestine: weakness of the anal sphincter, diarrhea, inflammation of the intestines.
Bladder: weakness of the sphincter of the bladder, nocturnal incontinence.

Parts of the body:

All the nerves injured; fingers: pain.
Lumbar area: lumbar vertebrae painful.
Lower limbs: weakness; knee (particularly upper medial part) pain; lower leg flaccid, without action; foot flaccid, toes flaccid, flexed or injured, painful.

Point of Weihe: Hypericum Perfoliatum. All injured or attacked nerves, fingers or crushed toes, from operation; shingles, inflammation of the nerves; injuries of face or hand; attacks on the spinal cord; pain in the lumbar area, lower leg, fingers or toes, burns.

GV-4 *mingmen* — gate of destiny

Lumbar area, midline: lower edge of the second lumbar vertebra. Between the second and third lumbar vertebrae (the upper edge of the fourth is slightly above the level of the iliac crest of the hip; the twelfth thoracic is slightly below the angle between the rib and the thoracic spine); two points: in the angle between the lateral upper edge of the vertebra and the muscular insertion.

Preceding point: *yaoyangguan* (GV-3); two FW below *xuanshu* (GV-5); two close FW medial to *sanjiaoshu* (BL-22).

When tonified:

Tonifies the governor vessel, sexual organs, cerebellum, inferior occipital lobes, eyes, kidney, lower leg same side, upper leg opposite.
Disperses the bladder.
Dispersing acts in the opposite way.

Direct effects:

All the crossing points go from below upwards to the opposite side through this point.
Lassitude, evolved man tired: moxa. Children: head shaking, body flexed backwards (Little's disease?): moxa; or meningitis, eclampsia, tetanus; epilepsy?
Fever of the internal organs: body burning without sweat; head as if broken.
Intestines: intestinal tuberculosis, intestinal hemorrhages, spasms and pain of the intestines, rectal prolapse, hemorrhoids.
Genital organs, particularly men: non-erection, testicles, seminal discharge.
Kidney: weakened, frequent needs, gets up many times in the night. Insufficient kidneys in old people. From insufficiency of the kidney, acute pain in the lumbar area, abdomen and lower limb, particularly when urinating.

Parts of the body:

Crossed coordination: lower limb same side and upper limb opposite.
Lumbar area and buttock: pain or weakness of the gluteal muscles, piriform, caput lateralis and medialis, crural neuralgia.
(Kuatsu) Massage or small repeated shocks revive drowned people; recovers from shock to the heart or brain.

Point of Weihe: Selenium. All exhaustion; sexual fatigue; debility of convalescence or old people; without hope or desire; extreme sadness; all work tires; bad sleep towards midnight and awakens early. Aging; aging of the genitourinary system. Selenium is a constituent of the bone and teeth. Hoarseness, particularly of singers; falling of the head hair from fat, and of the body hair; eruptions of the liver area; prostatitis; sexual atony.

GV-5 *xuanshu* — axis of suspension

Lumbar area, midline: lower edge of the first lumbar vertebra (between the first and second lumbar vertebrae). Two FW below the angle between the last rib and the thoracic spine; in the angle between the lower lateral edge of the first lumbar and the lateral edge of the median tendon; two points separated by the median tendon.

Two FW above *mingmen* (GV-4); three FW below *jizhong* (GV-6); one medial to *weishu* (BL-21).

When tonified:
  Tonifies the governor vessel, superior occipital lobes, primate, lumbar muscles of the back, gluteus medius and minimus, stomach, intestines, contracted caecum, liver; responds in *shanglian* (ST-37, IS *shangjuxu*), *zhongwan* (CV-12) and *tianzhu* (BL-10).
  Dispersing acts in the opposite way.

Direct effects:
  Always in a hurry, irrational impulses, dreams of snakes.
  Stomach: pain, does not digest.
  Large intestine: diarrhea, acute enteritis, old illnesses of the intestines.
  Uterus relaxed.

Parts of the body:
  Thoracic and lumbar muscles: contracture.
  Gluteus medius and minimus: stiffness, contracture.
  Crural neuralgia.

Point of Weihe: Argentum Nitricum. Always in a hurry, hasty, irrational impulses; dreams of snakes; headache with trembling and weakness. Eyes: weakness of the ciliary muscles, foggy, floating specs or spots, prurulent ophthalmia; desires sweets. Stomach: ulceration, gas. Intestines: gas, incontinence day and night; non-erection and rapid ejaculation; sensation as if strangled or of having a splinter.

GV-6 *jizhong* — middle of the vertebrae

At the bottom of the posterior thorax, midline: on the lower edge of the eleventh thoracic vertebra (which goes over the last rib); between the twelfth and eleventh thoracic vertebrae. In the angle between the lower edge of the vertebra (spinous process) and the lateral edge of the median tendon; two points: separated by a tendon.

Three FW above *xuanshu* (GV-5); three below *zhongshu* (GV-6A, IS GV-7); two medial to *pishu* (BL-20).

When tonified:
  Tonifies the governor vessel, posterior frontal lobes, cerebellum, spinal cord, large intestine, liver, bladder, throat, nose, palm, sole of foot.
  Disperses the kidney.

  Dispersing acts in the opposite way.

Direct effects:
  "Serious nervous trouble shaking the elbow and forearm to the point of breaking them: tonify."
  Parkinsonism? Multiple sclerosis? Epilepsy?
  Influenza.
  All disturbances from humidity?
  Stomach: lack of appetite.
  Large intestine: dysentery, intestinal hemorrhage; distended abdomen; all varieties of hemorrhoids. Children: prolapsed rectum falling to the knee.
  Jaundice with fullness of the abdomen and lack of appetite.
  Displaced kidney: pain: tonify.
  Congested prostate.

Parts of the body;
  Palm, sole: troubles of the skin.

Point of Weihe: Corallium Rubrum. Congested face after meals; nose: inflammation of the front of the nose and throat; sweat or ulcers of the genital apparatus; psoriasis of the palm or soles.

GV-6a *zhongshu* (IS GV-7) — central axis

A new point, discovered in Japan.

Back, midline: lower edge of the thoracic vertebra (spinous process); between the eleventh and twelfth thoracic vertebrae; in the angle between the lower edge of the vertebra and the lateral edge of the median tendon; two points separated by the median tendon.

Two FW above *jizhong* (GV-6); two under *jinsuo* (GV-7, IS GV-8); two FW medial to *danshu* (BL-19).

When tonified:
   Tonifies the governor vessel, esophagus, liver, large intestine.
   Dispersing acts in the opposite way.

Direct effects:
   Esophagus: spasms.
   Large intestine: spasms, contractions, pain.
   Heart: valves?
   Liver: contracted, in excess, pain.
   Children: tuberculosis.
   Prostate: congestion, too large: tonify.

Parts of the body:
   Back pain.

GV-7 *jinsuo* (IS GV-8) — contraction of the muscles

Back, midline: on the lower edge of the ninth thoracic vertebra (spinous process); between the tenth and ninth vertebrae; in the angle between the lower edge of the vertebra and the lateral edge of the median tendon; two points separated by the median tendon.

Two FW above *zhongshu* (GV-6a). Four FW beneath *zhiyang* (GV-8). *Ganshu* (BL-18) is found at two FW to either side.

When tonified:
   Tonifies the governor vessel, anterior frontal lobes, stomach, small intestine and kidneys.
   Dispersing acts in the opposite manner.

Direct effects:
   Nervous degeneration; excessive speaking, heart pains, vertigo. Loss of vitality. Epilepsy, also seizures brought on by fright. Tonic contractures.
   Eyes wide open?
   Stomach: spasms.
   Swollen appendix.
   Kidneys: insufficient urination leading to edema.
   Lumbar vertebrae: pain. Back and lumbar area: pain.

GV-8 *zhiyang* (IS GV-9) — maximum yang

Back, median line. On the inferior border of the seventh thoracic vertebrae. Between T7 and T8. In the angle of the inferior border of the vertebrae and the lateral border of the median tendon. Two points separated by the median tendon.

Four FW above *jinsuo* (GV-7, IS GV-8); two under *lingtai* (GV-9, IS GV-10); at two FW on either side is *geshu* (BL-17).

When tonified:
   Tonifies the governor vessel, anterior frontal lobes, evolved man, liver, stomach, large intestine, kidneys, sexual organs, back and lumbar area, opposite limbs.
   Dispersing acts in the opposite way.

Direct effects:
   Evolved man: weak, speaks with difficulty from insufficient energy or from discouragement.
   Stomach: cold or laziness: thinness, cannot eat; noises of the intestines; liver and gallbladder not emptying; diaphragm; jaundice.
   Kidneys: fever (nape stiff, lumbar area stiff, lower limbs numb).

Vagina: paralysis during orgasm?
Lung: pleurisy, intercostal neuralgia.

Parts of the body:
Sudden tonic (stiff) convulsions, pain in the heart and chest.
Limbs (opposite half of the body) heavy, lazy, tired.
Back, lumbar area: pain, ''in the middle of the back the energy rises and falls''; lumbar vertebrae: pain.

GV-9   *lingtai* (IS GV-10) — terrace of the immaterial

Back, median line: at the level of the mid-height between the spine of the scapula and its lower angle; on the lower edge of the sixth thoracic vertebra (spinous process). Between the seventh and sixth thoracic vertebrae; in the angle between the lower edge of the vertebra and the lateral edge of the median tendon; two points separated by the median tendon.

Two FW above *zhiyang* (GV-8, IS GV-9); two FW below *shendao* (GV-10, IS GV-11); at two FW on either side is *dushu* (BL-16).

When tonified:
Tonifies the governor vessel, medulla oblongata, spleen-pancreas, heart, arteries, lung.
Disperses the gallbladder.
Dispersing acts in the opposite way.
Influenza: preventive; pathogenic cold; nervous asthma: cannot sleep; bronchitis; pneumonia; pulmonary tuberculosis.
Heart: arteries: tonification contracts them; malaria, fever without sweat.
Jaundice; liver, gallbladder: tonification contracts and empties them.
Spleen-pancreas: fever (bluish complexion, nausea, heavy head, vertigo).

Point of Weihe: Osmium. Irritation of the respiratory tract, cough; eyes: foggy, glaucoma (intraocular high pressure with irridescent vision, pain above and below the orbit, green color around lights); pruritis, bumps, eczema; odor of onions in the axilla.

GV-10   *shendao* (IS GV-11) — way of the evolved man

Midline of the back: at the level of one third the distance from the spine of the scapula to its lower angle; on the lower edge of the fifth vertebra (spinous process). Between the sixth and fifth vertebrae; in the angle between the lower edge of the vertebra and the lateral edge of the median tendon; two points separated by the tendon.

Two FW above *lingtai* (GV-9, IS GV-10); four below *shenzhu* (GV-11, IS GV-12); at two FW on either side is *xinshu* (BL-15).

When tonified:
Tonifies the governor vessel, heart, anterior frontal lobes, evolved man, liver, eyes, maxilla, back, lumbar area.
Disperses the small intestine, gallbladder.
Dispersing acts in the opposite way.

Direct effects:
Evolved man: insufficient. Weakening of the brain and nerves.
Emotional. Loss of memory (amnesia). Convulsions of infants from shock. Epilepsy?
Swollen eyelids. Pterygion?
Asthma with fever.
Jaundice from tuberculosis. Chronic enteritis.
Heart: all troubles.

Parts of the body:
Maxilla, inflamation. Dislocated jaw?
Upper back weak. Stiffness of the lumbar vertebrae.
Intercostal neuralgia.

Point of Weihe: Tellurium. Negligent. Left corner of the mouth turns up when speaking. Swollen eyelids. Pterygion. Infiltration of the iris or the choroid. Middle ear: inflammation. Pain in the upper vertebrae, C7 through D5. Stinking foot-sweats. Ringworm.

GV-11 *shenzhu* (IS GV-12) — pillar of the body

Back, median line: at the level of the superior interior angle of the scapula. Lower edge of the third dorsal verte-bra (spinous process). Between the fourth and third vertebrae. In the angle between the lower edge of the vertebra and the lateral edge of the median tendon.

Four FW above *shendao* (GV-10, IS GV-11). Four FW under *taodao* (GV-12, IS GV-13). *Feishu* (BL-13) is two FW on either side.

When tonified:

Tonifies the governor vessel, brain, spinal cord, heart and triple warmer. Eyebrows, tongue, throat, bottom of the mouth, cutaneous brachial nerve and ancone.

Direct effects:

Brain, spinal cord, nerves: problems, or weaknesses. Hostility, phobias, hatred, wants to hurt to the point of tears. Delerium from fever, hallucinations. Fits from overexcitation. Fear at night.

Special point for all problems of infants.

Special point for convulsions. For epilepsy with hyperexciation, walking crazily. Congestive headache, cannot vomit?

All the pulses full, or advanced and blocked. Hypertension.

Tongue: inflammation. Great thirst. Throat swollen.

All causes of pain of the back and lumbar area. Bronchitis, contracted panting, heat in the chest. Tonification dilates the bronchioles and the lungs.

Parts of the body:

Eyebrows: all troubles.

Spinal cord: pain.

Arm: cutaneous brachial nerve.

Point of Weihe: Paris Quadrifolia. Constantly clears his throat, hoarseness without pain, mouth dry when waking up, bitter taste; eyes sunken, all problems of the eyebrows, occipital neuralgia, pain at the top of the head; imaginary bad smells; heaviness and fatigue of the nape and shoulder; fingers of the hand numb.

GV-11a [un-named] — third thoracic vertebra

When tonified:

Tonifies the governor vessel, sense organs, temporoparietal lobes.

It has a response in leg-*xialian* (ST-39, IS *xiajuxu*).

Eye: vision; ear: hearing; taste-smell; back of the throat, tongue, nose.

GV-12 *taodao* (IS GV-13 by name) — way of the ovens

Upper back, midline: on the lower edge of the second thoracic vertebra (spinous process). Between the second and third vertebrae and the lateral edge of the median tendon. [This location is different from the usual placement. See GV-13, *bailao,* below. — Trans.]

Four FW above *shenzhu* (GV-11, IS GV-12); two FW below *bailao* (GV-13, IS GV-14 *dazhui*); at two FW on either side is *fengmen* (BL-12).

When tonified:

Tonifies the governor vessel, heart, medulla oblongata, spinal cord, lung, upper limb, cubital nerve, teeth, throat, thyroid, eyes, palm, bladder.

Disperses the gallbladder.

Dispersing acts in the opposite way.

Exhausted from physical or mental effort; melancholy, timidity, searches for solitude and obscurity, loss of voice, hoarseness, short breath, needs alcohol and coffee; delusions without joy; repression and brooding over worries; insomnia from nervous debility.

Diplopia, lateral ocular muscles weakened.

Headache, head heavy, nape tight, eye troubles, painful, vertigo.

Frequent urination at night.

Ulnar nerve (ulnar side), ring-finger, little finger.

Point of Weihe: Coca. Nervous system exhausted from psychological or physical efforts; searches for solitude and obscurity; melancholy; timidity; insomnia from nervous debility; loss of voice; hoarseness, short breath; needs alcohol, coffee, tobacco; at high altitudes: troubles, palpitations, headache, buzzing; dental caries; nocturnal incontinence; diplopia.

GV-13 *bailao* (IS *taodao* by location, IS GV-14 by name) — hundred fatigues

Top of the back, midline: between the second and first thoracic vertebrae (the seventh cervical vertebra being the first which is prominent); two points; in the angle between the median tendon and the deep edge of the thoracic vertebra. Two points separated by the median tendon, each one commanding its side of the body.

Two FW above *taodao* (GV-12 [see preceding point for author's variant location — ed.]); one large FW under C7-pituitary (CV-13a); one medial to *dazhu* (BL-11); two FW inferior and medial to *jianwaishu* (SI-14).

When tonified:
> Tonifies the governor vessel (deep level of the pulse), all yang and yin meridians, conception vessel, opposite part of the brain, posterior upper limb, lateral lower limb, opposite eye, ear same side, nape.
> Dispersing acts in the opposite way.
> First point of the governor vessel, which is linked to the cerebral line starting from the thumb at *guiku* (MP-29a).

Direct effects:
> Strength exhausted, energy finished, sweats from emptiness, exhaustion, prostration, weakness, vertigo, back pain.
> Melancholy, apprehension, neurasthenia.
> Spinal cord: all trouble, degeneration of the spinal cord, spasms and weakness, ascending paralysis, false sclerosis.
> Brain: softening?
> Pernicious anemia.
> Influenza (fever, violent perspiration, weakness), fever from cold; malaise, agitation; tertian fever, great fever, heat of the bones.
> Opposite eye, eyelids same side.
> Ear same side: psychic buzzings?
> Lungs: all problems from tuberculosis, either atonic with exhaustion: tonify; or congestive with hemoptysis, epistaxis: disperse; emphysema, fullness of the sides.
> Gums: inflammation; teeth: the two large incisors dry.
> Vomiting, energy in the upper body, food irritates, jaundice.
> Kidneys: inflammation, urgent need to urinate at night: tonify; or uremia: disperse.
> Prostatitis, prolonged erections, vulvar pruritis.

Opposite effects:
> Skin: the whole body, face, extremities; vasoconstrictor. If pale or cold: disperse; if red, hot: tonify.

Parts of the body:
> Nape, posterior shoulder, anterior upper limb; pain; median nerve. Hands: sensation of puncturing; nape stiff, cannot look behind.
> Anterior thigh and knee.
> Contusions, bruises (important point).

Point of Weihe: Picricum Acidum. (Picric acid destroys colloids, breaks them up): exhaustion, prostration, weakness, vertigo, back pain, neurasthenia; softening of the brain; degeneration of the spinal cord; myelitis with spasms and prostration, contractures, ascending paralysis; pernicious anemia; conjunctivitis; buzzing; urgent needs to urinate at night, small amounts of urine; inflammation of the kidneys, uremia; prostatitis; priapism; vulvar pruritis; prickling of the extremities.

GV-13a IS *dazhui* (IS GV-14) — C7-pituitary

Lower nape, midline: between C7 and T1; in the angle between the lower edge of C7 (the seventh cervical vertebra is the first very prominent vertebra) and either edge of the median tendon. Two points; in a hollow.

One large FW above *bailao* (GV-13, IS *taodao*); one large FW under C6-parathyroids (GV-13b); one FW medial to *jianwaishu* (SI-14).

When tonified:
> Tonifies the pituitary (deficiency), its thirteen hormones and all the endocrines, vagus, adrenals, thyroids, parathyroids, kidneys, lungs, three nervous centers, testicles, ovaries.
> Disperses the pancreas.

Dispersing acts in the opposite way.

Tonifies the adrenals and thyroids through the sympathetic system. The anterior pituitary is dispersed by the ovaries; it increases through the testicles.

Insufficiency:

(From birth) arrogance, diplomacy; loose moral sense; childish mind; cries easily, distracted; lack of attention; asthenia, apathy (adrenalin -); falling hair, teeth; systolic hypotension.

Capillaries and vessels relaxed; (adrenalin -, vasopressin -, corticotropin -, parathyroid -, parasympathetic -), hands red.

Skin humid, sweats, thirst (sympathetic -) pale skin (vitiligo?) (intermedin -, adrenalin +).

Feet becoming flat.

(From birth) small head and mouth and extremities (growth hormone -).

(From birth) late dentition (insufficiency), loose teeth, coming forward, too close, falling.

(From birth) involuntary muscles relaxed, as well as ligaments; (urethra, uterus) little excitability, weak nerves (parathyroid +, corticotropin -, thyroid -, adrenalin -).

Large breasts (mammotropin +, sympathetic +).

Insufficient menses (gonadotropin -, luteotropin -, ovaries -).

Sterility (gonadotropin, estrone -, ovaries -).

Profuse urine, thinness, dehydration (antidiuretic -) from diabetes insipidis.

Becomes fat from work, thin from rest (ovaries -).

Basal metabolism - (thyrotropin -).

Excess:

Strong character; energetic; active; aggressive and masculine women (adrenalin +).

Vivacity, lightness, needs to act (adrenalin +) agitation (thyroid +).

Systolic hypertension.

Capillaries and vessels contracted, extremities cold (the same +).

Skin darkened, brown (from birth), (intermedin +, adrenalin -). Skin dry and sclerosed (sympathetic +). Goosebumps.

Big nose, chin and hands (growth hormone +). Prominent eyes (thyroid +, growth hormone +, adrenalin +).

(From birth) teeth spaced, large (growth hormone +).

Muscles excitable, contracted, cramps, trembling (parathyroid +, corticotropin +, adrenalin +).

Precocious puberty (ovaries +, testicles +), excess libido (gonadotropin +).

Small breasts (mammotropin -, ovaries +); abundant, frequent menses (gonadotropin, luteotropin +, ovaries +) (excess gonadotropin in the urine).

Fecundity (gonadotropin, estrone +, ovaries +).

Profuse urine, thirst (sugar diabetes, diabetogen +, adrenalin +).

Insufficient urine (antidiuretic +, pancreatin +).

Migraines (gonadotropin + in the urine).

Basal metabolism +.

GV-13b [un-named] — C6-parathyroid

Lower nape, midline: between C6 and C7; lower edge of C6; two points; in the angle at either edge of the median tendon; in a hollow.

One large FW above C7-pituitary (CV-13a); one large FW under C5-thyroid (GV-13c).

When tonified:

Tonifies the governor vessel, small intestine, parasympathetic, adrenals (adrenalin), liver, median nerve (thumb, index finger, middle finger); calcium.

Disperses the thyroid, all yang, phosphorus.

Dispersing acts in the opposite way.

It is tonified by small doses of vitamin D (liver -), pituitary, triple warmer (vitamin D is cholesterol that has been transformed into ergosterol by the sun and stored in the liver).

It is dispersed by large doses of vitamin D (liver +); pituitary insufficiency; triple warmer insufficiency; excess proteins, oxalates or citrates in the blood.

Insufficiency:

Excess phosphorus in the blood and urine (insufficient deionized calcium).

Cholesterol, vitamin D in high doses in the blood.

Excess of thyroid.

Insufficiency of the parasympathetic; slow action of adrenalin.

Crying or nocturnal tears. Horror of darkness; nightmares; sad, dispirited, mental instability, agitation.

Always hot.

Hypersensitivity; propensity to neuralgias; arm pain when pressed.

Itching, pruritis.

Trembling, tics, tickling, jerks, cramps, spasms.

Eclampsia, epilepsy, red face; saliva; convulsions.

Contracted muscles.

Stiffness, contracture.

Local edema; permeability of the cells.

Spasmodic hypertension; arterial spasms; vessels and heart contracted (from poisons of the capillaries).

Excess of NaCl stimulating the nervous and sensitive cells; salt poisoning; retracting gums (thyroid -); pyorrhea; loose teeth; saliva, thirst.

Deforming rheumatism?

Excess:

Excess calcium in the blood and urine (ionized calcium).

Cholesterol, vitamin D in low doses in the blood.

Insufficiency of thyroid.

Parasympathetic tonified: better action of adrenalin.

Good sleep.

Excess nitrogen in the blood.

Sometimes hot, sometimes cold.

Epilepsy with pale face, sudden falls.

Muscles soft, weakened.

Hypotonia of the vessels, capillaries and heart.

Liver, small intestine in excess.

GV-13c [un-named] — C5-thyroid

Nape, midline: between C5 and C6, on the lower edge of C5; in the angle on either side of the median tendon; two points.

One large FW above C6-parathyroid (CV-13b); one under *yamen* (GV-14, IS GV-15).

When tonified:

Tonifies (opposite side) thyroid, radial nerves (extensors, supinators); sympathetic system, pituitary, adrenals, governor vessel, small intestine, heart.

Dispersing acts in the opposite way.

Tonified by the pituitary (thyrotropin), parasympathetic.

Dispersed by the adrenals, sympathetic, parathyroids, insufficient iodine, zinc.

Its thyroxin stimulates all the cells (also the cerebral cells), the basal metabolism, phagocytosis and the metabolism of fats and proteins.

Insufficiency:

Understands slowly; apathy, weak intelligence; slow, insufficient memory.

Slow heart (parasympathetic +); hypotension.

Swelling under the eyes or face; obesity.

Hollow eyes, dull (parasympathetic +, sympathetic -); tinnitus or cold in the teeth.

Cold in the eyes; always cold.

Sensitive to the cold; skin cold or dry.

Subcutaneous edema with proteins.

Pale mucus, lips.

Retracted gums.

Dull nails, soft (parathyroid -).

Chronic coryza.

No appetite, slow digestion (parasympathetic -).

Insufficient menses, sterility (parasympathetic -).

Insufficient basal metabolism (pituitary, adrenals -).

(From birth); eyebrows spaced at the extremities; precocious white hair or baldness; children: late development; falling teeth, ossified.

In the extreme: myxedema, cretinism.

Excess:

Understands quickly, speaks rapidly, quick but superficial intelligence, easily angry, sensitive, passionate but unfaithful.

Rapid heart, anxiety, insomnia.

Trembling hands (sympathetic +, parasympathetic -).

Thinness.

Prominent eyes, bright (sympathetic +).

Always hot, sensitive to the heat, flushes of heat or perspiration (parasympathetic +).

Increased sensitivity to adrenalin.

Redness of the mucus, lips and skin.

Decalcified teeth, frequent caries.

Hard, bright nails (parathyroid +).

Spasmodic constipation, spasms (parathyroid -).

Large appetite (parasympathetic +).

Abundant menses, (parasympathetic, pituitary +).

Vulvar pruritis.

Raised metabolism (pituitary +, adrenals +).

(From birth) Tendency to goiter, to angina of the chest, to Basedow's disease, to a collapse of the heart. Prominent teeth; small abdomen; precocious development, young for a long time.

Instability gives some qualities of excess in an insufficiency, and vice versa: sudden congestions, sudden secretions, asthma, migraines, urticaria or uremia.

Point of Weihe: Lathyrus Sat.

GV-14   *yamen* (IS GV-15) — door of muteness

Nape, midline: between the fourth and third cervical vertebrae, on the lower edge of the third vertebra; in the angle of the median tendon; two points, separated by the tendon. [This is a variant location. The IS location is between the second and first cervical vertebrae. — Ed.]

One FW above C5-thyroid (CV-13c); one under *fengfu* (GV-15, IS GV-16).

When tonified:

Tonifies the governor vessel, spinal cord, temporoparietal lobes, fingers and toes, oblique muscles, transverse muscles, nose, larynx, tongue, back of the throat.

Dispersing acts in the opposite way.

Direct effects:

Speech (temporoparietal lobes) and tongue; spinal cord, four limbs.

Abundant energy in the upper body, all yang heat? Constant headaches; pain at the occiput; incessant nosebleeds; cerebral congestion; meningitis; inflammation of the spinal cord; convulsions; no resistance to fatigue.

Speech and making sounds difficult, speaks with effort, forms words with difficulty; tongue heavy, knotted, tight, contracted; swelling under the tongue.

Paralysis of the hyoidian muscle; sudden loss of ability to make a sound.

Cramps, agitation, trembling, tics.

Spinal cord: excess or insufficiency, inflammation; four extremities: temperature, sensitivity or motor function, cold in the extremities.

Parts of the body:

Painful, injured nerves.

Painful body: cannot twist; oblique and transverse muscles of the abdomen.

Posterior arm, dorsal forearm, radial nerve.

Point of Weihe: Menyanthes Trifoliatum. Agitation; involuntary movements; tics, cramps, discharge in the legs; icy cold extremities; headaches with pressure on top of the head; pains in the brain, nape, occiput; never thirsty; hunger leaves with the first mouthful; distended abdomen; diabetes; aggravated from tobacco.

GV-15 *fengfu* (IS GV-16) — workshop of the wind [neuralgias]

Nape, midline: between the third and second cervical vertebrae (the first is not visible); on the lower edge of the second vertebra; two points; in the angle on the lateral edge of the medial tendon. [This is a variant location. The IS location is in the depression directly below the external occipital protruberance. — Ed.]

One FW above *yamen* (GV-14, IS GV-15 by name); one under *naohu* (GV-16, IS GV-17 by name, IS GV-15 by location); one small FW medial to *tianzhu* (BL-10).

When tonified:

Tonifies the governor vessel, adrenals, anterior and central brain (vagus), cervical muscles, all yang producer meridians, lower limbs.

Disperses all yin distributor meridians, pancreas.

Dispersing acts in the opposite way.

Direct effects:

(Yin-yang, adrenals, pancreas; fever, flu, posterior surface of the arm and leg).

All mental troubles: desires to commit suicide; darting eyes; escapades (walks blindly without direction).

All sorts of fever.

Influenza (shivering, perspiration, fever, heat or cold, headaches, exhausted body).

Harmonizes yin and yang; hypertension: disperse; hypotension: tonify; nosebleeds, apoplexy.

Cerebral edema (pain and stiffness of the nape and occiput, headache, vertigo); throat: all trouble — pain or swelling, paralysis, energy going towards the heart.

Eyes same side: brown specks (from excess urea).

Ears same side.

Teeth: particularly incisors: loose.

Lower gums: pain.

Stomach: acidity one hour after pastries or jams and jelly: disperse (adrenals in excess inhibit the production of insulin in the pancreas and stimulate the liver to transform much more glycogen into sugar); sugar diabetes: disperse.

Phrenic nerve.

Parts of the body:

Upper shoulder same side: pain or stiffness, following a chill or fatigue; lower limbs same side, posterior surface: gives a lighter step.

Buttocks and lumbar area: pain, weakness.

Adrenals (right V superficial pulse): tonified by pituitary, thyroid, parathyroids, sympathetic system, spinal cord, calcium; dispersed by pancreas, potassium, parasympathetic system.

The adrenals tonify the pituitary, sympathetic system; they disperse the pancreas, thyroid, ovaries, parasympathetic system.

Their hormones are (from the cortex): estrogen, androgen, corticotropin (from the medulla), adrenalin. They are heat producing, antitoxic, circulation facilitating (except coronary arteries and brain) and hyperglycemic; they cause mydriasis and exophthalmia. Their prolonged use hardens the internal tissue of the arteries and artheroma. At 1/1000 dilution, they render the mucosa bloodless. They stimulate the tubules to reabsorb sugar and to diminish the absorption of potassium and urea (from adrenocortical hormones).

One adrenal can be insufficient and the other in excess.

Insufficiency:

Apathy (pituitary -, Na -, K +). Asthenia, no resistance to cold, to fatigue, to infections (pituitary -); slow recuperation (small intestine -); work difficult, slow, needs sleep, tired in the morning (spleen -); weak to painful muscles, myasthenia (pituitary -, parathyroid +); always cold, cold and wet extremities (pituitary -, parasympathetic +); thinness and weakness (pituitary -); cold in the eyes (small intestine -); slow coagulation of blood (liver, large intestine -).

Volume of blood increased.

Contracted coronary arteries, hypotension.

Permeability of the capillaries, edema (pituitary -).

Cutaneous arterioles relaxed (blue, red hands) (pituitary -), Raynaud's disease.

Heart slow or quick and small (K +).

Relaxed vessels.

Kidney filtration increased, reabsorption diminished, salt diminished.

Salt and sugar insufficient.

Urea, potassium in excess (and salt).
Excess insulin (injected) convulsions.
Atonic stomach (parasympathetic -).
Atonic gallbladder.
Slow and colored urine.
Large intestine relaxed.
Small intestine relaxed.
Insufficient ovaries, weak menses, big breasts (pituitary -).
Cervix contracted.
Frigidity of women.
Men: rapid ejaculation, weak erection.

Excess:
Active, energetic (pituitary +, Na +, K -).
Resistant to shock, fatigue, cold, infection.
Irritable, works without stopping, needs to act (pituitary +); no need of sleep.
Wakes soon.
Strong muscles (pituitary +, parathyroid -).
Always hot (pituitary +).
Hypertonic obesity, plethora.
Quick coagulation of blood (liver, large ingestine +)
Insufficient blood volume.
Dilated coronary arteries, hypertension.
Contracted capillaries (pituitary +).
Contracted cutaneous arterioles (pituitary +).
Energetic heart with blood volume.
Tone of vessels increased to sclerosis.
Kidney filtration diminished, reabsorption and salt increased.
Urea and potassium insufficient (and salt).
Salt and sugar in excess; cholesterol.
Acute edema of the lungs or blocked nose.
Burning of stomach one hour after food.
Insufficient insulin, hyperglycemia (pancreas -); eyes prominent, mydriasis (sympathetic +).
Esophagus, cardiac sphincter contracted, hiccoughs, vomiting, spasms of diaphragm.
Contracted stomach, acidity.
Gallbladder contracted and Oddi's sphincter relaxed.
Insufficiency of spleen. Kidneys: abundant, clear urine, contracted bladder, relaxed sphincter.
Large intestine contracted, spasms, constipation, anal sphincter relaxed.
Small intestine contracted, inflamed.
Stimulated ovaries, abundant menses, large fatty breasts.
Cervix relaxed, dilated.
Women: sexual obsession, vulvar pruritis.
Men: sexual hyperexcitation.

Point of Weihe: Cuprum Arseniatum or Arsenicosum. Arrhythmia, contractions, cramps in the calf after midnight; gangrene; cerebral edema, headaches, vertigo, insufficient kidneys; diabetes, diarrhea from tuberculosis; convulsions after gastroenteritis.

GV-16 *naohu* (IS GV-17 by name, IS GV-15 by location) — little brain barrier

Nape, midline: one large FW under the skull; between the first and second cervical vertebrae; two points; in the angle between the lateral edge of the medial tendon and the lower edge of the first vertebra (hardly perceptible); in a hollow.

One FW above *fengfu* (GV-15, IS GV-16 by name only); two under *qiangjian* (GV-17, IS GV-18 by name, GV-16 by location).

When tonified:
Tonifies the governor vessel, stomach, cerebellum, bladder, *zhongzhu* (TW-3), upper cheek same side, tonsils, lateral part of the eye same side, middle and internal ear, joints, skin opposite side.
Disperses the vessels and genital system.

Dispersing acts in the opposite way.

Direct effects:

Insomnia before midnight; extreme agitation; congestive headache, red face; cerebral congestion.

Eye, rheumatic iritis: swollen eyelids; orbits?

Ear: inflammation of the internal ear.

Teeth: seem long and loose, particularly upper.

Swelling and with pain: of the head, eyelids, nipples, vulva (with pruritis); of the fingers, feet at night; tumors.

Pains aggravated at night, in the evening, in the bed, from rest.

Joints, ligaments, tendons: rheumatism, pain.

Skin: red, swollen, itching, cellulitis, erysipelas, chicken pox.

Mucus.

Fibrous tissues?

Point of Weihe: Rhus Radicans, same as Rhus Tox (see *zhongji*, CV-3). Aggravated at night in bed, when at rest; rheumatic pains, joint pains, or tendons or ligaments or fibrous tissues; afflictions of the mucosa. Skin: red, swollen, itching, cellulitis, erysipelas, herpes, chicken pox; facial neuralgia aggravated at night; red nose; cellulitis of the orbit; iritis even with pus; swollen eyelids; painful gums; teeth seem long and loose, swelling of the breasts, swelling of the vulva with pruritis; swelling of the fingers; swelling of the feet in the evening; swelling of stomach; colored urine; extreme agitation; insomnia before midnight.

GV-17   *qiangjian* (IS GV-18 by name, IS GV-16 *fengfu* by location)   — stiff interval

Nape, midline: in the angle between the lower edge of the cranium and the lateral edge of the medial tendon; two points separated by the median tendon.

Two FW above *naohu* (GV-16, IS GV-17 by name, IS GV-15 by location); four below *houding* (GV-18, IS GV-19); one large FW below and medial to *yuzhen* (BL-9).

When tonified:

Tonifies all the energy of the governor vessel, medulla oblongata, superior occipital lobe, primate, inner ear, fallopian tubes, lower part of the sacrum, genital system, half-body opposite side.

Dispersing acts in the opposite way.

Direct effects:

Medulla oblongata (respiration, deglutition, saliva, vomiting, movement of eyes and eyelids. Tonifying nearly doubles the energy potential.

Insomnia; weakness of the nerves; hysteria? convulsions, convulsions of children; epilepsy, attacks without cause (convulsions, saliva, nausea), escapades (walks blindly without direction); vertigo, head spinning, headache, stiff nape, obscured vision.

Parts of the body:

Head feels as if pierced with a needle, nape as if torn out.

Opposite nape and lateral part of neck, cervical vertebrae, stiffness, cannot turn the head; movements of the head.

Angle of the maxilla and back molars.

Opposite upper and lower limbs.

GV-18   *houding* (IS GV-19)   — posterior summit of the head

Posterior top of the skull, midline: two FW posterior to the occipitoparietal suture; at the upper edge of a large protuberance; two points on either side of the vertical groove.

Four FW above *qiangjian* (GV-17, IS GV-18 by name, IS GV-16 by location); two tightened FW below *baihui* (GV-19, IS GV-20).

When tonified:

Tonifies the governor vessel, superior occipital lobe, primate, face (eye along the nose, corner of the lips, chin, throat); stomach, occiput, nape, posterior part of the shoulder same side, all articulations same side.

Dispersing acts in the opposite way.

Direct effects:

Yang heat (upper body, skin); insomnia; headache, migraine; facial neuralgia (line along the eyes, edge of the nose, corner of the lips, teeth, chin).

Hyperexcitation from attacks, insanity; cerebral congestion.
Convulsions, epilepsy, vertigo, dizziness.
Eyes: obscured vision.

Parts of the body:
Articular rheumatism, same side, with sweat and diarrhea.
Nape stiff and hard.

GV-19   *baihui* (IS GV-20) — hundred meetings

Head, posterior top: posterior fontanelle; midline; suture of the occiput and parietal bones. At the level of the posterior edge of two small rises; in a hollow; two points on either side of the groove.

Two FW above *houding* (GV-18, IS GV-19); two behind *qianding* (GV-20, IS GV-21); one large FW medial to *luoque* (BL-8).

When tonified:
Tonifies the governor vessel, conception vessel, superior occipital lobes, primate, all yang producer meridians, anterior midbrain, parasympathetic, face (line along eye, edge of the nose, corner of the lip, teeth, throat); anus, anterior part of thigh, opposite knee.
Dispersing acts in the opposite way.

Direct effects:
Awakens a response in leg-*shanglian* (ST-37, IS *shangjuxu*).
Cures all troubles, vegetal vitality, will to live; psychologically, primitive instincts, primate.
Energy of the posterior brain (primate, color).
Insufficiency: brain and nerves overtight, weakened; strength of mind diminished from too many worries and thoughts; forgets the past and neglects the future; loss of memory; difficult, constricted speech, melancholy, anxiety; depression, deranged mind, despondency, sadness, troubles with tears at night; loss of the sense of reality; delusions; insomnia; headache; cerebral anemia with weakness.
Excess: acute or chronic meningitis; hyperexcited children bending backwards; all nervous troubles; epilepsy (body bent backwards, bleating); hemiplegia?
After drinking, red face, congested brain, heavy head.
Facial neuralgia (eyes, along the nose, corner of the mouth, first molars, throat).
Upper eyelid (common occular motor nerve).
Facial paralysis (eyes cannot be closed: disperse; cannot be opened: tonify).
Inner ear, buzzing? psychological deafness.
Smell and taste (drink and food without taste).
Nose: all trouble, coryza (recent: disperse; old: tonify); nose blocked, headache, vertigo, flowing tears.
Anus: hemorrhoids, prolapsed rectum.
Testicles: attacks of swelling?

GV-20   *qianding* (IS GV-20) — anterior summit

Head, top, midline: mid-distance between the frontal and occipital bones; in a transverse fissure (sagittal plane); on the anterior edge of the posterior relief; two points on either side of the groove between the parietal bones.

Two FW in front of *baihui* (GV-19, IS GV-20); two behind *xinhui* (GV-21, IS GV-22); one large FW medial to *tongtian* (BL-7).

When tonified:
Tonifies the governor vessel, temporoparietal lobes; automaton-parrot, stomach, temples, cheekbone, corner of the mouth, tongue — all opposite; cervical vertebrae, opposite.
Dispersing acts in the opposite way.

Direct effects:
Awakens a response in leg-*xialian* (ST-39, IS *xiajuxu*).
Congestive headache (red face, heavy head, dizziness); cerebral congestion; cerebral anemia. (Acts on the temporoparietal lobes and memories); cervical vertebrae.
Children: tonic convulsions (with spasms); epilepsy? from sadness or despair.
Ear opposite.
Nose: coryza, abundant flow, nose blocked, sinusitis.
Edema?

Parts of the body:
 Face: temple, cheekbone, corner of the mouth, tongue; neuralgia and facial paralysis; face: swelling and redness.
 Head: swelling, pain, heat? pain at the top of the head.
 Cervical vertebra opposite side: nape, occiput.

GV-21   *chuanghui* (IS GV-22, IS *xinhui*) — meeting of the brain

Head, anterior top, midline: posterior edge of the frontal bone between the two parietal bones (fontanelles). Two points on either side of the groove between the parietal bones (acts on the opposite half of the brain).

Two FW in front of *qianding* (GV-20, IS GV-21); two FW behind *shangxing* (GV-22, IS GV-23); one large FW medial to *wuchu* (BL-5).

When tonified:
 Tonifies the opposite brain, all yin and yang meridians, whole face same side, fingers and dorsum of toes same side, tonifies the yang energy of the whole body.
 Disperses the conception vessel.
 Dispersing acts in the opposite way.

Direct effects:
 Awakens a response in *fenglong* (ST-40).
 Energy and vitality of the whole body, movements, heat.
 Anterior brain, true energy, vitality, evolved man, association of ideas, of sensations, of images; concentration, imagination. 1) Insufficiency: cerebral anemia, rapid fatigue of the brain, moments of weakness, foggy to the point of cerebral confusion; emotional agitation, deranged mind, bluish-white complexion, somnolence, weakness of the blood. 2) Excess: cerebral congestion, heat and pain in the brain as if broken, congested face, nosebleeds, vertigo, nose blocked. Congestion of face and head from drink.
 Excess blood.
 Psychological hearing: hears sounds, but comprehends the meaning poorly.[2]
 Hair: dry seborrhea, pellicle; swelling of the skin of the head.

GV-22   *shangxing* (IS GV-23) — superior star

Head, anterior top, midline, on the frontal bone: at about two FW in front of its suture with the two parietal bones (fontanelle); posterior (upper) edge of a slight rise on a plateau in a little hollow; two points on either side of the hollow.

Two FW in front of *xinhui* (GV-21, IS GV-22); two FW behind (below) *zhongting* (GV-23, IS GV-24); one FW medial and a little below *qucha* (BL-4).

When tonified:
 Tonifies the governor vessel, heart, vessels, liver, opposite cerebellum, eyeball same side, nostrils same side, mouth, gums and upper teeth.
 Disperses the small intestine, large intestine, triple warmer.
 Dispersing acts in the opposite way.

Direct effects:
 Energy rising to the head, face, eyes, throat.
 Eyes: glaucoma (congestion and hardness of the eyeball, pain of the pupil, headache, dizziness), myopia, trouble of the eyes, cataract, inflammation of the cornea (keratitis).
 Nose: coryza, clear or thick discharge, sensitive eyes, visual dizziness to the point where the nose is blocked, nosebleeds.
 Red face, easy congestion of the face, swelling and pain of the forehead, swelling of the face.
 Head: skin of the skull swollen.
 False croup.
 Hiccoughs.
 Intermittent fever, red face, shivering; fever without sweat?

GV-23   *shenting* (IS GV-24) — palace of the evolved man

Top of the forehead, midline: on the upper edge of the vertical medial relief (''Column of Life''); about mid-distance from the line of the eyebrow to the posterior (upper) edge of the frontal bone; two points separated by a narrow rise. They act on the opposite side.

Two FW in front of *shangxing* (GV-22, IS GV-23); on the forehead, four FW above *yintang* (GV-23a, IS M-HN-3); one large FW medial to head-*lingqi* (GB-11, IS GB-15).

When tonified:

Tonifies the gallbladder, opposite frontal lobes, evolved man, stomach, nose opposite side, opposite eye; bladder.

Dispersing acts in the opposite way.

Direct effects:

Awakens a response in *fenglong* (ST-40).

Psychological and cerebral hyperexcitation.

Excessive sadness, sobbing, pulls out the hair, cannot sleep, apprehension, anxiety; cerebral hyperexcitation, jumps up on tables, sings, takes off one's clothes (after malaria?); depression, tongue out.

Migraines (with) photophobia, nausea, vomiting.

Eyes swollen, veil over the eyes; catarrh of the lacrimal glands.

Nose: coryza, clear discharge, acute inflammation; bronchi: asthma.

Heart: palpitations.

Forehead: pain.

GV-23a   *yintang* (IS M-HN-3) — room of the seal

Between the eyebrows, midline: in the suture of the frontal and vomer bones; two points each in the angle of the upper edge between the extremity of the brow ridge and a vertical relief; acts on the opposite side.

About four FW below *shenting* (GV-23, IS GV-24); at the tip of the nose: *suliao* (GV-24, IS GV-25); one FW on either side of *zanzhu* (BL-2).

When tonified:

Tonifies the governor vessel (deep level), heart, lung, triple warmer, gallbladder, medulla oblongata, spinal cord, superior occipital lobe, primate, muscles of the opposite half-body.

Dispersing acts in the opposite way.

Direct effects:

Children: convulsions from high fever during dentition; all cramps, spasms, contractions from emotional agitation, etc., opposite side: disperse.

Acute or chronic meningitis (''cured if with great cries'').

Acute: disperse; chronic: tonify.

Violent sweating of the head.

Jiujitsu: knock-out point; yoga: chakra of the entrance of the brain, ''thousand petalled lotus'' [the ''thousand petalled lotus'' is traditionally above *baihui* (GV-19, IS GV-20) — Trans.].

GV-24   *suliao* (IS GV-25) — simple hole

Tip of the nose, midline: just above the small ball forming the tip of the nose; two points acting on the opposite sides.

Between the eyebrows: *yintang* (GV-23a, IS M-HN-3); above the upper lip: *shuigou* (GV-25, IS *renzhong*, GV-26). On either side between the nostrils and the tip is *bizhun* (MP-1). On the lateral edge of the nostril is *yingxiang* (LI-20).

When tonified:

Tonifies all the yin and yang meridians and governor vessel.

Dispersing acts in the opposite way.

''Can provide for all that has been neglected during a treatment.''

Dispersing can awaken from drunkenness.

Tears in excess.

Nose: abundant and clear discharge, nose blocked, often on one side; growths, abscesses in the nose.

Dyspnea, contracted respiration.

GV-25   *shuigou* (IS GV-26, IS *renzhong*) — drainage ditch (IS man's center)

Face, a little below the nose, midline: on the upper edge of a flat muscle (orbicular muscle of the lips); in a vertical groove of the upper lip; two points on either side of this groove.

On the tip of the nose, *suliao* (GV-24, IS GV-25); on the line of the upper lip, *duiduan* (GV-26, IS GV-27); one FW on either side is nose-*heliao* (LI-19).

When tonified:

Tonifies the governor vessel, large intestine, anterior and posterior frontal lobes, pituitary gland with C-8, conception vessel; general energy. Because of the sensitivity of the upper lip one should avoid needles and moxa; massage acts well, as does sonopuncture.

Disperses the kidney, same side.

Responds in *yangxi* (LI-5).

Direct effects:

General energy (potential energy as measured by apparatus). Massaging awakens from fainting from weakness: disperse for congestion; pituitary.

Moral and mental depression ("loss of one's laughter for a long time," "seized by ghosts"; hyperexcitation and instability, "alternates from sobbing to joy," "speaks without distinguishing respectable people from coarse people").

Acute or chronic meningitis; epilepsy? cerebral congestion; loss of smell (anosmia).

Diabetes (intense thirst, drinks endlessly): eyes unable to look.

Epidemic jaundice, whole body yellow.

Opposite effects:

Edema: tonify; generalized edema (anasarca).

Parts of the body:

Face: facial paralysis (of the facial nerve: mouth awry, corner flaccid, cannot speak): tonify the flaccid side, disperse the side which pulls; facial contraction (movements of the mouth and eye, lips trembling), jaw contracted, trismus.

Vertebrae: acute pain of the seventh cervical, paralysis or deviation of the thoracic spine, lumbar area curved, cannot straighten, acute pain from the lumbar area to the feet on the opposite side, pain and stiffness of all vertebrae on the opposite side (governor vessel).

Jiujitsu: knockout point.

GV-26 *duiduan* (IS GV-27) — prominent extremity

Upper lip (fold), midline: just at the upper edge of the red mucosal tissue. *Shuigou* (GV-25, IS GV-26 *renzhong*) under the nose; Gum-*yinjiao* (GV-27, IS GV-28) on the gum.

When tonified:

Tonifies the governor vessel, all yang meridians, midbrain.

Disperses all the yin meridians.

Dispersing acts in the opposite way.

Direct effects:

Clattering of the teeth, teeth contracted, saliva, epilepsy?

Nose: prolonged bleeding, nose blocked.

Jaundice?

Diabetes?

GV-27 *yinjiao* (IS GV-28) — crossing of the gums

Upper gum, midline: lower edge of the septum; between the two large incisors; two points.

Preceding point: *duiduan* (GV-26, IS GV-27). A branch going around the lips is connected to the conception vessel (at *chengjiang,* CV-24).

When tonified:

Tonifies the governor vessel, conception vessel, stomach, eyes, mouth, root of the nose, nape, maxilla.

Dispersing acts in the opposite way.

Direct effects:

Eyes: conjunctivitis (tears, oozing from the eyes, inflammation of the medial corner, pain, itching), keratitis, cataract.

Epidemics from hot or cold weather.

Teeth loose, alveolar pyorrhea, bleeding gums, falling teeth.

Nose blocked, abscesses of the nose, phagedenic abscesses.

Parts of the body:

Face: freckles; children: facial abscesses.

Mid-forehead, root of the nose: pain.

Mouth: pain, cannot open; maxilla: pain.

Nape: pain, as if torn out, tight.

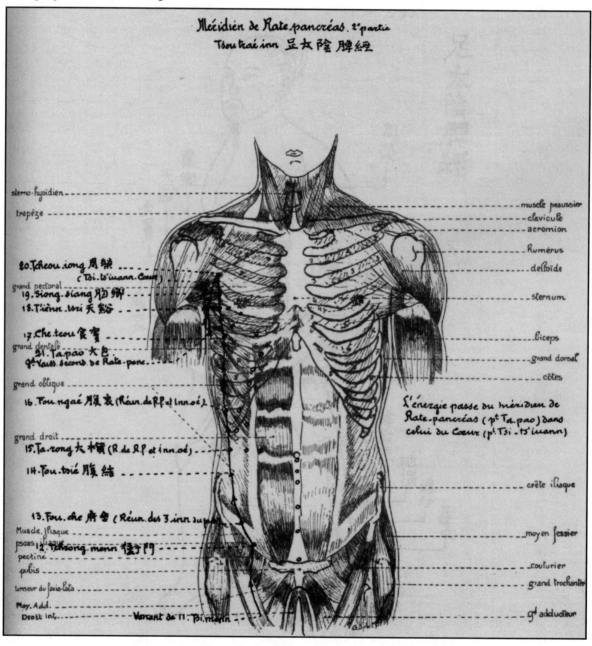

Meridian of the spleen-pancreas (part 2) (GSDM)

Notes

[1] The last works of the author seem to demonstrate that points BL-31, BL-32, BL-33, BL-34, BL-35 of the bladder meridian can be linked to the governor vessel between the points GV-2 and GV-3. — ed.

[2] This refers to psychological hearing impairment, as opposed to a physiological impairment. — Trans.

Part III

Points Outside The Meridians

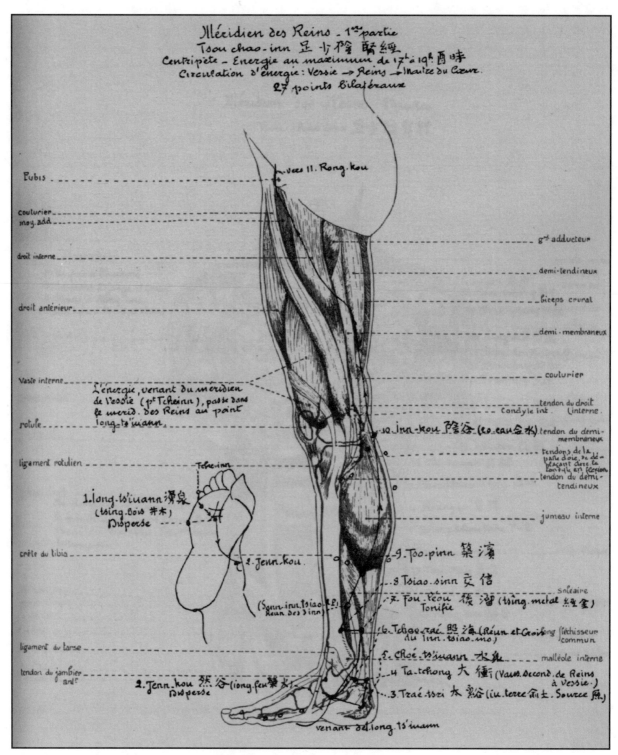

Meridian of the kidneys (part 1) (GSDM)

Jing Wai Qi Xue

"The Marvellous Points Outside the Meridians"

In addition to descriptions of the meridians and their points, the old tradition describes some points, discovered around the same time, called "marvellous points outside the meridians." It appears, after considering certain texts, that they wanted to keep the number of points on the meridians equal to a total of 365, the same as the number of days in the annual solar revolution.

However, after close examination of these "marvellous points," we find a certain number which are on the course of the meridians and which awaken a response in the meridian and the organ, in the upstream and downstream points and in the interrelated organs. They thus actually belong to the meridian on which they are located. Having no obligation to maintain the number 365 as the total for the points, we have decided that it is permissible to include them on the meridians. However, in respect for tradition, all the reasoning of which is probably not known, we have given them the letter "a" or "b" on the meridian.

The other points are really located "outside the meridians." We refer to them as MP (marvellous points). They act not only on a meridian and an organ, but also on either local or distant areas. Thus, *taiyang* of the temple (MP-3, IS M-HN-9) acts on the lateral edge of the thumb and the second and third cervical vertebrae.

We have classified them by areas, beginning the numbering from the head.

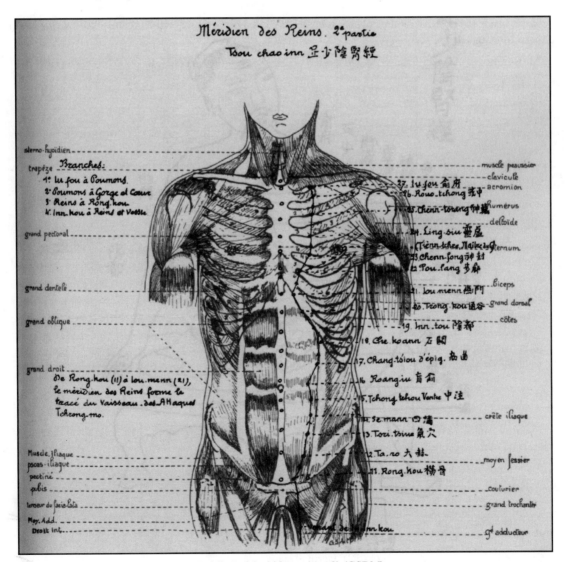

Meridian of the kidneys (part 2) (GSDM)

Chapter I
Marvellous Points of the Head

MP-1   *bizhun* — tip of the nose

Lateral tip of the nose: two points, each in the angle between the upper edge of the nostrils and the lateral edge of the medial cartilage.

One half FW on either side of *suliao* (GV-24, IS GV-25); one half FW on either side of the nostril is *yingxiang* (LI-20).

When tonified:
Tonifies the anterior frontal lobes, nose, eyes.
Dispersing acts in the opposite way.

Direct effects:
''Dissipates all manifestations of wine (drunkenness) on the nose.''

MP-2   *neiyingxiang* (IS M-NH-35) — smell of the internal perfume

Nose, inside the nostrils, on the concha: long needle; two points, one in either nostril: bleed the points (not very highly recommended).

Above *shuigou* (GV-25, IS GV-26, *renzhong*); on the nose: *suliao* (GV-24, IS GV-25), *bizhun* (MP-1).

Direct effects:
Eyes: violent pain and heat.

MP-3   *taiyang* (IS M-HN-9) — supreme yang

Temple: one FW above the lateral prominent angle of the eyebrow arch. In the inferior angle of a curve of the frontal-sphenoid suture, on the sphenoid; on the anterior edge of an arteriole.

Two FW under *touwei* (ST-1, IS ST-8); two above *chengqi* (ST-4, IS ST-1).

Just in front of the stomach meridian; two close FW anterior to *hanyan* (GB-4).

When tonified:
Tonifies the lower posterior frontal lobes, opposite eye, skin of the cheek, upper premolars, lateral side of the thumb.
Dispersing acts in the opposite way.

Direct effects:
Eyes red, swollen, to the point of headaches: bleed (disperse).
Skin from the cheekbone to the nose, upper premolars (trigeminal neuralgia).
Lateral side of thumb: long and short opposing abductors.

MP-4   *yuyao* (IS M-HN-4) — lumbar area of the fish

Eyebrow, mid-length, just on the lower edge of the crest of the eyebrow arch. In a hollow; on the lateral edge of the insertion of the muscle of the eyebrow: puncture towards the nose.

Two tight FW lateral to *zanzhu* (BL-2).

When tonified:
Tonifies the inferior occipital lobe, eye same side, levator palpebrae superioris, superciliary muscle.
Dispersing acts in the opposite way.

Direct effects:
Eye same side: cataract (''falling veil''), lacrimal canal.
Upper eyelid falling: tonify; cannot close: disperse; acts also on the lower lid and the orbicular muscle.
Superciliary muscle: eyebrows cannot be lifted: tonify; too lifted: disperse.

MP-5 *haiquan* (IS M-HN-37) — source of the seal

Tongue: inferior surface, mid-width, mid-length, "in the middle of the vessels."

When tonified:
Tonifies the pancreas, tongue.
Disperses the adrenals, posterior part of the liver.
Dispersing acts in the opposite way.

Direct effects:
Diabetes.
Swollen painful tongue.

MP-6 *jinzhen* [or *jinjin*] (IS M-HN-20b) — gold needle [or gold liquid]

Lower surface of the tongue, left side, "on the purple vessel," about mid-length; fold the tongue.

When dispersed:
Disperses the tongue, gullet.

Direct effects:
Larynx and opposite side of gullet: pain, swelling.
Tongue heavy, swollen, painful.

MP-7 *yuye* (IS M-HN-20a) — secretion of jade

Lower surface of the tongue: mid-length, right side, "on the purple vessel."

When dispersed:
Disperses the tongue, gullet.

Direct effects:
Larynx and opposite gullet: pain, swelling.
Tongue heavy, swollen, painful.

MP-8 *juquan* (IS M-HN-36) — rising source

Tip of the tongue, upper surface, mid-width, in a fine groove.

When dispersed:
Disperses the throat, bronchus, trachea.

Direct effects:
Cough and old asthma that remain uncured.

MP-9 *erjian* (IS M-HN-10) — point of the ear

Earlobe, anterior surface of the posterior edge, mid-height at the lower point of the cartilage.

When tonified:
Tonifies the inferior occipital lobes, superior frontal lobes, eyes same side, lumbar area, lower limb same side.

Direct effects:
Cataract starting on same side.
Lumbar area and lower limb same side: pain, sciatica and lumbar neuralgia.

Chapter II
Marvellous Points of the Upper Limb

MP-10 *jianzhugu* — bony column of the shoulder [acromion]

Extremity of the shoulder, on the lateral edge and mid-width to the bone (acromion).

In the articulation with the head of the humerus; in a hollow of the bone.

When tonified:
  Tonifies the lower posterior frontal lobes, large intestine (without acting on the kidney), triple warmer, lateral part of the neck, arm, dorsum of hand and fingers.
  Dispersing acts in the opposite way.

Direct effects:
  Ganglions.
  Arm-shoulder articulation.
  Arm cannot be lifted to the side from contracture or weakness; deltoid; supraspinatus and infraspinatus muscles (antagonists — posterior muscles: *jianzhen,* SI-9; anterior muscles: *binao,* LI-14).
  Hand cannot be lifted or moved; finger joints swollen, arthritic, or painful, contracted, or weak, flaccid.

MP-11 *zhoujian* (IS M-UE-46) — point of the elbow

Point of the elbow (the olecronon), elbow flexed, in a small hollow.

When tonified:
  Tonifies the posterior frontal and temporoparietal lobes.
  Disperses the lymph nodes of the neck, nape, armpit, anterior part of the neck and throat.
  Dispersing acts in the opposite way.

Direct effects:
  Lymph nodes on the lateral part of the neck, or nape or armpit same side.
  Submaxillary glands same side.

MP-12 *erbai* (IS M-UE-29) — two whites

Anterior surface of the forearm: four FW above the wrist; two points: 1) Radial point, on the inferior edge of the transverse mass and the radial edge of the flexor carpi radialis muscle; between it and the radial artery; in a hollow. 2) Ulnar point: on the inferior edge of the transverse mass and the ulnar edge of the medial tendons (flexors); in a hollow.

When tonified:
  Tonifies the lower posterior frontal lobes, palm of hand; anus.
  Dispersing acts in the opposite way.

Direct effects:
  Anus: hemorrhoids, fistulas, fissures, prolapsed rectum.
  Hand, palm (palmar aponeurosis).
  Radial point: thumb (flexor pollicis longus muscle) and the index finger (flexors: contracture, spasms or flaccidity, weakness).
  Ulnar point: ring and little finger (flexors: contracture, spasms or flaccidity, weakness).

Chapter III
Marvellous Points of the Hands and Fingers

MP-13 *wailaogong* (IS M-UE-23) — external palace of the fatigues

Dorsum of the hand, center: mid-length on the third metacarpal (middle finger), on the lateral edge (medial surface towards the fourth metacarpal of the ring finger), upper edge (posterior) of the insertion (of the third interosseus muscle); in a hollow.

Three FW above *zhongquan* (MP-14, IS M-UE-33); two FW posterior and medial to *shangdu* (MP-16, IS M-UE-23b); two FW above *xiadu* (MP-18, IS M-UE-23c); two FW under and lateral to *zhongzhu* (TW-3); three FW medial to *sanjian* (LI-3).

When tonified:
Tonifies the mid-brain, vessels, heart, lateral lower leg.
Disperses the triple warmer.

Direct effects:
Dispersing acts in the opposite way.
Hypertension: vessels and heart contracted: disperse.
Hypotension: vessels and heart weakened, cold at the extremities.
In winter: external body cold, congestion of the internal organs: tonify.
Hand contracted, fingers tightened: tonify.
A violent blow here can cause fainting.

MP-13a *weiling* — prestigious immateriality

Hand, palmar surface: lateral edge of the large muscle at the base of the thumb; thenar eminence; mid-length of the metacarpal of the thumb, the hand in supination.

Two FW under, in front of, and slightly lateral to *yuji* (LU-10); two FW from and level to *hegu* (LI-4).

Direct effects:
Massage point for children.
Acute meningitis of children.

MP-14 *zhongquan* (IS M-UE-33) — central source

Dorsal wrist, about mid-width: in the angle between the inferior (anterior) edge of the head of the radius and the medial edge (medial side of the little finger) of the tendon of the posterior radial muscle (insertion on the third metacarpal); in a hollow.

Three FW lateral and a little above *yangchi* (TW-4); two large FW medial to *yangxi* (LI-5); three FW above (behind) *wailaogong* (MP-13, IS M-UE-23).

Responds with *pianli* (LI-6), *wailaogong* (MP-13, IS M-UE-23), *shangdu* (MP-16, IS M-UE-23b), *zhongchong* (PC-9), and *shangyang* (LI-1).

Direct effects:
Anterior knee.
Heart: pains.
Large intestine: unbearable pains.
Wrist: pains, rheumatism or weakness.

MP-15 *dadu* (IS M-UE-23a) — great capital

Dorsum of hand: muscular articulation of the thumb and index finger; on the edge of the white skin; on the inferior edge of the first interosseus muscle, dorsal side; on the edge of an artery towards the index finger; in a hollow.

Two FW under (in front of) *hegu* (LI-4); one FW lateral to *sanjian* (LI-3): evokes a response in the large intestine meridian.

Direct effects:
Migraines, pain of the temple and eye.
Opposite teeth, particularly upper molars: pain.

MP-16   *shangdu* (IS M-UE-23b) — superior capital

Dorsum of hand: between the articulations at the base of the index and middle fingers; on the posterior edge of the interarticular ligament; in a hollow.

Three FW medial and inferior to *sanjian* (LI-3); two FW lateral and inferior to *wailaogong* (MP-13, IS M-UE-23); two FW lateral to *zhongdu* (MP-17, IS M-UE-23a).

Evokes a response in the index finger, lower posterior frontal lobe and *zhongchong* (PC-9), dorsum of the arch of the foot, *wailaogong* (MP-13, IS M-UE-23) and *pianli* (LI-6).

Direct effects:

Hand and forearm, redness and swelling; chilblains.

MP-17   *zhongdu* (M-UE-23a) — central capital

Dorsum of hand: between the articulations of the base of the middle finger and ring finger; upper (posterior) edge of the interarticular ligament; in a hollow.

Two FW medial to *shangdu* (MP-16, IS M-UE-23b); two lateral to *yemen* (TW-2) and a little more medial to *xiadu* (MP-18, IS M-UE-23c); two FW below *wailaogong* (MP-13, IS M-UE-23).

Evokes a response in the dorsum of hand, lower posterior frontal lobes, dorsum of the middle and ring fingers.

Direct effects:

Back of the hand and dorsum of the middle and ring fingers (redness and swelling), chilblains; acts on the extensors of the middle and ring fingers.

MP-18   *xiadu* (IS M-UE-23c) — lower capital

Dorsum of the hand: between the articulations of the base of the ring finger and little finger; upper (posterior) edge of the interarticular ligament; in a hollow.

One half FW medial (towards the little finger) to *yemen* (TW-2); two FW medial to *zhongdu* (MP-17, IS M-UE-23a); two large FW under *zhongzhu* (TW-3).

Responds in the lower posterior frontal lobes; dorsum of the hand, ring and little fingers.

Direct effects:

Dorsum of the hand, ring and little fingers: redness, swelling, chilblains; extensors of ring and little fingers.

MP-19   *dagukong* (IS M-UE-15) — hollow of the large bone [or "first tiger," IS M-UE-45a]

Dorsum of the thumb: in the distal interphalangeal articulation. With the thumb bent, between the two bones. On the lateral side the median bony point. In a hollow.

Shaoshang (LU-11) is found on the opposite side, toward the index finge. On the lateral edge is *guiyan* (MP-29b). At the center of the tip of the finger is the first of the *shixuan* (MP-25, IS M-UE-1).

Evokes a response in the opposite lateral eye, inferior occiput, triple warmer, and stomach; dorsal great toe.

Direct effects:

Lateral opposite eye: old problems; beginning of cataract. Acts on the lateral part of the eye.

Pains or contracture of the articulation of the thumb.

MP-20   [index-]*wuhu* (IS M-UE-45b) — second tiger

Index finger, dorsal surface, in the proximal interphalangeal articulation, about mid-width. Between the two bones. In the lateral hollow (towards the thumb) on the edge of the median bony point.

On the fingertip, at the level of the nail, is the second of the *shixuan* (MP-25, IS M-UE-2). Two FW under *erjian* (LI-2).

Direct effects:

Index finger: contracture or arthritis of the articulations; pain.

MP-21 *zhonggui* — central genii [or "third tiger," IS M-UE-45c]

Dorsum of the hand, middle finger: proximal interphalangeal articulation. On the lateral side (toward the index finger) of the median bony point of the articulation. In a hollow, with the finger flexed.

Two FW superior to *zhongchong* (PC-9), three FW superior to the third of the *shixuan* (MP-27, IS M-UE-3). Two FW inferior to *shangdu* (MP-16, IS M-UE-23b) and *zhongdu* (MP-17, IS M-UE-23a).

Direct effects:

Evokes a response in the stomach, *zhongwan* (CV-12); nose, opposite eye; small intestine, *zhizheng* (SI-7).

All types of stomach distress, indigestion, vomiting: disperse.

Congested eyes? Nasal congestion, poor breathing through the nose?

Warts and excrescences, particularly on the hands.

MP-22 [ring finger-]*wuhu* — fourth tiger

Dorsum of hand, ring finger: proximal interphalangeal articulation. On the lateral edge (toward the middle finger) of the median bony point. In a hollow, with the finger flexed.

Two FW above the fourth of the *shixuan* (MP-28, IS M-UE-4) and from *guanchong* (TW-1). Two FW below *yemen* (TW-2).

Direct effects:

Articulation of the fourth finger: contracture, pain; arthritis.

MP-23 *xiaogukong* (IS M-UE-17) — little hollow of the bone [or "fifth tiger," IS M-UE-45e]

Dorsum of the hand, little finger: in the distal interphalangeal articulation, with the finger flexed. On the lateral edge of the median bony point: in a hollow.

Two FW above the fifth *zhixuan* (MP-29, IS M-UE-5), *shaochong* (HT-9) and *shaoze* (SI-1).

Direct effects:

Lateral part of the opposite eye; medial part of the same side.

Lateral eye opposite: pain.

Articulation of the little finger: contracted, painful; arthritis.

Four toes opposite side, dorsae.

MP-24 *longxuan* — obscurity of the dragon

Dorsum of wrist: at the lower opening of the radial-ulnar joint. A little under and lateral to the ulnar styloid, on the line of the little finger.

One FW under and lateral to *yangchi* (TW-4); two FW medial to *zhongquan* (MP-14, IS M-UE-33).

Responds in the dorsum of the fingers.

Direct effects:

Pain of the joints, particularly the dorsal side of all the fingers.

Mid-dorsum of wrist: pain.

MP-25-29 *shixuan* (IS M-UE-1-5) — the ten advertisers

Dorsum of fingers: on each of the ten fingers; on the terminal phalanx, mid-width. At the tip of each finger, just under the nail.

Reponds in the tonsils, same side.

Direct effects:

Tonsillitis, same side. Inflamed throat: disperse.

MP-29a *guiku* — sobbing of ghosts

Hand, thumb, terminal phalanx: lateral surface (external, not towards the index finger, mid-width); in the angle between the inferior edge (towards the nail) of the swelling of the bone and the dorsal edge of the tendon (flexor pollicis longus); in a hollow.

At the level of *shaoshang* (LU-11); one FW lateral and under *dagukong* (MP-19, IS M-UE-15).

Direct effects:

Obsessions, obsessive remorse, delusions; epilepsy.

MP-29b   *guiyan* — eye of the ghost

Thumb, base of the nail, lateral corner: symmetrical to *shaoshang* (LU-11); between this point and *guiku* (MP-29a) at one half FW from the latter. There is also a point on the great toe called foot-*guiyan,* not to be confused with *yinbai* (SP-1).

Direct effects:

Epilepsy of babies and children.

MP-30   *gaogu* — elevated bone

Upper palm. One FW under (in front of) the thenar eminence. In the angle of the abductor pollicis and the flexor of the index finger.

Responds in the posterior frontal lobes (lower), thumb and index finger.

Direct effects:

Maladies of the hand?
Increases the pinch between the thumb and index finger.

MP-31-34   *sifeng* (IS M-UE-9) — the four seams

Palmar side of the fingers: one per finger; in the proximal interphalangeal joints, mid-width; does not exist on the thumb.

Responds in the opposite side of the throat, opposite side of the larynx, opposite lung; anterior part of mid-brain; opposite *tianzhu* (BL-10).

Direct effects:

''Babies: tuberculosis (of street urchins?) and others.''

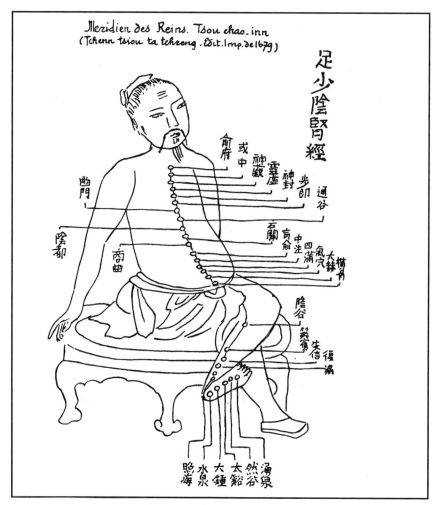

Meridian of the kidneys (DACH)

Chapter IV

Marvellous Points of the Trunk

MP-35   *zigong* (IS M-CA-18) — palace of children [uterus]

Lateral part of lower abdomen; approximately three FW on either side of the midline; one FW above the pubis.

About three FW on either side of *zhongji* (CV-3); between *guilai* (ST-29) and *qichong* (ST-30).

Responds in the genital system.

Direct effects:

Women who are childless for a long time.

MP-36   *yangdi* — base of the sack

In the crossing of the folds of the scrotum?

Direct effects:

Kidneys: abscess or neuralgia? All kidney illnesses?

Small intestine: spasms?

MP-36a   *pigen* (IS M-BW-16) — root of congestion of the spleen

Back: about four FW on either side of the upper edge of the second lumbar vertebra; under the twelfth rib. Posterior and lateral to *zhishi* (BL-47, IS BL-52).

Direct effects:

Congestion of the spleen-pancreas.

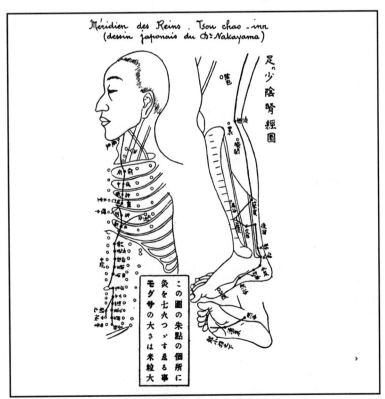

Meridian of the kidneys (Nakayama)

Chapter V

Marvellous Points of the Lower Limb

MP-37-38 *suigu* — bone with marrow

Anterior and superior knee: two points on each knee. 1) The medial point: in the angle between the medial edge of the median tendon and the inferior edge of the first fibers of the vastus medialis muscle; knee extended, one large FW above the knee cap. 2) The lateral point: two FW above and lateral to the patella; in the angle between the inferior lateral edge of the vastus lateralis and the external posterior edge of the femur.

Two FW on either side of *liangqiu* (ST-34).

Responds in: the medial line on the medial anterior surface of the lower limb; the lateral line on the lateral anterior surface of the lower limb.

Direct effects:

All problems of the lower limb?

MP-37a-38a *xiyan* — eye of the knee

Two points on each knee: knee, anterior surface; on either side of the patella, in the depressions which are the ''eyes of the knee.'' On either side in the angle between the head of the tibia and the patellar tendon.

The liver meridian passes through the median *xiyan,* which seems to have an effect on the liver.

Two FW on either side and above *dubi* (ST-35); lateral *xiyan* is three FW above leg-*sanli* (ST-36), medial *xiyang* is three FW above *yinlingquan* (SP-9), two FW in front of and slightly above *ququan* (LR-8).

Direct effects:

Arthritis of the knee; ligaments of the knee distended: apoplexy; beriberi.

MP-38b *kuangu* — bone and division

Thigh, posterior surface: mid-width; about five FW from the posterior fold of the knee; in the inferior angle between the large medial muscle (semitendinosis) and the lateral muscle (biceps); on the deep muscle (semimembranosis).

Direct effects:

Acute pain of the lower limb and foot.

MP-39-40 *lanmen* — door of the orchides

Knee, medial surface: two points on each knee; both points are on the same level, two large FW on either side of the angle between the head and body of the tibia. 1) Anterior point: on the anterior surface of the tibia, on the medial edge of the anterior tuberosity and under a rise. 2) Posteromedial point: in the posterior angle, medial to the head of the tibia, on the lower edge of the tuberosity of the insertion of the semimembranosis.

Two large FW on either side of *ququan* (LR-8).

Responds in the bladder and uterus.

Direct effects:

Bladder: spasms and painful crises?

MP-41 *waihuaijian* (IS M-LE-22) — point of the lateral malleolus

On the summit of the point of the lateral malleolus. In front of *kunlun* (BL-60).

Responds in the bladder meridian; lateral and dorsal surface of the foot; sprain of the lateral malleolus.

Direct effects:

Beriberi: cold and heat?

MP-42   *neihuaijian* (IS M-LE-17) — point of the medial malleolus

On the summit of the point of the medial malleolus.

Two FW above *zhaohai* (KI-3, IS KI-6); two FW behind and above *shangqiu* (SP-5).

Responds in the kidney meridian, medial surface of the foot and in front of the medial malleolus.

Direct effects:
  Beriberi: cold and heat?

MP-43   *bafeng* (IS M-LE-8) — the eight winds

Tradition names the four joints of the toes in this way. But the joint of the first and second toe has *xingjian* (LR-2), that of the second and third toes has *neiting* (ST-44), and that of the fourth and fifth toes has *xiaxi* (GB-43). There remains only the joint of the third and fourth toes.

Between *neiting* (ST-44) and *xiaxi* (GB-43).

Responds in the line of the metatarsophalangeal joints.

Direct effects:
  Swelling and redness of the foot.

MP-44   *duyin* (IS M-LE-18a) — yin only

Second toe, plantar surface: in the third and second phalangeal joint, mid-width, on the fold.

Responds in the abdomen and lower abdomen.

Direct effects:
  Small intestine: painful spasms.
  Dead fetus or placenta not descending by themselves; women: dry eructation or red vomit; menstrual blood irregular and not harmonious.

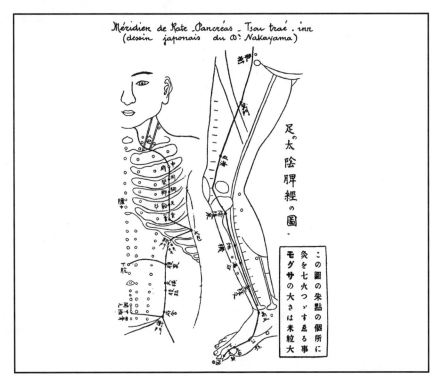

Meridian of the spleen-pancreas (Nakayama)

Volume V

Illnesses
and
Their Treatment

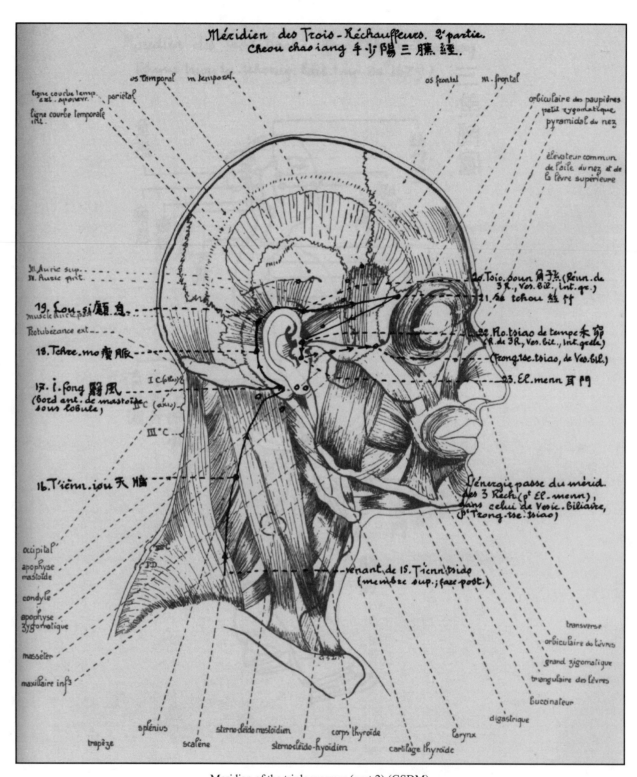

Meridian of the triple warmer (part 2) (GSDM)

Introduction

To make the best use of acupuncture treatment, the following principles must be kept in mind:

Acupuncture acts only in relation to the vital energy of the patient. It displaces the reserves of energy. Other than the atmospheric electricity carried by the needles (but not by moxa), it seems that it adds nothing by itself. The more exhausted the patient — without reserves of energy — the less clear and prolonged is the effect. Before expecting a favorable reaction, it is necessary for the acupuncture to hyperstimulate the assimilation functions and tonify the blood and energy; that is, it must facilitate and activate the circulation of energy, the balance of yin and yang. "Above all, the good doctor must uplift and regulate the energy of the patient." Let us add that beside a general microbe-terrain relativity there is the defensive organization of the leukocytes, which certainly depends on the general terrain, but can also be the only deficient part of a vigorous organism.

In an organism that is not yet exhausted, even serious recent functional problems are easily and quickly cured. This is the domain where acupuncture gives results that sometimes seem miraculous. Unless there has been an abuse of medicines or analgesics that retards the action, or recent X-rays, which kill the cutaneous reflexes for several months, if the organism is not tired and the beneficial effect of the needles stops quickly, then we must suspect an unnoticed lesion and inquire into it carefully. Organic lesions cannot be cured naturally in any way other than surgery. However, even an organic lesion always has a more or less congested and painful aspect with functional problems that can themselves be relieved. We must remember also that slight organic lesions can cause serious functional problems. In these cases acupuncture gives surprising and often lasting results.

*   *   *

The symptoms listed and the illnesses described in this volume must not be studied without taking the patient into account. For acupuncture, the real cause of the illness is a disruption of vital energy that involves a local or general failure of the defense in relation to the attack. The ancient Chinese or Japanese never gave lists of treatments. They feared that to appeal to the memory more than to observation and understanding would be to reduce the necessary effort that the physician must make to understand clearly the energy picture of the patient. Such lists would give the idea of formulae, which are sufficient for learning if we apply them to illnesses, but not sufficient for the patient. From century to century, the students or family of famous physicians have published the treatments for some illnesses that were noticed through the master's observations. They understood that if one can cure without medicines, it is because remedies and other material or immaterial medication (for even a word can kill or cure) only act as a stimulant for the organism, for a "service of repair" that is yet to be discovered.

For Europeans, the present classification is indispensable in order to have a picture of excess or insufficiency for each organ and to be able to find quickly, without years of study, the special point on each meridian that corresponds to the problems we see. As a matter of fact, all the points on the same meridian do not have the same effect on the organ. Each point has a more or less stronger action on one or the other of the organ functions, or on those organs to which it is related. Thus, for the liver, the functions of which are very numerous (Europe counts thirty-five), it is possible to show that certain points have a very clear action on one rather than another of its functions. *Ququan* (LR-8) particularly increases the bile. *Taichong* (LR-3) acts on swellings, the antitoxic functions and perhaps on the colloids. *Ligou* (LR-5) fights pruritis and sexual stimulations. *Dadun* (LR-1) acts on spasms. *Zhangmen* (LR-13) acts on the problems that follow the usual alimentary excesses, etc.

Many points on the different meridians may have some action on the same problem, acting either on the organ itself, or on a related organ. Thus, we must know how to choose. We should add that thanks to the possibility of acting on each of the functions of an organ, Europe could go beyond the ancient teachings by verifying the observations and thousands of years of experimentation in China and Japan, basing its understanding on modern instruments and proven tests. It has been possible, for example, to demonstrate the separate actions of the two branches of the so-called spleen-pancreas meridian. The right branch commands the spleen and the left commands the pancreas. It has been the same for the two branches of the kidney meridian, each one commanding the kidney located on the same side of the artery (hand in supination), as well as for the lungs and heart. Moreover, it has been possible to study separately the different functions of each organ.

Finally, we must not forget that each person can be ill in his own way, choosing or accentuating various symptoms of each illness. A patient can suffer from two or more illnesses at the same time. For example, an old malaria or colibacillus can be reactivated by an acute illness of the lungs or stomach, adding their symptoms.

Lastly, we must not forget that when a point is stimulated for its local or special effect, it stimulates the organ of its meridian simultaneously. Thus, *zanzhu* of the bladder meridian (BL-2), which acts especially on eye troubles, will also tonify the bladder, if it is tonified. Therefore, as soon as we touch a point, it is important to check the pulse, the function of the organ associated with that meridian, and, if the action on the point has deranged it, to return it to its normal pattern. The pulses must be checked constantly before the treatment to know which of the organs is affected, and during the treatment to know how the patient has responded, and if what is being done is giving a good result.

*   *   *

Generally it is necessary to obtain complete harmony among all the pulses. The perfect condition is that the whole right wrist (the wife) is a little weaker than the left wrist (the husband), and that the superficial pulses (the energy) are a little weaker than the deep pulses (the blood).

Among the many points that are indicated for curing each illness, choose points from the troubled meridian as shown at the pulse, then points on the meridians in relation to these. Finally, if the results are still not satisfactory, use points from the conception vessel and the triple warmer. This is mostly indicated in acute illnesses; in general, we must activate and facilitate the flow of energy; for that, balance yin and yang. To disperse, disperse the child meridian; to tonify, tonify the mother meridian.

For contracture, paresis, pain and swelling, it is often necessary to act locally. We should also mention that for contractures or neuralgias that are more than three weeks old there is always a secondary ankylosis that prevents the immediate release of the limb and this must be cured through mobilization and massage.

*   *   *

Regarding the methods of action, it is useful to review briefly the principal rules.

To tonify the vitality, to stimulate the function: 1) Gold needles penetrating just under the dermis into the subcutaneous tissue, about 2 mm. deep; leave them there until the skin does not grip them anymore; 2) Moxas, made with a cotton ball dampened in water taken boiling from the fire, touched very rapidly 40 to 50 times in sequence, on each point every morning.

Of moxa, it is known in Europe that hot water compresses relax spasms and help the circulation. But moxa by itself can either relax spasms (when done in numbers fewer than 15 to 20 at most), or activate the flow of energy, that is, tonify (when in numbers larger than 40 or 50). They are recommended for children and the elderly as being gentler than needles. They can and must be applied for some time, in fact until the cure is complete. The needles cause fatigue when they are used more than once every three or four days, except in acute cases, and for the point *gaohuangshu* (BL-38, IS BL-43) more than once a month.

To disperse and reduce excessive function, relieve congestion and stop pain: 1) Silver needles inserted into penetrate the subcutaneous tissue and retained as long as the skin grips them; 2) Moxa in small numbers (15 to 20 every evening).

For children at the beginning of tonsillitis or flu, or with insufficient function of the liver or stomach, normal function can be restored by simple massage with either the nail or the tip of the finger and repeated until the desired result is obtained.

*   *   *

While translating I have kept the descriptions and indications of antiquity in their original form. They are not always very clear or easy to translate into modern medical terminology. It is necessary to meditate to understand them, but they are never meaningless sentences.

Briefly, in order to obtain the best results with acupuncture it is advisable to:

1) Feel the pulses to find the one or more organs that have an excess or an insufficiency. This determines which of the meridians must be harmonized again, as well as the tonifying or dispersing action that must be taken.

2) From the particular quality of the troubled pulse, and through the special symptoms reported by the patient, determine the most efficient point to be used on each meridian.

3) With extreme attention look for the precise location of the point by using a guide that gives the exact center of the point, and by inquiring of the patient for the maximum sensation.

4) Puncture first the point related to the illness, the patient and the season, and then immediately verify at the pulse the changes that result. This allows us to see if the needle was exactly at the center of the point. Then, if the effect is insufficient, puncture the symmetrical point with the same precautions, as a mistake in location is very easy to make.

5) When all the pulses are harmonious, equal, and beating well, balance has been obtained. Daily moxa is necessary for old and serious cases or with weak patients.

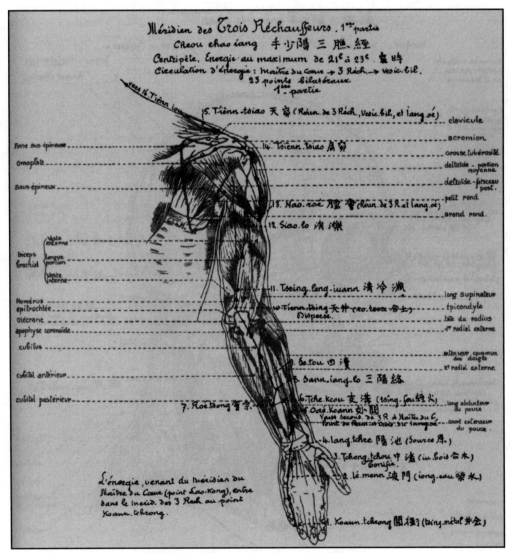

Meridian of the triple warmer (part 1) (GSDM)

Chapter I

Energy: The Yin and The Yang

I. The Energy (Qi) — II. The Yin-Yang Relativity — III. The Eight Points of the Extraordinary Meridians — IV. Points of Passage Between Yin and Yang — V. Vagus-Sympathetic

I. The Energy *(Qi)*

All diseases come from energy. (YIX I, 12v)

The hundreds of illnesses that are created all manifest through fullness or emptiness. (DACH V, 20 & 22v)

When there is emptiness, tonify; when there is fullness, disperse. (DACH V, 23r)

Energy *(qi)*, or healthy energy *(zheng qi)*, or ancestral energy *(yuan qi)* is the vital force drawn from food, air, sun, earth and night. The virulence of the disease is sometimes called perverse energy *(xie qi)*. Ancestral energy is yin; it is the energy of food and earth. Yang energy comes from the air and the lungs (see: Part IV, leg-*sanli* ST-36). Energy is dispersed and weakened by climates and temperatures that do not vary, that are always the same. It is tonified by extreme climates with differences between winter and summer, day and night. It is at maximum for two hours a day in each meridian and organ.

GB	11 p.m. - 1 a.m.	LR	1 a.m. - 3 a.m.	LU	3 a.m. - 5 a.m.	LI	5 a.m. - 7 a.m.
ST	7 a.m. - 9 a.m.	SP	9 a.m. - 11 a.m.	HT	11 a.m. - 1 p.m.	SI	1 p.m. - 3 p.m.
BL	3 p.m. - 5 p.m.	KI	5 p.m. - 7 p.m.	PC	7 p.m. - 9 p.m.	TW	9 p.m. - 11 p.m.

Disperse during the two active hours — tonify during the two hours following.

Emotions, according to their nature, act in an opposite way on the energy. But through their excess, they always injure the lungs and obstruct the energy. Then, the triple warmer no longer functions. The feelings that cause a fullness of energy (yang) are: dissatisfaction, worries, obsessions (thoughts), grief, as well as silence and laziness. They thicken and bind the energy; the fire abounds, overheats the humors and forms phlegm, accumulations of perverse energy and diseases of excess (pain and spasms). The accumulations and bindings must be dispersed and caused to circulate. If they are slight, exercise will cure.

The feelings that cause insufficiency and a lack of energy (yin) are: joy, apprehension, fear and also fatigue. "They disperse ancestral energy, creating internal emptiness, exhaustion, laziness, lack of strength, shortness of breath, insufficiency of respiration. Dissipation, lack of energy, must be tonified."

There is a constant relationship between vital energy and breathing, the sound of the voice. A strong loud voice means strong energy; a feeble voice means weak energy. Hurried breathing means unstable energy, anger, spasms, etc.

It is because of yin-yang relativity that energy presents itself with a yin or yang aspect. An excess of yin produces an insufficiency of yang and vice versa. Even so, there can be an excess or insufficiency of yin and yang at the same time. Therefore, we must study the different aspects of energy before studying the aspects that allow the treatment of excesses or insufficiencies of yin or yang.

The repression or paresis of energy depends on the lungs. (DACH IV, 15)

In general.

(DACH) Command of the energy: *hegu* (LI-4).
(YXRM I, 16v) The meeting point of all the energies that distribute themselves through the 12 meridians. The beginning and end of the ancestral energy: *shimen* (CV-5), herald point of the triple warmer.
(DACH IV 7v) All diseases of energy: *qihai* (CV-6).
(DACH) Meetings of the energy; diseases of energy are treated there: *shanzhong* (CV-17) *(GSdeM)*, especially the respiratory strength.
(YIX I, 7v) All kinds of infections of the energy: *gongsun* (SP-4).

Movements of energy.

(DACH) Energy in the upper body, yellow body, sometimes a slight fever: arm-*wuli* (LI-13).

(YXRM) Energy in the upper body, under the heart, swelling and pain; arm-*wuli* (LI-13).

Energy in the upper body causes cough (see: respiratory system).

Insufficiency and lack of energy.

(YXRM I, 46v) All emptiness: leg-*sanli* (ST-36), *guanyuan* (CV-4), *qihai* (CV-6), *gaohuangshu* (BL-38, IS BL-43), *shenshu* (BL-23).

(YXRM I, 46v) Emptiness of old people: *guanyuan* (CV-4); *(DACH X, 34r) sanyinjiao* (SP-6).

(DACH X, 31v) Women: all chills and exhaustion: *guanyuan* (CV-4).

(DACH) Emptiness, fatigue, chill, exhaustion: *xuanzhong* (GB-39), *guanyuan* (CV-4).

(DACH III, 25v) Emptiness, exhaustion: *tianshu* (ST-25).

(DACH) Lack of energy, lasting chill: *shenguan* (CV-8, IS *shenque*).

(DACH) Energy weak, insufficient: *shenmen* (HT-7), *ligou* (LR-5), *dazhong* (KI-6, IS KI-4).

(DACH) Little energy: *shaochong* (HT-9), *tongli* (HT-5), *ququan* (LR-8), *yongquan* (KI-1), *shenshu* (BL-23), *pang-guangshu* (BL-28).

(DACH) Little energy, agitation, fullness: *shaofu* (HT-8).

(DACH) Exhaustion of energy, outflowing of strength: *taodao* (GV-13, IS GV-14).

(DACH) Women: emptiness and chill of the lower abdominal functions; chill, exhaustion: *zhongji* (CV-3).

(DACH) Women: illnesses entering because of emptiness: *qimen* of thorax (LR-14).

(DACH) Remedies no longer effective: moxa at *guanyuan* (CV-4), *qihai* (CV-6), *zhongwan* (CV-12); *(GSdeM)* leg-*sanli* (ST-36).

(DACH) Emptiness of the face: *shangxing* (GV-22, IS GV-23).

Excess and fullness of energy.

Energy in counterflow: *(YXRM) feiyang* (BL-58); *(DACH) taibai* (SP-3); *(DACH X, 30r) quze* (PC-3); *(DACH) jianjing* (GB-21), *dushu* (BL-16), foot-*shangqiu* (SP-5).

(DACH) Women: counterflow of energy, vomits easily, food stays in chest: *youmen* (KI-21).

(YXRM) Energy in counterflow, hands suddenly blue, piercing pain though the heart: *fenglong* (ST-40).

(DACH) Energy in counterflow, sighing without stopping: *laogong* (PC-8).

(DACH) Energy in counterflow, groans, belches: disperse *shaohai* (HT-3).

(DACH) Energy in counterflow, yawning: *dazhong* (KI-6, IS KI-4, *taixi* KI-3 by location).

(DACH) Energy in counterflow, cannot sleep: *guanchong* (TW-1).

(DACH) Energy in counterflow, fits of vomiting: *yutang* (CV-18).

(DACH) Energy in counterflow, paralysis of the chest: *taiyuan* (LU-9).

(DACH) Fullness of energy: *lidui* (ST-45).

Excess energy, local.

(DACH) Counterflow at the top: *yinxi* (HT-6).

Energy pressing upwards: *(DACH)* disperse leg-*sanli* (ST-36), arm-*wuli* (LI-13), *shaochong* (HT-9).

Energy in the head: *tianzhu* (BL-10), *dazhu* (BL-11). If not better: foot-*tonggu* (BL-66), *shugu* (BL-65), *taibai* (SP-3).

Chest: *(DACH)* rising energy attacking the chest: leg-*shanglian* (ST-37, IS *shangjuxu*); energy piercing the two breasts: *(YXRM) taiyuan* (LU-9).

Energy in the chest, hiccoughs, fullness, as if obstructed: *shanzhong* (CV-17).

(DACH) Pain in the chest, the energy does not descend: *rugen* (ST-18); fullness in the center: *yinbao* (LR-9).

Energy in the heart: disperse *shenmen* (HT-7) and *daling* (PC-7).

Back: *(DACH)* In the middle of the back, the energy goes up and down: *zhiyang* (GV-8, IS GV-9).

Lungs: energy in the lungs, disperse *yuji* (LU-10), *taiyuan* (LU-9), *taixi* (KI-5, IS KI-3 by name, KI-4 *dazhong* by location).

Abdomen: energy in the stomach and intestines: disperse leg-*sanli* (ST-36), *zhongwan* (CV-12), *zhangmen* (LR-13); energy travelling through the abdomen: *guanmen* (ST-22).

Swelling of the energy: *(DACH) lidui* (ST-45).

Contractions of the energy: *(DACH III, 30v) taichong* (LR-3).

Energy from shock: *(DACH) tiaokou* (ST-38).

Emotiveness from energy: *(DACH) yinxi* (HT-6).

II. The Yin-Yang Relativity

As with everything, energy can only present itself with a yin or a yang aspect. In fact, this is a relativity, not a condition. The middle of the body is yin in relation to the upper body, but yang in relation to the lower body. A temperature of 15 (degrees) is yin in relation to 30° and yang in relation to 5°. There is a relativity of position (right: yang; left: yin; up: yang; down: yin, etc.) and a relativity of activity (heat: yang; cold: yin; activity: yang; laziness: yin).

Yin.

In the human body, the yin of position is left, down, inside, the "treasure organs," which act on blood and sex, but especially on the blood. The yin of activity is cold, flaccidity, weakness, laziness, sadness, the tendency for rest, sleep and death. It is the response to night through the diminution of vitality.

The ancestral energy is yin and comes from food and the earth through the stomach (see Part IV, leg-*sanli* ST-36). People with an excess of yin (insufficiency of yang), look for warmth and solitude (where yang can reform itself), but they have aggravations in the morning and the middle of the day. When the "treasure organs" (yin) are sick, the upper body is hot, but the lower body is too cold; the person looks for warmth and solitude.

The herald points, which command the insufficiency of ancestral qi (yin), are on the abdomen (yin). For yin illness (cold, depression) coming from feelings (yang) we have to look to the herald points.

> *If the yin energies cannot circulate, there are many problems of blood circulation and pains in the heart.*
> *(YXRM I, 9v)*

The heart governor meridian is the "mother" of the yin energy.
Yin depends on the kidneys and liver.
Insomnia always comes from an excess of yang and an insufficiency of yin.
Night-time aggravation of pain or agitation are an insufficiency of yin and an excess of yang.
Daytime aggravations are an excess of yin (insufficiency of yang).

In general:
Neiguan (PC-6) is the meeting and crossing point of the *yinwei mai,* which joins together all the yin energies.
Zhaohai (KI-3, IS KI-6) is the meeting and reunion point of the *yinqiao mai,* which acts on the yin.
Sanyinjiao (SP-6) rules the blood and yin (junction of the three yin meridians of the leg).

Emptiness of yin:
Emptiness of yin: internal heat through invasion of yang-heat, frequent need to urinate, weakness of the pulses, insomnia.
Insufficient yin energy: *(DACH)* leg-*sanli* (ST-36).
Emptiness of yin or yang in young people: *(DACH)* xinshu (BL-15).
Emptiness of yin, sudden suppression of yang, following illnesses: *(DACH)* qihai (CV-6).
Emptiness of "treasure organs" (yin): *qugu* (CV-2), *rangu* (KI-2) leg-*shanglian* (ST-37, IS *shangjuxu*).

Excess yin:
An abundance of yin: internal cold, sleep, desire for rest, heaviness, pulses "sunken" (hard without amplitude), desire for warmth and solitude: *(GSdeM)* disperse *sanyinjiao* (SP-6), leg-*sanli* (ST-36), *daling* (PC-7), add *shenmen* (HT-7) if the pulse is agitated and strong.

The heart governor meridian and the "door of destiny" (xin zhu, xin bao luo, shou jueyin).

> *It is not a material organ just as the triple warmer is not a material organ . . . it is the minister of unions. Men*
> *form sperm and women detach the ovum and have their menses through it — mother of the yin energy. (DACH)*

The right kidney is called "the door of destiny," *mingmen,* because of its importance for fertility in women; its function is related to that of the kidneys; it is nourished by the heart and animates it. Sadness wounds the heart governor (and the lung); its excess causes mental overexcitement; the antidote is joy, pleasure.

Insufficiency of the heart governor:

Physical symptoms: *(GSdeM)* fatigue, limbs heavy and weak, vertigo, low blood pressure, "sexual vigor without orgasm," pain in the ears, poor circulation.
Pulse of the heart governor (middle level of pulse III of the right wrist) soft, weak or even absent.

Pulse of the sexual organs (deep level of pulse III right); men, absent: no sexual desire; women: frigidity. For women this pulse is hardly perceptible (except for passionate women) from the end of the period to the ninth day, and from the twelfth day after to the seventh day before the next one.

Psychological symptoms: inactivity, mental indolence, melancholy, despondence.

To tonify:

Through the circulation of energy: *fuliu* (KI-7) — kidneys, the mother who nourishes; hand-*zhongzhu* (TW-3) — the triple warmer, the child who suckles.

Through the passage point: *neiguan* (PC-6) — heart governor to triple warmer.

Through the coupled yang organ: hand-*zhongzhu* (TW-3) — triple warmer.

Midday-midnight: *jiexi* (ST-41); stomach maximum from 7 a.m. to 9 a.m., the heart governor having its maximum from 7 p.m. to 9 p.m.

Husband-wife: *fuliu* (KI-7) — kidneys, the husband.

Has no herald point; *(GSdeM) qihai* (CV-6) seems to be the herald point.

By the direct meridian: *zhongchong* (PC-9) which tonifies, and *daling* (PC-7), the source point.

Excess of the heart governor:

Physical symptoms: urine feeble or difficult, high blood pressure, congestive headaches, internal fullness.

Pulse of heart governor (middle) hard, tense, expanding or contracting without expansion (ample or contracted without amplitude).

Pulse of sexual organs (deep) ample, hard, easy sexual excitation, or inflammation or congestion of sexual organs, or for women: pregnancy (round — boy, pointed — girl). For women this pulse is fairly strong between the ninth and twelfth day after the period (ovulation) and stronger and stronger from the seventh day before the period.

Psychological symptoms: oppression, preoccupation, anger, melancholy or bursts of laughter.

To disperse:

Through the circulation of energy: *rangu* (KI-2) or *yongquan* (KI-1), kidney, the mother who nourishes; *tianjing* (TW-10), the triple warmer, the child who suckles.

Through the passage point: disperse *waiguan* (TW-5), triple warmer to heart governor.

Through the coupled yang organ: *tianjing* (TW-10), triple warmer.

Midday-midnight: *lidui* (ST-45), stomach maximum 7 a.m. to 9 a.m., heart governor maximum 7 p.m. to 9 p.m.

Husband-wife: *rangu* (KI-2), *yongquan* (KI-1), kidney, the husband.

Association point: *jueyinshu* (BL-14).

Through direct meridian: *daling* (PC-7).

Yang.

In the human body the yang of position is right, top, back, exterior, the side of the limbs facing the sun. The yang activity is the psychological life, mental life, activity, warmth, life, gaiety, liveliness. It is energy; it is the response to the sun and the day. Yang energy comes from the air, the sun, through the lungs (see Part IV: leg-*sanli* ST-36). Excessively yang people (insufficiency of yin) look for coolness and company (in order to disperse the excess yang). When the workshop organs (yang) that transform the food (stomach, intestines, bladder, gallbladder), are in excess, there is internal cold and external heat. For yang illnesses (fever, agitation), especially coming from external agitation, it is necessary to look to the association points of the organs which are on the back (yang).

> *Excess yang, external heat; emptiness of yang, external cold. (DACH I, 7v)*

> *When the yang energies cannot circulate there is a lot of fever. (YXRM I, 9r)*

> *When the illness is in the workshop organs (yang) the person looks for coolness and company and the troubles are intermittent, mobile. (DACH I, 16r)*

> *Yang energy (and the skin) responds to the lung and the heart (both of them yin organs).*

In general:

Yang is ordered by the *yangqiao mai* for which the crossing and the meeting point is *shenmai* (BL-62).

Waiguan (TW-5) is the crossing and meeting point of the *yangwei mai* which joins all the yang energies.

Hegu (LI-4) orders the energy and the yang.

Yang illnesses in general: *(DACH) gongsun* (SP-4), foot-*linqi* (GB-41).

Meeting point of the three yang of the hand with the three yang of the foot: *bailao* (GV-13, IS *dazhui*), and *baihui* (GV-19, IS GV-20).

Meeting of the vessels of the three yang of the foot: *(DACH) zhongji* (CV-3).

Large secondary vessels of the three yang of the foot: *(DACH) xuanzhong* (GB-39).

(DACH) Meeting of the workshop organs, all their illnesses: *zhongwan* (CV-12).

(YXRM I, 18v) The workshop organs (yang) are in *qichong* (ST-30).

(JM) Any trouble or illness, chronic or acute, of the internal organs: leg-*sanli* (ST-36).

(DACH) The triple warmer is the "father of the yang energy."

Emptiness of yang:

With emptiness of yang there is external cold, somnolence, apathy (yin predominates).

(DACH) Loss of energy, deficiency of yang, sadness: leg-*sanli* (ST-36).

(YXRM I, 42v; YIX I, 2v) Feebleness or decline of yang energy: *gaohuangshu* (BL-38, IS BL-43).

(DACH III, 31r) Yang energy empty, declining: *zhongji* (CV-3).

(DACH) Desertion of yang, desire to die: *qihai* (CV-6).

(DACH) Emptiness and fatigue of yang: *(YXRM)* Emptiness of yang: *huiyang* (BL-35).

(DACH) Cold of energy of the workshop organs (yang); *xiawan* of epigastrium (CV-10).

Excess yang:

Abundance and excess yang manifests through external warmth, insomnia, pain, spasms, contractions, mental overexcitation (yin is insufficient in proportion).

(YXRM) Heat of all the yang: *houding* (GV-18, IS GV-19).

(DACH) If one punctures frequently, all the heat of the yang is dissipated: *fengmen* (BL-12).

(DACH) To puncture with a fine triangular needle disperses all the energy of yang heat and does not permit it to rise and attack the head and the eyes: *shangxing* (GV-22, IS GV-23).

(DACH) All the heat of the yang, abundance of energy: *yamen* (GV-14, IS GV-15).

The triple warmer meridian (sanjiao, shou shaoyang).
(father of the yang energy.)

> *The twelve organs separate from the twelve meridians. Joined, they form the triple warmer and this is only one: this is the origin. (DACH)*

The triple warmer especially makes the yang energy circulate; the others make the yin energy circulate.

"The triple warmer is the father of yang energy." *(DACH)*

(GSdeM) They correspond to the great functions: respiration, digestion and genitourinary.

"They have a name but no form." *(YXRM I, 18v)*

The upper warmer (respiratory functions) commands the yang energy that comes out of, or circulates in, the space between the skin and the muscle; it responds to *shanzhong* (CV-17). The middle warmer (digestive functions) commands the transformation of food and drink, of flavors, of the mysterious essence that rises up to the lungs after being mixed with the blood; it responds to *zhongwan* (CV-12). The lower warmer (genitourinary functions) commands the formation of urine and its evacuation as well as sexuality; it responds to *xuehai* (SP-10).

> *The herald point of all three warmers is **shimen** (CV-5). (DACH)*

> *The triple warmer uses **qichong** (ST-30) to distribute the energy of the stomach and of food to the twelve meridians. (YXRM I, 18)*

> *The pulse of the triple warmer combined with that of the heart and lungs indicates the function of the first warmer; combined with that of the stomach and spleen-pancreas it indicates the function of the second warmer; combined with that of the liver and kidneys it indicates the function of the third warmer. (YXRM)*

General command points of the triple warmer:

(DACH) Triple warmer not in harmony: *weidao* (GB-30, IS GB-28).

(GSdeM) Jiuwei (CV-15) acts on the triple warmer.

Insufficiency of the triple warmer:

Physical symptoms: *(DACH)* the energy goes to the lungs, in the center there is cold or congestion. In the extreme, urinary insufficiency, buzzing of the ears, limbs do not obey, fever without sweat, flushed or grey face, lassitude, everything is an effort. *(GSdeM)* Pulse of the triple warmer small, feeble, soft, without shape or even absent.

If there is insufficiency of the upper warmer, food does not enter (the stomach), painful stomach, nausea. If there is insufficiency of the middle warmer, food does not leave the stomach. If there is insufficiency of the lower warmer, food taken in the morning will be vomited in the evening; food taken in the evening will be vomited in the morning; urinary insufficiency, weakening of the genital functions. (YXRM V, 18v)

Psychological symptoms: depression, sadness, boredom, lacking zest and energy, lacking vivacity.

To tonify:

Through the circulation of energy: *zhongchong* (PC-9, the mother who nourishes) and *xiaxi* (GB-43, the child who suckles).

Passage point: *waiguan* (TW-5), triple warmer to heart governor.

Coupled organ (yin): *zhongchong* (PC-9).

Midnight-midday: foot-*dadu* (SP-2) of the spleen-pancreas, maximum from 9 a.m. to 11 a.m., triple warmer maximum from 9 p.m. to 11 p.m. Use during the yang hours and days (during the day, hot, clear).

Husband-wife: *zhiyin* (BL-67, husband meridian).

Herald points: upper warmer, *shanzhong* (CV-17); middle warmer: *zhongwan* (CV-12); lower warmer: *xuehai* (SP-10) and abdomen-*yinjiao* (CV-7); of all three warmers: *shimen* (CV-5).

Direct meridian: hand-*zhongzhu* (TW-3) and source point, *yangchi* (TW-4).

(DACH) For coldness of the warmers, tonify the lungs at *taiyuan* (LU-9) and the stomach at *jiexi* (ST-41); tonify *fuliu* (KI-7).

Excess energy of the triple warmer:

Physical symptoms: *(DACH)* lower pelvis hard, extreme difficulty in urination. In the extreme, first contraction then overflowing, the liquid comes; pain in the eyes as if they were being pulled out; pain in the jaw, behind the ear, in the shoulder, back, ring and little finger.

Accumulation of *zheng* and *jia, ma-zheng* eruptions (measles), pain from a great wind without knowing where; breath short, cannot speak (shortness of breath).

(GSdeM) Pulse of the triple warmer (superficial pulse III right) hard, ample, large or taut like a wire, or only slightly perceptible from excess tension.

Psychological symptoms: *(DACH)* extreme melancholy, upset, does not know where the pain is; sadness without joy; *(GSdeM)* very irritable, everything is a great effort; agitated, internalized emotions; insomnia.

To disperse:

Through the circulation of energy: *daling* (PC-7, the mother who nourishes) and *yangfu* (GB-38, the child who suckles).

Passage point: *neiguan* (PC-6), triple warmer to heart governor.

Coupled yin organ: disperse *daling* (PC-7).

Midday-midnight: foot-*shangqiu* (SP-5), spleen-pancreas maximum from 9 a.m. to 11 a.m., triple warmer maximum from 9 p.m. to 11 p.m.

Husband-wife: *shugu* (BL-65), bladder, husband.

Association point: *sanjiaoshu* (BL-22).

Direct meridian: *tianjing* (TW-10) and the source point: *yangchi* (TW-4).

Heat of the triple warmer:

(DACH III, 29r) Compressed heat abounding in the triple warmer: *guanchong* (TW-1).

(DACH IV, 5v) Energy and heat of the triple warmer compressing the upper warmer; bitter mouth, dry tongue: bleed *guanchong* (TW-1), and if the arms and hands are red and the wrist painful, increase the dispersion at *yemen* (TW-2) and *zhongzhu* of the hand (TW-3). When the wetness in the mouth returns, there will be recovery.

(DACH X, 33r) Heat attack of *shaoyang* (triple warmer-gallbladder): *taixi* (KI-5, IS KI-3 by name; IS KI-4 *dazhong* by location).

(DACH) The middle warmer holding heat: *xuanli* (GB-6).

(DACH, YXRM) Lower warmer bound, hot: *shuidao* (ST-28).

III. The Eight Points of the Extraordinary Meridians

The crossing and reunion points.

Eight points are described under the name "crossing and reunion points" of the eight extraordinary meridians. These points summarize the effects of the 66 antique points (see Volume II); these points in turn summarizing the effects of all the rest of the points on the body *(DACH VI, 4; YIX I, 9)*. Of these eight points, four are yang and four are yin. They are paired as "host and guest" or as "husband and wife," one yang with one yang and one yin with one yin. The second point acts when the first has been insufficient and vice versa.

Elsewhere, it is recommended that treatment of certain groups of illnesses be given one point at a time, adding other points according to the pulse and the state of the patient. The following four yang points are especially powerful for pain of the lumbar region, the back, for external troubles and troubles of the limbs.
Houxi (SI-3) for the governor vessel coupled with *shenmai* (BL-62) of the *yangqiao mai*. Start the treatment of the following illnesses with this point: neuralgia of the forehead and eyebrows; neuralgia from drunkenness; motor troubles of the extremities (see foot-*linqi*, GB-41); contraction of the throat and nape of the neck, or of the jaw; tetanus; red eyes, weeping; tonsillitis; paroxysm of toothache; cough and mucus; deafness.
Shenmai (BL-62) for the *yangqiao mai* (coupled with *houxi,* SI-3, which commands the governor vessel): contractions, hemiplegia; flaccid paralysis (see foot-*linqi*, GB-41); aphasia (loss of speech); pains in the nape of the neck and back; lumbago.
Waiguan (TW-5) for the *yangwei mai* (coupled with foot-*linqi*, GB-41 for *dai mai*). With this point begin treatment for: emptiness; tiredness; pain or swelling of the neck or nape, lymph nodes swollen at the nape; mumps; arthritis of fingers or toes; parulis, pain in the lower molars; headaches; pain or trouble in the eyes or ears.
Foot-*linqi* (GB-41) for the *dai mai* (coupled with *waiguan,* TW-5 of the *yangwei mai*). With this point begin treatment of: emptiness, tiredness; flaccid paralysis, or trembling or contractions of the hands and feet (see *houxi,* SI-3 and *shenmai,* BL-62); acute rheumatoid arthritis (acute articulatory rheumatism); arthritis of heels; redness or swelling of the wrists, knees, or lateral malleolus; pain in the back, shoulders, arms or lower limbs.

The following four yin points are especially powerful for problems of the internal organs and internal illnesses.
Lieque (LU-7) for the conception vessel coupled with *zhaohai* (KI-3, IS KI-6) of the *yinqiao mai*. With it begin treatment for: respiratory tract troubles, coryza, sneezing, bronchitis, asthma; alimentary intoxication; diabetes; excess heat; meningitis in children; paralysis from fear in children.
Zhaohai (KI-3, IS KI-6) for the *yinqiao mai* (coupled with *lieque,* LU-7, for the conception vessel). With it begin treatment for: tiredness in old people or women; constipation or toxic conditions in women. Pelvic region: spasms in the bladder, urine thick, frequent or bloody; loss of seminal fluid; women cannot retain the fetus; menstrual pain in virgins; abdominal pains after delivery; metritis.
Neiguan (PC-6) for the *yinwei mai* (coupled with *gongsun,* SP-4 of the *chong mai*). With it begin treatment for: amnesia, loss of words, anxiety, brain disorders; uncontrolled laughter; epilepsy; indigestion, fullness, spasmodic constipation, piles, abdominal pain.
Gongsun (SP-4) for the *chong mai* (coupled with *neiguan,* PC-6 of the *yinwei mai*). With it begin treatment for: any kind of heart pains, stomach troubles, aerogastria, pains, cramps, burning; any sort of malarial fever; any sort of jaundice.

The eight extraordinary meridians.

Although summarized here through the eight points, the eight extraordinary meridians have many other points (see Volume II). Each point has its own special effect that is important to mention so as to better understand the use of the eight crossing and reunion points (see: *DACH* II, 22v and *YXRM* I, 9r). The four yang extraordinary meridians respond to the shoulders, back, lumbar area, thighs and illnesses in the external sheaths. The four yin extraordinary meridians respond to the heart, abdomen, the sides, the ribs and internal illnesses.

(Yang) "governor vessel" *(du mai)* point of crossing and reunion: *houxi* (SI-3), coupled with *shenmai* (BL-62) of the *yangqiao mai*. Reunion of the yang meridians: corresponds to mental and physical strength, especially in men. Its illnesses are: stiffness of the vertebral column, lack of strength, depression, epilepsy, heat in the back, overexcitement, tendency to run away, hallucinations, pain in the eyes, acute pain in the seventh cervical vertebra. The governor vessel, the conception vessel and the *chong mai* originate at *qichong* (ST-30) *(DACH)*.

(Yang) *yangqiao mai,* "vessel of the hollow of the lateral malleolus," crossing and reunion point: *shenmai* (BL-62), coupled with *houxi* (SI-3) of the governor vessel. All agitations of yang, excess yang energy, insomnia, mental over-excitement, pain in the inner canthus, obsessions, boils.

(Yang) *yangwei mai,* "chain of yang," crossing and reunion point: *waiguan* (TW-5), coupled with foot-*linqi* (GB-41) of the *dai mai.* Joins all the yang energies; when they cannot circulate, there is a lot of fever, serious cold and heat, neuralgia, illnesses of the skin, pain and swelling of the joints, swelling of the heel.

(Yang) *dai mai,* "waist vessel," crossing and reunion point: foot-*linqi* (GB-41) coupled with *waiguan* (TW-5) of the *yangwei mai.* It joins all the meridians at the waist. Fullness, swellings of the abdomen, cold and slowness of the lumbar area.

(Yin) "conception vessel" *(ren mai),* crossing and reunion point: *lieque* (LI-7) coupled with *zhaohai* (KI-3, IS KI-6) of the *yinqiao mai.* The sea of yin meridians. If there is fullness, the skin of the abdomen is painful; if there is emptiness, pruritis; swelling and fullness of the abdomen, lassitude of the limbs, female illnesses, spasms in men, abscesses in the mouth and on the tongue, pain in the head and nape of the neck, on the vertex (see *chong mai*). Foot-*linqi* (GB-41) of the *dai mai* facilitates the flow of the conception vessel and *chong mai* and cures diseases of lactation and menstruation in women *(DACH).* In women when the conception vessel does not communicate: *zhigou* (TW-6). Conception vessel and governor vessel and the *chong mai* all take root in *qichong* (ST-30).

(Yin) *yinqiao mai* "vessel of the hollow of the internal malleolus," crossing and reunion point: *zhaohai* (KI-3, IS KI-6), coupled with *lieque* (LU-7) of the conception vessel. Contraction of yin, stiffness of the feet; sleep comes from excess energy in the *yinqiao mai.*

(Yin) *yinwei mai* "chain of yin," crossing and reunion point: *neiguan* (PC-6), coupled with *gongsun* (SP-4) of the *chong mai.* Joins all the yin energies. If they cannot move, there is poor blood circulation, heart pain, contraction in the chest, internal tension.

(Yin) *chong mai* "vessel of attacks," crossing and reunion point, *gongsun* (SP-4), coupled with *neiguan* (PC-6) of *yinwei mai.* Starts from the genital organs and surrounds the mouth and lips; home of blood for women having their periods; self-control, diseases of the heart, abdomen and the five treasure organs. Its diseases are linked to energies with internal contractions, leading to counterflow of energy. Women have no beard because the *ren mai* and *chong mai* do not join at the lips, and eunuchs lack one because the connection is cut at the origin. Foot-*linqi* of the *dai mai* (GB-41) facilitates the flow of the *chong mai* and the conception vessel and cures diseases of lactation and menstruation in women.

IV. Passage Points Between Yin and Yang

(GSdeM) Fifteen points are indicated under the name "fifteen *luo*" that have the function of helping the excess yang energy to pass into the yin and vice versa. We must tonify what is insufficient — what is in excess immediately diminishes proportionately. These points are very useful for making the excess energy pass into one or another of the coupled meridians (see Volume I).

Lung to large intestine	*lieque* (LU-7).
Large intestine to lung	*pianli* (LI-6).
Heart to small intestine	*tongli* (HT-5).
Small intestine to heart	*zhizheng* (SI-7).
Stomach to spleen-pancreas	*fenglong* (ST-40).
Spleen-pancreas to stomach	*gongsun* (SP-4).
Gallbladder to liver	*guangming* (GB-37).
Liver to gallbladder	*ligou* (LR-5).
Bladder to kidneys	*feiyang* (BL-58).
Kidneys to bladder	*dazhong* (KI-6, IS KI-4 by name, KI-3 *taixi* by location).
Triple warmer to heart governor	*waiguan* (TW-5).
Heart governor to triple warmer	*neiguan* (PC-6).
Great *luo* of Spleen-pancreas	*dabao* (SP-21).
Conception to governor vessel	*huiyin* (CV-1).
Governor to conception vessel	*changqiang* (GV-1) or *yaoyangguan* (GV-3).

V. Vagus — Sympathetic

(GSdeM) It is impossible for the mind not to compare yin-yang with the vagus-sympathetic systems. The sympathetic system dilates the heart, the lungs, spleen, liver and kidneys; it restrains and contracts the stomach, intestines, bladder and gallbladder. Yin energy animates the heart, lungs, spleen, liver and kidneys. The vagus system contracts and restrains those organs dilated by the sympathetic system; those which the sympathetic contracts and restrains, it activates. Yang energy acts in the same way as the vagus system.

The difference is as follows: yin energy tonifies, dilates, activates all the organs reflected on the deep pulses — the heart, lungs, spleen, liver, kidneys, and in addition, the sexual organs (deep III right pulses) and the vessels. The sympathetic system acts in the same way with the exception of what concerns the sexual organs, which it reduces when it activates and tonifies the triple warmer (right III superficial pulse) and the vessels.

Yang energy animates all the superficial pulses reflecting in the stomach, both intestines, bladder, gallbladder and additionally the triple warmer. The vagus system hardens and tightens the superficial pulses also, except for the triple warmer, but including the sexual organs (right III deep pulse) and the vessels.

For yin and yang, tonifying one diminishes the other. The vagus and sympathetic systems, however, react independently. Therefore, it is necessary to see if it is a matter of one of six possibilities: both in excess or insufficiency, vagus in excess with a normal or insufficient sympathetic, sympathetic in excess with a normal or insufficient vagus. Moreover, each of them can become unbalanced in parts — chest, abdomen, etc. On the contrary, the vagus, like the yin, dominates the night, lying down, the cold of winter (let us recall that it is stimulated by pilocarpine, phystostigmine, choline, and inhibited by atropine from belladonna). The sympathetic, like the yang, dominates the day, standing up, being in the heat, children (recall that it is stimulated by adrenaline from the suprarenal glands, which it restrains, and is inhibited by crataegus).

The vagus system responds to the point *tianzhu* (BL-10), which also acts on the glossopharyngeal nerve. The thoracic vagus responds to *feishu* (BL-13). The abdominal portion of the vagus responds to *zhongwan* (CV-12). The sympathetic system responds to *fengchi* (GB-20), also to *lieque* (LU-7) and hand-*zhongzhu* (TW-3). The thoracic portion of the sympathetic responds to *shanzhong* (CV-17), the abdominal sympathetic to *zhangmen* (LR-13).

Practically, when all the superficial pulses are tense, high, hard, and when the deep pulses are soft, there is an excess of yang on a weak yin: tonify *neiguan* (PC-6). When all the deep pulses are hard, excess yin: tonify *waiguan* (TW-5), and if that is inadequate, disperse *neiguan* (PC-6). When the superficial pulses are tense except the right III superficial and middle pulses, there is an excess of the vagus: disperse *tianzhu* (BL-10). When the deep pulses are tense and hard at a deep level except the right III deep, there is an excess of the sympathetic: disperse *fengchi* (GB-20).

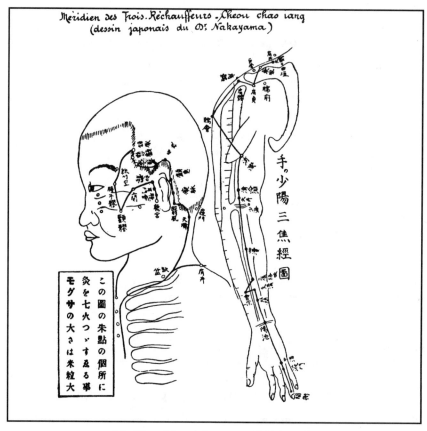

Meridian of the triple warmer (Nakayama)

Chapter II

Energy: The General Command Points

I. All Illnesses — II. Tonics — III. Internal Organs: Treasure Organs, Workshop Organs — IV. Reactions to the External Temperature

I. All Illnesses (Excess: Disperse; Insufficiency: Tonify)

Panaceas.

(DACH) Cures all illnesses; leg-*sanli* (ST-36).

(DACH) There is nothing that it cannot cure: *gaohuangshu* (BL-38, IS Bl-43).

(DACH) Cures the hundred illnesses: *baihui* (GV-19, IS GV-20), *zhongji* (CV-3), numerous moxa.

(YXRM I, 46r) Masters the hundred illnesses: *shenguan* (CV-8, IS *shenque*).

Acute or chronic illness.

(JM) All acute illnesses: *shenguan* (CV-8, IS *shenque*).

(JM) Chronic illness of all sorts: *sanjiaoshu* (BL-22).

Nervous system, energy.

(JM) All illnesses of the nervous system (and of the nerve fibers): leg-*sanli* (ST-36).

(DACH) Source of the vital centers: *jiuwei* (CV-15).

(DACH) Meeting point of all the energies distributed through the twelve meridians: *shimen* (CV-5).

(DACH) The stomach utilizes *qichong* (ST-30) in order to distribute the energy of the triple warmer to the twelve meridians.

(DACH) The twelve source points of the twelve meridians exit from *taichong* (LR-3) and *hegu* (LI-4).

Internal or external illnesses.

(YXRM I, 46r) Internal troubles: *tianshu* (ST-25).

(YXRM I, 46r) Internal troubles from external excitation: *feishu* (BL-13).

(YXRM I, 46v) External illnesses: *shenmai* (BL-62), *waiguan* (TW-5).

Mental illnesses.

(YXRM I, 46r) All central illnesses (mental or moral): *baihui* (GV-19, IS GV-20).

(DACH) The hundred illnesses for the head: *fengfu* (GV-15, IS GV-16).

(YXRM) The hundred illnesses with little energy (respiration): *feishu* (BL-13).

Local illnesses.

(DACH) For the upper body: *dabao* (SP-21).

(YXRM I, 39r) For the center: *tianshu* (ST-25).

(YXRM I, 46r) Illnesses of the center and lower body are all cured: *yinlingquan* (SP-9).

(DACH VII, 34r) Upper and lower body are harmonized through *waiguan* (TW-5) and foot-*linqi* (GB-41).

(JM) Local illnesses: *kongzui* (LU-6).

Yin or yang illnesses.

Yin illnesses (depression, weakness, cold) coming from feelings, i.e., from the interior (yin), must be cured through the herald points (yin).

Yang illnesses, coming from the exterior (fever, agitation), must be cured through the assent points (yang).

(DACH) Yang illnesses: *gongsun* (SP-4), foot-*linqi* (GB-41).

Illnesses of children.

(JM) Special point for all difficulties and illnesses of children: *shenzhu* (GV-11, IS GV-12).

Illnesses aggravated during the day or during the night.

(GSdeM) Illnesses aggravated during the day: *shenmai* (BL-62), tonify.

(GSdeM) Illnesses aggravated during the night: *zhaohai* (KI-3, IS KI-6), tonify.

Illnesses with attacks of contractions.

(DACH) Women: all illnesses with contraction and pain: *guanyuanshu* (BL-26).

II. The Tonics

(GSdeM) In cases of physical and nervous exhaustion, tonify *shaochong* (HT-9), *zhongchong* (PC-9), *zhongzhu* (TW-3), and, if life does not revive in the pulses, add *houxi* (SI-3) and leg-*sanli* (ST-36).

(GSdeM) In cases of anemia (neither pernicious nor cancerous): tonify *gaohuangshu* (BL-38, IS BL-43), which augments the number of red cells (around 500,000 to a million within 24 hours) and the hemoglobin level (10 to 20).

(GSdeM) Thinness: insufficiency of assimilation, lack of strength; tonify leg-*sanli* (ST-36) with 36 moxa every morning (in the evening the effect is reversed).

(GSdeM) Great fatigue in the morning with a better time from 5 p.m: tonify foot-*dadu* (SP-2).

(GSdeM) Fatigue of the aged: women — cold and exhaustion: *guanyuanshu* (CV-4).

(GSdeM) Mental fatigue, excess worries or work: mental tonic, moxa on *baihui* (GV-19, IS GV-20).

(JM) Weakness, emptiness and fatigue after flu: *guanyuanshu* (BL-26); thigh-*wuli* (LR-10).

III. Internal Organs: Treasure and Workshop Organs

(JM) All trouble or acute or chronic illnesses of the internal organs: leg-*sanli* (ST-36).

(JM) Internal organs weak and empty: *qugu* (CV-2).

(YIX I, 11v) Illnesses of the treasure and workshop organs: *zhaohai* (KI-3, IS KI-6).

(DACH) Contraction and pain of the treasure and workshop organs: *sanjiaoshu* (BL-22).

Treasure organs (yin): heart, lung, spleen, pancreas, liver, kidney.

(DACH I, 16r) When the illness is in the treasure organs (yin) we look for heat, solitude and silence. The illnesses are fixed and constant.

(DACH) All illnesses of the treasure organs, reunion of the treasure organs: *zhangmen* (LR-13).

(DACH IV, 5r) To stimulate the true energy of the treasure organs: *jianjing* (GB-21).

(DACH) Announces the energy of the treasure organs: *renying* (ST-9) on the left, ancient point corresponding to the left pulse.

(DACH) Emptiness, exhaustion of the treasure organs: leg-*sanli* (ST-36); *(YXRM)* *henggu* (KI-11).

(DACH) Emptiness and weakness of the treasure organs: *qugu* (CV-2).

(DACH) Cold and accumulations in the treasure organs: *guilai* (ST-29).

(YXRM) Energy of the treasure organs upset: *dazhu* (BL-11) and *tianzhu* (BL-10).

(DACH) Insufficiency of the energy of the treasure organs: leg-*shanglian* (ST-37, IS *shangjuxu*).

(DACH) Spasms running along the five treasure organs (yin), *shimen* (CV-5).

Workshop organs (yang): stomach, large intestine, small intestine, bladder, gallbladder.

(DACH I, 14r) When the illness is in the workshop organs, we look for coolness, company.

(DACH) All illnesses of the workshop organs, *zhongwan* (CV-12), reunion of the workshop organs.

Groups of organs.

(DACH) Illnesses of heart, stomach, spleen-pancreas, gallbladder: *neiguan* (PC-6).

(DACH) Illnesses of the kidneys, bladder, urethra: *shenshu* (BL-23).

IV. Reactions to the Exterior Temperature

The troubles of external origin: wind, cold, humidity, etc. with heat and agitation must be treated with the assent points of the back.[1]

(YXRM I 39r) All troubles from wind, cold, heat, humidity: hip-*juliao* (GB-28, IS GB-29).

(YIX I, 46r) Indisposed easily from wind or cold: *fengmen* (BL-12).

(YIX I, 11r) Illnesses of the skin and vessels from wind or cold: *waiguan* (TW-5).

(DACH) Has aversion to wind and cold: *sizhukong* (TW-21, IS TW-23).

(DACH) Wind or cold living in the pores: *fufen* (BL-36, IS BL-41).

(DACH) Cold having entered: *zhongwan* (CV-12), *qihai* (CV-6) ear-*erjian* (MP-9).

(DACH) Illness from cold: scarlet face: *qihai* (CV-6).

(DACH) Energy of the stoppage of function from cold: *zhongwan* (CV-12).

(DACH) Cold and humidity flowing down injuring the interior of the body: leg-*xialian* (ST-39, IS *xiajuxu*).

(DACH) Wind having entered, humidity also: leg-*sanli* (ST-36).

(DACH VI, 11r) Humidity having entered: *weishu* (BL-21), leg-*sanli* (ST-36).

(DACH) Trouble from humidity causing paresis, sweat, diarrhea: *qichong* (ST-30) and leg-*sanli* (ST-36).

(DACH) Illnesses from humidity: *jizhong* (GV-6); *(JM, 75) zhongwan* (CV-12), leg-*sanli* (ST-36), *xuanzhong* (GB-39), *huantiao* (GB-29, IS GB-30).

(DACH II, 19r) Cold from humidity, heat from humidity: *xialiao* (BL-34).

(DACH) Heat having entered: *dadun* (LR-1), *xiaochangshu* (BL-27).

(DACH I, 9r) Pains from hot and humid wind, from emptiness of blood: *baihui* (GV-19, GV-20), *huantiao* (GB-29, IS GB-30).

(DACH) Troubles from external heat: *zhongwan* (CV-12).

(DACH XI, 11v) Dryness having entered: *dachangshu* (BL-25).

(DACH) Epidemics of cold or hot weather: gums-*yinjiao* (GV-27, IS GV-28).

Influenza (gan mao).

Influenza prevention: *(JM) fengmen* (BL-12), *lingtai* (GV-9, IS GV-10), *ganshu* (BL-18 and *danshu* (BL-19).

Influenza: *lieque* (LU-7), *hegu* (LI-4), *shaoshang* (LU-11), *guanchong* (TW-1), foot-*qiaoyin* (GB-44), *dazhu* (BL-11), *fengmen* (BL-12) and *feishu* (BL-13).

Epidemic influenza: *hegu* (LI-4), *daheng* (SP-15).

Fever, whole body painful, tiredness, exhaustion, violent sweat: *(DACH) bailao* (GV-13, IS GV-14, *dazhui*) inhalations.

After influenza, emptiness and weakness: thigh-*wuli* (LR-10), *guanyuanshu* (BL-26).

Chills (shang han).

*In **shang han**, no sweat, feet and hands cold; it is the yin which is attacked. (Ci Yuan, ''Shang-han'')*

The same expression has been used from antiquity for typhoid fever.

(YXRM) Chills, heat abounds, malaise, vomiting: *bailao* (GV-13, IS GV-14, *dazhui*).

(DACH) Chills, incessant fever: *zhongwan* (CV-12).

(YXRM) Chills, body hot: *wenliu* (LI-7).

(DACH) Chills, four limbs hot: *weizhong* (BL-54, IS BL-40); *(DACH) yunmen* (LU-2). *yaoshu* (GV-2).

(DACH) Illness from chills, shivering, yawning; *chongyang* (ST-42).

(DACH IV, 11v) Chills, congestion of spleen-pancreas *(pi-qi),* knots in the chest, sweat not coming, makes the whole body sweat: *yongquan* (KI-1).

(DACH) Chills, great thirst: *hegu* (LI-4).

(DACH) Chills, heat in the chest: *zhongfu* (LU-10).

(DACH) Chills not dissipating, chest bound: *neiguan* (PC-6), *gongsun* (SP-4).

(DACH) Chills after drinking and eating too much: *qihai* (C-6).

(YXRM) Chills, nose blocked, headache, nape stiff, visual dizziness, epistaxis: *fengmen* (BL-12).

(DACH) Chills, cold of the yang, trouble of the yin: 300 moxa on *shenguan* (CV-8, IS *shenque*).

(DACH) Fever from chills: *erjian* (LI-2).

(DACH) Chills, water binding: *chengshan* (BL-57), *erjian* (LI-2).

(DACH IV, 4v) Chills, four limbs insufficient, counterflow cold, the energy of the pulses only comes from time to time and they must be searched for carefully; about 1.5 *cun* along the bone: *fuliu* (KI-7).

Malign wind *(e feng).*

(DACH) Malign wind, cold, emptiness, fever: *yuji* (LU-10).

Malign cold *(e han).*

Attack of fever from malign cold: *(DACH) hegu* (LI-4), *yinxi* (HT-6), *zhigou* (TW-6), *waiqiu* (GB-36), *mingmen* (GV-4), *wushu* (GB-27), *chengling* (GB-14, IS GB-18), *muchuang* (GB-12, IS GB-16).
(DACH) Malign cold, body hot, fullness of chest: *houxi* (SI-3).
(DACH) Malign cold, shock at the vertex: *houding* (GV-18, IS GV-19).
(DACH) Malign cold: *shangyang* (LI-1), *erjian* (LI-2), *tianjing* (TW-10), *qingling* (HT-2), *daying* (ST-8, IS ST-5).
(DACH) Malign cold, stuffed nose: *yuji* (LU-10).
(DACH) Malign cold, pain in maxilla: *shangyang* (LI-1).
(DACH) Malign cold, heat from the cold: *erjian* (LI-2).

Malign wind or cold.

(DACH, YXRM) waiqiu (GB-36); *(DACH) tianquan* (PC-2); *(DACH) tianchi* (PC-1).
Malign wind or cold: *(DACH)* malign wind or cold, vomiting: *tianchi* (PC-1).
Malign wind or cold, pain of the back: *(DACH) yiche* (BL-44, IS BL-49).
Malign wind or cold, body hot, dizziness: *(DACH) shugu* (BL-65).

Cold or heat; cold and heat.

(DACH) yanggu (SI-5), *jingmen* (BL-25); *(YXRM) tianwaishu* (SI-14), *jianzhongshu* (SI-15).
Cold and heat, swollen lymph nodes *(YXRM)*, cold and heat, swelling of the shoulder: *(DACH) naohui* (TW-13), *naoshu* (SI-10).
Intermittent cold and heat: *(DACH, YXRM) fuyang* (BL-59).
Heat and cold coming and going: *(JM) dushu* (BL-16).
Cold and heat, pain at the heart: *(DACH) dushu* (BL-16).
Cold and heat, pain of the arm, cannot lift: *(DACH) binao* (LI-14).
Cold and heat, neck and nape tightened, seized: *binao* (LI-14).
Cold and heat, alternating: *(DACH) lieque* (LU-7), *shiyang* (GV-8, IS GV-9).
Cold and heat, radiating pain from the vertebra: *(YXRM) pishu* (BL-20).
Cold and heat of the body: *(DACH) tiantu* (CV-22).
Cold and heat, body heavy: *(DACH) fengfu* (GV-15, IS GV-16).
Cold and heat, with perspiration: *(DACH) quepen* (ST-12).
Cold and heat, with no perspiration: *(DACH) shaoze* (SI-1); *(YXRM) muchuang* (GB-12, IS GB-16).
Cold and heat causing thirst: *(YXRM) quchi* (LI-11).
Cold and heat, fullness of the chest : *(DACH) tianliao* (TW-15).
Cold and heat, without limit: *(DACH) yinlingquan* (SP-9).
Cold and heat, swollen lymph nodes, pains in the front of the neck: *(YXRM) daying* (ST-8, IS ST-5).

Notes

[1] The six external causes of illness are: **1)** Cold *(han),* the group of illnesses comprised of cough, cholera, pain in the heart and spleen, pain in the belly; **2)** External heat *(shu),* causing fever or internal heat, or *(he),* causing intermittent fever and dysentery; **3)** Dryness *(xue),* external causing hyperexcitation, dry skin; internal causing constipation, oligura; **4)** Humidity *(shi),* causing congestion of the spleen-pancreas, diarrhea, acidity, icterus, edema, cystitis, lumbago, spasms, beriberi; **5)** Wind *(feng),* causing vertigo, internal headache, pain in the face, apoplexy, rheumatism, paralysis, eruptions; **6)** Fire *(hou),* causing pleurisy, seminal discharges in dreams, urethritis, retention, incontinence, rectal prolapse.

Chapter III

Energy: General Insufficiencies

I. Cold, Shivering from Cold — II. Emptiness, Weakness, Fatigue, Exhaustion — III. Heaviness, Numbness, Paresis, Flaccidity — IV. Infantile Paralysis (Poliomyelitis) — V. Vertigo, Syncope, Coma, Drowning, False Death

I. Cold, Shivering from Cold

Cold (han).

When the illness is from cold, tonify the yin meridians.

Emptiness of heart energy causes cold.

External cold: emptiness of yang.

Internal cold: excess of yin.

(DACH III, 32v) Can keep out cold as well as heat: *shenmai* (BL-62).

(YXRM I, 46v) All persistent cold; *(DACH XI, 14v)* all persistent cold from shock: *gaohuangshu* (BL-38, IS BL-43).

(YXRM I, 46v) Persistent cold, fullness of spleen-pancreas: *sanyinjiao* (SP-6).

(DACH) Extreme cold from emptiness: *qugu* (CV-2).

(DACH) Cold, emptiness, fatigue. *(DACH X, 31v)* Women: all cold and exhaustion — moxa; absolute cold, loss of strength — moxa. *(DACH)* Coldness, pain of knotty articulations: *guanyuan* (CV-4).

(DACH) Aversion to cold: leg-*sanli* (ST-36), *jingming* (BL-1).

(DACH) Desire to live in the heat, aversion to cold: *shenmen* (HT-7).

(DACH) Ill from cold, scarlet face; *(YXRM)* coldness attacking the heart; *(DACH X, 35r)* coldness, fragmented energy, mucus from insufficiency: *qihai* (CV-6).

(DACH) Emptiness, decline, prolonged cold: *shenguan* (CV-8, IS *shenque*).

(DACH) Energy of cold: *heyang* (BL-55).

(DACH) Cold in the body: foot-*shangqiu* (SP-5).

(DACH) Pain from cold: *juguan* (CV-14, IS *juque*).

(YXRM) A lot of cold, little heat: tonify *dazhong* (KI-6, IS KI-4).

(DACH) Cold in the bones: *fuliu* (KI-7).

(YIX I, 4v) Cold in the bones, icy cold in the marrow, goes to warm oneself by the fire: *lingdao* (HT-4).

(DACH) Cold in the marrow: arm-*shanglian* (LI-9), leg-*shanglian* (ST-37, IS *shangjuxu*).

(DACH) Cold: *fuai* (SP-16).

(DACH) Attacks of cold: *taichong* (LR-3).

(YXRM) Cold from shock: *juliao* (ST-6, IS ST-3), *gaohuangshu* (BL-38, IS BL-43).

(DACH) Cold under the heart: *huangshu* (KI-16).

(DACH) Little energy in the cold, heat in the palms: *jianshi* (PC-5).

Shivering in the bath (xian xi).

Xian: to shiver; *xi:* to wash or bathe.

(DACH) Shivering in the bath, fears the cold: *yinxi* (HT-6).

(DACH) Shivering in the bath, cold and heat: *fengchi* (GB-20), *shentang* (BL-39, IS BL-44).

(DACH) Shivering in the bath, stiffness of vertebrae and abdomen: *dazhong* (KI-6, IS KI-4).

(YXRM) Shivering in the bath, stiffness of vertebral column: *taodao* (GV-12, IS GV-13).

Shivering from cold (han chan, biao han).

(DACH) Shivering from cold *(han chan): shaoshang* (LU-11), *yuji* (LU-10), *lieque* (LU-7), *taiyuan* (LU-9), *erjian* (LI-2), *tianjing* (TW-10).

(DACH) Shivering from cold, energy in the upper body: *shenmen* (HT-7).

(DACH) Attacks of shivering: *zhongfeng* (LR-4).

(DACH) Shivering from cold with pain radiating to the pharynx: *neiting* (ST-44).

(DACH) Shivering from cold in the back and chest: tonify *lieque* (LU-7).

(YXRM) Illnesses with fever, no perspiration, shivering: *chongyang* (ST-42).

(YXRM, DACH) Intermittent fever, shivering: *shangxing* (GV-22, IS GV-23).

Shivering, pains in the sides: *(YXRM) qinglengyuan* (TW-11); *(DACH) qingling* (HT-2).

(DACH, YXRM) Shivering *(hanbiao),* occlusion of the larynx, swelling under the chin: *erjian* (LI-2).

(DACH) Shivering *(hanbiao): shengshan* (BL-57).

(DACH) Shivering, chattering of the teeth: *shaoshang* (LU-11).

(YXRM) Chattering of teeth in feverish illnesses; *(DACH X, 24v)* severe shivering, chattering of the teeth: *yuji* (LU-10).

II. Emptiness, Weakness, Fatigue, Exhaustion

Emptiness:

> *Weakness (**ruan**); insufficiency of energy and blood. (Ci Yuan, ''Xu'')*

Aging.

(YXRM I, 46v) Emptiness of old men: *guanyuan* (CV-4), *shenquan* (CV-8, IS *shenque*); *(DACH X, 34r)* emptiness of energy of old women: *sanyinjiao* (SP-6).

(DACH VII, 34r) Old people — exhaustion, emptiness, cramps of hands and feet, cannot twist or move: *shaohai* (KI-3, IS KI-6), foot-*linqi* (GB-41), *taichong* (LR-3), *chengshan* (BL-57), *yanglingquan* (GB-34), *chize* (LU-5), *hegu* (LI-4).

Emptiness.

(YXRM I, 46v) All emptiness: leg-*sanli* (ST-36), *qihai* (CV-6), *guanyuan* (CV-4), *gaohuangshu* (BL-38, IS BL-43), *shenshu* (BL-23).

(YXRM I, 39r) Emptiness, pain; *(YXRM I, 46r)* emptiness of face: *shangxing* (GV-22, IS GV-23).

(DACH) Emptiness, fatigue, cold, exhaustion: *xuanzhong* (GB-39).

(DACH III, 25v) Emptiness, exhaustion: *tianshu* (ST-25).

(YXRM) Emptiness, decline, prolonged cold: *shenguan* (CV-8, IS *shenque*).

(DACH) Emptiness, tuberculosis, fatigue, cold: *gaohuangshu* (BL-38, IS BL-43).

(DACH) Medicines no longer effective: moxa at *guanyuan* (CV-4), *qihai* (CV-6), *zhongwan* (CV-12).

(DACH VII, 34r) Emptiness, yang desertion: *xinshu* (BL-15), *shenshu* (BL-23), *zhongji* (CV-3), *sanyinjiao* (SP-6), *rangu* (KI-2).

(DACH) Emptiness, exhaustion, emaciation: moxa at *gaohuangshu* (BL-38, IS BL-43), needles at leg-*sanli* (ST-36).

(DACH) Extreme cold from emptiness: *qugu* (CV-2).

(DACH) Emptiness, beginning of anemia or tuberculosis: *gaohuangshu* (BL-38, IS BL-43), *bailao* (GV-13, IS GV-14, *dazhui*).

(DACH VII, 21v) All emptiness, the 100 exhaustions, limbs without strength: foot-*linqi* (GB-41) leg-*sanli* (ST-36), *guanyuan* (CV-4), *bailao* (GV-13, IS GV-14, *dazhui*), *gaohuangshu* (BL-38, IS BL-43), *xinshu* (BL-15).

(DACH) Women: illnesses entering because of emptiness: *qimen* of thorax (LR-14).

(DACH III, 31r) Emptiness and decline of the yang energy: *zhongji* (CV-3).

(YXRM I, 46r) Women: emptiness and cold of the lower abdomen, cold, exhaustion: *zhongji* (CV-3).

Laziness (tai, xia duo, lan duo, quan).

(GSdeM) Laziness, mostly in the morning, almost always comes from an emptiness of the spleen-pancreas (mostly the spleen). There is a maximum liveliness around 5 p.m: tonify foot-*dadu* (SP-2), mostly on the left foot (this point helps concentration and causes students to improve in mathematics).

(DACH) Laziness *(lan duo),* likes to rest: *shanqiu* (SP-5).

(DACH, YXRM) Laziness and slowness of the four limbs: *zhaohai* (KI-3, IS KI-6).

(DACH) Indolence, laziness *(tai duo); fenglong* (ST-40), *yanggang* (BL-43, IS BL-48).

(JM) Laziness, lassitude *(xuan tai): sanyinjiao* (SP-6).

(JM) Laziness of the four limbs: leg-*sanli* (ST-36); *(DACH) geshu* (BL-17), *zhangmen* (LR-13).

(JM) Four limbs heavy and lazy: *daju* (ST-27).

(JM) Four limbs lazy and tired: *zhiyang* (GV-8, IS GV-9).

Weakness (ruan).

Reunion of the muscles: tonify *yanglingquan* (GB-34).

(DACH) Weakness of force of the four limbs: *qihai* (CV-6).

(DACH) Outflowing of the strength, exhaustion of energy: *bailao* (GV-13, IS GV-14, *dazhui*).

(DACH) Paresis *(wei)* of strength, little energy: *yinshi* (ST-33).

(DACH VII, 21v) Four limbs without strength, all emptiness, the 100 exhaustions: foot-*linqi* (GB-41), leg-*sanli* (ST-36), *guanyuan* (CV-4), *bailao* (GV-13, IS GV-14, *dazhui*), *gaohuangshu* (BL-38, IS BL-43), *xinshu* (BL-15).

(GSdeM) Weak handshake: arm-*shanglian* (LI-9), tonify.

(DACH IV, 11v) Sits and stands like a decrepit old person: *yanglingquan* (GB-34), tonify.

(DACH) Enables one to sit confidently: *zhaohai* (KI-3, IS KI-6).

(DACH IX, 11v) If sitting, cannot stand up: *guangming* (GB-37), tonify.

(DACH) Body heavy: if sitting, cannot stand: *feiyang* (BL-58).

(YXRM) Paresis *(wei)*, deficiency *(xue):* if sitting, cannot stand up: *qiuxu* (GB-40).

(DACH) Pain of the lumbar area, cannot remain standing for a long time, if sitting cannot stand up: *fuyang* (BL-59).

(DACH) Hemiplegia, if kneeling cannot stand up: *shangliao* (BL-31).

(JM) Weakness and decline after flu: thigh-*wuli* (LR-10).

(JO) Weakness after illness with fever: *shaochong* (HT-9).

Fatigue (lao), exhaustion (sun).

(GSdeM) Fatigue and heaviness in the morning, better at 5 p.m.: foot-*dadu* (SP-2).

(DACH) Cold, fatigue, exhaustion, emptiness: *xuanzhong* (GB-39).

(YXRM) Fatigue, exhaustion, paresis *(wei):* *tianshu* (ST-25).

(GSdeM) Prevents and cures fatigue: moxa each morning on leg-*sanli* (ST-36) and *yanglingquan* (GB-34); can cause the arterial blood pressure to rise.

(YIX I, 5r) Fatigue, likes to lie down: *tongli* (HT-5) and *dazhong* (KI-6, IS KI-4).

(YIX I, 3V) Fatigue: *gaohuangshu* (BL-38, IS BL-43), and *bailao* (GV-13, IS GV-14, *dazhui*).

(DACH III, 32r) Fatigue, exhaustion of the body: *laogong* (PC-8).

(JM) Four limbs tired, lazy: *zhiyang* (GV-8, IS GV-9).

(YXRM) Shock from counterflow, four limbs exhausted: *fuliu* (KI-7).

(DACH) Exhaustion, emptiness, thinness: *gaohuangshu* (BL-38, IS BL-43).

(DACH X, 31v) Women: all cold and exhaustion: moxa on *guanyuan* (CV-4).

(DACH) Women: emptiness and cold of the lower abdomen, cold, exhaustion: *zhongji* (CV-3).

(DACH VII, 34r) Women: exhaustion, emptiness, emaciated appearance, white or red discharge: *zhaohai* (KI-3, IS KI-6), *sanyinjiao* (SP-6), *guanyuan* (CV-4), *bailao* (GV-13, IS GV-14, *dazhui*), *shenshu* (BL-23).

(DACH VII, 21v) The 100 exhaustions, all emptiness, four limbs without strength, foot-*linqi* (GB-41), leg-*sanli* (ST-36), *guanyuan* (CV-4), *bailao* (GV-13, IS GV-14, *dazhui*), *gaohuangshu* (BL-38, IS BL-43), *xinshu* (BL-15).

(DACH IV, 71) Teenagers — fatigue from change: *zhangmen* (LR-13).

(GSdeM) Cerebral fatigue: *baihui* (GV-19, IS GV-20): moxa on arm-*shanglian* (LI-9).

Inability to remain standing (astasia: nan li; see vertigo).

(DACH) Cannot remain standing for a long time: *chengshan* (BL-57).

Cannot remain standing for a long time: *(YXRM)* *chengshan* (BL-57); *(DACH)* leg-*sanli* (ST-36), *guangming* (GB-37), *tiaokou* (ST-38), *tianshu* (ST-25).

(DACH) Cannot remain standing for a long time, pain and numbness of the leg, cannot flex or extend the feet: leg-*shanglian* (ST-37, IS *shangjuxu*).

(DACH, YXRM) Body trembling, cannot remain standing for a long time: *jinmen* (BL-63).

(DACH) Prostrate, lying down, cannot remain standing for a long time: *dazhu* (BL-11).

(DACH) Numbness of the leg, cannot remain standing for a long time: *rangu* (KI-2).

(DACH) Coldness of the leg, cannot remain standing for a long time: leg-*zhongdu* (LR-6).

(DACH) Pain of the lumbar area, cannot remain standing for a long time, if sitting, cannot stand up: *fuyang* (BL-59); if sitting, cannot stand up, body heavy: *feiyang* (BL-58).

(DACH) Trembling, cannot remain sitting or standing for a long time: *feiyang* (BL-58).

(YIX I, 5r) Knee and lower leg without strength, difficulty to remain standing for a long time: *fengshi* (GB-31) and *yinshi* (ST-33).

Can neither walk nor remain standing (astasia-abasia, bu neng xing li).

(DACH) Panting respiration, can neither walk nor stand for a long time: leg-*shanglian* (ST-37, IS *shangjuxu*).

(DACH) Can neither walk nor remain standing: leg-*zhongdu* (LR-6).

(YXRM) Rheumatism from humidity, cannot remain standing or walking for a long time: *lougu* (SP-7).

Difficulty walking (abasia).

(YIX I, 4r, 5r; DACH IV, 7v) Great difficulty walking: *zhongfeng* (LR-4) and *taichong* (LR-3). *(YXRM I, 46r; DACH IX 2v)* Great difficulty walking. *(DACH III, 30v)* Difficulty walking, neither foot can walk: *taichong* (LR-3).

(YXRM) Difficulty walking: *taibai* (SP-3).

(DACH) Feet not able to walk: *lougu* (SP-7).

(GSdeM) Lack of strength for walking: *yanglingquan* (GB-34) tonify.

(DACH X, 32v) Walks without strength, acute pain. *(YXRM)* Feet as if bursting and cannot be put on the ground. *(DACH III, 30v)* Pain of the malleolae, feet cannot be lifted: *kunlun* (BL-60).

(DACH) Feet cannot press onto the ground: *yongquan* (KI-1), leg-*xialian* (ST-39, IS *xiajuxu*).

(DACH) Difficulty walking with shoes on: *heyang* (BL-55).

(GSdeM) Causes the knee and point of foot to lift: *liangqiu* (ST-34).

(YXRM) Slowness of the feet, relaxing of the hands: *fubai* (GB-16, IS GB-10).

(DACH) Feet cannot walk: *fengshi* (GB-31).

(DACH X, 30v) Feet heavy, sunken; articular rheumatism. *(YXRM I, 40r)* Difficulty moving both feet: *xuanzhong* (GB-39).

(DACH, YXRM) Paresis *(wei)* of the feet, cannot walk: *sanyinjiao* (SP-6).

(DACH) Paresis *(wei)* of the feet: *kunlun* (BL-60), *chongyang* (ST-42).

(DACH) Walks without lifting the feet, by shuffling. *(YXRM)* Paresis *(wei)* of the foot, loses his shoes, does not get them back. *(DACH)* In walking, shoes not gotten back on. *(DACH, YXRM)* Toes can neither extend nor flex: *feiyang* (BL-58).[1]

(DACH) Paresis *(wei)* of the feet, does not keep his shoes on: *fuliu* (KI-7) head-*wangu* (GB-17, IS GB-12).

(YXRM) Rheumatism from humidity, cannot remain standing or walking for a long time: *lougu* (SP-7).

(YIX I, 4v) Feet slow, difficulty walking: *xuanzhong* (GB-39), *tiaokou* (ST-38), *chongyang* (ST-42).

(YIX I, 5r) Feet cannot walk: foot-*shangqiu* (SP-5), *xingjian* (LR-2), *kunlun* (BL-60), *taichong* (LR-3), *yangfu* (GB-38), leg-*sanli* (ST-36).

III. Heaviness, Numbness, Paresis, Flaccidity

Heaviness.

(DACH) Body heavy, if sitting cannot stand: *feiyang* (BL-58).

(DACH, YXRM) Body heavy like water: *shenshu* (BL-23).

(DACH, YXRM) Body heavy, cannot lift the four limbs: *sanyinjiao* (SP-6).

(DACH X, 30v; YIZ, 44) Heaviness of the lower limbs, knee, lower leg, four limbs heavy, pain of lumbar area, cannot remain standing for a long time.

(DACH) If sitting cannot stand, pain of lumbar area, cannot remain standing for a long time: *fuyang* (BL-59).

(YXRM) Paresis *(wei)*, deficiency, if sitting cannot stand up: *qiuxu* (BL-40).

(YIX I, 8r; DACH IV, 11r) Four limbs heavy, redness of the face, cheeks, jaw, head: disperse *tongli* (HT-5).

(DACH, YXRM) Four limbs heavy, painful: *zhiyang* (GV-8, IS GV-9).

(DACH) Heaviness of the four limbs: *fuliu* (KI-7).

Numbness.

(YXRM) Acute pain and numbness of the muscles and bones: *jianyu* (LI-15).

(YXRM) Numbness of the bones, vomiting: *tinghui* (GB-2).

Paresis; flaccid paralysis.

Wei or *bi;* if serious, *ma bi,* same as *ma mu,* to the point of flaccidity.

> Same as **bi** — in the old times one differentiated them from one another. In the **Nei Jing,** there is a chapter: "Discussion on **Wei,**" and another, "Discussion on **Bi.**" In general, when the illness is in the exterior, we say **bi;** when it is in the interior, we say **wei.** First **bi,** then **wei.** The **Su Wen** explains **wei** through **bi.** The history of the Han dynasty says **wei** or **bi.** The two words are thus not different. (Ci Yuan, "Wei")

*When we speak of paralysis (**mamu**) of the skin, we say **ma**. When we speak of weakness of the muscles, we say **wei**. (Ci Yuan, ''Bi'')*

*When there is no pain, it is the **wei** and an emptiness. When there is pain, it is **bi feng** (shock of rheumatism) and fullness. (YXRM V, 38r)*

*The **wei** depends on the **yangming** (stomach-large intestine), which is the reunion of all the muscles. When the **yangming** is full, the muscles are smooth. (YXRM I, 38r)*

***Bi** can weaken the hands and feet like **wei**; but **wei** has an internal cause, which is emptiness of blood. **Bi** has an external cause: wind, cold or humidity. (YXRM I, 15r)*

*There are five **wei**. **Wei** of skin: the five treasure organs have received evil and form **wei** — sadness, decline, loss of decision, panting which rises, blood which descends, then heart hot and emptiness below. **Wei** of the vessels: muscles and vessels of the lower leg and knee are retracted, slow; they cannot be used freely; one has the air of being always preoccupied; too much sex and even masturbates all day, ''bitter-white licentiousness,'' then heat in the liver, excess bile. **Wei** of the muscles: vessels and muscles are dry, contracted in flexion, contracture. Occurs after living in a humid area. The flesh moves like worms, thirst plus heat of the spleen-pancreas, dryness of stomach. **Wei** of the flesh: flesh and skin are paralyzed (**mabi**) without action (**buren**); there is a tendency to walk to one side, great heat and thirst, then the yang energy attacks violently, the heat lodges itself in the kidney, water is no longer victorious over the fire, the marrow empties itself; black color; teeth dry. **Wei** of the bone: lumbar area, vertebra, knees do not lift. Those who are attacked by **wei** of the bone and who cannot lift themselves from their bed, die. (YXRM I, 38r)*

Wei fei: exhaustion through *wei*.

*When the lungs are injured, the body cannot be controlled. When the spleen-pancreas is injured, the four limbs cannot be used; it is **wei fei**. Some are from emptiness of blood or from emptiness of energy, or from an accumulation of blood causing an obstacle, or from humidity, or from heat. It is advisable to tonify these illnesses during the waxing moon (YXRM I, 38r).*

*Hands and feet attacked by **wei** that cannot be moved are called **buren**. (Ci Yuan, ''Ren'')*

(YXRM) Fatigue, exhaustion, paresis *(wei)*: pohu (BL-37 IS BL-42).
(DACH) Paresis *(wei)* of strength, little energy: yinshi (ST-33).
(YIZ, 47r) Paresis *(wei)* of the muscles: tonify xingjian (LR-2) and disperse taichong (LR-3).
(DACH X, 27r) Paresis *(wei)*, insufficiency: qiuxu (GB-40); *(DACH)* rangu (KI-2), zhongfeng (LR-4); *(DACH)* fuyang (BL-59).
(DACH) Paresis *(wei)*, lameness *(pi)*: guangming (GB-37).
(YXRM) Paresis *(weibi)* can neither extend nor flex: biguan (ST-31).
(DACH, YXRM) Paresis *(wei)*, deficiency, without action *(buren)*: weiyang (BL-53, IS BL-39).
(DACH) Paresis *(wei)*: jianyu (LI-15).
(YXRM) Paresis *(wei, bi, mamu)*: tianjing (TW-10).
(DACH IV, 11r) Paresis *(fengbi, wei)*, deficiency: dazhu (BL-11) and ququan (LR-8).
(YXRM) All trouble from paresis *(fengbi)*: weizhong (BL-54, IS BL-40).
(DACH) Paresis *(fengbi)*, irregular repetition: weizhong (BL-54, IS BL-40).
(DACH) Paresis *(fengbi)*, without action *(buren)*: yangfu (GB-38), fuyang (BL-58) knee-yangguan (GB-33).
(JM) Pain from paresis *(fengbi)* of the whole body: foot-linqi (GB-41).
(YIX I, 8r) Pain from paresis with paralysis *(ma)*: lieque (LU-7).
(DACH) Paresis from shock *(fengbi)*: chize (LU-5), xiguan (LR-7).
(DACH) Paresis *(fengbi)* without action *(buren)*, contracted muscles not functioning: yaoyangguan (GV-3).
(DACH) Paresis *(fengbi)*, thin elbow, without strength: quchi (LI-11).
(YXRM) Paresis *(fengbi)*, arm and hand not lifting: jianzhen (SI-9).
(YXRM I, 46v) Rheumatic paresis *(bifeng)*; *(YXRM)* paresis *(weibi)* of the limbs: hegu (LI-4).
(JM) Paralysis *(mabi)* of the whole body: zhongfeng (LR-4), wuyi (ST-15).
(JM) Paralysis *(mabi)* of the whole body: chize (LU-5).
(JM) Pain from paralysis *(mabi)* of the whole body: foot-linqi (GB-41).
(JM) Paralysis *(mabi)*: chengshan (BL-57).
(DACH) Reunion of the muscles, all illnesses of the muscles: yanglingquan (GB-34).

(DACH, YXRM) Body and constitution without action: *zhongfeng* (LR-4).
(DACH) Constitution without action *(buren)*: disperse *guangming* (GB-37).
(DACH, YXRM) Paresis *(bi)*: *xiaxi* (GB-43).
(DACH) Paresis *(weibi)*: *waiqiu* (GB-36).
(See Hemiplegia)

IV. Infantile Paralysis (Poliomyelitis) *(Nao Xing Xiao Er Ma Bi; Pian Gu)*

Infantile paralysis of a cerebral nature *(nao xing xiao er ma bi)*:

Origin — this illness appears in children from one to four years old from a difficult or premature delivery, or from whooping cough, typhoid, scarlet fever, measles, pneumonia, parotitis, etc. Symptoms: paralysis of the right side of the body; first, stiffness, suddenly the child has fever, vomits and is foggy. For half a day he has spasms of the whole body, he wakes from his unconsciousness and his body is half paralyzed. Then, a sort of hemiplegia of the left (tan). For a time, the foot is like a hoof of a horse, the lower limbs are crossed, the patella protrudes. There is opisthotonos, trembling, difficulty walking and an extraordinary posture. (JO, 70)

Treatments with needles:

fengchi (GB-20)	*3 fen*
tinghui (GB-2)	*1 fen*
jianyu (LI-15)	*4 fen*
tianzong (SI-11)	*2 fen*
quchi (LI-11) and *hegu* (LI-4)	*2 fen*
jianjing (GB-21)	*3 fen*
baohuang (BL-48, IS BL-53)	*5 fen*
zhibian (BL-49, IS BL-54)	*5 fen*
leg-zhongdu (LR-6)	*3 fen*
yanglingquan (GB-34)	*3 fen*
leg-sanli (ST-36)	*3 fen*
yangfu (GB-38)	*2 fen*
kunlun (BL-60)	*2 fen*
chengfu (BL-50, IS BL-36)	*5 fen.*

Treatments with moxa:

tinghui (GB-2)	*3 moxas*
bailao (GV-13, IS GV-14, *dazhui*)	*5 moxas*
jianyu (LI-15)	*5 moxas*
yangfu (GB-38)	*5 moxas. (JO, 70)*

Half of the body does not respond. (Ci Yuan, ''Pian-gu'' [lateral dryness])

If half of the body or only one limb does not respond, it is called pian gu. The speech is not changed, knowledge is not upset. The illness is in the interior of the dermis and the areolae; one lies down under covers and sweats. (YXRM V, 1r)

Pian gu: from apoplexy, half the body does not respond. One must make the blood and energy circulate. (DACH II, 25r)

In practice, this term ''lateral dryness'' is used for poliomyelitis and describes well the progressive atrophy on either one side or one limb.

Experiments conducted in France show that the sequelae can be effectively fought using tonifying moxa (twenty every morning) at *yanglingquan* (GB-34), reunion point of the muscles, and at *xuanzhong* (GB-39), both of which act on the tropism of the attacked limb, activating growth and again giving life to the muscles and bony structure. Hand-*wangu* (SI-4) acts more specifically on the forearm and the hand; *jianyu* (LI-15) acts on the whole upper arm. In addition, *fenglong* (ST-40) is indicated in atrophy of the lower leg.

V. Vertigo, Syncope, Coma, Drowning, False Death

Vertigo.

In Europe, "vertigo" can mean vertigo from heights, the sensation that everything whirls around oneself, the sensation that the earth is moving as if one were on a boat, or the onset of fainting. China uses several terms, exact equivalents for which do not seem to exist in Europe. Each one of these terms is described with the points which mention it and thus complete the description in the encyclopedia.

Xuan ("eyes turning"): Undoubtedly a matter of visual dizziness.

> *Eyes that do not constantly command, called in the vernacular "flowers-behind-the-eye"* **(mu xuan hua).**
> *(Ci Yuan, "Xuan")*

(DACH) Dizziness of the energy, swelling of the belly: *yixi* (BL-40, IS BL-45).

Xuan ("whirling, dizziness"): Undoubtedly related to great internal malaise.

> *Bent backwards, changes, whirling, sudden need to urinate, suspended like a bell. (Ci Yuan, "Xuan")*

(YXRM I, 39r) Without cause, head foggy and turbulent *(xuan)* (epileptiform vertigo): *shenmai* (BL-62), and *jinmen* (BL-63).

Feng xuan ("dizzied from shock"):
(DACH) chengguang (BL-6), *houding* (GV-18, IS GV-19).
(YXRM) tianzhu (BL-10), *yuzhen* (BL-9).
(DACH) shenmai (BL-62).

Yun:

> *Luminous halo around the sun or the moon, around all light sources; same as* **mu xuan** *(visual dizziness); used in the vernacular for troubles* **(hun).** *(Ci Yuan, "Yun")*

It is related to the onset of fainting, lipothymia or syncope.
(DACH III, 28r) Syncope *(yun)* under the needle: *shuigou* (GV-25, IS GV-26 *renzhong*).
(DACH) Point for awakening from fainting: arm-*sanli* (LI-10). *(GSdeM)* Massage this point strongly with the nail of the thumb, to revive persons who have fainted; do the same at *shaochong* (HT-9) and *shuigou* (GV-25, IS GV-26, *renzhong*).
(DACH) Fainting *(yun)* from metrorrhagia *(xue beng):* tonify *sanyinjiao* (SP-6) (disperse for metrorrhagia).

Mu xuan ("visual dizziness"):
(DACH) Head-*linqi* (GB-11, IS GB-15), *wuchu* (BL-5), *fengchi* (GB-20), *yangbai* (GB-10, IS GB-14), *houding* (GV-18, IS GV-19), *yanggu* (SI-5), *tongli* (HT-5), *yintang* (GV-23a, IS M-HN-3), *sibai* (ST-5, IS ST-2), *fengmen* (BL-12), *yixi* (BL-40, IS BL-45); *(JM) tonggu* (BL-66).
(DACH III, 18r; YIX I, 4) Zhizheng (SI-7), *feiyang* (BL-58).
(DACH II, 27v) Dizziness (morning and evening) from cramps: *chengshan* (BL-57) and *kunlun* (BL-60).
(JM) Morning and evening after illnesses with fever; *(DACH)* energy short morning and evening: *fengchi* (GB-20).
(DACH, YXRM) Eyes painful as if gouged out, morning and evening: *kunlun* (BL-60).

Tou xuan ("spinning of the head," "lightness of the head"):
(DACH) Spinning of the head: leg-*sanli* (ST-36).
(DACH) Spinning of the head, head dizziness: *neiguan* (PC-6), tonify.
(DACH X, 29v) Spinning of the head and eyes *(tou mu xuan),* acute pain, swelling of the skin, makes white spots [appear before the eyes?]: moxa at *chuanghai* (GV-21, IS GV-22, *xinhui*).
(YXRM) Spinning of the head; *(DACH)* lightness of the head: *luoque* (BL-8).
(DACH IX, 14r) Spinning of the head after meals: *weishu* (BL-21).
(DACH VII, 31r) Scarlet eyes, swollen, acute pain, headaches, pain joining the nape to the cheek, spinning of the head: foot-*linqi* (GB-41).
(DACH) Spinning of the head, pain of the eyes, *(YXRM).* Sight obscured, headaches, turning of the head: *tianzhu* (BL-10).

Xuan yun ("light halo"):

An illness which brings momentary confusion of consciousness and perception. It comes from an anemia to the point of lesion of the cerebellum, or from a weakness of the nerves. Is also found in vomiting, convulsions (jing lman), etc. (Ci Yuan, "Xuan yun")

(JM) Xuan yun: yinxi (HT-6), *shugu* (BL-65), *chengguang* (BL-6), *wuchu* (BL-5), *yuzhen* (BL-9), *xiaguan* of cheek (ST-2, IS ST-7).
(YIX I, 4r) Internal headache and *xuan yun: baihui* (GV-19, IS GV-20).
(YIZ, 38v) Xuan yun, fears the cold, wears a cap in spring and summer, has an attack when it is removed: *shangxing* (GV-22, IS GV-23), *baihui* (GV-19, IS GV-20), *fengchi* (GB-20), *fenglong* (ST-40).

Tou yun ("head dizziness"):

(DACH II, 30v) Visual dizziness *(mu xuan)* and *tou yun: fengchi* (GB-20).
(DACH VII, 32r) Tou yun, numbed, forgets everything, troubled and darkened eyes: *waiguan* (TW-5), *dadun* (LR-1), *baihui* (GV-19, IS GV-20), *ganshu* (BL-19).

Xue yun ("blood dizziness"):

(JM) Halo of blood after delivery: abdomen-*yinjiao* (CV-7).
(DACH II, 25r) Xue yun of women: *sanyinjiao* (SP-6), abdomen-*yinjiao* (CV-7).

Vertigo from heights:

(YXRM I, 46v) Falls when looking from a height: *qihai* (CV-6).
(Ling Shu XX) Spinning of the head and sudden weakness in the legs: *tianzhu* (BL-10).
(DACH) Spasms of energy, falling down: *ciliao* (BL-32).
(YXRM I, 46v) Spasms of energy: *zhubin* (KI-9).
(YXRM I, 46v) Feels like one is in a boat: *shenmai* (BL-62).

Syncope (jue).

The same as jue with the "illness" radical. Energy in counterflow; the energy is closed on itself; there is fog and syncope. (Ci Yuan, "Jue" [with the "roof" radical])

It is also written jue (with the "roof" radical): counterflow of the energy which closes on itself; suddenly one loses awareness, feelings, movement. (Ci Yuan, "Jue" [with the "illness" radical])

A distinction is made between hot and cold syncope. For the hot type, leave the needle in until coldness; three punctures in the yin for one puncture in the yang. For the cold type, leave the needle in until heat; three punctures in the yang for one puncture in the yin. If the illness is old, puncture deeply and leave for a long time. (DACH VI, 9r)

If hands and feet are cold, needles; if pulses are contracted or absent: moxa. (DACH X, 33v)

(GSdeM) Massage with the fingernail: arm-*sanli* (LI-10), if no result: *shuigou* (GV-25, IS GV-26, *renzhong*).
Cold syncope: *(YXRM, DACH) yangjiao* (GB-35); *(DACH II, 19r) yongquan* (KI-1); *(DACH, YXRM) yemen* (TW-2); *(DACH X, 27r) taiyuan* (LU-9) and *yemen* (TW-2).
Hot syncope: *(DACH II, 19r) yongquan* (KI-1).
Syncope: *(DACH IX, 11v)* disperse *guangming* (GB-37).
(DACH) Energy of the syncope under the umbilicus: *xiawan* (CV-10).
(DACH X, 27r) Syncope in counterflow (violent): *yangfu* (GB-38), foot-*linqi* (GB-41), *zhangmen* (LR-13).
(DACH) Energy of syncope attacking the upper body: *xiaxi* (GB-43).
Syncope of feet and hands (?): *(YXRM)* foot-*dadu* (SP-2).
Syncope of the four limbs: *(YIX I, 7v) neiting* (ST-44).
Syncope and cold of the four limbs: *(JM) sanyinjiao* (SP-6); *(JM)* after an illness with fever: *taixi* (KI-5, IS KI-3).

Coma (shi jue).

Under the general name of *shi jue*, "cadaverous syncope," it seems that from antiquity China has confused several problems which have a similar appearance, particularly catalepsia, complete loss of awareness, and apoplectic or diabetic comas.

❦ *Shi jue has the symptoms of sudden death: tightened mouth, deathlike inversion, recognizes no one.*
(DACH III, 31r)

Apoplectic coma: disperse *lidui* (ST-45), *yongquan* (KI-1), *shaoshang* (LU-11), *shenmen* (HT-7).

Diabetic coma: disperse *shangqiu* (SP-5) and *yamen* (GV-14, IS GV-15).

(DACH VI, 14v) Coma, syncope, but the pulse beats normally. The yin is at the top, the evil has risen in counterflow, the yang energy is troubled. The five secondary vessels (passage points) are closed and do not communicate; that is why the appearance is like a cadaver: *yinbai* (SP-1), *yongquan* (KI-1), *lidui* (ST-45), *shaoshang* (LU-11), *shaochong* (HT-9), *shenmen* (HT-7). At each extremity puncture three times; in serious cases moxa two times and puncture 2 *fen*.

(DACH IV, 9r; YXRM) Coma: *baihui* (GV-19, IS GV-20) and *yinbai* (SP-1).

(DACH III, 31r; DACH II, 26r) Coma: *zhongji* (CV-3), *xuanzhong* (GB-39).

(DACH) Coma: appearance of a cadaver: *dadun* (LR-1).

(DACH) Coma: *jinmen* (BL-63), *lieque* (LU-7), lip-*heliao* (LI-19).

(DACH) Coma: "running and flowing," *hunmen* (BL-42, IS BL-47).

(DACH) Baneful coma from depression: *zanzhu* (BL-2).

(YXRM) Coma, sunken into evil: *kunlun* (BL-60).

(DACH) Coma, face dark like coal: *yongquan* (KI-1).

(DACH) Coma, not reviving: 100 moxas on *shenque* (CV-8), and if he does not begin to revive, another 100 moxas.

Drowning.

(JO, 37) First, get the water out (by hanging the head down), then puncture deeply at *jiuwei* (CV-15), then fifteen moxas on *baihui* (GV-19, IS GV-20) and thirty moxas on *guanyuan* (CV-4). If men have the scrotum relaxed, if women have the mouth open, there is no possibility of reviving them.

(DACH) Death from drowning *(ni si)*, turn upside down (head down) to get the water out, puncture with tonification *huiyin* (CV-1); if he urinates, he will live.

False Death.

Sudden death *(cu si, bao si):*
(DACH XI, 14r) Sudden death: *dadun* (LR-1); *(YXRM)* *jinmen* (BL-63); *(YXRM I, 46r)* *shenque* (CV-8); *(DACH)* *huiyin* (CV-1), needles one *cun* deep.

(YXRM) Children: sudden death from meningitis: *hegu* (LI-4).

"Flying cadaver" *(fei shi):* plague?

(DACH) Evil symptoms of flying cadaver; *(YXRM)* sudden falling in cases of evil spells of flying cadaver: *tianfu* (LU-3).

(DACH) Following a flowing flying cadaver [after exposure to a po-animated pestilence?]: *zhongfu* (LU-1); *(DACH, YXRM)* *weiyang* (BL-53, IS BL-39).

Note

[1] The idea of not keeping shoes on seems to be that the feet cannot flex and thus cannot hold the shoes. — Trans.

Chapter IV

Energy: General Excesses

I. Heat, Fever, Malaria — II. Perspiration, Sweat, Odors — III. Pain, Contusions, Arthritis, General Rheumatism — IV. Agitation — V. Intermittent Contractions — VI. Prolonged Contractions, Contractures — VII. Fullness, Accumulations

I. Heat, Fever, Malaria

The distinctions among malaria, hyperthermia and fever are not clearly made. The ideogram pronounced *yo* indicates internal heat. The same ideogram pronounced *re* indicates heat emanating from the body or external heat.[1] The heat of the cutaneous covering is an excess of yang. The internal heat is an emptiness of yin, the interior being invaded by the yang as heat.

> When the energies of the yang meridians cannot communicate, there is a lot of fever. **Yangwei mai** *(point of crossing and reunion,* **waiguan,** *TW-5) links all the yang energies. (YXRM I, 9r)*

For fever and heat disperse the yang on the surface; tonify the yin (cold) on the left and disperse the yang (heat) on the right.

Heat (re).

(DACH) Can take out heat as well as cold: *shenmai* (BL-62).
(DACH) Extreme heat [even] in the shade: *jianyu* (LI-15), *waiguan* (TW-5).
(DACH VI, 14r) Agitating heat: *lidui* (ST-45).
(DACH) Puncturing frequently dissipates all yang heat: *fengmen* (BL-12).
(DACH) All yang heat and abundance of energy: *yamen* (GV-14, IS GV-15).
(YXRM I, 46r) Attack of heat over the whole body: *dazhu* (BL-11).
(YXRM I, 47r) Tides of heat and nocturnal sweats (violent): *xinshu* (BL-15).
(YXRM) Body hot like fire: *shaoshang* (HT-9).
(DACH) Body hot like fire, head aches as if broken: *mingmen* (GV-4).
(YXRM) Body hot like fire, palms hot, agitation, melancholia: *daling* (PC-7).
(DACH) Body hot without sweat: *shangwan* (CV-13).
(DACH) Sudden chill, inhibition, heat without end: *dazhu* (BL-11).
(YXRM) Heat of the body: *qucha* (BL-4); *(DACH) naokong* (GB-19), *shugu* (BL-65), *quze* (PC-3).

Fevers (ye).

(YXRM I, 46v) All fevers: *xuehai* (SP-10), *yixi* (BL-40, IS BL-45).
(YXRM) All types of heat from problems: *zhengying* (GB-13, IS GB-17).
(YXRM I, 46v) Prolonged fevers: *yixi* (BL-40, IS BL-45); *(YIX 7v) quchi* (LI-11).
(JM) Attacks of fever coming and going, entering and leaving: *shendao* (GV-10, IS GV-11).
(JO, 74) Fever: treatment with needles — *hegu* (LI-4) 4 *fen*; leg-*sanli* (ST-36), 8 *fen*; *zhaohai* (KI-3, IS KI-6), *zhongwan* (CV-12), 8 *fen*. If the fever is intense and serious at this moment, add: *shenmai* (BL-62), 3 *fen* and *chengshan* (BL-57), 4 *fen*.
(JM, 321) Fever: *bailao* (GV-13, IS GV-14, *dazhui*), *shenzhu* (GV-11, IS GV-12), *gaohuangshu* (BL-38, IS BL-43), leg-*sanli* (ST-36).
(YIX, 8v) Illness with fever is treated at the eighth reunion points: *zhangmen* (LR-13), *zhongwan* (CV-12), *xuanzhong* (GB-39), *yanglingquan* (GB-34), *geshu* (BL-17), *shanzhong* (CV-17), *taiyuan* (LU-9), *dazhu* (BL-11).
(YIX I, 4r) Attacks of fever: *zhongchong* (PC-9) and *quchi* (LI-11); *(DACH I, 19r) shaochong* (HT-9) and *quchi* (LI-11).
(YIZ, 40) Body hot, panting: *sanjian* (LI-3).
(JM) Fever from bad cold: *hegu* (LI-4), *yinxi* (HT-6), *zhigou* (TW-6), *waiqiu* (GB-36), *wushu* (GB-27), *danshu* (BL-19), *mingmen* (GV-4), *chengling* (GB-14, IS GB-18). *(DACH)* Fever from cold: *erjian* (LI-2).
(DACH) Fever, the whole body aching, exhaustion, violent sweat: *bailao* (GV-13, IS GV-14, *dazhui*).
(DACH) Fever with chattering of the teeth: *yuji* (LU-10).
(YXRM I, 46v) Fever from fatigue: *neiguan* (PC-6).

(JM) Attacks of fever: thigh-*wuli* (LR-10), *daling* (PC-7).

(DACH) Typhoid, excessive, continuous fever: leg-*sanli* (ST-36), *jianyu* (LI-15).

(DACH) Fever *(re)* from tuberculosis: *chize* (LU-5).

(GSdeM) Fever from flu: disperse *bailao* (GV-13, IS GV-14, *dazhui*) and *hegu* (LI-4).

(DACH) Fever from energy: *sanjian* (LI-3), same with stoppage of functions: *jiaoxin* (KI-8).

(DACH) Fever from melancholia, fullness of energy: *yixi* (BL-40, IS BL-45).

(DACH) Fever *(re)* from emptiness, blockage: *baihuanshu* (BL-30).

(DACH) Fever after delivery (puerperal): *ganshu* (BL-18).

(YXRM) Fever *(re)*, scarlet face: *neiguan* (PC-6).

(DACH VIII 32r) Fever *(re)* with a lot of sleep: *yangfu* (GB-38).

(YIX I, 4v, DACH V, 19r) Annual fever coming from time to time: *taodao* (GV-12, IS GV-13) and *feishu* (BL-13).

(DACH) Fever, pain in the bone: *pangguangshu* (BL-28).

(DACH) Illnesses from fever with shock, sweat not coming, middle of the palms hot, body hot like fire: *guanchong* (TW-1).

(DACH X, 33r) Body hot, sweats, feet unstable and cold: foot-*dadu* (SP-2).

(DACH) Puerperal fever: *ganshu* (BL-18).

Febrile illnesses, with or without sweating: see perspiration.

Fever of the organs.

> For example, to puncture the spleen-pancreas meridian for an illness of the liver, that of the heart for kidney troubles, that of the lungs for the heart, that of the liver for the lungs, or for an illness of the **taiyang** (bladder-small intestine), to disperse **yangming** (stomach-large intestine) will increase the counterflow of the energy; this kills. *(DACH I, 3r)*

It is necessary to take account of the flow of the energy and of the mother-child, husband-wife laws.

> For any fever of an organ, puncture the **rong** point of the meridian of this organ. *(DACH VI, 26v)*

Bladder: *(DACH)* Fever from the bladder: pain in the lumbar area, heaviness of head, sweats without cause, vertigo, foggy head, sweats constantly: *weizhong* (BL-54, IS BL-40), *jinmen* (BL-63), *shenmai* (BL-62).

(DACH I, 3r) If the fever starts in the head, puncture the bladder meridian at the nape (*tianzhu,* BL-10); when the sweat comes, cease.

Five Treasure Organs: fever of the five treasure organs: bleed *shaoshang* (LU-11) and *mingmen* (GV-4).

Gallbladder: *(DACH)* Fever from gallbladder, a little bit of cold and heat, cannot stand seeing people, apprehension, a lot of sweat: *xiaxi* (GB-43) .

Heart: *(DACH I, 3r)* In fevers of the heart, the whole face is scarlet first. *(DACH I, 2r)* First, no pleasure for whole days, then fever. It establishes itself, then violent pain in the heart, burning melancholia, vomits very easily, headaches, red face without sweat. Maximum at the *ren-gui* hours (7 to 11 a.m.), great sweat at *bing-ting* (3 to 7 p.m.). If there is a counterflow of the energy, death at *ren-gui* (7 to 11 a.m.); puncture the heart meridians (*rong* point *shaofu,* HT-8) and the small intestine (*qiangu,* SI-2).

(DACH) Great desire for cool water, palpitations: *shenmen* (HT-7), fevers of the heart: *yixi* (BL-40, IS BL-45).

Kidney: *(DACH I, 3r)* In fevers of the kidneys the chin is scarlet first. *(DACH I, 2r)* First, pain of lumbar area, lower legs numb, thirst with bitter taste, drinks a lot, body hot. If the fever is established, pain of the nape, lower legs cold and numb, heat on underside of the foot, does not want to speak. Maximum at the *wu-ji* hours (9 p.m. to 3 a.m.), great sweat at *ren-gui* (7 to 11 a.m.). If there is a counterflow of the energy, death comes at *wu-ji* (9 p.m. to 3 a.m.); puncture the kidney meridian (*rong* point, *rangu,* KI-2) and that of the bladder (*rong* point, BL-66, foot-*tonggu*); all sweat will be vanquished.

(DACH I, 3r) If the fever starts with heaviness of the body, pain of the bones, deafness, likes darkness, puncture the kidney meridian; if serious, 50 punctures. *(DACH)* Fever of kidneys: strong heat, vomits, shuts the door, pain of the lumbar area, numb lower legs, stiffness of the nape: *dazhong* (KI-6, IS KI-4), *taixi* (KI-5, IS KI-3), *zhiyang* (GV-8, IS GV-9).

Liver: *(DACH I, 3r)* In fevers of the liver the left cheek is scarlet first. *(DACH I, 2v)* Urine yellow, abdomen painful, sleeps a lot, pain and fullness of the sides, hands and feet agitated, cannot rest peacefully, headaches, vessels abound. Maximum at the *geng-xin* hours (3 to 7 a.m.), great sweat at *jia-yi* (11 a.m. to 3 p.m.). If there is a counterflow of the energy, death at *geng-xin* (3 to 7 a.m.); puncture the liver meridian (*rong* point, *xingjian* LR-2) and that of the gallbladder (*xiaxi* GB-43).

(DACH) Fevers of the liver: blue complexion, insufficient urine, fullness of the lower pelvic region, swelling of the bones of the knee: *taichong* (LR-3) and *zhongfeng* (LR-4).

Lungs: *(DACH I, 3r)* In fevers of the lungs the right cheek is scarlet first. *(DACH I, 2r)* First fatigued, ready to faint, evil wind or cold of the fine hairs, tongue yellow on the top, body hot. If the fever establishes itself then panting, cough, pain, chest agitated, cannot breathe deeply, unbearable headache, sweats and chills. Maximum at *bing-ding* hours (3 to 7 p.m.), great sweat at *geng-xin* (3 to 7 a.m.). If there is a counterflow of the energy, death comes at *bing-ding* (3 to 7 p.m.): puncture the lung meridian (*rong* point, *yuji,* LU-10) and that of the large intestine (*erjian,* LI-2); squeeze out blood as if milking a cow; cures immediately. *(DACH I, 3v)* If the fever starts from a pain of the arm and hand, puncture the large intestine and lung meridians. When the sweat is out, it will be finished. *(DACH)* Fever of the lungs: congestion, cough, emotiveness — *lieque* (LU-7).

Spleen-pancreas: *(DACH I, 3r)* In fevers of the spleen-pancreas the nose is scarlet first. *(DACH I, 2r)* First, heavy head and pain of the jaws; melancholia, agitation, bluish complexion, nausea, body hot. If the fever is established, pain of the lumbar area, cannot bend or get up, abdomen full, diarrhea, pain on both sides of the chin. Maximum at the *jia-yi* hours (11 a.m. to 3 a.m.), great sweat coming at *wu-ji* (9 p.m. to 3 a.m.). If there is a counterflow of the energy, death comes at *jia-yi* (11 a.m. to 3 p.m.); puncture the spleen-pancreas meridian (*rong* point, *dadu,* SP-2) and that of the stomach (*neiting,* ST-44).

(DACH) Fever of the spleen-pancreas: vomits and is depressed afterwards, heavy head, blue complexion, nausea: *gongsun* (SP-4), *shangqiu* (SP-5) and *lingtai* (GV-9, IS GV-10).

(DACH I, 3r) If the fever starts from the feet and lower legs, puncture the stomach meridian.

Alternations of cold and heat.

Sudden cold and sudden heat: *shaochong* (HT-9). *(DACH)* hand-*wangu* (SI-4), *taiyuan* (LU-9).

(DACH) Cold and heat alternating: *zhiyang* (GV-8, IS GV-9).

(DACH) Cold or heat of the lower leg and foot: foot-*linqi* (GB-41).

Malaria, tidal fever, intermittent fever (yo).

(YXRM I, 46r) All fevers; *(JM)* intermittent fever: *yixi* (BL-40, IS BL-45).

(YIX I, 9v) Malarial fevers; it cures them by itself: *neiguan* (PC-6).

(YXRM) All malarial fevers, body hot, back cold, sweat coming: *lieque* (LU-7).

(YXRM I, 46v) All fevers, all illness from blood: *xuehai* (SP-10).

(GSdeM) zhangmen (LR-13) on the left (homeopathic remedy — China).

(JM) Intermittent fever *(jian xie re):* *hegu* (LI-4), *sanjian* (LI-3), *yangshi* (TW-4); *(DACH) yangxi* (LI-5); *(JM) tai-yuan* (LU-9), *tianfu* (LU-3), *qingling* (HT-2), *neiting* (ST-44), foot-*linqi* (GB-41), *jinggu* (BL-64), *shugu* (BL-65), *xiangu* (ST-42), *bailao* (GV-13, IS GV-14, *dazhui*), *xuanli* (GB-6), *tianshu* (ST-25).

Fever in fourths (1, 4, 7, 10), every three days an attack: great cold, slight heat: *fuliu* (KI-7); slight cold, strong heat: *jianshi* (PC-5).

Fever in thirds (1, 3, 5, 7), an attack every two days: *bailao* (GV-13, IS GV-14, *dazhui*), *fengchi* (GB-20), *shaoshang* (LU-11), *ermen* (TW-23, IS TW-21), hand-*wangu* (SI-4), arm-*wuli* (LI-13), *qiangu* (SI-2), foot-*linqi* (GB-41), *xingjian* (LR-2), *mingmen* (GV-4), *yixi* (BL-40, IS BL-45), *shendao* (GV-10, IS GV-11), *tianchi* (PC-1).

(DACH) Fever in thirds, cold and heat: *shangyang* (LI-1), *taodao* (GV-12, IS GV-13).

(DACH) Fever in thirds, shivering: *shangxing* (GV-22, IS GV-23).

(DACH) Fever in thirds, vertigo: *dazhu* (BL-11).

Daily fever: *(DACH)* Attack every day (double fever): foot-*linqi* (GB-41).

Many attacks per day: *(DACH)* Malaria: *jinmen* (BL-63).

(YXRM) Malaria, two attacks per day: head-*linqi* (GB-11, IS GB-15).

Ice-cold malaria *(han nüe):* *(DACH) sanjian* (LI-3), *feiyang* (BL-58), *lidui* (ST-45), and does not eat: *gongsun* (SP-4).

(YXRM) Ice-cold malaria, sweat not coming out: *zhiyin* (BL-67), malaria, shivering: *xiangu* (ST-43).

(DACH) Old malaria, shivering, mucus; *guanmen* (GB-40).

(DACH) Malaria, shivering from cold, sweat: *yangfu* (GB-38).

Malaria, heat: *(DACH) baihuanshu* (BL-30), *zhongwan* (CV-12); *(YXRM) yindu* (KI-19), *rangu* (KI-2).

(DACH) Malaria, a lot of sweat: *kunlun* (BL-60).

(DACH) Malaria, heat returning when cold: *hegu* (LI-4).

Alternating fever: *(YXRM)* Malaria, either hot or cold: hand-*wangu* (SI-4).

(DACH) Malaria cold and hot: *hegu* (LI-4), *jianshi* (PC-5), *pianli* (LI-6), *yangxi* (LI-5), *tianfu* (LU-3), *tianshu* (ST-25), *yindu* (KI-19).

Hyperexcitation: *(DACH VI, 14r)* malaria, hyperexcitation: *lidui* (ST-45); *(YXRM) chongyang* (ST-42); *(DACH)* head-*wangu* (GB-17, IS GB-12), *feiyang* (BL-58).

Seasonal: *(DACH III, 29r; DACH IV, 5v)* Epidemic seasonal malaria, periodic attacks of malaria: *houxi* (SI-3).

Diverse: *(DACH)* malaria, little energy: *shenmen* (HT-7).

(YXRM) Malaria, vomiting, diarrhea, dysentery; *(DACH)* malaria causing thinness: *pishu* (BL-20).

(DACH) Malaria, pain in the heart: *gongsun* (SP-4).

(DACH) Malaria, takes food without tasting: *neiting* (ST-44).

(DACH) Malaria, attack when eating: *tianjing* (TW-10).

(DACH) Malaria from shock: *xiaohai* (SI-8).

(YIX I, 4r) Congestion of spleen-pancreas *(pi man)* after malaria: *zhangmen* (LR-13).

II. Perspiration, Sweat, Odors

Perspiration, sweat (han).

Weak energy with abundant elimination (kidney relaxed) results in scant perspiration. Abundant energy (from excess yang and insufficient yin) with weak renal elimination results in more copious perspiration.

Insufficient perspiration (sympatheticotonia):

(YXRM IV, 20v) Inability to sleep and sweat is commanded by the *yangming* (large intestine-stomach), nose dry often, pain in the eyes.

(YXRM I, 39r) To make sweat come, needle at *hegu* (LI-4). Put the needle in 2 *fen*, tonify with the number 9 X 9; number of punctures: 10 times; men on the left, women on the right. When puncturing we get the sweat (thus puncture many times). Then, use the dispersal method, the sweat stops; tepid body, then we can remove the needle. If the perspiration does not stop, puncture *yinshi* (ST-33), tonify *hegu* (LI-4).

(DACH X, 27r) Little sweat: tonify *hegu* (LI-4) and disperse *fuliu* (KI-7).

(DACH IV, 11v) Must sweat but cannot: tonify *hegu* (LI-4).

(DACH) Cannot sweat: leg-*xialian* (ST-39, IS *xiajuxu*).

(YXRM) Does not sweat: disperse *fengchi* (GB-20), which acts upon the sympathetic system.

(YXRM) Sweat not coming: *yuzhen* (BL-9), *zhonglüshu* (BL-29).

(DACH, YXRM) Body hot without sweat: *shangwan* (CV-13).

(DACH, YXRM) Shock, sweat not coming: *pianli* (LI-6), *daling* (PC-7).

Fever without sweat: *(DACH, YXRM) shangyang* (LI-7), *hegu* (LI-4), *qiangu* (SI-2), *yanggu* (SI-5), hand-*wangu* (SI-4), *yangchi* (TW-4), *zhigou* (TW-6), *zhongzhu* (TW-30), *jingqu* (LU-8), *kongzui* (LU-6), *daling* (PC-7), *laogong* (PC-8), leg-*sanli* (ST-36), *chongyang* (ST-42), *lidui* (ST-45), *xiangu* (ST-43), *xiaxi* (GB-43), *weizhong* (BL-54, IS BL-40), *dadu* (SP-2), *fengchi* (GB-20), *xuanli* (GB-6), *tianchi* (PC-1), *shangxing* (GV-22, IS GV-23).

(DACH, YXRM) Illnesses with fever, sweat not coming, sudden delirium: *guangming* (GB-37).

(DACH, YXRM) Fever without sweat, pain in the supraclavicular hollow: *tianliao* (TW-15).

Excess perspiration (hyperthyroidism, hypo-ovaria, vagotonia):

> *Emptiness, exhaustion and old illnesses have sweat without cause: the five internal organs are dry, mucus and saliva encumber and block, the energy passages do not communicate any longer . . . anger, discontent, energy tied up, closed . . . the kidneys respond to the heart. If fire abounds in the heart, then the small intestine tightens from heat, urination is difficult. (YXRM V, 28v)*

(DACH, X, 27r) A lot of sweat: disperse *hegu* (LI-4) and tonify *fuliu* (KI-7).

(GSdeM) Tonify *fengchi* (GB-20) and disperse *tianzhu* (BL-10).

(DACH VII, 31r) Chills, sweat without cause, external burning: *waiguan* (TW-5).

(DACH) Sweat flows without stopping; *(YXRM)* hot sweat flows without stopping; *(DACH IV, 11v)* sweat without reason and attacks of jaundice; *(DACH)* nocturnal sweat (or violent): *fuliu* (KI-7) tonify.

(DACH X, 27r) Lots of sweat: disperse *hegu* (LI-4).

(DACH) Sweat without cause: *(JM, DACH)* nocturnal sweat: *rangu* (KI-2).

(DACH VII, 27v) Sweat without cause, sweat flowing from the head: *shenmai* (BL-62).

(DACH, JM) Sweat without cause, nocturnal sweat *(YXRM)* body always wet: *geshu* (BL-17).

(DACH II, 25v) Nocturnal sweat *(YIX I, 4r)* nocturnal sweat coming in abundance: disperse *yinxi* (HT-6).

(YIX I, 10r) Nocturnal sweat: first disperse *houxi* (SI-3). *(DACH II, 10r)* Nocturnal sweat coming in abundance: disperse *houxi* (SI-3).

(YIX I, 4v) Nocturnal sweat: first disperse *houxi* (SI-3).

(YIX I, 4v) Nocturnal sweat: *jianshi* (PC-5); *(YIX I, 11r) waiguan* (TW-5); *(DACH) jiaoxin* (KI-8).

(YXRM I, 47r) Tides of heat, nocturnal sweat (violent): *xinshu* (BL-15).

(YXRM I) Sweeps up the sweat that flows: *qihai* (CV-6).

(DACH III, 32v) Attack of sweat without stopping: disperse *hegu* (LI-4).

(DACH) Sweat flows without stopping: tonify *fuliu* (KI-7).

(DACH X, 27r) Copious sweat: tonify *fuliu* (KI-7) and disperse *hegu* (LI-4); *(DACH, YXRM) daheng* (SP-15); *(JM) yuzhen* (BL-9); *(DACH VI, 15v)* foot-*qiaoyin* (GB-44), *hegu* (LI-4).

(YXRM) Body always wet: *geshu* (BL-17).

(YXRM) Sweat coming: *shaohai* (HT-3); the same with emptiness and thirst: *zhonglüshu* (BL-29).

(DACH III, 29v) Sweat from emptiness: *bailao* (GV-13, IS GV-14, *dazhui*).

(DACH) Great shock, sweat: moxa at *yixi* (BL-40, IS BL-45).

(DACH, YXRM) Sweat cold and flowing: *shaoshang* (LU-11).

(DACH) Moist head from sweat that does not extend below the shoulders: *quze* (PC-3). *(DACH VII, 27v; YIX, 10v)* Sweat flowing from the head: *shenmai* (BL-62); violent sweat (or nocturnal) in the area of the head: *yintang* (GV-23a, IS M-HN-3).

(DACH X, 33r) Body hot, sweat coming, cold and deficiency of the feet: foot-*dadu* (SP-2). *(YXRM)* Illnesses with fever, sweat coming: foot-*dadu* (SP-2); and feet cold: *taixi* (KI-5, IS KI-3), *daheng* (SP-15).

(DACH) A lot of heat and cold, sweat comes out: *gongsun* (SP-4).

(DACH) Shivering, heaviness, sweat coming out: *fengfu* (GV-15, IS GV-16).

(DACH XII, 26r) Children, massage can stop sweating: *yangchi* (TW-4).

(GSdeM) Sweats from the feet: disperse *xingjian* (LR-2).

Odors (chou).

(DACH XI, 11v) Odors depend on the heart meridian: disperse *shaochong* (HT-9).

(DACH) Zhang Ji cured stench and pruritis of the genital organs with *shaochong* (HT-9) after dissipating the sweat with *xingjian* (LR-2).

(DACH X, 26r) Eats a lot, body smells: *weishu* (BL-21), *pishu* (BL-20).

III. Pains, Contusions, Arthritis, General Rheumatism

Pains can have various origins: neuralgia, neuritis, rheumatism, childbirth, etc. "Pain is a fullness of yin energy; puncture deeply and return to the superficial level." *(YXRM V, 87v)*

However, it is constantly observed that neuralgias mostly cause a marked tension of the superficial pulses (yang) *(GSdeM)*. In fact, there are pains from excess of yang energy and pains from emptiness of yin blood. In order to differentiate them, it is necessary to remember that yin pains are fixed, constant, always in the same place, with aggravation during the day, and are based on a material problem. Yang pains are intermittent, not always in the same place and the excess yang has nightly aggravation. Thus, a pure sciatica has pain of the lower limb sometimes in one place and sometimes in another, while sciatica caused by a sacroiliac arthritis has constant and localized pain, mostly in the sacral area and ischia, and the thigh. In the first case the cure can be almost immediate; in the second we must evacuate the material deposit of the arthritis first, which requires several days; the immediate amelioration is partial. When pains do not succumb to the needle even partially or come back very quickly, there is surely a material lesion.

Neuralgia (pains of the nerves): *shen jing tong* includes pains without a material basis, simply hyperexcitation of one or many nerves, internal or external. Neuritis (lesion of the nerves: *shen jing shang*), includes material inflammation of the nerves, such as zona.

> Pain following the course of a nerve, numerous or rare attacks, piercing like a knife, or hammering like a club; they come and go . . . Caused either by nervous trouble or loss of blood, or by an infectious illness. They most often begin suddenly on the face or on the occiput or sacrum; after several months or years, they cure themselves.
> *(Ci Yuan, "Shen-jing-tong")*

Rheumatic pains are always accompanied either by a minor or major material modification — swelling, redness, etc. When the joints are painful, without the material modification being yet apparent, they are called arthralgia. When the articulation is already visibly inflamed, it is arthritis. The Chinese differentiate between rheumatism from inadequate food (or excess work) and rheumatism from too much food (and insufficient physical work). The Japanese, in order not to include the old regional ideas, have adopted the European name and call it *"liu ma chi se."* The old Chinese name is *tong feng,* "crossed by the wind," and when it is serious, "white-tiger." Arthralgias and arthritis are called either *li jie feng,* "wind of the different joints," or *rao guo feng,* "wind enveloping the joints."

> This word is an image, our country called it in the old days **tong feng** and also **li jie feng.**
> *(Ci Yuan, "Liu-ma-chi-se")*

Illness causing extreme pain in certain parts of the body. Those who like wine and meat a lot are easily attacked by this in their old age. At the painful places the skin is purplish; there are even points which come out as if burned. (Ci Yuan, "Tong-feng")

*For **tong feng** attacking the joints we differentiate between thin, weak people and strong, large people. For weak and thin people, the cause is internal: it is an emptiness of the blood (yin). For big and strong people, the cause is external: mostly wind or humidity (excess yang); they have an aggravation at night (yin), the time when the blood (yin) is in the yin (night). The pains, with or without swelling, are biting. When it bites like a tiger, it is called **bai hu tong feng**, "wind crossing the white tiger." (YXRM IV, 14)*

It is thus necessary to treat thin, weak people (emptiness of yin, thus tonify the yin and blood), and big strong people (excess yang, thus disperse yang) differently.

Pain (tong, dull pain; teng, acute pain).

(DACH IV, 10v; YIX I, 8r) If we want an analgesic, puncture there [at the painful point]. Groans with the least movement: *kunlun* (BL-60) disperse.

(DACH) For what is unbearable in the pain; *(DACH V, 5r)* cures especially pains that attack; *(DACH XI, 5r)* cures especially the energy pain of women: *qihai* (CV-6).

(JM) Pains of the nerves; *(JO)* pains of local illnesses: *wenliu* (LI-7).

(JM) All trouble or illnesses of the nervous system: leg-*sanli* (ST-36).

(YXRM I, 39v) Pains of energy: *taiyuan* (LU-9); *(DACH) yongquan* (KI-1).

(DACH) Pains of energy similar to sharp knives: abdomen-*yinjiao* (CV-7).

(DACH III, 32r) Malign acute pain from shock: *dubi* (ST-35).

Pain without fixed place:

(DACH, YXRM) Pain without fixed place: *yangfu* (GB-38); *(YXRM)* foot-*linqi* (GB-41); *(DACH, YXRM) xiaxi* (GB-43).

(DACH, YXRM) Great shock, stupifying, does not know what causes the pain: *tianjing* (TW-10), *zhaohai* (KI-3, IS KI-6).

Pains of the whole body:

(JM) Pain of the whole body: *yangfu* (GB-38); *(YXRM) chize* (LU-5); *(DACH)*: disperse *dabao* (SP-21).

(DACH) Extreme pain of the organism: *ququan* (LR-8)

(DACH) Unbearable pain and heaviness: *naokong* (GB-19).

(DACH) Pain and swelling of the body: *geshu* (BL-17).

Nighttime or daytime pains:

Night pains (excess of yang not transformed into yin): *(GSdeM)* tonify *zhaohai* (KI-3, IS KI-6) and disperse *shenmai* (BL-62).

Daytime pains (excess yin not transformed into yang): *(GSdeM)* tonify *shenmai* (BL-62) and disperse *zhaohai* (KI-3, IS KI-6).

Various pains:

(YXRM I, 39r) Pains of emptiness: *shangxing* (GV-22, IS GV-23).

(YXRM) Strangling pain: *qichong* (ST-30).

(YXRM) Sudden pain from contractions: *kunlun* (BL-60).

(DACH) Pains from tightness: *benshen* (GB-9, IS GB-13).

(YXRM I, 46v) Acute pains from tightened muscles: *hegu* (LI-4), *(YXRM I, 41r) zhigou* (TW-6).

(DACH VII, 31v; YIX I, 11v) Pain attacking bone and internal and external muscles, groin and back: *waiguan* (TW-5).

(YXRM) General pains, swelling and fullness under the ribs, hot lower abdomen: *guanyuan* (CV-4).

Pain like a necklace: *shangyang* (LI-1).

Pain like suspenders: *yangfu* (GB-38).

Contusions, injuries.

(DACH) Falling: bad blood staying in the abdomen: *rangu* (KI-2).

(DACH) Contusions *(pu shang): bailao* (GV-13, IS GV-14, *dazhui*), *jianjing* (GB-21).

Contusions, pains of intestines, pelvis, lumbar area: *(DACH) jianjing* (GB-21).

Lesions and exhaustion from blows and trembling: first the painful joints, then *chengshan* (BL-57).

Lesions from blows, pain of lumbar area and hips: *tianjing* (TW-10).

(DACH) Effort, bad blood from lifting heavy weights: *yinmen* (BL-51, IS BL-37).

Rheumatism, joint pain, arthralgia, arthritis.

One should differentiate insufficiency of blood (rheumatism of the poor, *wei*) and excess yang (rheumatism of the rich, *bi*)

Rheumatism, joint pain *(bi):*

> **Bi** *is a blockage of energy which no longer circulates. It can be either painful, itching, paralyzing* **(ma bi),** *or a weakening of the hands and feet, similar to* **wei,** *paresis. But the* **wei** *has an internal cause — the emptiness of blood — whereas* **bi** *has an external cause — wind, cold, humidity. (YXRM I, 15)*

> **Bi** *is caused by wind, cold or humidity. When the evil is deep, hands and feet, limbs and body are slowed down and weakened or painful. When there is pain, we know that it is* **bi,** *fullness and shock,* **feng.** *However, when there is no pain, it is* **wei** *and emptiness. The cause of* **bi** *being external stimulation, one should disperse. (YXRM I, 38)*

> *Three varieties of* **bi:**

> **Bi** *of the muscles: they are contracted, bound, painful, one cannot move. At the beginning of the illness the muscle is warm; this stops when the illness is finished. Puncture on the muscle; it is important to puncture in the intervals of the flesh but without touching the bones.*

> **Bi** *of the skin: the skin is completely painful, the affliction comes from damp cold; send the needle very deep, puncture the great and small divisions. It is necessary to tonify, but without causing injury to either the muscles or the bone because this would provoke abscesses. When all the divisions are warmed, the illness is finished.*

> *The* **Nei Jing** *says, ''* **Bi** *of the bones: the bones are heavy and cannot be lifted, bone and marrow have numb and dull pain. It comes from the energy of cold: puncture deeply, but it is important not to injure either the vessels or the flesh. The rule is that the illness is finished when the great and small divisions are warmed.'' (DACH I, 6r,)*

> *For all* **bi** *which come and go without fixed location, puncture under the skin at the painful place, but act according to the waxing and waning of the moon (one puncture at the new moon; fifteen at the full moon). (DACH I, 8v)*

For rheumatism, it thus seems that we must disperse those which attack muscles and on the contrary tonify the others. For the places to puncture, mostly the ''unfixed points,'' or ''center of pain points,'' are indicated; however, active points are indicated as well: *(GSdeM)* Disperse foot-*shangqiu* (SP-5) and *waiguan* (TW-5).
Generalized rheumatism *(zhou bi): yuji* (LU-10), *geshu* (BL-17); *(YXRM) quyuan* (SI-13); *(DACH) jianwaishu* (SI-14) and foot-*linqi* (GB-41).
(DACH) Rheumatism *(bi)* like a tempest: *tianfu* (LU-3) and *jingqu* (LU-8).
(DACH II, 31r; YIX I, 10v) Rheumatic pains, attacks of heat, arthritis, foot-*linqi* (GB-41).
(DACH) Rheumatism *(bi)* from cold, not following, rheumatism from humidity or shock: arm-*xialian* (LI-8), leg-*xialian* (ST-39, IS *xiajuxu*).
(YXRM) Rheumatism from humidity, cannot walk: leg-*zhongdu* (LR-6).
(DACH, YXRM) Rheumatism from humidity: *tiaokou* (ST-38).
(DACH IV, 11v; YIX I, 8r) Rheumatism *(bi)* from wind, cold, humidity; pain without movement from wind cold and humidity: *huantiao* (GB-29, IS GB-30).
(DACH III, 32r) Rheumatism from cold, decline of the kidneys: leg-*sanli* (ST-36).

Arthritis, articular rheumatism:

> **Guan jie yan** *(inflammation of the joints): generally comes after taking in humidity. The joints swell and are painful; if it comes frequently it becomes chronic. The joints of the hands, thighs and knees are like a balloon, growing and swelling. There is acute pain from movement; the bones of the arms or hands make noises which we can hear. On the whole, the symptoms are similar to those of chronic rheumatism, but the evil is localized in one or two joints instead of attacking all of them. (Ci Yuan, ''Guan-jie-yan'')*

> *Chronic articular rheumatism* **(man xing guan jie liu ma chi se).** *Origin: often comes from the sequelae of acute articular rheumatism, mostly in old people; external troubles, flu (gan mao), exposed to humidity.*

> *Symptoms: swelling of the joints, attacks of pain, difficult movements. The symptoms sometimes increase and sometimes decrease. The maximum is during spring and autumn.*

Treatment with needles and moxa:

yangxi (LI-5)	....	*3 fen,*
hunmen (BL-42, IS BL-47)	....	*5 fen,*
yanglingquan (GB-34)	....	*6 fen,*
yangfu (GB-38)	....	*3 fen,*
taichong (LR-3)	....	*4 fen,*
taixi (KI-5 IS location KI-4, IS name KI-3)		*3 fen;*
at each of the above points	....	*7 moxas. (JO, 33)*

(DACH) Start with foot-*linqi* (GB-41), finish with *waiguan* (TW-5).

(JM) Chronic arthritis: *tianfu* (LU-3).

(DACH VIII, 21r) Acute articular rheumatism *(li xie feng): feiyang* (BL-58); *(DACH) hanyan* (GB-4), 7 *fen.*

(DACH VII, 31r) Serious acute articular rheumatism *(bai hu li jie feng)* with acute pain: foot-*linqi* (GB-41), *weizhong* (BL-54, IS BL-40), *xingjian* (LR-2), *tianjing* (TW-10), *quchi* (LI-11), arm-*sanli* (LI-10), *hegu* (LI-4), *jianjing* (GB-21).

(DACH) Acute articular rheumatism with sweat: *houding* (GV-18, IS GV-19).

(JM) Articular rheumatism: *xiguan* (LR-7), *xiaoluo* (TW-12).

(GSdeM) Decalcification: tonify the upper edge of C6; excess calcification, disperse the same point.

Pain of the joints (arthralgia):

(DACH) Painful joints: *shangqiu* (SP-5).

(DACH, YXRM) Complete pain of all the joints: *yangfu* (GB-38); *(DACH)* pain and numbness of all the joints.

(YIX I, 11r; DACH VII, 31v) Acute pain and swelling of the joints of the limbs, cold knees: *waiguan* (TW-5).

(YIZ, 44r) All the joints painful, cannot walk: *yanglingquan* (GB-34), *xuanzhong* (GB-39), *zhongfeng* (LR-4), 50 moxas.

(DACH VII, 31v) Epidemic pains of all the joints: *waiguan* (TW-5), *xuanzhong* (GB-39), *mingmen* (GV-4), *hunmen* (BL-42, IS BL-47).

Muscular rheumatism *(jin rou liu ma chi se):*

Origins: flu (gan mao), exposure to humidity or other known evil causes.

Symptoms: the acute symptoms are mostly met in the trapezius muscle, the cervical or lumbar muscles. There is swelling, pain, contracture and tightness; attacks of nerve pain with heat, often accompanied by heat. In chronic cases, mostly the muscles of the nape, back and lumbar cannot be moved. There are attacks of pain which change place, with aggravation at dawn.

Treatments with needles:

lieque (LU-7)	....	*2 fen,*
hegu (LI-4)	....	*4 fen,*
taiyuan (LU-9)	....	*2 fen,*
shaohai (HT-3)	....	*3 fen,*
weizhong (BL-54, IS BL-40)		*5 fen,*
leg-sanli (ST-36)	....	*8 fen,*
yangfu (GB-38)	....	*3 fen,*
taibai (SP-3)	....	*5 fen,*
taixi (KI-5, IS KI-3)	....	*3 fen.*

Treatments with moxa:

lieque (LU-7)	....	*7 moxas,*
yangfu (GB-38)	.....	*7 moxas,*
leg-sanli (ST-36)	....	*10 moxas,*
taibai (SP-3)	....	*3 moxas,*
taixi (KI-5, IS KI-3)		*3 moxas. (JO, 32)*

(JM) Muscular rheumatism: *taiyin* (ST-23).

IV. Agitation

Agitation is differentiated as follows: internal agitation (*fan,* which causes interior disquiet; *zhong,* which acts precipitously and with difficulty); and external agitation (*zao,* which causes exterior disquiet).

Internal and external agitation:
(YXRM I, 46v) Internal and external agitation: tonify *neiguan* (PC-6).

Internal agitation:
(DACH) Anxiety, internal agitation of the mind, fullness: *xuanzhong* (GB-39).

External agitation:
(YXRM) Likes to move: tonify *jianshi* (PC-5).
(DACH) External agitation of the hands and feet: head-*qiaoyin* (GB-18, IS GB-11), foot-*qiaoyin* (GB-44).
(DACH) Children: emotiveness, deranged mind, cannot stay quiet: tonify *shaochong* (HT-9).
(DACH) Agitation from parasitic worms: tonify *fuliu* (KI-7) and *zhiyin* (BL-67).

V. Intermittent Contractions

1) Spasms. 2) Cramps. 3) Yawning. 4) Sneezing. 5) Chattering of the teeth. 6) Stuttering. 7) Nervous Shivering. 8) Ticks, Trembling, Chorea. 9) Clonic Convulsions. 10) Puerperal Eclampsia. 11) Tonic or Clonic Convulsions: *Jing lüan, Ji ju,* Contractions, Pains. 12) Epilepsy, Fugue.

Most intermittent contractions are from an excess of yang energy. There are also some from insufficiency of yin energy (see Yawning).

Spasms (shan).

In Europe the word "spasm" is applied to involuntary and intermittent contractions of the smooth muscle (spasms of intestines, of the stomach) as well as to the long-lasting, true contractures of the striated muscle (spasms of the jaws, trismus). It will be used here only in the sense of intermittent contractions. In China, in antiquity, this term was applied to various troubles. The term "the seven spasms" was used for the true spasms — hernia, orchitis, vaginismus, priapism, hydrocele, etc. The modern Chinese have retained the name *shan* for true intermittent spasms.

> Illness of acute or dull lumbar pain of the lumbar area, abdomen, etc., the varieties are numerous. Generally, if the smooth-muscle organs (**ping hua jin**) receive shock or blockage, then the muscles and flesh contract many times with the contractions tightening and relaxing, thus causing violent pain. Therefore, the stomach, intestine, biliary channels, urinary channels, uterus, etc., all have them. Pains from delivery in women are also a variety of **shan.** In the past it was said that communicable orchitis and swelling of the testicles were varieties of **shan.**
> (Ci Yuan, "Shan")

External muscular spasms are also called *ji,* "tightness," or more scientifically, *die dai jing lüan,* "intermittent contractions." This can come from hypoparathyroidism (hypocalcemia): tonify the upper edge of C6.
(YXRM I, 40r) All the seven spasms stop immediately: bleed *taichong* (LR-3), disperse *dadun* (LR-1).
(DACH IV, 6v; YIX I, 5r) The seven types of spasm; *(YXRM I, 46v)* master of all spasms: bleed *dadun* (LR-1).
(DACH) The seven spasms: *guanyuan* (CV-4), *guilai* (ST-29).
(DACH II, 27r) The seven spasms, pain in the lower abdomen: *zhaohai* (KI-3, IS KI-6), *sanyinjiao* (SP-6), *ququan* (LR-8); if not better: *qihai* (CV-6), *guanyuan* (CV-4).
(DACH XI, 35r) Spasm from cold, humidity, heat accumulation of mucus: needle at *taichong* (LR-3), *dadun* (LR-1) and *xuanzhong* (GB-39); moxa at *dadun* (LR-1) and *sanyinjiao* (SP-6).
(DACH) The five spasms: *yongquan* (KI-1).
Energy of spasms: *(YXRM I, 46r; DACH) sanyinjiao* (SP-6), *rangu* (KI-2), *yongquan* (KI-1), *dai mai* (GB-26); *(DACH III, 31r) zhongji* (CV-3).
Spasms of energy: *(YXRM I, 46v) zhubin* (KI-9).
Spasms of energy; energy falls: *ciliao* (BL-32).
Sudden spasms (like a storm): *(YXRM) zhaohai* (KI-3, IS KI-6); mostly at night: *(DACH X, 31v) taichong* (LR-3); *(DACH) jinmen* (BL-63); mainly in the daytime: *(DACH X, 27v) shenmai* (BL-62).
(DACH, YXRM) dadun (LR-1), *qiuxu* (GB-40).
Spasms *(YXRM) zhaohai* (KI-3, IS KI-6) (and all nocturnal contractions).
Spasms, accumulations *(jia): (DACH) fushe* (SP-13).
(DACH) Stormy pain from spasms: *guanyuan* (CV-4).
Pain from spasms: *(YXRM) xiaochangshu* (BL-27); *(DACH) baihuanshu* (BL-30).

(DACH) Energy of spasms flowing into the five treasure organs: *shimen* (CV-5). Spasms of children: *(JM) jinmen* (BL-63), *taichong* (LR-3), *hegu* (LI-4), *chize* (LU-5), *jugu* (LI-16), *qiangjian* (GV-17, IS GV-18), *qianding* (GV-20, IS GV-21).

Spasms or convulsions of children: *(JM) hanyan* (GB-4), *yintang* (GV-23a, IS M-HN-3).

Spasms of women: *(YXRM)* and accumulation: *yinlingquan* (SP-9).

Skin moving: *(DACH) shugu* (BL-65).

Involuntary movements of the skin: *(YXRM) zhongwan* (CV-12).

Cramps (zhuan jin).

Cramps are, in fact, local spasms, and this is the name the Japanese have given them. Although some cramps are felt only in one group of muscles, depending on the meridian going though them, there is a general tendency for cramps to come either in one area or another, or always in the same place. Most of them involve trouble of the kidney or bladder; they can come from hypoparathyroidism or from hypocalcemia.

Cramps: *(DACH) chengshan* (BL-57), *chengjin* (BL-56), *kunlun* (BL-60), *taibai* (SP-3), *qiuxu* (GB-40), *xingjian* (LR-2), *jiexi* (ST-41), foot-*qiaoyin* (GB-44), *rangu* (KI-2), *zhiyin* (BL-67); massage *jianshi* (PC-5) and *waiguan* (TW-5).

(JM) Local spasms: *chengshan* (BL-57), *yinlingquan* (SP-9), *fuyang* (BL-59), *fuxi* (BL-52, IS BL-38), *pucan* (BL-61), *jinmen* (BL-63), *zhigou* (TW-6), *taiyuan* (LU-9), *shuifen* (CV-9).

From hypoparathyroidism: tonify the point between C5 and C6 (see Cholera).

(JM) Local spasms; *(DACH)* cramps: *(DACH II, 30v)* painful cramps; *(YIZ, 40)* cramps and contracture: needle *chengshan* (BL-57).

(YIZ, 40) Old cramps not being cured: *chengshan* (BL-57), two courses of seven moxas (i.e., disperse twice).

(YIX I, 4r) Cramps: *jinmen* (BL-63), *qiuxu* (GB-40).

(DACH II, 19r) Cramps: *jinmen* (BL-63), *qiuxu* (GB-40), *yanggu* (SI-5), *xiaxi* (GB-43).

(YIX I, 4v) Cramps; flowery vision (in front of the eyes): *chengshan* (BL-57), *neihuaijian* (M-LE-17) (on the medial malleolus).

(DACH VIII, 27r) All illnesses with nocturnal contraction: *zhaohai* (KI-3, IS KI-6); daytime: *shenmai* (BL-62).

(DACH) Cramps, fullness of the four limbs: *xingjian* (LR-2).

(DACH, YXRM) Cramps of the four limbs: head-*qiaoyin* (GB-18, IS GB-11); *(YXRM)* foot-*qiaoyin* (GB-44).

(DACH XII, 28r) By massage, cramps: *jianshi* (PC-5) and *waiguan* (TW-5).

Yawning (ha jian, shi jian, jian shen).

*When we are very tired or deeply bored we involuntarily open the mouth very widely, inhaling and exhaling; this is **ha jian**. The cause is lassitude and decline of the nourishing energy in the chest; we yawn by inhaling in order to supply this deficiency. (Ci Yuan, "Ha-jian")*

*When there is fatigue and the energy is exhausted, we yawn **(jian)**; when the body is tired, we relax it **(shen)**. (Ci Yuan, "Jian shen")*

Opening the mouth widely in order to liberate the breath. (Ci Yuan, "Jian")

It is thus a matter of spasm from weakness or from sleep: we must tonify. Some yawning comes from the stomach or from boredom.

(DACH) Yawning *(ha jian): sanyinjiao* (SP-6); *(JM) xiangu* (ST-43).

(YIZ, 41r) (jian shen): xiaguan (ST-2, IS ST-7); *(JM) daying* (ST-8, IS ST-5).

(DACH) Frequent yawning and eructation: *taiyuan* (LU-9).

(DACH IX, 11v) Frequent yawning (emptiness of the secondary vessel from lung to the large intestine, much urination): *lieque* (LU-7).

(DACH IV, 10r) Frequent yawning, to the point of acute pain in the teeth: *neiting* (ST-44); yawning from the stomach.

Frequent yawning: *(DACH) tongli* (HT-5), yawning from boredom.

(DACH X, 25r) Energy from frequent yawning: *tongli* (HT-5), *neiting* (ST-44).

(DACH) Stiffness, yawning; *lougu* (SP-7).

(YIZ, 40v) Yawning: 200 moxa at *shanzhong* (CV-17).

(JM) Yawning. *(YXRM)* Energy of yawning. *(DACH)* A lot of energy from yawning: *fengchi* (GB-20); yawning from need for sleep.

(DACH) Yawning *(shi jian):* epigastrium-*tonggu* (KI-20), foot-*tonggu* (BL-66).
(YXRM) Frequent yawning: foot-*tonggu* (BL-66).
(DACH) Its movement is yawning: *ganshu* (BL-18).
(DACH) Children, habitual yawning: *yifeng* (TW-17).
(DACH) Habitual sadness and yawning: *yongquan* (KI-1).
(DACH X, 24v) Vomiting, yawning; *(JM)* yawning: *jingqu* (LU-8).
(DACH) Chill, yawning, shivering: *chongyang* (ST-42).

Sneezing (pen ti).

> *The breath comes out of the nose suddenly with noise, because the nasal mucosa is suddenly excited by the cold air,*
> *or is troubled by a foreign object. The cause is a sharp burning of the nerve of the nose; at this moment the air,*
> *after entering through the mouth, comes out violently through the nostrils and forms the sneeze.*
> *(Ci Yuan, ''Pen-ti'')*

(DACH IV, 6r) In sneezing, the energy is deep; disperse.
(DACH) Sneezes a lot; *(DACH IV, 6r)* sneezing; *(YIX, I, 5r)* sneezing, cough: *fengmen* (BL-12), numerous moxas.
(DACH) A good sneezer. *(YXRM)* Increased sneezing: *hanyan* (GB-4).
(DACH) Habitual sneezing: *chize* (LU-5).
(GSdeM) Sneezing: massage *yingxiang* (LI-20).
(DACH) Sneezing from visual dizziness or wind: *zanzhu* (BL-2).

Chattering of the teeth (gu han).

> *It is called this from the fact that during severe cold the jaw is trembling (Su Wen); caused also by the beginning of*
> *fever. It starts in the fine hairs; yawning, sneezing; it produces shivering and chattering of the teeth.*
> *(Ci Yuan, ''Gu-han'')*

(GSdeM) Excess: disperse; also from nervous crisis.
(DACH) Chattering of the teeth and cold; *(DACH X, 28v)* chattering of the teeth: *shaoshang* (LU-11).
(DACH, YXRM) Chattering of the teeth: leg-*sanli* (ST-36).
(YXRM) Chattering of the teeth from illnesses with fever; *(DACH X, 24v)* severe shivering, chattering of the teeth;
(DACH) shivering from cold, chattering of the teeth: *yuji* (LU-10).
(DACH) Chattering of the jaws *(gu han)*; *(JM)* teeth grinding *(dou ya)*: *duiduan* (GV-26, IS GV-27).

Stuttering.

(DACH) Speech rough, blocked: *yamen* (GV-14, IS GV-15), *tiantu* (CV-22), *zhejin* (GB-23); spasm of the throat:
neiting (ST-44).

Nervous shivering.

There are three types: 1) Shivering from cold *(zhen han, han li)* (c.f. Cold). 2) Shivering from emotiveness or
fear *(zhan li)*. 3) Shivering from nervous crisis, with which we shall occupy ourselves here:
(GSdeM) Nervous shivering: disperse *shaoshang* (LU-11).
(DACH) Shivering: disperse *tianjing* (TW-10).

Tics, Trembling, St. Vitus Dance.

Tics:
(YXRM) Involuntary movements of the skin; *(DACH)* involuntary movements, chills: *zhongwan* (CV-12).
(DACH) Interior of the skin moving: *shugu* (BL-65).

Trembling: *(zhan li, zhen zhan bing, zhi jing).*

The trembling itself, whatever the cause, is called *zhan li* and is differentiated from shivering from cold.

> *Trembling, shock, dizziness depend on the liver. (DACH I, 16r; DACH IV, 1r)*

> *Like convulsion-contractures **(jing lüan)**, but of an intermittent nature, coming unexpectedly in the hands or head,*
> *or from anger and discontent, or from fear, weakness and decline, or alcoholism, or lead poisoning. The patients*
> *have no vital troubles but they are not able to force their fingers to move. (Ci Yuan, ''Zhen-zhan-bing'')*

Treat the cause.

Parkinsonism:

> *The head is agitated, the eyes are prominent, the mouth is tightened, hands and feet are agitated, contracted, weak, head, nape and back are stiff; resembles convulsions, but does not stop. The pulse is sunken, slow, tight, thin. (YXRM IV, 8v, ''Zhi-jing'')*

The description of *zhi jing* is similar to the description of Parkinsonism more than to atherosclerosis. *YXRM* describes *zhi* thus:

> *The whole body stiff and hard is* **zhi** *. . . when the attacks begin with delirious speech, we call it firm; when it starts with cold in the limbs, it is called soft. (YXRM VI, 15v and IV, 8v)*

YXRM describes *Jing* thus:

> *Either the feet and hands are the only part attacked and move from the right to the left, or the chest is also attacked; there is contracture of the mouth and inarticulate sounds; when lying down, the patient does not feel the bed. (YXRM V, 35r)*

I still have not found the treatment for *zhi jing*. *Zhi* can be considered in the same way as tonic convulsions (see below), and *jing* like clonic convulsions. The Vessel of Attack *(chong mai)*, and its point of crossing and reunion, *gongsun* (SP-4), acts on all agitation and nervous crises.

Chorea, Saint Vitus dance *(tiao wu feng, wu ta bing)*:

> *Origin: disorder of the personality, anemia, acute rheumatism, illnesses of the heart valves, attacks of inversion; mainly little girls are attacked by this.*

> *Symptoms: the illness proceeds with an attack, the character changes, the face and four limbs do not respond to the mind. The muscles have some tight spots, and if they respond to the mind, the movements are especially weak. If serious, attacks of discontent, loss of laughter, easy tears.*

Treatment with needles:

xiaohai *(SI-8)*	2 fen,
yanglingquan *(GB-34)*	6 fen,
binao *(LI-14)*	5 fen,
arm-**sanli** *(LI-10)*	5 fen,
kunlun *(BL-60)*	4 fen,
shenzhu *(GV-11, IS GV-12)*	4 fen,
tianzong *(SI-11)*	5 fen,
fengchi *(GB-20)*	6 fen.

Treatment with moxa:

xiaohai *(SI-8)*	5 moxas,
huizong *(TW-7)*	7 moxas,
yanglingquan *(GB-34)*	7 moxas,
shenzhu *(GV-11, IS GV-12)*	10 moxas,
tianzong *(SI-11)*	7 moxas,
fengchi *(GB-20)*	10 moxas,
shenmen *(HT-7)*	7 moxas,
kunlun *(BL-60)*	7 moxas. *(JO, 42)*

(JM) Chorea: *yanglingquan* (GB-34), *huizong* (TW-7), *xiaohai* (SI-8); *(GSdeM)* jinmen (BL-63).

Colonic convulsions (chi zong, chou ni).

> *One of the symptoms of meningitis in children. At the beginning of the illness: sometimes contractions, and sometimes relaxation, pain on movement (ju) without rest. In the history of Han (Yi Wen Zhi, beginning of the Christian era) there are some prescriptions for* **chi zong.** *(Ci Yuan, ''Chi-zong'')*

> *There is the false* **chi zong** *without trismus or saliva, and the true* **chi zong** *with trismus and saliva. [Simple convulsions at the beginning of meningitis, or epilepsy?] (YXRM VI, 13r)*

Clonic convulsions *(chi zong):*

(YXRM, DACH) shaoze (SI-1), hand-*wangu* (SI-4), *lingdao* (HT-4), *lieque* (LU-7), *xiaohai* (SI-8), *quchi* (LI-11), *xingjian* (LR-2), *jinmen* (BL-63), foot-*dadu* (SP-2), *kunlun* (BL-60); *(YXRM)* and tightened muscles: *xuanzhong* (GB-39); *(YXRM) fuyang* (BL-59), *zhongfeng* (LR-4), *weiyang* (BL-53, IS BL-39), *jiexi* (ST-41), *chengshan* (BL-57), *tinghui* (GB-2), *yamen* (GV-14, IS GV-15), *qianding* (GV-20, IS GV-21), *kezhuren* (GB-3, IS GB-3 *shang-guan*), head-*wuchu* (BL-5), *luxi* (TW-19), *luoque* (BL-8), *qimai* (TW-18), *mingmen* (GV-4), *lianquan* (CV-23).
Clonic convulsions of children: *xiangu* (SI-5), *kunlun* (BL-60), *shangqiu* (SP-5), *xingjian* (LR-2), foot-*dadu* (SP-2), *yinbai* (SP-1), *jinmen* (BL-63), *jiuguan* (CV-14, IS *juque*), *jiuwei* (CV-15), *sizhukong* (TW-21, IS TW-23), *hanyan* (GB-4), *shenzhu* (GV-11, IS GV-12).
Children: clonic convulsions or spasms: *shenmai* (BL-62).
Clonic convulsions of babies, tongue stiff, does not suck: *yanggu* (SI-5); *(GSdeM)* massage *yintang* (GV-23a, IS M-HN-3).
Clonic convulsions without action: *wuyi* (ST-15), *yanggu* (SI-5).
Clonic convulsions, daytime attack: *shenmai* (BL-62).
Clonic convulsions from food: *jiuwei* (CV-15).
Clonic convulsions from emotional agitation: *tianjing* (TW-10), *yintang* (GV-23a, IS M-HN-3).
Clonic convulsions, muscles tight: *(DACH) xuanzhong* (GB-39).
Clonic convulsions, bent backwards: *(DACH) feiyang* (BL-58); *(YIX I, 6r) baihui* (GV-19, IS GV-20).

Clonic convulsions *(chou ni):*

The words *chou ni* seem to be used only in Japan.
Chou ni (JM): yanggu (SI-5), *jugu* (LI-16), *xingjian* (LR-2), *taixi* (KI-5, IS KI-3). *yinbai* (SP-1), foot-*shangqiu* (SP-5), *shendao* (GV-10, IS GV-11), *shenzhu* (GV-11, IS GV-12), *changqiang* (GV-1), *hanyan* (GB-4), *sizhukong* (TW-21, IS TW-23), *qimai* (TW-18).
(JM) chou ni of children: *jianshi* (PC-5), *chize* (LU-5), *jinmen* (BL-63), *chengshan* (BL-57), foot-*dadu* (SP-2), *qimai* (TW-18).

Clonic convulsions *(jing):*

> *Either the hands and feet are the only parts attacked and move from the right to the left, or the chest is attacked; there is contracture of the mouth and inarticulate sounds; lying down, [the patient] does not feel the bed. (YXRM V, 35r)*

(DACH) jing from shock; *(JM)* stiff and straight *jing: tianchong* (GB-15, IS GB-9).
(YXRM) All *jing* from shock: *lieque* (LU-7).
(YIX, I, 5r) Illness of *jing: luxi* (TW-19).

Puerperal eclampsia *(qi feng, zi xian, tai feng).*

> ***Qi feng*** *(umbilical shock): Pregnant women fall down with contractions; their sexual strength is not diminished. They awaken in a moment and recover their ordinary condition: it is also called **zi xian**, "epilepsy of children." (Ci Yuan, "Qi-feng")*

The name *qifeng* is sometimes given to umbilical inflammation from childbirth.

> ***Tai feng*** *(shock of the fetus): Pregnant women suddenly have nausea, contractions, mouth and eyes awry; short groans, cheeks red or blue; contracted jaws; salivation; contraction of the muscles, body stiffened; eyes closed. If the color is red between the eyebrows, she will live; if the color is purplish or black, she will die. (YXRM VI, 3r)*

(DACH XII, 26; YIZ, 5r) During delivery, eclampsia *(qi feng),* mouth tightened: *rangu* (KI-2), three moxa or needles 3 *fen* without bleeding: immediate cure.
(YIX I, 4r) Eclampsia *(qi feng): rangu* (KI-2).
(DACH) Women who have eclampsia with their first child *(qi feng)* and contracture of the jaw: *rangu* (KI-2).

Tonic or clonic convulsions *(jing, jing lüan, ji ju).*

> ***Jing:*** *Either hands and feet alone are attacked and move from the right to the left, or the chest is attacked; there is contracture of the mouth and inarticulate sounds. Lying down, [the patient] does not feel the bed. (YXRM V, 35r)*

> *Illnesses that stop and block the action of the muscles that command the skin or the large areas of the body. There are two sorts: continuous or intermittent.*

*Jing lüan of a stiff and straight nature (**qiang zhi xing**) is continuous. The muscles involved in the contraction are stiff and straight (beginning with incoherent speech, agitation; one must induce perspiration). The flaccidity begins with coldness of the limbs, slowness without sweat.*

*The intermittent **jing lüan (die dai xing)** has periodic muscle contractions. The brain, spinal cord and nerves which cause this illness do so periodically.*

Cases may be severe to the point of depression or epilepsy. (Ci Yuan, ''Jing-lüan'')

Jing:

(DACH IV, 11v; YIX I, 5v) The two *jing*, stiff *(gang)* and soft *(rou)*; mouth tightened, eyes crossed, red complexion, blood heat entering the lung: *shaoshang* (LU-11); if there is central fullness: *yinbao* (LR-9).
(YIX I, 5r) Illnesses of *qing*: *luxi* (TW-19).
(YXRM) Jing from shock of children: *lieque* (LU-7).

Jing lüan:

(JM) Local *jing lüan (ju suo; xian ju)*: *fuyang* (BL-59), *pucan* (BL-61).

Ji ju:

> *Name of an illness. Very violent clonic or tonic convulsions (**jing lüan**). The area of the chest and that of the abdomen generate acute pain. Even in serious causes, the awareness is not diminished. This illness is common in women. (Ci Yuan, ''Ji-ju'')*

(GSdeM) The accumulations known as *ji* and *ju* should not be confused with *ji ju*.

Troubles of the solar plexus? (Sympatheticotonia).
(DACH) Ji ju, accumulation in the abdomen and sometimes cutting pain, pain of the intestines, lack of appetite, eyes red at the inner canthus: *shangqiu* (SP-5).
(DACH) Ji ju, spasms, accumulation of energy, intestinal obstruction: *siman* (KI-14).
(DACH) Cold energy sometimes rising, attacking the heart, heat in the abdomen, knots and lumps in the lower abdomen, decline of the yang energy: *zhongji* (CV-3).
(DACH) Fullness under the ribs, diarrhea, pain in the vertebral column, jaundice, yawning, lack of appetite: *pishu* (BL-20).
(DACH) Ji ju of the treasure and workshop organs: *sanjiaoshu* (BL-22).
(DACH) Ji ju, hard like a bowl: *shangwan* (CV-13).
(DACH) Ji ju, accumulations of energy, all sorts of accumulations: *guanyuanshu* (BL-26).
(DACH) Ji ju and *jia* accumulations: *pangguangshu* (BL-28), *burong* (ST-19).
(DACH) Ji ju in the abdomen: *chongmen* (SP-12).

Epilepsy, escapades (walks blindly without direction)
(xian, dian xian, yang xian feng).

> *Nervous illness: comes mainly from alcoholic heredity. External shock on the head, very strong emotions; falls down as if dead, face white, frothing at the mouth, bites his tongue, urination, clonic convulsions, or contracture of the feet and hands. The attacks return; not easy to cure completely. (Ci Yuan, ''Dian-xian'')*

> *Nervous illness; falls suddenly, saliva from the mouth, cries like a sheep or pig, feet and hands agitated, popularly called ''**yang xian feng**.'' (Ci Yuan, ''Xian'')*

> *Also called **dian xian** or **yang xian feng**. The patients lose consciousness with convulsions (**jing**); saliva from the mouth; the cry sounds like bleating. The causes are various, heredity is the most frequent.*
> *(Ci Yuan, ''Yang-xian-feng'')*

> ***Xian** is similar to depression or hyperexcitation (**dian kuang**) but comes from time to time, then stops. The evil reaches into the five treasure organs. While in the depression or hyperexcitation, the meridians are ill and cannot be cured; it is an illness of the mind. Here, vertigo, sudden falls, feet and hands convulsed (**ju**), mouth clenched, eyes crossed, groaning shouts, expectoration of saliva or food; urination; then they wake up. When the body is hot, the pulse superficial and the face red before the attack, it is a yang epilepsy. It depends on the six workshop organs (stomach, both intestines, bladder, gallbladder, triple warmer). It is easy to cure. Yin epilepsy depends on the five treasure organs (heart, lungs, spleen-pancreas, kidneys, liver). Before the attack the body is cold, the pulse is*

sunken; awareness leaves the gaze, the eyes are glazed. If it lasts a long time, it surely depends on the treasure organs. It is difficult to cure.

Epilepsy of the five treasure organs (yin) includes: 1) Epilepsy of the liver: blue-black face, head shakes from fear or joy, cry of a cock; 2) epilepsy of the heart: red face, mouth wide open, shaking head, cry of a horse; 3) epilepsy of the spleen-pancreas: yellow face, diarrhea, tongue out, cries like a sheep; 4) epilepsy of the lungs: white face, saliva, swollen abdomen, cry of the ox; 5) epilepsy of the kidneys: black face, fixed look, cry of a pig. (YXRM V, 35v)

Dian xian. *Origin: heredity. The attack comes mostly from age fifteen or sixteen up to age twenty; it is called "epilepsy of the earlier heaven" [genetic epilepsy]* **(xian dian xian).** *For onset after age thirty, it is called "epilepsy of the later heaven" [acquired or postnatal epilepsy]* **(hou dian xian),** *coming when the constitution is fatigued from troubles or cerebral illnesses, alcoholism, or syphilis. Other causes include blockage of the digestion, emotions, illness, uterine problems or pregnancy. The true origin is not always clear.*

Symptoms: in epilepsy of an essential nature **(sun shuai)** *there are attacks of convulsions* **(jing lüan),** *loss of awareness and consciousness, and also from time to time a beginning of blockage of consciousness and thought. In slight epilepsy there is an attack consisting merely of a blockage of awareness and thought; face azure-white; vertigo. In epilepsy with series of attacks* **(lian fa cheng),** *the attacks of loss of awareness and thoughts are successive. In the large attacks: loss of awareness, vertigo, falls frontwards. At the same time there are attacks of convulsions either of a stiff and tense nature or of a clonic, often local nature; the tongue is bitten, the pupils are fixed; the back is bent backwards, respiration with snoring; after the attack, sleep.*

Treatment with needles:

yemen (TW-2) .... *3 fen,*
shuigou *(GV-25, IS GV-26,* **renzhong)** *3 fen,*
yanggu (SI-5) .... *3 fen,*
chongyang (ST-42) .... *3 fen,*
shenmen (HT-7) .... *3 fen,*
jianjing (GB-21) .... *6 fen.*

Treatment with moxa:

yemen (TW-2)........ *5 moxas,*
yanggu (SI-5) .... *5 moxas,*
chongyang (ST-42) .... *5 moxas,*
shenmen (HT-7).... *5 moxas,*
houxi (SI-3)........... *5 moxas,*
lidui (ST-45).......... *5 moxas,*
jizhong (GV-6) ...... *15 moxas. (JO, 43)*

Treatment of epilepsy with needles and moxa:

baihui *(GV-19, IS GV-20)* *1 fen,*
shenting *(GV-23, IS GV-24)* *1 fen,*
benshen *(GB-9, IS GB-13)* *1 fen,*
shuigou *(GV-25, IS GV-26,* **renzhong** *1 fen,*
tianzhu *(BL-10)* *5 fen,*
bailao *(GV-13, IS GV-14,* **dazhui)** *5 fen,*
shenzhu *(GV-11, IS GV-12)*............... *5 fen,*
xingjian *(LR-2)* *8 moxas*
yongquan *(KI-1)* .... *8 moxas. (JM)*

(GSdeM) Attacks suppressed during the day, come on at night: tonify *zhaohai* (KI-3, IS KI-6), disperse *shenmai* (BL-62).

(DACH II, 26v; DACH IV, 6r; DACH II, 29) For all types of epilepsy and for avoiding the return of the attacks:

jiuwei (CV-15).

Acute epilepsy of babies:

Origin: in babies under two years it often comes from emotions or cerebral problems, stomach and intestinal problems, intestinal worms, constipation, teething or beginning of an acute illness with fever.

Symptoms: first, disquiet, tears; suddenly, tonic spasms, dilated pupils, purplish face, frothing at the mouth.

Treatment with needles:

rangu (KI-2)	*2 fen,*
shenzhu (GV-11, IS GV-12) ..	*2 fen,*
zhongwan (CV-12)	*3 fen,*
jiuwei (CV-15)	*3 fen,*
liangmen (ST-21)	*3 fen,*
zhangmen (LR-13)	*3 fen,*
head-*linqi (GB-11, IS GB-15)*	*1 fen,*
benshen (GB-9, IS GB-13)	*1 fen,*
yangbai (GB-10, IS GB-14) ...	*1 fen,*
tongziliao (GB-1)	*1 fen,*
lieque (LU-7)	*1 fen.*

Treatment with moxa:

jiuwei (CV-15)	*5 moxas,*	
rangu (KI-2)...	*3-5 moxas,*	
jizhong (GV-6)	*5 moxas.*	*(JO, 68)*

The five epilepsies: (Therefore yin, and from the five treasure organs, difficult to cure): *(YIX I, 5r; DACH IV, 5; DACH II, 26)* *jiuwei* (CV-15), 7 moxas.

(YIX I, 40r) Laogong (PC-8); *(DACH) huizong* (TW-7), *meichong* (BL-3).

(YXRM I, 40r) Yongquan (KI-1), but first, *laogong* (PC-8).

(DACH IV, 7r; YIX I, 4r) Houxi (SI-3), *jiuwei* (CV-15), *shenmen* (HT-7).

(DACH VII, 26v) The five epilepsies with saliva coming out: *neiguan* (PC-6), *houxi* (SI-3), *shenmen* (HT-7), *xinshu* (BL-15).

(DACH XI, 9r; YIX I, 5v) Shangxing (GV-22, IS GV-23), *xuanlu* (GB-5), *jiuwei* (GB-15), *yongquan* (KI-1), *xinshu* (BL-15), *baihui* (GV-19, IS GV-20).

(DACH) The five epilepsies of adults and children: *shenmen* (HT-7).

(DACH) The five epilepsies during full attack: *guiku* (MP-29a).

(JM) Special for epilepsy: *shenzhu* (GV-11, IS GV-12).

(DACH X, 35r) Epilepsy *(xian)* all from fire and mucus: not useful to make a distinction between horse, pig, etc: moxa on *baihui* (GV-19, IS GV-20), *jiuwei* (CV-15), *kezhuren* (GB-3, IS *shangguan*), *shenmen* (HT-7), *shenmai* (BL-62), attacks during the day; *zhaohai* (KI-3, IS KI-6), attacks at night.

(DACH III, 30v) During the attack of epilepsy, depression or hyperexcitation: *houxi* (SI-3).

(JM) Epilepsy: *yemen* (TW-2), *yanggu* (SI-5), *shenmen* (HT-7), *jianjing* (GB-21), *taodao* (GV-12, IS GV-13), *shuigou* (GV-25, IS GV-26 *renzhong*), *chongyang* (ST-42).

(DACH) Epilepsy: *gongsun* (SP-4), *jiexi* (ST-41), *chongyang* (ST-42), *weiyang* (BL-53, IS BL-39), foot-*shangqiu* (SP-5), *waiqiu* (GB-36), *pianli* (LI-6), *xiaoluo* (TW-12), *baihui* (GV-19, IS GV-20), *houding* (GV-18, IS GV-19), *shuigou* (GV-25 IS GV-26 *renzhong*), *naokong* (GB-19), head-*wuchu* (BL-5), *tinggong* (SI-19), *lüxi* (TW-19), *changqiang* (GV-1), *jizhong* (GV-6), *xinshu* (BL-15), *huaroumen* (ST-24), *houxi* (SI-3).

(DACH) Attacks of epilepsy in children: *mingmen* (GV-4), *qianding* (GV-20, IS GV-21), *yintang* (GV-23a, IS M-HN-3).

(JM) Epilepsy of spleen-pancreas of children (cries like a sheep): *shangwan* (CV-13); *(JM)* Epilepsy of children with contractions: *kezhuren* (GB-3, IS *shangguan*).

(DACH) Children: epilepsy with convulsions: *kunlun* (BL-60).

(DACH) Epilepsy, emotiveness, fantastic visions: *lieque* (LU-7).

(YXRM I, 46v) Epilepsy with daytime attacks: *shenmai* (BL-62).

(DACH III, 32v; YIX I, 10v; DACH VII, 27v) Epilepsy *(xian dian)*, agitation of limbs and joints: *shenmai* (BL-62).

(DACH) All illness from epilepsy with nighttime attacks: moxa at *zhaohai* (KI-3, IS KI-6).

(YXRM) Epilepsy *(xian dian),* tongue out, chattering of the teeth, hyperexcited speech, sees ghosts, delusions, coma.

(DACH) Epilepsy, hyperexcited speech, sees ghosts: *pucan* (BL-61).

(DACH) Onset of epilepsy, chest and ribs responding: *lüxi* (TW-19).

(YXRM) Epilepsy: tongue out: *xiaohai* (SI-8).

(YXRM) Sudden epilepsy, like a storm; dizziness, hyperexcited speech, eyes looking up: *tianzhu* (BL-10).

(DACH) Epilepsy from hyperexcitation *(guang xian)* or depression *(tian xi),* does not sleep; attacks of epilepsy, clonic convulsions: *houding* (GV-18, IS GV-19).

Epilepsy from shock *(feng xian):*

(DACH) Baihui (GV-19, IS GV-20), *neiguan* (PC-6), *huizong* (TW-7), *shenting* (GV-23, IS GV-24).

(DACH) Epilepsy from shock, eyes lifted up, cannot recognize anyone, hyperexcitation, expectorates saliva, attacks without a fixed time: *sizhukong* (TW-21, IS TW-23).

(DACH) Epilepsy from shock, attacks of hyperexcitation: *shenzhu* (GV-11, IS GV-12).

(DACH) Children: epilepsy from shock, clonic convulsions from energy: seven moxas on *shendao* (GV-10, IS GV-11).

Epilepsy from fear (emotiveness — *jing xian*):

Epilepsy from fear in children: *(DACH)* shenzhu (GV-11, IS GV-12), foot-*linqi* (GB-41), *shenmen* (HT-7), *benshen* (GB-9, IS GB-13), *jinsuo* (GV-7, IS GV-8).

Epilepsy from fear, fantastic visions: *(DACH) lieque* (LU-7).

(YIX I, 6v) Epilepsy from fear in children: *baihui* (GV-19, IS GV-20) and *qimai* (TW-18), three moxas.

Epilepsy from grief *(liang xian):*

Epilepsy from grief: *(DACH)* qianding (GV-20, IS GV-21); *(DACH X, 26v)* guiyan (MP-29b); *(DACH)* xinhui (GV-21, IS GV-22).

Epilepsy from food *(shi xian):*

(YIX I, 5v; DACH XI, 9v) shaoshang (LU-11), *jiuwei* (CV-15), *zhongwan* (CV-12).

(YIX I, 6v) Zhongting (CV-16), three moxas.

Epilepsy from milk *(ru xian):*

(DACH X, 26v) Infantile epilepsy from milk: *guiyan* (MP-29b).

Fugue (escapades) *(guang zou,* lit. "manic flight"):

(DACH) Epilepsy: escapades (walking blindly without direction): *jiuwei* (CV-15), *zhongwan* (CV-12).

(DACH) Walks blindly without direction (escapades), scarlet lips: *xinshu* (BL-15).

(DACH) Climbs up, sings, throws off his clothes and walks about: *shenting* (GV-23, IS GV-24).

(DACH) Depression, walks blindly without direction: *yanggu* (SI-5), *taiyi* (ST-23).

(DACH) Walks blindly without direction: *fenglong* (ST-40).

VI. Prolonged Contractions; Contractures
(Tonic Convulsions; Prolonged Contractures; Tetanus)

Tonic convulsions (zhi, zhi bing, zhi jing).

> *The whole body stiff **(qiang)** and hard **(ying)**; this is **zhi**. Meridians and secondary vessels do not awaken with the sun. It is divided between firm **(gang)** and soft **(ruo)**. When the attack begins with delirious speech, it is called firm; one must induce perspiration. When it begins with coldness of the limbs, it is called soft; one must make the skin soft. (YXRM VI, 15v)*

> *When cold and humidity increase their shock, it becomes **zhi**. The diseases of the **taiyang** [BL-SI] come either from coryza or a chill, but if there is first the one and then also the other, **zhi** can be produced. The external symptoms are: cold and warm as if chilled, but the pulse has sunken and it is slow, tense and thin. The head shakes; the eyes bulge, the mouth is tightened, feet and hands are convulsed **(ju ni)**. If the head is thrown back as in epilepsy and the patient does not wake up the whole day, it is a special case. When [the attack] has come from shock and there is movement, it is the firm type, caused by increased shock from cold or humidity; therefore there is no sweat. When [the attack] has come from humidity, there is slowness; it is soft, primarily due to chill; therefore there is sweat. The firm types stand up for two or three days and seem to be hot; there is fullness of the chest as in **jie xiong** "contracted chest"; there is lack of desire, limping gait, inability to sleep. The soft type will not be ill for two or three day [periods, but will] perspire profusely. Cold weakens, muscles and vessels are contracted **(ju jin)**. It is dangerous, in that attacks can start and stop from moment to moment.*

*But there is still **zhi** where firm and soft are not distinguished: body hot, delirious speech, like in the firm type; weakness, fainting, varying desire, as in the soft type.*

*When there is perspiration and the urine is sometimes clear and sometimes spare, when the left eye, left hand and left foot are stretched and contracted, it is a **zhi** of the **shaoyang** [GB-TW].*

When the fingers are spread, and the eyes are rolled back in the head, with contracture from hemiplegia, perspiration like pearls, the body arched up from the bed a palm's width, or three finger widths for a child, it means death. (YXRM IV, 8v)

(YXRM) Spasms *(shan)* cold and warm, *zhi* to the point of being broken: *zhonglüshu* (BL-29).
(DACH II, 19r) The illnesses of *zhi (zhi bing)* cannot be cured without *lüxi* (TW-19).
(DACH) zhi hot or cold: *ganshu* (BL-18).
(YXRM) Fullness of the body, *zhi*, twisting of the body: *shiguan* (KI-18).
(YXRM) Zhi, twisting of the body: *shangliao* (BL-31).
(DACH) Zhi of the five poisons: *shangwan* (CV-13).
(YXRM I, 46v) Zhi with nighttime attacks: *zhaohai* (KI-3, IS KI-6).
(DACH, YXRM) Zhi, pain of the bones: *pishu* (BL-20).
(YXRM) Hot *zhi* radiating into pains of the bones: *pangguangshu* (BL-28).
(YXRM) Cold *zhi*: *changqiang* (GV-1).
(DACH) Sudden *zhi*, rebellion attacking the heart and chest: *zhiyang* (GV-8, IS GV-9).

Prolonged Contractures.

Contractures *(ju lüan, lüan, ji)*

Ju lüan:

*Feet and hands are seized, blocked, with attacks of violent pain, caused by an acute rheumatism (**tong feng**) or chronic rheumatism (**man xing luo ma chi se**), or by a nervous illness. (Ci Yuan, ''Ju-lüan'')*

Ju lüan: muscles and vessels are seized and bound. (DACH II, 2r)

(DACH IV, 7v; YIX I, 4r) Ju lüan of the muscles: *chize* (LU-5) needles.
(DACH VII, 12r) Ju lüan from apoplexy: hand-*zhongzhu* (TW-3), *yangchi* (TW-4), *quchi* (LI-11).
(YXRM) Ju lüan, pain and bad vomiting: *kunlun* (BL-60).
(DACH) Ju lüan with attacks of fever: foot-*linqi* (GB-41).

Lüan:

Curved [flexed] fist, cannot be extended. (Ci Yuan, ''Lüan'')

(YIZ, 47r) Muscle contractures *(lüan);* painful bones: tonify *hunmen* (BL-42, IS BL-47).
(YIZ, 47r) Muscle contractures, pain and tightening of the yin: *zhongfeng* (LR-4), 50 moxas.

Ji ''tightening.''
(DACH II, 29r) Chize (LU-5). (For contractures of hemiplegia, see Hemiplegia.)

Tetanus *(po shang feng).*

*Comes from a pathogenic bacteria that penetrates through an opening and gradually overcomes the entire body. The patient first feels a stiffness and hardness of the neck and head that reaches the four limbs to the point where the entire body is contracted. Respiration is tightened and contracted, the heart is numbed. Infantile eclampsia (**qi feng** of children) is of this type. (Ci Yuan, ''Po-shang-feng'')*

(YXRM I, 46v) Tetanus: *hegu* (LI-4), *dadun* (LR-1); *(YIX I, 11) waiguan* (TW-5), *chengshan* (BL-57).
(DACH VII, 27r; YIX I, 10r) Feet and hands paralyzed *(ma mu)*, flexible tetanus: *houxi* (SI-3).
(YIX, 5v) Tetanus, stiffness of the back, spasm, like a cadaver: *guanyuan* (CV-4), *dadun* (LR-1).
(DACH VII, 27v) Tetanus: *houxi* (SI-3), *hegu* (LI-4), *waiguan* (TW-5), *neiguan* (PC-6), *chengjiang* (CV-24).

(DACH VII, 27v) Tetanus or attacks of contracture *(ju)* for other causes, attacks of heat, stiff vertex: *houxi* (SI-3), *hegu* (LI-4), *shixuan* (MP-25-29, IS M-UE-1-5), *dadun* (LR-1), *xingjian* (LR-2), *tongziliao* (GB-1).

⊘ VII. Fullnesses; Accumulations

General fullnesses (shi, man).

Fullness, the description of which is given under different forms, is actually an excess of energy, either general or local, manifesting with a sensation of repletion, of swelling without swelling being visible, often accompanied by heat or redness. We must differentiate between fullness of both yin and yang, and those of either yin or yang. It is always necessary to disperse them; however, it is recommended to tonify swellings of the abdomen — aerogastria and aerocolia — at *gongsun* (SP-4).

(DACH) Disperse fullness: *gongsun* (SP-4), tonify for the swelling of the abdomen, disperse for the pains of the heart, stomach or intestines.

(DACH) Fullness without knowing the place: *yangfu* (GB-38).

(DACH VI, 14r) Fullnesses of the energy: *lidui* (ST-45).

(DACH) Good for energy accumulations *(ji)* and fullnesses: *guanmen* (ST-22).

(DACH) Agitation, fullness *(man)*: *xiabai* (LU-4).

(YXRM) Body hot, agitation, fullness without sweat: *xuanlu* (GB-5).

(YXRM) Fullness, agitation, or depression with bleating: *xuanli* (GB-6).

(DACH) Counterflow of the energy, fullness and agitation under the heart; *(YXRM)* energy in counterflow, fullness of the heart: *yindu* (KI-19).

(DACH) Fullness, does not desire to eat: *youmen* (KI-21).

(DACH) Fullness, internal contractions, body without quietness: *dazhu* (BL-11).

(YIX I, 9v) Internal fullness: *neiguan* (PC-6); *(DACH IV, 11v)* *yinbao* (LR-9).

Accumulations (ji).

Fullness has no defined form; on the other hand, accumulations have a distinct form. Cellulitis would have to be included among accumulations. Traditional China recognizes several types of accumulation. The difficulty of classify them according to the present European notions forces us to describe them by listing them one after the other.

Ji (yin energy accumulations):

> *Knots blood and mucus in order to form a shape; **ji** is yin energy. (Ci Yuan, ''Ji'')*

This term is used for congestion and inflammation of each of the internal organs *(yin)*; see each organ.

(YXRM I, 46v) Accumulations in lumps: *gongsun* (SP-4).

(YXRM) Pain from accumulations *(ji)*: *chongmen* (SP-12).

(DACH, YXRM) Energy of cold, accumulation *(ji)*: *tianzhu* (ST-25).

(DACH VII, 26r; YIX I, 9v) Accumulation *(ji)* in hard lumps, going crosswise on the ribs, piercing through: *neiguan* (PC-6).

(YXRM) Accumulation *(ji)* hard like a stone under the umbilicus, knots and lumps: *zhongji* (CV-3).

(YXRM) Accumulation *(ji)* of energy under the ribs: thorax-*qimen* (LR-14).

(YXRM) Obstruction (stopping of functions) from energy, accumulation *(ji)*, spasms of energy: *burong* (ST-19).

(YXRM) Accumulations *(ji)* of energy under the umbilicus, like stones: *ligou* (LR-5).

(DACH) Women who have thinness and accumulations *(ji)* from coitus near their periods: *sanyinjiao* (PC-6).

Zheng (hardened yin energy accumulations):

> *Accumulations (**ji**) suppressed for a long time are called **zheng**: hard lumps in the abdomen; comes from the sexual energy. If present for a long time, they form an accumulation of sexual energy. (Ci Yuan, ''Zheng'')*

(YXRM I, 46r) Accumulations *(zheng)* of food; *(DACH)* accumulations *(zheng)* in the intestines: *pishu* (BL-20).

(DACH X, 37) Accumulations *(zheng)* of food, does not dissipate, progressive thinness: *neiguan* (PC-6), hand-*wangu* (SI-4), *pishu* (BL-20), *gongsun* (SP-4).

Jia (yang energy accumulations):

These accumulations have shape but not hardness; they are not constant. Illness of the lower warmer (genitourinary functions) thus yang; often seen in women (q.v. *YXRM, Ci Yuan*).

(YXRM) Spasms of women and *jia* accumulations: *yinlingquan* (SP-9).

(DACH X, 37r) Jia accumulations in the abdomen: *shenmai* (BL-62).

(DACH) Spasms and *jia* accumulations: *fushe* (SP-13).

(DACH) Jia accumulations of blood, by pressing, as if boiling water were flooding the thigh: *ququan* (LR-8), *diji* (SP-8).

(DACH) Jia accumulation of energy in the uterus: *shuidao* (ST-28).

(DACH) Jia accumulations, contraction and pain in the genital system radiating down to the feet and into the hands without recourse: *taixi* (KI-5, IS KI-3).

Ju (yang energy excesses):

> *Exaggerated consequences of the normal energy.* **Ju** *is yang energy; it has neither roots nor fixed place: illness in the interior of the abdomen; illness of the middle warmer. This is the accumulation of the workshop organs. The pain is neither fixed in its location, nor constant, nor well defined. (Ci Yuan, ''Ju'')*

(YXRM, DACH) Ju accumulations: *pangguangshu* (BL-28).

Jia ju:

(YXRM) Jia ju accumulations (yang) of women; *(DACH) jia ju* accumulations of women; agitation, fullness, sweat does not come out: *pangguangshu* (BL-28).

Zheng and jia (yin and yang energy accumulations):

> *In the abdomen,* **ji** *accumulations in lumps; hard, they are* **zheng**. *Without material form, they are* **jia**.
> *(Ci Yuan, ''Zheng-jia'')*

(DACH) Intestines, bladder, kidneys: *zheng* and *jia* accumulations: bound lumps like a large bolus: *qihai* (CV-6).

(DACH) Women and girls: *zheng* and *jia* accumulations: blood bound in the form of lumps: *tianshu* (ST-25).

(DACH III, 31r) Women: accumulations *zheng jia* of blood energy; hardness; pressing: *zhongji* (CV-3).

Ji ju (see Contractions and Pains).

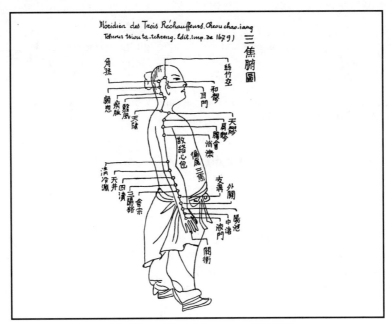

Meridian of the triple warmer (DACH)

Notes

[1] Both ancient and modern dictionaries give only one reading for this character, that being *re*. *Yo* may have been a local colloquialism in the author's time, or among his associates. — ed.

Chapter V

Nervous Centers, Endocrine Glands

I. Brain, Meninges — II. Spinal Cord — III. Nerves — IV. Vago-sympathetic System — V. Lymph Nodes, Adenitis — VI. Salivary Glands — VII. Pituitary Gland — VIII. Adrenal Glands — IX. Thyroid Gland — X. Parathyroid Glands — XI. Testicles — XII. Ovaries

(GSdeM) There are two important discoveries I have made regarding the nervous centers, from the point of view of acupuncture, which supplement the Chinese science. The first concerns the measure of the function of the three groups of nervous centers. A triple pulse gives these measures; it is located on the right wrist just proximal to the third pulse, and on the edge of a transverse muscle facing the hand. The superficial pulse indicates the spinal cord; the middle position indicates the medulla oblongata, pons and cerebellum; the deep position indicates the brain. For the middle and deep positions, the radial edge of the artery responds to and reflects the right half of the nervous centers. The medial half of the artery responds to the left half of the respective centers.

The second discovery, an extension of the first, has been the specification of the nervous centers on which indicated points act — according to the Chinese, on certain nervous functions; according to the Japanese, on the spinal cord or brain. The use of these points brought us, ultimately, to recognize the meaning of the difference in sizes of the bones of the skull, and to observe that overdevelopment of one bone or the other is significant. For example, a very developed frontal bone is always found in people who are highly conscientious and scrupulous; the evolved man dominates. An occipital bone rising up to the middle of the vertex is seen in people dominated by their instincts; the primate dominates. A right parietal bone passing the midline suggests a dominance of the ancestral talents, of the automaton, and also of the unconscious memory, of suggestibility. A very developed left parietal bone is found in people having instant and easy memory and speech, but without great depth; the parrot dominates. With this information, it is possible to act:

1) On the brain. Whole brain: *xinhui* (GV-21, IS GV-22). On the opposite half: *shaohai* (HT-3) and hand *wangu* (SI-4).

2) On the cerebellum, medulla oblongata and pons. Through the meridians of the gallbladder and liver, especially: *yanglingquan* (GB-34), *guangming* (GB-37), foot-*linqi* (GB-41), *ligou* (LR-5). It seems that *xuanzhong* (GB-39) acts mainly on the medulla oblongata and the pons.

3) On the spinal cord. Through the governor vessel and kidney, mostly: *yamen* (GV-14, IS GV-15), *bailao* (GV-13, IS GV-14, *dazhui*), *mingmen* (GV-4), *jiaoxin* (KI-8), *fuliu* (KI-7), *dazhong* (KI-6, IS KI-4).

I. Brain *(Nao);* Meninges

Brain.

Brain
(DACH X, 25v) Too many thoughts and worries, neglects the future, forgets the past, no more strength of mind: moxa *baihui* (GV-19, IS GV-20).
(GSdeM) Headache from cerebral fatigue: *shanglian* (LI-9).
(GSdeM) Facilitates intellectual work and concentration of the mind: tonify *dadu* (SP-2); the left point helps the understanding of mathematics.
(YIZ, 38v) Pain from the brain: moxa *xinhui* (GV-21, IS GV-22).
(GSdeM) Posterior, lateral half: *shaohai* (HT-3) — right for left and left for right; anterior, lateral half: *tongli* (HT-5) — right for left, left for right.
(DACH) After having drunk too much, the brain hurts as if broken: *xinhui* (GV-21, IS GV-22).
(YIZ, 38v) Coldness of brain: moxa at *xinhui* (GV-21, IS GV-22).
(DACH) Emptiness and coldness of the brain: *xinhu* (GV-21, IS GV-22).
(YIZ, 38v) Heat of the brain: *xinhu* (GV-21, IS GV-22), moxa.
(YIZ, 38v) Twistings *(xuan)* of the brain: *xinhui* (GV-21, IS GV-22).
(YXRM) Acute pain of the brain: *fengchi* (GB-20).
(DACH) Spinning of the head *(tou xuan);* pains in the brain: *tianzhu* (BL-10).

(JM) Pain in the nerves of the brain: *xuanlu* (GB-5).

(DACH) Abscess in the brain; *(YXRM I, 40r)* abscess coming out of the skull: *xuanzhong* (GB-39); *(DACH VII, 28r)* *shenmai* (BL-62), *weizhong* (BL-54, IS BL-40), *hegu* (LI-4), *bailao* (GV-13, IS GV-14, *dazhui*), *qiangjian* (GV-17, IS GV-18).

Cerebral anemia *(nao pin xue)*

(JM) Cerebral anemia: *yuji* (LU-10), *yangxi* (LI-5), *lidui* (ST-45), *xingjian* (LR-2), foot-*tonggu* (BL-66), foot-*qiaoyin* (GB-44), leg-*xialian* (ST-39, IS *xiajuxu*), *baihui* (GV-19, IS GV-20), *qianding* (GV-20, IS GV-21), *xinhui* (GV-21, IS GV-22), *shenque* (CV-8), *sanjiaoshu* (BL-22).

(JM) Cerebral anemia, groaning: *shaohai* (HT-1).

(JM) Cerebral anemia after delivery: *sanyinjiao* (SP-6).

Cerebral congestion *(nao chong xue)*

> *Nao chong xue:* the blood rises in counterflow: buzzing, headache, head red and hot; comes from excess drinking or from stomachache, or from heat stroke (**zhong shu**), or from excess desire or anger. Summer cases are easily cured; autumn cases are cured with difficulty. (JM)

(JM) Cerebral congestion: *hegu* (LI-4), *erjian* (LI-2), *shanglian* (LI-1), *shaoshang* (LU-11), *yuji* (LU-10), *wenliu* (LI-7), arm-*shanglian* (LI-9), *tianfu* (LU-3), *jinggu* (BL-64), foot-*tonggu* (BL-66), *yamen* (GV-14, IS GV-15), *houding* (GV-18, IS GV-19), *naohu* (GV-16, IS GV-17), head-*qiaoyin* (GB-18, IS GB-11), *benshen* (GB-9, IS GB-13), *shuigou* (GV-25, IS GV-26, *renzhong*), *xuanlu* (GB-5), *touwei* (ST-1, IS ST-8), head-*linqi* (GB-11, IS GB-15), *lüxi* (TW-19), *qianding* (GV-20, IS GV-21), *houding* (GV-18, IS GV-19).

(DACH) Heat stroke *(zhong shu, shu feng):* *xiatian* (LI-8), leg-*xialian* (ST-39, IS *xiajuxu*).

(DACH III, 32r) Energy pressing upwards: disperse leg-*sanli* (ST-36).

(GSdeM) Cerebral congestion: disperse *daling* (PC-7) leg-*sanli* (ST-36), *shenmai* (BL-62).

(DACH) After drinking wine, fire in the brain, scarlet face: disperse *baihui* (GV-19, IS GV-20).

(DACH) Attacks of burning heat at the vertex: *qucha* (BL-4).

Encephalitis *(nao feng)*

(DACH) Encephalitis: *shaohai* (HT-3), *naokong* (GB-19), *chengling* (GB-14, IS GB-18).

(DACH) Deranged mind, attacks of depression causing diplopia; *(YXRM)* encephalitis, eye pain, dizziness, buzzing, deafness: *naokong* (GB-19).

(DACH) Headache from encephalitis: arm-*shanglian* (LI-9).

Apoplexy, cerebral hemorrhage, hemiplegia *(zhong feng, bian feng):*

> Name of an illness, also called **nao chu xue** (cerebral hemorrhage). It comes from the rupture of an artery in the cerbral substance. The patient suddenly loses consciousness and falls down dazed, or he awakens and there is a change into paralysis (**ma mu**) of the nature of **tan** (left-side paralysis). The old medicine considered that the cause was a shock (**feng**), whence the name "shock-entered," **zhong feng.** (Ci Yuan, "Zhong-feng")

No mention is made of the causes: embolisms, thromboses or tumors.

Bian feng, lateral wind, is the general name for hemiplegia with contractures or flaccidity, right or left.

> **Bian feng** of the right is called **tuan,** that of the left is called **tan.** (DACH IV, 9v)

> Left hemiplegia with contracture: vessels and muscles are contracted; paralysis (**wei**) and lack of strength (**bi**) in the extreme, commonly called **zhong feng**, or **nao chu xue.** (Ci Yuan, "Tan")

> Emptiness of blood, then fire and mucus flow to the left: that is left hemiplegia, **tan**. The mouth cannot speak, the limbs cannot be lifted; this is weakness of blood. (YXRM V, 1v)

> Emptiness of energy, then fire and mucus flow to the right: that is **tuan** [right hemiplegia]. If the emptiness is extreme, there is incontinence of urine, snoring sounds, saliva. (YXRM V, 1v)

> Paralytic evil on the right and left, **tan tuan**; the limbs are paralyzed (**ma bi**) and do not obey. (Ci Yuan, "Tan")

> There are those who are truly stricken, those who are somewhat stricken, and those who seem stricken. In yang illnesses, the body is hot. In yin illnesses, the body is cool. In order to save people with stroke, pull out the hair of the vertex above the forehead, then use three to five large moxas on the earlobes; differentiate the type. (YXRM V, 1r)

Before the attack, intermittent limping:

> *One, two, three, four months or more before the apoplexy, there will be periodic, sudden heaviness with numbness, pain and paralysis in the leg and foot. After a moment this passes then recurs; this is the warning for apoplexy. Immediately stimulate leg-**sanli** (ST-36), three moxas, and **xuanzhong** (GB-39) three moxas (disperse). Boil together raw onion, mint, willow leaves, and si **wei** (four flavors), then bathe in it. Moxa causes the energy of the shock to leave through the opening of the blister. If it occurs during the transition from spring to summer or summer to autumn, use moxa until the two legs have blisters; it is wonderfully effective. If one lacks confidence in this method, and if eating and drinking are endless, if there is indulgence in excessive luxury, then sudden apoplexy will occur. Moxa can also be applied in seven places: two at leg-**sanli** (ST-36), two at **xuanzhong** (GB-39), two on the earlobes at **tinggong** (SI-19) and at **baihui** (GV-19, IS GV-20). For each point, three moxas — illness on the right, moxa on the left; illness on the left, moxa on the right. (DACH XI, 1r)*

(DACH) Apoplexy: feet and legs painful, cramps and contraction — *chengshan* (BL-57).

During the coma:

> **The Thousand Ounces of Gold** *says that during apoplexy the heart is contracted. In order to dissipate this contraction use 100 moxas at **xinshu** (BL-15). (DACH VIII, 20v)*

(DACH) Sudden apoplexy, does not recognize anybody: head-*linqi* (GB-11, IS GB-15).

(DACH) Apoplexy, blocked energy, rising saliva, no speech, serious syncope: *fengchi* (GB-20).

(DACH) Fury being transformed into apoplexy: *xuanzhong* (GB-39).

(DACH) Apoplexy, energy closed, no speech: *jianjing* (GB-21).

(DACH X, 32v) Apoplexy, the evil of the shock has entered into the workshop organs to the point where the hand and feet no longer respond: *baihui* (GV-19, IS GV-20), *gongsun* (SP-4), *jianyu* (LI-15), *quchi* (LI-11), *fengshi* (GB-31), leg-*sanli* (ST-36), *xuanzhong* (GB-39); moxa at the opposite of the paralysis. The paralysis of the feet and hands is the sign that the evil shock has entered the workshop organs: moxa on the left for illness of the right and on the right for illness of the left.

(DACH X, 32v) Apoplexy: the evil has entered the treasure organs to the point where the energy has become cold, saliva is compressed, no speech, danger of confusion: *baihui* (GV-19, IS GV-20), *fengshi* (GB-31), *jianjing* (GB-21), *quchi* (LI-11), leg-*sanli* (ST-36), *jianshi* (PC-5), on each moxa five times seven . . . agitation in the heart is felt, consciousness and thought are not peaceful, hands and feet are paralyzed *(yuan ma);* moxas mostly during spring and autumn.

(DACH X, 32v) Apoplexy, skin of the head swollen, vertigo, emptiness, shivering, eyes painful, cannot see at a distance; needles and moxa at *shangxing* (GV-22, IS GV-23).

(DACH IV, 5v) Apoplexy: first tonify, then disperse *zhongchong* (PC-9). If not in better condition; *shuigou* (GV-25, IS GV-26, *renzhong*).

(JM) Hegu (LI-4), *laogong* (PC-8), arm-*shanglian* (LI-9), *wenliu* (LI-7), *xingjian* (LR-2), *zhongfeng* (LR-4), *weizhong* (BL-54, IS BL-40), *xiyan* (MP-37a and 38a, IS M-LE-16), *huantiao* (GB-29, IS GB-30), *shangguan* (GB-3), *chengjiang* (CV-24), head-*wangu* (GB-17, IS GB-12).

(DACH) Apoplexy: cold from energy, saliva rising, fog, danger. *(DACH)* Apoplexy, muteness, dumbness, like hard lumps in the throat: *jianshi* (PC-5).

Hemiplegia (*bian feng, tan* on left, *tuan* on right):

(DACH IV, 9v) Hemiplegia of right or left *(tan, tuan):* *fengchi* (GB-20), needles, then seven moxas; leg-*sanli* (ST-36) disperse, and three times seven moxas; abdomen-*yinjiao* (CV-7), disperse, and three times seven moxas.

(DACH VII, 27v) Apoplexy *(tong feng),* hemiplegia of right or left *(tan tuan):* *shenmai* (BL-62), leg-*sanli* (ST-36), *wangu* (SI-4), *hegu* (LI-4), *xuanzhong* (GB-39), *xingjian* (LR-2), *fengshi* (GB-31), *sanyinjiao* (SP-6).

(DACH XI, 17r) Apoplexy, yang symptoms (right side of body): aphasia, feet and hand paralyzed: first puncture the healthy side, then the sick side; disperse then tonify *hegu* (LI-4), *jianyu* (LI-15), arm-*sanli* (LI-10), *baihui* (GV-19, IS GV-20), *jianjing* (GB-21), *fengshi* (GB-31), *huantiao* (GB-29, IS GB-30), leg-*sanli* (ST-36), *weizhong* (BL-54, IS BL-40), *yanglingquan* (GB-34).

Apoplexy: symptoms of yin (left side of the body), same treatment as for yang symptoms, but tonify first, then disperse.

(DACH XI, 1r) Apoplexy from heat stroke *(zhong shu):* comes during the summer or autumn from excess wine, anger, desire or external shock. Those which come at the beginning of summer are easy to cure; those which come during autumn are difficult to cure: *shuigou* (GV-25, IS GV-26, *renzhong*), *hegu* (LI-4), *neiting* (ST-44), *baihui*

(GV-19, IS GV-20), *zhongji* (CV-3), *qihai* (CV-6). If not better: *zhongchong* (PC-9), *xingjian* (LR-2), *quchi* (LI-11), *shaoze* (SI-1).

Hemiplegia: *(DACH) hegu* (LI-4), arm-*shanglian* (LI-9), arm-*sanli* (LI-10), *jianyu* (LI-15), *touwei* (ST-1, IS ST-8), *chongyang* (ST-42), leg-*shanglian* (ST-37, IS *shangjuxu*).

(JM) Half of body paralyzed: *yangxi* (LI-5).

Hemiplegia of right or left: *huantiao* (GB-29, IS GB-30); *(DACH) ciliao* (BL-32).

Hemiplegia with no improvement: *shenguan* (CV-8, IS *shenque*), 100 moxas.

Hemiplegia; heat stroke: *xialian* (LI-8).

Hemiplegia, half of the body not obeying: *yangxi* (LI-5), *lieque* (LU-7), arm-*sanli* (LI-10), *quchi* (LI-11), *weizhong* (BL-54, IS BL-40), *xiguan* (LR-7), *yanglingquan* (GB-34), thigh-*zhongdu* (GB-32), *jianjing* (GB-21), *chengjiang* (CV-24), *fengfu* (GV-15, IS GV-16), *xinshu* (BL-15), *tianchuang* (SI-16).

Hemiplegia; half of the body does not respond: *weizhong* (BL-54, IS BL-40), arm-*sanli* (LI-10); *(DACH)* special for half of the body not responding: *jianyu* (LI-15).

Hemiplegia; half of body not obeying *(JM, DACH)*: *yanglingquan* (GB-34); *(JM) yangxi* (LI-5); *(DACH) fengfu* (GV-15, IS GV-16).

(DACH) Hemiplegia, paresis *(wei)* of the lower limb, arch of foot not coming back into place: leg-*xialian* (ST-39, IS *xiajuxu*).

(DACH) Apoplexy, mouth closed, foot and hand not responding; arm-*sanli* (LI-10).

Hemiplegia or nervous spasmodic paralysis *(feng bi,* from shock): *chize* (LU-5), *tianjing* (TW-10), *xiguan* (LR-7); of the elbow joint: *zhouliao* (LI-12); of the whole body with flaccidity *(ma): lieque* (LU-7); not constant: *weizhong* (BL-54, IS BL-40); and without action: knee-*yangguan* (GB-33).

Practical treatment of apoplexy and hemiplegia:

1) During the attack, while comatose: disperse leg-*sanli* (ST-36) and *shenmai* (BL-62), which causes the energy to descend and decongests the top. Disperse *fengchi* (GB-20), which is a vasoconstrictor of the head and activates the heart. If the heart pulse is contracted, small, or if it is ample and hard, disperse *shenmen* (HT-7). If the pulse of the heart is weak and soft, tonify *shaochong* (HT-9). In all cases disperse *daling* (PC-7) in order to make the blood pressure drop, and *tianjing* (TW-10) in order to decrease the excess energy.

2) For established hemiplegia: if there is contracture, thus excess energy, tonify the yin (left and bottom of body, yin meridians) and disperse the yang (right, top, yang meridians). For flaccid hemiplegia, first tonify the right side (yang), then the sick side and if the flaccidity is in the right limbs, disperse the left side first.

In both cases:

1) **For the aphasia, disperse** *yamen* (GV-14, IS GV-15), *xinhui* (GV-21, IS GV-22) and *baihui* (GV-19, IS GV-20).

2) For the trismus, disperse *jiache* (ST-3, IS ST-6).

3) For the salivation, disperse *lianquan* (CV-23).

4) For mouth that is awry, disperse the side which pulls and tonify the relaxed side: *dicang* (ST-7, IS ST-4).

5) For shoulder and arm: *jianjing* (GB-21), *jianyu* (LI-15), *jianzhugu* (MP-10).

6) For the hand: *waiguan* (TW-5).

7) For the lower limbs: *yanglingquan* (GB-34).

8) For the arch of the foot: leg-*xialian* (ST-39, IS *xiajuxu*).

In order to hurry the recovery, 30 moxas daily at *shenque* (CV-8).

Aphasia:

(DACH VII, 3r) Apoplexy with aphasia, the most difficult to cure: *xinhui* (GV-21, IS GV-22), five moxas, *baihui* (GV-19, IS GV-20), first tonify, then disperse with seven moxas.

(DACH VII, 27v) Apoplexy, closed mouth not opening, difficult speech: *shenmai* (BL-62), *dicang* (ST-7, IS ST-4), *jiache* (ST-3, IS ST-6), *shuigou* (GV-25, IS GV-26, *renzhong*), *hegu* (LI-4).

(DACH) Apoplexy, tongue slow, no longer speaks: *fengfu* (GV-15, IS GV-16).

(JM) Heavy tongue, speech blocked, difficult; *(DACH)* Contracted tongue, does not speak: *yamen* (GV-14, IS GV-15).

Trismus:

(YIZ, 40) Mouth closed, tightened: *jiache* (ST-3, IS ST-6); mouth tight, bad shock, cannot chew; *jiache* (ST-3, IS ST-6), *quanliao* (ST-18).

(YIZ, 40) Mouth closed, cannot speak, corners of the lips not obeying: *hegu* (LI-4), *shuigou* (GV-25, IS GV-26, *renzhong*), *dicang* (ST-7, IS ST-4).

(DACH) Apoplexy, mouth closed, foot and hand not responding: arm-*sanli* (LI-10).

Salivation:

(DACH IV, 7v, YIX I, 5v) Apoplexy, mouth salivating: disperse *shuigou* (GV-25, IS GV-26 *renzhong*) and *jiache* (ST-3, IS ST-6).

(DACH) Saliva coming out, difficulty speaking, root of tongue bound: *lianquan* (CV-23).

(DACH) Apoplexy, saliva flowing in two threads: *dicang* (ST-7, IS ST-4).

(DACH) Apoplexy, depression, saliva: *benshen* (GB-9, IS GB-13).

Arm and hand:

(DACH IV, 10r) Hemiplegia, arm without strength, hand cannot be turned: *jianyu* (LI-15).

(DACH) Arm and hand cannot be lifted, elbow contracture, hand like a bow: *chize* (LU-5).

(DACH) Hemiplegia, arm and muscles slow, cannot hold objects, hand like a bow, afraid of combing the hair, contractures of the lumbar area and arm; *(DACH IV, 10v)* hand not moving: *quchi* (LI-11).

(YIZ, 40) Apoplexy, cannot lift the hand: *yangchi* (TW-4), needles and moxa.

(YIZ, 40) Apoplexy, wrist cannot be moved, cannot hold objects: *waiguan* (TW-5) needles and moxa.

(YIZ, 41) Apoplexy, elbow in contracture, fits of despair: *lieque* (LU-7); needles and moxa.

(DACH X, 29v) Apoplexy, elbow in contracture: *neiguan* (PC-6).

Lower limb:

(DACH) Apoplexy, walks with difficulty: *kunlun* (BL-60).

(DACH) Hemiplegia, paresis *(wei)* of the lower limb: leg-*xialian* (ST-39, IS *xiajuxu*).

(YIZ, 40) Apoplexy, arch of foot paralyzed, paralysis from cold, pain from cold: *yanglingquan* (GB-34).

(YIZ, 40) Apoplexy, knee and foot painful, in contracture with cramps: *chengshan* (BL-57).

❦ *Meninges (meningitis, jing feng, tian diao feng).*

> *Name of an illness of children: two kinds — acute and chronic. In fact, it is an illness of the brain. Formerly, it was said that the heart controlled emotivity, the liver controlled shocks. All children have a hot heart and abundant liver. If they are emotionally hurt or receive a shock, the illness starts. This is why it is called "emotion-shock." The acute cases are easy to cure, the chronic are difficult. The methods of treatment are not the same. (Ci Yuan, "Jing-feng")*

> *According to the old physicians, meningitis has eight warnings:*

> *1) **Ju** "contractions," that is, arms extending and retracting.*

> *2) **Ni** "gripping," that is, the ten fingers opening and closing.*

> *3) **Zhi** "holding," the shoulders retract towards one another.*

> *4) **Zhan,** "trembling," feet and hands are agitated.*

> *5) **Fan** "backward-bending," the body is bent backwards.*

> *6) **Yin,** "directed," the hand seems to take the shape of a bow.*

> *7) **Chuan** "avoidance," the eyes are fixed as if unhappy.*

> *8) **Shi** "fixing," the pupils are bulging and unresponsive.*

> *These are the eight warnings; acute and chronic meningitis are the same. (Ci Yuan, "Jing-feng Ba-hou")*

> *Acute meningitis; often has just seen a strange object or heard a strange noise. The consciousness is dispersed, the energy is troubled. General symptoms: appearance of fever, acute exterior agitation, red face, scarlet lips, mucus, rapid and compressed breath, trismus, needs to urinate twice in close succession. He needs calm and warmth. Prevent emotion in the patient in order to calm his consciousness. If the body is weakened, the illness will become chronic. (Ci Yuan, "Ji Jing-feng")*

> *Chronic meningitis; frequent illness with hereditary tuberculosis, or enfeebled from another cause. It is also called "inflammation of the envelope of the brain," of a tuberculous nature. The pulse is slow, retarded, weakened; neck and nape are stiff and straight, bent backward; torpor and continuous sleep. If it lasts for one or two months, there is no cure. Many children get this disease, as do adults. (Ci Yuan, "Man Jing-feng")*

The *Yi Xue Ru Men* (VI, 14r) gives some more detailed symptoms. *Zhen Jiu Da Cheng* (XI, 23r) specifies that acute meningitis is in the liver meridian, and chronic meningitis is in the spleen-pancreas meridian.

(DACH IV, 4r) For acute meningitis, disperse; chronic meningitis, tonify.

Meningitis: *(JM)* arm-*shanglian* (LI-9); *(DACH IV, 5r) zhongchong* (PC-9); *(JM) jinggu* (BL-64); *(JM)* head-*qiaoyin* (GB-18, IS GB-11); *(JM) luxi* (TW-19); *yamen* (GV-14, IS GV-15).

Meningitis: hyperexcited speech, clonic convulsions; *(DACH)* agitated melancholia, fingers contracted: *wangu* (SI-4).

Meningitis: mental shock, bent backwards like a bow, bleating, groaning, words not chosen, some attacks, then death: *(DACH, YXRM) baihui* (GV-19, IS GV-20).

Sudden meningitis in adults: *(DACH XI, 21v)* ten moxas at *zhongchong* (PC-9), *hegu* (LI-4), *yintang* (GV-23a, IS M-HN-3).

Acute or chronic meningitis in children: *(YXRM I, 40r) shaoshang* (LU-11), *shuigou* (GV-25, IS GV-26, *renzhong*), *yintang* (GV-23a, IS M-HN-3). Disperse, a little deeply, *baihui* (GV-19, IS GV-20).

(YXRM, 46v) dadun (LR-1); *(DACH IV, 4r)* 1 *fen* at *zanzhu* (BL-2) on the left, then on the right; cures if there are loud cries; if no cries, difficult. Disperse for acute meningitis; tonify for chronic meningitis.

Meningitis in children *(DACH XI, 23r) shaohai* (HT-3) massage (babies).

(DACH IV, 5v) zhongchong (PC-9), moxa; *(JM) mingmen* (GV-4), *dadun* (LR-1).

(DACH XII, 26r) Moxa at *jianjing* (GB-21), if no cure, 3 moxas at *zanzhu* (BL-2) and *shuigou* (GV-25, IS GV-26, *renzhong*) and 7 moxas at *chize* (LU-5).

Acute meningitis in children: *(DACH) xingjian* (LR-2) disperse.

Chronic meningitis in children: *(DACH) chize* (LU-5), *yinbai* (SP-1), tonify.

Meningitis in children, diarrhea, vomiting: treat on the left, to stop the vomiting; on the right to stop the diarrhea; the contrary for girls *(DACH XI, 23v): yongquan* (KI-1).

II. Spinal Cord *(Ji Sui)*

Inflammation of the spinal cord: *(JM) yamen* (GV-14, IS GV-15), *shuidao* (ST-28).

Illness of the spinal cord: *(JM) guangming* (GB-37), *ligou* (LR-5), *fuliu* (KI-7), *gaohuangshu* (BL-38, IS BL-43).

Lesions and illnesses of the spinal cord: *(JM) mingmen* (GV-4).

Tuberculosis of the spinal cord *(JM) guangming* (GB-37), *gaohuangshu* (BL-38, IS BL-43).

Reunion of the cord, all the illnesses of the cord are treated here: *(DACH) xuanzhong* (GB-39); *(DACH) yanglingquan* (GB-34).

III. Nerves *(Shen Jing)*

All illnesses of the nervous system of the nervous fibers: *(JM)* leg-*sanli* (ST-36).

Pain in the vagus nerve; paralysis of the sympathetic nerve: *(JM) fengchi* (GB-20).

Famous point for sensitive nerves and for motor nerves, vagus nerve, sympathetic nerve, glossopharyngeal nerve, brain: *(JM) tianzhu* (BL-10).

IV. Vagosympathetic System

Sympathetic system:

Excess: tachycardia, hot flashes, fever from infections, coagulates quickly, hypertension, headaches at the level of the eyebrow aggravated in the afternoon. Skin, mouth dry, digestion slow, solar plexus painful after food, atonic constipation, insufficient menses, excess renal filtration, pupils enlarged (mydriasis), eyes prominent, bright. The sympathetic system is hyperexcited by the adrenals (mostly the abdominal segments), the cervical sympathetic by the thyroid; slowed down by crataegus: *(chengman,* ST-20 on the right). In fact, the sympathetic system heats up the circulation and slows the digestion (saliva, stomach secretions, intestinal peristalsis) and skin.

Easily excited from 8 a.m. to 11 a.m. from excess of pancreas; hyperexcited by the pancreas (insulin), by pilocarpine; restrained by the ovaries and belladonna (atropine).

Fengchi (GB-20) and *shenzhu* (GV-11, IS GV-12).

Vagus system:

Excess: heart slow, arrhythmia, extra systoles, coagulates slowly, hypotension, headache in the morning, stops in the afternoon; nausea, excess of saliva, of sweat, mostly from emotion and of the hands; congestion of the liver; hyper-chlorhydria; diarrhea or spasmodic constipation; menses too abundant; eyes protruding, pupils constricted (miosis);

relaxation of the sphincters of the anus and bladder. In fact, the vagus system is concerned with assimilation through digestion, and the prevention of heating up the circulation; it activates the skin.
Tianzhu (BL-10).

IV. Ganglionitis *(Lou Li);* Adenitis
(Li Chuan, Li Chuang, Bai Zhua, Tong Li, Pan She Li)

*Lumps arise in the patient's flesh from swelling of the lymphatic ganglia (lin ba xian). If there is inflammation, pus appears; most often it comes on the side of the neck. After a long time it forms beads, which are called **li chuang**; these also appear in the axilla. (Ci Yuan, "Lou-li")*

*The nodes around the neck are called **pan she li** [coiled-serpent ganglia]. Ganglia appearing behind the chest and under the axilla are called **bai zhua tong li** [white-clawed Liana ganglia]. (DACH VII, 32r)*

***Li chuang** are abscesses of the ganglia." (DACH II, 19v)*

General treatment:
(GSdeM) Tonify *gaohuangshu* (BL-38, IS BL-43), (see Blood, Leukocytes).
(YIZ, 42r) Ganglia *(lou li):* moxa seven or two times seven at *zhoujian* (MP-11, IS M-UE-46) at the tip of the elbow, and in the area of the ganglia — an excellent method.
(DACH XI, 14r) Ganglia *(lou li): zhoujian* (MP-11, IS M-UE-46), illnesses on the right, moxa on the left; illness on the left, moxa on the right. If at the beginning there is pain on the left in men and on the right in women, moxa at *fengchi* (GB-20).
(DACH III, 29r) Ganglia and eruptions *(yin zhen): tianjing* (TW-10).
(YIX I, 4r) Ganglia *(lou li): tianjing* (TW-10), *shaohai* (HT-3).
(DACH) Ganglia *(lou li): binao* (LI-14).
(DACH X, 33r) Ganglia *(lou li):* moxas at *jianjing* (GB-21), *quchi* (LI-11), *daying* (ST-8, IS ST-5).
(DACH IV, 7v) Ganglia *(lou li): xiaohai* (SI-8).
(DACH) Ganglia *(lou li):* arm-*sanli* (LI-10), arm-*wuli* (LI-13); *(YXRM) jianyu* (LI-15).
(DACH) Yifeng (TW-17), *renying* (ST-9).
(DACH) Ganglia *(lou li,* cold and hot): *naohui* (TW-13).
(JM) Illness of the ganglia: *shaohai* (HT-3), *wuli* (LI-13).
(JM) Poison from illness of the ganglia: *kunlun* (BL-60).

Oozing ganglia (suppurative adenitis, *li chuang*):
(YXRM) zhigou (TW-6), *yangfu* (GB-38); *(DACH)* foot-*linqi* (GB-41), *tianjing* (TW-10), arm-*wuli* (LI-13), *binao* (LI-14).

At the neck and nape:
(YIZ, 37v; YIZ 42) zhoujian (MP-11, IS M-UE-46), *quchi* (LI-11).
(DACH VII, 32r) Ganglia around the neck, called *pan she li* (coiled-serpent ganglia): *waiguan* (TW-5), *tianjing* (TW-10), *zhoujian* (MP-11, M-UE-46), *fengchi* (GB-20), *quepen* (ST-12), *shixuan* (MP-25-29, IS M-UE-1-5).
(DACH IV, 4r) Ganglia at the nape: *yifeng* (TW-17); no dispersion with the needle and everything will relax.

Chest and axilla:
Bai zhua tong li (white-clawed Liana ganglia): *waiguan* (TW-5), *daling* (PC-7), *zhigou* (TW-6), *tianjing* (TW-10), *shanzhong* (CV-17), *yanglingquan* (GB-34).

Axilla (axillary adenitis):
(DACH VI, 15r) Swelling below the axilla: *zhongchong* (PC-9).
(JM) Inflammation of the glands under the axilla: *daling* (PC-7), *yangfu* (GB-38), *danshu* (BL-19), *jianshi* (PC-5).
(DACH) Inflammation of the axillary nodes as big as a shellfish: *xiaxi* (GB-43).
(DACH) Swelling and pain under the axilla: *qiuxu* (GB-40), *weiyang* (BL-53, IS BL-39), *chengjin* (BL-56), *chengfu* (BL-50, IS BL-36); *(DACH X, 30r) yanglingquan* (GB-34), *qiuxu* (GB-40), foot-*linqi* (GB-41); *(YIZ, 42r)* swelling under the axilla as big as a shellfish, almost a tumor; if he bites his tongue easily: *tianyou* (TW-16); if central swelling, cold and hot: foot-*linqi* (GB-41) and *qiuxu* (GB-40), 1 *fen* deep and five moxas, *taichong* (LR-3), 1 *fen* deep and three moxas; *(DACH II, 19r) weiyang* (BL-53, IS BL-39), *(DACH X, 31v) tianchi* (PC-1).
Children: swelling under the axilla: *yangfu* (GB-38) and *taichong* (LR-3).

Inguinal fold:
(JM) Inflammation of the inguinal ganglia; *(DACH)* swelling and pain in the inguinal fold: *jimen* (SP-11); abscess of the genital area: *xuehai* (SP-10).

VI. Salivary Glands

The salivary glands have an internal secretion [salivary amylase]; their extract has the same effect as insulin [pancreatic amylase]; they are second of all tissues for their richness in insulin [amylase]; 250 grams of extract per day causes a loss of five kilograms in weight per week.

Insufficiency: neuro-muscular asthenia; their removal causes hyperglycemia; activated through vagotonia, slowed through sympatheticotonia.
The glossopharyngeal nerve, stimulated, causes saliva and vomiting; acts on the glossopharyngeal nerve, etc: *(JM) tianzhu* (BL-10).
Sublingual glands: *(JM) huaroumen* (ST-24).
Vagotonia: *tianshu* (BL-10), tonification stimulates the vagus system.
Sympatheticotonia: *fengchi* (GB-20), tonification stimulates the sympathetic system.

VII. Hypophysis (Pituitary Gland)

Excess: excess development in height, lines of the face, nose, lips, extremities and sex; tachycardia, tachyarrhythmia, migraines, asthma, vertigo, headaches, neuralgia, deep wrinkles, prognathism, contraction of the uterus, hypertrichosis, dark skin, adrenal excitation, scoliosis, wet skin, intestinal hypertonia, hypertension, glycosuria, precocious puberty, genital erethism, masculinism, strong character, aggressive tendencies.

Insufficiency: obesity, blockage of development of height and sex, lowering of the temperature, hypotension, profuse sweat, relaxed ligaments, twisted ankles, apathy, asthenia, anguish, sleepiness, cries easily, moral deviations, tendency to steal, obstinacy, impulsiveness, quarrels, loss of memory, lack of concentration, very small extremities, overlapping of the teeth, small mouth, eyes near to each other, small head, dry skin, little pigmentation, bradycardia, hypotension, hypoasphyxia, oliguria, amenorrhea, metrorrhagia, puerility, hypoglycemia.

Treatments: (Abrams) upper edge of C7 increases the pituitary function. *(GSdeM)* In fact, it is the angle between the lower edge of C6 and C7 on the medial intervertebral ligament.
All articulations relaxed: tonify *dabao* (SP-21).
Joints relaxed, elbow useless: disperse *zhizheng* (SI-7).
Feet and hands especially small: tonify *guangming* (GB-37).
For the Chinese the organ of the moral senses, of concentration, and of growth is the spleen-pancreas: tonify foot-*dadu* (SP-2) or disperse *shangqiu* (SP-5).

VIII. Adrenals

The pulse of the adrenals is under (distal to, towards that of the liver) the kidney pulse, very close to it.

Excess: hyperasthenia, tics, plethora, under pressure, wakes up early, goes to sleep late, works without stopping, does not need sleep, danger of hypertension and arteriosclerosis, a little anxious, fits of mischievousness, extensive body hair, biliary lithiasis, asthma, edema of the lungs, glycosuria, good humor, will, courage.

Insufficiency: fatigue, asthenia, brown line on the abdomen, somnolence, abulia, sadness, fits of irascibility, dark spots on the upper gum above the incisors; if acute, agitation, nocturnal delirium and daytime torpor; convulsions, headaches; stimulated by the pituitary, pallor, thinness, weakness of the legs, cardiac insufficiency, hypotension; large breasts; diminution of energy, courage, will.

Adrenalin stimulates the production of sugar by the liver and depresses the production of insulin by the pancreas. The thyroid glands and the adrenals stimulate the sympathetic system. The production of adrenalin is depressed by insulin and potassium, reinforced by calcium (the secretion of insulin depends on the vagus system).

Treatments: Tonify *fuliu* (KI-7), *taixi* (KI-5, IS KI-3) to tonify the adrenals; disperse *rangu* (KI-2) and *yongquan* (KI-1) to depress the adrenals.
(Abrams) C2 and C3 raises the blood pressure. *Yamen* (GV-14, IS GV-15) is located between C2 and C3, *fengfu* (GV-15, IS GV-16) is between C1 and C2. Dispersing them decreases the blood pressure and the adrenal function.
Tonifying *dadu* of the right foot (SP-2) augments insulin.
Tonifying *tianzhu* (BL-10) augments the vagus system.

IX. Thyroid

Excess: bright and prominent eyes, thick eyebrows, abundant hair, agitation of hands and feet, hot flashes, always too hot, abundant perspiration, hypo-ovaria, ample nails, eats rapidly, tachycardia, likes warm drinks, cannot stop eating, gourmand, dark red lips, needs to act and to eat, always moving. Intelligent and understands quickly, voluble, excessive gaiety and sensitivity, anger, grumpy, impressionable, easily attached to people, altruistic, basal metabolism increased, very tall, persistent youthfulness, dental decalcification, sympatheticotonia.

Insufficiency: eyes sunken, dull; external extremity of the eyebrows deficient, slowness, slow development, slow movements, slow and thick speech, asthenia, easily tired, apathy, somnolence, puffed face, edema under the eyes, dyspepsia, constipation, obesity, sterility, rheumatism, hairlessness, hears buzzing, headaches, indifference, forget-fulness, indecisiveness, egotistical, sadness, absence of will and energy, basal metabolism diminishing, precocious senility, baldness, early whitening of hair, alopecia, always chilly, loosening of the teeth, lack of appetite, spasmodic coryza, vagotonia.

Instability: mixing or alternation of symptoms, shivering in children, agitation, not sleeping, red extremities, makes a scene from emotion, hits, involuntary movements, nightmares, thinness, fever; capricious, unstable, attacks of diarrhea, ridged nails.

Treatments: (JM) renying (ST-9) disperse or tonify.
(Abrams) The C6-C7 interval acts on exophthalmic goiter.
Basedow's disease, exophthalmic goiter, swelling of the thyroid: *(JM) renying* (ST-9).
Exophthalmia: *(JM) jiaosun* (TW-20).
Goiter: disperse *renying* (ST-9), and *tiantu* (CV-22).
The addition of potassium reinforces the action of the thyroid; calcium chloride blocks it.

X. Parathyroids

Excess: rheumatic pains, circumscribed bony rarification, hypercalcemia, hypophosphatemia, fibrocystic osteosis, neuromuscular hypotonia, increased excretion of phosphorus, nitrogen and calcium.

Insufficiency: spasms, cramps of the calves and toes, jerking, contractions, tics, blinking or batting of the eyelids, clenched teeth, fibrillary contractions, hysteria, eclampsia, epilepsy, tetany, troubles with hair, alopecia, troubles with the enamel of the teeth, of the nails, opacity of the lens, cataract, nocturnal terrors, secretive, small manias, scrupulous, bites his nails, coprolalia, agitation, sadness, worry, thirst, excess saliva.

Instability: Projection of the teeth of the lower jaw.

Treatments: Augmentation from stimulation of C6 (the C5/C6 interval).
Nocturnal terrors: *zhongchong* (PC-9), *baihui* (GV-19, IS GV-20).

XI. Testicles

Excess: early baldness, short legs, long thorax, initially abundant hair, fully developed sexual organ; sexual appetite. Calm, energetic character; artistic; cramps, pruritis. Hyperacusis.

Insufficiency: Abundant hair of the head, scarce body hair, small trunk and head. Atrophia of testicles, coldness. Phlegmatic character, pessimism, puerility, timidity, poor imagination, sadism, homosexuality.

Treatments: Tonify or disperse: *qichong* (ST-30), *xuehai* (SP-10), *mingmen* (GV-4); *(GSdeM) chongmen* (SP-12).

XII. Ovaries

Insufficiency: hot flashes, profuse sweat, buzzing, vertigo, palpitations, facial neuralgia, amnesia, nightmares, irritability, melancholia, boredom. With precocious menopause, there are stomach troubles, enteritis, asthma attacks; also cellulitis, cramps, numbness, crawling sensations, numb fingers. Enlarged breasts, long legs, late puberty, chlorosis, infantile uterus, painful and intermittent menses, leukorrhea, sterility. Psychological troubles at puberty, menses, pregnancy and menopause.

Excess: small in size, precocious development, small breasts, abundant lactation, precocious puberty, fecundity, amplified genital sensitivity.

Treatments: Tonify *sanyinjiao* (SP-6), *xuehai* (SP-10), *qixue* (KI-13), *guanyuanshu* (BL-26).

Chapter VI

The Psyche

I. The Psyche and Its Organic Connections — II. Intensity of the Psyche — III. Insufficiencies — IV. Excess — V. Alternations — VI. Hysteria — VII. Abnormal People

I. The Psyche and Its Organic Connections

The psyche.

The word "psyche" is used here in the sense of feelings as well as of thought, for morality as well as mentality. For Descartes it was "the thing which feels, which desires, which loves, which knows; which in one word, thinks." As we can see in this quotation, Descartes and after him the tradition of scholastic psychology, confused thought and feeling. For a long time these two have been viewed as separate from the body and have been thought to have an independent existence from the organs. Our modern medical psychology carefully distinguishes the involuntary impressions of the unconscious, the hardly perceived control of the subconscious and the picture of reality classified and compared by the conscious part. It has begun to teach the relation between the psyche and the endocrine glands and the organs.

The Chinese teach that the intensity of the psyche is primary and must be considered above all. This is described in its various aspects in section II.

The three planes of the psyche.

The experimental and nontheoretical science of China recognizes, as in Europe, three superimposed psychic planes. Our modern science, still affected by our scholastic traditions, distinguishes: 1) The unconscious, which has all the attributes of the psyche except consciousness. 2) The subconscious, which inhibits or activates the impulses of the unconscious. 3) Consciousness, which includes memory and judgement; all that is conscious without distinction between passion and judgement. The three planes of the Chinese are not exactly the same. The medical observations going back to the greatest antiquity and noted in the *Nei Jing* clearly expose these ideas by indicating how to act selectively on each of the three planes. We will follow the Chinese divisions as thoroughly as possible to understand and to treat the troubles of one or the other of the three planes.

It is important to specify some points: First, the psyche is yang and depends on the yang energy, that is, energy from air and light. At the same time it is nourished and fed by the yin energy, which is the original and vital energy (see Chapter I), and depends on food and the earth. Leaving aside the proportion and composition, the total intensity is first to be considered. On the other hand, these planes, as the organs among them, have a constant interpenetration. If the memory, for example, is the main attribute of the middle level, it is still the case that the lower level takes strength and profits from it. Judgement and reason, specific to the upper plane, act strongly on the lower and middle levels, and in their turn are either aided or unaffected. These are not three separate entities, but parts of a unity, the divisions allowing a better classification so as to avoid mistakes.

1) Motor level: po, the primate:

The lower level, the *po,* is life developing itself to the detriment of everything and everybody; it is captivation and desire-repulsion. This level is the deep motivation of the psyche, the source of feeling. It corresponds to the lower parts of the European idea of the unconscious. In the sixth century B.C., Confucius describes this level as follows:

> *What are called feelings in man are: joy or unhappiness, regrets or desire, fear, love or hate. We are capable of these seven feelings without studying them. But desire and repulsion are the great rulers of the heart; people have them hidden in the depths of their heart; we can neither fathom nor measure them. (Li Ji IV, 54, Kong-zi)*

The ancients have observed that the plant absorbs what is useful for it and rejects what is noxious. If it is very healthy, it can absorb a lot to the detriment of everything surrounding it. If it is weakened, it rejects almost everything and withers. They have observed this same grasping in newborn children and in adults, with the same variations of strength. Desire-repulsion constitutes the normal form of grasping. An excess of grasping becomes aggressivity, while insufficiency can reach the point of anguish.

This deep motor level of the psyche is called *po;* it is drawn with the two elements, "white-ghost." It is described through an image: it is the dark part of the moon that we perceive only slightly when the crescent shines; that is, the obscure and badly lit parts of ourselves. However, they are the most important, and determine whether or not we will act, and whether we will observe or reject. In fantastic tales there is often a cadaver animated by the *po,* which remains after the departure of the *shen* (consciousness) and the *hun* (unconscious, subconscious). The *po,* when it possesses enough vitality to prevent decomposition, which proves an excess of vitality, is given without limit to its aggressiveness and performs horrible crimes. For a fuller description of the *po,* see Volume II, Chapter III, Section II.

The *po,* for which there is more yin than yang, is said to have its home in the lungs, which are the yin organ for access to the yang energy of the air and stars. *Shanzhong* (CV-17) is the alarm point of the energy and for the respiratory function. But the *po* is even said to have its home — this time with the *hun* — at the point *tianshu* (ST-25) which, although a point of a yang organ, transforms the yin energy of food into yin blood. On the other hand, for an insufficiency of the *po* (anxiety) the heart and meridians have an action which no other meridian possesses, while for excess (aggressivity) the liver and spleen meridians dominate.

This motor level, finally, translates its excess or insufficiency into aggressiveness or anxiety on the moral level. It possesses a mental aspect of the greatest importance: astuteness or cleverness without scruples that goes towards its goal without worrying about the methods. Thus, astuteness and cleverness depend on the kidney function, which also acts on seduction and sex-appeal; these would thus be qualities of the *po.*

2) Level of the three memories: hun, the automaton:

The middle level, the *hun,* is the hereditary and acquired psyche of memory and constraint, which distinguishes the hunting dog from the sheep dog at birth, the man of quality from the brute. It is either the conscious or unconscious memory, or the possibility of repeating words and sentences without having learned or understood them. Here are stored the activating commands and the inhibiting defenses accumulated either from heredity, the unconscious or the conscious, coming from experience, education and studies of ancestors, and coming from the being at birth and perhaps before: the subconscious.

The term *hun,* used by the Chinese to designate this level, is formed by the characters "phantom" and "speech." It connotes the commands (and defenses) of ghosts, of heredity and parents, even after their death.

> The **shen** (consciousness) and the sexual energy of the human being . . . consciousness having penetrated the energy, forms the **hun.** (Ci Yuan, "Hun")

What has been recorded by the memory and has become unconscious or subconscious, blocking or activating the sexual energy, is the *hun.*

The constituents of this level are necessarily the unconscious memory of the hereditary commands and defenses, also the memory which is first conscious and then becomes partly unconscious of the environment at birth. The memory of words and expressions that are not understood but well established seems to depend on this level. It is well known that people who easily acquire ineradicable habits have a good memory while the people lacking habits have a bad memory. It corresponds quite well to the subconscious, as described by modern medical psychologists.

The *hun* dwells in the liver, which, according to the Chinese (and also from experiments done in France), is clearly indispensable to the sexual life. On the other hand, the liver is known for its action on the mind. However, the memory depends on the heart and it is mostly through tonification of the heart meridian that it is possible to fight against amnesia. The heart governor is equally powerful; the other meridians seem to tonify mostly the general state. Dreams seem to depend on this level. For memory the *Nei Jing* says: "When the *hun* and *po* are wounded, there is depression and forgetfulness." *(Ling Shu VIII, line 6)*

3) The upper level: shen, the evolved man:

The upper level is the *shen,* the psychic director of conscience and understanding, reason, judgement, common sense, the critical capacity and consciousness; the true intelligence that understands without having learned through simple comparisons. It draws on the perception of the external, changing moment and on the memory of the past furnished by the *hun* in order to harmonize the capacity to comprehend, the hereditary and acquired reactions and the possibilities of reality.

The ideogram pronounced *shen* is formed from the elements "what-falls-from-the-heavens-and-crosses-the-body." The commentators say: "the immaterial element of the astral energy, the cosmic force, the waves animating the form and giving it reason." The *Nei Jing* explains, "When the *hun* and *po* are wounded, there is depression and forgetfulness; but when there is no *shen,* one is no longer what a human being should be." *(Ling Shu VIII, line 6)*

The term is currently used to indicate remarkable people, geniuses, the guardian-spirits. Idiots and fools are said to be lacking *shen* (see Part II, Chapter III).

The *shen* has its home in the heart, the good function of which has been proven to be indispensable for the intellectual life and the equilibrium of the reason. However, experiments made in France on quite a number of children have demonstrated that the spleen (spleen-pancreas meridian on the left) has great importance for the consciousness. It is described as the minister who criticizes and speaks of justice. On the other hand, insufficiency of the spleen always corresponds with a great difficulty in resolving mathematical problems, even when the memory has clearly retained the course and the theorems. The kidneys also have a marked action on decision-indecision and on doubt; governor and conception vessels have an action on delusions, etc.

For Europeans, moral sense, consciousness and reason are in direct connection with the action of the pituitary gland. I was able to make an important discovery that adds much to the Chinese science concerning measurement and in consequence its regulation. By studying the system of Théodore de Bordeau (see historical section, Eighteenth Century), and guided by the experiments of Professor Leriche on the independence of the arterial segments, I have been able to observe that above (behind) the left III pulse there is a pulse which is modified according to the action of certain points on the psyche. Long experiments have specified the following facts:

1) Superficial pulse: responds to the evolved man. People gifted with reason, awareness and judgement in notable quantity have this pulse elevated, supple and clear. This pulse, when it is narrow and hard, indicates obsessions and unreasonable impulses. When absent, there is no reflection, cannot put two and two together to make four, lacks reason, judgement and awareness.

2) Middle pulse: on the radial side responds to the automaton, on the medial side to the parrot; measures the three memories.

3) Deep pulse: responds to the primate; its dominance indicates primitive instinct, cleverness and astuteness, deception.

The proportions of these three levels are not always the same in all human beings. Some people have a strong motor level with a weak conscious level, but a good memory. Others value only the memory with no comprehension or judgement and without any mental vitality. Students, faced with a composition, will transcribe without a single fault the questions relating to the course, but will not be able to resolve problems; others immediately solve the problems, but cannot reproduce the questions relating to the course. The predominance of memory generally disturbs understanding and does not allow the accomplishments that a dominance of comprehension gives. In order to judge an individual, it is important to observe carefully the proportion of intensities that he expresses in each of the three levels, and to look for the dominance or deficiencies which distinguish normal from abnormal people (see section VII below).

The qualities in each of the levels also have their importance. There are those who like to give happiness through courtesy, and sadistic people who contradict. The instinct of a hunting dog will not make a good sheep dog and vice versa. And it is also necessary to recognize the auditory or visual memory, or that of colors, shapes, faces, simple words and sentences, music, etc. In the same way, for understanding, it is possible to come across special comprehension, such as for secret numbers, idioms, mathematics, etc.

Interrelationship of the organs and the psyche.

The relations existing between the vitality of the different levels of the psyche and the functioning of each organ have been minutely observed by the Chinese. The palpation of the pulses, which gives the measure of the function of the internal organs, and the observation of the almost immediate effects of acupuncture, have given the Chinese an understanding of relationships that Western medicines, much slower in effect, have not given Europeans. It has thus been noticed that it is possible to act on the psyche through the organs and on the organs through the psyche.

Numerous experiments (controlled with instruments and made in France since I began teaching acupuncture) have permitted the verification and extension of Chinese knowledge on this point. Thus, the effects of the activation of the spleen on mental concentration and the understanding of mathematical problems are confirmed through the placements of students who have been treated for spleen insufficiency. In the same way we have confirmation of the effects of the tonification of the liver in cases of jealousy and envy.

The total vital energy (see Chapter I) as well as the energy of each organ can have an influence on the psyche in one or another of its divisions. In a contrary way, the psyche can cause fullness or emptiness either of the total energy or of the energy of certain organs. If it causes general fullness: unhappiness, worries, obsession, sadness, as well as silence and idleness. If it causes general insufficiency: pleasure, emotional agitation, apprehension, fear, as well as fatigue (see Chapter I).

The action of each feeling on a particular organ is described thusly:

> *The seven feelings bother the energy either by dispersing it or by making it more dense.*
>
> *Joy (xi) or pleasure (le) agitate (empty) the heart. The energy of the heart is dispersed. In excess, they cause amnesia. Joy can cure sadness; the antidote to joy is fear.*
>
> *Emotional agitation (qing) injures (empties) the gallbladder. Awareness is troubled and not fixed; the energy is overwhelmed. In excess it causes anxiety and loss of the decision-will. The antidote is habits or worries and regrets.*
>
> *Fear (kong) injures the kidneys. The sexual energy is flattened and does not rise; it descends. In excess the lower warmer (genitourinary function) swells and becomes full. Fear can cure joy. The antidote of fear is sadness or obsession. (Europeans know well the relaxing effect of fear on the large intestine as well as the depressing action of continual diarrhea.)*
>
> *Sadness (bei) or mourning (ai) injure (cause fullness of) the heart governor and the pulmonary artery. The contracted energy melts; there is acidity. Sadness can cure unhappiness and fear; the antidote to sadness is joy.*
>
> *Obsessions (si, thoughts) injure (cause fullness of) the spleen-pancreas, the energy of which is bound. In excess then there is congestion of the spleen (pi man); we must take out the heat. Obsessions can cure fear; the antidote to obsessions is unhappiness.*
>
> *Unhappiness (nu) or irritation (nao) injures (causes fullness of) the liver; the energy rises in counterflow. In excess, nausea and vomiting. Unhappiness can cure obsession; the antidote to unhappiness is sadness.*
>
> *Worries (you) or regrets (chou) injure (cause fullness of) the lungs, the energy of which accumulates. In excess, rapid panting; they can cure emotional agitation. The antidote is joy and pleasure. (YXRM I, 4v)*

Experiments pursued in France have allowed us to observe mental improvement obtained by treating each problem through its organ. Thus, the heart, when weakened by joy and pleasure, is susceptible to anxiety that is easily cured through tonification of *juque* (CV-14), herald point of the heart, or *shaochong* (HT-9) and the organs acting on the heart.

The heart governor and the circulation, being full from sadness or mourning, can be relaxed by dispersing *daling* (PC-7) or *tianjing* (TW-10).

The spleen-pancreas (actually the pancreas alone), being full from obsessions and thinking (if there is stomach acidity and nondigestion of starchy foods and jams), can be cured through dispersing *yamen* (GV-14, IS GV-15).

The liver, when it is contracted due to unhappiness, is cured, as is the unhappiness itself, by dispersing *xingjian* (LR-2).

The lungs, when they are bothered by worries and regrets, are cured as are the worries and regrets themselves, by dispersing *chize* (LU-5).

The kidneys, when they are weakened by fear, can be improved, as can the fear itself, by tonification of *fuliu* (KI-7) and *dazhong* (KI-6, IS KI-4).

The treatments for problems caused by feelings are as follows:

(DACH) Illnesses from the feelings must be cured with the herald points (which are all on the anterior surface of the trunk).

(DACH) In all illnesses coming from a problem with the seven feelings, the energy of the stomach no longer acts: leg-*sanli* (ST-36).

(DACH) Accumulations of energy from the seven feelings; repression of energy from the seven feelings: *zhizheng* (SI-7).

(DACH) Repression of feeling and ideas; *shenmai* (BL-62).

(DACH) All central illnesses (psychological): *baihui* (GV-19, IS GV-20); tonify in depression, disperse in hyperexcitation.

II. Intensity of the Psyche

An old proverb quoted in the *Yi Xue* says, "A good doctor is occupied most of all with the vitality." Another says, "A good horse is recognized through its energy." Indeed, all qualities are prized for the intensity of the energy animating them. Insufficiencies or excesses, or alternations of psychic intensities, can bear either on the totality of the mental life — and often depend then on a failure of the vital energy (see Chapter I) — or on one of the levels (see each of these). In Europe, the total insufficiencies are labeled neurasthenia, translated in Japan by "weakening of the nerves" or "of nerves and brain." Naturally, they are not all of the same intensity; in light cases only some symptoms appear, varying according to the individual.

For treatment it is useful to recall that the yin nourishes the yang. It is advisable to tonify the yin (heart, circulation, liver, blood, conception vessel), as much as the yang (triple warmer, small intestine, governing vessel). Having elucidated the treatments when describing the illness itself, the isolated symptoms will be described later. It is important to remember that each of these signs can either be a passing trouble or a symptom of an infirmity, or a psychic deformity constituting one of the psychopathological types described further on.

III. Insufficiencies

Insufficiences of the primate and automaton.

Depression; neurasthenia:

Depression (*dian,* state of depression; *dian bing* or *dian-ji,* illness from depression):

A variety of nervous illness; the ability to laugh is not frequent . . . errors, problems. (Ci Yuan, ''Dian'')

*The **Su Wen** says: Much pleasure causes depression **(dian)**. . . . Pleasure depends on the heart. . . . Through joy energy is dissipated; one follows its goals no longer. One comes to a point where he can no longer accumulate or hold back energy in order to make a decision. If the pleasure injures the heart, use unhappiness to dissipate it or fear to conquer it. . . . A yin excess can also cause depression. . . . But there is also depression from stupidity or from prolonged passion. This is emptiness of yin, little blood, lack of fire in the heart. There is falling with vertigo . . . confusion of language, tears and groaning. (YXRM V, 35v)*

***Dian bing** begins to manifest through a lack of joy in one's thoughts. One remains lying down, with fixed gaze. Both yin and yang, however, are abundant at all the pulses. We say **dian bing** when there are four or five attacks per month. Puncture all the divisions of the meridians; when there is no longer any cold, harmonize with the needle; the illness will be finished. (DACH I, 6r)*

Depression *(dian):*
(DACH) Qiangu (SI-2), *houxi* (SI-3), *yanggu* (SI-5), *quchi* (LI-11), *chize* (LU-5), *tianjing* (TW-10), *xiaoluo* (TW-12), *jinmen* (BL-63), *xingjian* (LR-2), *jiexi* (ST-41), *yongquan* (KI-1), *diji* (SP-8), *zhubin* (KI-9), *feiyang* (BL-58), *waiqiu* (GB-36), *houding* (GV-18, IS GV-19), *yamen* (GV-14, IS GV-15), *naokong* (GB-19), head-*wuchu* (BL-5), *tinggong* (SI-19), *taiyin* (ST-23), *jinsuo* (GV-7, IS GV-8), *changqiang* (GV-1).

Depression *(dian ji):*
(DACH) shuigou (GV-25, IS GV-26 *renzhong*); *(DACH II, 19r) shenzhu* (GV-11, IS GV-12) and *benshen* (GB-9, IS GB-13).
Depression, tongue out, nape bent, looks to the right and left, incoherent speech.
 (DACH) yanggu (SI-5); depression, tongue out *(DACH) shenting* (GV-23, IS GV-24).
 Depression, runs crazily: *(DACH) yanggu* (SI-5).
 Depression, strangeness: *(DACH) jianshi* (PC-5).
 Depression, frequent groaning: *(DACH) tongli* (HT-5).
 Depression, yawning: tonify *lieque* (LU-7).
 Depression, instability, falls down: *(DACH) wangu* (GB-17, IS GB-12).
 Depression, convulsions: *(DACH)* head-*wuchu* (BL-5).
 Depression, expectoration of saliva: *(DACH) benshen* (GB-9, IS GB-13), *duiduan* (GV-26, IS GV-27).
 Depression, counterflow, vomiting: *(DACH) houding* (GV-18, IS GV-19).
 Depression, loss of ability to make sound: *(DACH) tinggong* (SI-19).
 Depression, a lot of talking: *(DACH) juque* (CV-14), *pianli* (LI-6).
 Depression, internal headaches: *(DACH) weiyang* (BL-53, IS BL-39).

Illnesses of the vitality *(jing shen bing):*

Jing, ''sexual essence,'' *shen,* ''consciousness''

Vital activity is described under this name, a power of personality for which there is not an exact word in French. It is often used for liveliness, enthusiasm, gaiety, vivacity, ''pep.'' Dictionaries give, ''vital spirits, energy, ardor.'' Illnesses of the vitality: *(JM) yangxi* (LI-5), *zhizheng* (SI-7), *yemen* (TW-2), *tianjing* (TW-10), *shaohai* (HT-3), *tianfu* (LU-3), *xingjian* (LR-2), *yongquan* (KI-1), *zhubin* (KI-9), *fenglong* (ST-40), *lidui* (ST-45), *guangming* (GB-37), *pucan* (BL-61), *jiuwei* (CV-15), *yinjiao* (CV-7), *qihai* (CV-6), *huaroumen* (ST-24), *taiyin* (ST-23), *fujie* (SP-14), *luoque* (BL-8), *fengfu* (GV-15, IS GV-16), *shenzhu* (GV-11, IS GV-12), *jinsuo* (GV-7, IS GV-8).

Vitality corroded, dissipated: *(DACH) jiuwei* (CV-15).

Heat, somnolence, the vitality leaves: *(DACH) yangfu* (GB-38).

Weakening of nerves:

(JM) lougu (SP-7), *baihui* (GV-19, IS GV-20), *qiangjian* (GV-17, IS GV-18, GV-16 *fengfu* by location), *fengchi* (GB-20), *tianzhu* (BL-10), *jianjing* (GB-21), *gaohuangshu* (BL-38, IS BL-43), *jiuwei* (CV-15), *jiquan* (HT-1).

Weakening of the nerves and brain:

(JM) jianshi (PC-5), *zhizheng* (SI-7), *shenzhu* (GV-11, IS GV-12), *shendao* (GV-10, IS GV-11).

Various symptoms of depression and neurasthenia:

Aversion to noise, misanthropism, hypochondria:

Aversion to hearing human noises, likes silence, detests noise: *(YIX I, 7v) neiting* (ST-44).

Does not like to hear human voices: *(DACH) jiuwei* (CV-15).

Wants to close his door and keep out the world: *(DACH, YXRM) dazhong* (KI-6, IS KI-4).

Hates the houses of others, melancholia of the heart: *(DACH VI, 14r) lidui* (ST-45).

Dreads people: *(DACH)* arm-*ximen* (PC-4).

Hypochondria *(JM, 321) tianzhu* (BL-10), *fengchi* (GB-20), *shenzhu* (GV-11, IS GV-12), *yuji* (LU-10), *sanyinjiao* (SP-6).

Boredom-melancholia *(men, fan, fan men, yi yi)*, no joy, sadness:

> *This is boredom **(man)**, depression; it is popularly called **fan men**. (Ci Yuan, ''Men'')*
>
> *Melancholia-boredom **(men)**. (Ci Yuan, ''Man'')*
>
> *Worry **(you)** and boredom-melancholia **(men)**. (Ci Yuan, ''Yi-yi'')*

In general, an insufficiency of the liver, heart and small intestine.

Melancholia, boredom *(fan men, men): (DACH) shaochong* (HT-9), hand-*wangu* (SI-4), *zhigou* (TW-6), *chize* (LU-5), leg-*sanli* (ST-36), *yinlingquan* (SP-9), *dazhong* (KI-6, IS KI-4), *jiuwei* (CV-15), *juque* (CV-14), *shangwan* (CV-13), *zhongwan* (CV-12), *youmen* (KI-21), *jueyinshu* (BL-14), *xinshu* (BL-15).

Chest twisted by melancholia: *(DACH X, 35v) jianjing* (GB-21).

Melancholia, fullness of chest, cannot breathe: *(DACH) yangxi* (LI-5).

Melancholia, unhappiness, repression of worries: *(DACH) wuyi* (ST-15).

Melancholia, no joy, preoccupation *(yi yi): (DACH) ligou* (LR-5).

Preoccupation, melancholia *(yi yi)* without joy: *(DACH)* LR-1.

Melancholia in the heart: (DACH VII, 33v) *yinlingquan* (SP-9), and *neiguan* (PC-6).

Oppressive melancholia in the chest: *(YIX I, 4r) jianli* (CV-11) and *neiguan* (PC-6).

Melancholia from emptiness: *(DACH) tongli* (HT-5), if frightened, tonify; if melancholic, disperse: *laogong* (PC-8) and *daling* (PC-7).

Melancholia, fear: *(YXRM I, 46v) bailao* (GV-13, IS GV-14, *dazhui*).

Insipidness *(tan tan)* in the chest: *(DACH X, 29v) jianshi* (PC-5).

Loss of laughter for a long time: *(DACH) shuigou* (GV-25, IS GV-26, *renzhong*).

Many misfortunes, sitting on the edge of the road, cannot lift the head: *(DACH) ganshu* (BL-18).

Without joy: *(DACH)* foot-*shangqiu* (SP-5), *dazhong* (KI-6, IS KI-4).

Frenetic speech, without joy: *(DACH) daling* (PC-7).

Habitual sadness, without joy: *(DACH) zhaohai* (KI-3, IS KI-6).

Sighs *(tan, shen yin, yi, si):*

> *Very deep respiration. (Ci Yuan, ''Tan'')*
>
> *Popularly, when there is pain or illness, the sound which is emitted is called **shenyin**. (Ci Yuan, ''Shen-yin'')*
>
> *Sound of sighing from regrets **(chou tan)** or from pain or trouble. (Ci Yuan, ''Yi'')*
>
> *Respiration. (Ci Yuan, ''Si'')*

Does not stop sighing all day: *(DACH) taichong* (LR-3).

Deep sighs: *(DACH) xingjian* (LR-4), *yangfu* (GB-38), *qiuxu* (GB-40), *gaohuangshu* (BL-38, IS BL-43), *daheng* (SP-15).

Deep sighs, habitual sadness: *(YXRM) riyue* (GB-24), *zhejin* (GB-23).

Habitual deep sighs: *(DACH) gongsun* (SP-4), leg-*sanli* (ST-36), foot-*shangqiu* (SP-5).

Likes sighing *(yi): (DACH) taixi* (KI-5, IS KI-3), *xiangu* (ST-43).

Energy from sighs rising in counterflow: *(DACH) taiyuan* (LU-9).

Sighs, energy blocked at the diaphragm: *(DACH) wenliu* (LI-7).

His movement is sighing: *(DACH) xinshu* (BL-15).

Regrets *(chou):* **sadness** *(bei, qi, can):*

Worries:

Worries-memories **(you liu);** *chagrin-tears* **(bei ti).** *(Ci Yuan, "Chou")*

Sadness, restlessness, worries. (Dictionary of the Chinese Language)

Chagrin:

Pain which expresses itself through sound and not with tears. (Ci Yuan, "Bei")

The same as **bei.** *(Ci Yuan, "Qi")*

Face of acidity of the heart. (Ci Yuan, "Can")

Injuries from chagrin. (Dictionary of the Chinese Language)

Chagrin can cure discontentment or fear; joy and pleasure can cure chagrin.

Regrets, chagrin: *(DACH) zhizheng* (SI-7).

Regrets, chagrin, absolutely no joy: *(DACH) jiquan* (HT-1).

Regrets, maddening sadness: *(DACH) shendao* (GV-10, IS GV-11).

Chagrin: *(DACH) shaochong* (HT-9), *rugen* (ST-18).

Habitual sadness without joy: *(DACH) zhaohai* (KI-3, IS KI-6).

Problems of sadness without joy: *(DACH) tianjing* (TW-10).

Habitual deep sighs and sadness from the heart: *(DACH) riyue* (GB-24), *zhejin* (GB-23), foot-*shangqiu* (SP-5).

Speaks of sadness, then starts sniveling: *(DACH) xinshu* (BL-15).

Habitual sadness, tears, emotional agitation, fear: *(DACH) daling* (PC-7).

Chagrin, tears, emotional agitation from the heart: *(DACH) jiexi* (ST-41).

Chagrin, frequent groaning: *(DACH) tongli* (HT-5).

Chagrin, sobbing *(kou): (DACH) chize* (LU-5).

Chagrin and sobbing to the point of vomiting: *(YIX I, 5v) tianchong* (GB-15, IS GB-9) and *daheng* (SP-15).

Habitual sadness and yawning; *(DACH) yongquan* (KI-1).

Intense sadness, cannot sleep: *(DACH) tianjing* (TW-10).

Chagrin, maddening regrets, false ideas: *(DACH) shendao* (GV-10, IS GV-11).

Chagrin, fear, little energy: *(DACH) yuji* (LU-10).

Chagrin, fear, afraid of people: *(DACH) shaofu* (HT-8).

Chagrin, fear: *(DACH) shaochong* (HT-9), *tongli* (HT-5).

Chagrin and fear mutually supporting each other: *(DACH) lingdao* (HT-4).

Chagrin from the heat, energy in counterflow *(DACH) lougu* (SP-7).

Excessive sadness or laughter: *(DACH) shenmen* (HT-7).

Tears *(qi),* **sobbing** *(kou, geng ye):*

Noises of mourning; the great noise is **kou,** *the little noise is* **qi.** *(Ci Yuan, "Kou")*

Stifling chagrin, cannot speak. (Ci Yuan, "Geng-ye")

For tears from irritation of the eyes, see Tears.

Habitual tears, sadness, emotional agitation, fear: *(DACH) daling* (PC-7).

Tears, sadness, agitation of the heart: *(DACH) jiexi* (ST-41).

Pouring out torrents of tears from emptiness of the liver: *(DACH) ququan* (LR-8).

The 100 illnesses from tears at night: *(DACH) baihui* (GV-19, IS GV-20).

Nighttime tears in children: *(DACH) baihui* (GV-19, IS GV-20).

Sobbing to the point of vomiting: *(YIX I, 4r) tianchong* (GB-15, IS GB-9) and *daheng* (SP-15).

Sobbing from sadness: *(DACH) chize* (LU-5).

Pulls out his hair with sobbing or singing: *(YXRM) shenting* (GV-23, IS GV-24).

Likes to sob: *(DACH II, 19r) baihui* (GV-19, IS GV-20) and *shuigou* (GV-25, IS GV-26 *renzhong*).

Despair *(liang):*

Extreme sadness and affliction. (Ci Yuan, "Liang")

Despair, deranged mind, cannot sleep quietly: *(DACH) shenting* (GV-23, IS GV-24).
Despair, deranged mind: *(DACH) baihui* (GV-19, IS GV-20).
Extraordinary despair: *(DACH X, 26v)*. Despair in a storm: *xialian* (LI-8).
Apoplexy, attacks of despair: *(YIZ, 40v) lieque* (LU-7), needles and moxa.
Apoplexy, anxiety: *(DACH) tongli* (HT-5).
Despair, convulsions *(chi)*: *(DACH X, 26v) baihui* (GV-19, IS GV-20) and *houding* (GV-18, IS GV-19).

Suicidal impulse:
Desire to kill oneself: *(DACH) feishu* (BL-13).
Wants to kill oneself: *(DACH) fengfu* (GV-15, IS GV-16).
Wants to die: *(DACH) xingjian* (LR-2).
Depletion of yang, wants to die: *(DACH) qihai* (CV-6).

Insufficiency of the primate.

Anxiety is a reaction of self-denial, of despair in the face of desire, of freezing in the face of life and fight. This is a very clear insufficiency of the intensity of the motor level of the psyche. It includes fear with all its subtleties: apprehension, restlessness, dread, true fear, anxiety, anguish, with a starting point in emotional agitation. Modesty and timidity have their root in anxiety, and through a normal reversal of feeling can be transformed into pride that diminishes others in order to elevate oneself. Kindness, generosity and self-destructive qualities to the point of masochism are mental expressions of anxiety when they are not expressions of equivalent conceit.

Emotional agitation *(qing)*:

> *Afraid like a horse, fear, upset from everything which is surprising. (Ci Yuan, ''Qing'')*

> *Emotional agitation injures the gallbladder, the consciousness is then troubled and is no longer fixed. In excess, there is anxiety and loss of decision-will. (YXRM V, 4r)*

The antidote to emotional agitation is habits, also worries and regrets.

> *When the illness of the gallbladder is emotional agitation with derangement, depression or hyperexcitation, one must tonify the heart, which is the master. (DACH)*

Great emotional agitation: *(YXRM) erjian* (LI-2); *(DACH) jianshi* (PC-5).
A lot of emotional agitation: *(YXRM) liangqiu* (ST-34).
Emotional agitation: *(DACH) daling* (PC-7), *tongli* (HT-5), *jiexi* (ST-41), *danshu* (BL-19).
Habitual emotional agitation: *(DACH) shaochong* (HT-9), *sanjian* (LI-3); *(YXRM) yemen* (TW-2), *quze* (PC-3), *jinggu* (BL-64), *dazhong* (KI-6, IS KI-4).
Seizures from emotional agitation: *(DACH) yangxi* (LI-5); *(DACH II, 29r) yintang* (GV-23a, IS M-HN-3).
Acute emotional agitation of children: *(YXRM I, 46r) hegu* (LI-4).
Emotional agitation of artists: *(GSdeM) tongli* (HT-5), if pale and fearful, tonify; if flushed and agitated, disperse.
Emotional agitation, timidity, fear: *tongli* (HT-5).
Habitual emotional agitation, fear, tears, chagrin: *(DACH) daling* (PC-7).
Troubled, cannot sleep: *(DACH) qihai* (CV-6).
Likes to emote, can neither drink nor eat: *(DACH) jinggu* (BL-64).
Shock, emptiness, emotional agitation, fear: *(DACH) zhizheng* (SI-7).
Jumps up from noises, nightmares: *(GSdeM) lidui* (ST-45).
From emptiness of gallbladder and heart — emotional agitation, restlessness, anguish: *(DACH VII, 26v) neiguan* (PC-6), *tongli* (HT-5), *yinxi* (HT-6), *xinshu* (BL-15).
From cold of the gallbladder — emotional agitation, fear, sees ghosts in dreams: *(DACH IV, 6r) qihai* (CV-6) or *xinshu* (BL-15) or *baihuanshu* (BL-30).
Emotional agitation, deranged mind, mistakes in speech, confused speech: *(DACH VII, 26v) shaohai* (HT-3), *neiguan* (PC-6), *shaofu* (HT-8), *houxi* (SI-3), *xinshu* (BL-15).
Emotional agitation, then hyperexcitation, recognizes neither relatives nor strangers: *(DACH VII, 26v) shaochong* (HT-9) *neiguan* (PC-6), *shixuan* (MP 25-29, IS M-UE-1-5), *xinshu* (BL-15), *zhongwan* (CV-12).
Children: emotional agitation, deranged mind, disquieted, emptiness of the heart: *(DACH XI, 24r) shaochong* (HT-9).
Hyperexcitation from emotional agitation: *(DACH) yangjiao* (GB-35), *ganshu* (BL-18).
Emotional agitation, fear, pain in the heart, loss of ability to make sound: *(YXRM) yinxi* (HT-6).

Deranged mind *(qi):*

> *Emotional agitation, like the extremities of a belt. (Ci Yuan, "Qi")*

Deranged mind: *(DACH) tonggu* (BL-66).

Deranged mind, emotional agitation: *(DACH) tianjing* (TW-10), *jiuwei* (CV-15), *jijue* (CV-14), epigastrium-*tonggu* (KI-20), *daju* (ST-27), *xinhui* (GV-21, IS GV-22), *shendao* (GV-10, IS GV-11).

Deranged mind, emotional agitation, does not eat: *(YXRM) jinggu* (BL-64).

Deranged mind, emotional agitation, fear: *(DACH)* arm-*wuli* (LI-13), *shaofu* (HT-8); and with frenetic speech: *yemen* (TW-2).

Deranged mind, fear, numerous sighs: *(DACH) shenmen* (HT-7).

Deranged mind, emotional agitation, shock, melancholia: *(DACH) shangwan* (CV-13).

Deranged mind, despair: *(DACH) baihui* (GV-19, IS GV-20); and cannot sleep quietly: *shenting* (GV-23, IS GV-24).

Children, deranged mind, emotional agitation, not quiet: *(DACH) shaochong* (HT-9).

Deranged mind, incontinence of urine: *(YXRM) tongli* (HT-5).

Deranged mind, emptiness, trouble; *(DACH II, 29r)* tonify leg-*sanli* (ST-36).

Indecision, lack of will *(zhi bu zu):*

> *What fixes the heart, mind, the internal firm resolution, certitude; what is necessary for the archer to make decisions; judgement. (Ci Yuan, "Zhi")*
>
> *Decision is stored in the kidney. (DACH)*

Insufficiency of decision-will, weakness: *(DACH V, 23r) fuliu* (KI-7).

Loss of decision-will: *(DACH VIII, 29r) neiguan* (PC-6).

Loss of decision-will, stupidity: *(YIX I, 5v) shenmen* (HT-7), *baihui* (GV-19, IS GV-20), *jiuwei* (CV-15, *guiyan* (MP-29b), if not, gum-*yinjiao* (GV-27, IS GV-28), *chengjiang* (CV-24).

Doubt *(huo,* or *gu ji,* **illness from poisoning):**

> *Illness or trouble of the decision-will, doubt of mind. (Ci Yuan, "Gu-ji")*

The hundred illnesses from hyperexcited doubts *(kuang huo)* and from absurd errors: *(YXRM I, 46v) gaohuangshu* (BL-38, IS BL-43).

Fox-doubts *(hu huo): (DACH)* moxa at *guiku* (MP-29a).

Agitated mind *(chong):*

> *Agitated mind, acts with trouble and precipitation. (Ci Yuan, "Chong")*

Agitated mind: *(DACH) shangwan* (CV-13).

All day, agitated and empty mind: *(DACH IV, 5r) tongli* (HT-5).

Apprehension *(ti):*

> *Respect (qing), fear (ju). (Ci Yuan, "Ti")*
>
> *When the ears hear great noises, or the eyes see strange objects, or we seem to approach a danger, we feel apprehension (ti) through the emotions. In serious cases, the heart jumps; we seem to faint — the pulse is tight and bounding. There is emptiness of blood or emptiness of energy, or both. (YXRM V, 36r)*

Apprehension, restlessness: *(DACH) jianshi* (PC-5), *laogong* (PC-8).

Apprehension, cannot speak: *(GSdeM) jianshi* (PC-5) tonify.

Apprehension, hyperexcitation: *(DACH)* hand-*wangu* (SI-4).

Habitual apprehension, fear as if one were going to be captured: *(DACH) yongquan* (KI-1).

Apprehension, emptiness in the heart, disquietude of consciousness and thought: *(DACH VII, 26v) neiguan* (PC-6), *tongli* (HT-5), *rugen* (ST-18), *xinshu* (BL-15), *ganshu* (BL-18).

Restlessness *(chu):*

> *Fear, apprehension. (Ci Yuan, "Chu")*

Restlessness, apprehension: *(DACH) jianshi* (PC-5), *laogong* (PC-8).

Restlessness, disquietude: *(DACH) dazhu* (BL-11).

Fear *(kong):*

> *Fear* **(ju),** *emotional agitation and dread, painful apprehension. (Ci Yuan, ''Kong'')*

Fear: *(DACH) shaochong* (HT-9).
Habitual fear: *(DACH) dazhong* (KI-6, KI-4).
Habitual fear, little energy: *(DACH) zhangmen* (LR-13).
Habitual fear, apprehension, as if one were going to be captured: *(DACH) yanglingquan* (GB-34), *yongquan* (KI-1).
Fear and dread in the heart from emptiness of the gallbladder: *(DACH) xinshu* (BL-15).
Fear, emotional agitation: *(YXRM)* arm-*wuli* (LI-13), arm-*ximen* (PC-4); *(DACH) qimai* (TW-8).
Habitual fear and emotional agitation: *(DACH) tianchong* (GB-15, IS GB-9), *baihuanshu* (BL-30), *changqiang* (GV-1).
Shock, emptiness, emotional agitation, fear: *(DACH) zhizheng* (SI-7).
Emotional agitation, fear, pain in the heart, loss of ability to make sound: *(YXRM) yinxi* (HT-6).
Emotional agitation, fear, dreads people: arm-*ximen* (PC-4).
Chagrin, fear, little energy: *(DACH) yuji* (LU-10), *shaofu* (HT-8).
Fear and chagrin mutually supporting each other: *(DACH) lingdao* (HT-4).
Fear, unhappiness, great outrage: *(DACH)* leg-*sanli* (ST-36).
Fear, emotional agitation, deranged mind: *(DACH)* arm-*wuli* (LI-13), *shaofu* (HT-8), frenetic speech: *yemen* (TW-2).
Fear, emotional agitation, numerous sighs: *(DACH) shenmen* (HT-7).
Habitual fear, emotional agitation, chagrin, tears: *(DACH) daling* (PC-7).
Fear, melancholia: *(DACH) bailao* (GV-13, IS GV-14 *dazhui).*
Hearing a sudden noise, heart agitated from fear: *(DACH) lidui* (ST-45).
Illnesses from fear at night: *(JM) zhongchong* (PC-9).
Children crying at night: *(JM) zhongchong* (PC-9); *(DACH) baihui* (GV-19, IS GV-20).

Anxiety *(bu):*
Anxiety, fear: *(YXRM) shenmen* (HT-7).
Apoplexy, anxiety, despair: *(DACH) tongli* (HT-5).

Anguish *(cheng chong):*

> *Worry, chagrin, emotion of the heart. Previously it was said to be from insufficiency of the energy of the heart. (Ci Yuan, ''Cheng-chong'')*

> *When we feel as if someone were going to capture us, a feeling of anguish results; and when anguish lasts for a long time, there is obstinate forgetfulness. (YXRM V, 36v)*

> *Emotional agitation injures the gallbladder, the consciousness is troubled and no longer fixed. In excess, anguish and loss of decision. (YXRM V, 4v)*

> *When there is anguish, we must warm the gallbladder, which acts as master. Choose among the following points, tonifying them:* **xiaxi** *(GB-43),* **riyue** *(GB-24),* **qiuxu** *(GB-40). Obsessions cure anguish and fear; habits or worries and regrets cure emotional agitation and anguish. (YXRM I, 18v)*

Anguish: *(YXRM I, 46v) shaochong* (HT-9).
Anguish that prevents sleep, energy of cold impeding the heart: *(YXRM) qihai* (CV-6).
Anguish, agitation of the heart: *(DACH) yuji* (LU-10).
Anguish, emotional agitation: tonify *(DACH) tongli* (HT-5).
Anguish following apoplexy, aphonia, painful contracture of the elbow: *(YIZ, 40) tongli* (HT-5).
Fear as if one were going to be captured: *(DACH) yanglingquan* (GB-34), *yongquan* (KI-1).
Heart suspended as if from starvation: *(DACH) jianshi* (PC-5).
Remorse to the point of anguish: *(YIX I, 8r) tongli* (HT-5).
Anguish, emotional agitation, deranged mind: *(YIX I, 3v) yangjiao* (GB-35), *jiexi* (ST-41).
Anguish: *(DACH II, 34r) neiguan* (PC-6), shenmen (HT-7), *xinshu* (BL-15).

Restive, contrary children *(ke u):*

> *In* **ke u** *if the emotions receive a sudden shock, or if the child meets a visitor or unaccustomed object, it becomes restless; it is cold of the spleen-pancreas. (YXRM VI, 15r)*

Restive children *(ke u),* tonify: *(DACH) jianshi* (PC-5), *sanyinjiao* (SP-6), *yinbai* (SP-1).

Tonic convulsions *(chi)* of the mouth, fright penetrating, restive children: *(DACH XI, 14r)* moxa, boys on left, girls on right: *zhejin* (GB-23).

Insufficiency of the automaton.

Amnesia, loss of memory, forgetfulness:

Jian wang (obstinate forgetfulness); *shi ji* (loss of memory):

When joy agitates the heart, the energy is dispersed. In excess, obstinate forgetfulness . . . when anguish lasts for a long time, there is obstinate forgetfulness. (YXRM V, 4v)

In Europe, amnesia is considered as coming either from cerebral anemia or from fatigue, or from pituitary or ovarian insufficiency, etc.
Obstinate forgetfulness: *(DACH) shaochong* (HT-9), *shenmen* (HT-7), *shaohai* (HT-3), *lieque* (LU-7), *baihui* (GV-19, IS GV-20), *shendao* (GV-10, IS GV-11), *xinshu* (BL-15), *gaohuangshu* (BL-38, IS BL-43), *youmen* (KI-21).
Obstinate forgetfulness, insufficiency of consciousness: *(DACH) zhongchong* (PC-9).
Obstinate forgetfulness, apprehension, all mental trouble: *(DACH VII, 26r) neiguan* (PC-6).
Habitual forgetfulness, tears coming: *(DACH) tianfu* (LU-3).
Habitual forgetfulness: *(DACH) quchi* (LI-11).
Forgets immediately, habitual forgetfulness: *(DACH) yongquan* (KI-1).
Amnesia, stupidity, home of consciousness *(shen): (DACH) shaochong* (HT-9).

Insufficiency of the evolved man.

Consciousness *(shen):*
Home of consciousness — the heart: *shaochong* (HT-9).
Insufficiency of the energy of consciousness: *(YXRM) zhongchong* (HT-9), arm-*ximen* (PC-4).
Lassitude of the consciousness: *(DACH III, 29r) zhiyang* (GV-8, IS GV-9).
Children: insufficiency of consciousness, does not speak until several years old: *(DACH) xinshu* (BL-15).
Too many thoughts and worries, no more strength of mind, forgets the past, neglects the future: *(DACH X, 25v) baihui* (GV-19, IS GV-20).
Mental fatigue, consciousness without strength: *(GSdeM) shanglian* (LI-9).
Eyes with a lost look: *(YIX I, 6r) fengfu* (GV-15, IS GV-16).
Foxy evil of the consciousness giving attacks of hyperexcitation or depression: *(DACH) guiyan* (MP-29b).
Loss of consciousness (coma?): *(JM) yinbai* (SP-1).
Lack of moral sense, consciousness and reason: *(GSdeM)* tonify hypophysis between C6-C7.

Consciousness:
The spleen is the minister who shows the faults and who speaks of justice. Tonify on the left foot: foot-*dadu* (SP-2), *daibai* (SP-3), *sanyinjiao* (SP-6).

Cerebral fatigue:
Too many worries and thoughts, no more strength of mind, forgets the past, neglects the future: *(DACH X, 25v)* moxa at *baihui* (GV-19, IS GV-20).
Worries, obsessions: *(DACH) zhongwan* (CV-12).
Cerebral fatigue: *(GSdeM)* tonify *shenmai* (BL-62).
Headache from cerebral fatigue: *(GSdeM)* arm-*shanglian* (LI-9) tonify.

Stupidity *(xin feng, dai chi):*

Name of an illness: appears as if stupid (dai chi) or depressed (dian) but more mild; can come either from a weak constitution or [appear among] those who quickly lose the idea of things, or from a timid or defective temperament, having repressed their worries. (Ci Yuan, "Xin-feng")

All those not full of life are called dai. (Ci Yuan, "Dai")

Not keen; popularly, crazy people (feng dian) are called chi. (Ci Yuan, "Chi")

Especially cures turpitude *(YXRM I, 40v),* stupidity through the nature of the mind *(DACH);* slow-witted, not distinguishing between what is valuable and what is without value, insulting people.
(DACH IV, 5v) stupidity, laughs or wails; *(DACH III, 29r)* disperse *shenmen* (HT-7).
Stupidity, forgets things: *(DACH) shaochong* (HT-9).

To cure stupidity use: *(DACH II, 25v) dazhong* (KI-6, IS KI-4).
Does not recognize people: *(DACH)* head-*wuchu* (BL-5).

Somnolence *(duo min):*

> *To sleep a lot means an excess of yin (thus a relative insufficiency of yang). Even during the day it is not possible to conquer sleep . . . comes from a fullness of the liver. (YXRM V, 20v)*

If the liver is full and hot, we sleep too much: *(DACH)* disperse *xingjian* (LR-2).
Heat, a lot of sleep, the personality leaves: *(DACH VIII, 32r) yangfu* (GB-38).
Sleeps a lot: *(DACH) baihui* (GV-19, IS GV-20); acts on the yang: tonify.
Illness of somnolence: *(JM) xinhui* (GV-21, IS GV-22), tonify.
A lot of sleep: *(DACH) xinhui* (GV-21, IS GV-22), *tiantu* (CV-22).
Sulky, likes to sleep: *(DACH) taixi* (KI-5, KI-3).
Likes to sleep: *(DACH) sanjian* (LI-3), *sanyangluo* (TW-8), arm-*wuli* (LI-13), *zhouliao* (LI-12), *lidui* (ST-45), *yongquan* (KI-1), *fengmen* (BL-12).
Likes to sleep and not speak: *(YIZ, 40) geshu* (BL-17).
Likes to be in bed: *(DACH, YXRM) dadun* (LR-1).
Tired speech, wants to rest: *(YIX I, 4r) tongli* (HT-5) and *dazhong* (KI-6, IS KI-4).

Insufficient speech:

Mechanical troubles: see larynx, tongue and apoplexy. Speech can be insufficient or troubled either from physical trouble of the phonetic apparatus, from the tongue or from local muscles, from cerebral or bulbar problems, or simply from fatigue, loss of vitality or insufficiency of consciousness. It is only this last group that is studied here.
Children, insufficiency of the energy of the mind, does not speak for several years: *(DACH) xinshu* (BL-15).
Likes to avoid speaking: *(DACH) geshu* (BL-17).
Prefers to not speak: *(DACH) yongquan* (KI-1).
Short of energy, cannot speak: *(DACH) tianjing* (TW-10).
Little energy, speech difficult: *(DACH) zhiyang* (GV-8, IS GV-9).
Cannot speak: *(DACH) fubai* (GB-16, IS GB-10), *tianrong* (SI-17), *tiantu* (CV-22).
Speech not correct: *(DACH) chengjiang* (CV-24), *zhejin* (GB-23), *riyue* (GB-24).
Speech blocked, thick: *(DACH) yamen* (GV-14, IS GV-15).
No longer chooses his words: *(DACH) jiuwei* (CV-15).
Speech of a ghost *(gui yu): (DACH) sanyangluo* (TW-8).
Muteness in storms, cannot speak: *(DACH, YXRM) chengjiang* (CV-24); the same with pain in the throat: *(DACH) zhigou* (TW-6); the same and cannot eat: *(DACH)* tonify *tongli* (HT-5).
Muteness, cannot speak: *(DACH) hegu* (LI-4), *yongquan* (KI-1), *tiantu* (CV-22).
Energy of muteness: *(DACH) tianfu* (LU-3).

IV. Excesses

Excess of the primate and automaton:

Hyperexcitation *(kuang):*

> *Makes great decisions and great speeches. What is called **chi** (stupidity) or **dian** (depression).*
> *(Ci Yuan, ''Kuang'')*

> *The illnesses of hyperexcitation start to appear with less sleep and no hunger. One considers oneself to be an elevated and precious sage. One discourses on one's own talents; one laughs erroneously and likes to sing.*
> *(DACH I, 16v)*

> *The **Nan Jing** says: ''Increased yang causes hyperexcitation. The overexcited person is dangerous. Slightly attacked, they feel themselves to be elevated and correct; they like to sing and dance, to climb high. Seriously attacked, they tear off their clothes and run, scream and will commit murder.'' It is an excess of the heart; young people who have a disturbance of the heart meridian cannot be cured.*

> *The **Su Wen** says: ''Discontent causes overexcitation . . . so discontent comes from the liver . . . it is thus an excess of liver.''*

> *The stomach meridiun is also able to cause overexcitation. When the stomach and large intestine are full and hot, the fire accumulates and knots in the intestines; defecation is blocked.*

Drunkenness from sorghum causes hyperexcitation: to cause vomiting can ameliorate it.

Certain strong drugs cause overexcitation. (YXRM V, 35v)

Sadness and mourning injure the meridians, the energy is contracted. In excess, it causes overexcitation. (YXRM V, 4)

When the illness is in all the meridians — either hot or cold — it is called overexcitation. When the energy is disturbed, it is overexcitation. From the beginning, if there is one attack per year, it is incurable; if there is one attack per month, it is incurable. (DACH I, 6v)

For the 100 illnesses of overexcitation, there are thirteen points that must be known, in order to choose among them: *(DACH XI, 13v)* shuigou (GV-25, IS GV-26, *renzhong*), *jiache* (ST-3, IS ST-6), *chengjiang* (CV-24), *fengfu* (GV-15, IS GV-16), *houxi* (SI-3), *shaoshang* (LU-11), *daling* (PC-7), *laogong* (PC-8), *jianshi* (PC-5), *quchi* (LI-11), *huiyin* (CV-1), *yinbai* (SP-1), *shenmai* (BL-62).

Especially cures problems of the governor vessel, hyperexcitation or depression: *(DACH) houxi* (SI-3).

Hyperexcitation: *(DACH) lidui* (ST-45), *chongyang* (ST-42).

Sudden hyperexcitation *(DACH)*. Hyperexcitation, hallucinations, violent sweats: *(DACH IV, 11v) jianshi* (PC-5).

Attacks of hyperexcitation; *(DACH) shaohai* (HT-3), *gaohuangshu* (BL-38, IS BL-43), *jinque* (CV-14), *ququan* (LR-8); *(YIX I, 3v) shangwan* (CV-13) and *shenmen* (HT-7).

Overexcitation from emotional agitation: *(DACH) yangjiao* (GB-35), *ganshu* (BL-18).

Prolonged hyperexcitation, climbs up, sings, takes off his clothes, runs: *(DACH) lidui* (ST-45) *chongyang* (ST-42); *(YXRM, DACH) fenglong* (ST-40).

Hyperexcitation becoming apoplexy: *(DACH) xuanzhong* (GB-39).

Symptoms of hyperexcitation:

Excessive laughter *(kuang xiao)*:
Excessive laughter *(YXRM)* and singing and frenetic speech: *(DACH)* leg-*sanli* (ST-36).
Habitual laughter: *(DACH) lieque* (LU-7), *fenglong* (ST-40).
Excessive laughter or sobbing *(YXRM),* Excessive laughter or sadness: *(DACH) shenmen* (HT-7).

Internal agitation *(fan, chong)*:

Acts precipitously. (Ci Yuan, "Chong")

Internal and mental agitation. (Ci Yuan, "Fan")

Internal agitation *(fan)* and external agitation *(zao)*: *(YXRM I, 46v) neiguan* (PC-6).
(DACH) Remains bound with internal agitation and melancholia: *jueyinshu* (BL-14).
(DACH X, 25v) Internal agitation from emptiness, dry mouth: *feishu* (BL-13).
(DACH) Internal agitation and melancholia not allowing sleep: *taiyuan* (LU-9).
(DACH) Internal agitation of the mind, heart, boredom, trouble, nausea: foot-*dadu* (SP-2).
(DACH) Internal agitation of the mind, deranged mind: *baihui* (GV-19, IS GV-20), *gongsun* (SP-4).
(YXRM) Internal agitation, fullness: *zhongji* (CV-3).
(DACH) Body warm, internal agitation, fullness. *(YXRM)* Illnesses with fever, internal agitation, melancholia: *taibai* (SP-3).
(DACH) Internal agitation, fullness, sweat does not come: *taodao* (GV-12, IS GV-13), *qucha* (BL-4).
(DACH) Anxiety, internal agitation, fullness: *xuanzhong* (GB-39).
(DACH) Internal agitation of the mind, cough in counterflow: *zigong* (CV-19).
(DACH XI, 8r) The five internal agitations of the mind — heat, foggy eyes. Comes from fatigue after delivery, or excess zeal; virgins also have it. Yin and yang are not harmonized, energy and blood abound either from worries, regrets, obsessions, preoccupations: *hegu* (LI-4), *bailao* (GV-13, IS GV-14, *dazhui*), *yongquan* (KI-1), *laogong* (PC-8), *xinshu* (BL-15); if no improvement; *shaoshang* (LU-11), *quchi* (LI-11), *jianjing* (GB-21), *xinshu* (BL-15).
(DACH) The five internal agitations of the mind: *neiguan* (PC-6), *daling* (PC-7), *hegu* (LI-4), *shixuan* (MP-25-29, IS M-UE-1-5), *yongquan* (KI-1), *geshu* (BL-17), *ganshu* (BL-18).
(DACH) Not quiet *(bu an);* internal agitation; fullness or internal contraction: *dazhu* (BL-11).

Agitated mind:
(DACH) Agitated mind *(chong),* acts with trouble and precipitation: *shangwan* (CV-13).
(DACH IV, 5r) Every day, empty and agitated mind: *tongli* (HT-5).

Excess of the primate, aggressiveness:

Aggressiveness is an excess of a normal acquisitiveness, not held back by reason and an awareness of the external world. It includes jealousy, envy, unhappiness, sadism, anger, hate and the desire to kill when there is resistance to a desire or repulsion. It is good in all treatments to tonify for a long time and strongly the consciousness: *shaochong* (HT-9), *zhongchong* (PC-9), arm-*ximen* (PC-4).

Jealousy; envy *(du):*

The Chinese, though fine psychologists, only use one word to indicate two feelings that are in reality very different. Jealous people do not want anyone to touch what is in their possession, but do not envy what others have. Envious people, on the contrary, forgive no one for having what they do not have or even for having what they already have. Both of these feelings come from an insufficiency of the liver with spasms or inflammation of the gallbladder and are often accompanied by headaches. Tonify *ququan* (LR-8) and *taichong* (LR-3); disperse *yangfu* (GB-38) and use daily moxa continued for several months and repeated for a month around both the spring and autumn equinoxes.

Discontent *(nu):*

The ideogram *nu* is formed from the elements: "slave-heart."

> When the energy is excited, when the force is contracted, this is a bothersome excitation of the energy. *(Ci Yuan, "Nu")*

> Unhappiness injures (engorges) the liver; chagrin cures discontent; discontent can cure obsessions. *(YXRM V, 4r)*

Great unhappiness; eats the five bitternesses: *(DACH) ganshu* (BL-18).
Habitual discontent: *(DACH) xingjian* (LR-2).
Habitual discontent; a lot of talking: *(DACH) fuliu* (KI-7).
Habitual discontent; does not laugh for a long time: *(DACH) laogong* (PC-8).
Extravagant talking; discontent; insulting: *(DACH) zhubin* (KI-9).
Energy of unhappiness; difficulty speaking: *(DACH) zhiyang* (GV-8, IS GV-9).
Discontent, repression of worries, melancholia: *(DACH) wuyi* (ST-15).
Alternating joy and unhappiness: *(DACH) riyue* (GB-24).

Excess decision-will *(zhi):*

The decision-will depends on the kidneys.
Excess decision-will: *(DACH) rangu* (KI-2), *yongquan* (KI-1).

Anger, rage *(hui),* indignation:

> Hate **(hen),** discontent **(nu).** *(Ci Yuan, "Hui")*

Worry and rage in the heart: *(DACH) xuanzhong* (GB-39).
Anger easy and short: *(GSdeM) xingjian* (LR-2) disperse.

Wickedness, hatred *(hen),* impulse to say bad things about others, to say things that hurt, to do evil:

Detests people like fire: *(DACH) shenzhu* (GV-11, IS GV-12).
Extreme hatred: *(DACH) taiyuan* (LU-9).
Frenetic speech, foul mouth: *(DACH) taiyuan* (LU-9).

Desire to kill:

Detests people like fire, wants to kill: *(DACH) shenzhu* (GV-11, IS GV-12).

Excess of automaton.

Remorse *(ao nao, hui hen):*

> Remorse **(hui hen).** *(Ci Yuan, "Ao-nao")*

Often caused by insufficiency of the small intestine (which follows the heart in the flow of energy). Tonify *houxi* (SI-3).
Remorse progressing to anxiety: *(YIX I, 8r)* First, no more joy for several days, then remorse: *(DACH) tongli* (HT-5).

Repression of worries *(you yu cheng):*

Illness from repression of worries: *(JM) tianjing* (TW-10), *jianshi* (PC-5), *taodao* (GV-12, IS GV-13).

Repression of worries, discontent, melancholia: *(DACH) wuyi* (ST-15).

Obsessions *(xiong zhong huai, si, bao ji)*:

> *Xiong zhong huai: to keep in the chest.*
>
> *Si: thought, obsession.*
>
> *Bao ji: illness from holding in the chest. (Dictionary)*

Obsession cures anxiety; it fills the spleen-pancreas. Obsession is cured by discontent.

Obsessions *(xiong zhong huai):* *(DACH II, 32r)* shenmai (BL-62), disperse.

Obsessions *(bao ji):* *(DACH II, 26v) juque* (CV-14).

Worries, obsessions *(si): (YXRM) zhongwan* (CV-12).

Too many worries and thoughts *(si),* no more strength of mind, forgets the past, neglects the future: *(DACH X, 25v) baihui* (GV-19, IS GV-20).

Repression of feelings and ideas: *(DACH) shenmai* (BL-62).

Excess talking, hyperexcited:

A lot of talking: *(DACH X, 46r) baihui* (GV-19, IS GV-20); *(YXRM) riyue* (GB-24).

Depression, a lot of talking: *(DACH) pianli* (LI-6).

Frenetic speech *(kuang yan)*:

Frenetic speech: *(YXRM)* hand-*wangu* (SI-4); *(DACH)* arm-*xialian* (LI-8); *(YXRM)* leg-*sanli* (ST-36), *tianshu* (ST-25).

With agitation of the body: *(DACH)* leg-*sanli* (ST-36).

With internal agitation: *(DACH) gongsun* (SP-4).

With a depraved mouth: *(DACH) taiyuan* (LU-9).

With joyous laughter: *(YXRM) yangxi* (LI-5).

Habitual laughter: *(DACH) wenliu* (LI-7).

Without joy: *(DACH X, 26r) daling* (PC-7).

With hot body: *(YXRM) jinzheng* (SI-7).

Epilepsy, tongue out, chattering of the teeth, frenetic speech: *(YXRM) pucan* (BL-61).

Frequently looking back: *(YXRM I, 46r) yanggu* (SI-5) and *yemen* (TW-2).

Typhoid fever: *(DACH) tianshu* (ST-25).

Extravagant speech *(wang yan)*:

With troubled, deranged spirit: *(DACH) yemen* (TW-2).

With excessive laughter: *(DACH, YXRM): yanggu* (SI-5).

With hot body: *shenzhu* (GV-11, IS GV-12).

With insulting discontent: *(DACH) zhubin* (KI-9).

From violent fear, frenetic, extraordinary speech: *(YXRM)* leg-*xialian* (ST-39, IS *xiajuxu*).

Febrile delirium:

Frenetic speech *(kuang yan)* from typhoid fever: *(DACH) tianshu* (ST-25). Delirium from typhoid fever, cannot distinguish respectable people from coarse people: *(YIX I, 7v) quchi* (LI-11), *xuanzhong* (GB-39), *yongquan* (KI-1), *bailao* (GV-13, IS *taodao*).

Dreams *(meng)*:

It is admitted in China that dreams can be somatic (troubles with the body or internal organs), or psychological (giving images to feelings), or premonitory (announcing events in a figurative manner), or they can be communications with absent or dead people.

Dreams of water:

(Ling Shu, XLIII) To wade through a large body of water with fear and anxiety: emptiness of kidneys.

(YXRM I, 16r) Bamboo submerged in water: emptiness of kidneys.

(Ling Shu XLIII) To be in the middle of water: emptiness of kidneys.

(Ling Shu XLIII) To dream of urinating: emptiness of the bladder envelope.

Dreams of fire:

(Ling Shu, XLIII) A great fire which burns and scorches: excess yang.

Mountains that burn, fire, smoke: emptiness of heart.

Dreams of flying, gliding:
(Ling Shu XLIII) To fly, to glide: abundance in the upper body (yang).
(Ling Shu XLIII) To fly, to glide: excess energy of lungs or emptiness of lungs.

Vertigo:
(Ling Shu XLIII) To feel as if one were on the edge of an abyss, of an emptiness: emptiness of kidneys.
(Ling Shu XLIII) To fall, vertigo: abundance in the lower body (yin).

Dreams of the countryside:
(Ling Shu XLIII) Mountains, trees, forests: emptiness of the liver.
(Ling Shu XLIII) Rocky gorges, large ponds, houses in ruins under wind and rain: emptiness of the spleen-pancreas.
(Ling Shu XLIII) Uncultivated fields and countryside: emptiness of the large intestine.
(Ling Shu XLIII) Streets and narrow passages in a town: emptiness of the small intestine.

Dreams of eating:
(Ling Shu XLIII) Large meals: hunger.
(Ling Shu XLIII) Drinking and eating: emptiness of energy of the stomach.

Dreams of gestures, positions:
(DACH) Dreams of being upside down: *tianyou* (TW-16).
(YXRM I, 16v) Dreams it is difficult to untighten his belt: fullness of kidneys.
(Ling Shu, XLIII) Body heavy, cannot stand up: excess energy of the spleen-pancreas.

Dreams of movements:
(Ling Shu XLIII) Body heavy, cannot stand up: excess energy of the spleen-pancreas.
(Ling Shu XLIII) Runs without advancing or sinking into the earth: emptiness of legs (yin).
(Ling Shu XLIII) Bows, bends forward and rises: emptiness of the thighs and top of the arms (yang in the yin).

Dreams of the body:
(Ling Shu XLIII) Lumbar area and spine detached from the body, not connected: excess energy of the kidneys.
(Ling Shu XLIII) Relationship, copulation: emptiness of the genital system.
(Ling Shu XLIII) To have the head cut off: emptiness of the nape.

Dreams of fights:
(Ling Shu XLIII) Killing one another: excess of yin and yang.
(Ling Shu XLIII) Fights in the street, to split one's body oneself: emptiness of the gallbladder.

Dreams of music, songs:
(Ling Shu, XLIII) Songs, music, body heavy; excess energy of spleen-pancreas.

Dreams of children:
(Ling Shu, XLIII) Dreaming of children: one is full.

Dreams of objects, beings:
(Ling Shu, XLIII) Marvelous objects of gold or iron: emptiness of the lungs.
(YXRM V, 5v) Strange, marvelous beings: the mucus of heat causes panic in the heart.

Dreams of discontent, anxiety, fears:
(Ling Shu XLIII) Anxiety, tears, sobbing: excess of energy of lungs.
(Ling Shu XLIII) Discontent, disappointments: excess energy of the liver.

Nightmares *(meng yan).*
''Frightening dreams.'' *(Ci Yuan, ''Meng-yan'')*
(DACH) Nightmares without end: *lidui* (ST-45) *neiting* (ST-44).
(DACH) Dreams of ''nocturnal devils'' *(mo):* foot-*qiaoyin* (GB-44).
(DACH V, 7v) Nightmares, dreams of ghosts: foot-*shangqiu* (SP-5).
(DACH II, 19r) Nightmares without rest: *lidui* (ST-45) and *yinbai* (SP-1).
(DACH) Consciousness full of fear from ghosts and nightmares: *zanzhu* (BL-2).
(DACH) Cat-ghosts: *juque* (CV-14).

Hallucinations (*jian gui,* seeing ghosts; *xie sui,* baneful evil):

> To see and hear what is not there is called **xie sui.** Serious cases can describe speeches, vision, ghosts of five
> colors; everything which does not exist. This is either an emptiness of blood and energy, the consciousness no
> longer bright; or there is trouble from the pressure of fire and mucus. There are women whose excess

menstruation causes mental panic, or after delivery there can be mental trouble. When the consciousness and decision-will are lost, it is an emptiness of blood and a lack of consciousness.'' (YXRM V, 36v)

Sees ghosts: *(DACH X, 26v, YXRM) yangxi* (LI-5), *(DACH) wenliu* (LI-7). *Fenglong* (ST-40), *shenzhu* (GV-11, IS GV-12), *baihuanshu* (BL-30).

Hyperexcitation, sees ghosts: *(DACH) zhigou* (TW-6); suddenly falls in terror from being seized by ghosts: *shuigou* (GV-25, IS GV-26 *renzhong*).

Consciousness full of fear from ghosts and nightmares: *(DACH) zanzhu* (BL-2).

Sees ghosts in dreams: *(DACH) xinshu* (BL-15).

Epilepsy, tongue out, frenetic speech, sees ghosts, delusions: *(YXRM) pucan* (BL-61).

Speech of ghosts: *(DACH) tianfu* (LU-3).

Cat-ghosts (bewitched?): *(DACH) juque* (CV-14).

Fox-ghosts (haunted): *(DACH) guiku* (MP-29a).

Possession: (*hu mei shen xie,* evil consciousness from nightmares of foxes).

Possession: *(DACH X, 26v)* Three moxas at *guiyan* (MP-29b) and *yinbai* (SP-1).

Delusions (paranoia? *huang hu*):

Sees what is not. (Ci Yuan, ''Huang-hu'')

Delusions: *(DACH) taodao* (GV-12, IS GV-13), *shendao* (GV-10, IS GV-11), *zhongji* (CV-3), *tonggu* of epigastrium (KI-20).

Unremitting delusions: *(DACH) juque* (CV-14).

Joyless delusions: *(DACH) taodao* (GV-12, IS GV-13, see Part IV), *luoque* (BL-8), *tinghui* (GB-2).

Mind and consciousness with delusions: *(DACH) baihui* (GV-19, IS GV-20).

Delusions, energy of the mind troubled: *(DACH) xinshu* (BL-15).

Epilepsy, tongue out, teeth chattering, sees ghosts, delusions: *(DACH) pucan* (BL-61), to the point of coma.

Cures ghostly possessions, fox-doubts, delusions: *(YXRM I, 47v) guiku* (MP-29a).

The 100 illnesses of overexcited suspicions, and absurd errors: *(YXRM I, 46r) gaohuangshu* (BL-38, IS BL-43).

Oddities (*yao, tian yao*):

Depression-oddness: *(YXRM V, 40r) shuigou* (GV-25, IS GV-26, *renzhong*), *shangxing* (GV-22, IS GV-23).

Habitually purifies himself: *(DACH) yangfu* (GB-38).

Excess of the evolved man:

Insomnia (*bu min cheng, bu de wo*):

Insomnia is always caused by an excess of yang. (YXRM IV, 20v)

If there is cold and emptiness of the gallbladder, one cannot sleep and there is lassitude in the character; will and worry are not at peace. (DACH IX, 1v)

Insomnia is caused by excess energy in the **yangqiao mai** *(which unites all the yang energies), with emptiness in the* **yinqiao mai** *(which unites all the yin energies). (Ling Shu XXX, line 20)*

Not sleeping and not perspiring depend on the **yangming** *[LI-ST]; there is often pain in the eyes and a dry nose. (YXRM IV, 20v)*

Acts against insufficiency and the non-rising of yin and blood; corrects the inundation of the organs by the yang: *(DACH IX, 5r)* leg-*sanli* (ST-36).

Insomnia with mental agitation: *(GSdeM)* tonify *zhaohai* (KI-3, IS KI-6) and disperse *kunlun* (BL-60).

No sleep, apprehension, worries, emptiness of gallbladder: *(DACH VIII, 32r) xiaxi* (GB-43).

Sleeps little: *(DACH X, 34v)* tonify leg-*sanli* (ST-36) in the morning.

Does not sleep: *(JM) baihui* (GV-19, IS GV-20), *qiangjian* (GV-17, IS GV-18), *fengchi* (GB-20), *tianzhu* (BL-10), *taiyuan* (LU-9), *daju* (ST-27).

Melancholia, cannot sleep, agitation: *(DACH) taiyuan* (LU-9); *(DACH X, 26r) taiyuan* (LU-9), *gongsun* (SP-4).

Does not sleep, restlessness, emotional agitation: *(DACH) dazhu* (ST-27).

Intense sadness, cannot sleep, wants to sleep: *(DACH) tianjing* (TW-10).

Despair, deranged mind, cannot sleep quietly: *(DACH) shenting* (GV-23, IS GV-24).

Energy in counterflow, cannot sleep *(YXRM) guanchong* (TW-1).

Troubled, cannot sleep: *(YXRM) qihai* (CV-6). Little energy and breath, cannot sleep: *(DACH) zhongfu* (LU-1).

Panting, cannot sleep: *(DACH) yinbai* (SP-1), *yinlingquan* (SP-9), *sanyinjiao* (SP-6).

Cannot sleep: *(DACH) feishu* (BL-13).

Cannot sleep lying down: *(DACH) yingchuang* (ST-16); cannot sleep on the back [prone]: *qichong* (ST-30).

Cannot sleep for a long time: *(DACH) baihuanshu* (BL-30).

Cannot sleep from excess emptiness: *(DACH),* from exhaustion, fatigue, cannot sleep: *(YXRM) yixi* (BL-40, IS BL-45).

Cannot sleep quietly: *(DACH IX, 1v) danshu* (BL-19).

Fullness of chest, ribs, limbs, cannot sleep: *(DACH) zhejin* (GB-23).

Cannot sleep, cold legs, four limbs heavy, little energy, difficulty in speaking: *zhiyang* (GV-8, IS GV-9) and *sanyin-jiao* (SP-6).

Headache, body hot, cannot sleep: *(DACH) luxi* (TW-19).

Heaviness of head from lack of sleep: *(DACH) yuzhen* (BL-9).

Children crying during the night: *(JM) zhongchong* (PC-9).

(YXRM I, 46r) The 100 illnesses of tears at night; *(DACH X, 26r)* nocturnal tears of children: *taiyuan* (LU-9), *gong-sun* (SP-4), *yinbai* (SP-1), *sanyinjiao* (SP-6), *yinlingquan* (SP-9), *feishu* (BL-13).

Method of the needles for sleeping peacefully: *(JO, 76) zhongwan* (CV-12), 8 *fen, liangmen* (ST-21), 7 *fen, shenmen* (HT-7), 3 *fen.*

V. Alternations

Alternations:

Excessive laughter or excessive sobbing: *(DACH) shenmen* (HT-7).

Joy or happiness not constant: *(DACH) riyue* (GB-24).

Unhappy unless ceaselessly laughing: *(DACH) laogong* (PC-8).

Sometimes sobbing, sometimes joy: *(DACH) shuigou* (GV-25, IS GV-26, *renzhong*).

Either sings, laughs or cries: *(DACH II, 36) neiguan* (PC-6), *lingdao* (HT-4), *tongli* (HT-5), *xinshu* (BL-15).

Depression or hyperexcitation *(dian kuang)*:

Depression or hyperexcitation, instability: *(DACH) zhubin* (KI-9).

Depression or hyperexcitation: *shaochong* (HT-9); *(JM) qiangu* (SI-2); *yemen* (TW-2); *(YXRM) wenliu* (LI-7); *(DACH) zhizheng* (SI-7), *tianjing* (TW-10); *(YXRM) xiaohai* (SI-8); *(YXRM) jinggu* (BL-64); *(DACH VI, 15r) zhiyin* (BL-67); *(DACH) shugu* (BL-65); *(YXRM)* disperse *fenglong* (ST-40); *(DACH) fengchi* (GB-20), *luoque* (BL-8), *houding* (GV-18, IS GV-19), *baihui* (GV-19, IS GV-20); *(YXRM) tinghui* (GB-2); *(YXRM, JM) taiyin* (ST-25), *gui-yan* (MP-29b).

Shock: depression or hyperexcitation, streams of talking, neighing like a horse: *(DACH) juque* (CV-14).

Depression or hyperexcitation, vomiting: *(DACH) huaroumen* (ST-24).

Depression or hyperexcitation, fullness, agitation: *(DACH) fengchi* (GB-20).

Emotional agitation, shocks *(feng)* causing insufficiency or excess:

The ideogram represented by the sound *feng* indicates everything that is immaterial, which, however, often has serious effect. The class of illnesses placed under this heading includes neuralgia, nervous agitation, rheumatism, all that is aggravated by wind — nervous shock, emotions causing physical problems. Insanity is called *feng;* hysteria is a type of *feng.*

Soften bad news: *(YIX I, 7v) neiting* (ST-44).

Is used for curing shock: *(YIX I, 8v) fengfu* (GV-15, IS GV-16).

Great shock: *(DACH)* first tonify, then disperse *fengchi* (GB-20).

All shock: *(DACH) baihui* (GV-19, IS GV-20) and *fengchi* (GB-20).

Nature of the person blocked, held in from emotion: *(JM) zhishi* (BL-47, IS BL-52).

(DACH I, 6v) Great shock, pain of the neck and nape; puncture at *fengfu* (GV-15, IS GV-16); and if there is sweat, moxa at *yixi* (BL-40, IS BL-45).

Dissipates shock, conducts the energy and brings quietness: *(DACH IV, 11v) zhigou* (TW-6).

Hyperexcitation from shock:

Great shock, shock has entered, energy closed, saliva rising, danger of confusion, cannot speak: *(DACH) fengchi* (GB-20).

Great shock, dull, doesn't know what hit him: *(DACH) tianjing* (TW-10).

Great shock, counterflow of energy, a lot of cold: *(YXRM) daheng* (TW-15).

Acute evil pain from shock: *(DACH III, 32r) dubi* (ST-35).

Energy from shock: *(DACH) tiaokou* (ST-38).

Great shock; looks backwards: *(DACH)* head-*linqi* (GB-11, IS GB-15).

Great shock, sweat: *(DACH) yixi* (BL-40, IS BL-45), *zhongfu* (LU-1).

Great shock without sweat: *(DACH) pianli* (LI-6).

Old fevers from shock, without sweat: *(DACH)* moxa at *daling* (PC-7).

Energy in counterflow, hand suddenly blue, piercing pain of the heart: *(DACH) fenglong* (ST-40).

Shock in counterflow, four limbs swollen, feet blue, body wet and cold: *fenglong* (ST-40).

Shock in counterflow, four limbs swollen, tongue out: *(DACH) wenliu* (LI-7).

Depression from shock:

Shock in counterflow, four limbs exhausted: *(DACH) fuliu* (KI-7).

Shock, emotional agitation, deranged mind, melancholia: *(DACH) shangwan* (CV-13).

The *Nei Jing* says, in great shock, with the joints of the bones heavy, hair and beard falling, one should puncture the flesh for a hundred days and the bone and marrow for a hundred days, for a total of two hundred days. When the hair and beard grow back, stop puncturing. *(DACH 1, 6r)*

VI. Hysteria *(Ye Si Ti Li)*

Hysteria has been excluded from the scholastic textbooks as not being an organic evil entity, but rather a nervous syndrome. But as the clinicians and neurologists, such as Gilbert Robin, observe it, the problems classified under this name are as numerous as ever. Hysterical people are very dangerous for those who take care of them. It seems that the organic problems described in the preceding paragraph (emotions, shocks) are not without a connection to hysteria. But the question of neurosis is still quite confused and should not be mixed with that of hysteria.

> *Hysteria: name of an illness. Women who have an emptiness of blood (thus, a predominance of yang), if they have to bear worries, fear, restlessness or hyperexcitation of the character, are frequently attacked by it. There are delusions in the personality; joy or unhappiness are extreme. If serious, there is contracture and troubles of speech, similar to depression from shock (**feng dian**). (Ci Yuan, ''Ye-si-ti-li'')*

> *Origins: heredity, excessive emotions or pleasure, excess fatigue, degeneration of the whole organism. Alcohol or tobacco, poisoning from lead or mercury, troubles of the genital system, fear, difficult menstruation, obesity, stoppage of the periods. Weak women are primarily susceptible to it.*

> *Symptoms: changes in the being, of its appearance and reactions; stiffness and hidden tension of the attitude; cephalgia, vertigo, insomnia, palpitations, weak vision, diplopia, hard of hearing, buzzing in the ears; strangeness of tastes and odors, excessive saliva and fluids, counterflow of food, loss of feeling of warmth and ticklishness (often from the middle of the body), multiple sensations of the skin, contractures, tears, loss of laughter, yawning, sneezing, screams, attacks of spasms, instability of moods, diminution of the critical sense. (Ci Yuan,)*

(JM) Hysteria: *lingdao* (HT-4), *tongli* (HT-5) *ximen* (PC-4), *yangjiao* (GB-35), *zhaohai* (KI-3, IS KI-6), *dazhong* (KI-6, IS KI-4), *lougu* (SP-7), foot-*shangqiu* (SP-5), *jiexi* (ST-41), *fenglong* (ST-40), *zhubin* (KI-9), *qiangjian* (GV-17, IS GV-18), *bailao* (GV-13, IS GV-14, *dazhui*), *jiquan* (HT-1), *riyue* (GB-24), *ganshu* (BL-18).

(DACH) Face without expression, cannot eat: *tongli* (HT-5).

(DACH) Bent backwards, looks up: *ganshu* (BL-18).

Treatment with needles:

yamen (GV-14, IS GV-15).....................	*3 fen,*
shenzhu (GV-11, IS GV-12)..................	*3 fen,*
feishu (BL-13).......................................	*3 fen,*
gaohuangshu (BL-38, IS BL-43)...........	*3 fen,*
weishu (BL-21)	*5 fen,*
pishu (BL-20)	*5 fen,*
weicang (BL-45, IS BL-50)....................	*5 fen,*
shenshu (BL-23)	*7 fen,*
youmen (KI-21)	*5 fen,*
juque (CV-14)	*6 fen,*
zhongwan (CV-12)	*8 fen,*
*guanyuan (CV-4) and leg-**sanli** (ST-36)*	*each 1 **cun**.*

Treatment with moxa:

shenzhu (GV-11, IS GV-12).......	*7 moxas,*
feishu (BL-13)	*7 moxas,*
gaohuangshu (BL-38, IS BL-43)	*7 moxas,*
shenshu (BL-23)	*15 moxas,*
fengchi (GB-20)........................	*7 moxas,*
gongsun (SP-4)	*5 moxas. (JM, 41)*

VII. Abnormal People

In comparing the various types and numbers of abnormal people, there appear immediately two large groups: 1) Congenital, hereditary: abnormal people whose families present clear signs of mental or physical troubles. 2) Those who come from a healthy family and who are themselves healthy, but who have problems similar to the congenital ones, seeming to have acquired them through contagion or shock; perhaps from some sort of nervous predisposition. This is curable.

Doctor Vinchon makes a similar distinction between: 1) Psychotics who judge themselves as being perfect, and have thus never thought to cure themselves as they have lost their judgement and are almost completely alienated. 2) Neurotics who recognize themselves as being ill and look for a cure. Only the latter are curable. The subdivisions of these two large groups seem due to the infinite diversity of the composition of the psyche. However, the Chinese, basing themselves on the three-leveled concept of the psyche, divide into two opposite groups those people who are congenitally abnormal and those who are temporarily abnormal due to contagion or shock: 1) The psychically deformed who have an almost monstrous disproportion of the level of the primate and of "color," the two other levels being totally subordinate. 2) The mentally ill, with a serious insufficiency of the level of the primate and "color," either from excess cultivation of memory, or from an equally serious insufficiency of the level of judgement and consciousness of the "energy." In the two groups the varieties are infinite depending on the predominance or insufficiency of each one of the numerous qualities forming each of the three levels.

Psychically deformed people:

Paranoiacs (arrogant, egoistic, contradictory, defamatory, interpret everything, persecutors):

Paranoia from heredity or contagion affects up to eight tenths of the population on the continent to varying degrees (often, fortunately, very slightly). Even in the slightest degree, they are particularly dangerous for the happiness and success of their family, their associates and, in a manner of speaking, for their country. Heuyer writes: "They are domestic hangmen, familial tyrants." Gilbert Robin writes: "Many family dramas ignored for a long time by neighbors are planned and perpetrated, sometimes with cruel refinements, by paranoiacs." They are the more dangerous as they know very well how to pay careful attention to appearances in public, particularly towards those whom they torture. They know no limit when they have the upper hand; violent scenes or constant and humiliating hostility are followed by rare moments of approbation.

Their trait of habitual contradiction is enough to distinguish them; a speaker who contradicts them even without offensive intent will be branded as deceitful, an ignoramus, or a sot. They see their ability to insult others with impunity as a sign of their superiority. The universal devaluing of work and people, the lack of enthusiasm for beauty, grace and harmony, the satisfied smirk at stories of meanness; such are the signs which cannot exist in people other than paranoiacs. Egoistic people are always paranoid; they speak only of themselves, of their affairs, mostly of their health; they constantly provide gifts for themselves. They are inaccessible to rationality, to reason, when they have not inherited great intellectual talent or are not very developed in that way. Their sadistic cruelty dominates when they have not been raised in an environment of tenderness and love. The least attack from the shock of great disappointment (their only emotion), or from great danger — and at around 40 years — can reveal the gradual enlargement of their split. In the European view, they are considered candidates for alienation even when, in their youth, they seem far from being alienated.

Europeans describe three main qualities of this psychosis that is affecting more and more of the population: arrogance, malicious misinterpretation, and the need to cause and speak evil.

1. Arrogance, the father of all vices, can, with repeated shock, become delirious or insane arrogance. It consists of elevating oneself by debasing others. It thus consists of humiliation and debasement, and denigration of others, admiring nothing. This is the source of the contradiction and denigration, the certain signs of paranoia. Their desire to appear superior to everyone leads them always to clothe themselves carefully. The ridiculous ostentations of fashion would not continue if there were not so many paranoiacs. They judge and describe themselves as perfect; they have never committed the least error; they are always right. They are always misunderstood — poor, noble and courageous victims. When they are complaining like this, it is wise not to remind them of their false conduct or judgement; it would injure them to the quick. For them, all their troubles come from the malicious envy of others.

They have the greatest difficulty being thankful for a gift or a service, or information. Those who analyze themselves coolly say that, as they give only to affirm their superiority, to enslave, or to buy the right to insult, they cannot admit that it could be otherwise for others. Consequently, to be thankful is to show oneself as being taken advantage of. Any advice or information is an offense because those who give it prove themselves to be better informed and more intelligent, which is inadmissible. A loan of money is accepted with distrust and as if other loans are in view. If the lender asks only to be reimbursed, he should expect either insults or a lawsuit, and in any case the worst defamation.

Their contradictory mentality makes it difficult for another to propose a fact or an idea without them affirming the contrary. This is exacerbated to such a degree that in order to obtain something, those close to them will quickly refuse in advance what they in fact desire, and ask instead for what they want to have refused. Paranoiacs contradict themselves and do not at all know where the truth lies. When they do not contradict themselves, they have the art of looking sulky and disdainful which repudiates all validity.

Their unreasonable stubbornness, sustained by their arrogance, aggravates their contradictory mentality. When they have contradicted an idea and when their idea is complete nonsense, they stick to it obstinately, because to surrender would be to admit their error, and thus their inferiority. Nothing bothers them as much as asking their opinion before having expressed one's own thought. Then they hesitate, they are troubled, because in fact they have no judgement or opinion, other than contradiction.

To discuss business with them is not prudent because their contempt for the truth imbues them with surprisingly bad faith. Comments on any remarks which are badly supported are rejected, and the speaker accused of falsehood. Their tone is so convincing that an uninformed listener can be deceived. Moreover, their most precise written engagements are only kept if there is profit in it for them. It is not good to be their employee or associate. Their arrogance, which is so frequent, consists of an ''idolatry,'' an admiration which reaches the point of self adoration. Arrogant people constantly look at themselves in the mirror, turning and re-turning their head to better admire their image, fussing about their dress, their important attitude, their manner of walking on their heels, their way of being in society — either with silence and a closed face expressing contempt and mistrust, or with a contemptuous disturbing familiarity calculated to diminish others. If there is a smile, it is fixed, always the same, without nuance, without expansion of life or sympathy. Arrogant people cannot bear it if others have as much or more than they; they are generally tinged with envy for what they do not have and with jealousy when their devotees give their adoration to others.

2. Malicious misinterpretation: while correctly perceiving a portion of the facts, of speech, of gestures, they also attribute to others motives and intentions of a low and vile nature. It is derivative of their arrogance, which debases everything. With aging and shock, their abnormality is aggravated. Suddenly the same acts or speech are imbued with sinister intentions, personally aimed at him, that prove him to be already alienated; this nuance is associated with the persecution mania that so easily drifts into despotism.

The scholar P. de Tonquedec writes:

> To plead certain facts to one who misinterprets things, to try to push him into the contradiction, is a lost effort. Either he will interpret these facts in a manner favorable to his thesis, or he will drop them. . . . Intellectual lameness is fatal in him and his best can do nothing. All discussion with him is useless. . . . They often have penetrating, subtle, crafty minds; nothing escapes the acuity of their sight. The approximations that they establish are sometimes so numerous and ingenious that they impose themselves on people of healthy mind. . . . On the first plane, egocentrism, susceptibility, arrogance, spite and the spirit of vengeance are found.
> (Maladies Nerveuses ou Mentales, 166-168)

The precepts of Confucius contain many passages on malicious misinterpretation, one of which summarizes them all: ''Small people consider denigration and maliciousness to be perspicacity.'' So many people are attacked with this mental vice — the susceptible people who read into a look, a word, a gesture unkind intentions; jealous people, the least action of their spouse putting them in an alert state; litigious people. ''Misinterpretations,'' writes P. de Tonquedec, ''some of which are tangential to insanity, and some of which are fully in it, because not all mad people are interned, nor should they all be.''

3. The persecution mentality, which can go to the point of threatening death (for which we must intern the person), and even to the point of murder, deals with arrogance that cannot endure critics and at the same time with malicious misinterpretation that transform all acts, all speech, into perfidious intentions. Abnormal people like to persecute, and in order to justify their actions, they believe themselves to be persecuted.

The taste for domination becomes ambition, which is a desire for power. This only exists in proportion to the obedience on which it exerts itself; slavery is the sheath of power. Power does not bother the feelings of the slave. From the beginning, its exercise is an abuse in the hands of the paranoiac. The satisfaction in speaking and doing evil is manifest in the denigration of everything and everybody, which comes from arrogance and the need to crush all those who approach him, to humiliate them; that is, to do moral evil. From the domestic tyrant, the familial executioner, to the sadist, there is only a slight transition. It is useful to have interceded in some family dramas of paranoiacs in order to realize the danger to which mostly the wives are exposed, for whom the home, instead of being a refuge, becomes a true hell.

Paranoiacs retain an aura of mystery about their actions and thoughts, even to the smallest matters. To question them on this subject is to them an insult. Is it not an attack on their independence? One of them said, "My thoughts concern only myself; concerns of others do not interest me." It is through this aura of mystery that it is possible for them to say white or black and thereby obtain a small illicit advantage over others. So they have no conversation and when they do speak, their mind is fixed only on the detriment of others.

Their relationships are truly opposite those of conventional courtesy, which would have the person we are leaving be as satisfied as we are. Their teasing, passed off as innocent, is a mildly disquieting symptom. Moreover, there is a sort of teasing that makes people laugh, and another that makes them cry; this latter belongs to the persecution mentality. The French abroad have a reputation of greeting people by speaking in this way: "It's a long time since I've seen you. Perhaps you've been in prison?" "Oh, what a nice hat; where did you steal it?"

Physically, it has been remarked that this type always sports a sharp nose, and thin and tight lips with a hard look. The complexion is often "muddy" because alcohol is normal for them, even though the least aperitif gives them an attack of wickedness. Men make bad husbands whose sexual impulses quickly disappear. Women are generally frigid with their husbands, because it is the husband whom they need to humiliate and debase.

In spite of their dangerously vicious minds, their lack of real intelligence and thought, most of them possess a certain seductiveness. The Chinese explain this through a predominance of the primate level with its abundance of "color" (animal energy, sex appeal) and its astuteness-cleverness-deceitfulness with only two attitudes: servility or insolence.

They often succeed in business, not being distracted from their work by love or generosity, but being maintained in it by ambitious arrogance as well as by their greed for money, the instrument of power. They are always sure of their rights, even when they throw out their benefactors (hated for their acts of kindness) or ruin their associates who are overconfident. Do they not glorify themselves through deceit as others are glorified through good actions?

In Europe, "paranoia results from a constitutional predisposition and from a series of experiences the mechanisms of which have been elaborated by Freud. The constitutional predisposition explains why the subject becomes paranoid." Indeed, their families always present some specific hereditary signs: deafness, dental troubles, miscarriages, etc.

Neurologists advise one to escape from even the mild cases because any possibility of confident and sure happiness is impossible in their company, and because future emotions and life can only aggravate manifestations of their hostility.

The Chinese advise: against jealousy and envy, disperse *yangfu* (GB-38) and tonify *taichong* (LR-3). Against the excess of the primate, disperse *yongquan* (KI-1). Against the insufficiency of consciousness, judgement and sense of reality, tonify *dadu* (SP-2). Against malicious misunderstanding, disperse *guiku* (MP-29a), *baihui* (GV-19, IS GV-20), *taodao* (GV-12, IS GV-13). Against wickedness and the desire to do evil, disperse *shenzhu* (GV-11, IS GV-12).

The society of the seventeenth century, involved in religious and philosophical problems, called paranoiacs reprobates or fiends from hell, because they create hell around them and oblige those in their company to defend themselves by acting and speaking in a way which would otherwise be condemnable. The society of the eighteenth century, taking the social point of view, called them, with its freedom of language, "sticks of shit," which one cannot touch without becoming dirty.

Perverse or amoral people; protesting-aggressive people.

The varieties of paranoia are innumerable, according to the proportion of elements and according to the degree of intelligence and feeling, and also according to their education and milieu. It seems acceptable to include some types of psychically deformed people whom Europeans study separately, as they have done for those who are misinterpreters, persecutors, etc.

Dupré has described the complete type, but the incomplete forms are more frequent. Two elements are distinguished by Gilbert Robin: on the one hand moral indifference, lack of consciousness or moral sense; on the other hand, perverse tendencies. Some describe it as a dementia of protest encompassing hostility against the entire society. "The child from his first years is remarkable because of his anger; vindictive, cruel, vengeful, jealous. He is moreover undisciplined and disobedient. At puberty, the eroticism goes to the highest level. In excess, he soon indulges in vagrancy or stealing (a matter here of children from an unfortunate environment). They cannot look one in the eye. They judge people from the first glance and accept only those of their own 'climate'." For the Chinese, there is an excess of the primate with a detestable automaton, which makes all education useless.

Mentally ill people:

Distracted-dreamy people (schizoids).

Less numerous than the paranoiacs, schizoid people are dangerous only to themselves, or for those who are vainly awaiting direction, help or solace from them. They are always dependent on their family and are always the prey of businessmen with few scruples when they have not received a careful education. The most talented become great creative artists. The less intelligent content themselves with marvelous dreams through which they transform into gold the lead of their existence. To a lesser degree schizoids are those who are distracted, whose attention cannot be fixed for a long time, and whose look is vacant. If they are a little more serious, they become the dreamers who are awake. Their mind is constantly occupied with dreams in which they play a preponderant role. "They do not take into consideration the external reality; they live an internal life and adopt an attitude that gives the impression of indifference to the exterior. At a further stage, reality is increasingly neglected; the patient is inactive, inert, with an absent air. They are not interested in what goes on around them. However, the integrity of their intellectual faculties is intact."

They compensate for their low opinion of themselves, reflected from those around them, by having triumphant roles in their dreams. It very often seems as if their parents have not tried to socialize them, and have not gently corrected their predisposition to overimagination and their awkwardness due to lack of physical attention. Sometimes parents make fun of them, closing them off to external reality. Acupuncture can help, but not cure, by tonifying the consciousness: tonify *ximen* (PC-4), *shaochong* (HT-9) and *baihui* (GV-19, IS GV-20).

Mythomaniacs.

Mythomaniacs tell their dreams, their fantastic stories, with precise details and a convincing air. They are treated as liars, yet they affirm the reality of their story. They have lived their dream with such an intensity that they no longer distinguish it from the real facts that they have included. Most children are supposed to have a tendency to mythomania; many educators say that all children are liars. True mythomaniacs are only those who have passed the age of reason. They remain in the stage where judgement does not bring facts together, where the external attention is not always automatically awake in order to correct the imagination.

When the mythomaniac is slightly perverse as well, he accuses those who come within his range of vision or hearing of the most peculiar crimes, thus glorifying himself by attracting the attention of the people around him. Unlike the paranoid, he very rarely attacks those near him. The Chinese see in him a serious failure of the consciousness; treatment is thus the same as for schizoid types.

Chapter VII

Sense Organs

I. Taste — II. Smell — III. Touch — IV. Ears, Hearing — V. Eyes, Sight

I. Taste

Insufficiency of taste:

(DACH, YXRM) Does not recognize the taste of food: *qihu* (ST-13).
(DACH) Food and drink without taste: *baihui* (GV-19, IS GV-20).
(YXRM I, 47r) Yellow face, thin body, food without taste: *xinshu* (BL-15).
(DACH) No taste for food: *neiting* (ST-44).

Excess of taste:

(DACH) Ability to savor: *shangqiu* (SP-5).

II. Smell

Insufficiency, anosmia:

Bu shou chou xiang: ''Does not perceive either a stench or a perfume,'' *bi nei wu wen*, ''The inside of the nose perceives nothing.''
(DACH III, 30v; DACH III, 32r; DACH III, 29; DACH IV 3v; YIX I, 5r; YXRM, DACH) The nose does not smell either perfume or stench; *(YIZ, 40r)* stuffed nose, perceiving neither perfume nor stench: needle 1 *fen* under the skin upward, disperse a lot, tonify little, avoid moxa: *yingxiang* (LI-20).
(YXRM, 30r) Nose blocked, smells neither perfume nor stench: needle *yingxiang* (LI-20), *hegu* (LI-4).
(YXRM) Nose smells neither perfume nor stench: *shuigou* (GV-25, IS GV-26, *renzhong*); *(DACH IV, 19r, YIX I, 4r)* *tongtian* (BL-7).
(DACH) Nose blocked, smells neither perfume nor stench: *heliao* of nose (LI-19), *tianzhu* (BL-10), *xinhui* (GV-21, IS GV-22) *chengguang* (BL-6).
(YXRM) Nose smells neither perfume nor stench: *tianzhu* (BL-10).
(DACH X, 32v) Nose blocked, smells nothing — sometimes clear discharge: *xinhai* (GV-21, IS GV-22), moxas.
(DACH) With moxa on *xinhui* (GV-21, IS GV-22) improvement starts on the fourth day and the cure is complete on the seventh day.
(DACH) Nose blocked, smells neither perfume nor stench: *chengguang* (BL-6), *yuzhen* (BL-9).

Excess:

(DACH) Detests the smell of food odors: leg-*sanli* (ST-36).

III. Touch

(JM) Illness of perception of the fingertips: *laogong* (PC-8).
(JM) Illness of anomalies of the sensitivity and perception of the fingers (fingers or toes?): *diwuhui* (GB-42).
(YXRM I, 46v) All illnesses of the head, face, arm, wrist and five fingers: hand-*wangu* (SI-4).
(JM) Cold and lack of grip of the hand: *shaohai* (HT-3).

IV. Hearing, Ears

In general:

(YXRM I, 39r) Illnesses of the ear: *hegu* (LI-4).
(DACH) From pressure, radiates into the ear: *fengchi* (GB-20); *(JM)* (acts on the sympathetic and also the vagus systems); *(JM)* illness and troubles of the ear.

(JM) Motor-sensory nerves, glossopharyngeal nerve (sensitivity of the mucosa, tongue, pharynx, tympanic cavity, eustachian tube, vasodilation of the root of the tongue): *tianzhu* (BL-10), which acts on the vagus.
(GSdeM) When pressing, response in the inner ear: head-*qiaoyin* (GB-18, IS GB-11); *(JM)* the same for the pharynx: *yifeng* (TW-17); *(DACH) fengchi* (GB-20).
Middle ear: *(JM)* inflammation; *tinghui* (GB-2), head-*wangu* (GB-17, IS GB-12), *naohu* (GV-16, IS GV-17).
External ear: *(JM)* inflammation: *ermen* (TW-23, IS TW-21).
(YIX I, 4v) Ear: deafness, lymph nodes, pain, pruritis, abscess — disperse *tinghui* (GB-2), *yifeng* (TW-17).

Wax (ding, ding ning):

(JM, DACH, YXRM) Ear with wax: *ermen* (TW-23, IS TW-21), *tinggong* (SI-19); *(YIZ, 39r)* wax in the ear: *tinghui* (GB-2), *yifeng* (TW-17), *xiaguan* (ST-2, IS ST-7).

Pruritis of the ear:

(YIZ, 39r; DACH IV, 7v) Pruritis of the ear: disperse during eight inhalations *tinghui* (GB-2); *(YIZ, 39r)* needle *xiaxi* (GB-43) 5 *fen,* disperse during seven inhalations; *(YXRM) xiaxi* (GB-43).

Pain of the ear (otalgia, er tong):

> *Origin: tonsillitis, illness or troubles of the nose, pharynx, tongue, cartilage-which-presses-and-reunites* **(hui ya),** *from the articulation of the lower jaw, parotitis, or neighboring lymph nodes, or pain of the teeth. Symptoms: inflammation of the ear, pain of the ear, talks with difficulty, hears badly. (JO, 56)*

Treatment with needles:

xiaguan (ST-2, IS ST-7)...	*5 fen,*
ermen (TW-23, IS TW-21)	*6 fen,*
tinggong (SI-19)	*1 fen,*
leg-sanli (ST-36)..............	*1 cun. (JO, 56)*

Treatment with moxa:

tinggong (SI-19)	*5 moxas,*
ermen (TW-23, IS TW-21)	*5 moxas,*
leg-sanli (ST-36)..............	*7 moxas. (JO, 56)*

(YIZ, 39r) Pain in front of the ear: *shaoshang* (LU-11); same with pain in the ear: *quchi* (LI-11).
(DACH) Pain behind the ear; headaches: head-*wangu* (GB-17, IS GB-12); same with pain in the mastoid process: foot-*linqi* (GB-41).
(DACH) Pain behind the ear, at the shoulder and elbow: *tianjing* (TW-10).
(YIZ, 39r) Acute pain in the ear: disperse during eight inhalations. *(DACH IV, 7v)* Pain in the ear: *tinghui* (GB-2).
(YIZ, 39r) Acute pain in the ear: 5 *fen,* disperse during seven inhalations: *yifeng* (TW-17).
Pain in the ear: *(YIZ, 40v) guanchong* (TW-1); *(DACH) yemen* (TW-2); *(YXRM, JM) yangxi* (LI-5); *(YIZ, 40v) quchi* (LI-11); *(JM) pianli* (LI-6); *(JM) xiaguan* (ST-2, IS ST-7); *(YXRM; YIZ, 40v) ermen* (TW-23, IS TW-21), *(YXRM) kezhuren* (GB-3, IS *shangwan*); *(DACH) hanyan* (GB-4); *(YXRM) tianchuang* (SI-16).
(DACH VII, 23v) Pain inside the ear: *waiguan* (TW-5), *hegu* (LI-4), *kezhuren* (GB-3, IS *shangwan*), *tinghui* (GB-2).

Ear lobes:
(DACH XI, 4r) Ear swollen, red and painful: *tinghui* (GB-2), *hegu* (LI-4), *jiache* (ST-3, IS ST-6); if no improvement, leg-*sanli* (ST-36), *hegu* (LI-4), *yifeng* (TW-17).

Inflammation of the ear, otitis, abscess of the ear (er ting, er liu):

> *Also called* **er liu;** *it is an attack of catarrh of the inner ear; comes from an external lesion or an internal illness. Sometimes pus comes from the inside of the ear. (Ci Yuan, ''Er-ting'')*

(JM) Inflammation of the external acoustic meatus: *ermen* (TW-23, IS TW-21), *tinggong* (SI-19).
(JM) Inflammation of the middle ear: *tinghui* (GB-2), *wangu* (GB-17, IS GB-12), *naohu* (GV-16, IS GV-17, GV-15 by location).
(GSdeM) For the inner ear, *fengchi* (GB-20), head-*qiaoyin* (GB-18, IS GB-11), *yifeng* (TW-17), *qimai* (TW-18).

Otitis:

(DACH) Flowing from the ear *(er liu)*, pus coming out: *xiaguan* (ST-2, IS ST-7); the same with pain and pruritis: *tinghui* (GB-2).

> *Middle ear inflammation of a catarrhal nature.*
>
> *Origin: shivering, rhinitis, pharyngitis, tonsillitis, measles, etc.*
>
> *Symptoms: acute — fluids filling up the ear, which is sometimes blocked; there is a sensation of movement of fluids, pain of the ear, buzzing, diminution of hearing, attacks of chronic fever, difficulty hearing; the tympanum thickens, there is pus. (JO, 57)*

Treatment with needles:

tinghui (GB-2)	*5 fen,*
yifeng (TW-17)	*5 fen,*
qimai (TW-18)	*3 fen,*
head-**wangu** (GB-17, IS GB-12)	*5 fen. (JO, 57)*

Treatment with moxa:

fengshi (GB-31)	*7 moxas,*
neiguan (PC-6)	*7 moxas,*
qiangu (SI-2)....	*7 moxas. (JO, 57)*

(JM) Abscess in the ear: *ermen* (TW-23, IS TW-21).
(DACH XI, 4r) Ear forming an abscess with liquid and pus flowing: *yifeng* (TW-17), *hegu* (LI-4), *ermen* (TW-23, IS TW-21). If not better, *tinghui* (GB-2), leg-*sanli* (ST-36).

Buzzing (singing in the ear, er ming; cicada-songs, chan ming; great buzzings, hong; slight buzzings, liao, liao qiu):

> *Singing in the ears can be caused by: wax bound into stone from shock or heat, pus in the ears pushed upwards from shock or heat, occlusion of energy (can become deafness). There is singing in the ear with pain like insects in the ear, or with pain of dryness from wind; they come from shock, heat, fire or emptiness; some are from emptiness of the kidneys, some from anemia. In general, one must harmonize the energy and open the gates. (YXRM V, 12r)*
>
> *The singing in the ears come from an emptiness of the triple warmer branch entering from behind the ear. (YXRM I, 18)*
>
> *Insufficiency of the upper warmer and the triple warmer. (DACH)*

This condition can be caused by prolonged use of quinine or aspirin or from thyroid insufficiency. It can be a sign of interstitial, chronic nephritis (with small, red, contracted kidneys). The buzzing is on the side of the contracted and inflamed kidney *(GSdeM)*, or contracture of the muscles of the malleus (innervated by the inferior branch of the trigeminal nerve) that attracts the membrane of the tympanum and pushes the stapes into the fenestra vestibuli, causing compression and buzzing (the muscle of the stapes depends on the facial nerve), or from cephalic anemia (Hédon).

(GSdeM) Distinguish the noises as follows: 1) Great beating to the rhythm of the pulse, congestion; can be cured: disperse leg-*sanli* (ST-36), *shenmai* (BL-62), *daling* (PC-7). 2) Slight beating with a whistling end, cicada songs; difficult to cure: tonify *yifeng* (TW-16), *luxi* (TW-19), *shanzhong* (CV-17), *hegu* (LI-4). 3) Continued whistling, vapor which escapes; kidney trouble. For everyone, the high tones are the most difficult to cure.

In Europe: from an obstruction of the eustachian tubes, the tympanum bulges inward and pushes the stapes into the fenestra vestibuli.

> *Origin: problems or inflammation of the external or middle ear, sclerosis (hardening, **ying hua**) of the ear, problems of the vagus nerve or of the auditory nerve or of the brain, blood or heart. Symptoms: singing in the ear of high tones, various sounds, or close music, either intermittent or long lasting. Some of these are persistent and difficult to cure. (JO, 56)*

Treatment with needles:

xiaguan (ST-2, IS ST-7)...	**5 fen,**
ermen (TW-23, IS TW-21)	**6 fen,**
qimai (TW-18)	**3 fen,**
yangxi (LI-5)	**5 fen** *(JO, 56).*

Singing in the ear:

(JM) hegu (LI-4), *guanchong* (TW-1), *erjian* (LI-2); *(DACH, YXRM) yangxi* (LI-5), *yanggu* (SI-5); *(JM, YXRM)* hand-*wangu* (SI-4); *(YXRM) yemen* (TW-2); *(JM, DACH) pianli* (LI-6); *(YXRM) xiaxi* (GB-43); *(YXRM; DACH VI, 15r) zhiyin* (BL-67); *(DACH III, 39v; YXRM I, 30r)* disperse *shenmai* (BL-62); *(JM), ermen* (TW-23, IS TW-21); *JM, YXRM, DACH) yifeng* (TW-17); *(JM)* xiaguan (ST-2, IS ST-7); *(JM) tianyou* (TW-16); *(YXRM)* ear-*heliao* (TW-22, IS TW-21 *ermen* by location); *(JM, YXRM, DACH) hanyan* (GB-4); *(JM) luxi* (TW-19), *qimai* (TW-18), *fubai* (GB-16, IS GB-10); *(JM, YXRM, DACH) luoque* (BL-8); *(JM) chengqi* (ST-4, IS ST-1); *(JM, YXRM) tian-chuang* (SI-16).

(YIZ, 39v) Singing in the ear from emptiness (of kidneys): moxa *shenshu* (BL-23) and *taixi* (KI-5, IS KI-3).

(DACH XI, 4r) Singing in the ear from excess coitus or emptiness of kidneys: puncture *taixi* (KI-5, IS KI-3), leg-*sanli* (ST-36).

Cicada songs:

(DACH II, 26v) Leg-*sanli* (ST-36), and disperse or tonify *diwuhui* (GB-42). *(DACH) Ermen* (TW-23, IS TW-21); *(DACH) tinggong* (SI-19); *(DACH VII, 33v)* inside the ear, sounds of cicada: *lieque* (LU-7), *shaochong* (HT-9), *tinghui* (GB-2), *zhongchong* (PC-9), *shangyang* (LI-1); *(YIX I, 4r)* sounds of cicada in the ears: *tinghui* (GB-2), disperse during eight inhalations.

Hun dun dun:

(YIZ, 39r) Sining in the ear, *hun dun dun*, hears nothing; *(YXRM)* sining in the ear, *hun hun*: *waiguan* (TW-5); *(DACH) fubai* (GB-16, IS GB-10).

Chao chao nong nong:

(DACH) Chao chao nong nong in the ear and sounds of cicada: *tinggong* (SI-19); *(DACH)* great noise, *chao chao*, in the ears: ear-*heliao* (TW-22, IS TW-21 *ermen* by location).

Pain and buzzing:

(DACH I, 5v) Pain and singing in the ear: *luxi* (TW-19).

Buzzing and deafness:

(JM) houxi (SI-3); *YXRM baihui* (GV-19, IS GV-20); *(YIZ, 39r) tinghui* (GB-2); *(YIZ, 39r)* from shock: *shangyang* (LI-1), 1 *fen,* one respiration, three moxas; left for right, right for left; *(DACH) waiguan* (TW-5); *(JM, YXRM, DACH) kezhuren* (GB-3, IS *shangwan*); *fubai* (GB-16, IS GB-10). *(YIZ, 39r)* Singing in the ear, deafness: *yifeng* (TW-17), needle 5 *fen,* disperse during seven inhalations; *(DACH) tianrong* (SI-17).

Deafness (reng):

> Ears that do not hear, either from thickening of the tympanum or tearing out of the tympanum, etc; there are no longer vibrations that are related to the sound. Babies who are born deaf surely become mute. (Ci Yuan, ''Reng'')

> Deafness: left and right ears become deaf when the excess of flavor has troubled the fire of the stomach. The left becomes deaf when anger and malcontentment have troubled the fire of the gallbladder. The right becomes deaf when the fire of desire and licentiousness has troubled the fire of the consciousness. The most numerous are on the left from anger or unhappiness. Deafness is divided into new or old types, from emptiness or heat.

> New deafness has a lot of heat; the cause is abundant fire in the **shaoyang** [TW-GB] or in the **yangming** [LI-ST]. It is necessary to remove the heat, the shock and mucus, which are obstructive. Old deafness comes, for the most part, from an emptiness of the kidneys; one must assist and tonify them.

> The symptoms according to the pulses are through the pulses of the kidneys. Slow and soft: empty. Superficial and moving: fire. Superficial and ahead: shock. Sunken and rough: energy (anger, malcontentment). Numerous and full: heat. (YXRM V, 12r)

> When the perversity is in the secondary vessels of the **shou yangming** [LI], there is deafness; at times, not a single sound is heard. At the angle of the index finger nail puncture **shangyang** [LI-1], one puncture each. The person will hear immediately. If that does not work, puncture **zhongchong** [PC-9] at the angle of the nail of the middle

*finger at the joining of the flesh. For those who do not hear from time to time, one must not puncture on the right (side of energy); the energy is blocked, do not puncture. Those who have had a shock in the ear (**feng**) are punctured according to the numbers (6 x 6 to disperse, 9 x 9 to tonify), left for right, right for left. (DACH I, 8v)*

*For deafness, puncture on the meridian **shou yangming** (LI), and if there is no cure puncture the meridian that comes out in front of the ear (**ermen**, TW-23, IS TW-21). (DACH I, 9r)*

The sensitivity of the mucosa of the tympanic cavity and of the eustachian tube depends on the glossopharyngeal nerve.

(JM) Famous point for the glossopharyngeal nerve: *tianzhu* (BL-10).

It has been observed that sudden deafness often stops from one session with the needles; gradual deafness stops slowly and with difficulty.

In general:

(GSdeM) Old deafness; tonify *fuliu* (KI-7) and *taixi* (KI-5, IS KI-3), and local points.

(GSdeM) Recent deafness: disperse *hegu* (LI-4) and *tianjing* (TW-10), or *yangchi* (TW-4); disperse *ermen* (TW-23, IS TW-21 by name, SI-19 *tinggong* by location), and *tinghui* (GB-2).

Half-deafness:

(JM) Difficult hearing: *waiguan* (TW-5); *(DACH)* Indistinct hearing: *tianyou* (TW-16).

(DACH) Hears with difficulty or hears nothing: *ermen* (TW-23, IS TW-21); *(JM)* heavy sensation in the ear: nose-*heliao* (LI-19).

Deafness:

(DACH, JM, YIZ, 39v) Hegu (LI-4), seven moxas; *(JM, YXRM)* yemen (TW-2), *manggu* (SI-5); *(DACH, YXRM)* deafness; *(JM)* loss and sudden loss of hearing: *zhigou* (TW-6); *(JM)* deafness; *(DACH)* deafness, fullness of the secondary vessel, disperse; *(DACH I, 8v)* when the perversity is lodged in the secondary vessels of the large intestine (*pianli*, LI-6) this makes people deaf, from time to time they do not hear a sound: *pianli* (LI-6); *(JM) sanyangluo* (TW-8), *(JM) sidu* (TW-9), *tianjing* (TW-10); *(DACH VII, 31r; YIX I, 10v)* foot-*linqi* (GB-41); *(JM, DACH, YXRM) xiaxi* (GB-43); *(DACH VII, 27v; YIX I, 10v)* shenmai (BL-62); *(JM)* foot-*qiaoyin* (GB-44); *(JM, DACH, YXRM) shugu* (BL-65); *(JM, YXRM) ermen* (TW-23, IS TW-21); *(DACH) tinggong* (SI-19); *(DACH IV, 7v III, 29r; YIX I, 4r)* ear closed: needle 1.5 cun, do not wait, seven moxas — *tinghui* (GB-2); *(JM) xiaguan* (ST-2, IS ST-7); *(YXRM)* deafness: *yuzhen* (BL-9); *(JM)* deafness: *tianyou* (TW-16); *(JM, DACH, YXRM)) tianchuang* (SI-16), *kezhuren* (GB-3, IS *shangguan*), *shenshu* (BL-23).

Deafness in storms (sudden):

(YXRM) Sanyangluo (TW-8), *(YXRM)*, *sidu* (TW-9); *(DACH; YIZ, 39v)* deafness from the energy of storms: *sidu* (TW-9); *(YXRM I, 39r)* tonify foot-*linqi* (GB-41); *(DACH, YXRM)* foot-*qiaoyin* (GB-44); *(DACH)* deafness in storms; from energy, eyes not clear, ears no longer perceive: *tianyou* (TW-16); *(DACH)* deafness coming suddenly and unexpectedly: *yemen* (TW-2).

Deafness from energy:

(DACH, YXRM) Attacks of energy, blocked ears: *fengchi* (GB-20), *sidu* (TW-9).

Deafness from shock:

(YIZ, 39r) Deafness from shock with pain: *yifeng* (TW-17); *(YXRM)* deafness from shock: *luxi* (TW-19).

Deafness from closure of the energy:

(DACH III, 32r) Deafness from closure of the energy: *tinghui* (GB-2).

(DACH IV, 4r) Deafness from closure of the energy, pain and difficulty in speaking: *yifeng* (TW-17) disperse; *(YIX I, 4r) tinghui* (GB-2), *yifeng* (TW-17).

Deafness from emptiness of the kidneys:

(DACH) Deafness from emptiness of the kidneys: tonify *shenshu* (BL-23).

Deafness from chill or heat:

(DACH XI, 4r) Deafness coming from a chill or great heat: *tinggong* (SI-19), *tinghui* (GB-2), *yifeng* (TW-17); if no better: leg-*sanli* (ST-36), *hegu* (LI-4).

Deafness with pruritis or pain:

(DACH IV, 4r) Deafness from closure of the energy, pain and difficulty in speaking; *(YIZ, 39r)* deafness from shock with pain, seven moxas: *yifeng* (TW-17); *(DACH VI, 15v)* deafness, pain: *guanchong* (TW-1); *(YXRM)* ear painful, blocked: *luxi* (TW-19).

Deafness increasing *(chong):*

(DACH X, 28v) Deafness increasing, hears nothing: *ermen* (TW-23, IS TW-21), *fengchi* (GB-20), *xiaxi* (GB-43), *yifeng* (TW-17), *tinggong* (SI-19), *tinghui* (GB-2).

(DACH II 26v) Increasing deafness from chills: *jinmen* (BL-63) *tinghui* (GB-2).

Varied:

(JM) Loss and sudden loss of hearing: *huizong* (TW-7).

(JM) Difficulty of hearing, deafness: *waiguan* (TW-5).

V. Eyes, Vision

- *The bladder (**taiyang**), which has a lot of blood and little energy, passes into the internal corner of the eye; it also passes through the upper part. The gallbladder (**shaoyang**), which has little blood and a lot of energy, passes at the external corner of the eye. In the lower part is the stomach meridian (**yangming**), which has a lot of blood and little energy. (DACH XI, 12v)*

Zhang Zihuo states, ''The sexual energy of the five treasure organs and the six workshop organs flourishes in the five circles of the eyes; it is there that all the meridians rejoin.

*''The white depends on the lung (**jin,** metal). If the white circle becomes scarlet, the fire has risen to the lungs. The flesh depends on the spleen-pancreas (**tu,** earth); if the circle of flesh is scarlet and swollen, the fire has risen into the spleen-pancreas. The black, the consciousness, the luster depends on the water of the kidney (**shui,** water). (In Europe, on the sympathetic system.) If the black, the water, the consciousness and luster are veiled, the fire has risen to the liver and kidneys. The scarlet part depends on the heart (**huo,** fire); it depends also on the liver. If red vessels go through the eye, the fire is intense. The liver is connected to the arteries of the eyes; thus, if there is too much blood in the eye, there is fullness of the meridians of the bladder (**taiyang**) and of the stomach (**yangming**). If the blood does reach the eyes, the liver (**jueyin**) is empty. Consequently, if one must take out blood, it is from the meridians of the bladder (**taiyang**) and stomach (**yangming**). The gallbladder (**shaoyang**) must not be bled because it has little blood; bleeding the bladder and the stomach gives more clarity to the eyes. On the contrary, bleeding the gallbladder increases the fogginess of the eyes (i.e., one must not disperse the gallbladder meridian when the eyes are foggy, but rather tonify it, and likewise, one must disperse the bladder and stomach meridians)''* *(DACH IX, 12v).*

The eyes depend mainly on the general condition. Encephalic anemia causes accommodative asthenopia, floating spots before the eyes.

The common oculomotor nerve (third cranial nerve) innervates the levator palpebrae superioris, the sphincter of the iris, the ciliary muscle and all the muscles except the rectus lateralis and the orbiculus superior: *xuanlu* (GB-5), *yangbai* (GB-10, IS GB-14).

The lateral oculomotor nerve (sixth cranial nerve, nervus abducens) innervates the rectus lateralis: *hanyan* (GB-4).

The trochlear nerve (fourth cranial nerve) innervates the grand oblique muscle which pulls upwards and laterally.

The facial nerve innervates the depressor of the lower lid and the levator palpebrae inferioris: *daying* (ST-8, IS ST-5), *yifeng* (TW-17).

The suborbital branch of the facial nerve innervates the lower lid: *juliao* (ST-6, IS ST-3).

Cervical sympathetic nerves (dilator of the iris, exophthalmos): *fengchi* (GB-20).

In general:

Prophylactic for troubles and illnesses of the eyes: *(JM)* leg-*sanli* (ST-36).

(DACH IX, 11v; I, 12v) The arteries of the eyes depend on *tongli* (HT-5). The eyes depend on the liver meridian.

Tightness of the artery of the eyes, going to the interior, unbearable pain, external headache: *(DACH) yuzhen* (BL-9).

Contraction of the artery of the eyes, going to the interior, unbearable pain, external headache: *(DACH) yuzhen* (BL-9).

Master point for curing illnesses of the eye: *(JM) yangbai* (GB-10, IS GB-14), *jingming* (BL-1).

(DACH IV, 14v; YXRM) All illnesses of the eyes: moxa at *hegu* (LI-4); *(JM)* leg-*sanli* (ST-36).

(YXRM I, 38r; DACH III, 32v; YIX I, 10v) All illness or bitterness of the eyes, illnesses of the eye: puncture the needle and agitate at foot-*linqi* (GB-41).

(GSdeM) Important point for all illnesses of the eyes: *zanzhu* (BL-2), *tongziliao* (GB-1).

Illnesses of the eyes: *(YXRM I, 46v) erjian* (LI-2), *tianfu* (LU-3); *(DACH III, 30) xingjian* (LR-2); *(JM) taichong* (LR-3); *(YXRM II, 46r) shangxing* (GV-22, IS GV-23); *(JM) xuanli* (GB-6).

Eyes: *(JM) siman* (KI-14), *qixue* (KI-13), *dahe* (KI-12).

(DACH) Illnesses of the eye, face, etc.: *quchi* (LI-11).

For the internal corner of the eye: *(GSdeM) houxi* (SI-3), *qiangu* (SI-2), *jinggu* (BL-64).

For the external corner of the eye: *(GSdeM) waiguan* (TW-5), head-*linqi* (GB-11, IS GB-15).

Upper, outer corner of the eye: *dagukong* (MP-19); lower outer corner of the eye: *xiaogukong* (MP-23).

Medial and lateral corners: *yangfu* (GB-38), *tianjing* (TW-10).

Illnesses of eyes from energy: *(DACH III, 29v) kezhuren* (GB-3, IS *shangguan*).

(YIZ, 39r) Illnesses of the eyes, the majority from wind or heat or insufficiency of water of the kidney: disperse *sizhukong* (TW-21, IS TW-23), *shangxing* (GV-22, IS GV-23), *baihui* (GV-19, IS GV-20). If there is pain, moxa at *fengshi* (GB-20), *hegu* (LI-4).

(YIX I, 6r) The blood does not nourish the eye: tonify *ganshu* (BL-18), the assent point of the liver; disperse leg-*sanli* (ST-36).

Vision, sight, functional troubles:

It is advisable to differentiate:

1) Problems of accommodation, of focusing, which can come from encephalic anemia and manifest through a lack of clarity of the contours, either outside of a certain fixed distance (myopia, hyperopia), or outside of a fixed angle (astigmatism), or from a flickering of the vision mainly on waking (quivering of the ciliary muscles).

2) Problems of vision manifesting either with an undulation of straight lines (congestion of retina, beginning of detachment), or with black or brown spots and localized fog (local blindness), or with violet or white spots (hyperexcitation of the optic nerve), or double far vision in one eye.

3) Problems of coordination with the two eyes not superimposing exactly the same two images, or one eye sees smaller than the other, or the muscles of coordination function badly (encephalitic diplopia).

4) Excess or weakness of vision, either easy fatigue from weakness (amblyopia, amaurosis, hemeralopia, blindness) or sensitivity of the retina (dizzied, pained from light) or weakness of the sphincter of the iris.

5) Blindness for certain colors or for all colors (achloropsia, monochromatism).

6) Illnesses affecting vision — glaucoma, cataract, keratitis, albugo.

The apparatus:

1) Pupils *(jing)*, iris, sphincter of iris:

(YIX I, 11r) Redness of the pupils: *waiguan* (TW-5).

(JM) Holes of pupils incomplete or extraordinary: *qimai* (TW-18) (iritis?).

(YXRM) Tearing away of the pupil: *hegu* (LI-4).

(DACH IV, 4v) Both pupils red and swollen, aversion to sunlight: *tongziliao* (GB-1).

2) Retina *(yuan, gangmu)*:

Retinal hemorrhages can come from serious anemia.

(JM) Inflammation of retina: *tongziliao* (GB-1), *jingming* (BL-1).

(JM) Internal veil of the retina: *kezhuren* (GB-3, IS *shangwan*), *juliao* (ST-6, IS ST-3).

Weakness of the power of vision:

1) Amblyopia, amaurosis *(shi li jian fa, mu jing, pi lao)*:

(JM) Visual power tired: *muchuang* (GB-12, IS GB-16).

(JM) Fatigue and lack of vision: *touwei* (ST-1, IS ST-8) *jianzhongshu* (SI-15), *tianquan* (PC-2).

(JM) Power of vision and sight weakened: *zanzhu* (BL-2).

(JM) Power of vision diminished, tired: *wuchu* (BL-5), *qucha* (BL-4), *weishu* (BL-21).

(JM) Vision diminished: *fengchi* (GB-20).

(JM) Fatigue and exhaustion of the visual energy: *yanglao* (SI-6).

Vision foggy *(hun*, lack of clarity):

Vision foggy: *(DACH) xinshu* (BL-15); *(YXRM) qucha* (BL-4) and sight troubled: *shenshu* (BL-23); and face scarlet: hand-*zhongzhu* (TW-3); and heaviness of head: *luxi* (TW-19).

Fog and dizziness of head and eyes: leg-*sanli* (ST-36).

Attacks of foggy vision: *(DACH) dicang* (ST-7, IS ST-4).

(YIX I, 3v) Vision foggy from day to day: *yanglao* (SI-6), *tianzhu* (BL-10).

Obscured vision (*huang huang,* lackluster):

● *(DACH)* Puncturing in three sessions gives great clarity to the vision: *zanzhu* (BL-2), *muchuang* (GB-12, IS GB-16). *(DACH)* After the thirtieth year, if one uses moxa after needles, the vision will greatly increase in clarity; *(DACH)* after the thirtieth year, if one does not burn moxa, the energy rises and attacks the eyes: leg-*sanli* (ST-36).

Obscured vision: *(DACH) houding* (GV-18, IS GV-19), *taodao* (GV-12, IS GV-13), *zhengying* (GB-13, IS GB-17), *zanzhu* (BL-2), *jianzhongshu* (SI-15), *chengjiang* (CV-24), foot-*tonggu* (BL-66), *fuliu* (KI-7), *ququan* (LR-8), *yongquan* (KI-1), *kezhuren* (GB-3, IS *shangguan*), *neiguan* (PC-6), *pianli* (LI-6).

Eyes with obscure vision: *(DACH)* arm-*wuli* (LI-13), *tianzhu* (BL-10).

Obscured vision, not clear: *(DACH) tianquan* (PC-2), *tianchi* (PC-1).

Vision obscured, not seeing: *(DACH) jingming* (BL-1), *erjian* (LI-2), ear-*erjian* (MP-9), *yongquan* (KI-1), *xuanlu* (GB-5).

Vision obscured as in hemeralopia [nyctalopia?]: *(DACH) ganshu* (BL-18).

Vision obscured when coryza starts *(DACH) ganshu* (BL-18).

Vision obscured, does not see objects clearly: *zanzhu* (BL-2).

Vision obscured, heaviness of the head: *(DACH) luxi* (TW-19), *taodao* (GV-12, GV-13).

Vision obscured, generating cataracts: *qiuxu* (GB-40).

Vision troubled, obscured *(mi nu, huang huang): (DACH) pianli* (LI-6), *kezhuren* (GB-3, IS *shangguan*).

Vision obscured, eyes red: *zanzhu* (BL-2).

Eyes as if in an obscure cloud: *(DACH) baichong* (LR-3).

Eyes not seeing clearly: *(DACH) hegu* (LI-4).

Eyes not clear *(bu ming): (DACH)* leg-*sanli* (ST-36), *yanglao* (SI-6), *tianyou* (TW-16), *jianzhongshu* (SI-15), *qucha* (BL-4).

Looking and seeing as if darkened, as if at the stars: *(DACH) zhaohai* (KI-3, IS KI-6).

Grey or black veil in front of one or both eyes: *(GSdeM)* tonify *kezhuren* (GB-3, IS *shangguan*), *sibai* (ST-5, IS ST-2) *juliao* of cheek (ST-6, IS ST-3); disperse *zanzhu* (BL-20) or *jingming* (BL-1).

Eyes veiled, sees nothing: *juliao* of cheek (ST-6, IS ST-3).

(YIZ, 40) Black flowers in front of the eyes; facing the wind, cold tears, rheum: light moxa at *dagukong* (MP-19), *xiaogukong* (MP-23); needles at head-*linqi* (GB-11, IS GB-15), *hegu* (LI-4).

(YIZ, 40) Obscured, foggy vision: moxa at leg-*sanli* (ST-36); needle at *chengqi* (ST-4, IS ST-1); in addition: *ganshu* (BL-18), *tongziliao* (GB-1).

2) Nyctalopia (*ye mang,* "nightblindness," *jiao mu,* "sparrow eyes"):

Jiao mu: when night comes, one can no longer distinguish objects. *(DACH X, 29r)*

Nyctalopia, **jiao mu:** cannot see at night; comes from a lack of blood in the liver. One must not bleed, but tonify the liver and support the stomach. *(DACH XI, 12r)*

Ye mang. Origin: bad nutrition of the blood, strength diminished, icterus or heredity. Symptoms: during the day the strength and clarity of vision are in no way affected. At dusk, when the day falls, the vision diminishes. *(JO, 54)*

Treatment with moxa:

geshu *(BL-17)*	*7 moxas,*
ganshu *(BL-18)*	*7 moxas,*
gaohuangshu *(BL-38, IS BL-43)*	*7 moxas,*
jianzhongshu *(SI-15)*	*7 moxas. (JO, 54)*

(DACH) Cannot see in darkness: *xingjian* (LR-2).

(DACH) Blindness at night: *zanzhu* (BL-2).

(JM) Nyctalopia, *ye mang: (DACH, YXRM)* does not see anything at night or dusk: *yangbai* (GB-10, IS GB-14); *(DACH) chengqi* (ST-4, IS ST-1); *(DACH) dicang* (ST-7, IS ST-4); *(JM) ye mang; (DACH)* sparrow eyes: *jingming* (BL-1), *weishu* (BL-21).

Children: sparrow eyes, cannot see at night: *(DACH X, 29r) zhongchong* (PC-9); *(JM) weishu* (BL-21), *(JM) pishu* (BL-20).

3) Achloropsia, monochromatism (qing mang, shi mang):

*Green-blindness: one of the monochromatisms (**shi mang**). The patient cannot see green among all colors. In the past it was said those who had pupils but could not see were **qing mang** or **meng** (blind-from-nerve-illness). (Ci Yuan, "Qing-mang")*

Green-blindness: *(DACH) shangyang* (LI-1), three moxas, left for right, right for left; *(DACH) luoque* (BL-8), *kezhuren* (GB-3, IS *shangguan*).

(YIZ, 39v) Green-blindness: *juliao* (ST-6, IS ST-3), moxa, *ganshu* (BL-18), *mingmen* (GV-4), *shangyang* (LI-1).

Hypersensitivity, dizziness (mu xuan):

(DACH I, 16r; DACH IV, 1r) Dizziness, shocks, quivering depend on the liver.

Dizziness *(mu xuan): (DACH)* head-*linqi* (GB-11, IS GB-15), head-*wuchu* (BL-5). If with oppression: *fengshi* (GB-20); *(JM) yintang* (GV-23a, IS M-HN-3), *yangbai* (GB-10, IS GB-14), *houding* (GV-18, IS GV-19); *(JM, DACH, YXRM) yanggu* (SI-5); *(DACH, YXRM) xiaxi* (GB-43); *(YXRM)* foot-*dadu* (SP-2), *yongquan* (KI-1), *jinggu* (BL-64), *tonggu* (BL-66).

Painful dizziness: *(YXRM, DACH) kunlun* (BL-60).

(YXRM) Body hot, dizziness, sweat not coming: *ququan* (LR-8); dizziness from shock, wind: *(YXRM)* head-*linqi* (GB-11, IS GB-15); *(DACH) chengguang* (BL-6); *(YXRM) tianzhu* (BL-10); *(YXRM)* eyes cannot see anything: *hanyan* (GB-4).

(YXRM) Fog and dizziness of head and eyes: leg-*sanli* (ST-36).

Blindness (mang, meng):

(DACH) Qing mang: sees nothing: *juliao* of cheek (ST-6, IS ST-3), *tongziliao* (GB-1).

Eyes veiled, sees nothing: *juliao* of cheek (ST-6, IS ST-3).

Eyes not seeing: *(DACH) hanyan* (GB-4).

Blind eyes *(mang);* internal veil: *luoque* (BL-8).

Blind eyes *(mang): xingjian* (LR-2).

(YIZ, 39r) Sudden blindness; not seeing: *zanzhu* (BL-2), *jianjing* (GB-21), *bizhun* (MP-1).

(DACH) Sudden blindness: triple warmer meridian.

Eyes which cannot look: *shuigou* (GV-25, IS GV-26 *renzhong*).

(DACH II, 18v; YIX I, 3v) In the eyes, the desert: *zanzhu* (BL-2), *sanjian* (LI-3).

Physical problems of sight:
Myopia, presbyopia, astigmatism, diplopia, glaucoma, albugo, veils, cataract, keratitis:

Accommodation:

1) Myopia:

Looks closely *(jin shi): (DACH) jingming* (BL-1), *muchuang* (GB-12, IS GB-16).

Distance vision troubled *(yuan shi, huang huang):*

(DACH) tianfu (LU-3), *juliao* of cheek (ST-6, IS ST-3), *chengqi* (ST-4, IS ST-1), *tongziliao* (GB-1), *yangbai* (GB-10, IS GB-14), *dicang* (ST-7, IS ST-4).

Cannot see at a distance *(bu neng yuan shi):*
(DACH) shuiquan (KI-4, IS KI-5).

2) Presbyopia (yuan shi, bu neng jin shi):
(GSdeM) houxi (SI-3), hand-*zhongzhu* (TW-3), *quchi* (LI-11).

3) Astigmatism:
(GSdeM) Disperse *ningming* (BL-1), tonify *tongziliao* (GB-1), use daily moxa.

4) Coordination, diplopia:

(GSdeM) Sequelae of apoplexy: tonify *yangbai* (GB-10, IS GB-14) on the paralyzed side; disperse the other side.

(GSdeM) Sequelae of encephalitis: see arm-*shanglian* (LI-9), *naokong* (GB-19).

Illnesses affecting the vision:

1) Glaucoma (jiao mu shi zhi yan):

(JM) Inflammation and hardening of the cornea: *tongziliao* (GB-1).

(DACH IX, 9r) Eyes swollen, painful, the crystalline lens seems to want to come out: needles at *shenting* (GV-23, IS GV-24), *shangxing* (GV-22, IS GV-23), *xinhui* (GV-21, IS GV-22), *qianding* (GV-20, IS GV-21).

(DACH IX, 9r) Hegu (LI-4), *taichong* (LR-3), *waiguan* (TW-5), *neiguan* (PC-6).

(GSdeM) Fengchi (GB-20), tonify every day.

(YIZ, 39v) Eyes swollen and hardening, face swollen: *xiangu* (ST-43).

(DACH) Eyes swollen, painful: *shenmai* (BL-62).

2) Albugo, veils:

Floating spots before the eyes often come from encephalitic anemia.

In general:

(DACH) All sorts of albugo and veils: *sibai* (ST-5, IS ST-2); *(YXRM)* albugo, veils: *shangyang* (LI-1); *(DACH)* eyes generating albugo and veils, causing suffering for a long time: *zanzhu* (BL-2); *(DACH X, 19r)* from wind or fire eyes generating albugo, unbearable acute pain in both eyes: *jingming* (BL-1). *(DACH)* Veil of the eyes, sees nothing: *juliao* (ST-6, IS ST-3); eyes generating a veil: hand-*wangu* (SI-4).

Internal veil *(nei zhang):*

Veil in the interior of the pupils: *(DACH) shangyang* (LI-1).

(DACH XI, 2r; YIX I, 6r) Eyes; internal veil. Discontentment or fear has affected the liver; the blood is no longer at home; the water of the kidneys is dried up. Energy and blood is spread out; sex has been abused or there have been too many worries; difficult to cure (detachment of retina?): *tongziliao* (GB-1), head-*linqi* (GB-11, IS GB-15), *jingming* (BL-1), *hegu* (LI-4). If not better: *guangming* (GB-37), *tianfu* (LU-3), *fengchi* (GB-20).

(YIZ, 40) Internal veil, sees nothing: *luoque* (BL-8). *(YIZ, 40)* Internal veil: puncture the liver and kidney meridians and the *yangqiao mai.*

External veil *(wai zhang):*

(DACH XI, 2v; YIX I, 6r, 16r) External veil of the eye: *tongziliao* (GB-1), *jingming* (BL-1), *hegu* (LI-4), *xiaogukong* (MP-23). If not better; head-*linqi* (GB-11, IS GB-15), *zanzhu* (BL-2), leg-*sanli* (ST-36).

Pterygium *(mu sheng fu yi,* "eyes generate a veil of flesh").

(DACH III, 32r) Eyes invaded by additional flesh; *(DACH)* internal corner covering the pupil; "flesh of effort" covering the pupil; pupils generating a veil: *jingming* (BL-1).

(DACH) Eyes making a veil of flesh which covers the pupil: *sibai* (ST-5, IS ST-2), *jiaosun* (TW-20), *shaoze* (SI-1).

(DACH) Perverse flesh on the eyes: *juliao* (ST-6, IS ST-3).

(DACH I, 5) Additional flesh invading the pupil: *jingming* (BL-1), *tongziliao* (GB-1), *qimen* (LR-14). If not better: *fengchi* (GB-20), *tongziliao* (GB-1), *hegu* (LI-4), *qimen* (LR-14), *xingjian* (LR-2).

(DACH) Children from two to three years: corner of the eye protruding out: *hegu* (LI-4) three moxas.

(YIZ, 36v) Children with chancre of the eyes (tubercles): *hegu* (LI-4).

(DACH X, 29r) Scarlet eyes; veil of flesh: *taiyuan* (LU-9), *xiaxi* (GB-43), *fengchi* (GB-20), *zanzhu* (BL-2).

3) Cataract (yi, mu yi, mu zhang, bai muo):

Veil of the eye; used for white albugo which is generated by the crystalline lens (yinchu). (Ci Yuan, "Mu-zhang")

Eyes not clear; commonly known as the mu yi cataract. (Ci Yuan, "Muo")

The area of the beginning of the cataract indicates its origin: at the bottom, from the stomach; at the outside, the gallbladder; medially, the bladder; at the top, the small intestine. (DACH XI, 12v)

(JM) (Bai muo yan): shaoze (SI-1); *(YXRM) mu yi: guanchong* (TW-1); *(JM) yemen* (TW-2); *(JM) zhongzhu* (TW-3), *zhiyin* (BL-67). *(YXRM)* Cataract, white veil beginning at the left corner; *(DACH)* cataract: *jinggu* (BL-64); *(JM) qiuxu* (GB-40); *(JM, DACH) tongziliao* (GB-1), *zanzhu* (BL-2); *(YXRM)* head-*linqi* (GB-11, IS GB-15); *(JM) sizhukong* (TW-21, IS TW-23), *chengguang* (BL-6) *yinjiao* of gums (GV-27, IS GV-28); *(JM)* cataract: *(DACH, YXRM)* cataract covering the crystalline lens: *juliao* (ST-6, IS ST-3), *yindu* (KI-19), *huangshu* (KI-16), *siman* (KI-14).

Eyes generating cataract:

(JM, YXRM, DACH) hegu (LI-4); *(DACH) taiyuan* (LU-9), *dagukong* (MP-19); *(DACH, YXRM)* hand-*zhongzhu* (TW-3); *(DACH) zhiyin* (BL-67), *qiuxu* (GB-40), foot-*linqi* (GB-41), *sibai* (ST-5, IS ST-2), *yinjiao* of gums (GV-27,

IS GV-28), *tongziliao* (GB-1), *jingming* (BL-1); *(DACH)* eyes generating a cataract, does not see clearly: *guanchong* (TW-1); eyes causing suffering for a long time and generating a cataract: *zanzhu* (BL-2).

(DACH XI, 2r; YIX I, 6v) Eye generating a cataract *(yi muo)*. This illness is very deep; one cannot cure it in one session. One must puncture and re-puncture two or three times: *jingming* (BL-1),hegu (LI-4), *sibai* (ST-5, IS ST-2). If no better: *tongziliao* (GB-1), *guangming* (GB-37), *dagukong* (MP-19), *xiaogukong* (MP-23).

(YIX I, 17v) Eye generating a cataract: *jingming* (BL-1), *tongziliao* (GB-1), *hegu* (LI-4), *guangming* (GB-37); *(DACH X, 29r) tongziliao* (GB-1), *hegu* (LI-4), *shangyang* (LI-1), *ganshu* (BL-18), *mingmen* (GV-4).

(DACH, "Shen Ting") One can cause the retrogradation of the cataract and dissolve the swelling of the eye with: *shenting* (GV-23, IS GV-24), *shangxing* (GV-22, IS GV-23), *chuanghui* (GV-21, IS GV-24, *xinhui*), *qianding* (GV-20, IS GV-21).

Pain from cataract:

(JM) quanliao (SI-18).

4) Keratitis (jiao muo yan, "Inflammation of the corneal membrane"):

(JM) hegu (LI-4), *guanchong* (TW-1), *yemen* (TW-2), *zhongzhu* (TW-3), *houxi* (SI-3), *yangxi* (LI-5), *dadun* (LR-1), *qiuxu* (GB-40), *zanzhu* (BL-2), *jingming* (BL-1), *tongziliao* (GB-1), *sizhukong* (TW-21, IS 23), *sibai* (ST-5, IS ST-2), *juliao* (ST-6, IS ST-3), *jiaosun* (TW-20), *shangxing* (GV-22, IS GV-23), *yinjiao* (GV-27, IS GV-28), *yindu* (KI-19), *shangqiu* of epigastrium (KI-17), *huangshu* (KI-16), *henggu* (KI-11), *siman* (KI-14), abdomen-*zhongzhu* (KI-15), *qixue* (KI-13).

Veil of the cornea *(jiao muo yi):*

(JM) Hand *wangu* (SI-4), *juliao* of cheek (ST-6, IS ST-3), *tianyou* (TW-16).

Contractions, spasms, contractures (strabismus, nystagmus, etc):

Spasms:

Spasms of the ciliary muscles: *(JM) xuanlu* (GB-5).

Tightening of the artery (or nerve?) of the eye: *(YXRM) xiaxi* (GB-43); *(DACH)* same with continuing into the interior, unbearable pain: *yuzhen* (BL-9).

Contraction and tightening of the eye, fog, confusion: *yangbai* (GB-10, IS GB-14).

Strabismus, deviations:

Towards the top:

(Europe: up and laterally — paralysis of the trochlear nerve which innervates the superior oblique muscle.)

(DACH) Head-*wuchu* (BL-5), *yangbai* (GB-10, IS GB-14).

(DACH X, 24v; YIZ, 39v) The same and yellow: *sizhukong* (TW-21, IS TW-23).

(JM) Eyes turned looking upwards; *(DACH)* eyes turned, inverted, looking upwards: *jinsuo* (GV-7 SI GV-8).

(YIZ, 39v) Eyes pulled up, cannot look: seven moxas below the bone of the first dorsal (GV-13a, IS GV-14, *dazhui*) and above the fourth dorsal, *shenzhu* (GV-11, IS GV-12).

Towards the exterior, laterally (the same and downwards):

(Europe: paralysis of the common oculomotor nerve (trigeminal) that innervates the medial, superior and inferior rectus muscle and inferior oblique and also muscles of accommodation: or contracture of the rectus lateralis innervated by the lateral oculomotor nerve).

(DACH) Eyes pulled laterally from shock or cold, pain on the skull: *erjian* (LI-2), *hegu* (LI-4).

Towards the interior, medially (towards the nose):

(Europe: contraction of the internal rectus muscle (common oculomotor nerve) or paralysis of the rectus lateralis (external oculomotor nerve).

(GSdeM) Disperse *zanzhu* (BL-2), tonify *tongziliao* (GB-1).

(GSdeM) Disperse *yuzhen* (BL-9).

Eyes crossed:

(DACH) Zanzhu (BL-2), *dicang* (ST-7, IS ST-4), *chengqi* (ST-4, IS ST-1).

Does not look straight *(zhan shi bu zheng):*

(YIZ) Bleed laterally to the eye which is crossed: *tongziliao* (GB-1).

(DACH) Changqiang (GV-1).

Nystagmus (*diao yao shi zhan,* "gaze moves, trembles"):

(DACH) Eyes moving, cannot be stopped: *sibai* (ST-5, IS ST-2).

(DACH) Eyes blinking, move without stopping: *quanliao* (SI-18), ear-*heliao* (TW-22, IS *ermen* TW-21 by location).

(DACH) Gaze moving, flickering: *juliao* of cheek (ST-6, IS ST-3).

(YXRM) Eyes flickering: *dicang* (ST-7, IS ST-4) right for left, left for right, moxas.

The looks of mental disturbance:

(DACH) Looks to the right and left: *yanggu* (SI-5).

(DACH X, 26v; YIX I, 8r) Haggard look: *fengfu* (GV-15, IS GV-16).

Tears (lei):

Tears of sadness; weeping (qi):

(DACH X, 31v, YIX I, 5v) Nighttime tears of children: three moxas at *baihui* (GV-19, IS GV-20); *(JM) zhongchong* (PC-9).

(YXRM I, 46r) The 100 illnesses of tears at night: *baihui* (GV-19, IS GV-20).

Habitual sadness, tears, emotiveness, fear: *(DACH) daling* (P-7).

(DACH) Emotiveness of heart, sadness, tears: *jiexi* (ST-41).

(DACH) Talks about sadness, weeps: *xinshu* (BL-15).

(DACH) Liver empty, torrents of tears are poured out: tonify *ququan* (LR-8).

● *Narrow lacrimal duct:*

(JM) Narrow, contracted lacrimal duct: *shugu* (BL-65).

(YXRM) Medial corner of the eye injured: tears coming out: *qiangu* (SI-2).

Various causes:

Wind:

(DACH XI, 20) Eyes tear and fear the light, comes from wind during a voyage: *xiaogukong* (MP-23), *hegu* (LI-4), *erjian* (LI-2), *zanzhu* (BL-2). If not better: *jingming* (BL-1), *xingjian* (LR-2), *guangming* (GB-37).

(DACH VII, 32v) Eyes injured by the wind, cold tears: *waiguan* (TW-5), *zanzhu* (BL-2), *sizhukong* (TW-21, IS TW-23), *erjian* (LI-2), *xiaogukong* (MP-23).

(DACH XI, 2r, YIX I, 6v) Cold tears in the wind; comes from wind during drunkenness or redness or pain, comes from not avoiding sex or from eating spoiled organ meat. For women, often comes from lack of exercise after delivery, or having remained lying or sitting in the wind, or from troubled menses: *zanzhu* (BL-2), *dagukong* (MP-19), *xiaogukong* (MP-23). If not better: *ziaogukong* (MP-23) (wind after drunkenness); *sanyinjiao* (SP-6) (menstrual troubles); *zhonggui* (MP-21), three moxas.

(YIX I, 17r) Tears from cold or wind: *zanzhu* (BL-2), *xiaogukong* (MP-23), *dagukong* (MP-19), *hegu* (LI-4).

(DACH) Weeping eyes, exposed to the wind after drunkenness: *xiaogukong* (MP-23).

Catarrh of lacrimal glands:

(JM) Catarrh of lacrimal glands; inflammation of the lacrimal glands; *(DACH)* weeping and painful eyes: *shenting* (GV-23, IS GV-24).

(JM) Illness from flowing of tears, tears too abundant: *tongziliao* (GB-1).

(JM) Tears too abundant: hand-*wangu* (SI-4), *fengchi* (GB-20), *yinjiao* of gum (GV-27, IS GV-28), head-*linqi* (GB-11, IS GB-15), *zanzhu* (BL-2), *touwei* (ST-2, IS ST-8), *ganshu* (BL-18).

(YXRM) A lot of tears: head-*linqi* (GB-11, IS GB-15), *juliao* (ST-6, IS ST-3).

(DACH) Tears coming: *zanzhu* (BL-2), *tianfu* (LU-3), *tianzhu* (BL-10), *xingjian* (LR-2), *juliao* of cheek (ST-6, IS ST-3).

Tears coming, habitual forgetting: *quchi* (LI-11).

Tears coming, vision obscured: *ganshu* (BL-18).

Excess tears, no clarity: *(DACH) sibai* (ST-5, IS ST-2).

(DACH) Yellow, weeping eyes: *zhiyin* (BL-67).

(DACH) Cold tears from energy: *jingming* (BL-1), *ganshu* (BL-18).

(DACH) Eyes, pruritis, pain, tears coming: *sibai* (ST-5, IS ST-2).

(DACH II, 30v) Bleary eyes, tears coming: head-*linqi* (GB-11, IS GB-15); *(DACH) yinjiao* of gum (GV-27, IS GV-28).

Conjunctiva, eyelids, eyelashes:

Conjunctivitis (*jie muo yan*, "inflammation of the conjunctival mucosa"):

> *The mucosa connecting the eyelids to the eyes is red and swollen, tears and even pus flow. There is diphtheric conjunctivitis (die fu di li) and catarrhal conjunctivitis; often comes from contagious bacterias; serious cases can cause the loss of vision. (Ci Yuan, "Jie-muo-yan")*

(JM) Conjunctivitis and blenorrhagic ophthalmia: *tinghui* (GB-2), moxas.

(JM) Purulent conjunctivitis: *touwei* (ST-1, IS ST-8).

(JM) Conjunctivitis of babies: *jingming* (BL-1).

(JM) Conjunctivitis; *jingming* (BL-1), head-*linqi* (GB-11, IS GB-15), *taiyuan* (LU-9).

(DACH) Bleary eyes, tears: head-*linqi* (GB-11, IS GB-15).

(YIX I, 6v) Blinking, red, injured eyes; fearful of light and sun: *tongziliao* (GB-1).
Eyes painful and bleary: *yangbai* (GB-10, IS GB-14).

(YIZ, 40) Scarlet eyes, swelling of the blood vessels, fearful of light, rough, painful condition: *baihui* (GV-19, IS GV-20), *shangxing* (GV-22, IS GV-23), *zanzhu* (BL-2), *sizhukong* (TW-21, IS TW-23), *jingming* (BL-1), *tongliao* (GB-1), *hegu* (LI-4).

(DACH) Eyes suddenly red, swollen and painful: *xinhui* (GV-21, IS GV-22).

(DACH VII, 32v) Eyes suddenly red, swollen, acute pain: *waiguan* (TW-5), *hegu* (LI-4), *zanzhu* (BL-2), *yingxiang* (LI-20).

Conjunctival congestion: (*jie muo chong xue*, "blood flowing to the conjunctival mucosa"):

> *Origin: dust, wind, smoke, foreign objects, trouble with turned up eyelashes, intense light, excessive fatigue of the eye.*

> *Symptoms: influx of blood in the conjunctival mucosa, heat sensation of a foreign body, fearful of light. (JO, 55)*

Treatment with needles:

fengchi (GB-20)	*7 fen,*
tianzhu (BL-10)	*5 fen,*
jianjing (GB-21)	*6 fen,*
jianzhongshu (SI-15)	*5 fen,*
sizhukong (TW-21, IS TW-23)	*5 fen.* (JO, 55)

Treatment with moxa:

yuzhen (BL-9)	*5 moxas,*
tianzhu (BL-10)	*7 moxas,*
jianzhongshu (SI-15)	*7 moxas,*
qiangu (SI-2)	*5 moxas.* (JO, 55)

(GSdeM) Disperse *hegu* (LI-4) and *houxi* (SI-3).

Trachoma:

> *Origin: not clear.*

> *Symptoms: the part of the mucosa of the superior eyelid, then the eyelid has bubbles like rice grain of yellowish color. The conjunctiva are congested and have an unclean quality. If there is swelling, we can see nodes. After these bubbles, plaque-like scars remain. On the surface of the eyelid bubbles form like nipples. The bubbles, after forming, become soft like paste. What flows is contagious. (JO, 53)*

Treatment with needles:

jianzhongshu (SI-15)	*5 fen,*
head-*linqi* (GB-11, IS GB-15)	*3 fen,*
muchuang (GB-12, IS GB-16)	*3 fen,*
tongziliao (GB-1)	*6 fen,*
sizhukong (TW-21, IS TW-23)	*1 fen,*
zanzhu (BL-2)	*1 fen,*
yangbai (GB-10, IS GB-14)	*2 fen.* (JO, 53)

Treatment with moxa:

jianzhongshu (SI-15)	*10 moxas,*
muchuang (GB-12, IS GB-16)	*15 moxas,*
ge shu (BL-17)........................	*10 moxas,*
ganshu (BL-18)	*10 moxas. (JO, 53)*

(JM) Trachoma: *zanzhu* (BL-2).

Eyes open wide *(deng):*
(DACH) Eyes open wide: *jinsuo* (GV-7, IS GV-8).

Lagophthalmos (cannot close the eyes, sign of peripheral facial paralysis):
The muscle that lowers the lid, or orbicular muscle, is innervated by the facial nerve (see: *yamen* GV-14, IS GV-15, located after the Japanese) near the center of the closure of the eyelids. See the points acting on the facial nerve: head-*wangu* (GB-17, IS GB-12), *jingming* (BL-1), *kezhuren* (GB-3, IS *shangguan*), *xiaguan* of cheek (ST-2, IS ST-7).
(DACH) Eyes not able to close: *daying* (ST-8, IS ST-5), *dicang* (ST-7, IS ST-4).

Blepharoptosis, ptosis:
The muscle that lifts the lid is innervated by the common ocular motor nerve (trigeminal nerve, third pair) (see *xuanlu*, GB-5, and *yuyao*, MP-4).
(YXRM) Eyes closing: *chengjiang* (CV-24).
(DACH XII, 25r) Eyes closed: *tongziliao* (GB-1); *(DACH) hegu* (LI-4), *yingxiang* (LI-20), disperse.
(DACH) Eye not opening, pain in the head: *yongquan* (KI-1).
Blinking of the lids (spasms of the muscle that lowers the lid, innervated by the facial nerve — *run*, popularly, *tiao* or *yan lian run tong, run jian*).

> *Movements from spasms in the lateral part of the eye, popularly called* **tiao***. (Ci Yuan, ''Run'')*

(DACH) Eye blinking, moves without stopping: *quanliao* (SI-18), *dicang* (ST-7, IS ST-4), *(DACH)* Blinking eyes: *touwei* (ST-1, IS ST-8); *(YXRM)* same, movement without rest: *sibai* (ST-5, IS ST-2).
(JM) Eyelids blinking *(run lian): zanzhu* (BL-2), *daying* (ST-8, IS ST-5); *(DACH) xinshu* (BL-15).

Blepharitis (inflammation of the eyelid):

> *Yan lian yuan yan,* ''inflammation of the edge of the eyelids.''

> *Origin: illnesses of the lymph nodes, tuberculosis, anemia, damp eruptions of the face, illnesses of the lacrimal sac, uncleanliness, tobacco, heat, attack of chronic conjunctivitis. Symptoms: in sqamous blepharitis, at first the squama are of a grey-white color, when these are lifted away, there is a scarlet color. In inflammatory or purulent blepharitis, there is an invasion of redness and swelling. The sacs of the eyelids are surrounded with small inflammations and pus; there is disintegration; then the eyelids thicken or stiffen. (JO, 52)*

Treatment with needles:

zanzhu (BL-2).......	*1 fen,*
tongziliao (GB-1)..	*1 fen,*
erjian (LI-2)..........	*2 fen,*
hand-wangu (SI-4)	*5 fen. (JO, 52)*

Treatment with moxa:

tongziliao (GB-1).......	*7 moxas,*
dicang (ST-7, IS ST-4)	*7 moxas,*
erjian (LI-2)...............	*5 moxas,*
hand-wangu (SI-4).....	*5 moxas. (JO, 52)*

(JM) Inflammation of the edge of the eyelids: *yanglao* (SI-6), *tianjing* (TW-10).
(DACH) Both eyelids red, swollen, painful, fears light, burning hot: needle at *jingming* (BL-1), *tongziliao* (GB-1).

Entropion, ectropion (*yan jie mao dao*, ''eyelashes inverted''):
(YIZ, 40r; DACH X, 29v) Eyelashes inverted (entropion): *sizhukong* (TW-21, IS TW-23); *(JM)* the same, needling medially.

(YXRM) Eyelashes inverted *(dao jie): hegu* (LI-4).

(DACH) Eyelashes inverted: *hegu* (LI-4), leg-*sanli* (ST-36).

Styes:

(DACH) Eyes with repeated styes: tonify *zhizheng* (SI-7).

(DACH) Swelling or abscess of the face or eyes: *lieque* (LU-7).

Pain of the eyes, cold:

Pains:

Acute pain of the eyes: *(DACH VI, 15r) guanchong* (TW-1); *(DACH IV, 7v; YIX I, 4r) qinglengyuan* (TW-11); *(YIZ, 38r; DACH) xiaogukong* (MP-23); *(DACH III, 29v) tongziliao* (GB-1), *(DACH VI, 11v) jingming* (BL-1), *tongziliao* (GB-1).

(JM) Pain of nerves of the eye, pain of the eyeball: *sibai* (ST-5, IS ST-2), *yuzhen* (BL-9); pain of the eyeball: foot-*qiaoyin* (GB-44).

Pain of the eyes: *(YIZ, 39; DACH II, 30v) hegu* (LI-4) moxas; *(YXRM) sanjian* (LI-3), *yangxi* (LI-5); *(DACH IV, 8r)* foot-*dadu* (SP-2); *(YIZ, 40) dadun* (LR-1); *(DACH) zhiyin* (BL-67), head-*qiaoyin* (GB-18, IS GB-11); *(YXRM) yuzhen* (BL-9); *(DACH) yixi* (BL-40, IS BL-45).

(DACH) Prolonged pain of the eyes: *dagukong* (MP-19), *dicang* (ST-7, IS ST-4).

(DACH) Pain in the eye: *qianyou* (TW-16).

(DACH) Pain of the eyes as if they were pulled out: *yuzhen* (BL-9), *tianzhu* (BL-10).

(YXRM) Shooting pain in the eye so sudden that the patient stands, bends or lies down; detests wind and cold: *yuzhen* (BL-9).

Pain of pupils, dizziness: *shangxing* (GV-22, IS GV-23); *(DACH X, 29v) neiting* (ST-44).

Internal corner: *(DACH X, 29r)* pain and contraction of the internal corner of the eye: *sanjian* (LI-3); *(DACH I, 8v) yangqiao mai* causes great pain in the eye beginning at the medial corner: two punctures at *shenmai* (BL-62), right for left, left for right and walk five kilometers, it will be finished; *(DACH)* great pain of the internal corner of the eye: *zhiyin* (BL-67); *(DACH)* pain at the small medial corner (external?) of the eye: foot-*qiaoyin* (GB-44); *(DACH)* pain and redness of the medial corner of the eye: *jingming* (BL-1), *youmen* (KI-21); *(DACH)* same symptom: *yindu* (KI-19); *(DACH) siman* (KI-14); *(DACH) quxue* (KI-13).

(DACH) Eyes, internal corner scarlet, injured, tears coming: *shugu* (BL-65); *(YXRM) qiangu* (SI-2).

For the medial corner: *houxi* (SI-3), *qiangu* (SI-2), *jinggu* (BL-64).

External corner: *(DACH)* Pain of external corner of the eye; *(JM)* congestion of external corner of the eye: head-*linqi* (GB-11, IS GB-15).

For the external corner: *waiguan* (TW-5).

External and internal corners: *(JM, DACH)* pain at the external and internal corners of the eye: *yangfu* (GB-38); *(DACH) tianjing* (TW-10).

(DACH) Pain on one side of one eye: *kezhuren* (GB-3, IS *shangwan*).

(YIZ, 40v) Pain in the crystalline lens: *fengfu* (GV-15, IS GV-16), *fengchi* (GB-20), *tongli* (HT-5), *hegu* (LI-4), *shenmai* (BL-62), *zhaohai* (KI-3, IS KI-6), *dadun* (LR-1), foot-*qiaoyin* (GB-44), *zhiyin* (BL-67).

(YIX I, 6r) Acute pain between the eyebrows, on the bone of the eyebrows, vision foggy: *zanzhu* (BL-2) under the skin towards *touwei* (ST-1, IS ST-8).

(DACH) Pain in the eyes, bleary: *yangbai* (GB-10, IS GB-14).

(DACH) Contraction of the artery of the eye penetrating inside, unbearable pain: *yuzhen* (BL-9).

Cold:

Coldness of the eyes: hand-*wangu* (SI-4).

Congestion, swelling (yan qiu chong xue, "blood invading the eyeball"):

(JM) Blood invading the eyeball: *houxi* (SI-3), *yanglao* (SI-6), *tongli* (HT-5), *neiguan* (PC-6), *xiangu* (ST-43), *zhiyin* (BL-67), *youmen* (KI-21), *yindu* (KI-19), *shiguan* (KI-18), *shangu* (KI-17), *huangshu* (KI-16), *qixue* (KI-13), *dahe* (KI-12), *henggu* (KI-11), *zhongzhu* (KI-15), *shangxing* (GV-22, IS GV-23), *muchuang* (GB-12, IS GB-16), *sizhukong* (TW-21, IS TW-23), *xuanli* (GB-6), *tongziliao* (GB-1), *fengchi* (GB-20), *tianyou* (TW-16).

(DACH) Redness of pupil: *waiguan* (TW-5).

Eyes scarlet and painful beginning from the lateral corner: *huangshu* (KI-16), *henggu* (KI-11), *dahe* (KI-12), abdomen-*zhongzhu* (KI-15), *tonggu* of epigastrium (KI-20); *(DACH) jinggu* (BL-64); *(JM) yinjiao* of gum (GV-27, IS GV-28); redness and pain of the medial corner of the eye: *jingming* (BL-1).

External corner of the eye, redness and pain: *(DACH, YXRM) xuanli* (GB-6), head-*linqi* (GB-11, IS GB-15); external corner scarlet, eyes not clear: *zanzhu* (BL-2).

Eyes scarlet, pain in the heart: *neiguan* (PC-6).

(DACH X, 28v) Scarlet eyes, foggy brain: *zanzhu* (BL-2).

(DACH X, 29v) Eyes scarlet, injured from shock (wind): *yanggu* (SI-5).

Redness and swelling:

(YIX I, 6v) Redness and swelling inside the eye; pain: needle at *sizhukong* (TW-21, IS TW-23), *zanzhu* (BL-2). If there is pain between the eyebrows: *erjian* of index finger (LI-2), *zanzhu* (BL-2).

(DACH) Eyes suddenly red, swollen, painful: *xinhui* (GV-21, IS GV-22).

(DACH) Both pupils red, swollen, pain difficult to bear, fearful of light: *tongziliao* (GB-1).

(YXRM I, 39r) Swelling and redness of the eye, pain: bleed *yingxiang* (LI-20). If serious; disperse *taichong* (LR-3); and if the eyes are red, pupil swollen and painful with tears: bleed *taichong* (LR-3).

(YIX I, 4v; DACH IV, 7v) Swelling and redness of the eyes, oppression, eyebrows bushy: *sizhukong* (TW-21, IS TW-23), *zanzhu* (BL-2).

(YIZ, 29v) Swollen, red eyes; headaches: *tongziliao* (GB-1).

(DACH VII, 32r) Eyes suddenly swollen, red; acute pain: *waiguan* (TW-5), *hegu* (LI-4), *zanzhu* (BL-2), *yingxiang* (LI-20).

(DACH XI, 2v) Eyes, red, swollen, painful: *jingming* (BL-1), *xiabai* (ST-3, IS ST-2), head-*linqi* (GB-11, IS GB-15), *hegu* (LI-4).

(DACH VII, 27v) Eyes swollen, scarlet, obstructed; tears without stopping: *houxi* (SI-3), *xiaogukong* (MP-23), head-*linqi* (GB-11, IS GB-15), *zanzhu* (BL-2).

Swelling:

(DACH X, 28v) Swollen eyes: *muchuang* (GB-12, IS GB-16), *xiangu* (ST-43).

(YIZ, 40v) Swollen eyes, pain like a storm: *shenting* (GV-23, IS GV-24), *shangxing* (GV-22, IS GV-23), *xinhui* (GV-21, IS GV-22), *qianding* (GV-20, IS GV-21), *baihui* (GV-19, IS GV-20), bleed; add needle at *guangming* (GB-37) and *diwuhui* (GB-42).

(YIZ, 40) Eyes swollen, crying: *houxi* (SI-3).

(YIX, 39v) Eyes swollen, painful, [as if] the crystalline lens wants to come out: *hegu* (LI-4), *taichong* (LR-3), *neiguan* (PC-6), *waiguan* (TW-5) and the intervals between the ten fingers — bleed.

(DACH) Swelling and abscess of the eyes: *lieque* (LU-7).

(JM) Exophthalmia: *jiaosun* (TW-20) [see Basedow's disease: *renying* (ST-9)].

Pruritis, itching:

(JM) Pruritis of the eyeball: *jingming* (BL-1).

(DACH) Pruritis of the pupil: *zanzhu* (BL-2), *dicang* (ST-7, IS ST-4).

(DACH) Painful pruritis of the pupil: *yangbai* (GB-10, IS GB-14).

Pruritis of the pupil when looking up: *chengqi* (ST-4, IS ST-1).

(JM) Pruritis of the pupil. *(DACH)* Pruritis of the eye, painful pruritis of the eye: *sibai* (ST-5, IS ST-2).

(DACH, JM) Pruritis of the eye: *tongziliao* (GB-1); *(YXRM) juliao* of cheek (ST-6, IS ST-3).

(DACH) Pruritis of the medial corner of the eye: *tongziliao* (GB-1).

(DACH II, 25v) Pruritis and pain of the eyes: *guangming* (GB-37), *diwuhui* (GB-42).

External color of the eyes:

(DACH) Eyes circled with black: *ganshu* (BL-18).

Indeterminate problems:

"Frayed-rope wind" (lan xian feng):

(YXRM I, 39r) Disperse foot-*linqi* (GB-41), or *taichong* (LR-3) and *hegu* (LI-4).

(YIZ, 39v) Frayed-rope wind: *dagukong* (MP-19), 9 light moxas, *xiaogukong* (MP-23), 7 light moxas.

"Flesh of effort" (granulations) invading the pupil *(nu rou jin jing)*:

(YIX I, 6v) fengchi (GB-20), *jingming* (BL-1), *hegu* (LI-4), *tongziliao* (GB-1). If not better: *fengchi* (GB-20), thorax-*qimen* (LR-14), *xingjian* (LR-2), *tongziliao* (GB-1).

Granulations gripping the crystalline lens *(nu rou pan jing)*:

(YIZ, 39v) jingming (BL-1), *tongziliao* (GB-1), *fengchi* (GB-20), *qimen* (LR-14) bleed; *(YIX I, 6v) jingming* (BL-1), *tongziliao* (GB-1), *fengchi* (GB-20), *hegu* (LI-4).

(YXRM I, 39r) Granulations and entropion: leg-*sanli* (ST-36), *hegu* (LI-4).

Crystalline lens gripped: *(YIX I, 4r; DACH II, 18v)* *shaoze* (SI-1), *ganshu* (BL-18); *(DACH II, 32r)* *jingming* (BL-1).

Eyes swollen, painful, [as if] crystalline lens wants to come out: *(YIZ, 39r)* *hegu* (LI-4), *taichong* (LR-3), *neiguan* (PC-6), *waiguan* (TW-5).

> *It comes from an undissipated shock (wind) following coitus. The upper body abounds; the lower body is empty; energy and blood rise; or it comes from an external and not quickly cured headache, the blood traversing the pupils; or from energy injuring the liver, the fire of the heart rising; or, for women, after delivery, or coitus too soon after delivery injuring the heart and liver, or from limitless food and drink. It cannot be cured in one session. (DACH XI, 2v)*

Scarlet blindness *(chi xia):*

> *Eyes damaged, scarlet for a long time, popularly called* **chi xia**. *One must puncture with the triangular needle (cause bleeding) laterally to the damaged eye to disperse the humidity and heat. (DACH XI, 12v)*

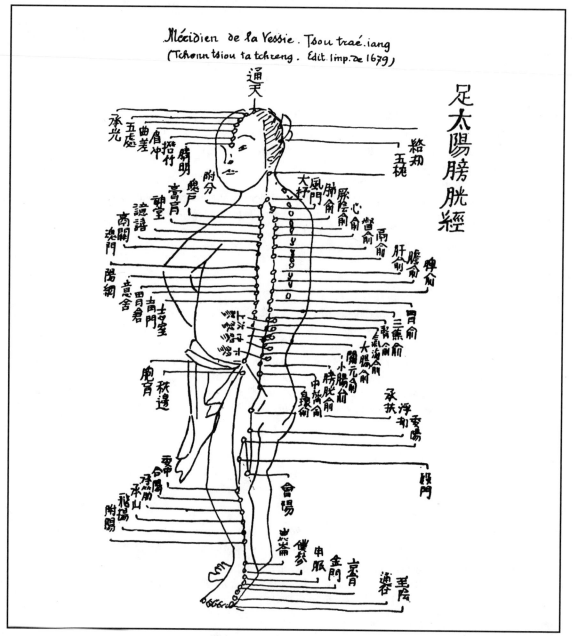

Meridian of the bladder (DACH)

Chapter VIII
Digestive System

I. Intoxication (From Drink, Food, Parasites or Poisons) — II. Fetid Breath — III. Eructations, Aerogastria — IV. Nausea, Vomiting — V. Saliva (Salivary Glands, Saliva) — VI. Lips — VII. Mouth — VIII. Gums — IX. Teeth — X. Tongue — XI. Root of the Tongue — XII. Epiglottis — XIII. Uvula — XIV. Tonsils — XV. Throat — XVI. Pharynx — XVII. Thirst — XVIII. Esophagus — XIX. Diaphragm — XX. Epigastrium — XXI. Stomach — XXII. Abdomen — XXIII. Small Intestine — XXIV. Large Intestine — XXV. Liver — XXVI. Gallbladder — XXVII. Icterus, Jaundice — XXVIII. Spleen-pancreas — XXIX. Diabetes, Glycosuria, Hyperglycemia — XXX. Beriberi

I. Intoxications (From Drink, Food, Parasites, Poisons)

Drink, drunkenness, dipsomania:

(GSdeM) Detoxifies and removes the need: disperse *shuaigu* (GB-8).

(YXRM I, 46r; DACH) Passion for alcohol: moxa *qihai* (CV-6) and take ginseng paste.

(DACH) Alcoholism: *yuji* (LU-10).

(JM) *zhongwan* (CV-12), *liangmen* (ST-21), leg-*sanli* (ST-36), *baihui* (GV-19, IS GV-20).

(YXRM I, 46r) Problems from alcohol, vomiting, mucus, dizziness: *shuaigu* (GB-8).

(YIZ, 40r) Headache after drunkenness; *(YXRM)* frontal bones painful after drunkenness: *shuaigu* (GB-8).

(YXRM, JM, DACH) All troubles following drunkenness: *shuaigu* (GB-8).

(DACH VII, 33v, I; YIX I, 11v) Accumulations *(ji)* from alcohol in the belly and under the umbilicus: *zhaohai* (KI-3, IS KI-6).

(DACH) Shock of drunkenness beginning on the nose: *bizhun* (MP-1).

(DACH) Icterus from alcohol: *danshu* (BL-19).

Food:

> Comes from impure food or drink. The patients have diarrhea or vomiting or both, the four limbs are weak and cold; there are some epidemic forms. In the past it was said to come from excess heat. We differentiate the black **(hei sha)** and the white **(bai sha)**. In the black variety there is fever, lumbar area and back are stiff. In the white variety there is cold, diarrhea, the ten nails are black. (Ci Yuan, ''Sha'')

(DACH VII, 33v) Black intoxication from food *(hei sha):* pain in the belly, cephalgia, fever, bad cold, lumbar area and back stiff and painful, cannot sleep: *bailao* (GV-13, IS GV-14 *dazhui*), *tianfu* (LU-3), *shixuan* (MP-25-29), *weizhong* (BL-54, IS BL-40).

(DACH VII, 33v) White intoxication from food *(bai sha):* pain in the belly, diarrhea and vomiting, four limbs cold and weak, the ten nails of the fingers black; cannot sleep: *bailao* (GV-13, IS GV-14 *dazhui*), *daling* (PC-7), *shixuan* (MP-25 - 29), *dadun* (LR-1).

(DACH XI, 10r, I; YIX I, 5v) Attacks of food-poisoning *(sha),* serious symptoms *(shuifen* CV-9, *bailao* GV-13, IS GV-14 *dazhui*), *daling* (PC-7), *weizhong* (BL-54, IS BL-40).

(DACH) Pain in the heart from food, piercing pain in the belly, stomach upset, body hot without sweat: *shangwan* (CV-13).

(DACH) All alimentary troubles: leg-*sanli* (ST-36).

(YXRM I, 46v) Women: food-poisoning *(shui gou):* *neiting* (ST-44).

Toxic substances:

(GSdeM) All toxic substances — opium, barbiturates, morphine, etc: detoxifies, removes the need and gives satisfaction with weaker and weaker quantities: disperse *shuaigu* (GB-8).

From parasitic worms (gu zhang):

> **Gu zhang:** There are many kinds of worms. But the poison produced by the worms in wine transforms it into vinegar in the same way as the worms act on the body. Face yellow, eyes yellow, no more strength, body painful, mucus, saliva, urine unclear or in drops, stools mixed with pus or blood, mouth and lips dry, chest and sides full, belly painful as if nibbled at by insects. Everything that the patient eats ferments. The worms invade the organs

and when all the organs have been invaded, there is death. In the past, in order to be sure of the existence of the poison, we made the patient spit into water. If the spit sinks, there are worms. (YXRM I, 30r)

(YXRM I, 30r) Poisoning from worms *(gu zhang):* three moxas at the ends of the fifth toe: *zhiyin* (BL-67).
(DACH, YXRM) Pain from ascaris worms *(hui)* and poisoning from worms *(gu zhang): juque* (CV-14).
(DACH) Agitation from parasitic worms: *fuliu* (KI-7).

From poisons *(gu du):*

''To poison a person and render unconscious.'' *(Ci Yuan, ''Gu-du'')*
(YIX I, 5v) Poisoning *(gu du)* of the treasure organs and descent of blood: *chengshan* (BL-57), *changqiang* (GV-1), *zhishi* (BL-47, IS BL-52), *pishu* (BL-20).
(DACH) Poisoning *(gu du):* leg-*sanli* (ST-36).
(DACH) Illnesses of the 100 poisons *(bai du bing): feishu* (BL-13).
(DACH) Tonic convulsions *(chi)* of the five poisons: *shangwan* (CV-13).
(JM) Saturnism, lead-poisoning: *zhubin* (KI-9).
(GSdeM) Intoxication with alcohol or drugs: *shuaigu* (GB-8).
(JM) Intoxication from fish *(hen zhu:* river-pork, tuna fish?).
(JO, 76) chize (LU-5), 3 *fen, shaoshang* (LU-11), 1 *fen, shuigou* (GV-25, IS GV-26 *renzhong),* 2 *fen, lieque* (LU-7), 3 *fen, quanshengzu* (Japanese point), 2 *fen.*

II. Fetid Breath *(Kou Chou)*

Europe: symptoms of chronic nephritis, of caries of the teeth, indigestion.
(YIX I, 5v) Stinking mouth, difficult to approach, comes from excess worries or fatigue or from organs retaining the food to the point of rotting: *chengjiang* (CV-24) gum-*yinjiao* (GV-27, IS GV-28), *jinjin* (MP-6, IS M-HN-20a) and *yuye* (MP-7, IS M-HN-20b).
(DACH IV, 7r) Very detestable stinking of mouth; fatigue of the heart from oppressiveness or from many feelings: disperse *daling* (PC-7), disperse *shuigou* (GV-25, IS GV-26 *renzhong).*
(DACH) Stinking mouth after reading for a long time: *zhongwan* (CV-12).
(YIZ, 40r, DACH) Rancidness and stinking in the mouth of adults and children: *laogong* (PC-8).

III. Eructations, Aerogastria

Eructations *(yue):*

''Air accumulated in the stomach goes out brusquely with a noise.'' *(YXRM)*
(YXRM) Eructations: *shangwan* (CV-13).
(YXRM) If one likes to burp: *jianshi* (PC-5).
(DACH) Habitual eructation: *shaoshang* (LU-11), leg-*sanli* (ST-36).
(DACH, YXRM) Counterflow eructations (attack): *wenliu* (LI-7).
(DACH) Eructations, sighs: *dadun* (LR-1).
(DACH) Counterflow of energy, groaning, eructations: *shaohai* (HT-3).
(YIZ, 37v, DACH) Women, dry eructations: *tuyin* (MP-44).

Eructations and vomiting:

(DACH) Eructations and vomiting: arm-*ximen* (PC-4), *taiyuan* (LU-9), *laogong* (PC-8), *daling* (PC-7), *taibai* (SP-3), *geguan* (BL-41, IS BL-46), *shiguan* (KI-18).
(DACH) Eructations, groaning, vomiting: *zhangmen* (LR-13).

Aerogastria *(fen tun):*

In aerogastria swelling of the stomach is produced after food, or suddenly at night; there is no reflex of swallowing air as in aerophagia.
(YXRM I, 46v) Swelling of energy of women: tonify. *(DACH)* Drum-swelling, emptiness of the secondary vessel from the spleen-pancreas to the stomach: tonify *gongsun* (SP-4).
(DACH IV, 10r; YIX I, 7v) Swelling of the epigastrium, all sorts of swelling from energy: leg-*sanli* (ST-36).
(YXRM I 46v) Swelling and fullness of the belly and sides: *yinlingquan* (SP-9).
(DACH, YXRM) Aerogastria, accumulations of the heart, eructations: *shangwan* (CV-13).
(YXRM) After reading a book, energy of aerogastria: *zhongwan* (CV-12).
(DACH, YXRM) Swelling of stomach: *xiaguan* of epigastrium (CV-10).

(YXRM I, 46v) Drum-swelling of the belly and umbilicus. *(DACH)* Aerogastria. *(YXRM)* Swelling of the belly, energy rising attacking the chest: *tianshu* (ST-25).

(DACH) Sudden swelling of the belly; when pressing, no penetration; *(YXRM I, 46v)* Drum-swelling of the epigastrium, pain in the sides.

(DACH) Aerogastria: *qihai* (CV-6).

(DACH III, 31r) Aerogastria pressing the heart: *zhongji* (CV-3).

(DACH) Aerogastria, aerogastria piercing the heart; *(YXRM)* aerogastria, energy entered into the lower pelvis: *guanyuan* (CV-4), *guilai* (ST-29).

(JM) Epigastrium swollen and ballooned: *youmen* (KI-21).

(YXRM) Swelling and fullness of the belly, cannot breathe: *luoque* (BL-7).

(DACH) Pain of aerogastria, aerogastria piercing the heart; *(YXRM)* energy of aerogastria rising from the belly; epigastrium full and hard; *shimen* (CV-5).

(YXRM) Aerogastria, pain in the belly; *(DACH)* aerogastria rising and descending: *siman* (KI-14).

Aerophagia (reflex of swallowing air):
(GSdeM) Dadun (LR-1), *taichong* (LR-3), *tianjing* (TW-10).

IV. Nausea, Vomiting *(Ou, Tu)*

Tu — *this is to fill up a washbasin without noise;* **ou** — *this is to fill a bowl with noise. . . . Nausea:* **e xin** *"bad heart," or* **xiang tu** *"thought of vomiting." (YXRM V, 31v)*

Desire to vomit, vomiting does not occur. (Ci Yuan, "E-xin")

(GSdeM) Nausea, bitter or bad taste in mouth when awakening: disperse *yangfu* (GB-38). If inadequate, also disperse *qiuxu* (GB-40), often accompanied with an insufficiency of liver.

(DACH) As if on a boat: *shenmai* (BL-62).

(DACH) Vomiting does not happen; headache: *shenzhu* (GV-11, IS GV-12).

Vomiting:
(GSdeM) The stimulation of the glossopharyngeal nerve causes saliva or vomiting: disperse *tianzhu* (BL-10).

(YXRM I, 39r) Vomiting *(tu)*: *neiguan* (PC-6), first tonify six times, then disperse three times. If the vomiting does not stop, tonify nine times four. At the thirty-third time the vomiting will stop; take out the needle and quickly close the hole. If it does not stop, tonify leg-*sanli* (ST-36).

(YXRM I, 3v) For treating vomiting *(tu)*: *zhongwan* (CV-12), *qihai* (CV-6), *shanzhong* (CV-17).

(DACH X, 33v) Vomiting *(ou tu)*: the illness has entered the interior from the exterior, mouth in order,[1] pulse sunken, rough, weak: moxa at *jueyinshu* (BL-14).

(DACH) All vomiting: leg-*sanli* (ST-36) and *neiting* (ST-44).

Vomiting: *shaoshang* (LU-11), *shaohai* (HT-3), *yinxi* (HT-6), *qiangu* (SI-2), hand-*wangu* (SI-4), *zhigou* (TW-6), *quze* (PC-3), *taixi* (KI-5, IS KI-3), *chongyang* (ST-42), *jinmen* (BL-63), *chengjin* (BL-56), *yinlingquan* (SP-9), leg-*sanli* (ST-36), *rangu* (KI-2), *shufu* (KI-27), *yuzhong* (KI-26), *shencang* (KI-25), *lingxu* (KI-24), *shengfeng* (KI-23), *bulang* (KI-22), *shanzhong* (CV-17), *shangwan* (CV-13), *zhongwan* (CV-12), *xiawan* (CV-10), *qihai* (CV-6), *burong* (ST-19), *youmen* (KI-21), *huaroumen* (ST-24), *tiantu* (CV-22), *jianli* (CV-11), *pohu* (BL-37, IS BL-42), *feishu* (BL-13), *fengmen* (BL-12), *jueyinshu* (BL-14), *bailao* (GV-13, IS GV-14 *dazhui*), *shenshu* (BL-23), *geshu* (BL-17), *weishu* (BL-21), *pishu* (BL-20), *xinshu* (BL-15), *danshu* (BL-19), *sanjiaoshu* (BL-22), *geguan* (BL-41, IS BL-46), *zhishi* (BL-47, IS BL-52), *shangliao* (BL-31).

Fits of vomiting: *wenliu* (LI-7), *tianfu* (LU-3), *dazhong* (KI-6, IS KI-4), foot-*dadu* (SP-2), *taichong* (LR-3), *tianrong* (SI-17), *zhongting* (CV-16), *juque* (CV-14), *zhangmen* (LR-13), *zhishi* (BL-47, IS BL-52), *jueyinshu* (BL-14), *feishu* (BL-13), *danshu* (BL-19); with sweat: *geshu* (BL-17).

Fits of vomiting, groaning, eructations; *shiguan* (KI-18).

(DACH) Nausea and vomiting without stopping: *hunmen* (BL-42, IS BL-47).

Counterflow of food *(shi ni)*:
(JM) Jingqu (LU-8), *shaohai* (HT-3), *tianquan* (PC-2), *taixi* (KI-5, IS KI-3), foot-*qiaoyin* (GB-44), *zhourong* (SP-20), *xiangqiang* (SP-19), *tianxi* (SP-18), *qihu* (ST-13), *gaohuangshu* (BL-38, IS BL-43), *yixi* (BL-40, IS BL-45), *geguan* (BL-41, IS BL-46).

Upset stomach (fan wei):

(DACH VII, 23v; YIX 9v) Upset stomach, difficulty in settling; *(YXRM)* Upset stomach, food stopped: *gongsun* (SP-4).

(DACH III, 29v, IV 5v, I; YIX 37r) Upset stomach, expectorates food: bleed *zhongkui* (MP-21, IS M-UE-16); *(YIX 4r) yinxi* (HT-6).

(DACH, YXRM) Upset stomach, vomiting, food not descending: *shangwan* (CV-13).

(YXRM I, 46r) Stomach upset, fullness of spleen; can cause in the stomach the beginning of energy that creates stiffness: *zhongwan* (CV-12). (Upset stomach of cholera).

(DACH) Stomach upset: *xiawan* (CV-10), *geshu* (BL-17).

(DACH) Does not want food, upset stomach, vomiting: *weishu* (BL-21).

Periods of vomiting:

(DACH) Vomiting acids at night: *zhejin* (GB-23).

(DACH) Vomiting and regurgitation of liquid acid at night: *riyue* (GB-24).

(GSdeM) Vomiting at night with painful attacks and spasms of the pyloric sphincter: *youmen* (KI-21).

(YXRM V, 34v) When the dryness is in the third warmer, the food from the morning is vomited in the evening, and that of the evening is vomited in the morning: *weidao* (GB-30, IS GB-28).

(DACH) Vomits immediately after eating: *zhangmen* (LR-13).

(DACH) Vomits immediately after eating; pain in shoulder and back; vomits after eating and drinking; food not digested; *sanjiaoshu* (BL-22).

(DACH) Food and drink go out immediately, fits vomiting: *zhangmen* (LR-13).

(DACH) Expectorates water after eating: *feishu* (BL-13); *(JM, DACH)* thorax-*qimen* (LR-14) 100 moxas, *xingjian* (LR-2), *sanyinjiao* (SP-6).

Returned substance:

Dry vomiting; *(DACH)* fits of dry vomiting: *xiabai* (LU-4); *(YXRM) jianshi* (PC-5), *jiquan* (HT-1); *(JM, DACH) lingdao* (HT-4); *(JM) guanchong* (TW-1); *(DACH) danshu* (BL-19).

Vomiting of water *(DACH)*. Vomits water, deep breathing: *(YIX I, 5v) juque* (CV-14). Expectoration of sour and cold water with heaviness in the heart: *(DACH VII, 25r)* moxa *xingjian* (LR-2). The mouth expectorates clear water, the stomach is blocked: *gongsun* (SP-4), *juque* (CV-14), *zhongwan* (CV-12), *lidui* (ST-45).

Vomiting of water after eating: *sanyinjiao* (SP-6), *xingjian* (LR-2), thorax-*qimen* (LR-14), *feishu* (BL-13).

Mucus: *(DACH)* Expectorates mucus after drinking: *sanyinjiao* (SP-6); vomiting of mucus: *taixi* (KI-5, IS KI-3); vomiting of cold mucus: *yutang* (CV-18).

Bile: *(DACH)* Vomiting of bile: *xingjian* (LR-2), same for sour and cold water.

Bitter: *(DACH)* Bitter vomiting: *tongli* (HT-5).

Acid: *(DACH)* Feels better after acid vomiting: thorax-*qimen* (LR-14).

Saliva: *(DACH) youmen* (KI-21), *lianquan* (CV-23), *shanzhong* (CV-17); *(DACH)* vomiting of saliva and mucus, heat: *juque* (CV-14); *(DACH, YXRM)* vomiting of saliva, dry tongue: *zhubin* (KI-9); *(DACH)* nausea and expectoration of saliva: *qiangjian* (GV-17, IS GV-18).

Blood (hematemesis):

> ***Tu xue*** *[vomiting of blood] is divided into:*
>
> 1)   *Abundance of yang: body hot, thirst; has a lot of accumulations, heat, unhappiness; caused by an excess acridity, heat, alcohol or by great unhappiness.*
>
> 2)   *Abundance of yin: body cool, no thirst; easy to cure; comes from sudden trouble of the strength of the heart. There is a knotting pain in the epigastrium, perspiration; comes either from cold with emptiness of energy or from a lesion from fatigue. First there is cough and mucus, then blood; this is a lot of fire. We must cool the blood and make the energy move. If first there is blood, then cough and mucus, this is emptiness of yin and movement of fire. One must tonify the blood. (YXRM I, 31r)*

(DACH VII, 32r) Expectorates blood, epistaxis; the yang dominates the yin; hot blood with disturbed circulation: *waiguan* (TW-5), *zhongchong* (PC-9), leg-*sanli* (ST-36), *sanyinjiao* (SP-6), *ganshu* (BL-18), *geshu* (BL-17).

(DACH VII, 32r) Expectorates blood, coolness of the blood. The yin dominates the yang; it is called vomiting *(ou)* of blood of the heart and lung meridian: *waiguan* (TW-5), *shaoshang* (LU-11), *shenmen* (HT-7), *sanyinjiao* (SP-6), *feishu* (BL-13), *geshu* (BL-17), *ganshu* (BL-18).

(DACH VII, 32r) Expectorates blood without stopping, five treasure organs bound with heat: *waiguan* (TW-5), *feishu* (BL-13), *xinshu* (BL-15), *geshu* (BL-17), *ganshu* (BL-18), *pishu* (BL-20), *shenshu* (BL-23).

(DACH VII, 32r) Expectorates blood, fog-vertigo, sexual vigor undiminished: *waiguan* (TW-5), *ganshu* (BL-18), *geshu* (BL-17), *tongli* (HT-5), *dadun* (LR-1).

(JM) Blood coming from the stomach: *yuji* (LU-10), *yinxi* (HT-6), arm-*ximen* (PC-4), *jugu* (LI-16), *zigong* (CV-19), *huaroumen* (ST-24), *xinshu* (BL-15), *pishu* (BL-20), *shenshu* (BL-23), *shimen* (CV-5).

Vomits blood *(DACH)*: *shenmen* (HT-7), *laogong* (PC-8), *daling* (PC-7), arm-*ximen* (PC-4), *taichong* (LR-3), *zhongwan* (CV-12), *zigong* of thorax (CV-19), *shangwan* (CV-13), *tianshu* (ST-25), *xinshu* (BL-15), *gaohuangshu* (BL-38, IS BL-43), *ganshu* (BL-18), *changqiang* (GV-1).

(DACH) Vomiting of blood, cough in counterflow: *xingjian* (LR-2).

(DACH) Numerous vomitings of blood not being cured: *qichong* (ST-30).

(DACH) Women: red vomiting: *tuyin* (MP-44).

(DACH) Heart broken, vomits blood: *jugu* (LI-16).

(DACH) Counterflow of energy, vomiting of saliva and blood: *quze* (PC-3).

Causes of vomiting:

(See cholera)

Sea sickness, car sickness *(yun chuan, gang yun e xin):*

> Seasickness is cured like nausea (**e xin**) if there is no thirst; this is emptiness or cold of stomach. If there is troubling thirst, it is an accumulation of heat or mucus. (YXRM I, 33r)

(DACH X, 35r) E-xin [nausea] either comes from mucus and heat or from emptiness: 1) No thirst, emptiness of stomach, or stomach cold: tonify at *geshu* (BL-17), *youmen* (KI-21), *shiguan* (KI-18), *shangqiu* (KI-17). 2) Thirst: heat or mucus — disperse at *weishu* (BL-21), *zhongwan* (CV-12), *yanggang* (BL-43, IS BL-48) and *youmen* (KI-21).

(DACH) As if on a boat: *shenmai* (BL-62).

(DACH) Violent nausea shaking the vertex: *houding* (GV-18, IS GV-19).

(GSdeM) In practice: tonify or disperse (according to the habitual whiteness or redness): *youmen* (KI-21); if not; leg-*sanli* (ST-36), *zhongwan* (CV-12).

(GSdeM) Mountain sickness: *jueyinshu* (BL-14).

(GSdeM) From excess alcohol, for alcoholics (fasting in the morning, bitter-tasting liquid mucus): *shuaigu* (GB-8), leg-*sanli* (ST-36).

(GSdeM) Cerebral vomiting (without effort, by sitting up from lying down): arm-*shanglian* (LI-9), *naohu* (GV-16, IS GV-17), *naokong* (GB-19).

(GSdeM) Vomiting of pregnancy: *youmen* (KI-21). Disperse if there is redness, tonify if there is whiteness.

Accompanied by:

Vomiting and diarrhea: *chize* (LU-5), *chengshan* (BL-57), *fuyang* (BL-59), *xingjian* (LR-2), *zhaohai* (KI-3, IS KI-6), *qimai* (TW-18), *fuxi* (BL-52, IS BL-38).

Vomiting and eructation: *taiyuan* (LU-9), *laogong* (PC-8), *daling* (PC-7), arm-*ximen* (PC-4), *taibai* (SP-3), *geguan* (BL-41, IS BL-46), *shiguan* (KI-18).

Vomiting and yawning: *jingqu* (LU-8).

Vomiting and perspiration: tonify *hegu* (LI-4), *geshu* (BL-17).

Vomiting followed by exhaustion: *gongsun* (SP-4).

Vomiting from repeated cough: *taiyuan* (LU-9), disperse.

Vomiting from spasms of the cardiac sphincter, babies regurgitating their milk as soon as it is taken: *zhongting* (CV-16).

V. Saliva (Salivary Glands, Mumps, Saliva)

Excitation of the glossopharyngeal nerve provokes saliva or vomiting: this nerve is commanded by *tianzhu* (BL-10).

Salivary glands, mumps:

Sublingual glands *(JM)*: *huaroumen* (ST-24).

Mumps, parotitis: *er xia xian yan,* "inflammation of the glands below the ear," *xia muo yan,* "frog epidemic," *zha sai zhang,* "evil serious swelling of the cheek." On the left, *hui dai li,* "bag of wisdom ganglia"; on the right, *feng wu li,* "bees' nest ganglia."

(DACH VII, 32v) Below the ear, painful and red swelling: *waiguan* (TW-5), *hegu* (LI-4), *yifeng* (TW-17), *jiache* (ST-3, IS ST-6).

(JM) Inflammation of the glands under the ear: *daying* (ST-8, IS ST-5), *heliao* (LI-19).

(DACH VII, 32r) Swelling of the gland under the left ear called ''bag of wisdom'': (TW-5), *houxi* (SI-3), *shoujian* (MP-11), *yifeng* (TW-17).

(DACH VII, 32r) Swelling of the gland under the right ear called ''bees' nest'': *waiguan* (TW-5), *houxi* (SI-3), *hegu* (LI-4), *yifeng* (TW-17), *jiache* (ST-3, IS ST-6).

Saliva:

Insufficient saliva:

(GSdeM) Tonify *tianzhu* (BL-10).

(DACH) Mouth dry, dry tongue: *fuliu* (KI-7), disperse.

(DACH) Mouth dry, empty, burns: *feishu* (BL-13).

(JM, DACH, YXRM) Dry mouth, chin swollen: *shangyang* (LI-1); with agitation and heat: *zhangmen* (LR-13); with heat in the stomach: *fuliu* (KI-7); with heat of chest: *shenzhu* (GV-11, IS GV-12), with agitating thirst: *quze* (PC-3).

(YXRM; YIZ, 40v) Mouth hot, mouth dry, saliva like gum: *shaoze* (SI-1), *taixi* (KI-5, IS KI-3); *(DACH)* white spit like gum: *zigong* (CV-19).

Excess saliva:

(GSdeM) Disperse *tianzhu* (BL-10).

(JM) Saliva too abundant: *lianquan* (CV-23), *yuzhong* (KI-26), *xiongxiang* (SP-19), *zhejin* (GB-23).

(YXRM) A lot of saliva: *lianquan* (CV-23), leg-*sanli* (ST-36), *geguan* (BL-41, IS BL-46), *hunmen* (BL-42, IS BL-47).

Saliva coming out: *(YIZ, 41r) lianquan* (CV-23); *(DACH)* same with relaxing of tongue; *(DACH, YXRM) rangu* (KI-2), leg-*xialian* (ST-39, IS *xiajuxu*), *geguan* (BL-41, IS BL-40), *kezhuren* (GB-3, IS *shangwan*).

Saliva flowing: *(JM) geguan* (BL-41, IS BL-46); *(YXRM)* leg *xialian* (ST-39, IS *xiajuxu*).

(JM) Saliva: *shaohai* (HT-3), *rangu* (KI-2), leg-*xialian* (ST-39, IS *xiajuxu*).

(DACH) Saliva coming out without being felt: leg-*xialian* (ST-39, IS *xiajuxu*).

(JM) Excess saliva flowing in streams: neck *futu* (LI-18).

(DACH III, 32r) Stops the flow of saliva which is in two threads: *dicang* (ST-7, IS ST-4).

(DACH) Children, vomiting and saliva: *luxi* (TW-19).

(DACH, YXRM) Vomiting of saliva: *lianquan* (CV-23), *youmen* (KI-21).

(YXRM) Eructates and spits a lot of saliva: *geguan* (BL-41, IS BL-46).

(DACH) Vomits and spits saliva: *shanzhong* (CV-17), *wenliu* (LI-7).

(YXRM) Spits saliva: *youmen* (KI-21).

(DACH) Saliva coming, dry lips: leg-*xialian* (ST-39, IS *xiajuxu*), *shaoshang* (LI-11).

(YIZ, 41v) Saliva falling, tongue relaxed: *yingu* (KI-10).

(DACH) Expectoration of saliva, cough and cold: *yangxi* (LI-5).

(DACH) Salivating, old women: *wuyi* (ST-15).

(DACH) Excess saliva from intestinal worms; from the three intestinal worms: *shangwan* (CV-13); *(DACH)* from ascaris: *zhongwan* (CV-12), *fuliu* (KI-7).

(YIX I, 11v) Strangling saliva, pain in the heart, chest, abdomen: *lieque* (LU-7).

(DACH) Spits a lot: *yuzhong* (KI-26), *shiguan* (KI-18), *zhejin* (GB-23); the same without stopping: *riyue* (GB-24), *sanjian* (LI-3).

(DACH) Likes to spit: *youmen* (KI-21).

(GSdeM) Nighttime salivation: *gongsun* (SP-4).

VI. Lips *(Chun);* Corners of the Lips *(Wu)*

Various:

(YIZ, 40v) Chews the lips (and cheek): *jinggu* (BL-64), *yanggu* (SI-5).

Colors:

(DACH, small intestine article) Blue-black lips with white edges (accompanied with excess urine) — emptiness of the small intestine: tonify *houxi* (SI-3), *guanyuan* (CV-4).

(DACH) Blackish lips, mouth blue — emptiness of the spleen-pancreas: tonify foot-*dadu* (SP-2).

(DACH) Scarlet lips: *xinshu* (BL-15).

Dry and cracked:

(DACH) Lips cracked, mouth split: *lidui* (ST-45).

(DACH) Cracked lips, mouth dry: *sanjian* (LI-3).

(DACH VII, 32r) Lips split, cracking, blood coming, dry, painful: *waiguan* (TW-5), *shaoshang* (LU-11), *guanchong* (TW-1), *chengjiang* (CV-24).

(DACH X, 29r) Dry lips, saliva coming out: leg-*xialian* (ST-39, IS *xiajuxu*), *fuliu* (KI-7).

Swelling:

(YXRM I, 39v) Swelling of the lips, cannot open them: disperse arm-*sanli* (LI-10); *(DACH II, 30r, X, 29v)* painful swelling of the lips: *yingxiang* (LI-20); *(DACH)* swelling of the lips: *yingchuang* (ST-16), *taichong* (LR-3).

(JM) Lips and cheeks, swelling congestion and pain; *(DACH)* lips and cheeks swollen: *juliao* (ST-6, IS ST-3).

(DACH) Troubles of the corners of the lips: *taichong* (LR-3).

Contractures:

(JM) Stiffness and hardness of the corners of the lips: *jiaosun* (TW-20), *ermen* (TW-23, IS TW-21); *(DACH)* *muchuang* (GB-12, IS GB-16), *zhengying* (GB-13, IS GB-17), *kechuren* (GB-3, IS *shangguan*); stiff and contracted: *(DACH)* *hegu* (LI-4), *shuigou* (GV-25, IS GV-26 *renzhong*).

(YIZ, 40v) Lips contracted, not able to open: *hegu* (LI-4), moxa, men on the left, women on the right; and *chengjiang* (CV-24), three moxas.

Paresis:

(YIZ, 40v) Lips and corners of the lips not obeying: aphonia, cannot speak; mouth closed: *hegu* (LI-4), *shuigou* (GV-25, IS GV-26 *renzhong*).

Acne, abscess:

(DACH) Abscess, pimples of the lips, tongue and mouth: *hegu* (LI-4).

(GSdeM) Tetter on the lips: *hegu* (LI-4); *(DACH X, 31v)* pimples coming out on the corners of the mouth and on the face: *hegu* (LI-4).

VIII. Mouth *(Kou, Zui)*

In general:

All trouble or illness of the mouth or throat: leg-*sanli* (ST-36), *hegu* (LI-4), and *quchi* (LI-11).

Heat, dryness:

Heat in the mouth: *(DACH, YXRM)* disperse *dazhong* (KI-6, IS KI-4).

Mouth hot, dry, thick saliva: *(DACH; YIZ, 44v)* *shaoze* (SI-1).

Mouth hot, dry, injured: *(YIZ, 40v)* *shaoze* (SI-1), *laogong* (PC-8), *sanjian* (LI-3), *taichong* (LR-3).

Heat of the mouth, pain of the tongue, acidity of the pharynx: *(YXRM)* *shaochong* (HT-9).

Dryness of the mouth: *(DACH)* *erjian* (LI-2), *burong* (ST-19), *chize* (LU-5), foot-*qiaoyin* (GB-44), *qimen* (LR-14).

Dryness of mouth and tongue: *(DACH)* *feishu* (BL-13), same with saliva coming out: *fuliu* (KI-7).

Mouth dry, chin swollen: *(DACH, YXRM)* *shangyang* (LI-1).

Mouth dry, heat of the stomach: *(DACH)* *fuliu* (KI-7).

Mouth dry, heat of the chest: *(YXRM)* *shenzhu* (GV-11, IS GV-12).

Mouth dry, agitating thirst: *quze* (PC-3).

Mouth dry, agitation, heat: *(DACH)* *zhangmen* (LR-13).

Mouth dry, lips cracked: *(DACH)* *sanjian* (LI-3).

Mouth cracked, lips split: *(DACH)* *lidui* (ST-45).

Tastes in the mouth:

Bitter taste in mouth (in the morning): *(DACH)* *yangfu* (GB-38).

Bitter taste in mouth, tongue dry: *(DACH IV, 5v)* *guanchong* (TW-1); *(DACH)* *danshu* (BL-19).

Bitter or bad taste in the mouth: *(DACH)* head-*qiaoyin* (GB-18, IS GB-11).

Bitter taste in mouth, pharynx useless: *(DACH)* *yanglingquan* (GB-34).

Bitter taste in mouth, habitual vomiting: *(DACH, YXRM)* leg-*sanli* (ST-36).

Pains:

Pain of mouth and tongue: *(YIZ, 14)* *wenliu* (LI-7).

Pain of the mouth, bites tongue: *(YIZ, 40r)* *jiexi* (ST-41).

Bites cheeks: *jinggu* (BL-64), *yanggu* (SI-5).

Inflammations, aphthae:

Inflammation of the mouth: *erjian* (LI-2), *yanggu* (SI-5), *wenliu* (LI-7), *shangyang* (LI-1), *taixi* (KI-5, IS KI-3), *dazhong* (KI-6, IS KI-4), *jiaosun* (TW-20), *feishu* (BL-13).
Rottenness of the mouth: *(DACH) laogong* (PC-8).
Rancidness and stench in the mouth of adults and children: *(DACH) laogong* (PC-8).

● **Abscess:**

Abscess of the mouth: *(DACH) lianquan* (CV-23), *chengjiang* (CV-24).
Abscess of the mouth, tongue and lips: *(DACH) hegu* (LI-4).
Mouth and teeth, gnawing chancre, swelling and abscess: *chengjiang* (CV-24).

Noma *(ya gan, zhuan sai feng)*:
Yagan: *(DACH)* gum-*yinjiao* (GV-27, IS GV-28), *chengjiang* (CV-24).

Thrush *(e kou chuang, "ox-mouth abscess")*:

> *Origin: comes from the bacteria of the mouth of the ox; this microbe develops particularly in the mucosa of the mouth and throat. The illness develops from giving the breast; it happens also in adults. Symptoms: the tongue and the mucosa covering the mouth show points and spots which spread and produce a grayish film. The interior of the mouth is hot and burns; acute pain, saliva flows. Treatment, through moxa:* **laogong** *(PC-8), three to five times. (JO, 69)*

VIII. Gums (Gingivitis, Alveolar Pyorrhea)

Pains:

Neuralgia of the dental alveoli: *(JM) muchuang* (GB-12, IS GB-16), *zhengying* (GB-13, IS GB-17), *jiache* (ST-3, IS ST-6).
Pain and noise when chewing: *(DACH) kezhuren* (GB-3, IS *shangguan*).

Swellings:

Swollen gums, teeth rotten: *(DACH) xiaohai* (SI-8).
Gums swollen, molars and incisors cannot be used for chewing: *(YIZ, 40v) jiaosun* (TW-20).

Inflammations *(che yin yan)*:

Inflammation of the dental alveoli: *(JM)* arm-*sanli* (LI-10).

Treatment with needles and moxa:

lip-**heliao** *(LI-19)*	*5 fen,* 9 moxas,
dicang *(ST-7, IS ST-4)*..	*3 fen,* 9 moxas,
xiaguan *(ST-2, IS ST-7)*	*7 fen,* 9 moxas,
jiache *(ST-3, IS ST-6)*...	*7 fen,* 9 moxas,
yifeng *(TW-17)*.............	*7 fen,* 9 moxas,
jianwaishu *(SI-14)*.......	*5 fen,* 9 moxas,
tianrong *(SI-15)*..........	*5 fen,* 9 moxas,
jianjing *(GB-21)*	*5 fen,* 9 moxas. *(JM, 315)*

Alveolar pyorrhea:

Blood coming out from between the gums, falling of the incisors, and even pain of the mouth, which cannot be opened, radiating up to the nose: *(YIZ, 41r)* needles and moxa to gum-*yinjiao* (GV-27, IS GV-28).
Wind from falling-of-frame: *(DACH) jiache* (ST-3, IS ST-6).
Gingival hemorrhage can come from serious anemia.

IX. Teeth *(Chi, Ya Chi)*

Generally, teeth are called *chi,* the molars *jiu chi* "mortar-teeth," or just *ya;* the incisors are called *men chi,* "door teeth," or just *chi.*

General commands:

Illnesses of the teeth *(ya): (YXRM I, 46v) erjian* (LI-2).

By pressing there is a response in:
All the teeth: *muchuang* (GB-12, IS GB-16), *neiting* (ST-44), *kunlun* (BL-60).
Molars and upper incisors: *muchuang* (GB-12, IS GB-16), *tinghui* (GB-2), *hegu* (LI-4), *quanliao* (SI-18).
Molars and lower incisors: *zhengying* (GB-13, IS GB-17).
Upper and lower incisors: *yanggu* (SI-5).
Upper incisors: *sanjian* (LI-3), *muchuang* (GB-12, IS GB-16), *tinghui* (GB-2), *ermen* (TW-23, IS TW-21).
Lower incisors: *shangyang* (LI-1), *erjian* (LI-2), *sanjian* (LI-3), *shenting* (GV-23, IS GV-24), *fengfu* (GV-15, IS GV-16).
Upper molars: *yanggu* (SI-5), *fubai* (GB-16, IS GB-10), *ermen* (TW-23, IS TW-21), cheek-*xiaguan* (ST-2, IS ST-7), *jiaosun* (TW-20).
Lower molars: *erjian* (LI-2), *lieque* (LU-7), *sidu* (TW-9), head-*wangu* (GB-17, IS GB-12), *jiache* (ST-3, IS ST-6), *jugu* (LI-16).

Pains:

(GSdeM) In general, *kunlun* (BL-60); lower incisors: *shangyang* (LI-1); lower molars; *erjian* (LI-2); upper incisors: *tinghui* (GB-2); upper molars: *fubai* (GB-16, IS GB-10).
Pain of all the teeth in the mouth: *(YXRM I, 39v) hegu* (LI-4) and foot-*linqi* (GB-41), disperse *yanggu* (SI-4).
Acute pain of the teeth: *(DACH IV, 5v)* like fire, *erjian* (LI-2); *(YIX I, 4v; DACH II 19v) ermen* (TW-23, IS TW-21) and *sizhukong* (TW-21, IS TW-23); *(YIX I, 4v) guanliao* (SI-18), *erjian* of index finger (LI-2); *(DACH VII, 39v) lieque* (LU-7); *(YXRM I, 46v) shenmai* (BL-62), *kunlun* (BL-60); *(DACH IV, 10v) neiting* (ST-44); *(YXRM) jiache* (ST-3, IS ST-6).
Pain of the teeth: *(YXRM) sanjian* (LI-3); *(JM, DACH, YXRM)* arm-*sanli* (LI-10); *(DACH) shangyang* (LI-1); *(JM) yangxi* (LI-5); *(YIZ, 46v) quchi* (LI-11), *waiguan* (TW-5), *pianli* (LI-6), *shaohai* (HT-3); *(DACH III, 30v), taixi* (KI-5, IS KI-3); *(DACH) jiexi* (ST-41); *(JM) wanyan* (GB-4), *(JM) dicang* (ST-7, IS ST-4), *ermen* (TW-23, IS TW-21), *yifeng* (TW-17), *fubai* (GB-16, IS GB-10), head-*wangu* (GB-17, IS GB-12), *(JM) chengjiang* (CV-24).
Pain of the teeth and mouth: *(DACH) wenliu* (LI-7); and cheek: *daling* (PC-7).
Pain of the teeth radiating into the ear: *(DACH) wenliu* (LI-7); and cheek: *daling* (PC-7).
Pain of the teeth radiating into the ear: *(DACH) ermen* (TW-23, IS TW-21).
Neuralgia of the dental alveoli: *(JM) muchuang* (GB-12, IS GB-16), *zhengying* (GB-13, IS GB-17), *jiache* (ST-3, IS ST-6).
Pain of the upper and lower teeth: *(YXRM I, 46v) yanggu* (SI-5).
Pain of the upper teeth: *(JM) quanliao* (SI-18); *(YIZ, 41v) yangchi* (TW-4) and *yangxi* (LI-5).
Pain of the lower teeth: *(YIZ, 41r)* pain of the lower teeth, bad cold, pain of jaw: *shangyang* (LI-1), *jugu* (LI-16); *(YXRM I, 39r) hegu* (LI-4), *xiaguan* (ST-2, IS ST-7).
Pain of the molars and incisors *(ya chi): (DACH, YXRM) houxi* (SI-3); *(YXRM I, 46v) kunlun* (BL-60); *(DACH) xuanlu* (GB-5); *(DACH), zhengying* (GB-13, IS GB-17), head-*wangu* (GB-17, IS GB-12).
Pain of the molars *(ya) (DACH)* and illnesses: *erjian* of index fingers (LI-2); *(DACH)* acute: *chengjiang* (CV-24); *(YXRM) jiaosun* (TW-20); *(YXRM)* acute: *jueyinshu* (BL-14).
Pain of the incisors *(chi): (DACH X, 29v; DACH, YXRM) shangyang* (LI-1), *(JM, DACH, YXRM) pianli* (LI-6); *(YIZ, 41r) sidu* (TW-9); *(JM) xuanlu* (GB-5); *(JM) tinghui* (GB-2), *zhengying* (GB-13, IS GB-17).
Pain of the upper molars: *(GSdeM) fubai* (GB-16, IS GB-10), *yanggu* (SI-5).
Pain of the lower molars: *(YXRM I, 39r) lieque* (LU-7), *sidu* (TW-9); *hegu* (LI-4), *erjian* (LI-2).
Pain of the upper incisors: *(JM) ermen* (TW-23, IS TW-21), *muchuang* (GB-12, IS GB-16), *tinghui* (GB-2).
Pain of the lower incisors: *(YXRM I, 46v) sanjian* (LI-3), *shangyang* (LI-1).

Pain from dental caries:

Caries of the incisors and molars, painful: *(YIZ, 41r)* head-*wangu* (GB-17, IS GB-12); *(DACH) yemen* (TW-2).
Pain of decayed incisors: *(YIZ 41r) hegu* (LI-4), *yemen* (TW-2); *(DACH) yanggu* (SI-5), *sanjian* (LI-3), *shaohai* (HT-3); *(JM, YXRM) chongyang* (ST-42); *(JM, DACH) fuliu* (KI-7); *(JM) tianrong* (SI-17), *duiduan* (GV-26, IS GV-27), *shangyang* (LI-1).

Pain of decayed molars: *(DACH) zhengying* (GB-13, IS GB-17), *hegu* (LI-4), *erjian* (LI-2).

Pain of upper decayed incisors: *(YIZ, 45) ermen* (TW-23, IS TW-21), *kezhuren* (GB-3, IS *shangguan*); *(DACH) zhengying* (GB-13, IS GB-17), *tinghui* (GB-2).

Pain of decayed lower incisors: *(YIZ, 41r)* cheek-*xiaguan* (ST-2, IS ST-7); *(DACH) sanjian* (LI-3), *(DACH) sidu* (TW-9), *shangyang* (LI-1).

Pain of decayed upper molars: *(YIZ, 41r) yangxi* (LI-5), *yanggu* (SI-5), *fubai* (GB-16, IS GB-10).

Pain of the lower molars, decayed: *erjian* (LI-2).

Caries of the teeth:

Caries of the teeth *(ju chi)*

(DACH) Meridian of the liver and, if this is ineffective, gum-*yinjiao* (GV-27, IS GV-28), *(DACH) hegu* (LI-4); *(YXRM) xiaohai* (SI-8); *(DACH)* foot-*linqi* (GB-41), *fuliu* (KI-7), *chongyang* (ST-42); *(YXRM) lidui* (ST-45); head-*wangu* (GB-17, IS GB-12); *(DACH) daying* (ST-8, IS ST-5).

Caries of the upper teeth: *lidui* (ST-45).

Caries of the lower teeth: *(DACH) hegu* (LI-4).

Caries of the lower molars: *(YIZ, 41r)* cheek-*xiaguan* (ST-2, IS ST-7).

Caries of the upper incisors: *(YIZ, 45) ermen* (TW-23, IS TW-21), *zhengying* (GB-13, IS GB-17); *(DACH) neiting* (ST-44).

Caries of the lower incisors: *(YIZ, 41r) xiaguan* (ST-2, IS ST-7).

Caries of the molars: *(DACH)* cheek-*xiaguan* (ST-2, IS ST-7).

Caries of the incisors: *(DACH) jiaosun* (TW-20); *(YXRM) qubin* (GB-7), *ermen* (TW-23, IS TW-21).

Children: rottenness and caries of the teeth: *laogong* (PC-8).

Dental inflammation:

(YIZ, 41v) Pain of the teeth, bad cold, swelling of the jaw: *shangyang* (LI-1).

(YXRM I, 39v) Decayed teeth, face swollen: *jiache* (ST-3, IS ST-6) and arm-*sanli* (LI-10); if all teeth are painful: *hegu* (LI-4) and foot-*linqi* (GB-41): disperse; if the lower teeth are painful: *hegu* (LI-4).

(DACH) Pain of the teeth and inflammation: *houxi* (SI-3), *tianchong* (GB-15, IS GB-9).

Inflammation of rotten teeth: head-*wangu* (GB-17, IS GB-12), *xiaohai* (SI-8).

Swelling of the cheekbone, pain of incisors: *quanliao* (SI-18).

(DACH) Decayed molars, swelling of the cheek: *xiaguan* (ST-2, IS ST-7).

(JM) Inflammation of upper teeth; decayed: *neiting* (ST-44).

(DACH) Pain of molars, swelling of the jaw: *daying* (ST-8, IS ST-5).

Dental abscess:

(GSdeM) Stops it at the beginning, decreases the swelling and duration if it is formed: disperse *shenmai* (BL-62), *kunlun* (BL-60). If it is the upper teeth, disperse *xiaguan* (ST-2, IS ST-7); if lower teeth, disperse *hegu* (LI-4) and *jiache* (ST-3, IS ST-6).

Loose teeth:

(GSdeM) Loose teeth from illness, fatigue or age: tonify the upper edge of C-6, *jiuwei* (CV-15); if insufficient, *zhubin* (KI-9). For lower incisors: *shangyang* (LI-1), disperse; lower molars: *erjian* (LI-2), disperse; upper molars: *fubai* (GB-16, IS GB-10); upper incisors: *tinghui* (GB-2 for location), *muchuang* (GB-12, IS GB-16) for upper teeth and *zengying* (GB-13, IS GB-17) for the lower teeth.

(DACH) Wind from falling-of-frame: *jiache* (ST-3, IS ST-6).

Various:

Grinding of the teeth at night (often a sign of parasitic worms): *(DACH) guangming* (GB-37), head-*linqi* (GB-11, IS GB-15).

Cold in the teeth: *(YIZ, 41r) shaohai* (HT-3); *(DACH)* Cold in the incisors: *pianli* (LI-6), *(DACH) bailao* (GV-13, IS GV-14 *dazhui*).

X. Tongue *(She)*

In general:

(JM) Famous point for the glossopharyngeal nerve (sensitivity of the tongue, tonsils, pharynx, tympanic cavity, eustachian tube; its stimulation produces saliva and vomiting, vasodilation of the base of the tongue, pharynx, motor function): *tianzhu* (BL-10).

(JM) Hypoglossal nerve (motor function of all the muscles of the tongue, vasoconstriction of the tongue): *wangu* (GB-17, IS GB-12), *renying* (ST-9).

(JM) Troubles of the tongue, near the middle for swallowing, breath, etc: *yamen* (GV-14, IS GV-15).

(JM) Illness of the mouth, tongue teeth, pharynx, etc: *hegu* (LI-4), *quchi* (LI-11).

Tongue and speech:

Hypoglossal nerve: head-*wangu* (GB-17, IS GB-12), *renying* (ST-9).

Glossopharyngeal nerve: *tianzhu* (BL-10).

(YIX I, 5v) Tongue slow, does not speak: *yamen* (GV-14, IS GV-15).

(DACH XI, 10r) Stiffness of the tongue, difficult speech: *fengfu* (GV-15, IS GV-16) and *yangquan* (CV-23).

(DACH) Apoplexy; tongue slow, no longer speaks: *fengfu* (GV-15, IS GV-16).

(JM) Paralysis of the hyoid muscles (bone of tongue): *yinxi* (HT-6), *tongli* (HT-5), *lingdao* (HT-4), *zhigou* (TW-6), *yongquan* (KI-1), *yamen* (GV-14, IS GV-15), *tiantu* (CV-22), neck-*futu* (LI-8), *tianding* (LI-17), *tonggu* (KI-20).

Paralysis of the tongue, cannot speak: leg-*sanli* (ST-36).

Spasms of the muscles of the glottis *(yin men):* *(JM)* *tiantu* (CV-22), *huagai* (CV-20), *dicang* (ST-7, IS ST-4).

Contraction of the voice muscles: *(JM)* *zhongfu* (LU-1).

Tongue tired, relaxed, retracted:

Tongue tired *(juan):* *(DACH)* *guanchong* (TW-1); *(YIZ, 40r)* *waiguan* (TW-5); *(YIZ, 41r)* *yemen* (TW-2), *erjian* (LI-2).

Tongue relaxed *(song):* *(DACH)* *rangu* (KI-2), *yingu* (KI-10), *lianquan* (CV-23).

Tongue retracted *(shuo, shu):* *(YIZ, 41v)* tongue retracted, saliva coming out in counterflow, slowness of the tongue: *yingu* (KI-10); *(DACH VII, 32r)* tongue retracted, difficulty speaking, called stiffness of yin: *waiguan* (TW-5), *xinshu* (BL-15), *shanzhong* (CV-17), *haiquan* (MP-5, IS M-HN-37).

Tongue heavy: *(DACH)* *yamen* (GV-14, IS GV-15), *hegu* (LI-4).

Pain of the tongue:

Pain of the tongue and mouth: *(DACH)* *wenliu* (LI-7); *(GSdeM)* *tianzhu* (BL-10).

Pain of the tongue and heat in the mouth, acidity of pharynx: *shaochong* (HT-9).

(DACH) Acute pain of the tongue: *jinjin* (MP-6, IS M-HN-20a) of the tongue, pain of the throat: *yuye* (MP-7, IS M-HN-20b), *lianquan* (CV-23) and *zhongchong* (PC-9), *jinjin* (MP-6, IS M-HN-20a) and *yuye* (MP-7, IS M-HN-20b).

Swelling, inflammation, abscesses of the tongue:

Swelling of the tongue:
Swelling of the tongue: *(YXRM)* *jiexi* (ST-41); *jinjin* (MP-6, IS M-HN-20a).

Tongue swollen, difficulty speaking: *(DACH XI, 3v)* linquan (CV-23), *jinjin* (MP-6, IS M-HN-20a), *yuye* (MP-7, IS M-HN-20b); If not better: *tiantu* (CV-22), *shaoshang* (LU-11).

Inflammation of the tongue:
Inflammation of the tongue: *(JM)* *wenliu* (LI-7), *huaroumen* (ST-24), *jinjin* (MP-6, IS M-HN-20a); *(JM, 315)* needles: *shenzhu* (GV-11, IS GV-12), *jianzhongshu* (SI-15), *dazhu* (BL-11). Moxa: twenty at *shenzhu* (GV-11, IS GV-12).

Swelling under the tongue:
Swelling under the tongue: *(JM)* *rangu* (KI-2), *lianquan* (CV-23).

Swelling and pain under the tongue: *(YIX I, 5v)* *lianquan* (CV-23) and *zhongchong* (PC-9).

(DACH) Swelling under the tongue, difficulty in speaking, abscess of mouth, tongue retracted, saliva coming out, root of the tongue retracted: *lianquan* (CV-23), 3 *fen:* wait for the energy and disperse, or use three moxas.

Inflammation of the sublingual glands: *(JM)* *huaroumen* (ST-42).

Abscess (sometimes due to excess energy of the small intestine):
(DACH) Abscess of the mouth, tongue, lips: *hegu* (LI-4).
(GSdeM) Abscess of tongue: *lianquan* (CV-23).

Heat and cold of the tongue:

Heat of mouth and tongue: *(DACH) shaochong* (HT-9).
Cold of the tongue, mouth dry, agitation of the heart: head-*qiaoyin* (GB-18, IS GB-11).

Trembling of the tongue:

Tongue dancing from right to left: *(DACH)* disperse arm-*sanli* (LI-10).

Dryness of the tongue:

(YXRM) Dry tongue: *chize* (LU-5); *(DACH, YXRM) dazhong* (KI-6, IS KI-4).
(DACH X, 29v; YIZ, 45) Dry tongue, saliva coming out; *(DACH II, 19r)* tongue dry, mouth dry: *fuliu* (KI-7).
(DACH) Tongue dry, swelling of the pharynx: *yongquan* (KI-1).

Lesions of the tongue:

Tongue torn: *(YXRM) hegu* (LI-4).
(DACH) Tongue split, bloody: *taichong* (LR-3), head-*qiaoyin* (GV-18, IS GB-11).
(DACH) Bites his tongue: *jiexi* (ST-41).
(DACH) Food pinching the tongue at the blue vessel of the seam, cannot descend: *tiantu* (CV-22).

Stiffness of the tongue:

Stiffness of the tongue: *(DACH X, 29v), yamen* (GV-14, IS GV-15), *shaoshang* (LU-11), *erjian* (LI-2), *zhongchong* (PC-9), *yingu* (KI-10), *rangu* (KI-2).
Stiffness of the tongue, difficulty in speaking: *fengfu* (GV-15, IS GV-16), *lianquan* (CV-23), *jinjin* (MP-6, IS *yuye* (MP-7, IS M-HN-20b).
Stiffness of the tongue, root of tongue bound: *zhongchong* (PC-9).
(DACH) Stiffness of tongue, pain in the ribs: head-*qiaoyin* (GB-18, IS GB-11).

Tongue protruding (see epilepsy):

(DACH) Tongue protruding, nape bent forward, looks to right and left: *yanggu* (SI-5).
(DACH) Tongue protruding, vomiting of saliva: *zhubin* (KI-9).
(DACH) Great shock, tongue protruding, four limbs swollen: *wenliu* (LI-7).

Colors, qualities:

(DACH) Tongue yellow, body hot, headache: *yuji* (LU-10).
(DACH) Top of the tongue producing albugo: *hegu* (LI-4), *ququan* (MP-8).

XI. Root of the Tongue *(She Gen, She Ben)*

(DACH) Enters and links the root of the tongue: *yamen* (GV-14, IS GV-15); *(DACH IX, 11v)* links the root of the tongue: *tongli* (HT-5).
(JM) Contracture or paralysis of all the muscles of the root of the tongue: *lianquan* (CV-23).
(YIZ, 41r) Root of the tongue bound and tightened: *lianquan* (CV-23).
(DACH) Pain and stiffness of the root of the tongue: foot-*shangqiu* (SP-5).
(YXRM) Pain of the root of the tongue: *guanchong* (TW-1); *(YXRM) daling* (PC-7).
(YXRM) Root of the tongue coming out: neck-*futu* (LI-18).
(DACH, YXRM) Root of the tongue bleeding: head-*qiaoyin* (GB-18, IS GB-11).

XII. Epiglottis *(Yin Men, Portal of Sound)*

(JM) Spasms of the portal of sound: *huagai* (CV-20).

XIII. Uvula (*I She*, Child-Tongue)

(DACH XI, 11r) Swelling of the uvula. If it becomes like a second tongue from bound heat, it is called *zi she zhang*, swelling of the uvula (edema of the uvula): *shaoshang* (LU-11), *hegu* (LI-4), *guanchong* (TW-1), *fengleng* (ST-40), *yongquan* (KI-1).

XIV. Tonsils (*Bian Tao Xian Yan*, Swelling of the Tonsils)

Popularly; butterflies of the larynx: *hou e, e feng;* milk butterflies: *ru e;* chronic: *hou bi*, rheumatism of the larynx.

*Acute tonsillitis comes from bad cold; attacks of fever. Balls appear on one or both sides of the throat. It is also called **hou e**, butterflies of the larynx. The chronic forms are called **hou bi**, rheumatism of the larynx. (Ci Yuan, "Bian-tao-xian Yan")*

*This may be an acute form of tonsillitis, **bian tao xian yan**. It is also called **ru e**, milk-butterfly. It appears to be a butterfly of the white silkworm, thus the name. There are the simple types (**dan**) and the double (**shuang**). The double types are mild, the simple are serious. (Ci Yuan, "Hou-e")*

*Also called **bian tao xian yan**: grows on the two sides of the throat. The two tonsils swell. Popularly called **hou e**, butterfly of the larynx. The chronic varieties are called **hou bi** and are difficult to cure. (Ci Yuan, "Ru-e")*

***Bian tao xian yan.** Origin: flu, catarrh of throat, inflammation of the inside of the mouth. Symptoms: bad cold, attack of fever, swelling of the tonsils with an attack of redness. Sometimes pus accumulates. One must distinguish it from diphtheria. (JO, 63)*

Treatment with needles:

***fengchi** (GB-20)*	*7 fen,*
*head-**wangu** (GB-17, IS GB-12)*	*5 fen,*
***tiantu** (CV-22)*	*6 fen,*
***fengmen** (BL-12)*	*5 fen,*
***shangyang** (LI-1)*	*1 fen,*
***shaochong** (HT-9)*	*2 fen,*
***rangu** (KI-2)*	*5 fen,*
***zhaohai** (KI-3, IS KI-6)*	*3 fen. (JO, 63)*

Treatment with moxa:

***tiantu** (CV-22)*	*7 moxas,*
***zhongting** (CV-16)*	*7 moxas,*
***fengmen** (BL-12)*	*7 moxas,*
***shangyang** (LI-1)*	*7 moxas,*
***shaochong** (HT-9)*	*7 moxas,*
***rangu** (KI-2)*	*7 moxas,*
***zhaohai** (KI-3, IS KI-6)*	*7 moxas. (JO, 63)*

Inflammation of the tonsils *(bian tao xian yan): (JM) yangxi* (LI-5), *guanchong* (TW-1), *yinxi* (HT-6), *sanjian* (LI-3), *shaoshang* (LI-11), *hegu* (LI-4), *shenmen* (HT-7), *tongli* (HT-5), *pianli* (LI-6), *yunmen* (LU-2), *zhongfu* (LU-1), *xiaguan* (ST-2, IS ST-7), *zhaohai* (KI-3, IS KI-6), *fubai* (GB-16, IS GB-10), *yangjiao* (GB-35), *xuanzhong* (GB-39), *lidui* (ST-45).

Simple milk-butterfly *(dan ru e): (DACH) shaoshang* (LU-11), *hegu* (LI-4), *lieque* (LU-7), *tianquan* (PC-6), *tianjing* (TW-10), *tiantu* (CV-22).

Double milk-butterfly *(shuang ru e): (DACH VII, 27r) houxi* (SI-3), *shaoshang* (LU-11); *(YXRM I, 46v) shaoshang* (LU-11).

(DACH) Simple tonsillitis of children: press *hegu* (LI-4) with the fingernail.

XV. Throat (*Yan Hou*, "Larynx and Pharynx," Popularly *Hou Yi*)

The deep level of the windings of the mouth; communicates with the esophagus and bronchi. (Ci Yuan, "Yan-hou")

*Same as **yan hou**. (Ci Yuan, "Yi")*

In general:

All sore throats: *(DACH)* seven moxas at *zhongkui* (MP-21, IS M-UE-16).
The five sore throats, swollen throat, painful: *(YIZ, 42r)*.
All illnesses of the throat: *(YIZ, 42r) fengfu* (GV-15, IS GV-16); *(DACH)* leg-*sanli* (ST-36).
For throat and lower pelvis: *(DACH) zhaohai* (KI-3, IS KI-6).

Sore throat, tonsillitis (hou bie; popularly, hou bi):

The word tonsillitis indicates an inflammation spreading to the tonsils, to the back of the throat, the pharynx and larynx. It is called *hou bie,* "paralysis of the larynx." The character *bie* is often changed erroneously into *bi,* "rheumatism," or *bi,* "closed." "This is chronic tonsillitis, *man xing bian tao xian yan. (Ci Yuan,* "Hou-bie" article)

> *Hou bie: bie, "paralyzed," this is bu ren, "without action." Popularly, it is written bi, "closed," which means sai, "closed." Fire commands swelling. The heat is established in the respiratory passages; the throat swells. (DACH XI, 12r)*

> *Name of an illness; pain and swelling of the pharynx and larynx, scarlet face and swelling of the cheek. At the extreme, the swelling spreads to the exterior. In the larynx, sensation as if there are lumps; even hot water is difficult to swallow; speech does not come out. Starts suddenly; aches, cold and hot. In the past it was said to come from an abundance of fire in the lungs and liver receiving wind and cold many times, which startle them. However, there are some which come from the vapors of alcohol in the two meridians of the heart and spleen-pancreas. These are called jiu tu hou bi, "alcoholic sore throat."*

> *(Ci Yuan, "Hou-bi" closure of the larynx article)*

Tonsillitis:

Hou bi: (DACH) hegu (LI-4), *guanchong* (TW-1), *sanjian* (LI-3), *yemen* (TW-2), *qiangu* (SI-2), *lieque* (LU-7), *tongli* (HT-5), *yangxi* (LI-5), *pianli* (LI-6), *wenliu* (LI-7), *rangu* (LI-2), *yongquan* (KI-1), leg-*xialian* (ST-39, IS *xiajuxu*), *yangfu* (GB-38), *xuanzhong* (GB-39), *lidui* (ST-45), *tianding* (LI-17), *fubai* (GB-16, IS GB-10), *tongziliao* (GB-1), *huagai* (CV-20), *zhongfu* (LU-1), *geshu* (BL-17).
Hou bie of old people: *(DACH IV, P. 14r) shaoshang* (LU-11), three moxas on the left for men and on the right for women.
Hou bie and swelling of the chin: *(DACH) shaoshang* (LU-11); of face: *yangjiao* (GB-35).
Hou bie, swelling of the bottom of the chin, pain in the back, shivering: *(YXRM) erjian* (LI-2).
Hou bie, sudden aphonia: *(DACH) fengleng* (ST-40).
Hou bie, energy in the upper body: *(DACH) chize* (LU-5).
Energy of *hou bie: (DACH) erjian* (LI-20), *chize* (LU-5).
Hou bie and tonsillitis *(ru e):* YIZ, 42) *shaoshang* (LU-11) 1 *fen, zhaohai* (KI-3, IS KI-6), *taichong* (LR-3) 3 *fen,* needle obliquely toward the back.
Hou bie, oppressed at the thought of death, cannot speak: *(DACH) quchi* (LI-11).
Hou bie, strangling: *(DACH) tiantu* (CV-22).
Hou bie, swelling of the throat, cannot breathe, food and drink not going down, singing in the larynx: *(DACH) tianding* (LI-17).
Hou bie (closure of the larynx): *(DACH VII, 33v, YIX,* 11v) zhaohai (KI-3, IS KI-6).

Catarrh of pharynx and larynx:

(JM) jianshi (PC-5), *sidu* (TW-9), *tianjing* (TW-10), *taixi* (KI-5, IS KI-3), *zhongdu* (LR-6), neck-*futu* (LI-18), *renying* (ST-9), *tianzhu* (BL-10), *fengchi* (GB-20), *danshu* (BL-19), *huagai* (CV-20), *tiantu* (CV-22).

Swelling of pharynx and larynx:

(JM) yamen (GV-14, IS GV-15), *tianzhu* (BL-10), *tianding* (LI-17), fengu (GV-14, IS GV-15), *lianquan* (CV-23), *shuitu* (ST-10), *qishe* (ST-11), *naohui* (TW-13), *rangu* (KI-2), *xiguan* (LR-7).
Swelling of the throat and chin: *(DACH) shaoshang* (LU-11).
Swelling and pruritis of the throat: hand-*zhongzhu* (TW-3).
Swelling of throat and heart: *(DACH IV, 10) taichong* (LR-3).

Pain in the throat, irritation:

(YXRM) Pain of the throat and pharynx: *laogong* (PC-8).
(DACH) Pain of pharynx and larynx: *xiguan* (LR-7).
(DACH) As if there were growths in the throat, neck contracted, tight: *ligou* (LR-5), *shaofu* (HT-8); *(DACH)* as if there were brambles in the throat; *(YIZ, 41v)* root of the throat: *tianrong* (SI-17).

(DACH) As if there were hard morsels in the throat; apoplexy, cannot pronounce a word: *jianshi* (PC-5).
(DACH) Swelling and pain in the throat: *fengfu* (GV-15, IS GV-16).

Contractions:

(DACH XI, 19r) Sensation as if a nut were going up and down in the throat and pharynx: several tens of moxas at *shanzhong* (CV-17), *qihai* (CV-6), leg-*sanli* (ST-36).
(YIZ, 42) Throat as if bound, bitter taste in mouth: *yanglingquan* (GB-34).
(JM) Contraction of the throat: *neiting* (ST-44); *(DACH) quepen* (ST-12).
(JM) Great difficulty in swallowing: *xiongxiang* (SP-19).

Dryness of the throat:

Dryness of pharynx and larynx: *(DACH, YXRM) pianli* (LI-6).
Dryness of throat, agitating thirst: *(DACH) xingjian* (LR-2).
Dryness of the throat, energy in the upper body: *(DACH) yongquan* (KI-1).
Dryness of the throat and pharynx: *(DACH) zhaohai* (KI-3, IS KI-6).

Abscess in the throat:

Abscess and swelling of the pharynx and larynx: *(DACH) shuitu* (ST-10), *renying* (ST-9).
Abscess of pharynx: *(YXRM)* foot-*tonggu* (BL-66); *(DACH) xuanji* (CV-21).
See also all abscesses: *shenmai* (BL-62), *xuehai* (SP-10), *shugu* (BL-65), *rangu* (KI-22), foot-*qiaoyin* (GB-44), *taichong* (LR-3), *fengmen* (BL-12).

XVI. Pharynx *(Yan, Yan Tou)*

In general:

(DACH) Illnesses and shocks in the pharynx: *zhaohai* (KI-3, IS KI-6).
(YIZ, 42r) All sore throats: *shaoshang* (LU-11), *fengfu* (GV-15, IS GV-16), leg-*sanli* (ST-36).
(DACH) The five sore throats: *zhaohai* (KI-3, IS KI-6).
(JM) Glossopharyngeal nerve (sensitivity of the mucosa and motor function of the pharynx): *tianshu* (BL-10).

Pains of the pharynx:

Pain of the pharynx: *(YXRM) yangxi* (LI-5); *(DACH) danshu* (BL-19); *(YXRM) neiting* (ST-44).
Pain of pharynx and throat: *(DACH) laogong* (PC-8).
Pain of the pharynx; muteness in storms: *(YXRM) tianchuang* (SI-16).
Pain of the pharynx, cannot eat food: *(DACH) yongquan* (LI-1).
As if there were brambles in the pharynx: *(DACH) sanjian* (LI-3).
Pain and swelling of the pharynx: *(DACH) fengfu* (GV-15, IS GV-16).

Inflammation, swelling of the pharynx:

Acute pharyngitis *(ji xing yan tou yan)*:

> *Origin: flu, measles, scarlet fever, whooping cough; or irritation from medicines, tobacco, alcohol; or laryngitis, rhinitis, etc. Symptoms: headache, head heavy, unaccustomed sensations of dryness and heat in the pharynx, pain upon swallowing, noisy coughing fits, progressively accumulating mucus, lymph nodes at the inferior maxillary angle swollen, painful. (JO, 60)*

Treatment with needles:

tianyou (TW-16)	*5 fen,*
shuitu (ST-10)	*4 fen,*
jiache (ST-3, IS ST-6)..................	*5 fen,*
tiantu (CV-22)	*5 fen,*

lianquan (CV-23) .... 5 *fen,*
fengchi (GB-20) .... 5 *fen,*
head-*wangu* (GB-17, IS GB-12) . 5 *fen,*
bailao (GV-13, IS GV-14 **dazhui**) 5 *fen,*
shangyang (LI-1) .... 1 *fen. (JO, 60)*

Treatment with moxa:

shangyang (LI-1)   5 *moxas,*
tianzhu (BL-10) ..   7 *moxas,*
fengchi (GB-20)..   7 *moxas,*
jianjing (GB-21) .   7 *moxas,*
lianquan (CV-22)   7 *moxas,*
sidu (TW-9).........   7 *moxas. (JO, 60)*

Chronic pharyngitis *(man xing yan tou yan):*

> Origins: for many, the sequelae of acute pharyngitis or sinusitis. Chronic fatty rhinitis, nasal blockage, difficulty breathing through the nose; tobacco, alcohol, dust, dryness. Irritation from inhaled particles, excess heat from drink, abuse of speech or singing, troubles of the stomach or intestines. Symptoms: in the area of the pharynx, dryness and redness of the posterior surface of the pharynx, phlegm and mucus; when coughing, redness of the face and tears. (JO, 61)

Treatment with needles:

tiantu (CV-22) .... 5 *fen,*
tianyou (TW-16) .... 5 *fen,*
shuitu (ST-10) .... 4 *fen,*
fengchi (GB-20) .... 7 *fen,*
head-*wangu* (GB-17, IS GB-12) . 5 *fen,*
bailao (GV-13, IS GV-14 **dazhui**) 5 *fen,*
lianquan (CV-23) .... 5 *fen,*
jiache (ST-3, IS ST-6).................. 5 *fen,*
shangyang (LI-1) .... 1 *fen. JO, 61)*

Treatment with moxa:

shangyang (LI-1)   5 *moxas,*
tianzhu (BL-10) ..   7 *moxas,*
fengchi (GB-20)..   7 *moxas,*
jianjing (GB-21) .   7 *moxas,*
lianquan (CV-23)   7 *moxas,*
sidu (TW-9).........   7 *moxas. (JO, 61)*

Swelling of the pharynx: *(DACH)* hand-*zhongzhu* (TW-3); *(YXRM)* *qiangu* (SI-2); *(YXRM)* *naohui* (TW-13); *(DACH)* *tiantu* (CV-22); *(YXRM, DACH)* *taixi* (KI-5, IS KI-3); *(DACH VII, 31r; YIX)* foot-*linqi* (GB-41).
Swelling of pharynx and internal headache: *(DACH)* *kongzui* (LU-6).
Swelling of the pharynx, liquids do not pass: *huagai* (CV-20).
Swelling of pharynx, cannot swallow saliva and sometimes cannot get it out: *(DACH)* *rangu* (KI-2).
Swelling of pharynx that does not go away: *(DACH)* *qishe* (ST-11).
As if there were brambles in the pharynx, food and drink not passing: *(DACH)* *sanjian* (LI-3).
Difficulty in swallowing: *(DACH)* *chengman* (ST-20).
Pharyngitis (catarrh of the pharynx): *(JM)* *qishe* (ST-11), *renying* (ST-9).
External swelling of the pharynx as if there were growths inside: *(YIZ, 40)* *yemen* (TW-2).
As if there were appearances of growths in the pharynx: *(DACH)* *sidu* (TW-9).
See also Inflammation of the Throat.

Dryness of the pharynx:

See also Dryness of the Throat and Mouth.
Dryness of pharynx: *(DACH) shenmen* (HT-7), *taiyuan* (LU-9), *pianli* (LI-6).
Pharynx, throat dry: *(DACH) zhaohai* (KI-3, IS KI-6).

Abscess of the pharynx:

See also Abscesses of Throat and All Kinds of Abscesses.
Abscess of pharynx: *(DACH) tonggu* (BL-66); *(DACH) xuanji* (CV-21).

XVII. Thirst *(Ke)*

(See also Diabetes, Alcoholism, Dry Mouth.) Hemorrhages produce thirst, as does heavy sweat.
Thirst of mouth: *(YXRM I, 46v) jianshi* (PC-5), *(YXRM) yinbai* (SP-1).
Thirst of mouth, emptiness of blood: *(YIX I, 4v) shaoshang* (LU-11), *quze* (PC-3).
Agitating thirst: *(DACH) laogong* (PC-8), and mouth dry: *quze* (PC-3), *jiquan* (HT-1), and throat dry: *xingjian* (LR-2), *(JM) xuanlu* (GB-5), *shenzhu* (GV-11, IS GV-12), *daju* (ST-27).
Drinks a lot: *(DACH) gongsun* (SP-4).
Habitual thirst: *(YXRM) laogong* (PC-8); *(DACH) zizheng* (SI-7), *yongquan* (KI-1); *(DACH, YXRM) taichong* (LR-3).
Ability to drink, dryness of pharynx and throat: *(YXRM) zhongfeng* (LR-4).
Delights in drinking: *(DACH) zhourong* (SP-20) and heat of the belly; *(YXRM) zhongwan* (CV-12).
Drinks too much water: *(DACH) tianshu* (ST-25).
Drinks without being able to quench the thirst: *(DACH III, 33r) zhaohai* (KI-3, IS KI-6), diabetes.
Intense thirst, diabetes: *(DACH) shuigou* (GV-25, IS GV-26 *renzhong*).
Agitation of the heart, at the extreme, desire for cold drinks: *(DACH) shenmen* (HT-7).
Thirst, if he drinks he sweats; if he does not drink, skin dry: *(DACH) quchi* (LI-11).

XVIII. Esophagus *(She Dao)*

In general:

(JM) Esophagus: *shufu* (KI-27), *yuzhong* (KI-26), *geshu* (BL-17), *weishu* (BL-21).

Inflammation of the esophagus (she dao yan), esophagitis:

Origin: from ingestion of chemical substances, or from utensils; or from spicy foods; or catarrh of throat or stomach, measles, smallpox, scarlet fever. Symptoms: the problem increases during sleep or during the passage of food. Upon swallowing, and during downward passage, one feels an acute, sometimes burning pain behind the sternum. It is difficult to swallow. (JO, 13)

Treatment with needles:

yingchuang (ST-16)	5 *fen,*
wuyi (ST-15)	5 *fen,*
geshu (BL-17)	5 *fen.* *(JO, 13)*

Treatment with moxa:

xinshu (BL-15)	7 *moxas,*
geshu (BL-17)	7 *moxas.* *(JO, 13)*

Dilated esophagus:

If on an X-ray the esophagus presents a dilated, enlarged pocket, acupuncture can do nothing. The most it can do is to relax the spasm of the cardiac sphincter, which is generally the cause.

Esophagism, spasm of the esophagus (she dao jing lman):

Spasms of the esophagus:

Treatment with needles and moxa:

tianzhu (BL-10)	*5 fen,* 8 moxas,
fengchi (GB-20)	*5 fen,* 8 moxas,
jianzhong (SI-15)	*5 fen,* 8 moxas,
jianwai (SI-14)	*5 fen,* 8 moxas,
jianjing (GB-21)	*5 fen,* 8 moxas,
tianchi (PC-1)	*5 fen to 1 cun,* 8 moxas,
thorax-*qimen (LR-14)*	*5 fen to 1 cun,* 8 moxas,
riyue (GB-24)	*5 fen to 1 cun,* 8 moxas,
ganshu (BL-18)	*5 fen to 1 cun,* 8 moxas,
arm-*sanli (LI-10)*	*3 fen,* 8 moxas,
hegu (LI-4)	*3 fen,* 8 moxas. *(JM, 315)*

Spasms of the esophagus, counterflow of food, vomiting: *(JM) jingqu* (LU-8).
Spasms of the esophagus: *(JM) renying* (ST-9), *geguan* (BL-41, IS BL-46), *zigong* (CV-19).
Nervous spasms of the esophagus: *(JM) zhongshu* (GV-6a, IS GV-7).

Narrowed, contracted esophagus; esophagospasm (she dao jie zhai):

Origin: purulent irritation of the esophagus; ingestion by mistake of hard objects or false teeth; swelling of the thyroid gland; arterial tumors pressing on the esophagus from outside; cancer of the esophagus, etc. Symptoms: difficulty in swallowing and making the food descend; attacks of vomiting, blockage of the food at an exact point in the esophagus. If the narrowing is serious, even liquids no longer go through. (JO, 14)

Treatment with needles:

geshu (BL-17)	*5 fen,*
bishu (BL-20)	*5 fen,*
yingchuang (ST-16)	*5 fen,*
wuyi (ST-15)	*5 fen. (JO, 14)*

Treatment with moxa:

shaoshang (LU-11)	5 moxas,
gongsun (SP-4)	5 moxas,
zigong (CV-19)	5 moxas,
xinshu (BL-15)	10 moxas,
geshu (BL-17)	10 moxas. *(JO, 14)*

(JM) erjian (LI-2), *zhongkui* (MP-21, IS M-UE-16), *shaoshang* (LU-11), *dazhong* (KI-6, IS KI-4), *xuanji* (CV-21), *zigong* (CV-19), *shanzhong* (CV-17), *zhongting* (CV-16), *zhourong* (SP-20), *xiongxiang* (SP-19), *xinshu* (BL-15), *geshu* (BL-17), *danshu* (BL-19), *geguan* (BL-41, IS BL-46), *pishu* (BL-20), *hunmen* (BL-42, IS BL-47).

Ge ye, "suffocation of the diaphragm":

Ye is closure of the pharynx; ge is closure of the stomach. Food does not go down, digestion cannot take place. Atrophy (ku) of the first warmer: food does not descend; as soon as the patient is able to vomit, the pain stops; atrophy of the second warmer; the food goes in but does not come out; atrophy of the third warmer: food, vomited twelve hours later. (YXRM V, 18v)

The three yang bound, this is ge. (YXRM V, 18v)

Ge ye: (DACH) *gaohuangshu* (BL-38, IS BL-43).
The five *ye:* (DACH) *tiantu* (CV-22), *zhongkui* (MP-21, IS M-UE-16).
Energy of *ye: tiantu* (CV-22), *shanzhong* (CV-17).
Ye, obstructing; *(YXRM) tiantu* (CV-22), *zhongting* (CV-16).

Ye, vomiting: *(YXRM I, 46v) sanyinjiao* (SP-6).

Ye, acute pain of the epigastrium and abdomen: *(DACH VII, 32v) lieque* (LU-7).

Ye, in the pharynx there is much suffocation, cannot make the food go down: *(YXRM) dazhong* (KI-6, IS KI-4), tonify.

Ye of food: *(DACH) rugen* (ST-18).

Ye in the chest, melancholia: *(DACH) geguan* (BL-41, IS BL-46).

Food or drink not descending:

Food not descending: *(DACH)* leg-*sanli* (ST-36), *danshu* (BL-19).

Food not descending; vomiting: *(DACH) yinbai* (SP-1), *(DACH)* and the body is warm: *sanjiaoshu* (BL-22).

Food and drink not descending: *zhongting* (CV-16); *(DACH, YXRM) zhongfu* (LU-1); *(DACH) chengman* (ST-20); *(DACH, YXRM) zigong* (CV-19); *(DACH) qimen* of thorax (LR-14), *youmen* (KI-21), *xuanji* (CV-21), *zhourong* (SP-20), *shufu* (KI-27), *laogong* (PC-8), *shaoshang* (LU-11), *weicang* (BL-45, IS BL-50), *yishe* (BL-44, IS BL-49), *yanggang* (BL-43, IS BL-48), *geguan* (BL-41, IS BL-46), *hunmen* (BL-42, IS BL-47).

Great difficulty in swallowing: *(JM) xiongxiang* (SP-19).

Food and drink does not go in: *(DACH) zhongwan* (CV-12).

XIX. Diaphragm *(Ge)*

Harmonizes the diaphragm: *(DACH) zhongwan* (CV-12).

Pains of the diaphragm: *(DACH) shidou* (SP-17).

Thunderous sounds in the interval of the diaphragm; there is always the noise of water: *(DACH, YXRM) shidou* (SP-17).

Inflammation of the diaphragm: *(JO) shaochong* (HT-9).

Swelling of the diaphragm (fullness of the secondary vessels: *(DACH) tongli* (HT-5).

Useless diaphragm: *(DACH) juque* (CV-14).

Agitation of the diaphragm: *(YXRM I, 46v) gaohuangshu* (BL-38, IS BL-43).

Spasms of the diaphragm (hiccoughs):

> *From insufficiency or emptiness of yin, bluish face, weakness of stomach and spleen-pancreas after an illness. Women have it after delivery, at night. If it is from a yang excess, there is great anger; it follows a feast; chills with fever; these are easy to cure. (JM)*

(JM) taixi (KI-5, IS KI-3), *qishe* (ST-11), *qihu* (ST-13), *riyue* (GB-24), *juque* (CV-14), *jianli* (CV-11).

Hiccoughs *(e ni),* sometimes caused by a dilation of the stomach:

(YXRM I, 46v) Agitation of the diaphragm; *(DACH XI, 14r; YXRM I, 46v; YIX I, 2v)* hiccoughs: *gaohuangshu* (BL-38, IS BL-43).

(GSdeM) Hiccoughs: *zhongwan* (CV-12) and from cerebellar troubles: arm-*shanglian* (LI-9), disperse.

Counterflow when eating; hiccoughs: *shangqiu* (KI-17).

The C4/C5 interval is the origin of the phrenic nerve.

XX. Epigastrium *(Xin Fu)*

In general:

Illnesses of epigastrium: *(YIX I, 9v) gongsun* (SP-4), *lieque* (LU-7).

Pains of the epigastrium:

Pains attacking the epigastrium: *(YXRM) tianshu* (ST-25).

Pains in the hollow of the stomach: *(JM) dadu* (SP-2), *taibai* (SP-3).

Pains in front portion of the stomach; saddening food: *(DACH) zhongfeng* (LR-4).

Pains of the epigastrium and sides: *(DACH) fushe* (SP-13).

Epigastrium painful, firm, hard: *(YXRM) shimen* (CV-5).

Contracture of the epigastrium:

Stiffness of the epigastric muscles *(JM) chengman* (ST-20).

Cold or emptiness:

Cold or emptiness of the epigastrium: *(JM) yinlingquan* (SP-9).
Cold, emptiness or ballooning of the epigastrium and umbilicus: *(JM) dadun* (LR-1).

Swelling:

See Aerogastria.
Tonify *gongsun* (SP-4), disperse *youmen* (KI-21).
Swelling and fullness of the epigastrium: *(DACH) sanyinjiao* (SP-6), *xuanzhong* (GB-39).
Fullness and pain of the epigastrium: *(DACH) tinggong* (SI-19).
Fullness and congestion of the pancreas *(bi man): (YXRM I, 39v) yinlingquan* (SP-9), on the right.
Swelling and fullness of epigastrium: *(DACH) lidui* (ST-45).
Swelling and fullness of the epigastrium: *(DACH).* Swollen drum in the epigastrium; *(YXRM)* leg-*sanli* (ST-36).
Swollen drum in epigastrium and pain of the sides: *(DACH) qihai* (CV-6).
Swelling and pain under the heart, energy in the upper body *(DACH)* arm-*wuli* (LI-13).
Counterflow of energy rising and pinching the epigastrium, cannot breathe: *(DACH) qichong* (ST-30).
Interior contracted: *(DACH) youmen* (KI-21).

XXI. Stomach *(Wei)*

Although the stomach is a yang workshop organ, the energy which it extracts from food, thus from the earth, is yin: it is the original energy, upon which everything depends. (See Volume III, leg-*sanli*, ST-36). The stomach is a workshop organ, yang, linked to the spleen-pancreas treasure organ, which is yin. Flow of energy: large intestine, stomach, spleen-pancreas. The energy here is at its maximum from 7 to 9 a.m. and from April to May. In correspondence, the heart governor has its maximum from 7 to 9 p.m. Feelings injure the stomach; it is possible to tonify the stomach through joy, activity, mildness.

The meridian (zu yangming).

Insufficiency of energy (particularly in November):

The stomach pulse is soft, small, without shape or absent. If it is swollen, big or long, there is ballooning, aerogastria and somnolence after a meal.
Physical symptoms: swelling of the stomach after meals, slow digestion, belching, gas; face and eyes empty, superficial; cold feet after meals.
Psychological symptoms: hates people, wants to be alone, door closed, near the window, jerks at the least noise, dreams of abundant meals, of eating and drinking or being hungry.
By the main meridian: tonify *jiexi* (ST-41) and the source point *chongyang* (ST-42).
By the herald point: tonify *zhongwan* (CV-12).
By the circulation of energy: tonify large intestine (the mother who feeds): *quchi* (LI-11); tonify the child who suckles (spleen- pancreas); foot-*dadu* (SP-2).
Coupled yin organ: tonify the spleen-pancreas: foot-*dadu* (SP-2).
By the passage point: tonify *gongsun* (SP-4), spleen to stomach, if there is aerogastria; *fenglong* (ST-40) if spleen-pancreas is abundant.
By the midday-midnight correspondence: stomach, maximum 7-9 a.m.; pericardium, maximum 7-9 p.m.; tonify *zhongchong* (PC-9).
By husband-wife: regulate the gallbladder: *qiuxu* (GB-40).

Excess energy (particularly in May):

If the pulse of the stomach is hard and small: stomach cramps; hard and big: inflammation of the stomach; hard and sharp, along with the small intestine pulse: pyloric spasm; ample and firm without hardness indicates a good appetite and rapid digestion.
Physical symptoms: lips and mouth dry, yellow complexion, swelling and pain of the armpit, cramps, pains, acidity, burning.
Psychological symptoms: nightmares, lassitude, heaviness, sad and sharp visions with people and things, impatience.
By the main meridian: disperse *lidui* (ST-45) and the source point, *chongyang* (ST-42).
By the association point: disperse *weishu* (BL-21).
By the circulation of energy: disperse the large intestine (the mother who feeds), *sanjian* (LI-3); disperse spleen-pancreas (the child who suckles), *shangqiu* (SP-5).

By the coupled yin treasure organ: spleen-pancreas, *shangqiu* (SP-5).

By the passage point: disperse *fenglong* (ST-40) stomach to spleen-pancreas.

By the midday-midnight correspondence: stomach maximum 7-9 a.m.; pericardium maximum 7-9 p.m.; disperse *daling* (PC-7) during the night, rain and cold (yin).

By husband-wife: disperse the gallbladder, *yangfu* (GB-38).

(GSdeM) Disperse the pancreas (right *shangqiu,* SP-5), and small intestine, *xiaohai* (SI-8).

In general.

Master points of the stomach: *(DACH) zhongwan* (CV-12), *xiawan* (CV-10), *weishu* (BL-21).

Stomach: *(JM) shufu* (KI-27), *yuzhong* (KI-26), *shencang* (KI-25), *lingxu* (KI-24), *shenfeng* (KI-23), *bulang* (KI-22), *tianshu* (ST-25), *xinshu* (BL-15), *ganshu* (BL-18), *weishu* (BL-21), *sanjiaoshu* (BL-22).

Illnesses of the stomach: *(DACH) chengman* (ST-20); *(JM) tianzhu* (BL-10), *dushu* (BL-16), *pishu* (BL-20).

(YXRM) Decline of the stomach: leg-*sanli* (ST-36).

Inflammatory illnesses of the stomach: *(JM) taiyin* (ST-23), *huaroumen* (ST-24).

(DACH) Joy, malcontentment, worries, fear can block the function of the stomach: leg-*sanli* (ST-36); however, joy also can activate the stomach.

Lower esophageal sphincter: *(JM) shangwan* (CV-13), *yutang* (CV-18).

Pyloric sphincter: *(JM) youmen* (KI-21), *zhongting* (CV-16).

(YXRM V, 34v) Pyloric sphincter: *youmen* (KI-21).

> Food and drink are able to leave the stomach through the pyloric sphincter. Indeed, when they have stayed for a long time in the stomach, they come out through the pyloric sphincter which is linked to the stomach. It is through this passage that the food and drink go into the small intestine. When its action is blocked by **lanmen,** ''screen gate'' of the lower warmer (ileocecal valve), the morning meal is vomited at night; the nighttime meal is vomited at dawn. The **lanmen** is below the umbilicus; it is the grill and the knot distributing liquids or solids between the bladder and large intestine.

Stomach and abdomen not harmonious, cannot eat: *(DACH) xiawan* (CV-10).

All chronic illnesses of the stomach and intestines: *(JM) tianshu* (ST-25), *sanyinjiao* (SP-6).

Internal trouble of the stomach and spleen-pancreas: *(YXRM I, 46r) pishu* (BL-20), *tianshu* (ST-25).

Illnesses of the stomach, small intestine, liver and kidneys: *(DACH) weicang* (BL-45, IS BL-50).

When the energy of the stomach descends and the five energies of the intestines are troubled, stimulate *yuji* (LU-10) and *shenmen* (HT-7).

Connections with the coupled treasure organ (yin), spleen and pancreas:

> When the stomach is the host and the spleen-pancreas is the guest: the abdomen collects melancholy of the heart; thoughts of sadness; detests people like fire, detests lamplight. If the ears hear a noise, the heart is agitated, anxious; epistaxis, lips are to the side, a return of tidal fever, throws off his clothes, heat on the body, abundant mucus, pain of the feet, abscesses, pruritis, expansion of the energy, chest and thighs painful, difficult to calm: **chongyang** (ST-42), source point of the stomach and **gongsun** (SP-4), passage point from spleen-pancreas to the stomach.

> When the spleen-pancreas is the host and the stomach is the guest: stiffness of the root of the tongue, vomiting, pain and upset of the stomach, the energy of the intestines rises and obstructs; sighs, difficult to calm, pruritis, body hot, spleen-pancreas agitating the heart, no appetite, paludism, hidden icterus, palms hot, internal surface of the thigh and knee swollen and painful: **taibai** (SP-3), source point of the spleen-pancreas, and **fenglong** (ST-40), passage point from the stomach to the spleen-pancreas. (DACH VII, 21v)

Troubles of the stomach meridian:

> When this meridian is ill, there are cramps of the second toe and on the anterolateral surface of the leg, arch of the foot; stiffness and swelling in front of the hip joint; emaciation, spasms, contractions of the muscles of the abdomen up to the cheek with tightened mouth. If there are contractions, the eyes are not coordinated. If there is heat, the eyes do not open, the muscles are relaxed. If there is cold of the jaw and shoulder, there is contraction up to the jaw. If the mouth is hot, the muscles are slow, not obeying. (DACH XI, 12)

Illnesses of the energy of the stomach:

> When the stomach is troubled, Li Gao [Dongyuan, twelfth century] advises:
> Bad digestion from emptiness: tonify leg-**sanli** (ST-36).

*Bad digestion from fullness: disperse leg-sanli (ST-36) and **qichong** (ST-30).*

*If the excess energy comes from the heart: disperse **shenmen** (HT-7) and **daling** (PC-7).*

*If the energy comes from the liver: disperse **yuji** (LU-10) and **taiyuan** (LU-9) [Perhaps a mistake? Comes from the lungs?]*

*If the energy is in the intestines: disperse **tianzhu** (BL-10), **dazhu** (BL-11), also **tonggu** (BL-66), **shugu** (BL-65).*

*If the energy is in the arm and the feet; disperse **erjian** (LI-2), **sanjian** (LI-3), **neiting** (ST-44), **xiangu** (ST-43). (DACH XI, 10v)*

Insufficiency of stomach energy.

(Lack of appetite, aerogastria, slow digestion, weakness of stomach, cold of stomach, hyposecretion, muscular atony of the stomach, indigestion, dilation of the stomach, ptosis.)

Lack of appetite:

Lack of appetite in babies: *(DACH, YXRM)* tonify *xuanzhong* (GB-39); *(GSdeM)* leg-*sanli* (ST-36).

Does not desire food: *(DACH)* guanchong (TW-1); *(DACH)* xuanzhong (GB-39), chongyang (ST-42), taixi (KI-5, IS KI-3), diji (SP-8), burong (ST-19), bulang (KI-22), jianli (CV-11), guanmen (ST-22); *(DACH, YXRM)* shangqiu (KI-17); *(DACH)* weidao (GB-30, IS GB-28), feishu (BL-13).

Does not desire food; face swollen (inflammation of the stomach): *(YXRM I, 39v)* lidui (ST-45).

Does not desire to eat, fullness: *(DACH)* youmen (KI-21), shimen (CV-5).

Even though starved, does not desire food: *(DACH)* yongquan (KI-1).

Appetite diminished: *(JM)* guanchong (TW-1), zhongkui (MP-21, IS M-UE-16), shenmen (HT-7), gongsun (SP-4), chongyang (ST-42), sanyinjiao (SP-6), diji (SP-8), zhongfeng (LR-4), leg-*sanli* (ST-36), leg-*xialian* (ST-39, IS xiajuxu), zhongwan (CV-12), guanmen (ST-22), liangmen (ST-21), xiawan (CV-10), shufu (KI-27), shencang (KI-25), lingxu (KI-24), bulang (KI-22), weidao (GB-30, IS GB-28), shenfeng (KI-23), shuifen (CV-9), zhiyang (GV-8, IS GV-9), yanggang (BL-43, IS BL-48), yishe (BL-44, IS BL-49), jizhong (GV-6), geshu (BL-17).

Illness of emptiness, cannot eat: *(YIX I, 7v; DACH IV, 10v)* neiting (ST-44).

No taste for food: *(DACH)* neiting (ST-44).

Raging hunger: bleed *rangu* (KI-2).

Is not pleased by food: *(DACH)* tianjing (TW-10).

Does not think about food and drink: *(DACH, YXRM)* liangmen (ST-21).

Emaciation, can neither drink nor eat: *(DACH)* sanjiaoshu (BL-22).

Does not eat: *(YXRM)* shanzhong (CV-17), geshu (BL-17), ganshu (BL-18).

Does not eat; if he eats, then pain: *(YXRM)* geshu (BL-17).

Does not eat; heat in the stomach: *(DACH X, 26r)* leg-*xialian* (ST-39, IS xiajuxu).

Does not eat, attacked by cold: *(DACH)* chongyang (ST-42).

Without strength, does not eat: *(YXRM)* juque (CV-14).

Swelling and fullness which prevents eating: *(DACH)* zhongwan (CV-12).

Habitual hunger, but cannot eat: *(YXRM I, 46)* weishu (BL-21); *(DACH, YXRM)* zhongji (CV-3).

Saddening food, pain in the umbilicus; *(DACH)* zhongfeng (LR-4).

Detests smelling the odor of food: *(DACH)* leg-*sanli* (ST-36).

Aerogastria (ben tun):

(See abdominal swelling, wei zhang; aerocolia, xin fu gu zhang).

In aerogastria, the painful swelling of the stomach is produced either after eating or suddenly at night. There is no reflex of swallowing air as in aerophagia. It stops at an altitude of 800 meters, through hyperglobulinemia.

> *Bursting in the lower abdomen and rising up under the heart, jumping from here to there like a white pig (**tun**), now up and now down with no fixed duration. If not cured for a long time, it causes people to have attacks of panting, bone paresis, little energy. (DACH I, 16v)*

Aerogastria (stomach balloons after eating, or sudden attack of swelling at night): tonify *gongsun* (SP-4); chronic cases: tonify *gaohuangshu* (BL-38, IS BL-43) which increases the blood cells; disperse *youmen* (KI-21), which opens the pyloric sphincter.

Sudden swelling of the abdomen; when pressing it does not go in; pain and coldness of the energy below the umbilicus; sudden swelling of the epigastrium: *qihai* (CV-6).

Throbbing pain of epigastrium; accumulated wind; obstruction from energy: *(DACH VII, 26v)* neiguan (PC-6), laogong (PC-8), arm-*sanli* (LI-10), fengmen (BL-12), shanzhong (CV-17).

Swelling and fullness from the umbilicus to the heart; fits of eructation, malaise, coldness of the lower warmer: moxa at *zhangmen* (LR-13) and *qihai* (CV-6).

Air which rises up is generated in the stomach: *(DACH X, 14v) zhongwan* (CV-12).

Swollen drum in the epigastrium: *(DACH)* leg-*sanli* (ST-36).

Ben tun: (DACH) abdomen-*yinjiao* (CV-7), *qihai* (CV-6), *qixue* (KI-13), *siman* (KI-14), *qichong* (ST-30), *zhangmen* (LR-13), *shangwan* (CV-13), *tianshu* (ST-25), *yinlingquan* (SP-9).

(YXRM I, 46v) Expansion of the energy in women; *(DACH)* swollen drum, emptiness of the secondary vessel from the spleen-pancreas to the stomach: tonify *gongsun* (SP-4).

(DACH IV, 10r; YIX I, 7v) Swelling of the epigastrium, all types of swelling from energy: leg-*sanli* (ST-36).

(YXRM I, 40v) Swelling and fullness of the abdomen and sides: *yinlingquan* (SP-9).

(DACH, YXRM) Aerogastria, accumulation in the heart, eructations: *shangwan* (CV-13).

(YXRM) After reading a book, energy of aerogastria: *zhongwan* (CV-12).

(DACH, YXRM) Swelling of the stomach: *xiawan* (CV-10).

(YXRM I, 40v) Swollen drum of the abdomen and umbilicus; *(DACH)* aerogastria; *(YXRM)* swelling of the abdomen, energy rising to assail the chest: *tianshu* (ST-25).

(DACH III, 31r) Aerogastria piercing the heart: *zhongji* (CV-3).

(DACH) Aerogastria, heart pierced; *(YXRM)* aerogastria, energy coming into the lower abdomen: *guanyuan* (CV-4), *guilai* (ST-29).

(JM) Epigastrium swollen and ballooned: *youmen* (KI-21).

(YXRM) Swelling and fullness of the abdomen, cannot breathe: *luoque* (BL-8).

(DACH) Pain from aerogastria, aerogastria piercing the heart; *(YXRM)* energy of aerogastria rising from the abdomen, epigastrium full and hard: *shimen* (CV-5).

(YXRM) Aerogastria, pain in the abdomen; *(DACH)* aerogastria rising and descending: *siman* (KI-14).

Aerophagia (reflex of swallowing air):

(GSdeM) dadun (LR-1), *taichong* (LR-3), *tianjing* (TW-10).

● *Digestion slow or stopped (slow digestion, bad digestion):*

Slow digestion:

➤ *(GSdeM)* Tonify *jiexi* (ST-41) and leg-*sanli* (ST-36).

Food is not digested: *(DACH) taibai* (SP-3), foot-*shangqiu* (SP-5), *zhangmen* (LR-13), epigastrium-*tonggu* (KI-20), *dachangshu* (BL-25), *baohuang* (BL-48, IS BL-53).

Cereals not digested, not being transformed: *(DACH) xiawan* (CV-10); *(YXRM)* cereals and food not digested: *xiawan* (CV-10); *(DACH, YXRM) liangmen* (ST-21).

Cereals and liquids not digested: *(DACH) sanjiaoshu* (BL-22); *(DACH, YXRM) xuanshu* (GV-5), *baohuang* (BL-48, IS BL-53), *weicang* (BL-45, IS BL-50).

Accumulation *(zheng)* of food: *(DACH) pishu* (BL-20); accumulation in the stomach: *xuanji* (CV-21).

Digests with difficulty, accumulation in the sides: *(DACH) neiguan* (PC-6).

Food squeezed, not passing: *chengshan* (BL-57).

Eats without digesting: *(DACH, YXRM) ganshu* (BL-18), *sanjiaoshu* (BL-22).

Food going down with difficulty and not being digested: *(YXRM) danshu* (BL-19).

Difficult digestion: *(DACH)* leg-*shanglian* (ST-37, IS *shangjuxu*).

Bad digestion:

> *Bad digestion of a nervous nature. Origin: neurasthenia, hysteria, tobacco, anemia, illness or trouble of the genital system or lungs. Symptoms: eructation, agitation of the stomach, nausea, vomiting, swelling and fullness of the stomach area with heaviness, headache, vertigo, bitter melancholia in the pit of the stomach, palpitations, insomnia; suppression of worries and of the personality. (JO, 25)*

Treatment with needles:

zhongwan (CV-12)	*8 fen,*
liangmen (ST-21)	*8 fen,*
tianshu (ST-25)	*8 fen,*
daheng (SP-15)	*8 fen,*
abdomen-yinjiao (CV-7)	*8 fen,*
qihai (CV-6)	*8 fen,*
guanyuan (CV-4)	*1 cun,*
youmen (KI-21)	*6 fen,*

pishu (BL-20) .... *8 fen,*
sanjiaoshu (BL-22) .... *8 fen,*
leg-sanli (ST-36) .... *1 cun. (JO, 25)*

Treatment with moxa:

gaohuangshu (BL-38, IS BL-43)   *10 moxas,*
geshu (BL-17) .... *10 moxas,*
pishu (BL-20) .... *10 moxas,*
sanjiaoshu (BL-22) .... *10 moxas,*
tianshu (ST-25) .... *10 moxas,*
xiawan (CV-10) .... *10 moxas,*
guanyuan (CV-4) .... *10 moxas,*
leg-sanli (ST-36) .... *10 moxas. (JO, 25)*

Bad digestion of a nervous nature:

Treatment with needles and moxa:

tianzhu (BL-10) .... *2 to 5 fen, 8 moxas,*
fengchi (GB-20) .... *2 to 5 fen, 8 moxas,*
pishu (BL-20) .... *1 to 2 cun, 8 moxas,*
sanjiaoshu (BL-22) .... *1 to 2 cun, 8 moxas,*
yishe (BL-44, IS BL-49)......... *1 to 2 cun, 8 moxas,*
weicang (BL-45, IS BL-50).... *1 to 2 cun, 8 moxas,*
huangmen (BL-46, IS BL-51) *1 to 2 cun, 8 moxas. (JM, 315)*

(DACH XI, 10v) Bad digestion from emptiness: tonify; bad digestion from fullness: disperse *ligou* (LR-5), leg-*sanli* (ST-36).

Bad digestion *(JM):* taibai (SP-3), shangqiu (SP-5), yinlingquan (SP-9), leg-*sanli* (ST-36), fuai (SP-16), zhongwan (CV-12), xiawan (CV-10), jianli (CV-11), shimen (CV-5), tonggu (KI-20), daheng (SP-15), zhangmen (LR-13), chengman (ST-20), qishe (ST-11), weishu (BL-21), pishu (BL-20), hunmen (BL-42, IS BL-47), yishe (BL-44, IS BL-49), zhishi (BL-47, IS BL-52), sanjiaoshu (BL-22), yanggang (BL-43, IS BL-48).

Fullness of the stomach, diaphragm heavy after meals, weighing on the stomach: *gongsun* (SP-4).

Vertigo after meals: *(DACH) weishu* (BL-21).

Weakness of stomach (or emptiness of spleen-pancreas and stomach):

Emptiness of spleen-pancreas and stomach *(wei pi xu):*

> *Name of an illness, it is also called weakness of the stomach **(wei juan).** It is a laziness in the stomach, bad diges-*
> *tion; little by little the vital strength diminishes; headache, body tired, sometimes feels bored and satiated, attacks*
> *of eructation, nausea or vomiting. (Ci Yuan, ''Wei-bi xu'')*

(DACH) Emptiness and weakness of the stomach and spleen-pancreas *(wei bi xu juan);* troubles from humidity, becomes paresis; perspiration, great diarrhea, avoids food: bled leg-*sanli* (ST-36) and *qichong* (ST-30). If sweat does not stop, bleed leg-*sanli* (ST-36) and leg-*xialian* (ST-39, IS *xiajuxu*); avoid wine and sticky pastries.

Emptiness of energy of the stomach: *(DACH) zhongchong* (PC-9), *jiexi* (ST-41).

Coldness of the stomach (wei han).

(DACH IV, 10v) Stomach cold: tonify leg-*sanli* (ST-36); *(DACH IV, 7v; YIX I, 5v)* stomach cold: *xiawan* (CV-10).

Extreme coldness of the stomach *(JM).* Energy of the stomach cold *(DACH): zhiyang* (GV-8, IS GV-9).

Cold of stomach with mucus, stopping of the digestion, food and drink not descending: *(DACH XI, 11v) geshu* (BL-17).

Cold and emptiness of the stomach: *(JM) shangqu* (KI-17), *huangshu* (KI-16), *fuai* (SP-16).

Weakness of the stomach: *(JM)* thorax-*qimen* (LR-14), *weishu* (BL-21), *pishu* (BL-20), *yishe* (BL-44, IS BL-49), *shuifen* (CV-9).

Emptiness and weakness of stomach and spleen-pancreas: *sanyinjiao* (SP-6).

Emptiness and weakness of stomach and intestines: *(DACH) shuifen* (CV-9).

Hyposecretion (stomach juices empty and tired):

(JM): burong (ST-19).

Eats a lot, thin body: *(DACH) weishu* (BL-21), *pishu* (BL-20), *dachangshu* (BL-25).

Eats without assimilating; thin: *tianshu* (ST-25).

Food and drink form neither flesh nor skin: *(DACH, YXRM)* lougu (SP-7).

Thinness of children, not forming flesh: *(DACH)* weishu (BL-21).

Food entering but not digested: *(DACH)* shimen (CV-5).

Fears cold food and sexual fatigue: *(DACH)* changqiang (GV-1).

Muscular atony of the stomach (wei jin zhang li shuai ruan):

Origin: difficult digestion, ptosis of the stomach, stomach ulcers, chronic gastritis, sequelae of narrowing of eso-phagus, swelling or ulcers of the intestines, gallstones; also nervous troubles of hysteria. Symptoms: ballooning of the stomach; decrease of appetite; eructations; headaches; vertigo; sometimes comes with asthma from difficult digestion; the sound of water is heard on percussion. (JO)

Treatment with needles:

juque (CV-14)	*6 fen,*
riyue (GB-24)	*6 fen,*
shangwan (CV-13)	*1 cun,*
liangmen (ST-21) ..	*1 cun,*
taiyin (ST-23)	*1 cun,*
zhongwan (CV-12)	*1 cun,*
tianshu (ST-25)	*1 cun,*
leg-sanli (ST-36) ...	*1 cun. (JO)*

Treatment with moxa:

shangwan (CV-13)	*10 moxas,*
xiawan (CV-10)	*10 moxas,*
guanmen (ST-22) ..	*10 moxas,*
riyue (GB-24)	*10 moxas,*
leg-sanli (ST-36) ...	*10 moxas,*
geshu (BL-17)	*15 moxas,*
ganshu (BL-18)	*15 moxas,*
pishu (BL-20)	*15 moxas. (JO)*

Indigestion (shi ji):

Accumulations of food from internal shock and congestion of the spleen-pancreas: *(YXRM I, 40r)* arm-*sanli* (LI-10).

Accumulation in the stomach: *(DACH II, 26v)* xuanji (CV-21), arm-*sanli* (LI-10).

Counterflow of energy from fullness after meals which are too big: *(DACH II, 29r)* arm-*sanli* (LI-10).

Shivering from eating or drinking in excess: *(DACH)* qihai CV-6).

Cold during meals, acute pain of the epigastrium: *(DACH XI, 4v)* daling (PC-7), neiguan (PC-6), *quze* (PC-3). If not better: *zhongwan* (CV-12), *shangwan* (CV-13), arm-*sanli* (LI-10).

Troubles from alimentary excess: *(DACH X, 27r)* zhangmen (CV-13); food and drink not digested: *(YXRM)* zhongwan (CV-12).

Illnesses from obstructions to food and drink, contractions and pain, sounds in the stomach and intestines, from wine or food: *(DACH VII, 23v; YIX I, 9v)* gongsun (SP-4).

Cannot eat; if he eats, pain and vomiting: *(DACH)* geshu (BL-17).

Dilation of the stomach (wei guo zhang):

Food and drink are stopped and accumulated in the stomach. The body of the stomach swells and increases little by little. There is fatigue and decline of strength. The appetite diminishes, there is vomiting, attacks of hiccoughs. For treatment: choose food and drink carefully; cleanse the stomach. In serious cases, massage, and even remove the distended part. (Ci Yuan, ''Wei Guo-zhang'')

Origin: narrowing of the pyloric sphincter from scarring of an ulcer, from thickening of the muscles of the pyloric sphincter, or from spasms of the pyloric sphincter; atony of the stomach, inflammation of the neighboring organs; habitual great eaters. Symptoms: ballooning and fullness of the area of the stomach; abnormal appetite; eructa-tions; hyperchlorhydria; agitation of the stomach; nausea; vomiting attacks; prolapse of the lower edge of the stomach; one hears the sound of agitated water; becoming thin; habitual constipation. (JO, 17)

Treatment with needles:

zhongwan (CV-12).......	*8 fen,*
shangwan (CV-13).......	*8 fen,*
juque (CV-14)	*6 fen,*
burong (ST-19)	*5 fen,*
chengman (ST-20).......	*5 fen,*
qimen (LR-14)	*5 fen,*
geshu (BL-17)	*5 fen,*
ganshu (BL-18)............	*5 fen,*
yishe (BL-44, IS BL-49)	*5 fen. (JO, 17)*

Treatment with moxa:

zhongwan (CV-12).......	*10 moxas,*
chengman (ST-20).......	*10 moxas,*
qimen (LR-14)	*10 moxas,*
ganshu (BL-18)............	*10 moxas,*
yishe (BL-44, IS BL-49)	*10 moxas,*
danshu (BL-19)............	*10 moxas,*
leg-sanli (ST-36)	*10 moxas. (JO, 17)*

Dilation of the stomach, relaxing of the muscles of the stomach:

Treatment with needles and moxa:

pishu (BL-20)	*2 cun, 10 moxas,*
weishu (BL-21)......	*2 cun, 10 moxas,*
sanjiaoshu (BL-22)	*2 cun, 10 moxas. (JM, 315)*

(GSdeM) Dilation of the stomach: *shenque* (CV-8), 20 daily moxas in the morning.
(DACH IV, 10r; YIX I, 4v) Food remains in the stomach, tonify: leg-*sanli* (ST-36) and *xuanji* (CV-21).
Sounds of water in a bag: *(DACH) dai mai* (GB-26).
Water accumulating and not descending: *(DACH) xuanji* (CV-21).
Liquid remaining, accumulation of food; yawning: *(DACH) zhongkui* (MP-21, IS M-UE-16).
Lumbar area and abdomen relaxed, stomach mucus, drinks remaining, accumulation and stoppage of digestate: *(DACH) tonggu* of the epigastrium (KI-20).
Liquids remain: *(DACH)* foot-*tonggu* (BL-66).
Dilation of stomach: *(JM) zhongkui* (MP-21, IS M-UE-16), *xuanzhong* (GB-39), *juque* (CV-14), *zhongwan* (CV-12), *xiawan* (CV-10), *tonggu* of the epigastrium (KI-20), *ganshu* (BL-18), *weishu* (BL-21).

Ptosis of the stomach:
Ptosis of the stomach: *(JM) shenque* (CV-8), daily moxas.

Excess energy of the stomach.

(Bulimia, heat, acidity, burning, hyperchlorhydria, hypersecretion, gastritis, pains, cramps, ulcerations, ulcers, cancer.)

Bulimia (shi pi, "morbid appetite for food"):
Bulimia: spleen-pancreas hard *(pi kuai)*, counterflow of energy; fullness from excessive meals: *(DACH II, 29r)* leg-*sanli* (ST-36).
Bulimia: fragmented energy: *(DACH II, 26v)* arm-*sanli* (LI-10) and leg-*sanli* (ST-36).
Excessive digestion, always hungry, would digest bone: *(DACH) lidui* (ST-45).

False hunger (excess thyroid):
Always hungry but cannot eat: *(DACH) weishu* (BL-21).
Starved, but cannot eat: *(DACH) zhongji* (CV-3).

Stomach heat:
Stomach heat: *(YIZ 40v) xuanzhong* (GB-39).
Stomach heat, does not eat: leg-*xialian* (ST-39, IS *xiajuxu*).
Stomach and large intestine heat: *qichong* (ST-30).

To dissipate stomach heat: *(DACH, 7r; Nei Jing))* qichong (ST-30), hip-*wushu* (GB-27), leg-*sanli* (ST-36), leg-*shanglian* (ST-37, IS *shangjuxu*), leg-*xialian* (ST-39, IS *xiajuxu*).

Acidity, hyperchlorhydria:

Acidity *(tun suan):*

Often comes from an insufficiency of the pancreas, either from inflammation (the pulse of the pancreas is swollen and hard, burning after jams and cakes, bad digestion of beans, chestnuts): *(GSdeM)* disperse *yamen* (GV-14, IS GV-15) or from weakness; then tonify: foot-*shangqiu* (SP-5) and foot-*dadu* (SP-2).
Acidity: *(DACH)* xuanji (CV-21), burong (ST-19), fuai (SP-16), youmen (KI-21).
All acidity with nondigestion and accumulation: *(YXRM I, 39v)* leg-*sanli* (ST-36) and *neiting* (ST-44).
Acidity, energy of suffocation: *(YIX I, 4v; DACH):* shanzhong (CV-17), seven moxas.

> Swallowing and vomiting acid always come from humidity and heat. The Book says, "all vomiting comes from heat." It also says, "When **shaoyang** (GB) dominates, we vomit acid"; but this acid comes from the liver. If there is a lot of humidity, then there will be acidity and diarrhea; if there is a lot of heat, then there will be vomiting and constipation. If hot drinks are taken, there will be temporary relaxation. *(YXRM V, 22r)*

Hyperchlorhydria *(wei suan guo duo)* (see Acidity above);

> Perversity from excess acidity of the stomach. Origin: frequently from twenty to forty years old, mostly men; excess fatigue of vitality; repression of worries; chronic troubles of the intestines, blocking of the biliary flow; drinks wine, eats salted meat, fasts too much. Symptoms: worries and weight in the stomach, acidity, agitation of the stomach; comes two or three hours after the meal; abdomen empty, acute pain; remission one hour after the meal. *(JO, 18)*

Treatment with needles:

geshu (BL-17).........	*5 fen,*
ganshu (BL-18)	*5 fen,*
pishu (BL-20)	*5 fen,*
zhongwan (CV-12) .	*8 fen,*
shiguan (KI-18)......	*8 fen,*
shangqiu (KI-17)....	*8 fen,*
leg-sanli (ST-36).....	*1 cun,*
taibai (SP-3)	*5 fen,*
xuanzhong (GB-39)	*6 fen. (JO, 18)*

Treatment with moxa:

zhongwan (CV-12) .	*10 moxas,*
shiguan (KI-18)......	*10 moxas,*
shangqiu (KI-17)....	*10 moxas,*
leg-sanli (ST-36).....	*10 moxas,*
xuanzhong (GB-39)	*10 moxas. (JO, 18)*

Hyperchlorhydria: *(JM)* taibai (SP-3), gongsun (SP-4), youmen (KI-21), weishu (BL-21).

Hypersecretion (xiao hua guo duo):

Excessive digestion: *(JM)* lidui (ST-45).
Nocturnal vomiting, regurgitates liquid acids: *(DACH)* disperse *riyue* (GB-24).
Vomits acids at night: *(DACH)* zhejin (GB-23).

Acute or chronic gastritis, catarrh of stomach; inflammation of stomach (wei yan, wei feng, wei jia da er, shang shi):

> Also called **wei jia da er,** catarrh of the stomach. There are two types: acute and chronic. The acute type comes particularly from having eaten spoiled food or having drunk something too hot or too cold. The patient feels that the food does not advance, the limbs are not at ease; from time to time, vomiting. It is necessary to regulate the diet or fast for one or two days. The chronic form is almost the same, but difficult to cure. (Ci Yuan, "Wei-yan")

> **Wei jia da er,** catarrh of the stomach. Origin: eats or drinks a lot, eats unclean food; drinks or eats things that are too hot or too cold, unripe fruits, rotten meat; or enteritis, parasitic worms, flu, emotions. Symptoms: diminishing of the appetite, nausea, vomiting, acidity, agitation of the stomach, eructation, ballooning of the stomach, pains in the stomach, headaches, vertigo, attacks of fever, tongue white to yellow, constipation, rarely diarrhea. *(JO, 15)*

This is an acute catarrh of the stomach. The patient disdains nourishment; he is timorous, weakened, fatigued; there is nausea; heavy pain beneath the heart; constipation; a white tongue engendering a white fur; periodic acid counterflow. If the condition becomes chronic, it is even more difficult to cure. (Ci Yuan, "Shang-shi")

Chronic gastritis *(wei feng):*

*Also called chronic catarrh of the stomach, **man xing wei jia da er**. The patient becomes thin; his face and appearance are dried out. This is a transformation from an acute catarrh of the stomach. (Ci Yuan, "Wei-feng")*

Chronic catarrh of the stomach. Origin: ulcers of the stomach, cancer of the stomach, dilation of the stomach; troubles of the liver, heart or lungs; catarrh of the stomach from intoxication; also comes from insufficient chewing, from drinking wine in excess, from smoking in excess or from insufficient physical exercise. Symptoms: diminishing of appetite, counterflow of food, no taste, agitation of stomach, eructations, ballooning of abdomen, vomiting; constipation, blockage of assimilation, repression of worries. (JO, 16)

Inflammation of the stomach *(wei yan):* (JM) *guanyuan* (CV-4), *weishu* (BL-21).

Acute gastritis *(ji xing wei jia da er):*

Treatment with needles:

shangwan (CV-13)	*8 fen,*
zhongwan (CV-12)	*1 cun,*
xiawan (CV-10)	*1 cun,*
liangmen (ST-21)..	*5 fen,*
tianshu (ST-25).....	*8 fen,*
taibai (SP-3)..........	*5 fen,*
shangqiu (SP-5)....	*3 fen,*
daling (PC-7)........	*3 fen. (JO, 15)*

Treatment with moxa:

juque (CV-14).......	*10 to 15 moxas,*
zhongwan (CV-12)	*10 to 15 moxas,*
yangmen (ST-21)..	*10 to 15 moxas. (JO, 15)*

Treatment with needles and moxa:

danshu (BL-19).................	*1.5 **cun**, 10 moxas,*
pishu (BL-20)....................	*1.5 **cun**, 10 moxas,*
weishu (BL-21)	*1.5 **cun**, 10 moxas,*
sanjiaoshu (BL-22)...........	*1 to 1.5 **cun**, 10 moxas,*
yishe (BL-44, IS BL-49).....	*1 to 1.5 **cun**, 10 moxas,*
weicang (BL-45, IS BL-50)	*1 to 1.5 **cun**, 10 moxas,*
burong (ST-19)	*on the left 1 **cun**, 10 moxas,*
chengman (ST-20)	*on the left 1 **cun**, 10 moxas,*
*arm-**sanli** (LI-10) ....*	*5 **cun**, 10 moxas,*
hegu (LI-4)	*5 **cun**, 10 moxas. (JM, 315)*

(JM) *Xuanji* (CV-21), *taiyin* (ST-23), *burong* (ST-19), *jiuwei* (CV-15), *sanyinjiao* (SP-6), *daling* (PC-7), *jianshi* (PC-5).

Chronic gastritis *(man xing wei jia da er):*

Treatment with needles:

shangwan (CV-13)	*8 fen,*
zhongwan (CV-12)	*8 fen,*
xiawan (CV-10)	*1 cun,*
liangmen (ST-21)..	*8 fen,*
tianshu (ST-25).....	*8 fen,*
jianshi (PC-5).......	*3 fen,*
*leg-**sanli** (ST-36)...*	*8 fen,*
sanyinjiao (SP-6)..	*5 fen. (JO, 16)*

Treatment with moxa:

geshu (BL-17) ...	*10 moxas,*
pishu (BL-20)	*10 moxas,*
leg-sanli (ST-36)	*10 moxas,*
ganshu (BL-18) .	*10 moxas. (JO, 16)*

For acute gastritis, include these points:

Treatment with needles and moxa:

pishu (BL-20)	*2 cun, 10 moxas,*
weishu (BL-21)	*2 cun, 10 moxas,*
sanjiaoshu (BL-22)	*2 cun, 10 moxas. (JM, 315)*

(JM) Shangwan (CV-13), *xiawan* (CV-10), *zhongwan* (CV-12), *jiuwei* (CV-15), *yangmen* (ST-21), *pishu* (BL-20), *ganshu* (BL-18), *guanyuanshu* (BL-26), *foot-tonggu* (BL-66), *xuanli* (GB-6).

Pain, cramps of the stomach (xin fu tong, wei guan tong, wei jing):

*Attacks of pain in the stomach, **jing** or **lman** type contractures; popularly called **wei guan tong**, stomach pain. The patient first feels nausea and violent headache, then under the heart in the chest and ribs there are piercing or burning pains. Generally, people who are empty of blood have it often. (Ci Yuan, "Wei-jing")*

***Wei jing lman:** stomach pain of a nervous origin. Origins: illness or troubles of the stomach; tuberculosis of the spinal cord; hysteria, neurasthenia; ascaris worms; illness and troubles of the uterus. Symptoms: sudden pains or heaviness of the stomach, nausea, attacks of headache, pain in the back, body bent forward, complexion bluish-white, four limbs cold, occasional vomiting. (JO, 19)*

Acute or dull pains in the epigastrium come from an accumulation or from a chill with food ... or from excess after hunger, or damp from the rain or from wind, or after coitus: the food does not digest. (DACH XI, 4v)

*When in troubles of the stomach, the middle of the stomach in front of the heart is painful, as well as the four limbs and two sides; when the diaphragm and pharynx do not communicate; when drink and food do not descend, tonify leg-**sanli** (ST-36). (DACH XI, 10r, quoting Li Gao)*

(DACH II, 25r) Stomach pain, cold of the spleen-pancreas: disperse *gongsun* (SP-4).

(DACH) Stomach pain: disperse *xuanji* (CV-21), *burong* (ST-19).

Pain in the hollow of the stomach: *(JM) taibai* (SP-3); *(DACH) foot-dadu* (SP-2).

Pain attacking the epigastrium: *(YXRM) tianshu* (ST-25).

Stomach pain to the point of a pain in the heart: *(DACH III, 30v) laogong* (PC-8).

Pain and swelling of the stomach: *(DACH X, 25v) geshu* (BL-17).

Food descends with difficulty, stoppage of the digestion; immediately after drinking it, wine irritates: *(DACH VII, 26r; YIX I, 9v) neiguan* (PC-6).

Pain in the stomach, heart, liver, spleen-pancreas; internal troubles *(DACH) zhongwan* (CV-12).

Pain in the epigastrium from an excess after hunger, or wet from rain or shock or after coitus; the food does not digest: *(DACH XI, 4v) neiguan* (PC-6), leg-*sanli* (ST-36), *zhongwan* (CV-12). If not better, *guanyuan* (CV-4), *shuifen* (CV-9), *tiantu* (CV-22).

Shooting pain in the heart and stomach, acute pain in the ribs and sides: *(DACH VII, 26v) neiguan* (PC-6), *qihai* (CV-6), *yanglingquan* (GB-34), *xingjian* (LR-2).

Treatment with needles *(wei jing lman)*:

zhongwan (CV-12) .	*6fen,*
liangmen (ST-21) ...	*6fen,*
huaroumen (ST-24)	*6fen,*
xiawan (CV-10)	*6fen,*
daheng (SP-15)	*6fen,*
tianshu (ST-25)	*6fen,*
juque (CV-14)	*6 fen,*
burong (ST-19)	*5 fen,*
riyue (GB-24)	*5 fen,*
guanyuan (CV-4) ...	*1 cun. (JO, 19)*

Treatment with moxa *(wei jing lman):*

juque (CV-14).......	*10 moxas,*
zhongwan (CV-12)	*10 moxas,*
yangmen (ST-21) ..	*10 moxas,*
tianshu (ST-25).....	*10 moxas,*
riyue (GB-24)........	*10 moxas. (JO, 19)*

Treatment with needles and moxa *(wei jing lman):*

weishu *(BL-21)*	*2 **cun,** 20 moxas,*
sanjiaoshu *(BL-22)*...........	*2 **cun,** 20 moxas,*
yishe *(BL-44, IS BL-49)*.....	*1 **cun,** 20 moxas,*
weicang *(BL-45, IS BL-50)*	*1 **cun,** 20 moxas,*
hegu *(LI-4)*	*3 to 5 **fen** 20 moxas,*
leg-**sanli** *(ST-36)*	*3 to 5 **fen,** 20 moxas. (JM, 315)*

(JM) wei jing lman: quchi (LI-11), *dadu* (SP-2), *taibai* (SP-3), *diji* (SP-8), leg-*sanli* (ST-36), *juque* (CV-14), *zhongwan* (CV-12), *xiawan* (CV-10), *shiguan* (KI-18), *shangqiu* (KI-17), *huangshu* (KI-16), *yangmen* (ST-21), *fuai* (SP-16), *huaroumen* (ST-24), *chongmen* (SP-12), *dushu* (BL-16), *ganshu* (BL-18), *weishu* (BL-21), *pishu* (BL-20), *yanggang* (BL-43, IS BL-48), *yishe* (BL-44, IS BL-49), *hunmen* (BL-42, IS BL-47), *huangmen* (BL-46, IS BL-51). Pain from spasms attacking the chest and stomach to the point of death, without recognizing anyone: *zhongwan* (CV-12).

Ulcerations, ulcers (wei hui yang, wei yong):

The name given in Japan to **weiyong.** *(Ci Yuan, ''Wei-hui-yang'')*

Also called **wei hui yang,** *it comes from an ulceration (***fu lan***) of the internal mucosa of the stomach. The patient has a sweet taste in the mouth; the stomach is hot. After having vomited, bubbly saliva the color of dark blood is secreted. In serious cases it goes to the point of perforating the stomach lining, then it cannot be cured. At the beginning it is advisable to take food mixed with noodles which give a coating; foods of the sweetening type; feed especially with peptonized [enzyme converted] food. . . . Vomits immediately after meals, pains several hours after meals, vomiting of blood. (Ci Yuan, ''Wei-yong'')*

Inflammatory illness of the stomach: *(JM)* *taiyin* (ST-23), *huaroumen* (ST-24).
Ulceration of the stomach, ulcer: *(JM)* *fuai* (SP-16), *tianxi* (SP-18); *(Wetterwald)* *yindu* (KI-19).
Vomits after drinking and eating: *(DACH)* *sanjiaoshu* (BL-22), *zhangmen* (LR-13).
Numerous vomitings of blood, not being cured: *(DACH)* *qichong* (ST-30).
Counterflow vomiting, food and drink immediately come back up: *(DACH)* *zhangmen* (LR-13).

Cancer of the stomach (wei yan, wei ge):

It is a swelling of cancer generated by the stomach. People from forty to fifty years and more who are of strong constitution and who are great eaters are sometimes attacked. In the beginning, pain of the stomach; eats and drinks less and less; loses sleep; then expels a dark red fluid through the mouth. The body becomes thin; food and drink no longer move; the cancer grows; there is decline and death: it is also called **wei ge.** *The pulse of cancer is slow with missed beats. (Ci Yuan, ''Wei-yan'')*

Cancer of the stomach: *(JO)* *burong* (ST-19), *zhongwan* (CV-12), *geshu* (BL-17) *weishu* (BL-21).

XII. Abdomen, Intestines

In general.

All illnesses of the abdomen: *(DACH IV, 14v; YXRM* I, 39v) without equal for all illnesses of the abdomen (with *neiting,* ST-44): leg-*sanli* (ST-36).
Illness of the abdomen: *(DACH)* *xiangu* (ST-43).
Appeases and strengthens permanently for all illnesses in the abdomen: *(DACH IV, 5r)* *neiguan* (PC-6).
For the abdomen: *(YIX* I, 7v) *neiting* (ST-44).
All illness below the umbilicus: *(DACH III, 25v)* *gongsun* (SP-4).
Illnesses staying in the abdomen: *(DACH)* *xuanshu* (GV-5).
Illnesses of the umbilicus and abdomen: *(DACH, 11r)* *ququan* (LR-8); energy in the abdomen, small and large intestines: *(DACH)* *xingjian* (LR-2).

Energy running through the abdomen: *(DACH, YXRM) guanmen* (ST-22).

Energy of accumulation rising and going down within the abdomen: *(DACH) xuanshu* (GV-5).

All chronic illness of the stomach and intestine: *(JM) tianshu* (ST-25), *sanyinjiao* (SP-6), *sanjiaoshu* (BL-22).

Intestines: *(JM) tianshu* (ST-25), *wailing* (ST-26), *geshu* (BL-17), *weishu* (BL-21), *sanjiaoshu* (BL-22).

(JM) Yamen (GV-14, IS GV-15) is close to the center controlling peristalsis of the stomach and intestines.

All illnesses of the intestines: *(DACH VII, 34v) gongsun* (SP-4) and foot-*linqi* (GB-41); *(JM) taiyi* (ST-23).

Illness and troubles of the intestines: *(JM) tiaokou* (ST-38).

(DACH VII, 4v, quoting Li Gao) When the energy of the stomach descends, when all the energy of the intestines is troubled: *yuji* (LU-10).

Pain of the abdomen and intestines.

All abdominal pains: *(DACH III, 32v) kunlun* (BL-60); *(YXRM I, 39) gongsun* (SP-4).

Slight abdominal pains: *(YXRM I, 39v)* leg-*sanli* (ST-36).

Acute abdominal pain, the blood rises and attacks the heart: *(DACH) shiguan* (KI-18).

Abdominal pain: *(DACH) neiguan* (PC-6), *zhongquan* (MP-14, IS M-UE-33), *gongsun* (SP-4), leg-*sanli* (ST-36); *(YXRM) ligou* (LR-5), *taibai* (SP-3), leg-*shanglian* (ST-37, IS *shangjuxu*), *yongquan* (KI-1); *(YIX I, 7v) chengshan* (BL-57), *fuai* (SP-16), *shangqiu* (KI-17), *huangshu* (KI-16), *dazhu* (BL-11), *baohuang* (BL-48, IS BL-53), *dushu* (BL-16), *dachangshu* (BL-25), *pangguangshu* (BL-28).

Abdominal pain from cold or humidity with an excess of food: *(DACH IX, 5r) tianshu* (ST-25).

Abdominal pain and fullness of the chest: *(DACH III, 25v) neiguan* (PC-6).

Acute abdominal pain, fragmented energy; if there is constipation, disperse: *(YIX I, 4v) neiguan* (PC-6).

Abdominal pain with vertebral pain: *(DACH) chengshan* (BL-57).

Pain of the abdomen and sides: *(DACH, YXRM) taixi* (KI-5, IS KI-3).

Pain of the abdomen and sides; fullness, runs madly: *(DACH) xialian* (LI-8).

Abdominal pain, little energy: *(YXRM I 46v; DACH) juque* (CV-14).

Abdominal pain, obstruction from mucus: *(DACH) sanyinjiao* (SP-6).

Pain on one side of the abdomen: *(DACH) zhaohai* (KI-3, IS KI-6).

Piercing pains of the abdomen and chest: *(DACH) fenglong* (ST-40).

Exhausting pain of the abdomen, heart as if suspended: *(DACH) wailing* (ST-26).

Pain and hardness of the abdomen radiating into the genitals: *(DACH)* abdomen-*yinjiao* (CV-7).

Pain rising from the genitals to the abdomen: *(DACH) wushu* (GB-27).

Pain of the abdomen even without taking food: *(DACH, YXRM) yuji* (LU-10).

Pain around and below the umbilicus:

Pain below the umbilicus: *(DACH) zhongfeng* (LR-4).

Pain below the umbilicus: *(YXRM) zhongfeng* (LR-4); *(DACH) shuifen* (CV-9), *shenque* (CV-8); *(JM)* acute pain: *qihai* (CV-6); *(DACH, YXRM)* cutting pain: *tianshu* (ST-25); strangling pain: *dachangshu* (BL-25), *fujie* (SP-14).

Pain below the umbilicus, acute pain in the abdomen, swelling of the sides: *(DACH VII, 23v; YIX I, 9v) gongsun* (SP-4).

Pain pinching the umbilicus, abdomen and sides: *(DACH)* leg-*shanglian* (ST-37, IS *shangjuxu*).

Pain knotting below the umbilicus, flowing and entering into the genitals, coming without a fixed time: *(DACH) guanyuan* (CV-4).

Spasmodic pain surrounding the umbilicus, cannot breathe: *(YXRM) shimen* (CV-5).

Cutting pains below the umbilicus, shivering: *(DACH) siman* (KI-14).

Pain in the abdomen and the middle of the umbilicus: *(DACH) dadun* (LR-1).

Contracting pain tightening the umbilicus: *(DACH, YXRM) guanmen* (ST-22).

Pain and cold below the umbilicus: *(DACH III, 31r) zhongji* (CV-3).

Skin of the abdomen:

Pain of the skin of the abdomen: *(DACH) huiyin* (CV-1); inflammation of the omentum: *(JM) shimen* (CV-5).

Intestines:

Intestinal pain (cutting pain): *(DACH)* disperse *gongsun* (SP-4).

Cutting intestinal pain and thunderous sounds: *(DACH)* leg-*shanglian* (ST-37, IS *shangjuxu*).

Intestinal pain, heat and pain at the sides of the lower pelvis: *(YXRM) zhaohai* (KI-3, IS KI-6).

Acute pain in the intestine; energy at the top: *(DACH) jianli* (CV-11).

Pain in the intestine: *(GSdeM) sanjian* (LI-3); *(YXRM) pangguang* (BL-28).

Intestinal neuralgia: *(JM)* leg-*shanglian* (ST-37, IS *shangjuxu*), *yinlingquan* (SP-9), *taibai* (SP-3), *sanyinjiao* (SP-6), *ququan* (LR-8), *shaochong* (HT-9), *qihai* (CV-6), *taiyin* (ST-23), *jingmen* (GB-25).

Pain of the superficial nerves of the intestines: *(JM) xiangu* (ST-43).
Pain in the stomach and intestines: *(DACH) xuanshu* (GV-5).
Pain from spasms of the intestines (see Spasms).

Abdominal and intestinal pain and swelling.

Abdomen:
Abdominal pain and swelling: *(YXRM) kunlun* (BL-60), *weishu* (BL-21), *sanjiaoshu* (BL-22), *dadun* (LR-1), *juque* (CV-14).

Intestines:
Ballooned intestines: *(JM) chongyang* (ST-42).

Abdominal and intestinal swelling.

(See Aerogastria.)

Abdomen:
Men — similar to ascites; women — similar to pregnancy: *(DACH, YXRM) yingu* (KI-10).
Illness of women, false pregnancy; "pregnant look" in men: *(DACH III, 32r) yongquan* (KI-1).
Sudden swelling of the abdomen, the evil has entered: *(DACH) zhongwan* (CV-12).
Abdomen swelling from energy attacking the top: *(DACH)* leg-*sanli* (ST-36).
Abdominal swelling: *(DACH) chize* (LU-5), *jiexi* (ST-41), *xingjian* (LR-2), *dadun* (LR-1); *(YXRM) tianshu* (ST-25), *zhongji* (CV-3), *zhangmen* (LR-13), *chengman* (ST-20); *(DACH) zhongfu* (LU-1), *(DACH) yufu* (KI-27), *zhongliao* (BL-33).
Ballooned abdomen: *(DACH III, 30v) neiting* (ST-44); *(JM) lougu* (SP-7), *chongyang* (ST-42), *jizhong* (GV-6); *(DACH) dachangshu* (BL-25), *weishu* (BL-21).
Ballooned abdomen, sounds in intestines, no need to go to the toilet: *(DACH) shangqiu* (SP-5).
Drum-swelling (tympanism: *gu zhang*): *(JM) yingu* (KI-10), *jiexi* (ST-41), thigh-*wuli* (LR-10), *chengman* (ST-20), *jianli* (CV-11); *(JM) weicang* (BL-45, IS BL-50), *zhangmen* (LR-13).
Drum-swelling of the abdomen and umbilicus: *(YXRM I, 46r) tianshu* (ST-25).

Intestines:
Swelling of the intestines, ballooned intestines: *(JM) chongyang* (ST-42).
Drum-like intestine: *(JM) jizhong* (GV-6), *jingmen* (GB-25), *chongmen* (SP-12).
Ballooned abdomen, drum-like intestine: *(JM) dachangshu* (BL-25).
Fullness in the intestines: *(DACH)* thigh-*wuli* (LR-10).
Swelling and sounds in the intestines:
(YXRM, DACH) sanyinjiao (SP-6); *(DACH) sanjiaoshu* (BL-22), *chengman* (ST-20) *weishu* (BL-21).
Abdominal swelling and fullness: *(DACH) lougu* (SP-7); *(DACH, YXRM)* and cannot breathe: *yingu* (KI-10); *(YXRM) yinbai* (SP-1), *youmen* (KI-21).
Abdominal fullness: *(DACH) sanjian* (LI-3), *xiangu* (ST-43), *burong* (ST-19).
Swelling-obesity of the abdomen: (Fuji) *dachangshu* (BL-25).
In cold, swelling of the abdomen and fullness of the sides: *(YXRM) yinlingquan* (SP-9).
Swelling and fullness of the abdomen and sides: *(YXRM I, 46r) yanglingquan* (SP-9).
Swelling of the abdomen and fullness of the sides: *(DACH X, 27r) yanglingquan* (GB-34).
Swollen abdomen, pain of the sides: *(DACH) zhonglüshu* (BL-29).
Abdomen and sides swollen; pasty diarrhea: *(DACH);* abdominal pain, swelling from energy, pasty diarrhea *(YXRM): diji* (SP-8).
Counterflow of energy, abdominal swelling *(DACH),* counterflow of energy, swelling and fullness *(YXRM): xuehai* (SP-10).
Swollen abdomen, little energy: *(DACH)* thigh-*futu* (ST-32).
Abdominal swelling after delivery: *(YXRM I, 46r) shenque* (CV-8), (cf. *qugu*, CV-2).
Children, thinness with a big belly: *(DACH)* moxa at *zhangmen* (LR-13).

Hardness of the abdomen and intestines.

Abdomen:
Hardness of the abdomen: *(DACH) zhongwan* (CV-12).
Epigastrium with abdomen firm and hard: *(DACH) shimen* (CV-5).
Hard accumulation as if there were a stone below the umbilicus: *(DACH) zhongji* (CV-3).
Abdomen hard and large: *(DACH) chongyang* (ST-42).
Abdomen hard, tight: *(DACH) baohuang* (BL-48, IS BL-53).
Pain and hardness of the abdomen radiating to the genitals and preventing one from lifting things: *(DACH)* abdomen-*yinjiao* (CV-7).
Abdomen hard and agitated: *(DACH) xiawan* (CV-10).
Fullness of the abdomen, paresis *(wei),* emptiness, little energy: *(YXRM) yinshi* (ST-33).

Intestines:
Hardness of the intestines: *(DACH) xiawan* (CV-10).
Fullness in the intestines: *(DACH)* thigh-*wuli* (LR-10).
Accumulations in the intestines: *(DACH) pishu* (BL-20).

Spasms of the abdomen and intestines.

Abdomen:
Nervous spasms of the omentum: *(JM) huangshu* (KI-16).
Contractions above, around and over the umbilicus: *(DACH VI, 15v) dadun* (LR-1).
Pain from spasms surrounding the umbilicus, cannot breathe: *(YXRM) shimen* (CV-5).
Knotting pain below the umbilicus, flowing and entering into the genitals, without fixed periods: *(DACH) guanyuan* (CV-4).
Pain from spasms below the umbilicus: *(DACH) siman* (KI-14).

Intestines:
Spasms of the intestines: *(JM) ququan* (LR-8), *shangwan* (CV-13), *shuifen* (CV-9), *wailing* (ST-26), *henggu* (KI-11), *fujie* (SP-14), *fushe* (SP-13), *tianshu* (ST-25), *siman* (KI-14), *chongmen* (SP-12), *guanmen* (ST-22), *qihaishu* (BL-24).
Sudden spasms of the intestines of a nervous type: *(JM) qiuxu* (GB-40).
Intestinal contractions, colic: *(GSdeM)* disperse *sanjian* (LI-3).
Spasms of the inter-intestinal nerves: *(JM) shangqiu* (KI-17).
Pains from spasms in the intestines: *(JM) xiangu* (ST-43), *xingjian* (LR-2), *ligou* (LR-5), *dadun* (LR-1), *tianshu* (ST-26), *shuifen* (CV-9), *guanmen* (ST-22), *zhongwan* (CV-12), *siman* (KI-14), *huantiao* (GB-29, IS GB-30), *taiyin* (ST-23), *mingmen* (GV-4), *xiaochangshu* (BL-27), *zhonglüshu* (BL-29).

Cold or heat of abdomen and intestines.

Abdomen, cold:
Extreme coldness of the abdomen: *(JM) chengman* (ST-20), *fujie* (SP-14).
Cold in the abdomen: *(YXRM) yinbai* (SP-1); *(DACH, YXRM) huiyang* (BL-35).
Cold in the abdomen; does not enjoy eating; fullness: *(DACH) yinlingquan* (SP-9).
Cold of the abdomen: *(DACH, YXRM) fujie* (SP-14).
Cold of the abdomen; fullness of energy: *(DACH) chongmen* (SP-12).
Painful coldness below the umbilicus: *(DACH III, 31r) zhongji* (CV-3).
Ballooning, cold, emptiness of the area of the abdomen: *(DACH) chongmen* (SP-12).

Intestines, cold:
Cold of the intestines: *(DACH) zhonglüshu* (BL-29).
Cold and heat of the small and large intestine: *(DACH) xiaochangshu* (BL-27).

Abdomen, heat:
Heat below the umbilicus: *(DACH, YXRM)* abdomen-*yinjiao* (CV-7).
Heat in the abdomen: *(DACH) zhongji* (CV-3).
Extreme heat in the abdomen attacking the heart: *(YXRM) qichong* (ST-30).
Heat of the abdomen; wants to run: *(YXRM) daheng* (SP-15).
Heat of the abdomen, heat of the body: *(DACH)* leg-*sanli* (ST-36).
If one is without food, heat of the abdomen: *(YXRM)* leg-*sanli* (ST-36).
Heat of the abdomen; enjoys drinking: *(YXRM) zhongwan* (CV-12).

Inflammation, ulceration, abscess.

Inflammation:
Inflammation of the omentum: *(JM) shimen* (CV-5).

Ulcerations:
Intestinal ulcerations: *(JM) ququan* (LR-8).
Urine and blood in the intestines: *(DACH) guanyuan* (CV-4).
Shock entering the intestines *(chang feng),* loss of blood, interior contracted: *(YXRM);* shock in the intestines, loss of blood: *(YXRM I, 46v) gongsun* (SP-4), *mingmen* (GV-4).
Shock entering the intestines, constant or frequent descent of blood; peculiar energy in the diaphragm; nucleus of invading energy: *(DACH VII, 33r; YIX I, 11v) zhaohai* (KI-3, IS KI-6).
Shock entering the intestines: *(DACH) yongquan* (KI-1).

Abscess:
Abscess of the intestines with putrefaction: *(JM)* leg-*zhongdu* (LR-6).
Abscess of the large intestine; 100 moxas and the pus will descend: *(DACH II, 19v) zhoujian* (MP-11, IS M-UE-46).

Intestinal tuberculosis.

Intestinal tuberculosis: (Fuji) *shenque* (CV-8).
From tuberculosis, diarrhea after meals, food not digested: *(DACH)* leg-*shanglian* (ST-37, IS *shangjuxu*).
Diarrhea after meals: *(DACH) xialian* (LI-8), *zhongliao* (BL-33), *yinlingquan* (SP-9).

Paralysis, muscular atony of the intestines.

Paralysis of the abdominal muscles: *(JM) fushi* (SP-13).

XXIII. Small Intestine *(Xiao Chang)*

🌢 An essential organ due to its various functions (the duodenum and jejunum having mostly functions of digestive transformation, the ileum of absorption); stimulated by the parasympathetic system; depressed by the sympathetic system.

For the Chinese, it adds a vital element to the dead food which characterizes the blood. Europeans specify that it decomposes the large albumin molecules down to their amino acids. From these it reformulates a smaller molecule which is correctly and rigorously specific for the blood and tissues of each individual. It synthesizes neutral fats as well. Although important for the Europeans, these two types of synthesis are vital for the Chinese.

Action on the pancreas: its secretin increases the pancreatic secretions which are essential for digestion. Its enteropeptidase makes the pancreatic sugar active. Its erepsin activates and splits the peptones into amino acids; its hyperacidity activates and inflames the pancreas to the point where insulin does not function.

Action on the liver: the flow of the bile is regulated by a duodenal reflex produced by the peptones extracted from meat, especially animal fats. This reflex commands Oddi's sphincter (gallbladder), the common bile duct canal.

Action on the kidneys:

> *The flow of urine coming from the kidneys depends on the small intestine and the third warmer. The small intestine makes the division between fluids and solids, sending the one to the kidneys and the other to the large intestine.*
> *(DACH VIII, 18r)*

The more active it is and the less liquid and solid wastes there are, the better the digestion. Europeans specify that a resection of the nerves of a portion of the small intestine causes a considerable influx of liquid into the intestinal cavity produced by the transudation of the blood vessels of the mucosa. The same phenomenon is produced by great or repeated emotions, producing either diarrhea from fear or abundant and pressing urination (as has been observed during the war). Nervous inhibition of the small intestine for the Chinese results in a flow of troubled energy (heart, small intestine, bladder).

Action on the heart: if the small intestine is insufficient, the heart weakens and the blood pressure decreases. Tonifying the small intestine tonifies the heart.

The meridian (shou taiyang).

The meridian of the small intestine is yang, centripetal (rising). It is linked to the meridian of the heart, yin treasure organ, which precedes it in the flow of energy. The energy is at its maximum from 1 to 3 p.m., corresponding to the liver (yin), which has its maximum from 1 to 3 a.m.

Insufficiency of energy of the small intestine:

In case of insufficiency of function of the small intestine, the pulse (I superficial, left wrist) is either abolished, soft, small, proximal, or without shape.

Physical symptoms: face without color, bluish lips with white edges, swelling under the chin, abundant or frequent urine; at the extreme, undigested diarrhea, liquid mucus.

Psychological symptoms: sadness, regrets, remorse, dreams of streets or narrow lanes in towns.

Through the main meridian: tonify *houxi* (SI-3) and the source point *wangu* (SI-4).

Through the herald point: *guanyuan* (CV-4).

Through the circulation of energy: tonify the heart (mother who feeds), *shaochong* (HT-9) and the bladder (the child who suckles) *zhiyin* (BL-67).

Through the coupled yin organ: *shaochong* (HT-9).

Through the passage point: tonify *zhizheng* (SI-7), from the heart to the small intestine.

Midday-midnight rule: at night, or during cold, dark times, tonify the liver which is the corresponding organ (midnight-midday rule).

Husband-wife rule: tonify the large intestine, *quchi* (LI-11).

Excess energy of the small intestine:

The pulse of the small intestine is large, ample, distal or hard. If it is agitated, there is a probability of intestinal parasites of the small intestine, often of *Giardia lamblia.*

Physical symptoms: anuria, sometimes pain in the urethra, red face. If there is contracture, diarrhea with undigested food; abscess of the mouth or tongue.

Psychological symptoms: happy, laughs a lot.

Through the main meridian: disperse *xiaohai* (SI-8) and the source point *wangu* (SI-4).

Passage point: tonify *tongli* (HT-5), from the small intestine to the heart.

Assent point: disperse *xiaochangshu* (BL-27).

Through the coupled yin treasure organ: disperse the heart at *shenmen* (HT-7).

Through the circulation of the energy: disperse the heart (*shenmen*, HT-7), the mother who feeds and the bladder (*shugu*, BL-65), the child who suckles.

Midnight-midday law: at night, or cold, dark times, disperse the liver, which is the correspondent.

Husband-wife law: disperse the large intestine at *sanjian* (LI-3) and *erjian* (LI-2).

Hernia is popularly called ''energy of the small intestine.''

In general.

> In the illnesses of the small intestine, it is advisable to make the pancreas, which is the master, unctuous.
> (DACH XI, 10r, quoting Li Gao)

Duodenum: *(JM) ganshu* (BL-18).

Insufficiency of the energy of the small intestine, face without color: *(DACH)* leg-*xialian* (ST-39, IS *xiajuxu*), arm-*xialian* (LI-8).

Insufficiency of the small intestine: tonify pancreas, foot-*dadu* (SP-2) on the right.

Heat of the small intestine: *(DACH) fuxi* (BL-52, IS BL-38).

Energy in the small and large intestine: *(DACH) xingjian* (LR-2).

Illnesses of the small intestine, stomach, liver, kidneys: *(DACH) weicang* (BL-45, IS BL-50).

All illnesses of the intestines: *(DACH VII, 34v) gongsun* (SP-4) and foot-*linqi* (GB-41); *(JM) taiyin* (ST-23).

Pain of the small intestine.

Pain of the small intestine: *xiaohai* (SI-8).

Pains from energy of the small intestine (see hernia): *(DACH III, 27r) sanyinjiao* (SP-6), *(DACH IV, 7v) guilai* (ST-29); *(YIX, 4r) guilai* (ST-29), *zhongliao* (BL-33).

Pain of the small intestine linked with umbilicus: *(DACH IV, 10v; YIX I, 4r)* yinlingquan (SP-9) and yongquan (KI-1); *(YIX, 4r),* changqiang (GV-1) and dadun (LR-2).
(See also pains around the umbilicus.)
Pain of the superficial nerves of the intestines: *(JM)* leg-shanglian (ST-37, IS shangjuxu).

Spasms of the small intestine and pylorus.

Spasms of the small intestine, vivid pain of the abdomen and umbilicus, urine escaping: *(DACH III, 32r)* dadun (LR-2).
Spasms of the small intestine: *(YXRM I, 46r)* disperse xiaxi (GB-43) and sanyinjiao (SP-6).
Reflex dilation of the pyloric sphincter: right edge of L5.
Spasms of the pyloric sphincter: *(GSdeM)* youmen (KI-21).

Swelling (see also swelling around the umbilicus).

Swelling of the small intestine: *(DACH)* leg-sanli (ST-36).
Noisy small intestine, fullness of energy: *(DACH)* shimen (CV-5).

Duodenal ulcer.

Local pain two hours after a liquid meal and four hours after a solid meal radiating to the right shoulder: *(GSdeM)* disperse fuai (SP-16) mostly on right, gongsun (SP-4); and if the pancreas is inflamed, disperse yamen (GV-14, IS GV-15).

Hernias (shan qi).

> It is popularly called **xiao chang qi,** *energy of the small intestine. (Ci Yuan, ''Shan-qi'')* Causes violent pain in the umbilical area. There are some types which makes one testicle swell laterally. The types are numerous.
> *(Ci Yuan, ''Xiaochang-qi'')*

(See also pain around the umbilicus, energy of the small intestine): *(DACH)* leg-sanli (ST-36).
Hernia from childbirth, pain prevents suckling: *(DACH)* zhubin (KI-9).

> Fox-hernia *(hu shan):*
>
> *Appears like a round tile; when one lies down, it enters into the lower abdomen like a fox enters his den at night. (YXRM V, 35v)*

(DACH) Fox-hernia coming and going, pain of the lower abdomen, cannot bend or get up: shangqiu (SP-5).
Fox-hernia coming out when one coughs: *(DACH)* juque (CV-14). Hernia of the small intestine, sudden pain, pain of the umbilicus and abdomen, four limbs no longer lifting, granular or blocked urine, body heavy, feet paralyzed; needle 3/10 *cun,* three moxas at sanyinjiao (SP-6).
Scrotal hernia, pain of the lower pelvis: *(DACH)* qugu (CV-2).

XXIV. Large Intestine *(Da Chang)*

The peristalsis of the large intestine and the relaxation of the anal sphincter are activated by the parasympathetic system and depressed by the sympathetic system.

Connection with the liver: if the liver is insufficient in bile, there is constipation, or in case of inflammation, there is pale diarrhea. Excess bile causes dark diarrhea:

> *In illnesses of the large intestine, it is advisable to harmonize the liver, which is the master. If the liver is ill, facilitate the function of the large intestine. (DACH XI, 10r)*

The throat and rhinopharynx depend on its function and are commanded by its points.

Respiratory passages: in case of inflammation of the lungs, disperse the the large intestine.

The meridian (shou yangming).

The energy is at its maximum from 5 to 7 a.m. and during the month of May. It corresponds with the kidney meridian, maximum from 5 to 7 p.m. It is a yang workshop organ, centripetal (rising). The coupled yin treasure organ is that of the lung *(shou taiyin).* Dispersing the lungs decreases spasms in the large intestine.

Insufficient energy of the large intestine:

The pulse of the large intestine is either abolished, or small and soft. If it is soft and without shape, there is either a recent laxative, habitual relaxation or a noticeable atony.

Physical symptoms: cold, heat slow to return, pain in the cheek bones, atony with diarrhea or atonic constipation (mostly in old people, obese women, sedentary people) with slow and hard stools; flaccid abdomen, tongue thickened and yellow at the back; acidity and coolness; tonify.

Psychological symptoms: lack of vitality; dreams of fields and uncultivated country.

Through the main meridian: tonify *quchi* (LI-11) and the source point, *hegu* (LI-4).

Through the circulation of energy: tonify the lungs (the mother who feeds) at *taiyuan* (LU-9) and the stomach (the child who suckles) at *jiexi* (ST-41).

Alarm point: *tianshu* (ST-25).

Passage point: *lieque* (LU-7) from the lungs to the large intestine, disperse; or disperse *pianli* (LI-6).

Coupled yin organ: lungs, tonify *taiyuan* (LU-9).

Husband-wife rule; tonify the small intestine at *houxi* (SI-3).

Midnight-midday rule: the large intestine has its maximum from 5 to 7 a.m.; at night and during cold, rainy times tonify the kidney (maximum from 5 to 7 p.m.) at *fuliu* (KI-7).

Excess energy of the large intestine:

The pulse of the large intestine will be hard and large. If it is hard and large proximally there is retention in the large intestine. If it is hard and narrow, there is pain, colic and spasms. If it is agitated distally, towards the thumb, there are hemorrhoids. If the whole pulse is agitated and large, there are intestinal parasites, usually oxyures. If it is agitated proximally, there is the possibility of colibacillosis.

Physical symptoms: spasmodic constipation, stools like ribbons or thin like a pencil, sometimes with mucus; large intestine hard on palpation, pain or colic. The path of the meridian (mostly on the shoulder) is hot and sensitive. There is the possibility of rheumatism of the shoulder.

Psychological symptoms: agitation, irritability. Children who have worms are nervous, choleric, always crying; they frequently rub their nostrils.

Through the main meridian: disperse *sanjian* (LI-3) and *erjian* (LI-2) and the source point *hegu* (LI-4).

Through the circulation of energy: disperse the lungs (the mother who feeds) at *chize* (LU-5) and the stomach (the child who suckles) at *lidui* (ST-45).

Coupled yin treasure organ: disperse the lungs at *chize* (LU-5).

Passage point: disperse *pianli* (LI-6) from the large intestine to the lungs, or tonify *lieque* (LU-7).

Midnight-midday rule: disperse the kidney at night or cold, dark times (correspondent from 5-7 p.m.).

Husband-wife rule: disperse the small intestine at *xiaohai* (LI-8).

In general.

(See all illnesses of intestines) *Tianshu* (ST-25), *wailing* (ST-26), *geshu* (BL-17), *weishu* (BL-21), *sanjiaoshu* (BL-22).

(GSdeM) Arm-*shanglian* (LI-9) is painful when there is diarrhea; arm-*sanli* (LI-10) when there is constipation.

(DACH) This point sends the energy to the large intestine: lip-*heliao* (LI-19).

> In large intestine illnesses, it is advisable to harmonize the liver, which is the master. If the liver is ill, facilitate the functions of the large intestine. *(DACH XI, 10r)*

Intestinal gas, aerocolia, flatulence, intestinal sounds.

(See also swelling of belly and intestines; aerogastria.)

Intestinal sounds: *(DACH) sanjian* (LI-3); disperse leg-*sanli* (ST-36), *xiangu* (ST-43), *zhaohai* (KI-3, IS KI-6), *lougu* (SP-7), *chengman* (ST-20), *yindu* (KI-19), *zhiyang* (GV-8, IS GV-9), *yanggang* (BL-43, IS BL-48), *ciliao* (BL-32), *xialiao* (BL-34), *weishu* (BL-21).

Thunderous sounds in the intestines: *(DACH) chengman* (ST-20), *yindu* (KI-19), *sanjian* (LI-3), *baohuang* (BL-48, IS BL-53), *dachangshu* (BL-25), leg-*shanglian* (ST-37, IS *shangjuxu*), *fuliu* (KI-7).

Thunderous sounds in the intestines rising and attacking the heart: *(DACH) shuifen* (CV-9).

Painful intestinal sounds: *(YXRM) xiangu* (ST-43).

Thunderous sounds in the abdomen: *(DACH)* leg-*sanli* (ST-36), *hunmen* (BL-42, IS BL-47).

Intestinal sounds, diarrhea, prolapsed rectum: *(DACH VII, 26r; YIX 9v) neiguan* (PC-6).

Intestinal sounds; pains of energy running and flowing: *(DACH) xialian* (LI-8).

Aerocolia of the lower belly: *(DACH) guilai* (ST-29).

Intestinal sounds and swelling of the abdomen: *(DACH, YXRM) sanyinjiao* (SP-6), *chengman* (ST-20), *weishu* (BL-21).

Sounds from emptiness in the abdomen: *(DACH) burong* (ST-19).

Intestinal sounds, sudden pain: *(DACH)* energy running through the abdomen *(DACH, YXRM) guanmen* (ST-22).

Feces.

Large intestine, slippery feces: *(DACH) liangmen* (ST-21), *yishe* (BL-44, IS BL-49).

Defecates, but dry: *(DACH, YXRM) huangshu* (KI-16), abdomen-*zhongzhu* (KI-15).

Defecation, hard: *(DACH) huangmen* (BL-46, IS BL-51), *buxi* (BL-52, IS BL-38).

Constipation (da bian bu yi, bu tong).

Acupuncture is not efficient in cases of megacolon or dolichocolon. In constipation, I have found that arm-*sanli* (LI-10) is very painful.

> *Origins: lack of exercise, influence of one's profession on the vitality, irregularities of life, gastritis, ulcer of the stomach, cancer of the stomach, nervous illness of the stomach, intestinal ptosis, neurasthenia, etc.*
>
> *Symptoms: in constipation of a transitory nature, defecation is simply blocked. In chronic constipation, the abdomen is heavy and presses somewhat. There are sensations of contraction, of ballooning, of fullness. The appetite is diminished; nausea, eructation, cephalalgia accompanied with vertigo. It is impossible to pass stool without medicine. The stools are in lumps and remain a long time in the rectum. (JO, 34)*

Treatment with needles:

dadun *(LR-2)*	*2 fen,*
yanglingquan *(GB-34)*	*6 fen,*
leg-**sanli** *(ST-36)*	*1 cun,*
abdomen-**zhongzhu** *(KI-15)*.......	*7 fen,*
shiguan *(KI-18)*	*8 fen,*
gaohuangshu *(BL-38, IS BL-43)*	*1 cun,*
zhigou *(TW-6)*	*3 fen. (JO, 34)*

Treatment with moxa:

dadun *(LR-2)*	*5 moxas,*
zhigou *(TW-6)*	*7 moxas,*
yanglingquan *(GB-34)*	*7 moxas,*
leg-**sanli** *(ST-36)*	*10 moxas,*
shiguan *(KI-18)*	*10 moxas,*
gaohuangshu *(BL-38, IS BL-43)*	*10 moxas. (JO, 34)*

Habitual constipation:

Treatment with needles and moxa:

dachangshu *(BL-25)*	*2 cun, 10 moxas,*
xiaochangshu *(BL-27)*	*2 cun, 10 moxas,*
abdomen-**zhongzhu** *(KI-15)*	*1 cun, 10 moxas,*
daju *(ST-27)*	*1 cun, 10 moxas,*
wailing *(ST-26)*..................	*1 cun, 10 moxas,*
fushi *(SP-13)*	*1 cun, 10 moxas (JM).*

(GSdeM) Most constipation comes from an insufficiency of the liver: tonify *ququan* (LR-8) and use ten daily moxas at the same point (the stools have little color, the blood coagulates slowly, bruises easily, patient digests chocolate and eggs badly).

(GSdeM) Constipation from muscular atony of the intestine (sympatheticotonia): tonify *quchi* (LI-11), *hegu* (LI-4), *yanglingquan* (GB-34); disperse *fengchi* (GB-20).

(GSdeM) Constipation from insufficient stools (sympatheticotonia): the some points as for atony.

(JM) Paresis of the abdominal muscles: *fushe* (SP-13).

(GSdeM) Spasmodic constipation (vagotonia): disperse *sanjian* (LI-3) and *erjian* (LI-2). Otherwise, disperse *tianjing* (TW-10) and *dadun* (LR-2), and tonify *fengchi* (GB-20).

(DACH) Difficult defecation: *taixi* (KI-5, IS KI-3), *yongquan* (KI-1), *taichong* (LR-3), *dazhong* (KI-6, IS KI-4), *taibai* (SP-3), *jiaoxin* (KI-8), *chengshan* (BL-57), thorax-*qimen* (LR-14), *yindu* (KI-19), *dachangshu* (BL-25), *pangguangshu* (BL-28), *xiaochangshu* (BL-27), *zhongliao* (BL-33).

(DACH) Difficult defecation; abdominal fullness; *pangguangshu* (BL-28).

(DACH) No need to defecate: *shangqiu* (SP-5).

(JM) Habitual, constant constipation: *zhigou* (TW-6), *yanglingquan* (GB-34), *shangqiu* (KI-17), *huangshu* (KI-16), *huangmen* (BL-46, IS BL-51).

Defecation blocked *(da bian bi)*: *(JM)* *xingjian* (LR-2), leg-*sanli* (ST-36), *taibai* (SP-3), *dazhong* (KI-6, IS KI-4), *fenglong* (ST-40), *fuxi* (BL-52, IS BL-38), *dadun* (LR-1), *taixi* (KI-5, IS KI-3), *zhaohai* (KI-3, IS KI-6), *jiexi* (ST-41), *jiaoxin* (KI-8), *chengshan* (BL-57), *chengjin* (BL-56), *bingfeng* (SI-12), *shiguan* (KI-18), *shimen* (CV-5), *daheng* (SP-15), *fushe* (SP-13), *zhongzhu* (KI-15), *huangshu* (KI-16), *shangliao* (BL-31), *ciliao* (BL-32), *zhongliao* (BL-33), *xialiao* (BL-34), *dachangshu* (BL-25), *xiaochangshu* (BL-27), *pangguangshu* (BL-28), *baihuanshu* (BL-30), *baohuang* (BL-48, IS BL-53), *huiyin* (CV-1), *weicang* (BL-45, IS BL-50); *(DACH II, 27r)* *zhigou* (TW-6), *zhaohai* (KI-3, IS KI-6).

Defecation blocked from emptiness: *(YXRM I, 40r)* tonify *zhigou* (TW-6), disperse leg-*sanli* (ST-36).

Defecation blocked from heat or energy: disperse *dadun* (LR-1), *chengshan* (BL-57), *yanglingquan* (GB-34) and if there is vomiting, *yinlingquan* (SP-9).

Defecation blocked, grainy: *(DACH II, 27r)* *dadun* (LR-1).

Defecation blocked from heat or cold: *(DACH XI, 6r)* first tonify then disperse *zhangmen* (LR-13), *taibai* (SP-3), *zhaohai* (KI-3, IS KI-6).

Defecation not passing: *(YXRM I, 39r)* *sanyinjiao* (SP-6) men on left, women on right; *(DACH)* *chengshan* (BL-57), *qihai* (CV-6), *(DACH)* *shangliao* (BL-31).

Women — defecation blocked: *(DACH VII, 34r)* *zhaohai* (KI-3, IS KI-6), *shenmai* (BL-62), *taixi* (KI-5, IS KI-3), *sanyinjiao* (SP-6), *yinlingquan* (SP-9).

Defecation not passing, accumulation of energy in the abdomen: *(YIX I, 5r)* disperse *neiguan* (PC-6).

Defecation not passing; lumbar area seized: *(DACH)* *chengjin* (BL-56).

Defecation not passing, from fullness of the spleen-pancreas: *(DACH)* *shangqiu* (SP-5).

Intestinal obstructions, intestinal occlusions:

(GSdeM) arm-*wuli* (LI-13), *sanjian* (LI-3), *dadun* (LR-1).

Obstruction, occlusion *(chang bi)*: *(JM)* arm-*wuli* (LI-13), *shugu* (BL-65), *fuliu* (KI-7), leg-*zhongdu* (LR-6), *heyang* (BL-55), *huiyang* (BL-35), *siman* (KI-14).

Obstruction, occlusion, stools bloody, descent of blood: *(DACH)* *huiyang* (BL-35).

Spasms-obstructions *(shan bi)*: *(DACH X, 27v)* *yinlingquan* (SP-9), *taixi* (KI-5, IS KI-3), *qiuxu* (GB-40), *zhaohai* (KI-3, IS KI-6).

Also cures vomiting with constipation: *(YXRM I, 40r)* disperse *yinlingquan* (SP-9), leg-*sanli* (ST-36).

Large intestine bound, hard feces: *(DACH)* *fuxi* (BL-52, IS BL-38).

Causes dilation of the intestines and liver: (Abrams) L11 and L12, *jizhong* (GV-6).

Stoppage of functions (leng bi).

Large and small grainy stools (blocked): *(DACH)* *xuanzhong* (GB-39).

Defecation and urination are difficult, unproductive: *(DACH)* *taichong* (LR-3), *diji* (SP-8), *lougu* (SP-7), *sanyinjiao* (SP-6), *jiaoxin* (KI-8), *fenglong* (ST-40), *yongquan* (KI-1), *dazhong* (KI-6, IS KI-4), *shimen* (CV-5), *zhongji* (CV-3), *shuidao* (ST-28), *ciliao* (BL-32), *zhongliao* (BL-33), *xialiao* (BL-34), *baihuanshu* (BL-30), *dachangshu* (BL-25), *changqiang* (GV-1).

Defecation and urination blocked, not passing: *(DACH)* *shuidao* (ST-28), *weishu* (BL-21), *baohuang* (BL-48, IS BL-53), *huiyin* (CV-1).

Defecation and urination impossible: *(DACH)* *baohuang* (BL-48, IS BL-53).

Stoppage of function *(leng bi)*: *(DACH)* *xingjian* (LR-2) disperse, *dazhong* (KI-6, IS KI-4), *ququan* (LR-8).

Energy from stoppage of function *(bi)* from cold: *(DACH)* *zhongwan* (CV-12).

Pain like a storm from stoppage of function *(leng)*: *(YXRM)* *zhongfeng* (LR-4).

Stoppage of function *(leng bi)*, swelling of lower part: *(DACH)* *baohuang* (BL-48, IS BL-53).

Diarrhea, enteritis, catarrh of intestines.

Diarrhea *(xie li, xie xie; bai li,* white dysentery):

> *Name of illness: what comes out flows as a liquid and spreads; these days it is called* **xie xie.** *(Ci Yuan, ''Xie-li'')*

Enteritis, catarrh of intestines *(chang jia da er):*

> *Swelling and inflammation of the intestinal mucosa. Acute form: pains of the abdomen and very violent diarrhea. Chronic form: pains in the abdomen, diarrhea or stoppage of feces. (Ci Yuan, ''Chang-jia Da-er'')*

Acute enteritis:

> *Origin: drink and food which contains no life; duodenal worms; poisoning; contagious illnesses (typhoid, dysentery, malaria, anemia), extreme coldness of the abdomen, flu, acute gastritis, acute peritonitis.*
>
> *Symptoms: lower part of the abdomen swollen, ballooned, intestinal sounds, pain of abdomen, diarrhea, decrease of urine; attack of fever from time to time; numerous stools, sometimes the bile colors the stool, but in general grey-white; the smell is very bad. (JO, 20)*

Chronic enteritis:

> *Origin: it is a continuation of acute enteritis or a repressing of the blood from the lungs, heart or liver; gastritis, dilation of the stomach, atony of stomach, intestinal tuberculosis, parasitic worms.*
>
> *Symptoms: constipation or diarrhea alternating with peculiar sensations; after defecation, the sensation that the stool still remains; at each defecation acute or dull pain; liquid mucus comes out, intestinal sounds, pains of the abdomen, drum-like abdomen (tympanism), headaches, vertigo, lessening of the appetite, skin dry and atrophied, repression of anxieties, disturbed vitality. (JO, 21)*

Arm-*xialian* (LI-8) is very sensitive to pressure in cases of diarrhea or enteritis. Distinguish carefully between diarrhea from emptiness and atony and that from inflammation.

All illnesses in the intestines: *(DACH VII, 34v) gongsun* (SP-4) and foot-*linqi* (GB-41); *(GSdeM)* from inflammation: *gongsun* (SP-4), from emptiness *guanyuan* (CV-4) and *tianshu* (ST-25).

Diarrhea responds immediately: *(DACH VII, 23v; YIX I, 9v);* diarrhea, intestinal sounds, swelling of abdomen: *(YXRM) gongsun* (SP-4).

All diarrhea and illnesses of the abdomen: *(YXRM I, 29v)* leg-*sanli* (ST-36) and *neiting* (ST-44).

Controls diarrhea: *(DACH) yingchuang* (ST-16).

Diarrhea: *(YIX I, 4v) tianshu* (ST-25) moxa; *(YXRM I, 46r) guanyuan* (CV-4); diarrhea without control *(DACH) shimen* (CV-5); *(DACH X, 31v) shenque* (CV-8), *shuifen* (CV-9), *lieque* (LU-7), *yinbai* (SP-1), *rangu* (KI-2), *jiaoxin* (KI-8), *qimai* (TW-18), *huiyang* (BL-35); *(JM) fujie* (SP-14), *pangguangshu* (BL-28), *yaoyangguan* (GV-3), *dachangshu* (BL-25).

Enteritis; catarrh of the intestines: *(JM) sanjian* (LI-3), *jiaoxin* (KI-8), *qihai* (CV-6), *guanyuan* (CV-4), *zhongzhu* (KI-15), *guanmen* (ST-22), *liangmen* (ST-21), *zhongwan* (CV-12), *xiawan* (CV-10), *siman* (KI-14), *weidao* (GB-30, IS GB-28), *juliao* (GB-28, IS GB-29), *pishu* (BL-20), *weishu* (BL-21), *geshu* (BL-17), *geguan* (BL-41, IS BL-46), *huiyang* (BL-35), *dachangshu* (BL-25), *sanjiaoshu* (BL-22), *xiaochangshu* (BL-27), *zhonglüshu* (BL-29).

Enteritis of children: *(JM) sanjiaoshu* (BL-22).

Catarrh of small intestine: *(JM) huangshu* (KI-16).

Acute enteritis:

Treatment with needles:

tianshu (ST-25)...........	*8 fen,*
yindu (KI-19)..............	*8 fen,*
guanyuan (CV-4)........	*1 cun,*
qihai (CV-6)................	*8 fen,*
siman (KI-14)	*6 fen,*
daheng (SP-15)...........	*8 fen,*
zhongwan (CV-12)	*8 fen,*
leg-sanli (ST-36).........	*1 cun,*
sanyinjiao (SP-6)........	*5 fen,*
dachangshu (BL-25)...	*1 cun,*
xiaochangshu (BL-27)	*1 cun. (JO, 20)*

Treatment with moxa:

shenque (CV-8) ..	*20 to 50 moxas,*
tianshu (ST-25)...	*15 moxas,*
guanyuan (CV-4)	*15 moxas,*
leg-sanli (ST-36)	*10 moxas. (JO, 20)*

Treatment with needles and moxa:

leg-sanli (ST-36)	*5 fen, 15 moxas,*
sanyinjiao (SP-6)	*5 fen, 15 moxas,*
weishu (BL-21)	*5 fen, 15 moxas,*
sanjiaoshu (BL-22)	*5 fen, 15 moxas,*
qihaishu (BL-24)	*5 fen, 15 moxas,*
dachangshu (BL-25) ..	*5 fen, 15 moxas,*
guanyuanshu (BL-26)	*5 fen, 15 moxas. (JM, 316)*

Treatment with moxa:

shangqiu (KI-17)	*20 moxas,*
daheng (SP-15)	*20 moxas. (JM, 316)*

Chronic enteritis:·

Treatment with needles:

weishu (BL-21)	*5 fen,*
pishu (BL-20)	*5 fen,*
guanyuan (CV-4)	*1 cun,*
dachangshu (BL-25)	*1 cun,*
pangguangshu (BL-28)	*1 cun,*
xiawan (CV-10)	*8 fen,*
tianshu (ST-25)	*8 fen,*
daheng (SP-15)	*8 fen. (JO, 21)*

Treatment with moxa:

leg-sanli (ST-36)	*10 moxas,*
dachangshu (BL-25)	*15 moxas,*
pangguangshu (BL-28)	*15 moxas,*
xiawan (CV-10)	*15 moxas,*
guanyuan (CV-4)	*15 moxas,*
daheng (SP-15)	*15 moxas,*
qihai (CV-6)	*15 moxas. (JO, 21)*

Treatment with needles:

sanjiaoshu (BL-22)	*1.5 to 2 cun,*
qihaishu (BL-24)	*1.5 to 2 cun,*
dachangshu (BL-25) ...	*1.5 to 2 cun,*
guanyuanshu (BL-26)	*1.5 to 2 cun,*
xiaochangshu (BL-27)	*1.5 to 2 cun,*
zhongzhu (KI-15)	*2 to 5 fen,*
daju (ST-27)	*2 to 5 fen,*
leg-sanli (ST-36)	*2 to 5 fen,*
sanyinjiao (SP-6)	*2 to 5 fen. (JM, 316)*

(JM) Shangwan (CV-13), *shuifen* (CV-9), *shenque* (CV-8), *shimen* (CV-5), *shangqiu* (KI-17), *daheng* (SP-15).
Diarrhea to the point of staying near the toilet *(tong xie): (DACH) sanjian* (LI-3); *(DACH) kunlun* (BL-60), *daheng* (SP-15); and with undigested food: *dachangshu* (BL-25), *changqiang* (GV-1); and with sounds in the intestines; pain radiating into the hip joint: *jingmen* (GB-25); serious diarrhea: *qihai* (CV-6).
Diarrhea without eating: *(DACH) guanmen* (ST-22); *(YXRM, DACH) hunmen* (BL-42, IS BL-47).
Diarrhea that does not stop: *(DACH) guanyuan* (CV-4), *qixue* (KI-13), *tianshu* (ST-25), shenjue (CV-8), *geguan* (BL-41, IS BL-46); *(DACH II, 6r; YIX I, 5r)* moxa at *zhongwan* (CV-12), *tianshu* (ST-25), *zhongji* (CV-3); *(DACH XII, 25r)* with interior contractions, then heaviness: *gongsun* (SP-4), *zhaohai* (KI-3, IS KI-6), *xiawan* (CV-10), *tianshu* (ST-25); with pain in the intestines and abdomen: *(DACH VII, 32r)* lieque (LU-7), *tianshu* (ST-25), *sanyinjiao* (SP-6), *neiting* (ST-44).
Diarrhea coming out without being felt: *(YIZ, 45v) zhongwan* (CV-12).
Sudden diarrhea: *(DACH) yinbai* (SP-1), *yinlingquan* (SP-9), leg-*xialian* (ST-39, IS *xiajuxu*).

Diarrhea after eating: *(DACH) yinlingquan* (SP-9), leg-*xialian* (ST-39, IS *xiajuxu*), leg-*shanglian* (ST-37, IS *shangjuxu*), arm-*xialian* (LI-8), *zhongliao* (BL-33).

Diarrhea with fever: *(DACH) pishu* (BL-20).

Diarrhea rising to pierce the heart: *(DACH) fujie* (SP-14).

Diarrhea and hemorrhoids: *(DACH) shugu* (BL-65).

Diarrhea of old people and those who are empty, cured like magic with: *(YXRM I, 46r) shenque* (CV-8).

Diarrhea of children: *(YIZ) shenque* (CV-8).

Diarrhea from illness of the spleen-pancreas: *(DACH) sanyinjiao* (SP-6).

Pasty diarrhea: *(DACH) taichong* (LR-3); *(YXRM I, 39r) sanyinjiao* (SP-6).

Pasty diarrhea finishing as liquid: *(YXRM) taichong* (LR-3).

Thick diarrhea of undigested food: *(DACH, YXRM) sanyinjiao* (SP-6).

Liquid diarrhea: *(DACH) xuanzhong* (GB-39), *ququan* (LR-8); and without stopping: *(DACH) tianshu* (ST-25); flow of diarrhea, diarrhea descending: *sanjiaoshu* (BL-22).

Diarrhea of bile: *(JM) pishu* (BL-20), *changqiang* (GV-1).

Diarrhea of undigested food: *(DACH)* leg-*sanli* (ST-36); *(YXRM) tianshu* (ST-25), *sanyinjiao* (SP-6); during cold times: *shenshu* (BL-23).

Paralysis of small intestine causing diarrhea of undigested food; *(YXRM V, 28v)* tonify *houxi* (SI-3).

Dysentery (hong li, chi li, bian xue, li ji).

In serious cases of li (diarrhea), a tiny being multiplies in the large intestine and causes the mucus covering the intestine to come down. Then the feces are mixed with pus and blood; there is pain. This is hong li, "red dysentery." It is a very violent contagious disease. Each time a dysentery begins, press below the umbilicus with your finger on the median line, but a little to the left; if there is acute pain, it is red dysentery. (Ci Yuan, "Li")

Contagious illness, contracted from food and drink; pain in the abdomen; strong and frequent diarrhea. What is vomited is similar to minced meat. (Ci Yuan, "Hong-li")

A very serious contagious illness. It is also called hong li, red dysentery. It is always contracted through food and drink or objects infected by stools infected with the illness. It starts with a bad chill and attack of fever. Pain in the abdomen; the contraction comes but without stool; only pasty fluid and blood comes, and that 20 to 60 times in 24 hours. The odor is very bad. The anus burns and is painful as if slashed. After one or two weeks there is improvement. The chronic form is difficult to cure. (Ci Yuan, "Chi-li")

Red dysentery: *(JM) zhongdu* (LR-6).

Red or white dysentery: *(DACH)* leg-*sanli* (ST-36), *zhongwan* (CV-12), *zhonglüshu* (BL-29), *tianshu* (ST-25).

Blood dysentery: *(JM) tianshu* (ST-25); abounds in autumn: *(DACH) changqiang* (GV-1).

Dysentery with descent of blood, accumulation in intestines: *(DACH) huiyang* (BL-35).

Fresh blood from the intestine: *(YIX I, 4r) qihai* (CV-6) and *sanyinjiao* (SP-6).

Scarlet or white dysentery; chill and pain in the abdomen: *(DACH VII, 32r) lieque* (LU-7), *shuidao* (ST-28), *qihai* (CV-6), *wailing* (ST-26), *tianshu* (ST-25), leg-*sanli* (ST-36), *sanyinjiao* (SP-6).

Diarrhea with pus and blood: *(DACH)* leg-*xialian* (ST-39, IS *xiajuxu*), *youmen* (KI-21).

Intestinal hemorrhages.

Intestinal hemorrhages: *(JM) taibai* (SP-3), *heyang* (BL-55), *qihai* (CV-6), *guanyuan* (CV-4), *fuai* (SP-16), *geshu* (BL-17), *ganshu* (BL-18), *shenshu* (BL-23), *dachangshu* (BL-25), *xialiao* (BL-34), *changqiang* (GV-1).

Shock of the intestines, loss of blood: *(DACH) gongsun* (SP-4), *mingmen* (GV-4), *changqiang* (GV-1).

Shock of the intestines, ejection of fresh blood: *(DACH II, 19r) changqiang* (GV-1), *chengshan* (BL-57).

Intestinal hemorrhages, shock of the intestines, a lot depends either on the stomach or the large intestines: *(DACH X, 34r)* needles at *yinbai* (SP-1), moxa at leg-*sanli* (ST-36).

Pulses full, descent of blood: *(DACH) guanyuan* (CV-4).

Scarlet defecation and urination: *(DACH) xiawan* (CV-10).

Urine and blood in the intestine: *(DACH) guanyuan* (CV-4).

Intestinal worms (ji sheng chong: parasites).

Oxyuriasis (hao):

*An animal in the form of **hui** (ascaris) but very small; the females have a length of 6 mm. (3 **fen**); the males have a length of 2 mm. (1 **fen**); white color, round shape; the extremities are curved. Lives in the intestines of people; comes from swallowing their eggs. Sometimes they come out through the anus; causes pruritis and swelling of the anus which can become inflamed; causes pain in the abdomen, internal headache, nausea, vomiting. They are expelled with vermifuge and enemas. (Ci Yuan, "Hao")*

Squirms in the large intestine; often causes hemorrhoids, and if serious, pruritis, abscess and even epilepsy. (YXRM V, 39v)

(Europe) Copulates and lays eggs at the new moon.

Ascaris (hui, hui hui):

An animal similar to an earthworm, but without a ring; white in color. The two extremities are very pointed. It develops and lives mainly in the small intestines of children. Patients have pain in the abdomen, vomiting, diarrhea. The females are about 30 cm. long; the male is from 15 to 20 cm. long. (Ci Yuan, "Hui")

Various:

*There are nine varieties of parasitic worms: 1) **hui chong** (ascaris); 2) **hao chong** (oxyuris); 3) **fu chong**, ("hookworm"), about 4 **cun** long (10 cm.) maximum; 4) **rou chong** ("meat worms"), shaped similar to orchids, they cause malaise, fullness, boredom; 5) **bai chong** ("white worms"), 2.5 cm. long long (1 **cun**); mother and offspring propagate and squirm; can cause death; 6) **fei chong** ("lung worms"), shaped like a silkworm; they cause coughing; 7) **wei chong** ("stomach worms"), they cause vomiting, hiccoughs; make one eat clay or raw rice, carbon or other objects; 8) **ruanzhong** ("weak worms"), or **gechong** ("diaphragm worms"), similar to a melon tendril, cause a lot of saliva, abscesses, furuncles and hemorrhoids; 9) **chi chong** ("scarlet worms"), similar to raw meat; cause sounds in the intestines. (YXRM V, 39v)*

We should add: *shi er zhi chang chong* ("duodenal worms") and parasitic worms in general: *ji sheng chong; wu mei* ("black prunes"), flukeworms.

Toxins coming from parasites (gu zhang):

The same as the poison coming from the worms in wine that transform it into vinegar; likewise, in the body the poisons produced by worms act the same. They cause a yellow face, yellow painful body, no strength at all, mucus, saliva, urinary troubles, mouth and lips dry. . . . If the spit sinks in water, there are worms. (YXRM V, 39v, "Gu-zhang")

Intoxication from intestinal worms *(gu zhang)*:
Cures all intoxications from intestinal worms *(gu zhang) (DACH VI, 11v; YXRM V, 30r)* three moxas at *zhiyin* (BL-67).
Intoxication from intestinal worms: *(YXRM) juque* (CV-14).
Abundance of saliva from the three intestinal worms: *(YXRM) shangwan* (CV-13); *(DACH) zhongwan* (CV-12).
Agitation from intestinal worms, saliva comes out: *(DACH) fuliu* (KI-7).
Pain from intestinal worms, ascaris: *(DACH) juque* (CV-14).
Sudden pain in the heart from the two intestinal worms: *(DACH) shangwan* (CV-13).
Pain in the heart from worms: *(YIZ, 43v)* needle thorax-*qimen* (LR-14).
Pain in the heart from ascaris *(hui): (DACH)* foot-*dadu* (SP-2).
All worms *(GSdeM)*: causes parasites to be ejected, prevents their reproduction: ten moxas four days before and after the new moon at *zhiyin* (BL-67).
Abdominal pain from worms constantly nibbling, expectoration of ascaris. If prune-black (flukeworm?) they are difficult to combat; death in nine to ten days.
Zhongwan (CV-12) re-establishes the energy of the stomach: *(DACH IV, 11v).*
Worms in the treasure organs and workshop organs, nibbling the flesh: *(DACH IV, 11v) dicang* (ST-7, IS ST-4).
Parasitic worms *(ji sheng chong): (JM) sanyangluo* (TW-8), *tiantu* (CV-22), *zhongwan* (CV-12), *burong* (ST-19), *tianshu* (ST-25), *daheng* (SP-15), *zhangmen* (LR-13).
Duodenal worms: *(JM) tianshu* (ST-25), *ganshu* (BL-18), *weishu* (BL-21).

Cold, emptiness, atony of the large intestine.

Large intestine does not return (flaccid, atony): *(DACH) waiqiu* (GB-36).

Extreme coldness of the large intestine: *(JM)* leg-*shanglian* (ST-37, IS *shangjuxu*).

Cold of the large intestine; diarrhea, not digesting cereals: *(DACH) liangmen* (ST-21), leg-*shanglian* (ST-37, IS *shangjuxu*).

Energy of the large intestine dispersing (and prolapse of the rectum): *(DACH) baihui* (GV-19, IS GV-20).

Large intestine cold, empty: prolapsed rectum cannot be drawn in: *(DACH VII, 26v) neiguan* (PC-6), *baihui* (GV-19, IS GV-20), *mingmen* (GV-4), *changqiang* (GV-1), *chengshan* (BL-57).

Atony of the large intestine: *(GSdeM)* tonify *quchi* (LI-11) and *hegu* (LI-4).

Fullness, heat of the large intestine.

Heat in the large intestine: *(DACH) qichong* (ST-30).

In the abdomen, extreme heat attacking and overrunning: *(YXRM) qichong* (ST-30).

Fullness of the large intestine; heat, occlusion, unable to urinate: *(DACH)* thigh-*wuli* (LR-10).

Energy of the large intestine: *(DACH)* arm-*shanglian* (LI-9).

Energy from large and small intestines: *(DACH) xingjian* (LR-2).

When defecating, heaviness below: *(DACH) yongquan* (KI-1).

Pain of the large intestine, spasms, accumulations, water.

(See pain in the abdomen and intestine)

Pain in the large intestine; unbearable pain below the umbilicus: *(DACH) sanyinjiao* (SP-6).

Spasms; intestinal peristalsis is activated by the vagus nerve: *tianzhu* (BL-10).

Accumulations in the large intestine: *(YIZ) guanyuan* (CV-4).

Water in the large intestine: *(DACH) siman* (KI-14).

Ulcerations, abscesses.

Intestinal ulcerations: *(JM) ququan* (LR-8).

Abscess of the large intestine: *(DACH) zhoujian* (MP-11, IS M-UE-46), one hundred moxas.

Pus and blood in the feces: *(DACH)* leg-*xialian* (ST-39, IS *xiajuxu*), *ququan* (LR-8), *fuai* (SP-16), *youmen* (KI-21).

Abscess and putrefaction in the large intestine: *(DACH)* leg-*zhongdu* (LR-6).

Pruritis of the rectum: *(JM) huiyin* (CV-1).

Peritonitis, appendicitis.

Peritonitis (*fu mo yan*, "inflammation of the membrane of the abdomen"):

> *The illness causes violent pain in the abdomen. It comes either from injuries or flu or illness of the stomach at intestines. There is swelling of the abdomen; sometimes diarrhea or constipation; high temperature. (Ci Yuan, "Fu-mo-yan")*

Peritonitis: *(JM)* leg-*sanli* (ST-36), *yinlingquan* (SP-9), *xuehai* (SP-10), *xingjian* (LR-2), *yinbai* (SP-1), *jinmen* (BL-63), *shangwan* (CV-13), *chengman* (ST-20), thorax-*qimen* (LR-14), *zhonglüshu* (BL-29).

Chronic peritonitis:

Treatment with needles and moxa:

weishu *(BL-21)*	*1.5 to 2 **cun,** 10 moxas,*
sanjiaoshu *(BL-22)*	*1.5 to 2 **cun,** 10 moxas,*
shenshu *(BL-23)*	*1.5 to 2 **cun,** 10 moxas,*
weicang *(BL-45, IS BL-50)....*	*1.5 to 2 **cun,** 10 moxas,*
huangmen *(BL-46, IS BL-51)*	*1.5 to 2 **cun,** 10 moxas,*
zhishi *(BL-47, IS BL-52)*	*1.5 to 2 **cun,** 10 moxas. (JM, 316)*

(JM) Xuehai (SP-10), *zhongwan* (CV-12), *qihai* (CV-6), thorax-*qimen* (LR-14).

Appendicitis (*huang chang yan*, "inflammation of the cecum"):

> *Origins: irritation from drugs or from heat or from the intestinal fluids not flowing, or from foreign objects (seeds, etc.); from intestinal worms or parasites; contagion from urethritis, constipation, etc.*

Symptoms: in general, constipation and acute pain in the right iliac fossa; attacks of swelling, pain when moving or dressing. There is hardness along the line from the umbilicus to the lower part of the iliac bone; bad chill and attacks of heat, appetite disappears, nausea, vomiting, stools blocked; drum-swelling of the abdomen. (JO, 23)

Treatment with needles:

guanyuan (CV-4)	*1 cun,*
ganshu (BL-18) ..	*5 fen,*
danshu (BL-19) ..	*5 fen,*
pishu (BL-20)	*8 fen. (JO, 23.)*

Treatment with moxa:

ganshu (BL-18)	*25 moxas,*
danshu (BL-19)	*25 moxas,*
pishu (BL-20)	*25 moxas,*
jinsuo (GV-7, IS GV-8)	*25 moxas,*
zhongshu (GV-6a, IS GV-7)	*25 moxas. (JO, 23.)*

(JM) Chronic appendicitis: *shimen* (CV-5), *qihai* (CV-6).
(DACH) Pain in the intestine, heat and pain on one side: *zhaohai* (KI-3, IS KI-6).

Rectal prolapse (tuo gang, tuo chang).

Prolapsed rectum: *(YXRM I, 46v) gongsun* (SP-4); *(DACH) erbai* (MP-12, IS M-UE-29); *(YXRM I, 46r; JM, DACH) baihui* (GV-19, IS GV-20); *(YXRM I, 46r) mingmen* (GV-4); *(JM) chongmen* (SP-12), *changqiang* (GV-1), *jizhong* (GV-6).
Prolapsed rectum in children: *(DACH) baihui* (GV-19, IS GV-20); *(JM) shenque* (CV-8).
(DACH III, 27r) jiuwei (CV-15) and *baihui* (GV-19, IS GV-20) moxa.
Prolapsed rectum, intestinal sounds, diarrhea: *(DACH VII, 26r; YIX I, 9v) neiguan* (PC-6).
Difficult defecation; if forced, the rectum prolapses: *(DACH VII, 26v) neiguan* (PC-6), *zhigou* (TW-6), *baihui* (GV-19, IS GV-20), *zhaohai* (KI-3, IS KI-6).
Prolapse of the rectum which cannot be brought back; cold and emptiness of the large intestine: *(DACH VII, 26v) baihui* (GV-19, IS GV-20), *changqiang* (GV-1), *mingmen* (GV-4), *chengshan* (BL-57).
Prolapsed rectum and old hemorrhoids: *(DACH XI, 6v; YIX I, 5v) baihui* (GV-19, IS GV-20), *changqiang* (GV-1), *erbai* (MP-21, IS M-UE-29), *zhishi* (BL-47, IS BL-52).
Prolapsed rectum: *(DACH IV, 19v; Zhenjiu Juying) baihui* (GV-19, IS GV-20), *wuyi* (ST-15).

Anus (gang).

The relaxation of the anal sphincter is activated through the vagus nerve.
Anus: *(JM, Fuji) shenshu* (BL-23), *xiaochangshu* (BL-27).
Spasms of all the muscles of the anus: *(JM) baihuanshu* (BL-30).
Inflammation of all the muscles of the anus: *(JM) baihuanshu* (BL-30).
Pruritis of the anus (anal itching): *(DACH) huiyin* (CV-1).
Pain responding front and back: *(JM) huiyin* (CV-1).
Contractions or contractures of the anal sphincter: *(GSdeM) huiyang* (BL-35), *baihuanshu* (BL-30).
When pressing, responds in the anus: *taixi* (KI-5, IS KI-3).

Hemorrhoids (chi, chi chuang, chi he, nei chi, wai chi).

*Painful and burning swelling of the anus. The causes are various: constipation, inflammation of the rectum, repeated purges, frequent intestinal pain, illness of the heart and lung, interrupted circulation of the blood, remaining sitting or standing for a long time. In women it comes from swelling of the uterus which presses and weighs down, or from pregnancy disturbing the circulation; intestinal worms. When the vessels of the anus swell like tumors of blood, **lou,** they are called **chi he,** ''nut-hemorrhoids.'' (Ci Yuan, ''Chi, Chi-chuang'')*

(GSdeM) In congestive and hypertensive people, begin by lowering the blood-pressure: disperse *daling* (PC-7) and *shenmen* (HT-7); the hemorrhoids serve as a safety-valve. Often, they have as an initial cause a pronounced insufficiency of the liver; tonify *ququan* (LR-8) and *taichong* (LR-3).
Special master point for hemorrhoids: *(JM) changqiang* (GV-1).
Changqiang (GV-1) is the root of hemorrhoids; avoid cold *(DACH).*

The five hemorrhoids: *(DACH) changqiang* (GV-1); naturally caused by heat of the blood *(DACH IV, 11v; Juying) chengshan* (BL-57).

All hemorrhoids: *(YXRM I, 46r) mingmen* (GV-4).

Hemorrhoids: *weizhong* (BL-54, IS BL-40); *(DACH VI, 15r) zhiyin* (BL-67); *(DACH) chengshan* (BL-57), *chengjin* (BL-56); *(DACH V, 19v)* foot-*shangqiu* (SP-5); *(JM) sanyinjiao* (SP-6); *(DACH) zhengfu* (BL-50, IS BL-36), *(DACH) changqiang* (GV-1); *(JM) feiyang* (BL-58).

Old hemorrhoids, chronic: *(JM; YIZ, 45) changqiang* (GV-1); *(DACH III, 32r) chengshan* (BL-57); *(DACH) hui-yang* (BL-35); *(JM) huiyin* (CV-1).

Pain of hemorrhoids: *(DACH, YXRM) weizhong* (BL-54, IS BL-40), *feiyang* (BL-58).

Attack of swelling of the five hemorrhoids: *(DACH) zhibian* (BL-49, IS BL-54), swelling from hemorrhoids: *(DACH) chengshan* (BL-57).

Hemorrhoids; swelling during defecation: *(DACH VII, 32v; YIX I, 11v) lieque* (LU-7).

Hemorrhoids; pains, loss of blood: *(YXRM) xiaochangshu* (BL-27).

Hemorrhoids; bleeding after defecation: *(DACH) fuliu* (KI-7).

Hemorrhoids; serious with flow of blood: *(YXRM) shangqiu* (SP-5).

Hemorrhoids with a loss of blood: *(YXRM) shangqiu* (SP-5).

Hemorrhoids with a loss of blood: *(DACH XI, 21v)* needle 2 *fen* and seven moxas at *changqiang* (GV-1); *(YXRM) xiaochangshu* (BL-27).

Pains in the lumbar area from hemorrhoids: *(DACH) qihaishu* (BL-24).

Hemorrhoids inflamed, pain from the lesion: *(YXRM) feiyang* (BL-58).

"Hemorrhoids of cock-pheasants" (pederasts?): *(YXRM) feiyang* (BL-58).

Hemorrhoids and diarrhea: *(DACH) shugu* (BL-65).

Hemorrhoids, difficulty in defecation: *(DACH IV, 10v; YIX I, 8r) chengshan* (BL-57).

Hemorrhoids either oozing, bleeding or pressing into the interior; heaviness, itching, pain, the five hemorrhoids: *(YIZ, 40v; YIX, 5v) chengshan* (BL-57), 2.5 cun, tonify during one expiration; seven moxas.

Hemorrhoids:

Treatment with needles and moxa:

dachangshu *(BL-25)*	*2 to 2.5* **cun,** *10 moxas,*	
xiaochangshu *(BL-27)*	*2 to 2.5* **cun,** *10 moxas,*	
zhibian *(BL-49, IS BL-54)*	*2 to 2.5* **cun,** *10 moxas,*	
changqiang *(GV-1)*	*5* **fen,** *10 moxas,*	
huiyang *(BL-35)*	*5* **fen,** *10 moxas,*	
shangqiu *(SP-5)*	*5* **fen,** *10 moxas,*	
xuanzhong *(GB-39)*	*5* **fen,** *10 moxas. (JO, 316)*	

Hemorrhoids, external, tumor of blood *(lou)*: *(YIX I, 5v) shangqiu* (SP-5).

Hemorrhoids, accumulation of blood: *(DACH) xuanzhong* (GB-39).

Anal fistulae (chi lou).

> *If they are around the hole from which a lot of pus and fluid flows, the hemorrhoids are called* **chi lou**.
> *(Ci Yuan, "Chi-chuang")*

Fistulae: *(YXRM 46v) chengshan* (BL-57); *(DACH II, 19v; Juying) shangqiu* (SP-5); *(YXRM I, 46r) changqiang* (GV-1); *(DACH) qihaishu* (BL-24); *(DACH) erbai* (MP-12, IS M-UE-29), *tianchuang* (SI-16).

Fistulae of the intestines; thickening of the blood: *(DACH) xuanzhong* (GB-39).

Bleeding fistulae, pruritis, pain: *(YIZ, 46r) chengshan* (BL-57); *changqiang* (GV-1), one *cun*, disperse; three moxas.

Old oozing fistulae: *(DACH) changqiang* (GV-1).

Hemorrhoids communicating among themselves: *(DACH IV, 6r) huiyin* (CV-1).

The nine kinds of fistulae: *(DACH IV, 6r) chengshan* (BL-57), *changqiang* (GV-1).

Typhoid fever (ancient: shang han, bai he; Japanese: chang tie fu si).

Experience has shown that typhoid treated at the beginning can be cured in one week: disperse *hegu* (LI-4), *san-jian* (LI-3), *erjian* (LI-2).

> *In the past called* **shanghan**. *It is a contagious illness which is propagated through the typhus bacteria. The body is exhausted, lazy; bad chill, attack of fever, cephalalgia, vertigo; swelling and ballooning of the abdomen and*

intestines. At the beginning there is constipation, then diarrhea. Awareness is cloudy, there is even delirium. The patient expels a lot of poison from the illness through the urine and feces. (Ci Yuan, "Chang-tie [fu-si]")

At the beginning cephalalgia, the nape is stiff; bad chills, attack of fever. The tongue is covered with a thick coating; defecation and urination are blocked; one can think neither of eating nor drinking. Then the illness changes its nature; the fever does not diminish; there is trouble of the awareness and from time to time delirium. If the dangerous symptoms aggravate, the cure is difficult. Ancient medicine said that it was a pair of illnesses, one hot the other cold, and called it **shang han.** *Western medicine makes of it a single illness of the intestines, and the Japanese transcribe the European name by* **tie fu si.** *" (Ci Yuan, "Shang-han")*

In the cold **shang han,** *if the cold of yin reaches the vessels, one must use moxa. For the attacks of fever, there is cold fever, fever from anguish which comes and goes; feverish illness without sweating. (DACH X, 34r)*

"Bai he: this is shang han . . . pulse slow, elevated typhoid fever." (YXRM I, 22v)

(JM) Typhoid fever: disperse *hegu* (LI-4), *sanjian* (LI-3), *erjian* (LI-2).
(DACH IV, 11v) Typhoid *(bai he shang han),* very difficult to cure, mouth closed, eyes closed, medicine does not go down: *hegu* (LI-4).

(YIX, 6v) For *shang han:*

On the first day puncture *fengfu* (GV-15, IS GV-16), then stimulate the necessary yin or yang meridians.

Second day: *erjian* (LI-2) and *neiting* (ST-44), *rong* points of the *yangming.*

Third day: foot-*linqi* (GB-41) and hand-*zhongzhu* (TW-3), *shu* points of the *shaoyang.*

Fourth day: *yinbai* (SP-1) and *shaoshang* (LU-11), *jing* points of the *taiyin.*

Fifth day: *taixi* (KI-5, IS KI-3) and *shenmen* (HT-7), *shu* points of the *shaoyin.*

Sixth day: *zhongfeng* (LR-4) and *jianshi* (PC-5), *jing* points of *jueyin.*

If on the sixth day there is no sweat, puncture thorax-*qimen* (LR-14) and leg-*sanli* (ST-36); this is an ancient method.
If there is only a yin illness (cold), moxas at *guanyuan* (CV-4) are marvellous.
For sweat, vomiting and diarrhea: *hegu* (LI-4), *neiguan* (PC-6), *sanyinjiao* (SP-6): there is no other way. For abundant sweat, disperse *hegu* (LI-4) 2 *fen,* nine times nine, turning the needle ten times to the left on the right side and to the right on the left side. After obtaining the energy, disperse; the sweat will stop. When the temperature is normal, take out the needle. If the sweat has not stopped, disperse *yinshi* (ST-33) and tonify *hegu* (LI-4). For vomiting, needles at *neiguan* (PC-6) 3 *fen.* First, tonify six times and disperse three times. Make the energy rise, then push and agitate one time. After the patient breathes ten times, all will be finished. If the vomiting does not stop, tonify during thirty-six respirations. When the vomiting stops, slowly take out the needle and quickly cover the hole. If the vomiting still does not stop, tonify leg-*sanli* (ST-36). For diarrhea, needles at *sanyinjiao* (SP-6) 3 *fen* — men on the left, women on the right. Make the respiration shallow; puncture and disperse thirty-six times when the patient breathes in. If the diarrhea is not stopped, needle *hegu* (LI-4).
(DACH XI, 8-9; YIX I, 7r) Shang han:
For headaches: *daling* (PC-7), *laogong* (PC-8), *shanzhong* (CV-17), *qimen* (LR-14).
For pains in the sides: *zhigou* (TW-6), *zhangmen* (LR-13), *yanglingquan* (GB-34), bleed *weizhong* (BL-54, IS BL-40).
For cold and headaches: *hegu* (LI-4), *zanzhu* (BL-2), *tongziliao* (GB-1).
For pains of the ribs and sides: *daling* (PC-7), *laogong* (PC-8), *shanzhong* (CV-17), *qimen* (LR-14).
If the great fever does not recede, disperse *hegu* (LI-4), *quchi* (LI-11), *bailao* (GV-13, IS GV-14 *dazhui*), leg-*sanli* (ST-36), *xuanzhong* (GB-39), *yongquan* (KI-1).
If the fever has receded, but is still there: *hegu* (LI-4), *fengmen* (BL-12), *xuanzhong* (GB-39), *xiangjiao* (LR-2).
Delirious, cannot distinguish between respectable people and coarse people: *quchi* (LI-11), *qimen* (LR-14), *qihai* (CV-6); or *quchi* (LI-11), *bailao* (GV-13, IS GV-14 *dazhui*), *xuanzhong* (GB-39), *yongquan* (KI-1).
Attack of tonic convulsions: *quchi* (LI-11), *hegu* (LI-4), *shuigou* (GV-25, IS GV-26 *renzhong*), *fuliu* (KI-7).
Defecation not passing: *zhigou* (TW-6), *zhangmen* (LR-13), *zhaohai* (KI-3, IS KI-6), *taibai* (SP-3).
Urine not passing: *yingu* (KI-10), *yinlingquan* (SP-9).
Icterus of typhoid: hand-*wangu* (SI-4), *waiguan* (TW-5), *shenmai* (BL-62), *yongquan* (KI-1).
The six pulses are absent; the yin symptoms are numerous: *hegu* (LI-4), *fuliu* (KI-7), *zhongji* (CV-3).
The pulses are superficial: *xuanzhong* (GB-39); if cold, tonify, if hot disperse.
Sunken pulses, thin: tonify *xuanzhong* (GB-39).

Intestinal tuberculosis (chang lao, chang xie he).

> Intestinal tuberculosis, **chang xie he,** is also called **chang lao.** The patient has an attack of fever each day from 3
> to 5 p.m. The abdomen is painful; there is diarrhea. The appetite is lost little by little, the flesh thins and disap-
> pears.'' (Ci Yuan, ''Lao'')

(Europe) Diarrhea after meals, etc.

Intestinal tuberculosis (chang xie he): (JM) mingmen (GV-4), shenque (CV-8).

Tuberculosis; diarrhea after meals; intestinal cold; intestinal pain; difficult digestion: (DACH) leg-shanglian (ST-37,
IS shangjuxu).

Diarrhea after meals, abdomen painful: (DACH) xialian (LI-8).

Diarrhea after meals, swollen abdomen, the six extremes, the seven troubles of the five kinds of tuberculosis:
(YXRM, DACH) zhongliao (BL-33).

Serious diarrhea, emptiness, swelling: (DACH) guanyuan (CV-4).

(GSdeM) Tonify gaohuangshu (BL-38, IS BL-43), leg-sanli (ST-36) and daily moxas at shenque (CV-8) and leg-
sanli (ST-36).

Cholera (huo luan bing).

Cholera: (DACH, YXRM) leg-sanli (ST-36), kunlun (BL-60), yuji (LU-10), yinxi (HT-6), zhigou (TW-6); (GSdeM)
hegu (LI-4), sanjian (LI-3), ququan (LR-8).

(DACH) For cholera with energy in counterflow, stimulate leg-sanli (ST-36) and it will descend.

Cholera, diarrhea, vomiting: (JM) zhongwan (CV-12); (DACH) cholera, vomiting, cramps, diarrhea: zhigou (TW-6).

Cholera, stomach upset: (YXRM) zhongwan (CV-12).

Cholera, first pain in the abdomen, then diarrhea: (DACH) zhongwan (CV-12).

Attack of vomiting from cholera: (JM, DACH) renying (ST-9).

Vomiting from cholera: (DACH) tianshu (ST-25); (DACH X, 26v) zhigou (TW-6).

Cholera: first pain at the heart or first vomiting: (DACH). Cholera, vomiting of mucus and saliva: (DACH IV, 7v).

Cholera, acute pain at the heart, vomiting of mucus and saliva: (YIX I, 4v) juque (CV-14), moxas.

Malign cholera, dry vomiting: (DACH) jianshi (PC-5).

Cholera, cramps, vomiting, coma: (DACH) pucan (BL-61).

Cholera, pains, agitation, cramps: (YXRM) pucan (BL-61).

Cramps from cholera: (DACH) zhigou (TW-6); (YXRM I, 46v; DACH IV, 10r) needle 7 fen, five moxa at chengshan
(BL-57); (DACH) chengjin (BL-56); (YXRM I, 46v) yanglingquan (GB-34); (DACH, YXRM) jinmen (BL-63);
(YXRM I, 46v); cholera, cramps of feet and hands: taichong (LR-3); (YXRM) cramps from cholera: jiexi (ST-41),
fuyang (BL-59); (DACH) fuxi (BL-52, IS BL-38); (DACH) yongquan (KI-1).

Cholera, cramps, the four emptinesses: rugen (ST-18).

Spasms and accumulations from cholera: (DACH) yinlingquan (SP-9).

Cold:

Cholera, cold: (DACH) guanchong (TW-1).

Cholera, cold of the extremities: (DACH) sanyinjiao (SP-6).

Syncope:

Cholera, loss of consciousness, of sound, of energy: (DACH) arm-sanli (LI-10).

Cholera, energy of emptiness: (DACH) fushe (SP-13).

Drinks a lot, emptiness of the gallbladder, energy of emptiness, counterflow rising, then cholera: (DACH) gongsun
(SP-4).

Cholera, cold syncope: (DACH) yongquan (KI-1).

Pains:

Cholera, strangling pains of the abdomen: (DACH X, 33v) weizhong (BL-54, IS BL-40).

Panting:

Attacks of panting from cholera: (YXRM) yinlingquan (SP-9).

XXV. Liver (Gan)

The medial edge (towards the median line) of the artery corresponds to the posterior lobes and to the antitoxic
function; skin, blood, pruritis, eczema. The lateral edge (towards the radius) corresponds to the interior lobes and to
the bile function — constipation or diarrhea. The left meridian mostly acts on the anterior lobes and bile. The right
meridian acts on the posterior lobes and the antitoxic function.

Pulse: left wrist, middle pulse (there is no deep position) at the level of the radial styloid process. The right edge seems to correspond to the posterior lobes and to action on the skin (blood, pruritis, acne). The left edge would then correspond to the anterior lobes and action on the bile and constipation. The right meridian would mostly act on the posterior lobes and the left on the bile.

The upper edge of T11 (*jizhong*, GV-6) causes a reflex dilation of the liver; L2, a reflex contraction. The liver holds the *hun* (memory level, automaton, parrot) *(DACH)*; it holds the blood *((DACH)*. Shocks, trembling, dizziness, depend on the liver *(DACH IV, 1r; I, 16r)*. Sexual energy accumulates in the liver *(DACH)*. Even a slight retention of the biliary salts in the blood causes pruritis. The liver flourishes in the nails *(DACH)*. Unhappiness injures, stimulates the liver (and cures obsessions); sadness cures malcontentment *(YXRM V, 4r)*.

The liver is at its lowest level at the spring (March) and autumn (September) equinoxes; summer congests it. It is the only organ which produces sugar; when the movement of blood into the liver is slowed down, the blood is charged with sugar. The production of sugar by the liver is stimulated by adrenalin (hyperadrenalism).

The gallbladder *(zu shaoyang)* is the yang workshop organ of the liver *(zu jueyin)* yin treasure organ. A tightened gallbladder blocks the liver. The gallbladder acts as regulator of the liver.

(DACH XI, 10r) In fullness of the liver, it is advisable to facilitate the function of the large intestine; if the large intestine is ill, regulate the liver. If the lungs are ill, the liver is in danger: tonify it. If the liver is empty, tonify the heart. *(DACH III, 31v)* If the liver is ill, tonify the spleen-pancreas, which is in danger. Emptiness of the spleen-pancreas empties the liver. *(DACH III, 31v)* In emptiness of the liver, tonify the water of the kidney, which is the mother — then the liver meridian will thrive.

Liver and the psyche: insufficiency of the liver with irritation of the gallbladder can cause either the trio — migraines, asthma and returning eczema — if the director level of the psyche dominates; or a fit of jealousy, envy or paranoid wickedness if the motor level dominates.

The dermatoses which are attributed to an insufficiency of the liver are: pruritis (retention of the biliary salts) gout, typhus (insufficient elaboration of purines), purpura (due to blood coagulation problem), xanthoma, or xanthelasma. But all others are improved or cured by tonifying the liver.

The meridian (zu jueyin):

Insufficiency of energy (hepatic insufficiency):

Pulse of the liver abolished or soft, without shape, or small and soft without amplitude, proximal; if big and soft, the liver overflows.

Physical symptoms: waxy complexion, upper eyelids bluish, sees badly at night or at dusk; eyes troubled or tearing; grinds the teeth at night; stools more or less discolored, badly formed; the blood of scratches takes a long time to dry; it causes easy, marked bruising. Subject to eczema, asthma, migraines, eruptions, urticaria or pruritis; nailbiting; muscular asthenia, weakness, awkwardness. Less than 20 to 30 grams of urea in the urine, ammonia more than 0.70. Diminution of glycemia; presence of lactic acid; diminished urine, anuria.

Psychological symptoms: apathy, lassitude, lack of buoyancy, sadness, irritability, awkwardness; dreams of mountains, trees and forests; or pours out torrents of tears, fits of stubbornness, ill-will, slander, calumny; jealousy, envy.
Through the main meridian: tonify *ququan* (LR-8) and the source point, *taichong* (LR-3).
Through the circulation of the energy: tonify the gallbladder, *xiaxi* (GB-43) if the gallbladder is not tight or swollen (in which case disperse it, because the circulation of "the mother who feeds" is not occurring). Tonify the lungs (the child who suckles) at *taiyuan* (LU-9).
Through the herald point of the liver: tonify *qimen* (LR-14).
Yin and yang coupled organs: tonify (or disperse) the gallbladder (*xiaxi* GB-43, or *yangfu* GB-38).
Husband-wife rule: tonify the spleen-pancreas, *dadu* (SP-2).
Midday-midnight correspondence: the liver (maximum energy from 1 to 3 a.m.) responds to the small intestine (maximum energy from 1 to 3 p.m.); tonify the latter at the yang time (during the day, hot): *houxi* (SI-3).
Through the passage point: tonify *guangming* (GB-37) in spring and summer, *ligou* (LR-5) in autumn and winter.
To tonify the heart: *shaochong* (HT-9).
To tonify the liver: acrid flavors (radishes), asarum *(xi xin)*, orange, ginger, chicken, wheat, heat.

Excess of liver energy:

Pulse of the liver: hard, ample, big or distal. The liver is congested, hyperexcited, big, painful. If the pulse is small and hard, the liver is contracted or the volume is diminished or hardened, as in sclerosis.

Physical symptoms: right side and right back painful, stiffened; yellow-brown complexion, brown spots; corners of the eyes swollen, painful. Stools darkened to the point of being blackish; hot breath; painful point below and anterior to the lower angle of the right scapula; urine abundant and frequent.

Psychological symptoms: unhappiness, oppressiveness, anger; sleepiness; dreams of disappointment and unhappiness.

Through the main meridian: disperse *xingjian* (LR-2) and the source point *taichong* (LR-3).

Through the assent point: disperse *ganshu* (BL-18).

Through the circulation of energy: disperse the gallbladder (the mother who nourishes) at *yangfu* (GB-38); disperse the lung (the child who suckles) at *chize* (LU-5).

Coupled yin and yang organs: disperse the gallbladder, the coupled yang workshop organ: *yangfu* (GB-38).

Passage point: disperse *ligou* (LI-5) in autumn and winter, *guangming* (GB-37) in spring and summer.

Midday-midnight correspondence: liver (maximum energy from 1 to 3 a.m); small intestine (maximum at 1 to 3 p.m.); disperse the latter during yang hours and days (during the day, hot and sunlit).

Husband-wife rule: disperse the spleen-pancreas at *shangqiu* (SP-5).

Disperse and drain the liver: coolness, acidity (lemons), angelica, peony root, rhubarb.

In general:

Illnesses of the liver: *(JM) youmen* on the right (KI-21), *qimen* (LR-14); *(JM) hunmen* (BL-42, IS BL-47); *yanggang* (BL-43, IS BL-48), *yishe* (BL-44, IS BL-49).

Illnesses of the liver, stomach, small intestine and kidney: *(JM) weicang* (BL-45, IS BL-50).

Liver pain:

Pains of the liver: *(JM) shidou* (SP-17).

Pain of the liver, anterior lobes above the large intestine, left branch of the meridian, *xingjian* on the left (LR-2). Posterior lobe and back, right branch of the meridian: *(GSdeM) xingjian* on the right (LR-2).

Pain in the liver and heart, bluish complexion as if dead, cannot breathe at all during the day: *(DACH) xingjian* (LR-2); pain in the liver and heart: *(DACH) taichong* (LR-3).

Hepatic colic: (Wetterwald) T9 and T10: *jinsuo* (GV-7, IS GV-8).

Congestion, inflammation:

Congestion of the liver: *(GSdeM) xingjian* (LR-2) disperse.

Liver full of blood: *(DACH IV, 7v; YIX I, 4v) ganshu* (BL-18) disperse.

Congestion of the liver; pain in the sides: *(JM) qiuxu* (GB-40), *xiadu* (GB-32, IS *zhongdu*).

Illness of the liver: a lot of blood, eyes obscured, flowery vision: *ganshu* (BL-18), numerous moxas, leg-*sanli* (ST-36) disperse many times and if there is blood, it is not a mistake. *(DACH IV, 6r)*

Liver big and fat: *(JM) shenshu* (BL-23) and *weishu* (BL-21); inflammation of the liver: *(JM) fenglong* (ST-40).

XXVI. Gallbladder *(Dan)*

Maximum energy in the organ and the meridian from 11 p.m. to 1 a.m., and in February. Contains much energy and little blood. Liver and gallbladder are troubled in spring *(DACH); (GSdeM)*. The gallbladder is easily irritated at the spring equinox (March) and at the autumn equinox (September). The gallbladder has a regulating function on the liver: when it is tight and contracted, the liver becomes insufficient; when it is swollen and soft, the liver is generally congested or too big.

In Europe it is specified: between digestions when the biliary excretions are called for and during fasting, the bile accumulates in the gallbladder because of the contraction of Oddi's sphincter (which closes the common bile duct) whence comes nausea in the morning if the contraction continues. The flow of bile into the duodenum through the common bile duct and the emptying of the gallbladder are regulated through a duodenal reflex activated by peptone (a substance extracted from meat), mostly by fats as well as by acidity (which activate the secretions of the pancreas to the point of inflammation). The removal of the gallbladder does not suppress the spasm of Oddi's sphincter nor the nervous command of the duodenal reflex (the splanchnic nerves of the solar plexus which open it and the vagus nerves which close it).

> The gallbladder holds the influx of the sexual energy. It is the master of internal integrity; decisive choices depend on it. All the eleven other organs take their decisions from the gallbladder. All the organs make waste; only the gallbladder does not produce it. This is why the gallbladder is called pure. It holds audacity, courage. *(DACH VIII, 32v)*

In Chinese, intrepid, audacious people are called "big gallbladders" *(YXRM V, 4r)*. It is upon its function that combativity depends. Emotional agitation injures and empties the gallbladder, troubles the consciousness and, if in excess, causes anguish and loss of decision. Habit can cure emotiveness; worries and regrets can also do this. The gallbladder is the yang workshop organ of the liver, which is a yin treasure organ.

Relationship with the heart (midday-midnight rule) *(YXRM I, 18v)*: when illnesses of the gallbladder take the form of trembling *(zhan biao)* or depression or hyperexcitation, it is advisable to tonify the heart, which is master. The gallbladder nourishes the heart. The gallbladder endangers the stomach (husband-wife rule). The lung and large intestine endanger the gallbladder.

The meridian (zu shaoyang):

Insufficiency of energy:

Pulse of the gallbladder (left wrist II, superficial) abolished or without amplitude, shape, or soft, proximal.

Physical symptoms: eyes without luster, foggy; tremblings.

Psychological symptoms: agitation, unstable will, constant worries, lack of character, insomnia, depression or hyperexcitation; dreams of street-fights, of splitting one's body oneself.

Through the main meridian: tonify *xiaxi* (GB-43) and the source point, *qiuxu* (GB-40).

Through the herald point: *riyue* (GB-24) and *zhejin* (GB-23).

Through the circulation of energy: tonify the triple warmer (the mother who feeds) at *zhongzhu* (TW-3) and the liver (the child who suckles) at *ququan* (LR-8).

Through the passage point, if the liver is strong enough: tonify *guangming* (GB-37).

Through the coupled yin treasure organ: tonify the liver at *ququan* (LR-8).

Through the midday-midnight correspondence: the gallbladder (maximum energy from 11 p.m. to 1 a.m.) corresponds to the heart (maximum from 11 a.m. to 1 p.m.). Tonify the latter at the yang hours (during the day, hot, sunny).

Husband-wife rule: tonify the stomach at *jiexi* (ST-41).

Excess energy:

The pulse of the gallbladder is ample and hard, big, distal. If the pulse is big and hard, there is the probability of stones, the size of which will be in proportion to the size of the pulse. If the pulse is hard and narrow like a wire, there is nervous tightening, irritability and spasm of the gallbladder.

Physical symptoms: bitterness in mouth, mostly on waking, to the point of nausea. Dusty complexion, eyes circled with black, painful eyebrows, headache on the temples, vomiting of bile; "sometimes causes one to see horizontal objects as vertical." Cramps on the lateral surface of the leg, contractures of the calves, swelling under the knee. "Eyes cannot look to the right or the left, corresponding to the opposite foot."

Psychological symptoms: likes silence, easily unhappy, irritable character, apprehensive without reason, fear as if he were seized, feelings of insecurity, tendency to envy, jealousy, to say and do bad things.

Through the main meridian: disperse *yangfu* (GB-38) and the source point *qiuxu* (GB-40).

Through the assent point: disperse *danshu* (BL-19).

Through the circulation of energy: disperse the triple warmer (the mother who feeds) at *tianjing* (TW-10); disperse the liver (the child who suckles) at *xingjian* (LR-2). Very often, we must on the contrary tonify the liver which has been blocked by the gallbladder for a long time (or the gallbladder has become inflamed through vain efforts to activate the insufficient liver).

Through the passage point: in winter tonify *ligou* (LR-5), in summer tonify *guangming* (GB-37).

Yin and yang coupled organs: according to the case disperse or tonify the liver (coupled yin treasure organ, *ququan* (LR-8) or disperse *xingjian* (LR-2).

Husband-wife rule: disperse the stomach, *lidui* (ST-45).

Midnight-midday rule: tonify the heart during the hours and days of sun and heat.

In general:

Illnesses of the gallbladder: *(JM) danshu* (BL-19).

Gallbladder: *(JM) feishu* (BL-13), *ganshu* (BL-18).

Reflex of evacuation of the gallbladder (Abrams): T7, *zhiyang* (GV-8, IS GV-9), contracts the gallbladder.

Secondary vessel of the gallbladder going to the two yin (genitals and anus): *(DACH) xiadu* (GB-32, IS *zhongdu*).

Emptiness:

Emptiness of the gallbladder, attacks of eructation, vomiting, heat, energy at the upper body: *(DACH X, 26r) qihai* (CV-6).

Emptiness of the gallbladder from a lot of drinking: *(DACH) gongsun* (SP-4).

Apprehension, worries, insomnia from emptiness of the gallbladder: *(DACH VIII, 32r) xiaxi* (GB-43).

Emptiness of the heart-mind from emptiness of the gallbladder: *(DACH IV, 5v) shaochong* (HT-9) 3 *fen*, no moxa.

Excess:

Bitter mouth, called *dan dan* — it is cured by the herald point: *riyue* (GB-24) or the assent point of the gallbladder, *danshu* (BL-19) *(DACH I, 5r)*.

Bitter and bad taste in the mouth, mostly in the morning: *(GSdeM) yangfu* (GB-38); *(DACH)* head-*qiaoyin* (GB-18, IS GB-11).

Heat of the gallbladder, counterflow vomiting: *(DACH) zhongfu* (LU-1).

Pain and swelling of the gallbladder: *(GSdeM)* disperse *yangfu* (GB-38) and *qiuxu* (GB-40).

Spasms of the Oddi's sphincter: disperse *yangfu* (GB-38) and *dadun* (LR-1) and *xiaohai* (SI-8).

Stones:

Causes the stones to come out if they are not large (after X-ray): disperse *xingjian* (LR-2), *yangfu* (GB-38) and *qiuxu* (GB-40).

XXVII. Icterus, Jaundice *(Dan, Huang Dan)*

The patient's epidermis, dermis and sclera are yellow; headaches, vertigo (dizziness-fainting); vomiting which stimulate one another. The food will not go in, constipation or diarrhea. If serious, there is sometimes delirium or even blindness, comes from the bile entering the blood; it is also called **huang dan bing.**''
(Ci Yuan, "Huang-dan")

Two types of **huang dan** *which include the five types of icterus — the damp* **(shi)** *and the dry* **(gan).** *In the damp type, boiling heat, humidity dominates: hot blood; eyes, face and even the nails have the color of the earth; slippery stools (diarrhea); the whole body is painful. In the dry type, heat dominates: clear yellow color, dry and blocked defecation (constipation). (YXRM V, 22)*

Five types of icterus are differentiated by the ancient authors:

Name of the illness: There are five types of icterus: 1) **huang dan** *(the true type); 2)* **jiu dan** *(icterus from wine); 3)* **gu dan** *(icterus from cereals); 4)* **nu lao dan** *(icterus from tuberculosis of women); 5)* **huang pang** *(yellow obesity)" (Ci Yuan, "Huang-dan")*

It is called **jiu dan** *(wine icterus) when the heart is anxious, there is nausea without eating, abdomen like water, soles of the feet hot. It is called* **gu dan** *(icterus from cereals) when after meals the head bobs and the body swells. It is called* **nu lao dan** *(icterus of tuberculosis in women) when there is sweat, the palms and soles are hot, there is strong heat, attacks at dusk and insufficiency of urine and bladder. (YXRM V, 22v)*

Also called **gan huang** *(yellow of chancre or tuberculosis); comes from a decrease of the red cells in the blood, almost the same as the illness of blood emptiness (anemia). The patients have skin which is azure-white with yellow. The face is a bit swollen; the heart is unsettled with palpitations. Inspiration and expiration are not harmonious, sometimes headaches. (Ci Yuan, "Huang-pang")*

Icterus:

(GSdeM) Disperse the small intestine (*xiaohai*, SI-8); gallbladder (*yangfu*, GB-38) and *qiuxu* (GB-40), the pancreas, foot-*shangqiu* on the right (SP-5). Tonify the liver at *ququan* (LR-8), increase the red cells (tonify *gaohuangshu* (BL-38, IS BL-43). Tonify the blood at *xuehai* (SP-10) and *weiyang* (BL-53, IS BL-39).

Icterus: *(DACH III, 30v) wangu* (SI-4); *(DACH II, 19r; Ju Ying; YXRM) laogong* (PC-8); *(JM) shaoshang* (LU-11), *zhongfeng* (LR-4); *(JM, DACH) shangqiu* (SP-5), *fengfu* (GV-15, IS GV-16), *feishu* (BL-13); *(DACH) xinshu* (BL-15); *(JM) danshu* (BL-19); *(YXRM I, 46r) dazhu* (BL-11); *(JM, DACH III, 29r; DACH IV, 7r; DACH IV, 6r; YIX I, 4r) zhiyang* (GV-8, IS GV-9), first tonify, then disperse; *(JM) riyue* (GB-24), *yindu* (KI-19), *zhangmen* (LR-13); *(DACH X, 9r) shimen* (CV-5); *(DACH) juque* (CV-14); *(JM) huangshu* (KI-16); *(DACH)* mouth-*yinjiao* (GV-27, IS GV-28).

The five icterus, congestion of spleen-pancreas *(pi man):* *(YXRM I, 46r) zhiyang* (GV-8, IS GV-9), first tonify, then disperse.

Epidemic icterus; the whole body yellow: *(DACH) shuigou* (GV-25, IS GV-26 *renzhong*).

Epidemic icterus with fever: *(DACH) taichong* (LR-3).

Icterus, stoppage of the intestines: *(DACH) yongquan* (KI-1).

Cures icterus over the whole body: *(DACH, 9r) yingchuang* (KI-1).

Icterus from wine *(DACH XI, 9r) yinlingquan* (SP-9), *danshu* (BL-19).

Icterus from tuberculosis of women; body and eyes yellow, attack of fever, severe cold, insufficient urine: *(DACH XII, 26r) gongsun* (SP-4), *guanyuan* (CV-4), *shenshu* (BL-23), *zhiyang* (GV-8, IS GV-9), *rangu* (KI-2).

Icterus of tuberculosis: *(DACH) shenshu* (BL-23).

Icterus from cereals: *(DACH) zhaohai* (KI-3, IS KI-6).

Icterus from excess food: *(DACH X, 27r) zhangmen* (LR-13).

Icterus — much heat and little cold: *(DACH) taixi* (KI-5, IS KI-3).

Icterus — fullness of the abdomen, does not desire food: *(JM, DACH) jizhong* (GV-6).

Icterus — accumulation of yellow *(DACH)*; body yellow *(YXRM)*: *zhangmen* (LR-13).

Icterus, paresis *(wei) (YXRM) biguan* (ST-31).

Icterus, angina of the chest, body heavy *(YXRM I, 46r; Fuji)*; icterus, easy yawning: *(DACH) pishu* (BL-20).

Icterus, epistaxis: *(DACH) lidui* (ST-45).

Treatment with needles:

huangmen *(BL-46, IS BL-51)*	2 *cun,*
zhishi *(BL-47, IS BL-52)*	2 *cun,*
burong on right *(ST-19)*	1 *cun,*
qimen *(LR-14)*	1 *cun,*
riyue *(GB-24)*	1 *cun,*
zhangmen *(LR-13)*	1 *cun.* *(JM, 316)*

Treatment with moxa:

huangmen on right *(BL-46, IS BL-51)*	8 *moxas,*
zhishi *(BL-47, IS BL-52)*....................	8 *moxas.* *(JM, 316)*

Icterus, upset stomach, vomits food: *(YIX I, 4v)* needles at *wangu* (SI-4); moxa at *zhongwan* (CV-12).

XXVIII. Spleen and Pancreas

Ancient and modern Chinese and Japanese authors teach that there is a meridian of the spleen *(pi)* and do not mention a meridian for the pancreas. However, both the spleen and pancreas were anatomically known from the greatest antiquity. On the other hand, clinicians who have written on the actions of the meridian named after the spleen no longer make a distinction between the two organs. Were they frequently joined among the Chinese as is sometimes observed in the present? There is, however, one pulse for the spleen and another one for the pancreas.

Ultimately, the properties of the two organs are completely mixed; no indications allow us to differentiate one from the other. On the other hand, numerous well-controlled observations have allowed me to observe that the right branch of the meridian named after the spleen corresponds to the function of the spleen itself and alone, while the left branch reflects the modification of only the pancreas.

The functions of the spleen and the pancreas as we know them in Europe allowed me to control the different actions of these two branches. This is not the least of the contributions which Europe will have brought to acupuncture. Having thus divided the functions as described by the Chinese, I have observed that there are some which the Europeans do not mention. Prolonged experiments have allowed me to attribute some to the spleen and others to the pancreas. Our European knowledge is thus richer than before. Subsequent important work will allow our successors to perfect and increase these observations. But for now, we must study separately the two branches of the meridian named after the spleen, which I call the spleen-pancreas meridian. There are some uncertainties which make it necessary for there to be repetitions which the future will have to clarify.

The Spleen *(Pi)*

The action upon the blood that the Europeans attribute to the spleen is clearly described in the *Nei Jing* in these terms *(Ling Shu X):* ''The spleen harmonizes and transforms the blood in order to deliver it to the other organs.'' It destroys the used blood cells and makes new ones; it produces white cells.

Old China observed an action on intelligence for the spleen which experiments made in Paris have recognized and specified. The *Da Cheng* says: "The spleen accumulates imagination (ideas, *yi*) and knowledge (intelligence, *zhi,* knowledge with speech)." It has indeed been observed in Paris in many children and young people that with an insufficiency of the spleen there was always a correspondence with very poor performance in their studies, mostly in mathematics in the higher classes. After the spleen was tonified, we found them at the head of the class. Good function of the spleen allows quick and prolonged concentration of the intellectual focus. The synthetic mind replaces the analytic, dispersed memory.

In the course of these experiments we have observed, on the physical level, that people with an insufficiency of the spleen are heavy and tired in the morning, becoming suddenly normal and well towards five in the evening. This tendency disappears as soon as the spleen is sufficiently tonified. Dr. Gilbert Robin has found that this fatigue in the morning, with improvement around 5 p.m., is associated with an increase of the urinary pH and the blood alkalinity. Although still insufficient in number, the experiments on this phenomenon indicate an association with an insufficiency of the spleen and the disappearance of the problem when the spleen is well-tonified. This tendency has been associated with a stimulation of the parasympathetic system through the rhythmic excess of insulin observed from 7 a.m. to 2 p.m.

Finally, the Chinese have observed that the intensity of the awareness, of discrimination between good and bad, of feelings of reciprocity, is in close connection with the activity of the spleen. The *Da Cheng* expresses it as follows: "The spleen *(pi)* is the minister who shows errors *(jian)* and who speaks of equity *(yi).*" Observations on this issue are not easy; however, several families have observed a noticeable improvement when the spleen of their children was functioning well, and a decrease when the other symptoms of insufficiency newly manifested. If it were possible to be sure of this action of the spleen, the treatment of many abnormal people would be facilitated, the absence of awareness and equity being the dominant trait of abnormal people, even the least dangerous.

"Mucus often comes from the spleen." The mononuclear leukocytes, in fact, are produced by the spleen.

Let us note finally an extremely frequent connection between an insufficiency of the spleen and that of the liver. Dutch and English doctors who have had the occasion of seeing the difference between vaccinated and unvaccinated children (vaccination is free and encouraged in Holland and England) attribute these insufficiencies of the liver and spleen to the numerous vaccinations imposed these days.

Moreover, the Chinese have observed *(YXRM V, 4v)* that obsession *(si)* and worries *(lü)* injure and engorge the spleen (or the pancreas), the energy of which is then bound, causing an excess *pi man* "fullness and obstruction": then the heat must be expelled. Obsession, which cures anxiety, is cured by unhappiness.

The pulse of the spleen is on the right wrist, middle position (styloid process) at the deep level under the stomach (upper level) and the pancreas (middle level).

The meridian (zu taiyin), left branch.

The energy is at its maximum from 9 to 11 a.m., corresponding to the triple warmer, which has its maximum from 9 to 11 p.m. It is preceded in the circulation of energy by the stomach and followed by the heart. It is a yin organ: the flow goes up the lower limb (left). The coupled yang workshop organ is the stomach.

Insufficiency of energy of the spleen:

Pulse of the spleen (II deep right) is either abolished, or soft and without amplitude, without shape, proximal, small. A large and soft pulse indicates insufficiency and swelling. A very large and hard pulse can indicate insufficiency from a serious inflammation.

Physical symptoms: blue mouth, lips like cinders; becoming thin, sometimes rheumatism; fatigue in the morning, limbs heavy, better after 5 p.m; easily subject to neuralgia. The liver is generally insufficient.

Psychological symptoms: bad intellectual work, cannot concentrate for a long time, distracted, lazy, lassitude, with no vitality or gaiety, wants to rest; dreams of rocky gorges, large ponds, of houses in ruins in the wind and rain.

Through the main meridian: tonify *dadu* on the left (SP-2) and the source point, *taibai* (SP-3) on the left.
Through the herald point: *zhangmen* on the left (LR-13).
Through the passage point: tonify *fenglong* (ST-40) in the summer and *gongsun* (SP-4) in the winter on the left; and the great *luo* of the spleen: *dabao* (SP-21) on the left.
Through the circulation of the energy: tonify the stomach at *jiexi* (ST-41, the mother who feeds); tonify the heart at *shaoshang* (HT-9, the child who suckles).
Coupled yin-yang organs: tonify the stomach at *jiexi* (ST-41).

Husband-wife rule: tonify the liver at *ququan* (LR-8).

Midday-midnight rule: the spleen (maximum from 9 to 11 a.m.) corresponds to the triple warmer (maximum from 9 to 11 a.m.). Tonify the latter at night and in cold or cloudy weather.

Excess energy of the spleen:

Pulse of the spleen is hard and contracted, tense and without amplitude, or very ample and hard. If it is large and hard there is insufficiency from inflammation. If it is simply distal, there is a slight excess.

Physical symptoms: somnolence, body hot and heavy as if swollen; does not think about food, swelling of the abdomen. In women: insufficient menses; excess destruction of red cells and production of white cells.

Psychological symptoms: mind numb; tired, discouraged; dreams of songs, of music, of the body so heavy it cannot stand up.

Through the main meridian: disperse *shangqiu* (SP-5) on the left and *taibai* (SP-3) on the left, the source point.

Through the assent point: *pishu* (BL-20).

Through the circulation of the energy: disperse the stomach at *lidui* (ST-45) (the mother who feeds) and the heart at *shenmen* (HT-7) (the child who suckles).

Through the coupled yin and yang organs: disperse the stomach, the coupled workshop organ at *lidui* (ST-45).

Through the passage point: disperse *gongsun* (SP-4) in summer and *fenglong* (ST-40) in winter.

Husband-wife rule: tonify the liver (husband) if it is weaker than the spleen.

Midnight-midday rule: the spleen (maximum from 9 to 11 a.m.) corresponds to the triple warmer (maximum from 9 to 11 p.m.): disperse it during yin days and times, cold, dark and at night.

In general:

All illnesses of the spleen (and pancreas?): *(DACH IV, 5r) jianshi* (PC-5); if cold, tonify; if hot, disperse; *(DACH) sanyinjiao* (SP-6).

Illnesses of the spleen (and pancreas?) are numerous; from upset stomach and icterus: *wangu* (SI-4), *zhongwan* (CV-12). For chills without sweat: *fuliu* (KI-7) disperse 3 *fen* under the skin, then towards the bone 1 *cun;* with a lot of sweat: disperse *hegu.* (LI-4) *(DACH IV, 6v)*

Illnesses of the spleen (and pancreas?): *(YIX I, 4v) qixue* (KI-13), *hegu* (LI-4), *sanyinjiao* (SP-6).

Illnesses of the spleen (and pancreas?): *(YXRM I, 40r; YIX I, 4v; DACH IV, 10v)*, from energy: *hegu* (LI-4). In order to increase the blood: *sanyinjiao* (SP-6). If there are lumps: leg-*sanli* (ST-36): hot needles (moxa on the point of the needle.)

Illness of the spleen (and pancreas?), thick diarrhea: *(DACH) sanyinjiao* (SP-6).

Internal troubles of the spleen and stomach: *(YXRM I, 46r) pishu* (BL-20), *tianshu* (ST-25).

Cold and heat affecting the spleen (and pancreas?) *(YIX I, 5r) jianshi* (PC-5).

Emptiness of the spleen; cold of the spleen:

Emptiness of the spleen (and pancreas?): *dadu* (SP-2) on the left.

Illness from cold of the spleen (and pancreas?): *(YXRM I, 46v) jianshi* (PC-5).

Cold of the spleen (and pancreas), acute pain of the stomach: *(YXRM I, 46v) gongsun* (SP-4).

Weakness and emptiness of the spleen and stomach: *(DACH) sanyinjiao* (SP-6); from humidity: leg-*shanglian* (ST-37, IS *shangjuxu*).

Emptiness of the spleen (and pancreas?), undigested food, swollen abdomen: *(DACH X, 26r; YIZ, 40)* leg-*sanli* (ST-36).

Relaxing of the spleen from emptiness, several moxas: *(DACH IV, 7r) tianshu* (ST-25); *(DACH III, 29r; Ju Ying)* the same from misfortune or emotion: *tianshu* (ST-25).

Excess, heat of spleen, congestion, inflammation:

Heat of the spleen: *(DACH) shangqiu* (SP-5) on the left, disperse.

Inflammation of the spleen: *(JO) fushe* (SP-13).

Occlusion of the spleen: *(DACH) juque* (CV-14).

Pain of the spleen:

Acute pain of the spleen (and pancreas?): *(YXRM I, 46r) jianshi* (PC-5); *(DACH) shangqiu* (SP-5); *(DACH IV, 7r; YIX I, 4r) jianjing* (GB-21), *zhongwan* (CV-12).

Pain of the spleen, heaviness of the body: *(DACH) sanyinjiao* (SP-6).

Pain of the spleen and contractions, following the sides, rising, descending, piercing the heart: *(DACH) fushe* (SP-13).

Pain of the spleen (and pancreas?) and heart: *(YIX I, 5r) shangwan* (CV-13); *(YIX I, 4r) gongsun* (SP-4); *(DACH IV, 7v; YIX I, 46r) zhongwan* (CV-12).

Tuberculosis of the spleen (pi gan):

> *Swelling and enlargement of the spleen; comes from anemia or microbes. The spleen hardens and compresses the neighboring organs, ashen complexion; respirations pressed, constrained, difficult to cure. (Ci Yuan, "Pi-gan")*

It is treated with *gaohuangshu* (BL-38, IS BL-43), tonify; left *taibai* (SP-3), left *gongsun* (SP-4), *jianshi* (PC-5), *pishu* (BL-20), disperse.

Congestion of the spleen following malaria (pi, pi kuai re mu):

The ideogram *pi* is composed of "illness" and "isn't it?" *Pi kuai* ("lumps of congestion-of-spleen"):

> *Common name for **pi**, congestion of the spleen. (Ci Yuan, "Pi")*

> *Name of an illness; swelling and chronic growth of the spleen. In the abdomen it is as if hard lumps were being produced. From this it is also called **pi kuai**, "lumps-of-congestion of the spleen." It always overcomes the patient following malaria. From this it is called **re mu**, "mother of fever." (Ci Yuan, "Pi")*

> *When the lines and canals where the sexual energy, the consciousness and the energy of the blood enter and exit, flow and circulate, are blocked and closed, there is formed under the heart a cold congestion of the spleen (**pi**). There is no pain upon pressure. It is different from **zhang man**, swelling-fullness, which takes the form of contraction or swelling. But when the chest is full and painful, it is **jie xiong**, bound chest. (YXRM V, 20v)*

> *Inside soft; outside hard. If it lasts for a long time, it then becomes **zhang man**, swelling-and-fullness, and it cannot be cured. In summary, **pi** and **xian pi** (angina of the chest) are the alarms of the chest and diaphragm. They are an illness of the upper and central warmers. (DACH XI, 21r)*

The same sound is given for another ideogram often used for what has just been described. It is formed from "illness" and "obstruction."

Pi, "congestion-of-spleen":

Pi of the blood and accumulation of food *(shi ji):* in the abdomen, hidden pain: *(DACH VII, 26r) neiguan* (PC-6), *weishu* (BL-21), *qihai* (CV-6), *xingjian* (LR-2).

Pi of blood, the five accumulations, fragmentation of energy, accumulation of blood: *(DACH VII, 26r) neiguan* (PC-6), *geshu* (BL-17), *ganshu* (BL-18), *dadun* (LR-1), *zhaohai* (KI-3, IS KI-6).

Pi, the lumps dissolve by puncturing: *zhangmen* (LR-13). *(DACH XI, 22r*

Pi kuai: (YXRM I, 46r) zhangmen (LR-13) moxa mostly on the left; *(YXRM I, 40r) arm-sanli* (LI-10); *(DACH XI, 20v) zhongwan* (CV-12), needles and moxa.

Pi kuai connected with agitation and energy of emptiness above the umbilicus: *(DACH) xiawan* (CV-10).

All forms of *pi kuai: (DACH XI, 14r) pigen* (MP-36a, IS M-BW-16). Many moxas on the left; and if there is pain on both sides, then moxas on left and right.

All *pi kuai* and food accumulations: *(YXRM I, 40r) arm-sanli* (LI-10), leg-*sanli* (ST-36).

Pi kuai, on the side of the stomach, large accumulation like a bowl: *(DACH XI, 20v)* moxas at *zhongwan* (CV-12).

Pi qi:

Pi qi, "energy of congestion of the spleen":

> *Accumulations of the spleen, and on the right, accumulations of the stomach, are called **pi qi**. That is, the yang energy is fed by humidity, causing icterus and laziness; food and drink no longer form flesh. (YXRM V, 30v)*

> *Accumulations of the spleen (**pi zhi qi**) are called **pi qi**. The bottom of the stomach swells like a balloon. If it lasts for a long time, it causes the four limbs not to come back; it causes icterus. There is a desire for food, and flesh is not formed. In the sack or large curve of the stomach there is swelling like a large bowl. If this lasts, the four limbs cannot be bent (aerogastria?). (DACH I, 16v)*

Pi qi, takes out the shock and brings relief: *(DACH IV, 11v) zhigou* (TW-6).

Pi qi of women, poisoning either of blood or water from energy or stones: *(DACH VIII, 34r) zhaohai* (KI-3, IS KI-6), then *xingjian* (LR-2) for the blood, *gongsun* (SP-4) for the energy, *neiting* (ST-44) for the stones; then *sanyinjiao* (SP-6), leg-*sanli* (ST-36), *shanzhong* (CV-17), *qihai* (CV-6), *guanyuan* (CV-4), *zhigou* (TW-6).

Pi man:

Pi man ("fullness from congestion of the spleen"):

> *The energy blocked above the diaphragm brings on vomiting with effort, cough. (YXRM V, 30v)*

> **Pi man:** *it is first of all important to know if defecation is easy or difficult. If it is difficult or blocked there is fullness; if it is easy or copious there is emptiness. It is cured like **shang han** [chills; also typhoid fever].*
> *(YXRM V, 20v)*

Pi man: if serious on the right, moxa on the left; if serious on the left, moxa on the right: *(YXRM I, 46r)* neiting (ST-44).

Pi man: after malarial fever: *(YIX I, 5r) zhangmen* (LR-13).

Pi man of chest and diaphragm: *(YIX I, 4v; DACH IV, 10v)* abdomen-*yinjiao* (CV-7), *chengshan* (BL-57).

Zhang man: "swelling and fullness":

Zhang man: (DACH) taichong (LR-3).

Young people — *pi man* from fatigue of growth: *(DACH IV, 7v) zhangmen* (LR-13).

Pancreas

(In ancient times called *yi* and *gan rou jing*. Popularly called *jia gan*, "double-liver." Modern term: *cui*.)

> **Cui** *is a word created by the Japanese. It is now used in physiology. In the past, our country used the word **gan rou jing**, meridian of sweet meat. See the "Cui-chang" article. (Ci Yuan, "Cui")*

> *A physiological term; also called **yi** and popularly called **jia gan**, "double-liver." It is flat like a beef tongue, yellow-white in color. It rests horizontally under the stomach in the interval of the duodenum. It touches the spleen. Inside of it there are glands like grapes; exteriorly there is a thin membrane. The glands form the pancreatic secretions which flow out through small canals into the duodenum and help digestion.*
> *(Ci Yuan, "Cui-chang")*

> *Name of an organ; in Japan called **cui**. In the past we have translated it as **gan rou jing**, "meridian of sweet meat." In the old days, during the winter, women dissolved the pancreas of pork in alcohol and spread it on the face and hands in order to prevent them from becoming chapped; from this it happens that soap, **fei zao**, is called **yi zi**. (Ci Yuan, "Yi")*

Although ancient and modern China recognize a different pulse for the spleen and pancreas, they know of only one meridian for the two organs. The many experiments pursued in Paris have allowed us to understand something which has escaped the Chinese and Japanese. The right branch of the spleen meridian *(zu taiyin)* reflects the function of the spleen; the left branch reflects the function of the pancreas. This important discovery allows us to study the problems of the pancreas for which the Europeans have only a chemical idea, and to distinguish those problems which depend on the spleen and those which depend on the pancreas. These problems are enumerated under the name for each point of this double meridian.

Europeans consider the pancreas to be indispensable organ for digestion on the one hand, and for the metabolism of sugar on the other hand. The pancreatic secretions, through trypsin, digest meat (proteins and albumins), through amylopsin digest carbohydrates (beans, chestnuts), and through lipase digest fat. The internal secretion produces insulin, which is indispensable for the liver to form glycogen transformed from sugary foods, and the liver stores the glycogen in order to retransform it into sugar according to need.

The small intestine, through its secretin, stimulates the pancreatic secretions, and activates them through enteropeptidase. The adrenal glands can reduce the production of insulin through an excess of adrenalin. Insulin slows down adrenal activity. We should add that adrenalin stimulates the production of sugar by the liver while reducing the production of insulin, which activates the transformation of the sugar into glycogen in the liver. We should note also that the liver is the only organ which produces sugar (through the transformation of glycogen) and all the tissues contain it. The secretion of insulin by the pancreas depends on the vagus nerve and stimulates it. Excess insulin in the daily rhythm from 7 a.m. to 2 p.m. (with hypoglycemia) is in relation to a rhythmic excess of the vagus nerve.

The meridian (zu taiyin), right branch.
(Meridian of the spleen-pancreas, zu taiyin, right branch.)

The pulse of the pancreas is at the middle level on the second pulse of the right wrist. Its energy is at its maximum from 9 to 11 a.m. and corresponds with the triple warmer, the maximum of which is from 9 to 11 p.m.

Preceded in the circulation of energy by the stomach, followed by the heart, it is a yin treasure organ. Its flow goes up the right lower limb. Its coupled yang workshop organ is the stomach.

Insufficiency of energy of the pancreas:

Pulse of the pancreas: swollen and soft (insufficiency through inflammation of the pancreas, frequent case; often a sign of diabetes or glycosuria; the pancreas is then painful and its swelling is perceptible). Linked to hypertension, it comes from an excess of the adrenals. In this case it is advisable to treat the cause of the inflammation by dispersing the adrenals. True insufficiency from atony with diabetes is rare; the pulse is either abolished or small and flaccid and proximal: tonify the organ.

Physical symptoms: pockets under the eyes, acidity or burning of the stomach about one hour after eating jam, sugar, chestnuts and beans. In general, patients have an aversion to this type of food. They take a little sugar in their drinks (coffee, tea). Meat is not completely digested, but does not cause obvious pain. Often carbohydrates (noodles, macaroni, etc.) are badly digested and patients do not like them. There is often frequent urination and the total urine is relatively abundant. If the insufficiency is serious, the stools are shining, slippery, fatty (steatorrhea) after the ingestion of fats or fried foods; analysis shows an augmentation of the blood urea and sometimes the glycemic level; cramps; eyes foggy.

Psychological symptoms: sadness, discouragement, fatigue; sleepiness after eating; easily fatigued, weakness, sensation of mental heaviness; cannot work continuously for a long time; constantly forgets.
Through the main meridian: tonify *dadu* (SP-2) on the right, and the source point *taibai* (SP-3) on the right.
Through the herald point: *zhangmen* (LR-13) on the left; alarm point of the pancreas.
Through the passage point: tonify *fenglong* (ST-40) in summer, and in winter *gongsun* (SP-4), both on the right.
By circulation of energy: tonify the stomach (*jiexi*, ST-41), the mother who nourishes, and the heart (*shaochong*, HT-9), the child who suckles.
Through the yin and yang coupled organs: tonify the stomach at *jiexi* (ST-41).
Husband-wife rule: tonify the liver (*ququan*, LR-8).
Midday-midnight rule: the pancreas (maximum from 9 to 11 a.m.) corresponds to the triple warmer (maximum from 9 to 11 p.m.). Tonify the latter at sunset and during cold or cloudy weather: *zhongzhu* (TW-3).

Excess energy of the pancreas:

The pulse of the pancreas is ample, hard and distal, or small, hard and contracted. Inflammation of the pancreas causing insufficiency is generally indicated by an ample and soft pulse.

Physical symptoms: hunger pangs, nausea, migraines. If serious, convulsions and loss of consciousness. Sometimes there is hemianopia. Blood analysis reveals hypoglycemia from an excess production of insulin.

Psychological symptoms: anguish, phobias, attacks of hostility against those around them, and even maniacal attacks.
Through the main meridian: disperse *shangqiu* (SP-5) on the right and *taibai* (SP-3) on the right.
Through the assent point: disperse *pishu* (BL-20) on the left.
Through the herald point: disperse *zhangmen* (LR-13) on the left.
Through the passage point: disperse *gongsun* (SP-4) on the right; tonify *fenglong* (ST-40) on the right.
Through the circulation of energy: disperse the stomach: *lidui* (ST-45), the mother who nourishes; and disperse the heart at *shenmen* (HT-7), the child who suckles.
Through the coupled yin and yang organs: disperse the stomach at *lidui* (ST-45).
Husband-wife rule: tonify the liver at *ququan* (LR-8) and *taichong* (LR-3).
Midday-midnight rule: the pancreas (maximum from 9 to 11 a.m.) corresponds to the triple warmer (maximum from 9 to 11 p.m.). Disperse the latter at *tianjing* (TW-10) during night hours on cold, dark and rainy days.

In general.

(*GSdeM*) Insufficiency of the pancreas from inflammation, pulse big and hard, digests beans and chestnuts poorly, burning of the stomach with jam and sugar: disperse *yamen* (GV-14, IS GV-15).
All illnesses of the pancreas (and spleen?): (*DACH IV, 5r*) *jianshi* (PC-5), if cold, tonify; if hot, disperse.
The illnesses of the pancreas (and spleen?) are many. From upset stomach and icterus: hand-*wangu* (SI-4), *zhongchong* (PC-9); from chills without sweat: *fuliu* (KI-7) disperse 3 *fen* under the skin, then toward the bone 1 *cun;* with a lot of sweat: disperse *hegu* (LI-4). (*DACH IV, 6v*)
Illnesses of the pancreas (and spleen?): (*YXRM I, 40r; YIX I, 4v; DACH IV, 10v*) through energy: *hegu* (LI-4); to lift up the blood: *sanyinjiao* (SP-6). If there are lumps: leg-*sanli* (ST-36) hot needle, (moxa on the tip of the needle).
Illnesses of the pancreas (and spleen?), thick diarrhea (*DACH*) *sanyinjiao* (SP-6) on the right.

Cold and heat attacking the pancreas (and spleen?): *(YIX I, 5r) jianshi* (PC-5).

Internal trouble of pancreas (and spleen?) and stomach: *(YXRM* I, 46r) *tianshu* (ST-25), *pishu* (BL-20) on the right.

Emptiness, cold, weakness of the pancreas.

Emptiness of the pancreas: *(DACH)* foot-*dadu* (SP-2) on the right; *(GSdeM) taibai* (SP-3) on the right, *sanyinjiao* (SP-6), *gongsun* (SP-4) on the right.

Emptiness of the pancreas (and spleen?), abdomen swollen, nondigested food: *(YIZ 40; DACH X, 26r)* leg-*sanli* (ST-36).

Relaxation of the pancreas (and spleen?) from emptiness: several moxas *(DACH IV, 7r)* at *tianshu* (ST-25); *(DACH III, 29r)* the same from misfortune or emotion: *tianshu* (ST-25).

Illnesses from cold of the pancreas (and spleen?): *(YXRM I, 46v) jianshi* (PC-5).

Cold of the pancreas (and spleen?), acute pain of the stomach: *(YXRM I, 46v) gongsun* (SP-4).

Excess, heat, congestion, inflammation of the pancreas.

Heat of the pancreas; *(DACH)* foot-*shangqiu* (SP-5) on the right, disperse.

Inflammation of the pancreas (and spleen?) *(JO) fushe* (SP-13) on the right.

Occlusion of the pancreas (and spleen?) *(DACH) juque* (CV-14).

Contraction of the pancreas (and spleen?) and heart: *(DACH IV, 7v) gongsun* (SP-4).

Congestion, inflammation of the pancreas: *(GSdeM)* foot-*shangqiu* (SP-5), *gongsun* (SP-4), *fushe* (SP-13), all on the right; *fushe* (SP-13) on the left acts especially on the stomach.

Pain of the pancreas.

Pain of the pancreas: *(GSdeM)* foot-*shangqiu* (SP-5) on the right, *gongsun* (SP-4) on the right, *taibai* (SP-3) on right, disperse all; *yamen* (GV-14, IS GV-15).

Acute pain of the pancreas (and spleen?): *(YXRM I, 46r) jianshi* (PC-5); *(DACH)* foot-*shangqiu* (SP-5); *(DACH IV, 7r; YIX I, 4r) jianjing* (GB-21), *zhongwan* (CV-12).

Pain and contraction of the pancreas (and spleen?) following the side, rising and descending, piercing the heart: *(DACH) fushe* (SP-13) on the right.

Pain of the pancreas (spleen) and heart: *(YIX I, 4r) gongsun* (SP-4); *(YIX I, 5r) shangwan* (CV-13); *(DACH)* thorax-*qimen* (LR-14).

Acute pain of the pancreas (spleen) and back: *(DACH IV, 7v)* disperse hand-*zhongzhu* (TW-3).

Internal troubles; acute pain of the pancreas (and spleen?) stomach, heart, liver: *(YXRM I, 46r) zhongwan* (CV-12).

XXIX. Diabetes, Glycosuria, Hyperglycemia *(Tang Niao Bing, Xiao Ke, San Xiao)*

Europeans distinguish two types of problems in this category:

1) Glycosuria, (sugar in the urine) without hyperglycemia (sugar in the blood), resulting from a problem in the kidney function which allows more sugar than normal to pass; and

2) Hyperglycemia, (excess sugar in the blood, more than 1.7 grams) from which is observed many problems — insufficient production of insulin by the pancreas (whence comes an insufficient transformation of sugar in glycogen by the liver); over-production of sugar transformed by the liver. The causes can be: a) excess of the adrenals, the adrenalin of which has the double property of stimulating the production of sugar by the liver and slowing down the production of insulin by the pancreas (the insulin being indispensable for the liver to be able to transform the sugar into glycogen and to store it; the production of insulin is stimulated by the vagus nerve); b) excess of the pituitary gland which stimulates the adrenals; c) insufficiency of the breakdown of sugar in the tissues (glycolysis), mostly in the muscles from a lack of exercise; d) excess of the sympathetic system which stimulates the kidneys and the adrenals; e) slowing down of the blood flow through the liver, the blood taking up more and more sugar; f) insufficiency of the small intestine, which stimulates the pancreas with its secretion, or an excess which causes inflammation.

Instead of tonifying or dispersing the organ, the Europeans treat hyperglycemia (with or without glycosuria) with injections of insulin. According to European knowledge, acupuncture would have to regulate the troubled organs in the following manner:

1)   For glycosuria without hyperglycemia: regulate the function of the kidney (verify on the pulses); if insufficient from excess or if actually in excess, disperse *yongquan* (KI-1), *rangu* (KI-2), *taixi* (KI-5, IS KI-3); if truly insufficient, tonify *fuliu* (KI-7), *taixi* (KI-5, IS KI-3) and *sanyinjiao* (SP-6).

2)   For hyperglycemia, accompanied or not by glycosuria, regulate the pancreas; if insufficient from inflammation (the organ will be sensitive to pressure), disperse *shangqiu* (SP-5) on the right foot, right *taibai* (SP-3), right *gongsun* (SP-4) and *jianshi* (PC-5); if truly atonic and without life, tonify right *dadu* (SP-2), right *taibai* (SP-3) and right *gongsun* (SP-4).

Inflammation of the pancreas with insufficiency can be due to an excess of the adrenals or to an excess of the small intestine, which increases the production of the pancreatic secretions with its secretion and can cause an irritation of the gland; disperse it at right hand-*wangu* (SI-4), which will be painful under pressure, and at right *xiaohai* (SI-8). If at the same time there is insufficiency of the pancreas and small intestine, tonify the latter at *houxi* (SI-3) and hand-*wangu* (SI-4) on both hands.

For the liver: the Chinese regulate the excess production of sugar and the insufficient transformation into glycogen and the congestion slowing down the blood flow through the liver at the same time by dispersing *xingjian* (LR-2). It is necessary to verify if the anterior lobe (corresponding to the left edge of the pulse) or the posterior lobe (right edge of the pulse) are different, in which case we must stimulate one side and disperse the other.

The Chinese differentiate two types of diabetes: one from inflammation of the organs by the adrenals, the other from atonia or nondevelopment.

The adrenals can be slowed down by dispersing *fengfu* (GV-15, IS GV-16), and *yamen* (GV-14, IS GV-15) (C2 and C3 of Abrams). The parasympathetic system can be stimulated by tonifying *tianzhu* (BL-10), and the sympathetic system by dispersion of *fengchi* (GB-20). Glycolysis must be increased by physical exercise. Inflammation of the pancreas is treated through *fushe* (SP-13). The C6/C7 interval disperses and calms the pituitary gland.

In a general way, it is sufficient to disperse *yamen* (GV-14, IS GV-15).

> It is an illness of sugar in the urine: **tang niao bing.** *In the past there were three varieties: upper, middle and lower. These were the three fusions,* **san xiao.** *(Ci Yuan, ''Xiao-ke'')*

> *There is a certain proportion of sugar taken from the body in the urine. The capacity to transform sugar diminishes due to a disorder of the digestive system. Sugar in the blood increases and comes out through the urine. At the beginning, there is headache, insomnia, bad digestion; then an increase in the quantity of urine. The dryness increases the thirst. One should eat meat, fish and eggs, and avoid pasta and noodles, rice, carbohydrates and beans. In the past it was called* **xiao ke.** *(Ci Yuan, ''Tang-niao-bing'')*

> **San xiao,** *the three fusions, do not have the same symptoms: 1)* **xiao pi** *''shrinking spleen (pancreas).'' Emptiness of stomach; bushels of food will not satisfy the hunger. 2)* **xiao zhong,** *''shrinking-center.'' Drinking 100 cups will not satisfy the thirst. 3)* **xiao shen,** *''shrinking-kidney.'' Having sex does not fulfill the desire. (DACH VII, 33r)*

> *There is always fire and inflammation. In upper fusion the heat is in the upper warmer (respiratory functions); heart and lung are dry and agitated, the tongue is scarlet, the lips red, little appetite. Central fusion is habitual hunger; there is neither urine or feces. The heat invades the middle warmer (digestive function: spleen-pancreas and stomach); urine is red and copious; in the fusion of the kidney urine is thick, with stiffness of the penis. The heat dominates the lower warmer as well as the sexual energy. Thirst forces one to take water in order to relieve it; then the urine comes out, troubled, thick, unctuous, a type of urethritis. Thighs and knees atrophy, become thin, the face becomes grayish-black. The ears are burnt and thinly shaped. People who become thinner day by day will not be cured. Protect the lungs and appease the kidneys, then the pancreas will move by itself. The root is in the kidneys (adrenals). Feed the spleen (the pancreas) and the fluids will be produced by themselves. (YXRM V, 26v)*

(GSdeM) Disperse *yamen* (GV-14, IS GV-15), *fengfu* (GV-15, IS GV-16), *fengchi* (GB-20), *xingjian* (LR-2); tonify *houxi* (SI-3), *shaochong* (HT-9), *fuliu* (KI-7), *dadu* (SP-2) on the left, *jianshi* (PC-5), *zhongchong* (PC-9), *taiyuan* (LU-9), *tianzhu* (BL-10).

Japanese treatment:
(Dr. Nakayama): Moxa at *ganshu* (BL-18) which acts on the liver; *pishu* (BL-20) which acts on the spleen and pancreas (on the left), *shenshu* (BL-23) which acts on the kidneys. Regime: 70 percent cereals, 30 percent vegetables; special meal: 30 percent pumpkin, 70 percent soya — each day one meal of this.

Chinese treatment:
(DACH II, 19r; YIX 4r & 5r) yongquan (KI-1), which disperses the kidneys and adrenals, *xingjian* (LR-2) which disperses the liver.

(DACH VII, 33r) Diabetes; the three fusions: *lieque* (LU-7), union and crossing point of the conception vessel, *shui-gou* (GV-25, IS GV-26, *renzhong*), *guanchong* (TW-1) which takes out the compressed heat of the warmers, *zhongwan* (CV-12) herald point of the central warmer, *pishu* (BL-20) ascent point of the pancreas, leg-*sanli* (ST-36), *gongsun* (SP-4), *zhaohai* (KI-3, IS KI-6) which acts on the thirst, and *taixi* (KI-5, IS KI-3) for impotency.

Diabetes; enjoys eating: *(JM) zhizheng* (SI-7).

Cures the problem of eating without the hunger being satisfied: *(DACH III, 33r)* leg-*sanli* (ST-36).

Eats a lot and remains thin: *(DACH) pishu* (BL-20).

Diabetes, enjoys drinking: *(DACH) xingjian* (LR-2).

Cures the problem of drinking without the thirst being satisfied, diabetes: *(DACH III, 33r) zhaohai* (KI-3, IS KI-6).

Habitual thirst: *(DACH) zhizheng* (SI-7).

Diabetes, dry mouth: unbearable, emptiness, fatigue: *(DACH) xiaochangshu* (BL-27).

Diabetes, dry mouth: *(DACH) yangchi* (TW-4).

Diabetes, intense thirst, drinks endlessly: *(DACH) shuigou* (GV-25, IS GV-26 *renzhong*).

Diabetes, intense thirst: *(DACH) chengjiang* (CV-24).

Diabetes, yellow face, scarlet eyes, wants to drink: *yixi* (BL-40, IS BL-45).

Diabetes; cures house-fatigue that is no longer responding to desires: *(DACH III, 33r) taixi* (KI-5, IS KI-3).

Removes the exhaustion of the kidneys: *(DACH) zhaohai* (KI-3, IS KI-6).

Glycosuria: *(JM) yangchi* (TW-4), *xingjian* (LR-2), *dadun* (LR-1), *rangu* (KI-2), *chengjiang* (CV-24), *shenshu* (BL-23), *zhonglushu* (BL-29).

Glycosuria, intense thirst: *(JM) shuigou* (GV-25, IS GV-26 *renzhong*).

Diabetes: *(DACH) yangchi* (TW-4); *(DACH) rangu* (KI-2); *(YXRM I, 46r) zhaohai* (KI-3, IS KI-6), *lougu* (SP-7); *(DACH, JM) yinshi* (ST-33); *(YXRM I, 46r) juque* (CV-14); *(JM) qimen* (LR-14); *(DACH) shenshu* (BL-23), *zhonglushu* (BL-29); *(DACH) haiquan* (MP-5, IS M-HN-37), *chengjiang* (CV-24), *duiduan* (GV-26, IS GV-27).

Diabetes, body hot: *(DACH) yanggang* (BL-43, IS BL-48).

Convulsions from excess insulin: *(GSdeM)* disperse left *shangqiu* (SP-5); left *taibai* (SP-3).

XXX. Beriberi (*Jiao Qi;* Formerly *Jue; Jue Ji; Huan Feng*)

The Su Wen calls it jue ji; emptiness illness. During the Tang Dynasty (seventh to tenth centuries), they began to call it jiao qi. Both feet are slightly swollen. In the armies and schools the contagion from it is frequent and dangerous. In antiquity it was said to come from humidity on top of an emptiness of the kidneys. Dong Qi of the Song Dynasty has written General Rules for the Method of Curing Beriberi. Modern medicine relates this illness to rice-eating countries because this illness is frequent there; it is said that if the rice is husked in such a way that the silver coating is removed, then the blood lacks strength (vitamins). Those who eat unpolished rice do not have this problem. (Ci Yuan, ''Jiao-qi'')

Jiao qi was called jue, ''lack,'' in the Nei Jing, and huan feng, ''moderate wind,'' under the two Han dynasties (second century B.C. to third century A.D.). First, there is pain in the feet, then in the humid form swelling or abscesses on the leg; the pulse is large and weak. In the hot form, the pulse is changing, retracted, tightened; pain and atrophy; it comes from food, wind and cold. (YXRM V, 26r)

The fire-needles are forbidden for beriberi; they increase the pain and swelling. (DACH V, 19v)

Beriberi. Origins: comes either from an inflamed swelling or from ingested poison, or from poison from rice, or from a lack of B vitamin, or from contagion. What causes it is not fixed with certainty. Students, soldiers, groups of workers, people who sit a lot and women after delivery are easily attacked by it. Its maximum is seen from the last month of summer to the last month of autumn.

Symptoms: 1) Nervous beriberi — laziness and fatigue of the lower limbs. Extension of the calf muscles has a response in the lower abdomen. The medial surfaces of the four limbs, the fingers, the lips have a changed sensation. The medial surfaces of the legs swell slightly. The ligaments of the patella are lost little by little. Moreover, there is palpitation, rapid pulse and constipation. 2) Paralyzing beriberi — flesh and muscles decrease and become thin. The skin thickens and loses its brightness. The fingers and the anterior surface of the forearm, the toes and the medial surfaces of the lower limbs and the lower abdomen all have the sensation of paralysis; their movements are blocked. Soon the feet and hands lose their freedom of movement. 3) Edematous beriberi — in the beginning, slight swelling occurring in the lower limbs from time to time. The whole body slows down. There is a bitter melancholia in the pit of the stomach. Respiration is difficult; urine is diminished; constipation. 4) Cardiac beriberi — first weak palpitations, bitter melancholia in the pit of the stomach; constrained and difficult respiration; nausea, attacks of vomiting. The patient lies on his bed and groans. Appearance of bitter melancholia; anxiety. (JO, 34)

Treatment with needles:

tianshu (ST-25)	*8 fen,*
guanyuan (CV-4) ..	*1 cun,*
geshu (BL-17)	*5 fen,*
ganshu (BL-18)	*5 fen,*
pishu (BL-20)	*5 fen,*
yinlingquan (SP-9)	*5 fen,*
lougu (SP-7)	*5 fen,*
sanyinjiao (SP-6) ..	*5 fen,*
zhubin (KI-9)	*5 fen,*
xuehai (SP-10)	*5 fen,*
jimen (SP-11)	*5 fen. (JO, 34)*

Treatment with moxa:

taichong (LR-3) ..	*7 moxas,*
sanyinjiao (SP-6)	*7 moxas,*
geshu (BL-17)	*7 moxas,*
ganshu (BL-18) ..	*7 moxas,*
pishu (BL-20)	*7 moxas. (JO, 34)*

Beriberi: *(DACH)* leg-*sanli* (ST-36), *qimen* (SP-11), *xiyan* (MP-37a & 38a, IS M-LE-16), *yinlingquan* (SP-9), *lougu* (SP-7), *sanyinjiao* (SP-6), *xuanzhong* (GB-39), *kunlun* (BL-60), *fuliu* (KI-7), leg-*shanglian* (ST-37, IS *shangjuxu*), *chengjin* (BL-56), *xiadu* (GB-32, IS *zhongdu*), *jianjing* (GB-21), *taiyin* (ST-23), *fujie* (SP-14), *dachangshu* (BL-25).

Beriberi: *(DACH) xuanzhong* (GB-39), *sanyinjiao* (SP-6), leg-*sanli* (ST-36).

Beriberi, insufficiency, sinks into heaviness: *(DACH)* leg-*xialian* (ST-39, IS *xiajuxu*).

Beriberi, rising to the upper body: *(DACH) tianjing* (TW-10), *jianjing* (GB-21).

Beriberi, the type which attacks the heart: *(JM) jianjing* (GB-21).

Beriberi, swelling and fullness: *(DACH) yinshi* (ST-33).

Beriberi, head swollen: *(DACH)* thigh-*futu* (ST-32).

Beriberi, pruritis or paralysis of the whole body: *(DACH) fengshi* (GB-31).

Beriberi, pain of the lumbar area and coccyx: *(DACH) kunlun* (BL-60).

Beriberi, pain of the knee and leg: *(DACH) xuanzhong* (GB-39).

Beriberi, swelling of the leg: *(JM) tiaokou* (ST-38).

Beriberi, swelling of the knee: *(DACH) pucan* (BL-61), *juliao* (ST-6, IS ST-3); *(DACH IV, 10v; YIX I, 8r) chengshan* (BL-57). If there is pus, it cannot be cured: *dubi* (ST-35).

Beriberi, swelling of the feet: *(DACH) chengshan* (BL-57).

Beriberi from cold and humidity: *(YXRM I, 46v)* leg-*sanli* (ST-36); *(DACH IV, 4v)* leg-*sanli* (ST-36) and *sanyinjiao* (SP-6).

Notes

[1]This may be a typographical error in the French text, ''ordre'' instead of ''ordure.'' ''Stinking'' or ''malordorus'' fits the medical context. — Trans.

Chapter IX

The Respiratory System

I. Respiratory System — II. Chills, Cold and Heat, Evil Cold, Evil Wind, Penetrating Cold — III. Nose, Rhinopharynx — IV. Throat — V. Larynx — VI. Trachea, Bronchus — VII. Lungs — VIII. Cough — IX. Hemoptysis — X. Abscess of Lungs — XI. Pulmonary Congestion — XIII. Pleura, Pleurisy, Pleuritis — XIII. Pneumonia — XIV. Asthma, Panting, Dyspnea, Breathlessness — XV. Emphysema — XVI. Pulmonary Tuberculosis (General Treatments, Types) — XVII. Pulmonary Plague

I. The Respiratory System

In general.

Illnesses of the respiratory system: *jueyinshu* (BL-14).
Cannot breathe deeply, weakness of the respiratory muscles *(GSdeM): shanzhong* (CV-17).

The meridian (shou taiyin).

The meridian named after the lungs *(fei jing)* in fact commands all the respiratory passages: larynx, trachea, bronchi and lungs. This yin meridian has as its yang coupled meridian the large intestine meridian, to which it is linked "like the outside and inside of the cloth." The nose mostly depends on the large intestine. Dispersing the lungs decreases spasms of the large intestine.

Excess energy of the lung can act on the kidneys and cause abundant and numerous urinations. Its energy is at its maximum from 3 to 5 a.m. It corresponds to the meridian of the bladder, which has its maximum from 3 to 5 p.m. The flow goes down the upper limbs. The flow of energy comes from the liver and goes into the large intestine.

Insufficiency of energy:

The pulse of the lungs (right wrist, near the thumb, deep) is abolished or soft and without amplitude, without shape, small or proximal. We should note that the function of the two lungs is not always equal; when the heart, particularly the right heart, is tired, the left lung is generally atonic.

Physical symptoms: weak respiration, underdeveloped thorax, shortness of breath, mercurial complexion, shoulders and back cold, weakness, cannot breathe in (stoppage of empty lungs).

Psychological symptoms: sudden depression, dreams of anxiety, tears and sobs.
Through the main meridian: tonify *taiyuan* (LU-9), which is also the source point.
Through the herald point: tonify *zhongfu* (LU-1).
Through the circulation of the energy: tonify the liver (*ququan,* LR-8), the mother who nourishes and the large intestine (*quchi,* LI-11), the child who suckles.
Passage point: tonify *lieque* (LU-7) on cold, cloudy days and in winter, and *pianli* (LI-6) in summer and on hot, sunny days.
Husband-wife rule: tonify the heart (*shaochong,* HT-9), the pulse of which must be stronger than that of the lungs.
Midday-midnight rule: during afternoon hours tonify the bladder, which corresponds to it.
Coupled yang workshop organ: tonify the large intestine (*quchi,* LI-11). When the large intestine is ill and disturbs the lungs, the nose has a clear discharge; angina, pain in front of the shoulder: tonify *hegu* (LI-4), source point of the large intestine, and *lieque* (LU-7), passage point.

Excess energy of the lungs:

The pulse of the lungs is hard, ample, large, long and distal. If it is hard proximally (near the styloid process), there is emphysema or asthma. The base of the lung is encumbered. If it is hard and near the thumb (ahead, distal) the throat, larynx or the trachea are involved; the bronchi are towards the middle.

Physical symptoms: internal fullness, shoulder and back painful, numerous and abundant urination, perspiration, cold, yawning, cannot breathe out (stoppage of the lung in fullness); cough, mucus.

Psychological symptoms: emotional, tender, cries easily, melancholia or great gaiety, dreams of gliding, of flying.
Through the main meridian: disperse *chize* (LU-5) and the source point (*taiyuan,* LU-9).

Through the assent point: disperse *feishu* (BL-13).

Through the circulation of the energy: disperse the liver (*xingjian,* LR-2), the mother who feeds, and the large intestine (*sanjian,* LI-3), the child who suckles.

Through the passage point: disperse in winter *pianli* (LI-6) and in the summer, *lieque* (LU-7).

Through the coupled yang workshop organ: large intestine (*sanjian,* LI-3).

Husband-wife rule: tonify the heart (*shaochong,* HT-9).

Midnight-midday rule: the lungs, maximum from 3 to 5 a.m. correspond to the bladder, maximum from 3 to 5 p.m. Disperse the latter in the afternoon and on sunny and hot days.

Lung host, large intestine guest: panting, cough, mucus: disperse *taiyuan* (LU-9) and *pianli* (LI-6).

Emptiness, cold, insufficiency of lungs.

Emptiness, exhaustion and paresis of the lungs: *(DACH) pohu* (BL-37, IS BL-42).

Cold of the lungs: *(YXRM) kufang* (ST-14).

Little energy, insufficient for breathing: *(DACH) lieque* (LU-7).

Energy (respiration) short: *(DACH) shanzhong* (CV-17), *dabao* (SP-21).

Fullness, heat, accumulation.

Accumulation in the lung, fullness of the chest, panting, contracting: *(DACH) quepen* (ST-12).

Fullness of lungs and respiratory system: *(YIX I) chize* (LU-5), *feishu* (BL-13).

Pain in the sides, rises up and attacks: *(DACH) quepen* (ST-12).

Swelling in the supraclavicular fossa, then fullness and heat of the chest: *(DACH) quepen* (ST-12).

Weakness of respiration.

Cannot breathe deeply, weakness of the exterior respiratory muscles, thorax and diaphragm: *(GSdeM)* tonify *shanzhong* (CV-17).

❂ II. Chills, Cold and Heat, Evil Cold, Evil Wind, Penetrating Cold
(Shang Han, Han Re, E Han, E Feng, Zhong Han)

The word *shang han* is also used for typhoid fever: *(YXRM V, 32v)* ''When there is no sweat in *shang han,* and the feet and hands are cold, it is the yin which is attacked.''

Chills *(shang han):*

Chills: *(DACH) fengchi* (GB-20), *shendao* (GV-10, IS GV-11), *jingqu* (LU-8).

Chills, heat abounds, malaise, vomiting: *(DACH) bailao* (GV-13, IS GV-14, *dazhui*).

Chills, fever not stopping: *(DACH)* leg-*sanli* (ST-36), *zhongwan* (CV-12), *quchi* (LI-11).

Chills, body hot: *wenliu* (LI-7); without end: *yunmen* (LU-2).

Chills, four limbs hot: *weizhong* (BL-54, IS BL-40).

Chills, heat in the chest: *zhongfu* (LU-1).

Fever from chills: *erjian* (LI-2).

Chills, shivering, yawning: *chongyang* (ST-42).

Chills, cold of the four limbs in counterflow: *neiting* (ST-44).

Chills, nose blocked, headache, nape stiff, eyes blind, cough, short and agitated breath, lungs and back painful: *fengmen* (BL-12).

Chills, cold of the yang, trouble of the yin: 300 moxas at *shenque* (CV-8).

Chills, great thirst: *hegu* (LI-4).

Chills not dissipating; chest knotted: *neiguan* (PC-6).

Chills, chest knotted: *gongsun* (SP-4), *neiguan* (PC-6), *zhigou* (TW-6), *jianshi* (PC-5).

Chills, from having drunk and eaten too much: *qihai* (CV-6).

Chills, hyperexcited speech: *tianshu* (ST-25).

Chills, water knotted: *chengshan* (BL-57), *erjian* (LI-2).

Pain in the ribs after chills: thorax-*qimen* (LR-14).

Chills, cutting pain in the heart: thorax-*qimen* (LR-14).

Cold and heat *(han re):*

Cold and heat: *(DACH) yanggu* (SI-5), *tianjing* (TW-10), *naoshu* (SI-10), *naohui* (TW-13), *jianwaishu* (SI-14), *jianzhongshu* (SI-15), *jinmen* (BL-63).

Cold and heat coming and going: *(DACH) shendao* (GV-10, IS GV-11); *(JM) dushu* (BL-16).

Cold and hot interweaving: disperse *lieque* (LU-7) *(DACH).*

Cold and heat, bad cold: *hegu* (LI-4).

A lot of cold and heat, sweat comes out: *(DACH) gongsun* (SP-4).

Cold and heat from time to time: *(YXRM, DACH) fuyang* (BL-59).

Attacks of cold and heat: *(DACH) fubai* (GB-16, IS GB-10).

Cold and heat, pain in the arm, cannot lift: *(DACH) binao* (LI-14).

Cold and heat, stiff nape: *(YXRM) naokong* (GB-19).

Cold and heat, radiating into pain of the vertebrae: *(DACH) pishu* (BL-20).

Cold and heat, energy at the top: *(DACH, YXRM) tianchi* (PC-1).

Sometimes hot, sometimes cold: *(DACH) shaochong* (HT-9), *taiyuan* (LU-9).

Cold and heat of the body: *(DACH) tiantu* (CV-22).

Cold and heat, body heavy: *(DACH) fengfu* (GV-15, IS GV-16).

Cold and heat, sweat comes out: *(DACH) quepen* (ST-12).

Cold and heat, sweat not coming: *(DACH) shaoze* (SI-1), *muchuang* (GB-12, IS GB-16).

Cold and heat causing thirst: *(YXRM) quchi* (LI-11).

Cold and heat without measure: *(DACH) yinlingquan* (SP-9).

Cold and heat, fullness of chest: *(YXRM, DACH) tianliao* (TW-15).

Cold and heat, pain in the front of the neck: *(DACH) daying* (ST-8, IS ST-5).

Cold and heat, lymph nodes swollen: *(YXRM) daying* (ST-8, IS ST-5).

Cold and heat, stiffness of the column: *(DACH, YXRM) taodao* (GV-12, IS GV-13).

Evil wind or cold *(e han feng):*

Evil wind or cold: *(YXRM, DACH) waiqiu* (GB-36); *(DACH) tianquan* (PC-2), *tianshi* (PC-5), *chengling* (GB-14, IS GB-18).

Face, evil wind or cold, jaw swollen, painful: *(DACH) tianchuang* (SI-16).

Evil cold *(e han):*

Evil cold: *(JM) qingling* (HT-2), *tianliao* (TW-15); *(DACH) daying* (ST-8, IS ST-5); *(YXRM) ciliao* (BL-32).

Attack of fever from evil cold: *(JM) chengling* (GB-14, IS GB-18), *hegu* (LI-4); *(JM) xinxi* (HT-6), *zhigou* (TW-6); *(JM) mingmen* (GV-4); *(JM) muchuang* (GB-12, IS GB-16); *(JM) waiqiu* (GB-36).

Evil cold, back and vertebrae cannot be bent forward or backward: *(DACH, YXRM)* bad cold, can neither bend nor straighten: *waiqiu* (GB-36).

Evil cold, tightening of the shoulder and back, pain radiating to the supraclavicular fossa: *(DACH, YXRM)* pain like a necklace; *(GSdeM) shangyang* (LI-1).

Evil cold, intense cold: *(YIX I, 4r) erjian* (LI-2).

Evil cold, pain in the jaw: *(YIZ, 41r) shangyang* (LI-1).

Evil cold and shock *(DACH)* at the vertex *(YXRM): houding* (GV-18, IS GV-19).

Evil wind *(e feng):*

Evil wind, cold, emptiness, fever: *(DACH) yuji* (LU-10).

Penetrating cold *(zhong han):*

Penetrating cold: *(YXRM) zhongwan* (CV-12).

For cold which has penetrated, quickly warm the bladder with an onion cake, and moxas at *qihai* (CV-6), also warm the extremities: *(YXRM V, 2r) qihai* (CV-6).

Cold having entered, bad cold: *(YIX I, 5v)* ear-*erjian* (MP-9, IS M-HN-10).

III. Nose, Rhinopharynx

In general.

All illnesses of the nose: *(DACH X, 15v) fengmen* (BL-12).

Prolonged illnesses of the nose: *(YXRM I, 46r) baihui* (GV-19, IS GV-20).

Nose: *(JM) yingxiang* (LI-20).

Rhinopharynx: *(GSdeM) hegu* (LI-4).

Smell, anosmia (see organs of sense).

Sneezing (pen-ti).

(DACH) The energy is in the depths for sneezing — disperse.

Sneezing; energy is in the depths for sneezing — needles: *(DACH IV, 6r) fengmen* (BL-12).

A lot of sneezing: *(DACH) fengmen* (BL-12).
Ability to sneeze: *(DACH) chize* (LU-5), *hanyan* (GB-4).
Sneezing from dazzling light or wind: *(DACH) zanzhu* (BL-2).

Pain.

Pain in the nose: *(DACH) naokong* (GB-19).
Pain in the root of the nose and the middle of the forehead: *(YXRM)* gum-*yinjiao* (GV-27, IS GV-28).
Nose and eyes acid in the interior: *(DACH) ganshu* (BL-18).

Pain and swelling, swelling, mucus.

Pain and swelling at the tip of the nose: *(DACH) juliao* (ST-6, IS ST-3).
Swelling of the nose: *(DACH)* ear-*heliao* (TW-22, IS TW-21 *ermen* by location).
Inflammation of the nose of a fatty type: *(JM) yingxiang* (LI-20), *qucha* (BL-4).
Shock on the face, swelling of the nose and cheek: *(DACH) juliao* (ST-6, IS ST-3).

Cold, heat, dryness.

Cold of the nose: *(DACH) qiangu* (SI-2).
Heat and numbness of the nose after an illness: *(DACH) ganshu* (BL-18).
Dryness of the nose: *(DACH, JM) xuanzhong* (GB-39).
Useless nose: *(DACH) jinggu* (BL-64).

Cold in the head, coryza, catarrh of the nose, rhinitis

Gan mao; popularly *shang feng;* anciently *qiu, qiu ti.*

> *Illness from chills; the nose is blocked. (Ci Yuan, ''Qiu'')*

> *The clear or thick* **qiu** *are distinguished; little fever. (YXRM, 12v)*

> *Begins like catarrh of the nose* **(bi jia da er);** *the nose is blocked and flows; there is sneezing. The slight cases cure themselves in a few days. (Ci Yuan, ''Shang-feng'')*

> *In* **shang feng** *the first symptoms are catarrh of the nose, sneezing, hot feet and hands, does not dislike food. It is the blood which is troubled; the cause is wind. This is the popular name for* **gan mao.** *(YXRM V, 6v)*

> *When coryza lasts a long time (***qiu, bi yuan** *and others) the cause is a deficiency of the blood, a lack of kidney fluids nourishing the blood: one tonifies the kidneys. (YXRM, VI, 13r)*

> *Nasal catarrh; the most frequent of the illnesses of the nose. Acute and chronic types are differentiated: the acute type comes from a slight illness (***gan mao,** *flu) or from a contagion; swelling of mucosa, nostrils blocked, flow of liquid abundant; it can be cured without treatment. The chronic type comes from having inhaled some foreign bodies or vapors which cause irritation; or it comes after a nervous crisis. The mucosa is either fatty and thick or thin and dry. The first mucus secretions are thick like pus. The second have a thick flow with a bad odor; the mucus is transformed by drying into a crust which is fixed to the mucosa; if they are removed, the blood flows. It can spread into the ears and eyes. It is not easily cured. (Ci Yuan, ''Bi-ji-da-er'')*

Acute rhinitis *(ji xing bi yan):*

> *Origins: measles, scarlet fever, whooping cough, mercury poisoning, contagious illnesses, flu, dust, acidity, vapors, the breathing of poisons, nasal lesions, etc. Symptoms: swelling of the mucosa, blocked nose, sneezing, bad cold, the whole body tired, lazy, restlessness, heavy forehead, a lot of discharge, headache, often fever. (JO, 57)*

Chronic rhinitis *(man xing bi yan):*

> *Origin: change from acute rhinitis; or dust, coal; a scratch from a brick or a tile; smoking tobacco; drinking a lot of alcohol; illness of the lymph nodes. It often comes from syphilis. Symptoms: nose blocked, closed, abundant nasal discharge; diminished smell; pharynx obstructed, dry and burning; sometimes a bad smell. (JO, 58)*

Disperse for those who easily have diarrhea, abundant urine, eruptions, sweat; tonify for those who hold their toxins, who have great fever, serious types with complications.

Shang feng (''damaging wind''):

Shang feng, face scarlet, headache, fever: *(DACH VII, 32v) lieque* (LU-7), *tongli* (HT-5), *quchi* (LI-11).
Shang feng, nose with clear discharge: *(DACH XI, 29r) shangxing* (GV-22, IS GV-23) *shuigou,* (GV-25, IS GV-26 *renzhong), fengfu* (GV-15, IS GV-16). If *shang feng* is not removed, and there is cough and mucus and the inside

head is painful: *baihui* (GV-19, IS GV-20), *fengchi* (GB-20), *fengmen* (BL-12), *bailao* (GV-13, IS GV-14 *dazhui*): all points, 2 *fen*.

Shang feng, four limbs ill at ease, fever, cephalalgia: *(DACH VII, 32r) lieque* (LU-7), *jingqu* (LU-8), *quchi* (LI-11), *hegu* (LI-4), *weizhong* (BL-54, IS BL-40). *Shang feng,* upset from cold, cough or fullness from cough: *(DACH VII, 32r) lieque* (LU-7), *shanzhong* (CV-17), *fengmen* (BL-12), *fengfu* (GV-15, IS GV-16), *hegu* (LI-4).

Coryza *(qiu):*
Coryza, discharge from the nose: *(YXRM) hegu* (LI-4).
Coryza, clear discharge: *(DACH) fengmen* (BL-12), *zhiyin* (BL-67), foot-*tonggu* (BL-66).
Coryza, painful eyes: *(DACH IV, 3v) shangxing* (GV-22, IS GV-23).

Acute catarrh of the nose:
Acute catarrh of the nose: *(JM) shenting* (GV-23, IS GV-24), nose-*heliao* (LI-19), *lidui* (ST-45); *(JM) yingxiang* (LI-20).

Acute or chronic catarrh of the nose:
Acute or chronic catarrh of the nose: *(JM) juliao* (ST-6, IS ST-3).

Nose with clear discharge:
Nose with clear discharge: *(YIZ, 40r) shangxing* (GV-22, IS GV-23,) moxa, disperse 2 x 7; *(YXRM I, 39r)* prolonged: *shangxing* (GV-22, IS GV-23).
Coryza and clear discharge: *(DACH) fengmen* (BL-12), *zhiyin* (BL-67), foot-*tonggu* (BL-66), *tonggu* of the epigastrium (KI-20).
Nose, a lot of clear discharge: *(DACH) chengguang* (BL-6); *(YXRM)* incessant discharge: nose-*heliao* (LI-19); *(DACH)* not able to be stopped: *baihui* (GV-19, IS GV-20).

Nose with thick discharge:
Nose with thick discharge: *(YIZ, 40r) shangxing* (GV-22, IS GV-23), disperse.
Nose with thick discharge without fever: *(DACH VII, 33v) shangxing* (GV-22, IS GV-23), *quchi* (LI-11), *lieque* (LU-7), *neiguan* (PC-6), *hegu* (LI-4).
Nose with thick discharge without stopping, ending in continuous coryza: *(DACH) xuanlu* (GB-5).

Nose with clear, thick discharge:
Nose with clear, thick discharge; *(YXRM I, 39r) hegu* (LI-4), *taichong* (LR-3).

Catarrh of the nose:

Treatment with needles and moxa:

tianzhu (BL-10)	2 to 5 *fen,* 7 moxas,
fengchi (GB-20)	2 to 5 *fen,* 7 moxas,
head-*wangu* (GB-17, IS GB-12)	2 to 5 *fen,* 7 moxas,
zanzhu (BL-2)	2 *fen,* 7 moxas,
dazhu (BL-11)	2 *fen,* 7 moxas,
fengmen (BL-12)	2 *fen,* 7 moxas,
quchi (LI-11)	2 *fen,* 7 moxas,
hegu (LI-4)	2 *fen,* 7 moxas. *(JM, 317)*

Acute rhinitis:

Treatment with needles:

yingxiang (LI-20)	5 *fen,*
nose-*heliao* (LI-19)	2 *fen,*
tianzhu (BL-10)	3 *fen,*
shenzhu (GV-11, IS GV-12)	3 *fen. (JO, 57)*

Treatment with moxa:

fengchi (GB-20)	7 moxas,
tianzhu (BL-10)	5 moxas,
baihui (GV-19, IS GV-20)	7 moxas,
mouth-*yinjiao* (GV-27, IS GV-28)	3 moxas. *(JO, 57)*

Chronic rhinitis:

Treatment with needles:

yingxiang (LI-10)	*5 fen,*
baihui (GV-19, IS GV-20)	*2 fen,*
shangxing (GV-22, IS GV-23)	*2 fen,*
nose-heliao (LI-19)	*2 fen,*
tianzhu (BL-10)	*5 fen,*
shenzhu (GV-11, IS GV-12) ...	*3 fen. (JO, 58)*

Treatment with moxa:

tianzhu (BL-10)	*10 moxas,*
shenzhu (GV-11, IS GV-12)	*10 moxas,*
yingxiang (LI-20)	*5 moxas,*
baihui (GV-19, IS GV-20) ...	*7 moxas,*
lidui (ST-45)	*3 moxas. (JO, 58)*

Sinusitis, blocked nose, nose encumbered.

Sinusitis (zhu neng zheng, "pus-production illness"):

Origin: the maxillary sinus is hollowed out and produces pus; there is inflammation of the membrane of the bones of the roots of the teeth; influenza; measles; scarlet fever; mercury poisoning. Or the maxillary sinus is hollowed out and produces pus; there is acute inflammation of the hollow of the maxillary sinus. Often it comes from rotten teeth.

Symptoms: in the acute cases where pus is produced in the maxillary sinuses, the average patient has fever attacks and facial spasms. The maxillary bone and its area is swollen, compressed to the point of acute pain. There is cough when they bend forward, and the pain is aggravated. In many cases, if the pus comes out, the pain diminishes or stops. In chronic cases the nose is blocked, there is headache, decreases of vitality and the memory is diminished; vertigo. When bending forward a foul smell escapes from the nose and there is a discharge flowing inside the septum. The cases of purulent transformation of the hollow of the maxillary sinuses accompany flu with acute illnesses of the nose. There is pain in the front of the forehead and this pain is mostly strong before midday and at noon. Moreover, there is pain from compressing the front of the forehead or by tapping lightly. In chronic cases there is continued pain in the forehead aggravated by drinking alcohol, by coughing, etc.

Treatments with needles:

tianding (LI-17)	*3 fen,*
quchi (LI-11)	*7 fen,*
fengchi (GB-20)	*6 fen,*
sibai (ST-5, IS ST-2)	*3 fen,*
juliao (ST-6, IS ST-3)	*4 fen,*
yangbai (GB-10 IS GB-14)	*2 fen,*
yingxiang (LI-20)	*3 fen,*
quanliao (SI-19)	*6 fen,*
yintang (GV-23a, IS M-HN-3)	*2 fen,*
fengmen (BL-12)	*5 fen,*
geshu (BL-17)	*5 fen,*
hegu (LI-4)	*5 fen.*

Treatment with moxa:

tianding (LI-17)	*7 moxas,*
yintang (GV-23a, IS M-HN-3)	*5 moxas,*
head-linqi (GB-11, IS GB-15)	*15 moxas,*
geshu (BL-17)	*7 moxas,*
duiduan (GV-26, IS GV-27) ...	*3 moxas. (JO, 59)*

Sinusitis: *(JM) hegu* (LI-4), *yingxiang* (LI-20), *xiabai* (ST-5, IS ST-2), head-*linqi* (GB-11, IS GB-15), *muchuang* (GB-12, IS GB-16), *qucha* (BL-4), *juliao* (ST-6, IS ST-3), *qianding* (GV-20, IS GV-21); nose-*heliao* (LI-19).
Inflammation of the sinus: *(JM)* nose-*heliao* (LI-19).
Nose, yellow mucus: *(YXRM) jinggu* (BL-64).

Nose blocked, smells nothing *(DACH);* pain at the base of the nose and middle of forehead: *(YXRM, DACH) yinjiao* (GV-27, IS GV-28).

Useless nose, yellow discharge: *(DACH) lidui* (ST-45).

Sinusitis *(bi yuan, nao liu, nao sha):*

> *Name of an illness: from the nostrils there comes out a yellow, thick discharge from time to time. If it is not cured for a long time there flows from the nose a putrescent, bloody liquid. There is vertigo and syncope. It is also called* **nao liu,** *"discharge-from-the-brain." (Ci Yuan, "Bi-yuan")*

> *One must distinguish between* **bi yuan,** *thick discharge with high fever, and* **nao sha,** *with inflammation of the brain, yellow and stinking discharge and a painful skull. (YXRM VI, 12v)*

Bi yuan: thick discharge, painful eyes, anosmia, headaches: *(YIX I, 5r)* tonify *yingxiang* (LI-20), disperse *shangxing* (GV-22, IS GV-23).

Bi yuan: nosebleeds, emptiness: *(YXRM I, 39r)* tonify particularly *shangxing* (GV-22, IS GV-23).

Blocked nose (bi sai, nao sha):

Nostrils blocked *(JM).* Nose blocked *(YXRM).* Nose blocked, useless *(DACH): qiangu* (SI-2). Nostrils blocked *(JM);* nose blocked *(YXRM): zhiyin* (BL-67); *(YXRM) chenguang* (BL-9), *qucha* (BL-4). Nose blocked *(YXRM): bulang* (KI-22); *(DACH) duiduan* (GV-26, IS GV-27), nose-*heliao* (LI-19); *(JM) baihui* (GV-19, IS GV-20).

Nose blocked: *(JM, YXRM, DACH) tongtian* (BL-7); *(YXRM)* head-*linqi* (GB-11, IS GB-15).

Nose blocked, nosebleeds: *(DACH) shenmen* (HT-7).

Nose blocked, smells neither perfumes nor stench: *(YXRM) hegu* (LI-4), nose-*heliao* (LI-19).

Nose blocked, fullness of chest: *(YXRM I, 38r) shenmai* (BL-62), *xinhui* (GV-21, IS GV-22), *yuzhen* (BL-9), *tianzhu* (BL-10).

Nose blocked, head heavy: *(DACH) zhiyin* (BL-67).

Coryza, nose blocked: *(DACH) chengling* (GB-14, IS GB-18), *feiyang* (BL-58).

Nose blocked, tears flowing: *(YXRM) baihui* (GV-19, IS GV-20).

Nose blocked, smells nothing; from time to time, clear discharge: moxa *(DACH X, 32v) xinhui* (GV-21, IS GV-22).

Nose blocked, bad cold: *(DACH)* head-*linqi* (GB-11, IS GB-15).

Nose blocked, internal headaches: *(DACH) meichong* (BL-3), *shangxing* (GV-22, IS GV-23).

Nose blocked, discharge from the nose; *(JM, DACH)* blockage or discharge with redness of the face: *(YXRM I, 46r) shangxing* (GV-22, IS GV-23).

Nose blocked, swelling of the face: *(YXRM) shangxing* (GV-22, IS GV-23).

Nose encumbered (ni):

(JM) yingxiang (LI-20), nose-*heliao* (LI-19), *qucha* (BL-4), ear-*heliao* (TW-22, IS TW-21 *ermen* by location), *baihui* (GV-19, IS GV-20), *chengguang* (BL-6).

Blockage of the nose: *(JM)* nose-*heliao* (LI-19).

Ozena:

Fetid discharge from the nose, dissipation of the brain: *(DACH X, 29r) qucha* (BL-4), *shangxing* (GV-22, IS GV-23).

Cold of the brain, foul-smelling discharges; comes from an infection from inhalant medicines: *shangxing* (GV-22, IS GV-23), *qucha* (BL-4), *hegu* (LI-4); if not better: *shuigou* (GV-25, IS GV-26 *renzhong*), *yingxiang* (LI-20).

Nose is so malodorous that one recoils: *(JM)* nose-*heliao* (LI-19), *tianzhu* (BL-10), *shenfeng* (KI-23), *bulang* (KI-22), *lingxu* (KI-24).

Obturation of the nose; foul odor so that one recoils: *(JM) yingxiang* (LI-20).

Fissures of the nose (bi chi):

Fissure of the nose; bad smell on the left, moxa on the right; bad smell on the right, moxa on the left. When something like a piece of dry bone comes out of the nose, the energy of the stench cures itself: *(YXRM I, 46r) tongtian* (BL-7).

Fissure of the nose and fetid discharge: *(DACH XI, 3r) shangxing* (GV-22, IS GV-23), *fengfu* (GV-15, IS GV-16). If not better, nose-*heliao* (LI-19), *fengchi* (GB-20), *shuigou* (GV-25, IS GV-26 *renzhong*), *baihui* (GV-19, IS GV-20), *bailao* (GV-13, IS GV-14 *dazhui*), *fengmen* (BL-12).

Fissure of the nose, clear or thick discharge: *(YXRM I, 39r)* disperse *taichong* (LR-3), *hegu* (LI-4).

Abscesses, ulcers.

Swelling of the tip of the nose: *(DACH)* ear-*heliao* (TW-22, IS TW-21 *ermen* by location).

Abscess of the nose: *(JM, DACH) qucha* (BL-4); *(GSdeM) shenmai* (BL-62), *tongtian* (BL-7).

Abscess of the nose: gum-*yinjiao* (GV-27, IS GV-28), *(YXRM, JM)* yingxiang (LI-20).
Abscess gnawing at the nose: *(DACH, YXRM)* gum-*yinjiao* (GV-27, IS GV-28).

Growths (si ru).

Growth in the nose: *(DACH)* gum-*yinjiao* (GV-27, IS GV-28), *yingxiang* (LI-20), nose-*heliao* (LI-19), *suliao* (GV-24, IS GV-25).
Growths, nose obstructed, no longer functioning: *shangxing* (GV-22 IS GV-23), *yintang* (GV-23a, IS M-HN-3), *yingxiang* (LI-20), *fengmen* (BL-12).
Growths with cold and nosebleeds: *fengchi* (GB-20), *fengfu* (GV-15, IS GV-16), *shuigou* (GV-25, IS GV-26 *renzhong*), nose-*heliao* (LI-19).
Growth in the throat, short of breath: *(DACH) sidu* (TW-9).

Hay fever.

(GSdeM) The liver is generally deficient; tonify *ququan* (LR-8), then disperse *hegu* (LI-4), *fengmen* (BL-12), and *fengfu* (GV-15, IS GV-16).
Asthma from hay fever: the same points, then disperse *feishu* (BL-13) and *yuzhong* (KI-26), and tonify *shanzhong* (CV-17).

Nosebleeds, epistaxis (nue, nue xue).

> *Blood comes out from the nose. If serious, there are headaches and buzzing. Women for whom the menses does not arrive often have this problem. (Ci Yuan, "Nue-xue")*

> *Comes from great heat or from cold, or from prolonged coryza. It is necessary to balance the emptiness. (YXRM V, 31v)*

Europeans see here a possible connection with hemorrhages in the brain or elsewhere when there is occasional or enduring high blood pressure; it comes also from relaxing of the tissues and hemophilia.
Ghost pinching the nose and extracting blood: *(DACH)* abdomen-*yinjiao* (CV-7).
Nosebleeds *(JM, YXRM, DACH) ququan* (LR-8), *xuanzhong* (GB-39), *dadun* (LR-1), *jinggu* (BL-64), *zhiyin* (BL-67); *(JM) neiting* (ST-44), *qiangu* (SI-1), *zhongwan* (CV-12), *xuanlu* (GB-5), *shangxing* (GV-22, IS GV-23); *(JM) yamen* (GV-14, IS GV-15); *(DACH X, 29r) shangxing* (GV-22, IS GV-23), *xinhui* (GV-21, IS GV-22), *xuanzhong* (GB-39).
Coryza, nosebleeds: *erjian* (LI-2), *hegu* (LI-4), *sanjian* (LI-3), *pianli* (LI-6), *kunlun* (BL-60), *chengshan* (BL-57), *chengjin* (BL-56).
Nosebleed, scarlet face: *(DACH) xinhui* (GV-21, IS GV-22).
Nosebleeds, not stopping: *(DACH) laogong* (PC-8); *(JM, DACH) hegu* (LI-4), *yongquan* (KI-1), *neiting* (ST-44), *weizhong* (BL-54 IS BL-40); *(YXRM, DACH) yamen* (GV-14, IS GV-15), nose-*heliao* (LI-19).
Blood coming from the nose and mouth without stopping: *(DACH) shangxing* (GV-22, IS GV-23), *tianfu* (LU-3).

IV. Throat (Yan Hou, Yi)

Speech, sound, hoarseness.

Loss of speech from cerebral troubles (see Apoplexy and Hemiplegia).
Loss of speech from emotional agitation, weakness, cerebral insufficiency (see Insufficiency of energy of the consciousness).
Here, we only consider loss of speech from troubles of the vocal system; larynx, hoarseness, etc.
Hoarse voice, loss of ability to make sound: *(DACH) kongzui* (LU-6); *(JM) tinggong* (SI-19); *(JM) yongquan* (KI-1).
Hoarse voice: *(JM) jiache* (ST-3, IS ST-6).
Broken sound: *(DACH) tiantu* (CV-22).

Loss of ability to make sound.

Loss of ability to make sound, aphonia, muteness (shi yin; yin):
Loss of ability to make sound: *(DACH) shenmen* (HT-7), *kongzui* (LU-6); *(YXRM) tinggong* (SI-19); *(DACH, YXRM) jiache* (ST-3, IS ST-6).
Loss of ability to make sound, knotted tongue: *(DACH) yongquan* (KI-1).
Loss of ability to make sound, no longer speaks: *(YXRM) yuji* (LU-10); *(DACH) dicang* (ST-7, IS ST-4).

Loss of ability to make sound, emotional agitation, fear: *(YXRM) yinxi* (HT-6).

Loss of ability to make sound; gibberish; stops himself: *(DACH II, 19r; YIX I, 4r) tianding* (LI-17), *jianshi* (PC-5).

Sudden loss of ability to make sound, speech and sound difficult: *(DACH IV, 3r) yamen* (GV-14, IS GV-15).

Aphasia and aphonia in storms: *(DACH) sanyangluo* (TW-8).

Aphonia, sudden muteness in storms, no longer speaks: *(DACH) lingdao* (HT-4), *zhigou* (TW-6); *(YXRM) sanyangluo* (TW-8); *(DACH) chengjiang* (CV-24).

Sudden aphonia and aphasia, cannot speak: *(DACH) tonggu* of the epigastrium (KI-20).

Aphonia, cannot speak: *(DACH) yongquan* (KI-1); *(DACH) hegu* (LI-4); *(DACH) tiantu* (CV-22).

Cannot speak: *(JM) dicang* (ST-7, IS ST-4), *tianrong* (SI-17); *(DACH) fubai* (GB-16, IS GB-10); *(JM) tiantu* (CV-22).

Sudden aphonia, hardened energy: *(DACH) tianding* (LI-17), neck-*futu* (LI-18).

Aphonia in storms, face without expression, cannot eat: *(DACH IV, 11r; YIX I, 8r)* tonify *tongli* (HT-5).

Speech tired, wants to rest: *(DACH II, 19r) tongli* (HT-5) and *dazhong* (KI-6, IS KI-4).

Aphonia and aphasia: *(DACH X, 24r) jianshi* (PC-5), *zhigou* (TW-6), *hegu* (LI-4), *yuji* (LU-10), *yingu* (KI-10), *fuliu* (KI-7).

Muteness in storms, cannot speak: *(DACH)*. And pain of the throat: *(YXRM) zhigou* (TW-6).

Sadness, timidity, not a sound comes out: *(YIZ, 40) tongli* (HT-5), needles and moxa.

Aphasia, no longer speaks (muteness: *bu yu; ya; ya ba*):

Does not speak, slowness of the tongue: *(DACH II, 19r; YIX, 4v; Ju Ying) yamen* (GV-14, IS GV-15), *guanchong* (TW-1).

(For aphasia after apoplexy, see Apoplexy.)

Blocked speech, becoming thick: *(JM) yamen* (GV-14, IS GV-15); speech rough, blocked: *(JM) tiantu* (CV-22).

Muscles, nerves, vocal organs:

Master point of the glossopharyngeal nerve (motor function of the pharynx, sense function of the mucosa of the pharynx and larynx): *(JM) tianzhu* (BL-10).

Paralysis of the hypoglossal nerve (motor function of the tongue): *(JM)* head-*wangu* (GB-17, IS GB-12), *renying* (ST-9).

Spasms of the throat: *(JM) neiting* (ST-44).

Contractions of the muscles of sound: *(JM) zhongfu* (LU-1).

Spasms of the muscles of the "door-of-sound" *(yin men)*: *(JM) tiantu* (CV-22), *huagai* (CV-20), *dicang* (ST-7, IS ST-4).

Contracture or paralysis of all the muscles of the region of the root of the tongue *(she gen)*: *(JM) lianquan* (CV-23). Linked to the root of the tongue: *(DACH) shangqiu* (SP-5).

Paralysis of the hyoid muscles (bone of the tongue, *she gu*): *(JM) yinxi* (HT-6), *tongli* (HT-5), *lingdao* (HT-4), *zhigou* (TW-6), *yongquan* (KI-1), *yamen* (GV-14, IS GV-15), *tiantu* (CV-22), neck-*futu* (LI-18), *tianting* (LI-17), *tonggu* of the epigastrium (KI-20).

(See also Tongue.)

Mouth slow, does not come back, cannot speak: *(DACH) daying* (ST-8, IS ST-5), *dicang* (ST-7, IS ST-4), *chengqi* (ST-4, IS ST-1).

(See also Stuttering.)

Children who do not start to speak for many years; insufficiency of consciousness: *(DACH)* tonify *yinshu* (BL-15).

(See also Excess speech)

V. Larynx *(Hou; Hou Tou)*

(See also Hoarseness, Loss of Ability to Make Sound.)

In general.

All illnesses of the larynx: *(YIZ, 41r) fengfu* (GV-15, IS GV-16), *shaoshang* (LU-11).

The five sore throats *(yan hou)*: *(DACH) zhongkui* (MP-21, IS M-UE-16).

All illnesses of the throat *(yan hou)*: *(DACH) fengfu* (GV-15, IS GV-16), leg-*sanli* (ST-36).

Vocal cords (sheng dai).

Relaxed: tonify; contracted, inflamed: disperse: *(GSdeM) renying* (ST-9).

Laryngitis, catarrh of the larynx, inflammation of the larynx (hou feng, hou tong, hou tou jia da er).

The mucosa of the larynx have attacks of heat with itching of the larynx, much coughing, dribbles of white mucus; the sounds become softer and softer. Among children who are attacked by it, it often changes into **ma bi feng**. *(Ci Yuan, ''Hou-tou-jia-da-er'')*

There are many varieties: 1) Acute laryngitis, **ji hou feng** *or* **jin hou feng**. *It comes from eating too much strong-flavored food, accumulating heat in the stomach and in the lungs; this heat rises, crowding and attacking the throat. It is violent and sudden at first: the throat becomes red and swollen, with acute or dull pain. Even hot water will not go down; mucus and saliva crowd and obstruct. The voice is as if drawn over a saw.*

2) Chronic laryngitis, **man hou feng**. *It comes from an emptiness in the constitution, or from violent unhappiness, or from eating too much of the five acrid [flavors], or from fretfulness, excess worries or thoughts. It is slow in the beginning, the complexion is slightly accentuated, there is slight swelling and the pharynx is dry.*

3) Laryngitis from muteness, **ya zhang**, *or from tongue throat-wind,* **neng she hou feng**. *It resembles acute laryngitis, but the jaws are contracted and one cannot speak. The voice is dull, the speech rough; the tongue is not retracted but comes out and is agitated from time to time. The patient always wants to touch it with his finger.*

4) Laryngitis which strangles, **chan hou feng**. *A type of acute laryngitis, but with swelling obvious externally. This illness is often more serious than the others. (Ci Yuan, ''Hai-u-feng,'' ''Hou-feng'')*

A serious illness of the throat: mucus and saliva enveloping the interstices of the larynx, with internal and external swelling and occlusion. Even hot water will not go down. The **hou feng** *laryngitis is popularly called* **hou tong,** *''laryngeal pain.'' (Ci Yuan, ''Chan-hou-feng'')*

Name of an illness; children between one and seven years of age are frequently attacked. It begins with a light cough; bouts of fever, no peace. Three to five days later, inhalation and exhalation are pressed and hurried. The sound of the cough is like the chirping of chicks or the barking of a dog. An oppressive anxiety irritates the chest, and the body turns without rest; then, little by little the patient weakens and tires until the moment when, near death, he seems to sleep peacefully with neither anguish nor pain. (Ci Yuan, ''Ma-bi-feng'' [Horse-spleen Wind])

When cold remains for an extended time at **feishu** *(BL-13), it is transformed into heat, which produces mucus, panting, hiccoughs, swelling of the lungs and sneezing. This is popularly called* **ma bi feng**. *If there is only mucus, cough, attacks of convulsions and the nature is robust, it is curable. (YXRM VI, 15r, ''Ma-bi-feng'')*

(See also Angina.)
Hou tong (laryngitis): *(DACH IV, 14r) shaoshang* (LU-11); *(YIX I, 5v) yuji* (LU-10).
Catarrh of the throat *(yan hou jia da er): (JM) yuji* (LU-10).
Catarrh of the larynx:
(JM) kongzui (LU-6), *xiguan* (LR-7), *tongziliao* (GB-1).
Hou feng (laryngitis): *(DACH III, 26v) tiantu* (CV-22); *(YXRM I, 38r) zhaohai* (KI-3, IS KI-6).
Hou feng of old people: *(DACH) shaoshang* (LU-11) three moxas; on the left for men, on the right for women; *(DACH) dagukong* (MP-19, IS M-UE-15), three moxas.
Swelling of the larynx: *(DACH) lieque* (LU-7).
Inflammation of the larynx: *(JM, 315) shenzhu* (GV-11, IS GV-12) twenty moxas.
Inflammation of the throat: *(JM) rangu* (KI-2), *fengfu* (GV-15, IS GV-16), *shaoshang* (LU-11), *jiuwei* (CV-15).
Heat in the larynx: *(YXRM) tiantu* (CV-22).
In the larynx, obstruction, like the ''honk-honk'' noise of a duck: *(DACH, YXRM) tiantu* (CV-22), neck-*futu* (LI-18).
Larynx constricted by blood: *(DACH) tiantu* (CV-22).
''Root-foot throat,'' repeated attacks: *(YIZ, 41v) tianrong* (SI-17), 7 to 2 x 7 moxas.
Singing sounds in the larynx: *(DACH, YXRM) dazhong* (KI-6, IS KI-4), tonify; *(YXRM) taichong* (LR-3), *tinggong* (SI-19), *shaoshang* (LU-11).
Singing sounds in the larynx, energy in the upper body: *(DACH) shanzhong* (CV-17); *(YXRM) tianchi* (PC-1).

Pains in the larynx.

Pain in the larynx: *(YXRM) guanchong* (TW-1), *xiguan* (LR-7), *yemen* (TW-2), *yuji* (LU-10).
Pain in the larynx, muteness, cannot speak: *(DACH) tianchuang* (SI-16).
Pain and swelling of the throat: *(YIZ, 42r) shaoshang* (LU-11).

Spasms of the larynx.

Muscle spasms at the ''gate of sound'': *(JM) tiantu* (CV-22), *huagai* (CV-20), *dicang* (ST-7, IS ST-4).
Larynx asleep: *(DACH) sanyangluo* (TW-8).

Dryness.

Dryness of the larynx: *(DACH)* tonify *yuji* (LU-10).
Dryness: *(DACH) pianli* (LI-6), *zhaohai* (KI-3, IS KI-6).

Abscess of the larynx:

Abscess of the larynx, nothing passes: *(YXRM) tiantu* (CV-22); *(DACH) hegu* (LI-4), *renying* (ST-9), *xuanji* (CV-21).

Various illnesses of the larynx (hou xian, hou gan, hou liu).

Hou xian, "laryngeal exanthem," or *tian bai yi*, "sky-white ants":

> *Name of an illness also called **tian bai yi**. At first, from time to time one feels pruritis in the larynx. Then there is an exanthem of dark red color produced. The dryness is intense. A stinking saliva is ejected, preventing one from drinking or eating. For the patient it is advisable to purify the mind and to become empty of desires, to avoid strong flavors. If he does not improve, then the putrescence will become established. On the sides small holes are formed as if nibbled by white ants (termites). Many cases cannot be helped. (Ci Yuan, "Hou-xian")*

Treatment is achieved through the general points of the larynx and throat and with *yuji* (LU-10), which acts against the dryness.

Hou gan, "tuberculosis (or chancre) of the larynx":

> *In the beginning, the pharynx and larynx are dry, as if body hair or straw are constantly piercing the larynx and as if a hard object is blocking the bottom of the pharynx. There is vomiting of acid water. Sweet, slightly red saliva is brought up by eructations; a little swelling, a little pain. Then the color becomes a dark violet, like frozen persimmons. In the past it was said to come from a deficiency of the kidney and from an inflammation rising counterflow. If pain and swelling increases from day to day, there is putrefaction and fetid disintegration which prevents the patient from eating and drinking. Many cases cannot be helped. (Ci Yuan, "Hou-gan")*

Treatment is achieved through the general points for the larynx, and leg-*sanli* (ST-36).

Hou liu, "laryngeal tumor":

> *On the side of the larynx there is produced a fleshy tumor, **ying**, like the hole in a coin. Red threads crisscross there; either simple or double. In the past it was said to come from heat pushed back into the lung meridian; at the same time there is excess speech, which exhausts the energy." (Ci Yuan, "Hou-liu")*

False croup (heng bi, "mooing occlusion").

False croup of children, mucus, cough: *(YIX I, 4v) feishu* (BL-17), *tiantu* (CV-22), *jinsuo* (GV-7, IS GV-8).
False croup, it unbinds by itself; the two hands are numb, they hold objects with difficulty: *(DACH IV, 7v) hegu* (LI-4), *quchi* (LI-11), *jianyu* (LI-15). Disperse *hegu* (LI-4) and leg-*sanli* (ST-36).

Diphtheria.

Zou ma hou bi, "galloping-horse laryngitis"; *hou sha,* "laryngeal infection"; popularly, *bai hou,* "white larynx." Japanese transcription: *tie fu di li,* or *ge lu bu.*

> *Angina which comes suddenly and causes death is called **zou ma hou bi**. (DACH XI, 12r)*

> *Called in Japan **tie fu di li**, popularly called **bai hou**. In Europe, called croup **(ge lu bu)**, it is contagious with extreme rapidity. Caused by a pathogenic bacteria which is first transmitted into the larynx. The tonsils become red and swollen, producing cinder-grey pellicules, a painful pharynx, difficult deglutition, a strangled voice, laryngeal constriction; the voice is similar to barking; whistling respiration which is very difficult. The patient sleeps more and more heavily, as if dead. These serious cases are frequently found in children. (Ci Yuan, "Hou-sha")*

Zou ma hou bi: *(DACH XI, 12r) shaoshang* (LU-11), *hegu* (LI-4), *guanchong* (TW-1), *fenglong* (ST-40), *yongquan* (KI-1).
All the general points of the throat, mainly *fengfu* (GV-15, IS GV-16), *zhongkui* (MP-21, IS M-UE-16), leg-*sanli* (ST-36), *zhaohai* (KI-3, IS KI-6), *shaoshang* (LU-11).

VI. Trachea, Bronchi

It seems that the Chinese, curing all inflammations of the different parts of the upper respiratory passage with the same points, did not distinguish between tracheitis and bronchitis. These problems are classified as mucus illnesses (see below), causing cough and expectoration. The Japanese, and certain experiments made in Paris, now enable us to specify the effects of certain points; later experiments will do this even more precisely.

Trachea, tracheitis *(shang qi guan yan, jia da er):*
Trachea: *(GSdeM)* zigong (CV-19).
Tracheitis: *(GSdeM)* kongzui (LU-6), disperse *lieque* (LU-7), *tiantu* (CV-22).

Bronchi, bronchitis *(qi guan yan, jia da er):*
Bronchi: *(JM) wuyi* (ST-15), *feishu* (BL-13), *geshu* (BL-17), *ganshu* (BL-18).
Bronchitis: *(GSdeM)* disperse *lieque* (LU-7); *(GSdeM) taiyuan* (LU-9). *(JM) houxi* (SI-3), *(JM) wenliu* (LI-7), *chize* (LU-5), *tianjing* (TW-10), *tianfu* (LU-3), *feishu* (BL-13), *fengmen* (BL-12), *dazhu* (BL-11), *geshu* (BL-17), *gaohuangshu* (BL-38, IS BL-43), *lingtai* (GV-9, IS GV-10), *tianjing* (GB-21), *jianzhongshu* (SI-15), *quepen* (ST-12), *shufu* (KI-27), *yuzhong* (KI-26), *shencang* (KI-25), *lingxu* (KI-24), *shenfeng* (KI-23), *kufang* (ST-14), *yingchuang* (ST-16), *lianquan* (CV-23), *zigong* (CV-19), *shanzhong* (CV-17), *juque* (CV-14), *shangwan* (CV-13), *youmen* (KI-21).
Acute bronchitis: *(JM) quepen* (ST-12), *quze* (PC-3), *bulang* (KI-22).
Chronic bronchitis: *(JM) tongtian* (BL-7), *qihu* (ST-13).
Intercostal neuralgia from bronchitis: *(JM) bulang* (KI-22), *ganshu* (BL-18).
Bleeding bronchi: *(JM) taiyuan* (LU-9).
Abscess of bronchi causing nosebleeds: *(YXRM)* head-*qiaoyin* (GB-18, IS GB-11).
Bronchitis: *(JM)* with needles — *dazhu* (BL-11), *fengmen* (BL-12), *feishu* (BL-13), *jueyinshu* (BL-14), *ganshu* (BL-18), *geshu* (BL-17), *fufen* (BL-36, IS BL-41), *pohu* (BL-37, IS BL-42), *gaohuangshu* (BL-38, IS BL-43), *geguan* (BL-41, IS BL-46), arm-*sanli* (LI-10), *xiaohai* (SI-8); with moxa — *ganshu* (BL-18), *danshu* (BL-19), *pishu* (BL-20).
Bronchitis *(tan yin)*, at the beginning, difficulty speaking, suffocation and also mucus, cough: *(DACH IV, 5v; YIX I, 5r) lieque* (LU-7), *taiyuan* (LU-9); cough, tan yin: *(DACH) taiyuan* (LU-9).
Bronchitis *(tan yin)*, chest and sides full, oppressed, painful: *(YIZ, 45) gongsun* (SP-4).
Bronchitis *(tan yin)*, body swollen, breathes with shoulders: *(DACH) chengman* (ST-20).
Bronchitis *(tan yin)*, expectorates water: *(DACH) juque* (CV-14).

VII. Lungs *(Fei)*

*The lungs are the home of the **po** (unconsciousness, level of the instincts). (DACH)*

The lungs dominate (through their troubles) in autumn. (DACH X, 16v)

They are the minister of exchanges . . . they give life to the skin and body hair. (DACH VIII, 2r & v)

Worrying and regret (which cure emotiveness and anguish) injure the lungs; in excess they cause asthma, which is cured through joy.

Choking back the energy or paresis of energy depends on the lungs. (DACH IV, 1r)

Europeans feel that the lungs have several internal functions. The main is the metabolism of fatty substances. They stop the emulsified fats which the chyliferous lymphatics have collected in the intestines; they attack the fats and make them disappear into the interior itself of the capillaries through a veritable intravascular digestion (Roger and Binet).

Relations of the organs: circulation of energy — liver, maximum from 1 to 3 a.m., then the lung from 3 to 5 a.m., then large intestine from 5 to 7 a.m.

The coupled yang workshop organ for the lungs (yin treasure organ) is the large intestine.

In illnesses of the lungs, one must tonify the large intestine if the lungs are weakened, and disperse it if the lungs are inflamed. (DACH)

The lungs are dominated by the heart *(DACH I, 16v)*. The illnesses of the heart are transmitted to the lung; the illnesses of the lung are transmitted to the liver.

Meridian: see the beginning of this chapter.

If to the right of the umbilicus, there are movements of energy and if by pressing it we cause an acute pain, there is trouble of the lung. (DACH VI, 18r)

In general.

Illnesses of the respiratory system: *(JM) jueyinshu* (BL-14).

Master point of all illnesses of the lung: *(JM) feishu* (BL-13); all illnesses of lung: *(JM) fengmen* (BL-12).

Lung: *(JM) feishu* (BL-13), *xinshu* (BL-15), *qihu* (ST-13).

Unites the vessels of the lung, larynx, chest and diaphragm: *(YXRM I, 38r) lieque* (LU-7).

Activates the pulmonary artery: *(YIX I, 9r) lieque* (LU-7).

Pulmonary artery tightened: *(DACH) zhongfu* (LU-1).

(GSdeM) Shanzhong (CV-17) commands the exterior muscles of respiration, thorax and diaphragm; cannot breathe deeply.

Insufficiency of energy of the lungs.

Emptiness, exhaustion, paresis of the lung: *(DACH) pohu* (BL-37, IS BL-42).

Cold of the lung: *(YXRM) kufang* (ST-14).

Little energy, not enough for breathing: *(DACH, YXRM) lieque* (LU-7).

Energy (respiration) short: *(DACH) shanzhong* (CV-17), *xingjian* (LR-2), thorax-*qimen* (LR-14), *dabao* (SP-21).

Paresis *(wei)* of the lungs: *(DACH) feishu* (BL-13).

Paresis of the lungs, respiration stopped: *(GSdeM)* disperse *kunlun* (BL-60).

Excess energy of the lungs.

Oppression of the lungs: *(DACH) shanzhong* (CV-17).

Cold and heat in the lungs: *(DACH) zhongfu* (LU-1).

Accumulations in the lungs *(fei zhi ji, si fen)*: *(DACH) quepen* (ST-12).

Fullness of the lung, abundant urination: disperse *chize* (LU-5) and *feishu* (BL-13).

Controls the heat in the chest *(YIZ, 30)*: *(DACH) shenzhu* (GV-11, IS GV-12); heat and agitation: thorax-*qimen* (LR-14); *(DACH VI, 15r) zhongchong* (PC-9), *yinlingquan* (SP-9), *yinbai* (SP-1).

Burning of the chest: *qimen* (LR-14).

Pain in the chest: *yinbai* (SP-1) and *yuji* (LU-10).

Fullness of the chest, sides and limbs.

Energy rising and attacking the chest: leg-*shanglian* (ST-37, IS *shangjuxu*).

Fullness of the chest: *sanjian* (LI-3), *quchi* (LI-11), *neiguan* (PC-6), *yangjiao* (GB-35), foot-*linqi* (GB-41), *zhongfu* (LU-1), *tianchi* (PC-1).

Fullness and pain of the chest: *tianxi* (SP-18), *zhongfu* (LU-1).

Fullness of chest, cannot breathe: *tianrong* (SI-17).

Fullness of chest, panting on exhalation, cannot inhale: *renying* (ST-9).

Fullness and swelling of the chest: *waiqiu* (GB-36), *weiyang* (BL-53, IS BL-39).

Fullness of chest, breath short: *zhongfu* (LU-1), *yingchuang* (ST-16).

Fullness and agitation below the heart, energy in counterflow: *yindu* (KI-19).

Fullness of chest and sides: *qiuxu* (GB-40), *taibai* (SP-3), foot-*tonggu* (BL-66), *zhangmen* (LR-13), *yanglingquan* (GB-34).

Chest bound, not loosening: *neiguan* (PC-6).

Fullness of the sides: *yishe* (BL-44, IS BL-49).

Fullness of the last ribs and the limbs: foot-*linqi* (GB-41).

Fullness of heart and chest, central fullness: *neiguan* (PC-6).

Fullness of the chest, sides, limbs: *laogong* (PC-8), *xiaxi* (GB-43), *xiangu* (ST-43), *huagai* (CV-20), *zigong* (CV-19), *xuanji* (CV-21), *zhongting* (CV-16), *qihu* (ST-13), *kufang* (ST-14), *yuzhong* (KI-26), *lingxu* (KI-24), *bulang* (KI-22), *xiongxiang* (SP-19), *zhourong* (SP-20), *zhiyang* (GV-8, IS GV-9), *weishu* (BL-21).

Chest full, obstructed, pain and malaise of chest: *zhongfu* (LU-1).

Ballooning of chest: *jinggu* (LU-8).

Fullness of chest, cannot breathe: (GB-16, IS GB-10), *yutang* (CV-18), *tianfu* (LU-3).

Fullness of chest and abdomen: *sanjian* (LI-3).

Fullness of chest, pain in the abdomen: *neiguan* (PC-6).

VIII. Cough *(Ke Sou)*

This is the apparent symptom of a problem in the respiratory tract on inhalation or exhalation. There is thick mucus; or from certain types of air, there is stimulation of the mucosa of the respiratory passages; then there is noise and cough in the larynx. (Ci Yuan, "Ke-sou")

Qi Bo answered, "Not only the lungs, but all the organs can cause cough. Cough of the lungs: panting, respiration, noise; if serious, hemoptysis. If the cough of the lung does not stop, there is cough of the large intestine with relaxation. Cough of the heart: pain in the heart, tongue knotted, hard; if serious, pharynx swollen, angina. Cough of the liver: pain at the base of the two sides; if serious, cannot turn backwards because of fullness of the base of the two sides. Cough of the spleen-pancreas: pain below the right side (left?). When one coughs, the pain spreads to the shoulder and back; if serious, one cannot move without serious coughing. Cough of the kidney: when coughing, pain in lumbar area and back. If serious, coughs saliva. If the cough of the kidney does not stop, there is cough of the bladder with incontinence of urine when coughing. If the cough of the heart does not stop, there is cough of the small intestine with loss of energy. If the cough of the liver does not stop, there is cough of the gallbladder with vomiting of bile when coughing. If the cough of spleen-pancreas does not stop, there is cough of stomach with vomiting. If the cough lasts a long time, the triple warmer is attacked. Then we do not want to eat any longer. We treat the cough of each treasure organ at the **shu** *point of each meridian:* **taiyuan** *(LU-9),* **shenmen** *(HT-7),* **taichong** *(LR-3),* **taibai** *(SP-3),* **taixi** *(KI-5, IS KI-3). One treats the cough of each workshop organ at the* **he** *point of each meridian:* **quchi** *(LI-11),* **xiaohai** *(SI-8),* **yanglingquan** *(GB-34),* leg-**sanli** *(ST-36),* **weizhong** *(BL-54, IS BL-40)." (DACH I, 4r, quoting the Nei Jing)*

In general.

To treat cough: *(YIX I, 3v)* moxa at *feishu* (BL-13), *fengmen* (BL-12).
To stop cough: *(DACH IV, 6v)* shenzhu (GV-11, IS GV-12).
Stops all coughs: disperse *tiantu* (CV-22).
Cough: *tiantu* (CV-22), *shanzhong* (CV-17), *juque* (CV-14), *taiyuan* (LU-9), *kongzui* (LU-6), *quepen* (ST-12), *kufang* (ST-14), *wuyi* (ST-15), *rugen* (ST-18), leg-*sanli* (ST-36), *chengman* (ST-20), *qishe* (ST-11), arm-*wuli* (LI-13), *qiangu* (SI-2), *taixi* (KI-5, IS KI-3), *yongquan* (KI-1), *shencang* (KI-25), *dazhu* (BL-11), *xinshu* (BL-15), *fujie* (SP-14).
Coughing fits (cough in counterflow): *zigong* (CV-19), *shanzhong* (CV-17), *juque* (CV-14), *yuzhong* (KI-26), *shenfeng* (KI-23), *qimen* (LR-14), *fujie* (SP-14), *kongzui* (LU-6), *xiabai* (LU-4), *jianjing* (GB-21), head-*qiaoyin* (GB-18, IS GB-11), *pohu* (BL-37, IS BL-42), *jueyinshu* (BL-14), *geshu* (BL-17).

Old cough.

Old coughs which are not being cured; comes from cured meat injuring the lungs or from alcoholism, or chronic bronchitis: *(DACH XI, 7v; YIX I, 5v)* fengmen (BL-12), *feishu* (BL-13), *quepen* (ST-12), *shanzhong* (CV-17), *rugen* (ST-18), arm-*sanli* (LI-10).
Chronic bronchitis, frequent cough; if treated for a long time and not cured, tuberculosis is established: *(DACH IV, 6r)* for cough, *feishu* (BL-13); for mucus, *fenglong* (ST-40).
Old cough: *(YIZ, 40)* juquan (MP-8, IS M-HN-36), seven moxas. If it is a hot cough, mix sulphur of arsenic with the artemisia of the moxa. If it is a cold cough, mix with tussilago.
Old cough, difficulty in swallowing: *(DACH)* chengman (ST-20).
Old cough not being cured, spits bloody mucus when coughing: *(DACH VII, 33r)* lieque (LU-7), *taiyuan* (LU-9), *fengmen* (BL-12), *shanzhong* (CV-17).
Old cough: *(DACH)* shaoshang (LU-11), *tianzhu* (BL-10).

Cough, particular symptoms.

Cough, fever, scarlet face: *(DACH X, 34v)* zhigou (TW-6).
Cough, energy in the upper body: *(DACH)* lianquan (CV-23), *shanzhong* (CV-17), *tiantu* (CV-22).
Cough, energy in the upper body, short of energy, cannot speak: *(DACH)* tianjing (TW-10).
Energy of cough, energy in the upper body, agitation of the heart: *(DACH)* yutang (CV-18).
Coughing fits, energy in the upper body: *(DACH)* jingqu (LU-8), *qishe* (ST-11), neck-*futu* (LI-18), *tiantu* (CV-22), *xuanji* (CV-21), *shufu* (KI-27), *qihu* (ST-13), *wuyi* (ST-15), *zhourong* (SP-20), *zhongfu* (LU-1), *huagai* (CV-20), *juque* (CV-14).
Cough, panting: *(DACH)* shaoshang (LU-11), *laogong* (PC-8), *burong* (ST-19); with cold and heat: *(DACH)* tianrong (SI-17).
Coughing fits, panting: *(DACH)* pohu (BL-37, IS BL-42), *huagai* (CV-20).

Cough and panting after food: *(DACH XI, 16v) geshu* (BL-17).

Cough, panting, spits saliva which drops, then blood: *(YXRM) wuyi* (ST-15).

Cough, panting, chest and back radiating pain: *(YXRM) burong* (ST-19).

Coughing fit, energy of panting, pain of back and chest: *(DACH)*. Cough, shortness of breath, agitated, lungs and back painful: *(YXRM) fengmen* (BL-12).

Coughing fits, pain radiating into the chest: *(DACH) bulang* (KI-22).

Coughing fits, fullness of chest and sides: *(DACH) tianquan* (PC-2).

Cough from cold: *(DACH)* tonify *hegu* (LI-4), disperse *sanyinjiao* (SP-6).

Cough, body hot: *(DACH, YXRM) yongquan* (KI-1).

Cough from cold and heat: *(DACH) taixi* (KI-5, IS KI-3); *(YXRM) quepen* (ST-12).

Cough from cold injuring the stomach: *(DACH III, 29r) fengmen* (BL-12).

Coughing fits, pain radiating into the chest: *(DACH) tianquan* (PC-2).

Cough from cold: *(DACH)* tonify *hegu* (LI-4), disperse *sanyinjiao* (SP-6).

Cough, body hot: *(DACH, YXRM) yongquan* (KI-1).

Cough from cold and heat: *(DACH) taixi* (KI-5, IS KI-3); *(YXRM) quepen* (ST-12).

Cough from cold injuring the stomach: *(DACH III, 29r) fengmen* (BL-12).

Coughs to the point of not being able to breathe: *(DACH) qihu* (ST-13).

Cough contracted, tightened, as if there are growths in the throat: *(DACH) ligou* (LR-5).

Coughing fits when looking up: *(DACH) rugen* (ST-18).

Sudden cough, pain in the lumbar area and back: *(DACH IV, 6r) shenzhu* (GV-11, IS GV-12).

Cough, panting, fullness, lumbar area and interior of spine conducting the pain: *(DACH) kunlun* (BL-60).

Cough provoking pain in the coccyx, urine comes out: *(DACH) yuji* (LU-10).

Cough radiating to the two sides with tightening pain, cannot breathe: *(DACH IV, 5r) ganshu* (BL-18).

Pain when coughing: *(DACH) xuanzhong* (GB-39).

Cough when drinking water: *(DACH X, 24r) taiyuan* (LU-9).

Cough, eructations: *(DACH) yuji* (LU-10).

Cough from the throat: *(GSdeM) tianding* (LI-17); from the larynx: *tiantu* (CV-22). From the bronchus: *lieque* (LU-7), *taiyuan* (LU-9); from the lungs: *chize* (LU-5), *shanzhong* (CV-17).

Whooping cough.

Bai ri ke, "cough of a hundred days," *ke sou lian sheng,* "cough connected with a noise," *dun sou,* "prostrating cough."

> Whooping cough; in the past called **dun sou**. The Japanese call it **bai ri ke**. Children get it easily. The cough comes in fits; it has a prolonged sound. In serious cases the cough is followed by vomiting with spasms during the cough; aggravation at night and in the morning. In the saliva, there are rod-like microbes.
> (Ci Yuan, "Bai-ri-ke")

> Cough of a hundred days. Origin: contagion from a microbe. Mostly small children are attacked. After the illness, avoid contagion. Symptoms: prostration which lasts about a week. A period of catarrh which lasts about two weeks, catarrh of the nose, congestion of the conjunctiva, cough, hoarseness. Spasmodic cough for several weeks with vomiting after the cough. The attacks are more frequent at night. In one day from one to a few dozen attacks. In the recovery period, the cough diminishes and is then cured. (JO, 68)

Treatment with needles:

shangqiu (SP-5)	*3 fen,*
fengmen (BL-12)	*3 fen,*
feishu (BL-13)	*3 fen,*
shenzhu (GV-11, IS GV-12)	*3 fen.*

Treatment with moxa:

feishu (BL-13)	*7 moxas,*
shenzhu (GV-11, IS GV-12)	*7 moxas.*

Cough connected with a sound: *(YIX I, 4r; DACH II, 19r; Ju Ying) tiantu* (CV-22), disperse, *feishu* (BL-13), disperse.

Cough of a hundred days: *(JM) tiantu* (CV-22), *shuitu* (ST-10), *huagai* (CV-20), *qihu* (ST-13), *fengmen* (BL-12), *feishu* (BL-13), foot-*shangqiu* (SP-5).

Cough with mucus (see bronchitis, tracheitis, etc.); mucus.

Cough and mucus from cold: *(DACH III, 30v; IV, 5v)* disperse *lieque* (LU-7).

Cough, a lot of spit: *(DACH)* leg-*sanli* (ST-36).

Cough, thick spit: *(DACH) chize* (LU-5).

Cough, saliva and spit in the mouth and larynx: *(DACH) shaoze* (SI-1).

Cough, thick or clear spit: *(DACH, YXRM) zhongfu* (LU-1).

Cough, counterflow expectoration, sudden pains: *(DACH) kunlun* (BL-60).

Coughs and spits mucus: *(DACH IV, 7v, yang) feishu* (BL-13), moxa.

Cough, spit, counterflow of energy: *(DACH) dazhong* (KI-6, IS KI-4).

Coughs mucus: *(JM) shuaigu* (GB-8).

Coughing fits, mucus and saliva: *(DACH, YXRM) fubai* (GB-16, IS GB-10).

White spit like paste: *(DACH) zigong* (CV-19) and *shaoze* (SI-1).

Mucus:

> (Respiratory mucus, *tan;* stomach mucus, *yin*).

> *Thick **tan** mucus which blocks the vessels is expelled through the lungs and spit out. When it blocks the spleen-pancreas, the saliva flows from the corners of the mouth. **Yin** liquid mucus produced in the stomach is expelled through the esophagus. (YXRM V, 6r)*

> *Mucus which accumulates in the lungs is secreted by them and comes out from the mucosa of the internal surface of the respiratory tract and larynx. In the past it was said that mental illnesses **(feng dian, kuang xian)** were illnesses from mucus. (Ci Yuan, "Tan")*

> *It is not sufficiently understood that much of the mucus is produced in the spleen-pancreas (the mononuclear leukocytes are indeed produced by the spleen, the polynuclear leukocytes coming from the bone marrow).*

> *Mucus is divided into old or new, from external or internal causes. The newer type is mild, of a white or bluish color, tasteless. The energy is diminished, thinned. The old type is serious, knotted like paste or porridge. It is thick, yellow and difficult to expel. Little by little it forms a bad acidic or astringent taste, salty or bitter.*

> *Illnesses with mucus which start with headaches and fever attacks have an external origin. What remains with coughing fits and nighttime aggravations have an internal cause, a fire from the yin.*

> *Mucus from humidity causes exhaustion of the four limbs, laziness, pain in the abdomen with swelling, diarrhea. The alimentary mucus causes an accumulation of food, thickening of the blood and even congestions of the spleen. Mucus from fire remains in the stomach with vomiting, acid belching, agitation rising in assault, head and face hot. The mucus from alcohol, when drinking wine, gives dry eructations, belching, pain of the sides and arms. The mucus of dryness rises to the lungs with dry hair, bluish face, dry pharynx, dry mouth, cough, oppressed panting. Mucus from energy remains a long time; it causes a lot of mucus in old people. Moreover, mucus obstructs the pharynx and diaphragm from the seven feelings. There is fullness of the spleen **(pi man)**, of the sides and chest. The mucus from heat causes panic in the heart, great anxiety, depression and hyperexcitation, dreams of peculiar or marvelous beings. The mucus from wind (shock) causes movements of the liver, a lot of vertigo, headaches, eyes fixed or with troubled or rough movement; pruritis of the ear lobe, painful swelling of the sides and ribs; hemiplegia on the right or left, anesthesia; legs collapsing, limping or extraordinary symptoms. The mucus from cold or emptiness accumulates in the kidneys; a lot of acidity, weakness of knees and feet, lumbar area, back stiff and painful. Articulations cold or with paresis, pain of the bones. . . . In all cases one must first conquer and expel the mucus, then harmonize the remainder. (YXRM V, 5v)*

In order to reactivate the leukocytes; tonify *dadun* (SP-2) on the right and *xuanzhong* (GB-39).

In order to puncture for mucus: *(YIX I, 3v) zhongwan* (CV-12) and leg-*sanli* (ST-36).

Energy from mucus: *(DACH, YXRM) shaochong* (HT-9).

Abundance of mucus, spits saliva: *(DACH) shangwan* (CV-13).

Mucus, saliva crowding and obstructing: *(YXRM I, 38r) zhaohai* (KI-3, IS KI-6).

Overflowing of mucus: *(YXRM) jinggu* (BL-64).

Mucus from shock, internal headaches: *(YIZ, 38) fenglong* (ST-40).

Mucus and saliva often welling upward: *(DACH) lieque* (LU-7).

Running flow from the three *(DACH)* or five *(YXRM)* doors: *pohu* (BL-37, IS BL-42).

Obstruction from mucus, accumulation of energy: *(DACH) burong* (ST-19).

Illnesses with mucus: *(DACH) gaohuangshu* (BL-38, IS BL-43), which increases the red cells and leukocytes.

Mucus, panting: *(DACH) tiantu* (CV-22).

All the mucus in the middle and lower body: *(DACH) yinlingquan* (SP-9)

Mucus oppressing the chest and diaphragm: *(DACH) gongsun* (SP-4).

Mucus after drinking: *(DACH) sanyinjiao* (SP-6).

Mucus with fire, pain of the heart and chest: *neiguan* (PC-6).

Fullness of mucus like paste in the mouth: *(DACH) taixi* (KI-5, IS KI-3).

Vomits and expectorates cold mucus: *(YXRM) yutang* (CV-18).

All mucus from energy, energy of cold: *(DACH X, 25v) qihai* (CV-6).

Tan yin:

> *Name of the illness: knotted mucus inside the interior of the bronchus so that inhalation and exhalation are not easy. There are several types:* **tan yin** *with energy abolished,* **feng tan** *with panicky melancholia. In the past it was said that there were five yin. . . . (Ci Yuan, "Tan-yin")*

> **Tan yin:** *the water stops in the intestines, stomach or abdomen and makes a noise, "luo luo"; sometimes causes thinness, sometimes fatness. (YXRM V, 6r)*

IX. Hemoptysis
Ke Xue, "Coughing Blood";
Sou Tan Dai Xue, "Cough and Mucus with Blood."

Cough and mucus with threads of blood depend on the spleen-pancreas. When the cough depends on the lungs, there is difficulty in swallowing. Blood which comes after the spit comes from the kidneys. (YXRM I, 3v)

Coughing red mucus if it remains for a long time is a sign of pulmonary tuberculosis. It comes from desires and energy in excess; spleen-pancreas and kidneys are injured. The fire rises and injures the liver. The blood is no longer normal and forms mucus which penetrates the lungs. Tonify: **bailao** *(GV-13, IS GV-14* **dazhui**) *feishu (BL-13),* **zhongwan** *(CV-12), leg-***sanli** *(ST-36); if not better,* **feishu** *(BL-13),* **shenshu** *(BL-23),* **rugen** *(ST-18). (DACH XI, 7; YIX I, 5r)*

Coughing blood: *(DACH X, 24r) lieque* (LU-7), arm-*sanli* (LI-10), *bailao* (GV-13, IS GV-14 *dazhui*), *fengmen* (BL-12), *feishu* (BL-13), *rugen* (ST-18).

Unequalled for relieving expectoration of blood: *(YXRM I, 40r) chize* (LU-5).

Coughs and spits blood: *(YXRM) taiyuan* (LU-9); *(DACH) yongquan* (KI-1), *rangu* (KI-2), *dazhong* (KI-6, IS KI-4); *(DACH) jiuwei* (CV-15), *tianzongshu* (SI-15), *xinshu* (BL-15).

Blood in the bronchus: *(JM) taiyuan* (LU-9).

Accumulation in the lungs, expectoration of blood: *(YXRM) juque* (CV-14).

Spits blood: *(YXRM) taixi* (KI-5, IS KI-3).

Spits blood, stops the panting: *(DACH III, 32r)* tonify *chize* (LU-5).

Spits blood, breathes with the shoulders: *(DACH) chengman* (ST-20).

Spits blood, expectorates blood: *(YXRM) tianshu* (ST-25).

Internal exhaustion, spits blood: *(DACH) diwuhui* (GB-42).

Panting, cough, mucosa bleeding: *(YXRM) rangu* (KI-2), *taiyuan* (LU-9).

Numerous expectorations of blood which are not being cured: *(DACH) qichong* (ST-30).

Expectorates blood: *(DACH)* arm-*wuli* (LI-13), *ganshu* (BL-18).

Coughs blood: *(JM, DACH, YXRM) kongzui* (LU-6), *feishu* (BL-13).

Spit is red, blood weak, coughs mucus: *(YIX I, 11v) lieque* (LU-7).

Tuberculosis, coughs and spits blood: *(GSdeM) chize* (LU-5), tonify. Expectorates blood from tuberculosis, emptiness: *(YXRM, DACH) shangwan* (CV-13).

Expectorations of blood from a broken heart, accumulation of blood in the chest: *(DACH) jugu* (LI-16) from 4 *fen* to 1.5 *cun*.

X. Abscesses of the Lungs *(Fei Yong)*:

Abscess of the lungs: *(YXRM I, 46v, JM) feishu* (BL-13), *shanzhong* (CV-17).

Abscess of the lung, spits pus and blood: *(YXRM) tiantu* (CV-22).

Abscess of the lung, fever, cough, panting: *(DACH I, 15v) quepen* (ST-12).

Coughs and spits pus: *(DACH, YXRM) tianjing* (TW-10); *(DACH) zhourong* (SP-20).

Spits pus and blood, saliva turbid: *(DACH) kufang* (ST-14).

Cough, panting, spits saliva, pus and blood: *(DACH) wuyi* (ST-15).

Cough, abscess of the lungs, comes from internal or external chills not dissipating; coughs without stopping and spits pus and blood; this is a lung abscess: *(DACH XI, 7r; YIX I, 5v) feishu* (BL-13), *fengmen* (BL-12), *zhigou* (TW-6), *daling* (PC-7), *shanzhong* (CV-17), arm-*sanli* (LI-10).

XI. Pulmonary Congestion[1]
Fei Chong Xue, "Abundant Blood in the Lungs"; *Fei Feng*, "Shock of the Lungs."

In the beginning, generally without fever, chest full: disperse: *(GSdeM) lieque* (LU-5) and *taiyuan* (LU-9); if insufficient, add *chize* (LU-5) and even *sanjian* (LI-3) and most of all *feishu* (BL-13).

Pulmonary congestion *(fei chong xue): (JM) xiaxi* (GB-43), *qiuxu* (GB-40), *yufu* (KI-27), *yuzhong* (KI-26), *shencang* (KI-25), *zigong* (CV-19), *kufang* (ST-14), *yingchuang* (ST-16), *yunmen* (LU-2), *xiongxiang* (SP-19), *shidou* (SP-17); *(GSdeM) jueyinshu* (BL-14).

Pulmonary congestion *(fei feng): (YXRM, DACH III, 30v);* with acute pain of the brain *(YXRM);* with scarlet face, swelling of the face, eye troubles, stiff nape, nosebleeds that do not stop *(YXRM);* with apoplexy of the lungs *(fei chong feng): (YXRM I, 46r) fengchi* (GB-20).

Pulmonary congestion *(fei chong feng),* fullness of the chest when lying down: *(DACH) feishu* (BL-13).

Return of blood to the chest: *(DACH, YXRM) jugu* (LI-16).

Energy rising and attacking the chest: *(DACH)* leg-*sanli* (ST-36), leg-*shanglian* (ST-37, IS *shangjuxu*).

XII. Pleura, Pleurisy, Pleuritis
China: *Xie Tong*, "Pain of the Sides";
Japan: *Lei Mo Yan*, "Inflammation of the Membrane of the Lungs."

*This is inflammation of the pleura, **lei mo yan**. Respiration is difficult, pain of the sides, intercostal neuralgia, moderate fever, cough, occasional fits of suffocation, white mucus. (Ci Yuan, "Xie-tong")*

Pleura *(lei mo): (JM) feishu* (BL-13), *geshu* (BL-17).

Pleurisy: *(JM) wenliu* (LI-7), *shaohai* (HT-3), *chize* (LU-5), *erjian* (LI-2), hand-*wangu* (SI-4), *zhigou* (TW-6), *quchi* (LI-11), *gongsun* (SP-4), *taixi* (KI-5, IS KI-3), foot-*qiaoyin* (GB-44), *qiuxu* (GB-40), *yanglingquan* (GB-34), *yinlingquan* (SP-9), *xuanzhong* (GB-39), *waiqiu* (GB-36), *shufu* (KI-27), *yuzhong* (KI-26), *shencang* (KI-25), *lingxu* (KI-24), *shenfeng* (KI-23), *bulang* (KI-22), *quepen* (ST-12), *qihu* (ST-13), *wuyi* (ST-15), *yingchuang* (ST-16), thorax-*qimen* (LR-14), *shidou* (SP-17), *feishu* (BL-13), *fengmen* (BL-12), *geshu* (BL-17), *danshu* (BL-19), *hunmen* (BL-42, IS BL-47), *yishe* (BL-44, IS BL-49), *fenglong* (ST-40), thigh-*wuli* (LR-10), *huagai* (CV-20), *zigong* (CV-19), *yutang* (CV-18).

Pleurisy *(xie tong):* left for right, right for left: *(YIZ, 42r) xuanzhong* (GB-39), foot-*qiaoyin* (GB-44), *waiguan* (TW-5), arm-*sanli* (LI-10).

Pleurisy: *(YIZ, 41v) yanglingquan* (GB-34), *qimen* (LR-14).

Pleurisy from chills: *(YIZ, 42v) zhigou* (TW-6), *yanglingquan* (GB-34).

Pleurisy, energy of malcontentment: *(YIZ, 42v) xingjian* (LR-2).

Pleurisy, coughing fits, cannot breathe: *(DACH)* foot-*qiaoyin* (GB-44).

Pleurisy, pain of the chest: *(YIZ, 42r) qimen* (LR-14), *zhigou* (TW-6), *danshu* (BL-19), 5 *fen* under the skin.

Pleurisy, pain of the lumbar area: *(YIZ, 42v) huantiao* (GB-29, IS GB-30), *zhiyin* (BL-67), *taibai* (SP-3), *yangfu* (GB-38).

(JM, 318) With needles — *zhongfeng* (LR-4), *wuyi* (ST-15), *zhongting* (CV-16), *qimen* (LR-14), *zhangmen* (LR-13), *feishu* (BL-13), *ganshu* (BL-18), *danshu* (BL-19), *hunmen* (BL-42, IS BL-47), *weishu* (BL-21), *sanjiaoshu* (BL-22). With moxa — *sanshu* (BL-18) and *danshu* (BL-19), 15 moxas each.

Pleuritis *(lei mo shen jing tong),* "neuralgia of the pleura" or pleurodynia, rheumatism of the muscles of the rib cage): *(JM) shufu* (KI-27), *yuzhong* (KI-26), *shencang* (KI-25).

Pleurisy, pain of the chest: *(JM) yangjiao* (GB-35).

XIII. Pneumonia
Fei Zang Yan: "Inflammation of the Lung-Organ"; *Fei Yan*

Due to a pneumococcus, thus contagious. First, a stitch in the side, stiffness, shivering, then dyspnea and rust-colored sputum, rattling rales, fever suddenly drops on the fifth day. It comes in overworked and alcoholic people; benign except for alcoholics.

We cannot always know the origin. It comes from inflammation of the small bronchioles which are hair-thin. This is why it is also called bronchial inflammation of the lungs. It follows smallpox, whooping cough, typhoid, epidemic flu, also follows bronchitis. There are also some pneumonias caused by foreign objects which come when breathing in, etc. Mostly children and old people are attacked.

Symptoms: inflammation of the capillary bronchioles which open with difficulty, high fever with sudden rises and drops; cough; rusty mucus; pains of the chest; oppressed and difficult respiration. On auscultation the top has a noise like a drum which becomes dull as we move downwards and while listening there is at the top the sounds of small bubbles of water which can be distinguished from the bronchiole noise.

Treatment with moxa:

fengmen (BL-12)	*20 moxas,*
feishu (BL-13)	*20 moxas,*
jueyinshu (BL-14).....................	*20 moxas,*
gaohuangshu (BL-38, IS BL-43)	*20 moxas,*
arm-wuli (LI-13)	*5 moxas. (JO, 5)*

Inflammation of the body of the lungs. At the beginning the patient has a bad cold, shivering, fever, fatigue with no joy, frequent cough, expectoration with bloody or rusty threads; weak and discontinuous voice. It can be transmitted by contagion. (Ci Yuan, "Fei-yan")

(YXRM V, 7) Fei yan: it is cured like all mucus — *lieque* (LU-7), *taiyuan* (LU-9), *chize* (LU-5), *feishu* (BL-13). Catarrh of the point of the lungs: *(JM) wenliu* (LI-7), *jianjing* (GB-21), *fufen* (BL-36, IS BL-41).
Pneumonia: *(JM)* arm-*wuli* (LI-13), *qiuxu* (GB-40), *fengmen* (BL-12), *feishu* (BL-13), *jueyinshu* (BL-14), *pohu* (BL-37, IS BL-42), *qihu* (ST-13), *tianxi* (SP-18), *qimen* (LR-14), *dabao* (SP-21), *shidou* (SP-17).
Pneumonia of a catarrhal type: *(JM) dabao* (SP-21), *tianxi* (SP-18).
Purulent pneumonia: *(JM) shidou* (SP-17).

XIV. Asthma, Panting, Dyspnea, Breathlessness
(China: *Xiao Chuan*; Japan: *Chuan Xi*)

In order to understand and use the Chinese treatments for asthma it is necessary to clarify the European understanding of this problem and its causes. First of all, it is advisable to restrict this expression to its proper significance and to separate the analogous, but different, problems, such as breathlessness (or dyspnea from effort) from going up stairs, from walking quickly up a hill, etc., breathlessness which is caused by weakness of muscles of the heart, and weakness caused by a long illness or physical or intellectual work or emotions.

This breathlessness can be easily and quickly cured by tonifying *shaoshang* (HT-9) in proportion to the illness. We must separate out also panting, which keeps bronchitis patients from breathing after meals, temporary congestion because of digestion and which adds to the congestion of the illness. In these cases great improvement is obtained by tonification of *gongsun* (SP-4), which prevents all swellings of the stomach, aerogastria, etc., treating at the same time the illness itself by dispersing *chize* (LU-5), *feishu* (BL-13), *sanjian* (LI-3) or *wenliu* (LI-7).

It is accepted that true asthma has (besides attacks of temporary or continuous suffocation at certain times or without any particular time) a characteristic whistling observed on auscultation and the expectoration of special sputum resembling grains of tapioca. It has been observed through the diagnosis of the Chinese that all asthmatic people suffer from an old insufficiency of the liver. There have been migraines, eczema, pruritis, distaste of chocolate, eggs and fats, etc. This would be the cause of the chemical trouble observed in Europe (toxemia, uremia, excess carbon dioxide), an insufficiency of the liver causing a defective function of the kidneys. The Chinese add: linked to a marked insufficiency of the spleen. This insufficiency of the liver, spleen and kidneys can be corrected and cured by tonifying *ququan* (LR-8) and *sanyinjiao* (SP-6), which acts on the spleen, liver and kidneys. Among the most effective Chinese points against asthma, we find kidney points *shufu* (KI-27) and *yuzhong* (KI-26).

In these patients, Europeans additionally recognize as a cause an excess of the parasympathetic system which inhibits the smooth muscles of the bronchus, the motor muscles, the glottis (through the inferior laryngeal nerve, efferent motor passage), the larynx (through the superior laryngeal nerve, sensory afferent passage). During the asthma attacks, there are spasms of the smooth bronchiole fibers from which comes retention of air in the alveoli; difficult exhalation; distention. The parasympathetic is commanded by *tianzhu* (BL-10), which is dispersed. Tonify the sympathetic nerves in opposition through *fengchi* (GB-20) until the oculocardiac reflex no longer slows the heart. The phrenic nerve is commanded by the C3-C4, C4-C5 intervals.

In the somewhat complicated terminology of the old Chinese texts it is possible to rediscover analogous notions. Asthma is properly called *xiao chuan* "whistling contractions." The contraction *(chuan)* is in fact the dyspnea, the suffocation. The *xiao* is asthma with special mucus. The Japanese use for asthma and dyspnea the word *chuan xi*, "panting respiration."

*In **chuan** inhalation and exhalation are oppressed and contracted, but we must know that if an illness has been present for a long time, the respiration is short. This resembles **chuan** without being it. Such are people with tuberculosis after a walk, people who become hot after food, people loaded with mucus, those who cough, spit or vomit. In **xiao** there is noise in the larynx (and bronchus). This is **chuan** with mucus of a serious type and through attack. (YXRM V, 22v)*

For both of these we must distinguish fullness from emptiness:

*For **chuan**, one distinguishes whether there is fullness of the lungs: then the energy is accumulated in the chest, the body is hot, the feces are hard. If there is emptiness in the lungs, then the energy is tired, the body is cool or cold; mucus is like water. For **xiao**, either there is fullness and one spits mucus, or there is emptiness and one does not spit. (YXRM V, 22v)*

Tonifying or dispersing incorrectly will lead to failure.

Remember this advice for mucus:

We do not know with certainty that much of the mucus comes from the spleen-pancreas. Lasting mucus provokes coughing fits and aggravation at night and arises from troubles of an internal origin, the fire of the yin. (YXRM V, 5v)

For dyspnea without mucus, if there is fullness (or with water-like mucus if there is emptiness) the following distinctions are indicated:

*For **chuan** (dyspnea from fullness):*

1) If there is fire and inflammation, it comes from the lungs and stomach. It comes suddenly and leaves in the same way. Food increases the inflammation and panting (dyspnea of food?).

2) If the energy has been compressed by the seven internal emotions, there is no noise. Fear, sadness, anger, or worries make the respiration compressed without mucus or noise (neuropathic dyspnea?).

3) If an external stimulation has caused the attack, it is because wind and cold cause swelling of the lungs, counterflow and panting. If there is swelling from water, the swelling of the lungs and dyspnea will always generate each other. But if the dyspnea is caused by the lungs, the swelling comes later, while if there is first swelling, then panting, it is the spleen-pancreas which causes swelling from water. However, the origin is always anuria (edema of the lungs?). (YXRM V, 5v)

*For **chuan** from emptiness:*

1) If there is emptiness of yin, there is emptiness of blood. The yang does not know where to place itself and rises (anemia, exhaustion and nervous congestion?). There are dyspneas which come from a violent rising, from inflammation of the lower abdomen (hysterical dyspnea?).

2) If there is cold of the kidneys, energy and respiration cannot be brought together. There is panting; attacks of panting at night come from an evil energy of the kidneys troubling the lungs (toxemia, uremia?).

3) If there is emptiness of the stomach in the extreme, there is sudden rising of the energy and panting.

4) If there is panting with fear of falling (vertigo), the evil energy of the liver troubles the spleen-pancreas.

5) If the perversity has troubled the six workshop organs, the body is hot; one cannot lie down. (YXRM 5, 5v)

*For all forms of asthma (**xiao chuan**), one must avoid astringent drugs; do not create cold, but bring the energy outside. Eat only slightly strong flavors. One must purify the lungs and rectify the energy. (YXRM 5, 22v)*

*Bronchial asthma, respiration panting (**chuan xi**) of the bronchus. Origin: in this illness, the difficulty in breathing is often hereditary, coming from illnesses or troubles of the nose, ears, stomach, intestines, heart, kidneys, uterus, etc. Moreover, perfumes, intoxication, emotions and shocks to the vitality cause attacks. Symptoms: when there is an attack, the respiration becomes difficult with the sound of a flute; there is also groaning, the chest is oppressed, the pulse accelerates, the physiognomy shows fear. (YXRM V, 22v)*

Treatment with needles:

***youmen** (KI-21)*	*8 fen,*
***shangwan** (CV-13)*	*8 fen,*
***juque** (CV-14)*	*6 fen,*
***zhongwan** (CV-12)*	*8 fen,*
***tiantu** (CV-22)*	*6 fen,*
***geshu** (BL-17)*	*4 fen. (JO, 4)*

Treatment with moxa:

tiantu (CV-22)	7 moxas,	
zhongfu (LU-1)	7 moxas,	
geshu (BL-17)	20 moxas. (JO, 4)	

Asthma **(chuan xi)** *for respiratory passages and heart:* **fufen** *(BL-36, IS BL-41),* **pohu** *(BL-37, IS BL-42),* **shentang** *(BL-39, IS BL-44),* **gaohuangshu** *(BL-38, IS BL-43),* **yixi** *(BL-40, BL-45),* **dazhu** *(BL-11),* **fengmen** *(BL-12),* **feishu** *(BL-13),* **jueyinshu** *(BL-14),* **xinshu** *(BL-15), all 5 to 8* **fen.** *For the parasympathetic and sympathetic systems:* **tianzhu** *(BL-10),* **fengchi** *(GB-20),* **wangu** *(GB-17, IS GB-12), all 5 fen or ten moxas. In addition, for the small and large intestines:* **xiaohai** *(LI-8), five moxas;* **hegu** *(LI-4), seven moxas. (JM, 318)*

In Europe, the best results have been obtained through taking account of fullness (disperse) or emptiness (tonify) with the following points:

1) For the respiratory passages themselves: *feishu* (BL-13), *jueyinshu* (BL-14); and if there is irritation of the rhinopharynx with mucus flowing into the bronchus at night, *fengmen* (BL-12) and *hegu* (LI-4).

2) For the heart, *shaochong* (HT-9) gives better results in cases of emptiness, *xinshu* (BL-15) in the case of fullness.

3) For the parasympathetic system, *tianzhu* (BL-10), C3-C4 and C4-C5 intervals, disperse. For the sympathetic system, *fengchi* (GB-20), tonify.

4) In order to harmonize the energy, *shanzhong* (CV-17), tonify or disperse according to the energy, and tonify *zhongzhu* (TW-3) if there is depression, or disperse *tianjing* (TW-10) if there is nervous hyperexcitation.

Asthma and dyspnea are the external manifestations of internal poisoning of any one or several of the internal organs. Each of the meridians has several points which are able to act on the problem of the organ which causes the asthma. The list is long; for greater clarity, I have classified them according to analogous symptoms.

Hong chuan, "groaning-panting:"

(DACH IV, 7r) Groaning, panting, cough and abundant mucus: *shufu* (KI-27), *rugen* (ST-18) and if the panting comes from bronchitis *(feng tan)* which has reduced little by little without going away: thorax-*qimen* (LR-14), first tonify, then disperse. If the energy of panting suddenly attacks the chest and diaphragm, disperse leg-*sanli* (ST-36) and *fenglong* (ST-40).

(DACH VII, 33r) Panting, groaning, fullness of the breath, swollen lungs, cannot sleep: *lieque* (LU-7), *taiyuan* (LU-9), *shufu* (KI-27), *shanzhong* (CV-17), *zhongfu* (LU-1), *fengmen* (BL-12), leg-*sanli* (ST-36).

Tan chuan "mucus-panting" (phlegm? catarrh of old people? chronic bronchitis?):

Mucus accumulated in the bronchi; inhalation and exhalation are not easy. The patient gets to the point of "panting-respiration" **(chuan xi),** *heart jumping, attacks of perspiration, extraordinary oppressive melancholia. It frequently attacks old people who smoke and drink. . . . In* **tan xuan,** *there is always a noise of the mucus like that of ducks eating. (Ci Yuan, "Tan-chuan")*

Panting-mucus: *(DACH II, 32r) tiantu* (CV-22).
Panting-mucus: emptiness of energy or emptiness of yin: *(DACH X, 35) tianfu* (LU-3), *zhongfu* (LU-1), *huagai* (CV-20), *feishu* (BL-13), *yinmen* (BL-51, IS BL-37).

Xiao "whistling":

Whistling **(xiao),** *rumbling* **(hong),** *cough* **(hou),** *panting* **(chuan).** *It comes from hot drinks or spicy food, from fish, from acids. This has its own variety of evil shock: bronchitis* **(tan yin)** *spreading into the lungs, or unhappiness which injures the liver; just after this unhappiness the food is not digested; or from coitus after endless drinking. This illness has many varieties:*

1) **Shui xiao yin** *"water-mucus-whistling," which appears with water.*

2) **Qi xiao** *"whistling from energy," which is caused by unhappiness, with abundant mucus.*

3) **Yan xiao** *"whistling-from-salt" which comes from eating cured meat or dried foods.*

First, **shufu** *(KI-27),* **tiantu** *(CV-22),* **zhongwan** *(CV-12),* **feishu** *(BL-13), leg-***sanli** *(ST-36). Then,* **gaohuangshu** *(BL-38, IS BL-43),* **rugen** *(ST-18),* **qihai** *(CV-6),* **guanyuan** *(CV-4). (YIX I, 5v; DACH XI, 7v)*

Asthma in general (*xiao chuan;* Japanese, *chuan xi*):

With panting: *(YXRM I, 46v)* leg-*sanli* (ST-36); *(JM) chize* (LU-5); *(YXRM I, 46) shanzhong* (CV-17); *(JM)* cannot eat: *yuzhong* (KI-26); has internal fullness: *(YXRM) fubai* (GB-16, IS GB-10).

Energy rising and attacking the chest: *(YXRM)* leg-*shanglian* (ST-37, IS *shangjuxu*).

Energy knotted, panting: *(DACH) zhongji* (CV-3).

Energy knotted to the point of being subdued: *zhongwan* (CV-12).

Attacks of panting; energy at the top: *huagai* (CV-20).

Attacks of panting: *(DACH) kunlun* (BL-60).

Great panting; can neither extend nor sit: thorax-*qimen* (LR-14).

Panting *(chuan)* in general: *qize* (LU-5), arm-*shanglian* (LI-9), *jingqu* (LU-8), *diji* (SP-8), *yangjiao* (GB-35), *taixi* (KI-5, IS KI-3), *qimen* (LR-14), *burong* (ST-19), *jiuwei* (CV-15), *xuanji* (CV-21), *jianzhong* (SI-15), *zhongting* (CV-16), *chengling* (GB-14, IS GB-18).

Nocturnal attacks of asthma or panting:

Asthma, cannot rest, short breath on inhalation and exhalation: *(DACH) shuitu* (ST-10).

Asthma very difficult to cure, cannot rest at night, energy contracted: *(DACH IV, 6v) tiantu* (CV-22), *shanzhong* (CV-17); *(YIX I, 5v)* moxa at the same points.

Asthma, attacks coming, cannot sleep: *(DACH IV, 11v; YIX I, 4v, Ju Ying) fenglong* (ST-40) 3 *fen.*

Panting; does not sleep; burning oppressiveness and worries day and night: *(DACH IV, 6v; YIX I, 5v) xuanji* (CV-21), *qihai* (CV-6) moxa.

Panting, cannot sleep: *yinlingquan* (SP-9).

Panting, cannot sleep: moxas at *lingtai* (GV-9, IS GV-10).

Panting, fullness, cannot rest peacefully: *(DACH) yinbai* (SP-1).

Energy short, fears resting, cannot sleep: *danshu* (BL-19).

Aggravation from food or drink:

Cough, panting after food: *geshu* (BL-17).

Panting, cough, cannot get the food to go down: *shanzhong* (CV-17).

Asthma, does not eat: *tianding* (LI-17), *chengman* (ST-20).

Asthma like a storm which prevents eating: *yongquan* (KI-1).

Panting, cannot eat: *yuzhong* (KI-26).

Pharynx spreading the asthma: neck-*futu* (LI-18).

Drinks, then pants: *yongquan* (KI-1).

Aggravation from cold:

In cold, panting, cannot breathe: *(DACH) taiyuan* (LU-9).

Asthma from cold or humidity: *hegu* (LI-4), *taiyuan* (LU-9).

Little energy (breath) in cold; heat in the palms: *(DACH) jianshi* (PC-5).

Aggravation on movement:

Asthma, cannot lift the arms: *bulang* (KI-22).

Asthma, cannot walk: *(DACH)* arm-*xialian* (LI-8).

Asthma, cannot walk, cannot remain standing for long: *(DACH)* leg-*shanglian* (ST-37, IS *shangjuxu*).

Panting, cannot walk: foot-*linqi* (GB-41).

Asthma with mucus (fullness, disperse):

Panting, mucus from shock, accumulating little by little; first tonify, then disperse: *(DACH) IV, 7r)* thorax-*qimen* (LR-14).

Mucus, panting: *(DACH III, 32r) tiantu* (CV-22).

Asthma, mucus, vomiting, vertigo: *(YXRM I, 46r) fenglong* (ST-40).

Energy from asthma, there is noise: *(DACH) qihu* (ST-13).

Cannot loosen the mucus: *(GSdeM) zigong* (CV-19), *shaoze* (SI-1), *taixi* (KI-5, IS KI-3).

Asthma and panting with cough:

Fits of coughing, panting: *(DACH) shaoshang* (LU-11), *pohu* (BL-37, IS BL-42), *huagai* (CV-20), *yunmen* (LU-2).

Fits of coughing, energy from panting, pain in back and chest: *(DACH) fengmen* (BL-12); *(YXRM) burong* (ST-19).

Asthma with fever:

Asthma with fever: *(DACH) shenmen* (HT-7); *(YXRM) shendao* (GV-10 IS GV-11).

Asthma from hay:

(GSdeM) Tonify the liver, which is always deficient: *ququan* (LR-8) and *taichong* (LR-3), disperse *feishu* (BL-13), *fengmen* (BL-12), *jueyinshu* (BL-14), *hegu* (LI-4).

Asthma with swollen legs:

(DACH I, 7r) Panting in counterflow from the lungs, cannot rest; below, swelling of the leg or abdomen; swelling from the kidneys; energy of water remaining; this is the way of the kidneys: thigh-*futu* (ST-32).

(GSdeM) For asthma with swelling of the ankles and feet: tonify the heart at *shaochong* (HT-9), disperse the kidney at *rangu* (KI-2) and *taixi* (KI-5, IS KI-3), and 7 moxas daily at *yongquan* (KI-1).

Panting contracted, sounds in the larynx, cough: *(YXRM) dazhong* (KI-6, IS KI-4), secondary vessel from kidney to bladder.

(DACH VII, 34r) Panting from simple ascites of the abdomen: *zhaohai* (KI-3, IS KI-6), *xingjian* (LR-2), *sanyinjiao* (SP-6), leg-*sanli* (ST-36), *qihai* (CV-6), *shuifen* (CV-9), *shanzhong* (CV-17).

Asthma and panting from emptiness:

Panting from emptiness: *(DACH II, 26v)* leg-*sanli* (ST-36).

Asthma with prostration: *(DACH II, 26v)* foot-*linqi* (GB-41), *zhaohai* (KI-3, IS KI-6).

Asthma, cannot lift the arms: *(DACH) bulang* (KI-22).

Asthma and panting from fullness:

Asthma, fullness of chest, side and limbs: *(DACH) sanjian* (LI-3).

Asthma, uncontrolled breathing:

Inhalation and exhalation difficult, tiring: *(DACH) sanjian* (LI-3), *qiuxu* (GB-40), foot-*linqi* (GB-41), *fubai* (GB-16, IS GB-10).

Not enough energy for inhalation and exhalation: *(DACH) bulang* (KI-22).

Inhalation and exhalation occur without being able to draw a full breath: *(DACH) kufang* (ST-14).

Breath short, not enough energy for inhalation and exhalation: *(DACH) shuitu* (ST-10).

Panting at exhalation: *(DACH) ququan* (LR-8), *renying* (ST-9).

Panting, exhalation without energy: *(DACH) rangu* (KI-2).

Panting, breathes without result: *yingxiang* (LI-20), gum-*yinjiao* (GV-27, IS GV-28).

Panting contracted: *(YXRM I, 40r) lieque* (LU-7), leg-*sanli* (ST-36); *(YXRM) yinbai* (SP-1); *(DACH) lianquan* (CV-23), *qihu* (ST-13), *chengling* (GB-14, IS GB-18), *pishu* (BL-20), *yixi* (BL-40, IS BL-45), *suliao* (GV-24, IS GV-25).

Panting contracted, energy at the top: *huagai* (CV-20).

Panting contracted, swelling of the chest: *dazhong* (KI-6, IS KI-4), *quepen* (ST-12).

Panting contracted: *jingqu* (LU-8), neck-*futu* (LI-18), *shenzhu* (GV-11, IS GV-12).

Panting contracted, thinness: *xuanji* (CV-21).

Energy knotted, panting to the point where the energy is subdued: *(DACH X, 25r) zhongwan* (CV-12).

Energy from panting: *(YXRM) chize* (LU-5), *lingxu* (KI-24), *tianxi* (SP-18), *dabao* (SP-21).

Panting: *sanjian* (LI-3), foot-*linqi* (GB-41), *kunlun* (BL-60); *(DACH) qihai* (CV-6).

Attacks of panting from energy: *(DACH) tiantu* (CV-22).

Panting, swelling of the abdomen: *(DACH) tianshu* (ST-25).

Panting without taking in a breath:

Panting without result: *(DACH) yingxiang* (LI-20); *(DACH) tongtian* (BL-7), gum-*yinjiao* (GV-27, IS GV-28), *suliao* (GV-24, IS GV-25).

Asthma with no result: *(DACH) chengling* (GB-14, IS GB-18).

Respiration weak and insufficient:

Respiration weak, insufficiency of breathing: *(DACH) lieque* (LU-7), *shenmen* (HT-7), *dazhong* (KI-6, IS KI-4), *ligou* (LR-5), *kunlun* (BL-60).

Energy (respiration) short: thorax-*qimen* (LR-14), *jiuwei* (CV-15), *dabao* (SP-1), *shanzhong* (CV-17).

Little energy, speech difficult: *zhiyang* (GV-8, IS GV-9).

Shortness of energy, dizzying worries: *feishu* (BL-13), the same in all illnesses with little energy (breath).

Shortness of energy, fullness of chest: *yingchuang* (ST-16), *yuanye* (GB-22).

Little energy (breath): *chize* (LU-5), *ququan* (LR-8), *yongquan* (KI-1), *juque* (CV-14).

XV. Emphysema
Fei Zhang, "Swelling of the Lungs;" *Fei Qi Zhong* "Swelling of the Lung Energy."

*Also called **fei qi zhong**. It begins with swelling of the lobules of the lung: comes from irritation through catarrh of the bronchus; compressed breath in the patient; he coughs mucus containing bubbles. It is much aggravated by cold weather. Singers and orators are often affected. (Ci Yuan, "Fei-zhong")*

(GSdeM) quepen (ST-12) is painful in emphysema.

For Europeans, swelling of the lungs, panting, edema, can come from an insufficiency of the urine, or from the beginning of epithelial chronic nephritis (with enlarged white kidneys) with sudden edema of the face: moxas at *yongquan* (KI-1) and *taixi* (KI-5, IS KI-3).

Emphysema *(fei zhang): (DACH) feishu* (BL-13), *bailao* (GV-13, IS GV-14 *dazhui*).

Emphysema *(fei qi zhong): (JM) bailao* (GV-13, IS GV-14 *dazhui*), *jueyinshu* (BL-14), *zhongfu* (LU-1), *liuwei* (CV-15), *yindu* (KI-19).

Emphysema *(fei zhang):* rumbling, panting, fullness of energy, cannot sleep: *(DACH VII, 33r) lieque* (LU-7), *taiyuan* (LU-9), *fengmen* (BL-12), *shufu* (KI-27), *zhongfu* (LU-1), *shanzhong* (CV-17).

Swelling and ballooning of the lung: *(DACH) chize* (LU-5).

Swelling and ballooning of diaphragm and chest, energy short: *(DACH) X, 25r) hegu* (LI-4) arm-*sanli* (LI-10), thorax-*qimen* (LR-14), *rugen* (ST-18).

Lungs enlarged and swollen: *(DACH) taiyuan* (LU-9).

Energy in the chest full as if blocked: *(DACH) shanzhong* (CV-17).

XVI. Pulmonary Tuberculosis
Lao, Fei Lao, Fei Xie He, Chuan Shi, Lao Zhai; Children: *Gan*

The tuberculosis microbe seems to have been known from before the sixteenth century. In fact, the *Da Cheng* of 1578 *(XI, 14r, "gui yan")* says, "especially cures the tuberculosis insect *(lao chong),"* and the *Yi Xue Ru Men* of the sixteenth century *(V, 39r)* notes, "By sustaining, by rectifying, we remove the perversity, the microbes die." Since antiquity, the Chinese have possessed lenses of rock-crystal which were very powerful, and from which eyeglasses were also made.

Today we write **lao** *(with the radical for illness, exhaustion) for* **lao** *(exhaustion),* **fei lao** *or* **fei xie he**.
(Ci Yuan, "Fei-lao")

Illness-exhaustion: this is pulmonary tuberculosis **(fei xie he)**, *also called* **fei lao**. *The special confirmation is the bloody sputum which is coughed up; it contains tiny bacteria. When the sputum has dried, the bacteria fly up, spread and invade humans through the respiration. Then the lungs generate tubercles and show lesions. Of those who are attacked, many are not cured. The lungs of young people, being of a delicate nature, are easily affected.*
(Ci Yuan, "Lao")

Called this because it can be transmitted through contagion to people close to dead people; it is called "transmitted-from-cadaver" **chuan shi;** *this is pulmonary tuberculosis,* **fei lao bing**. *(Ci Yuan, "Chuan-shi")*

The **Sheng Jing** *says: the quality of old tuberculosis is: heat of the palms and soles of the feet, nocturnal sweats, tried and weakened strength, pains in the joints, cough in the beginning; later, expectoration of pus and blood; thinness; yellow face, lessening of appetite, little strength. (DACH XI, 15r)*

Lao zhai*: when lao is extreme, it is called* **zhai**. *One must first distinguish yin and yang:*

1)Tuberculosis with fever is a yang illness: mouth dry, abscess of tongue, pharynx painful; tears and sputum are thick; palms and soles of feet are painful; urine yellow-red; feces dry and knotted.

2)Tuberculosis from emptiness is a yin illness: mucus and white sputum, counterflow of the stomach, bad breath; digestion of food and drink are difficult; the urine is turbid and contains a lot of whitish deposits; great difficulty in bending backwards or in extending. However, there are illnesses which are both yin and yang at the same time.

Many cases come from the fact that from fifteen to sixteen years of age, when the blood and energy are not yet stable, the taste for alcohol ruins the sexual energy and blood.

Many of these cases which depend on the yin come from external causes. When there is a prolonged fever, prolonged cough, they depend on the yang. In tuberculosis with fever, if there is an abscess of the pharynx and loss of ability to make sound, these people die. In tuberculosis from emptiness (yin) if the diarrhea does not stop, there is death.

For yin and yang, the evolution and care are not the same.

Whether they are yin or yang, they can all be transformed and transmitted. . . .

Benign or serious cases are discerned from the sweat, the cough and the diarrhea. . . . If the legs are numb and the lumbar area seized up, it comes from the kidneys.

If one coughs blood with a lot of sweat, with emotional agitation and palpitation, and abscesses of the mouth and tongue, the perversity is in the heart.

When there is panting with coughing of blood, with the skin dry and the nose cold, the voice deep, the perversity is in the lungs.

When there are deposits with pain in the sides, great unhappiness, and ''kernels'' on the nape, the perversity is in the liver.

When there is diarrhea with pains in the abdomen, swelling of the spleen-pancreas, drink and food without flavor, and the four limbs are exhausted, the perversity is in the spleen-pancreas.

One must calm and harmonize according to the location of the evil. First, one must open or close the stomach.

For emptiness of yang, one should not in error use pungent cloves and other foods of the same type. For emptiness of yin, do not use bitter by mistake, or cold, or cypress, and others.

In order to open the gates of yang illness: purify the fever, give support to excretion; when urine becomes abundant, the illness goes away. In order to open the gates of the yin illness, cause the mucus to circulate and support the energy. When the energy is purified, and the mucus diminished, the illness is regressing. When the illness is old, we must always tonify; then the fire calms itself. . . .

By sustaining, by rectifying, we remove the evil; the microbes die **(chong wang)**. *In fact, the microbes develop in the accumulation of blood from the stoppage of the energy and the blood and in mucus as well. By tonifying and balancing energy and blood, we master them.*

In spite of what has been said about transmission from the cadaver, we should not consider this too deeply, but remember that tuberculosis often comes from alcoholism which has enriched the energy but damaged the heart and blood.

The ancients, when this illness multiplied, buried the utensils and objects of the dead people because they were convinced that the illness was transmitted through the air. They also said: of the thirty-six types of tuberculosis, only the virtue of yin can cure them; the patients either retired to the forest or the mountains or lived in a detached building, immobile and purifying their heart, burning perfume and cleaning their teeth; they took special food, avoiding their desires in order to cut the root of the illness. (YXRM V, 39r)

Before twenty years, it is called **gan,** *chancre; after twenty years, it is called* **lao.** *(YXRM VI, 19r)*

The five tuberculoses: those which attack one or the other of the five treasure organs.

General treatment.

In Europe, the best results have been obtained by tonifying *gaohuangshu* (BL-38, IS BL-43), which greatly increases the blood cells (gold needle, one time per month) and the tonification of leg-*sanli* (ST-36) every day in the morning with ten moxas, thus regulating the insufficient or excess organs and tonifying the triple warmer.

All tuberculoses: *(YIX, 2v) bailao* (GV-13, IS GV-14 *dazhui*).

Tuberculosis *(fei xie he): (JM) wenliu* (LI-7), *shaohai* (HT-3), *chize* (LU-5), *quze* (PC-3), *xiaohai* (SI-8), *zhongfu* (LU-1), *youmen* (LU-2), *qihu* (ST-13), *zigong* (CV-19), *bailao* (GV-13, IS GV-14 *dazhui*), *gaohuangshu* (BL-38, IS BL-43), *lingtai* (GV-9, IS GV-10), *naokong* (GB-19), *pohu* (BL-37, IS BL-42).

Tuberculosis *(chuan shi): (DACH III, 29r) gaohuangshu* (BL-38, IS BL-43), *feishu* (BL-13).

Tuberculosis *(lao): (DACH) gaohuangshu* (BL-38, IS BL-43); *(YXRM) feishu* (BL-13); *(DACH IV, 6r) yongquan* (KI-1).

The seven troubles of the five tuberculoses: *(DACH, YXRM) bailao* (GV-13, IS GV-14 *dazhui*); *(YXRM I, 47r)* moxa at *xinshu* (BL-15); *(YXRM, DACH) shenshu* (BL-23). The same with the six extremes: *(DACH, YXRM) zhongliao* (BL-33); *(DACH, YXRM) jianjing* (GB-21); *(DACH)* leg-*sanli* (ST-36).

The five tuberculoses, the four limbs weak and empty: *(DACH) zhizheng* (SI-7).

All tuberculoses: one moxa per year of age, plus one at twenty (21 moxas); *(DACH III, 27r) xinshu* (BL-15).

Types of tuberculosis.

Tuberculosis from shock *(feng lao):*
(DACH, YXRM) arm-*wuli* (LI-13), *zhouliao* (LI-12); the same symptoms, with heavy body *(YXRM) xuanzhong* (GB-39); *(DACH, YXRM)* thigh-*wuli* (LR-10), *bailao* (GV-13, IS GV-14 *dazhui*), *fengmen* (BL-12), *guanyuanshu* (BL-26), *pangguangshu* (BL-28).

Tuberculosis from shock, lung and arms without action: *(YXRM) fufen* (BL-36, IS BL-41).

Tuberculosis of children *(xia er gan chong,* ''microbes of tuberculosis of children''): *(JM) shaoshang* (LU-11), *shaoze* (SI-1), *guanchong* (TW-1), *laogong* (PC-8), hand-*wangu* (SI-4), *zhongchong* (PC-9), *qiangu* (SI-2), *yangxi* (LI-5), *xinhui* (GV-21, IS GV-22), *shenzhu* (GV-11, IS GV-12), *zhongshu* (GV-6a, IS GV-7), *wuyi* (ST-15), *shuifen* (CV-9), abdomen-*yinjiao* (CV-7).

Emptiness from tuberculosis: *(DACH II, 29v) gaohuangshu* (BL-38, IS BL-43).

Tuberculosis from emptiness, exhaustion from tuberculosis: *(DACH) pohu* (BL-37, IS BL-42).

Fever from tuberculosis: *(DACH) chize* (LU-5), *feishu* (BL-13); *(YXRM I, 46v) neiguan* (PC-6); and tuberculosis of bones: *danshu* (BL-19).

Cough from tuberculosis: *(DACH II, 25v);* and body hot: disperse *pohu* (BL-37, IS BL-42); *(DACH) dazhu* (BL-11). Thinness from tuberculosis, loss of strength; thinness from the five types of tuberculosis *(YXRM I, 40r);* thinness of the five types of tuberculosis, emptiness and fatigue from the seven troubles *(DACH III, 30v; Ju Ying; Hua Tuo in YXRM)*. Fullness, shape wasted from tuberculosis: *(DACH, Li Gao)* leg-*sanli* (ST-36).

Hemoptysis from tuberculosis: *(GSdeM) chize* (LU-5), tonify. Expectoration of blood from tuberculosis, emptiness: *(DACH, YXRM) shangwan* (CV-13). *Gaohuang* (BL-38, IS BL-43) is absolutely forbidden in all cases of hemoptysis because it causes bleeding (See IX: Hemoptysis).

Icterus from tuberculosis: *(DACH) shenshu* (BL-23).

Tuberculosis with inflamed lymph nodes: *(DACH XI, 10r, "luo li xie he") jianjing* (GB-21), *tianjing* (TW-10), *quchi* (LI-11), *sanyangluo* (TW-8), *yinlingquan* (SP-9).

First beginning (tuberculotic, and previously, lymphatic) adenitis, ganglia, frequent caries, pain in the mastoid process, pain without fixed place, thinness, weakness, shivering in the bath: *(DACH)* tonify foot-*linqi* (GB-41) (and daily moxa).

XVII. Pulmonary Plague (*Fei Shi*, "Flying Death")

Evil symptoms of flying death: *(DACH) tianfu* (LU-3); falls suddenly under a terrible evil influence from flying death: *(YXRM) tianfu* (LU-3); flying death running and following: *(DACH) weiyang* (BL-53, IS BL-39), *zhongfu* (LU-1).

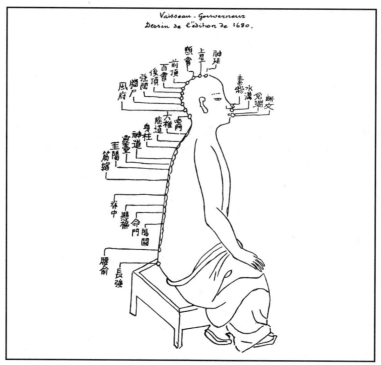

Governor vessel (DACH)

Notes

[1] Martinet (898, second edition): "The ancient idea of congestion of the chest described a thoracic inflammatory condition which includes the muscles (pleurodynia), the nerves (neuralgia), the pleura (pleurisy), the lung (pneumonia, inflammatory congestion). If the syndrome has disappeared from our texts, it has not stopped appearing in the clinic."

Chapter X

Circulatory System

I. Heart — II. Arteries, Veins — III. Blood

The circulatory system is commanded by two meridians: the heart, which will be described in this chapter, and the heart governor, which we must not forget although it has been described in the beginning of this book in the chapter on energy, and whose action is considerable on the arteries and veins as well as on the nervous commands which produce hyper- or hypotension. Moreover, the heart governor is represented by two pulses on the third segment of the right wrist. The middle level corresponds to the sexual life and genital organs. All assessment of circulation must begin with the evaluation of the two pulses of the heart governor immediately after assessing the pulses of the heart.

I. Heart

The pulse of the heart is at the first segment (near the thumb) on the left wrist at the deep level. Its normal quality must be ample, supple, regular at its location and with a rounded form when the hand is supinated. The left edge (radial side) represents the left heart and general circulation. The right edge of the artery corresponds to the right heart and the lesser pulmonary circulation. When the right edge is very weak, the left lung (and the left edge of the pulse of the lung) is without activity, insufficient (or both lungs may be).

The heart is a yin treasure organ, the coupled yang workshop organ of which is the small intestine. The flow of energy goes down the upper limb. It comes from the spleen-pancreas through the point *dabao* (SP-21) into the point *jiquan* (HT-1) and passes into the small intestine from the point *shaoshang* (HT-9) into the point *shaoze* (SI-1). The maximum energy is found in the heart from 11 a.m. to 1 p.m. It corresponds with the gallbladder (from 11 p.m to 1 a.m.).

The heart is the great master of all the organs. It is the home of consciousness, of sexual energy and of vitality. When this organ is firm and strong, illnesses do not enter easily. This is why all illnesses first come into the heart governor meridian. (DACH VIII, 16r)

The heart holds consciousness. (DACH VIII, 16r.)

In the past it was said that the heart governs thought and worries. Everything thought and worried was called the heart. (Ci Yuan, ''Xin'' [heart])

Joy injures the heart, slows down and disperses the energy [the antidote to joy is fear]. (YXRM)

The heart reigns (is at its maximum activity) during the summer. (DACH I, 10v)

Relations of organs:

Kidneys:

If the illness is transmitted from the kidney to the heart, danger. (DACH V, 20r)

Liver:

If the illness is transmitted from the liver to the heart, the intermediary organs (spleen-pancreas and kidney) live. In emptinesses of the heart, tonify the liver and gallbladder. (DACH V, 20r.)

Gallbladder:

The heart and the gallbladder are related. When anguish is the illness of the heart, it is advisable to tonify the gallbladder. When illness of the gallbladder causes derangement, depression or hyperexcitation, it is advisable to tonify the heart, which is the master (midday-midnight rule). (DACH V, 25r)

Small intestine:

If the heart is ill, also stimulate the points of the small intestine (according to the flow of energy). (DACH I, 24v)

Spleen-pancreas:

If the heart is ill with fever, disperse the stomach and spleen-pancreas (according to the flow of energy). (DACH V, 25v)

In general.

Master point for illnesses of the heart (and assent point of the heart): *(JM) xinshu* (BL-15).
Heart: *(JM) feishu* (BL-13).
Illnesses of the heart: *(JM);* and troubles: *daling* (PC-7), *zhongchong* (PC-9). *(DACH II, 25v; III, 32v)* Illnesses of the heart and chest: *daling* (PC-7).
Illnesses of the heart: *(JM) xiaohai* (SI-8); *(JM) xiabai* (LU-4); *(JM) yunmen* (LU-2); *(JM) zhongfu* (LU-1). *(JM) jinggu* (BL-64); *(JM) shengfeng* (KI-23); *(JM) jueyinshu* (BL-14); *(JM) geshu* (BL-17); *(JM) shentang* (BL-39, IS BL-44), *chengguang* (BL-6).

Meridian of the heart (shou shaoyin).

Insufficiency of energy.

Pulse of the heart: abolished, or soft, small, without form, without amplitude or with emptiness or hesitation.
Physical symptoms: breathlessness on walking fast or when going up stairs, without strength, fears cold water, energy and blood unequal (right and left pulses different), urine clear.
Psychological symptoms: moral depression, attacks of sadness, anxiety, anguish, chagrin, sees the dark side of everything, dreams of mountains on fire, of smoke, of fire; false ideas, timidity, fear. (Children: immobility, fatigue, fear.)
Through the main meridian: tonify *shaochong* (HT-9) and the source point, *shenmen* (HT-7).
Through the herald point: tonify *juque* (CV-14).
Through the circulation of energy: tonify spleen-pancreas (the mother who nourishes) at foot-*dadu* (SP-2) and the small intestine (the child who suckles) at *houxi* (SI-3).
Through the coupled organ: tonify the small intestine at *houxi* (SI-3).
Through the passage point: *tongli* (HT-5).
Midday-midnight rule: heart, maximum from 11 a.m. to 1 p.m.; corresponds with the gallbladder, maximum from 11 p.m. to 1 a.m. Tonify the gallbladder on dark, cold days and at night.
Husband-wife rule: disperse the lung (wife) at *chize* (LU-5).
To facilitate the return circulation: tonify thigh-*futu* (ST-32) *(GSdeM).*

Insufficiency:
Prevents paralysis (rheumatism?) from the heart: *(JM) geshu* (BL-17).
Emptiness of the heart; unbearable pain in the heart: *(DACH II, 19r) yongquan* (KI-1).
Pulse slow (bradycardia): *(DACH) shaoshang* (LU-11); the same with pain in the heart: *(DACH) taibai* (SP-3).
Pulse slow: *(GSdeM) shaochong* (HT-9), *fengchi* (GB-20); *(DACH) shaoshang* (LU-11).

Arrhythmia:
(GSdeM) Tonify *shaochong* (HT-9), *neiguan* (PC-6), *zhongzhu* (TW-3), leg-*sanli* (ST-36).
Weakness and decline of the heart:

Treatment with needles:

feishu (BL-13)....	*1 cun,*
xinshu (BL-15)...	*1 cun,*
geshu (BL-17)	*1 cun,*
tianzhu (BL-10)..	*9 fen,*
fengchi (GB-20).	*9 fen,*
arm-*sanli (LI-10)*	*9 fen. (JM, 317)*

Treatment with moxa:

ganshu (BL-18)	*15 moxas,*
danshu (BL-19)	*15 moxas,*
pishu (BL-20)...	*15 moxas. (JM, 317)*

Excess of energy.

Pulse of the heart: ample, hard, big, distal, agitated, rapid.
Physical symptoms: either fever or red cheeks; mouth dry, palpitations, physical agitation. (Children: sobbing, calls, agitation of feet and hands, drinking water.)

Psychological symptoms: hyperexcitation, acts inappropriately, laughter or sobbing, delirium, dreams of audacity and of laughing at danger.

Through the main meridian: disperse *shenmen* (HT-7).

Assent point: *xinshu* (BL-15). Through the circulation of energy: disperse the spleen-pancreas (the mother who nourishes) at *shangqiu* (SP-5) and the small intestine (the child who suckles) at *xiaohai* (SI-8).

Through the passage point: tonify *zhizheng* (SI-7) or disperse *tongli* (HT-5).

Through the yang coupled organ: disperse the small intestine at *xiaohai* (SI-8).

Midday-midnight rule: heart, maximum from 11 a.m. to 1 p.m., corresponds with the gallbladder, maximum at 11 p.m. to 1 a.m. Disperse the gallbladder at *yangfu* (GB-38) during dark and cold days or at night.

Husband-wife rule: disperse the lung at *chize* (LU-5).

Accumulation in the heart *(fu liang)*: *(DACH) shenmen* (HT-7), *zhongwan* (CV-12).

Tachycardia: *(DACH)* disperse *shenmen* (HT-7). *(GSdeM)* Often symptomatic, between 90 and 120, of chronic nephritis or Bright's disease: *taixi* (KI-5, IS KI-3), *rangu* (KI-2), *yongquan* (KI-1).

Agitation of the heart *(xin fan)*, hyperexcited speech: *(DACH) gongsun* (SP-4).

Agitation of the heart: *(DACH)* foot-*qiaoyin* (GB-44), *guanchong* (TW-1), *daling* (PC-7), head-*wangu* (GB-17, IS GB-12).

Extreme agitation of the heart: *(DACH) shenmen* (HT-7).

Agitation of the heart, fullness below the heart: *(DACH, YXRM) shaoshang* (LU-11), *tianshu* (ST-25); and with anguish: *(DACH) yuji* (LU-10).

Palpitation of nervous origin: *(JM) shaochong* (HT-9), *shenmen* (HT-7), *yinxi* (HT-6), *tongli* (HT-5), *xiabai* (LU-4), *xingjian* (LR-2), *dazhong* (KI-6, IS KI-4), *shenting* (GV-23, IS GV-24), *burong* (ST-19) *shendao* (GV-10, IS GV-11), *naokong* (GB-19).

Heart suspended as if from hunger: *(DACH, YXRM) jianshi* (PC-5).

Rheumatism of the heart, prevents it: *(JM) geshu* (BL-17).

Rheumatism of the heart: *(DACH) yuji* (LU-10).

Heart enlarged and swollen (exists in chronic epithelial nephritis with enlarged white kidneys): *(JM) shaoze* (SI-1), *qiangu* (SI-2), *qucha* (BL-4), *taiyin* (ST-23), *huangshu* (KI-16), *jueyinshu* (BL-14), *xinshu* (BL-15), *geshu* (BL-17).

Swelling and ballooning of the heart, yellow complexion: *(DACH) zhongwan* (CV-12).

Swelling and fullness of the heart: *(DACH) danshu* (BL-19).

Swelling of the heart, pain in the pharynx: *(DACH III, 25v) taichong* (LR-3).

Women: blood disturbing the heart: *(DACH) gongsun* (SP-4).

Fever of the heart (palpitations, malaise, agitated, great desire for cold water): *(YXRM I, 39v) shenmen* (HT-7).

The five heats of the heart: *(DACH) yixi* (BL-40, IS BL-45).

Inflammation of the muscle of the heart (myocarditis): *(JM) neiguan* (PC-6), *jiuwei* (CV-15).

Inflammation of the heart: *(JM) zhongchong* (PC-9), *daling* (PC-7), *neiguan* (PC-6), *jianshi* (PC-5), *quze* (PC-3), *rangu* (KI-2), *yongquan* (KI-1), *jinggu* (BL-64), *gongsun* (SP-4), *jiuwei* (CV-15), *huangshu* (KI-16), *jiquan* (HT-1).

Inflammation of the internal and external membrane of the heart (endocarditis and pericarditis): *(JM) zhongchong* (PC-9), *feishu* (BL-13).

Inflammation of the internal membrane of the heart (endocarditis): *(JM) neiguan* (PC-6), *lingdao* (HT-4), jianshi (PC-5), *quze* (PC-3), *tianquan* (PC-2), *jiquan* (HT-1), foot-*linqi* (GB-41), *taixi* (KI-5, IS KI-3), *yunmen* (LU-2), *burong* (ST-19), *tianchi* (PC-1), *dabao* (SP-21), *xuanli* (GB-6), *feishu* (BL-13), *xinshu* (BL-15), *yixi* (BL-40, IS BL-45), *hunmen* (BL-42, IS BL-47), *yanggang* (BL-43, IS BL-48).

Inflammation of the external membrane of the heart (pericarditis): *(JM) zhongchong* (PC-9), *daling* (PC-7), *neiguan* (PC-6), *feishu* (BL-13), *jueyinshu* (BL-14).

Illnesses of the valves of the heart: *(JM) yuji* (LU-10), *xiabai* (LU-4); pericardium large and fat: *(JM) huangshu* (KI-16).

Pains of the heart.

Acute pain in the heart: *shaohai* (HT-3); *(DACH VII, 34v) neiguan* (PC-6); *(DACH) gongsun* (SP-4); *(DACH) xingjian* (LR-2); *(DACH) zhongwan* (CV-12).

Unbearable pain in the heart, emptiness of the heart: *(DACH II, 19v) yongquan* (KI-1).

Pain in the heart, cardiac neuralgia: *shenmen* (HT-7); *(YXRM) tianjing* (TW-10), *xiabai* (LU-4), *daling* (PC-7); *(JM) taixi* (KI-5, IS KI-3); *(DACH)* foot-*linqi* (GB-41), *dadun* (LR-1); *(JM) shanzhong* (CV-17); *(JM) jiuwei* (CV-15), *juque* (CV-14); *(DACH IV, 5r) shangwan* (CV-13).

Pain in the heart as if pierced by an awl to the heart and vessels; in serious cases, feet and hands are cold into the joints; if there is panting, death: *(DACH) taixi* (KI-5, IS KI-3).

Pain in the heart as if pierced by an awl: *(DACH, YXRM) rangu* (KI-2).

Pain piercing the heart, hands suddenly blue, counterflow of energy: *(YXRM) fenglong* (ST-40).

Pain in the heart, numbness of the shoulders and arms: *(YXRM) guanchong* (TW-1).

Sudden pain in the heart, palms hot, chest full, ballooned, hands contracted; pain in the arm, which can neither be extended nor flexed, swelling under the axilla, face red, yellow eyes, easy laughter: *(YIZ, 40) zhongchong* (PC-9).

Sudden pain in the heart: *(DACH, YXRM) jianshi* (PC-5); *(DACH) zhigou* (TW-6); *(DACH)* leg-*sanli* (ST-36); *(DACH III, 28r) xingjian* (LR-2); *(DACH, YXRM) qihai* (CV-6).

Sudden pains in the heart, fullness of chest, sides, limbs: right for left: *(DACH IV, 15v) yongquan* (KI-1).

Sudden pain in the heart, coma: *(DACH) juque* (CV-14).

Women; sudden pain in the heart: *(DACH III, 27r) xinshu* (BL-15).

Hot pain in the heart: *(YXRM I, 39r) laogong* (PC-8); *(YXRM) yongquan* (KI-1).

Pain in the heart, heat: *(YXRM) zhongwan* (CV-12).

Heat in the heart, agitation, thirst: *(DACH X, 25v) quze* (PC-3).

Cold pain in the heart: *(YXRM I, 39v)* tonify *shaoze* (SI-1).

Pain in the heart generating cold, can neither bend forward nor backward: *(DACH) zhongwan* (CV-12).

Pain in the heart, cold and heat: *(DACH) dushu* (BL-16).

Pain in the heart, short of energy: *(DACH) xiabai* (LU-4).

Pain in the heart, hands trembling: *(DACH II, 26v) shaohai* (HT-3).

Pain in the heart, fullness of the chest: *(YXRM)* foot-*linqi* (GB-41).

Pain in the heart, mouth dry, pain in both the shoulder and the back: *(DACH) burong* (ST-19).

Stabbing pain in both the heart and back: *(DACH) tiantu* (CV-22).

Acute pain in the vertebrae behind the heart: *(DACH IV, 15v) guanchong* (TW-1).

Pain in the interval between the vertebrae behind the heart: *(DACH III, 32r) zhongzhu* (TW-3).

Pain in the heart linked to the back: *(DACH) kunlun* (BL-60); and in the chest: *(DACH) hunmen* (BL-42, IS BL-47).

Pain in the heart; pain alternating between the back and the heart: *(YXRM) zhongwan* (CV-12).

Pain in the heart radiating to the chest and back: *(YXRM I, 47r) yinshu* (BL-15).

Pain in the heart and chest, mucus with fire: *(YXRM, 46v) weiguan* (PC-6).

Pain in the nerves of the heart and chest: *(JM) xialian* (LI-8).

Pain in the heart, chest, sides: *(YXRM I, 46r) geshu* (BL-17).

Fullness and pain in the heart and abdomen: *(YXRM) tinggong* (SI-19).

Pain in the heart, panting: *(DACH, YXRM) zhangmen* (LR-13).

Pain in the heart, dazzling: *(YXRM) jinggu* (BL-64).

Pain in the heart, multiple swellings: *(DACH, YXRM) juque* (CV-14).

Pain in the heart, swelling of the face and head: *(YXRM) gongsun* (SP-4).

Interior of the heart as if bound: *(DACH) yongquan* (KI-1).

Pain in the heart and liver: *(DACH) taichong* (LR-3); and complexion blue as if dead; cannot breathe all during the day: *(DACH) xingjian* (LR-2).

Pain in the heart and spleen-pancreas:

(DACH IV, 7r) Acute pain in the heart and pain in the spleen-pancreas: *shangwan* (CV-13). *(DACH IV, 5r)* The nine varieties of pain in the heart to the point of acute pain in the spleen-pancreas: *shangwan* (CV-13); *(YIX I, 4r).* Acute pain in the heart, pain in the spleen-pancreas: *yinbai* (SP-1).

Pain in the heart and stomach:

Pain in the heart and stomach: *DACH) taibai* (SP-3).

Pain in the heart from food: *(DACH VI, 14r) shangwan* (CV-13); *(DACH) yindu* (KI-19).

Pain in the stomach to the point of pain in the heart: *(DACH III, 30v) laogong* (PC-8).

Pain in the heart from intestinal worms:

Sudden pain in the heart from the two intestinal worms: *(DACH) shangwan* (CV-13).

Pain in the heart from ascaris worms: *(DACH)* foot-*dadu* (SP-2).

Pain in the heart and kidney: *(GSdeM) rangu* (KI-2) *yongquan* (KI-1).

Angina of the chest.
Zhen xin tong, xin shan, xin feng, xian bi.

Xian bi: there are also false types. This is the name of an admirable mystery — insoluble, suspended, absolute, hidden, closed. (DACH XI, 21v)

*Name of an illness: sudden pain in the heart and chest; also called **zhen xin tong**, "true pain in the heart." In the past called **xin shan**, "spasms of the heart." These days we also say **xin xiong jiao zhai**, "contracting and strangling of the heart and chest." (Ci Yuan, "Xian-bi")*

True angina (zhen xin tong).

*When there is only pain in the heart, so the feet and hands become blue, it is called **zhen xin tong**; often dead the same day in this case. (DACH I, 16v)*

True pain in the heart, like an awl piercing the heart and vessels. If serious, feet and hands cold including the articulations. If there is panting, death: *(DACH) taixi* (KI-5, IS KI-3).

True pain in the heart *(YXRM)*; sudden pain in the heart; seized by a ghost: *(DACH) zhigou* (TW-6).

Vessels deviated, piercing the heart: *(DACH) zhongji* (CV-3).

Pain in the heart, numbness of shoulder and arm: *(DACH) guanchong* (TW-1).

Sudden pain in the heart (see above: Pains of the heart).

Heart-shock *(xin feng): (DACH X, 25v)* moxa at *xinshu* (BL-15) and *zhongwan* (CV-12).

Xian bi, true or false angina.

Angina of the chest *(xianbi)* like a saber piercing, unbearable: *(DACH)* arm-*xialian* (LI-8).

Xian bi, seized by a ghost *(DACH III, 27r); xian bi*, fullness, swelling: *(YXRM I, 39v)* leg-*sanli* (ST-36).

Xian bi, cold and hot, cough, lack of appetite: *(DACH, YXRM) taixi* (KI-5, IS KI-3).

Xian bi, cold in the abdomen, energy in counterflow: *(DACH, YXRM) sanyinjiao* (SP-6).

Xian bi, gripping, energy of cold: *(DACH) lougu* (SP-7).

Xian bi, fullness of the abdomen, expectorates blood: *(DACH) burong* (ST-19).

Xian bi, fullness of chest: *(DACH)* epigastrium-*tonggu* (KI-20).

Xian bi, contraction-pains, swelling under the sides: *(DACH) pishu* (BL-20).

Xian bi, icterus, body heavy: *(YXRM I, 46r) pishu* (BL-20).

Xian bi, stoppage of digestion: *(DACH) geshu* (BL-17).

Vertigo from arteries, pain in the heart: *(DACH) taichong* (LR-3).

II. Arteries, Veins

Reunion point of the vessels (mostly arteries): *(DACH) taiyuan* (LU-9).

Reunion point of arteries and veins (mostly veins): *(DACH)* thigh-*futu* (ST-32).

Arteries
(Dong mai, "moving vessels.").

Illnesses of vessels (mostly arteries) are treated here: *(DACH) taiyuan* (LU-9).

Paresis *(bie)* or rheumatism *(bi)* of the upper and lower vessels: *(DACH, YXRM) zhiyin* (BL-67).

Illnesses of skin and vessels from wind or cold: *(DACH VII, 31v; YIX I, 11r) waiguan* (TW-5).

Vertigo from the arteries, pain in the heart: *(DACH) taichong* (LR-3).

Heat and apoplexy of the hand: *(DACH) neiguan* (PC-6).

Vessels deviated, piercing the heart: *(DACH) zhongji* (CV-3).

(DACH) The arteries of the eye depend on *tongli* (HT-5).

Artery of the eye contracted: *(DACH) xiaxi* (GB-43).

Arteries of the lungs contracted: *(DACH) zhongfu* (LU-1).

Muscles of the vessels contracted, tightened: *(YXRM) weishu* (BL-21).

Arteriosclerosis
Dong mai ying hua zheng, "Illness of hardening of the arteries"

Origin: excessive movement, neurasthenia, nervous illnesses of the heart, syphilis, obesity, deficient contracted kidneys, alcohol, tobacco, coffee, tea, lead poisoning; invades old people frequently.

Symptoms: diminution of the strength of the vitality, from time to time stoppage of the heart. The terminal arteries are hard; on palpation the pulses are hard, dilated, slow, retarded. The left ventricle of the heart is fat and large. The beats of the tip of the heart are exaggerated; the sound of the second great artery is strong, abundant; there is vertigo.

Treatments with needles:

fengchi (GB-20)..................	*6 fen,*
jianjing (GB-21)	*6 fen,*
wangu (GB-17, IS GB-12)...	*5 fen,*
jianyu (LI-15)	*8 fen,*
quchi (LI-11)	*6 fen,*
weizhong (BL-54, IS BL-40)	*1 cun,*
leg-sanli (ST-36)	*1 cun.* (JO, 12)

Treatment with moxa:

leg-sanli (ST-36)	*9 moxas,*
weizhong (BL-54, IS BL-40)	*5 moxas*
shenmai (BL-62).................	*5 moxas.* (JO, 12)

Arteriosclerosis: *(JM) laogong* (PC-8), *jianyu* (LI-15), *shenmai* (BL-62), *xuanzhong* (GB-39), *sanyinjiao* (SP-6), leg-*sanli* (ST-36), *yanglingquan* (GB-34), thigh-*juliao* (GB-29, IS GB-30), head-*wangu* (GB-17, IS GB-12), *baihui* (GV-19, IS GV-20), *shenque* (CV-8).

Hypertension.
Xue ya kang jin, "excessive augmentation of the blood pressure."

Hypertension can come from several causes, which must be differentiated: contracted kidneys, inflammation of the adrenals, inflammation of the liver or pancreas, etc.; contraction of the arteries, contraction of the capillaries from hyper-pituitary function; irritability of the heart from coffee or tobacco, or exaggerated eating with good wines, emotional agitation, arteriosclerosis. There is no single cause of hypertension. The points which have been experimented with and which give some results are:

Daling (PC-7): dispersed (the longer the silver needle is left in place, the more the tension drops); acts on the contraction of the arteries (nervous command of the arterial muscles?); lowers mainly the diastolic pressure.

Tianjing (TW-10): dispersed, lowers the pressure when it has a purely nervous cause, and acts on the general nervous commands.

Shenmen (HT-7): dispersed, calms and slows down the heart (acts often on the systolic pressure).

(GSdeM) From excess of the adrenals (pulse of the kidney hard, of the liver big, swollen; of the pancreas hard and big). Disperse *fengfu* (GV-15, IS GV-16), *yamen* (GV-14, IS GV-15).

Rangu (KI-2), *taixi* (KI-5, IS KI-3) and *yongquan* (KI-1) diminish or make disappear the congestion, the hardness, and the hyperactivity of the kidney and adrenals (and interstitial chronic nephritis with small red kidneys).

Gongsun (SP-4) acts on hypertension from aerogastria compressing the kidney (alkalosis, flocculent urine, nighttime salivation). It acts much better when tonified.

Fengchi (GB-20) may disperse the sympathetic system; *tianzhu* (BL-10) may tonify the parasympathetic system. High blood pressure from arteriosclerosis will not stop if the cause is still there.

Thigh-*futu* (ST-32) acts on the venous system and facilitates the return circulation when this is the cause of the high blood-pressure.

(JM) Hypertension and arteriosclerosis: *sanyinjiao* (SP-6), leg-*sanli* (ST-36), *laogong* (PC-8), *jianyu* (LI-15).

Pulse large from alcohol: *(DACH) qihai* (CV-6).

When the pulses are all huge or distal or compressed: *(DACH) shenzhu* (GV-11, IS GV-12).

Hypotension.

Hypotension can come from many causes. The points are:

Shaochong (HT-9): tonifies the weakness of the muscles of the heart and increases their impulsion.

Taiyuan (LU-9): seems to act on the arteries by tonifying the muscular envelope.

Gaohuang (BL-38, IS BL-43): acts on anemia, weakness of the blood, red cell insufficiency, hemoglobin, etc.

Yamen (GV-14, IS GV-15): when tonified the adrenals are stimulated.

Zhongchong (PC-9): tonifies the circulation and seems to contract the arteries.

Fengchi (GB-20): tonifies the sympathetic system; *tianzhu* (BL-10) disperses the parasympathetic system.

Fuliu (KI-7): tonifies the kidneys as does *taixi* (KI-5, IS KI-3).

Taibai (SP-3) is indicated for a slow pulse, heavy body and pain in the heart *(DACH)*.

(DACH) For abolition of the pulse: moxa at *jianshi* (PC-5) and *fuliu* (KI-7); the latter is indicated for pulses thin and occasionally imperceptible *(DACH)*.

Aortitis: see *taiyuan* (LU-9).

(DACH) Swelling of the subclavicular fossa; external ulceration, then heat and fullness in the chest: *quepen* (ST-12).

(DACH VI, 15v) Acute intervertebral pain behind the heart: *guanchong* (TW-1).

(DACH III, 32v) Acute pain behind the heart in the vertebral column: hand *zhongzhu* (TW-3).

Arthritis, intermittent limping:

*Comes one, two, three, four months or more before an apoplectic stroke. From time to time there comes suddenly in the leg and foot a heaviness with pain, numbness or insensitivity. After a time it stops only to come again. This is the warning for apoplectic stroke. Quickly use (disperse) leg-sanli (ST-36) with three moxas, and **xuanzhong** (GB-39) three moxas. The moxas allow the departure of the perverse energy through their openings. If it is during the transition from spring to summer or from summer to autumn, use moxas every day and if the legs have blisters, its effect will be admirable. Then take a raw onion, mint, leaves of willow and **si wei** (four flavors); bring to a boil and bathe in it. If these methods are not used, and if one eats and drinks without limit, there will be sudden stroke. (DACH XI, 1r)*

(DACH) Muscles tight, painful. *(YIZ, 40)* Apoplexy, pain from knee to feet: *chengshan* (BL-57).

Local asphyxia (Raynaud's disease?) *(mai bi feng)*:

''In *mai bi feng*, ''vessel paralysis-shock,'' the vessels are closed; humidity contracts them.'' *(YXRM V, 15)*

(DACH) Arm and hand red, swollen with acute and dull pain. It comes from non-circulation of blood and thickened energy: arm-*sanli* (LI-10), *quchi* (LI-11), *tongli* (HT-5), *zhongzhu* (TW-3). If not better *hegu* (LI-4), *chize* (LU-5).

(DACH, YXRM) Paralysis of the vessels: *zhiyin* (BL-67).

Veins (jing mai, "tranquil vessels").

Varicosity (jing mai zhong zhang).

(GSdeM) Thigh-*futu* (ST-32) clearly acts on the venous tissue.

(DACH) Reunion point of the arteries and veins: thigh-*futu* (ST-32).

(GSdeM) Acts on the pain from varicosity and on varicosities not yet completely distended; can cure the varicosity.

(DACH V, 19v) *Liu* (blood tumors): foot-*shangqiu* (SP-5).

(Wetterwald) Internal varicosity; periphlebitis: *ququan* (LR-8), *zhubin* (LR-9), *sanyinjiao* (SP-6).

The liver is generally insufficient in cases of varicosity: tonify *ququan* (LR-8).

III. Blood

The blood is formed by a transformation of the essence of food and drinks . . . the blood circulates by following the energy. If the energy flows, the blood flows; if the energy stops, the blood stops. Thus, in order to refresh the blood, we must purify the energy . . . we know that the hundred illnesses come from the energy, but we do not know that the blood is the body (the fetus) of the hundred illnesses . . . for everything to do with the blood we must discern which meridian is involved. Then if there is counterflow and circulation upwards, we must encourage the downwards circulation . . . protect the pancreas and stomach and one will live for a long time. (YXRM V, 5r)

The water clock falls for nearly two quarters of an hour, during which the blood makes a complete circuit of the body and comes back to the wrist (in Europe, 23 minutes). (YIX 3r & 3v, citing the Nei Jing)

Knowing the meridian where the blood abounds, we must act on the energy of this meridian; with the energy refreshed, the blood will again flow by itself. If there is thickened blood or impeded blood, we must first clear away the accumulation and then act on the energy. (YXRM V, 5r)

Blood coagulating slowly: insufficiency of the liver.

Blood coagulating too quickly: excess of the sympathetic system.

In general.

(DACH) Governs the blood: always tonify *sanyinjiao* (SP-6); *(GSdeM)* (except in cases of hypertension).
(DACH I; YIX I, 8v) Reunion point of the blood: *geshu* (BL-17).
All illnesses of the blood: *(DACH, YXRM I, 46r) geshu* (BL-17). Start with *geshu* (BL-17). However, used alone, it can trouble the intestine and impede the cure; if the patient has less than one year of age, it means death. Also add *xinshu* (BL-15) and *ganshu* (BL-18). All illnesses of the blood: *(YXRM I, 46v) xuehai* (SP-10).
Illnesses of the blood: *(DACH VIII, 32r; YIX I, 11v) lieque* (LU-7).
One punctures here for illnesses of blood and all are corrected: *(YXRM) weizhong* (BL-54, IS BL-40).
Route of the blood: *(DACH) juliao* (GB-28, IS GB-29).
(GSdeM) *Weizhong* (BL-54, IS BL-40) acts on all illnesses of skin and eruptions.
(GSdeM) *Gaohuang* (BL-38, IS BL-43) increases the blood cells by about one million in twenty-four hours.
(GSdeM) Foot-*dadu* (SP-2) on the left increases the action of the mononuclear leukocytes (which are produced by the spleen).
Xuanzhong (GB-39) acts on the polynuclear leukocytes (which are formed by the red bone marrow).

Anemia (pin xue, xue xu).

> *"Emptiness of blood," an illness also called* **pin xue,** *"poor blood." (Ci Yuan, "Xue-xu")*

The body becomes thin and weak, white or bluish complexion; comes from problems with digestion or from excess fatigue. Also classified with tuberculosis *(YXRM I, 40)*, for which it indicates the beginning.

> *Name of an illness, comes from the small number of red cells in the blood. A lot of similarity to, and few differences from anemia,* **pin xue.** *The patient has azure-white skin striped with yellow; slight swelling of the face; palpitations, heart trembling, disharmonious respiration, sometimes headache. It is also called* **huang pang,** *"yellow obesity." (Ci Yuan, "Gan-huang" [yellow of tuberculosis])*

Serious anemia can cause: dyspnea with or without effort, encephalitic anemia with giddiness, accommodative asthenopia, floating spots before the eyes, buzzing, severe headache, mental cloudiness. There is a frequent coincidence between anemia and retinal hemorrhage and gingivitis, etc.

Anemia *(pin xue, xue xu):* two types, from an insufficiency of red cell production and from an excess destruction of the red cells by the spleen.

1) *(GSdeM)* Tonify *gaohuangshu* (BL-38, IS BL-43). In 24 hours the number of red blood cells is increased by one million, hemoglobin is augmented, etc. It is also good to tonify leg-*sanli* (ST-36), because otherwise some people feel heat-flushes immediately.

2) From an excess of the spleen: disperse *shangqiu* (SP-5).

(JM, 314) Anemia *(pin xue):* with needles: *weishu* (BL-21), *sanjiaoshu* (BL-22), *huangmen* (BL-46, IS BL-51), *zhishi* (BL-47, IS BL-52), two *cun* for each, arm-*sanli* (LI-10) and leg-*sanli* (ST-36). With moxa: eight moxas on the preceding points and additionally at *dadun* (LR-1) and *lidui* (ST-45).
(YIX I, 2v) Emptiness of blood: *bailao* (GV-13, IS GV-14 *dazhui*), *gaohuangshu* (BL-38, IS BL-43).
(YIX I, 4r) Anemia *(xue xu),* thirst in the mouth: *shaoshang* (LU-11), *quze* (PC-3).
(GSdeM) Pohu (BL-37, IS BL-42) causes a quite clear increase in the number of red cells.

Heat; blood heavy, thick, impeded, bound.

Heat of the blood:
The five hemorrhoids naturally caused by the heat of the blood: *(YIX I, 7v) chengshan* (BL-57).
Panic from the blood, fainting from blood: *(DACH VII, 33v) shuigou* (GV-25, IS GV-26, *renzhong*).
Ballooning from blood: *(DACH III, 30v)* thorax-*qimen* (LR-14).
Bad blood, from having lifted heavy weights, accumulation of blood: *(DACH, YXRM) yinmen* (BL-51, IS BL-37).
Falls, bad blood in the abdomen: *(DACH) rangu* (KI-2).

Thickened blood *(yu xue):*

> *Problems and forgetfulness as in mental depression, malaise in the chest, sides, lower belly. The blood, which must be liquid, is thick. Either one must sweat, but has not done so (so the fluids are thickened), or one has*

mistakenly caused perspiration (so the fluids have been troubled). Or there is too much urine; the blood is heated and forms an evil thickening. Or there is obsession, habitual worries: the blood thickens. Or one has eaten too much fried food: the hot blood becomes thick. (YXRM IV, 10r)

Without fever, chest full, lips dry, saliva not entering the pharynx, fullness of the lower abdomen, abundant urine, black feces. It is a thickening of the blood. (YXRM IV, 15r)

Blood thick in the chest and abdomen: *(YXRM)* leg-*sanli* (ST-36).
Thickening of blood: *(DACH) xuanzhong* (GB-39).
Blood thickened in the chest: *(DACH, YXRM) jugu* (LI-16).
Thick blood remaining in the chest and diaphragm: *(DACH II, 19r) shenshu* (BL-23).

Hemorrhages, hemophilia (xue jian).

"Arrows of blood": name of an illness. The blood comes out from the pores of the hair follicles and springs out like an arrow. (Ci Yuan, "Xue-jian")

Blood in the urine and feces, constant epistaxis: *(DACH) laogong* (PC-9). Troubles of emptiness; hands suddenly blue: *(DACH) fenglong* (ST-40). Vessels suddenly bluish: *(DACH) tiantu* (CV-22).
To act on the liver, tonify *ququan* (LR-8) and *sanyinjiao* (SP-6); on the arteries, tonify *taiyuan* (LU-9), and on the veins, tonify thigh-*futu* (ST-32).
(See above: Anemia.)

Septicemia.

(GSdeM) Tonify right *dadu* (SP-2) (the spleen produces mononuclear leukocytes), and *xuanzhong* (GB-39). (The red bone marrow produces the polynuclear leukocytes.) Tonify *gaohuangshu* (BL-38, IS BL-43) which will increase the red cells by approximately one million in 24 hours, increase the white cells, and raise the proportion of hemoglobin.

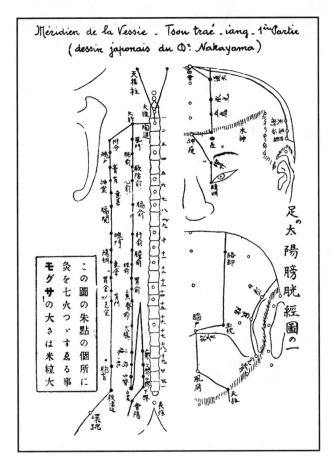
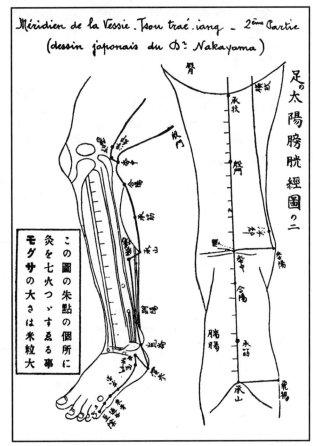

Meridian of the bladder (Nakayama)

Chapter XI

Genital System

Sheng Zhi Qi, Yin Qi, Yin

I. In General — II. Genitality, Sexual Pleasure, Frigidity, Impotence, Hyperexcitation, Fatigue — III. Men — IV. Women

> *The special mechanism of reproduction in moving beings. Thus, in females there are ovaries (**luan chao**) and the uterus (**zi gong**); in males there are testicles (**gao wan**) and the penis (**yin geng**), etc. (Ci Yuan, "Sheng-zhi-qi")*

The genital system is a secondary vessel of the liver meridian *(zu jueyin)*, the liver nourishing the genital activity *(DACH XII, 11v)*.
Ming men, "door of destiny," a branch of the heart governor meridian, the pulse of which is at the deep level of the third segment of the right wrist, represents the genital system.
The innervation of the genital system depends on the caudis equinus (third, fourth and fifth sacral and coccygeal nerves).

I. In General

Illnesses of the genitourinary system: *(JM) qixue* (KI-13), *mingmen* (GV-4).
All illnesses of the genital system: *(JM) qichong* (ST-30), *(JM) guilai* (ST-29); *(DACH) qihai* (CV-6). *(DACH, YXRM)* All illnesses of the interior of the genital system: *huiyin* (CV-1).
Genital system: (Fuji) *dahe* (KI-12).
Alarm point of the third warmer (genitourinary functions): *(DACH) xuehai* (SP-10).
All the illnesses of the area of the groin: *(DACH) futu* (ST-32).
Men — illnesses of the male genital system: *(JM) mingmen* (GV-4).
Women — all illnesses of the female genital system: *(JM) sanyinjiao* (SP-6).
Illnesses of women: *(JM) guanyuanshu* (BL-26), *xiaochangshu* (BL-27), *baihuanshu* (BL-30), *baohuang* (BL-48, IS BL-53), *zhibian* (BL-49, IS BL-54), *daimai* (GB-26), thigh-*futu* (ST-32); *(DACH III, 32r) yongquan* (KI-1).

Swellings:
Swelling of the genital organs: *(DACH) ququan* (LR-8), *(DACH) zhishi* (BL-47, IS BL-52); *(DACH X, 27v) ququan* (LR-8), *sanyinjiao* (SP-6), *taixi* (KI-5, IS KI-3), *dadun* (LR-1), *shenshu* (BL-23); pain and swelling of the genital apparatus: *(DACH) kunlun* (BL-60).
Genital apparatus contracted, internal swelling: *(DACH) rangu* (KI-2).
Inflammation of the genital organs: *(YXRM) heyang* (BL-55).

Abscess, chancre:
Inflammation of the inguinal lymph nodes *(JM)*; swelling and pain in the inguinal nodes: *(DACH) jimen* (SP-11).
All abscesses of the genital system: *(JM) zhishi* (BL-47, IS BL-52).
Abscess *(chuang)* of the genital area: *(YIX I, 23v) xuehai* (SP-10).
Genital system generating abscesses: *(DACH) pangguangshu* (BL-28).
Abscess of the lower area: *(YIZ, 38r)* 2 x 7 moxas: *xuehai* (SP-10).

Chancre *(xia gan)*:

> *A type of venereal disease (**hua liu bing**, "illness of flowers and willows"). It is divided into soft and indurated: the indurated chancre (**ying xing xia gan**) is the first stage of syphilis (**mei du**, "plum tree poison"): first bound, hard, then open and raw; the soft chancre (**ruan xing xia gan**) shows first in fine grains which later open; the surrounding is soft. They reach the lymph nodes and produce buboes. Both types occur on the male or female genitals, or in the mouth, or elsewhere. It comes from a contaminated contact. (Ci Yuan, "Xia-gan")*

Women: chancre *(xia gan)* sweat, scarlet discharge: *(YXRM) xialiao* (BL-34).
Raw chancre (phagedenic) *(YXRM)* of the genital region: *(DACH) changqiang* (GV-1).

Pain in general:
Pain of the genital system: *(DACH) yinlingquan* (SP-9); *(DACH, YXRM) dadun* (LR-1), *taichong* (LR-3); *(YXRM) heyang* (BL-55); *(DACH) shaofu* (HT-8); *(YXRM) henggu* (KI-11); *(DACH) zhongji* (CV-3).
Pain of the genital system; pain in the back: *(DACH) zhishi* (BL-47, IS BL-52).

Pain in the genital system, pain in the abdomen: *(YXRM) zhishi* (BL-47, IS BL-52).

Pain in the genital nerves: *(JM) guilai* (ST-29).

Pains and hardness of the abdomen radiating into the genital organs and preventing urination: *(DACH)* abdomen-*yinjiao* (CV-7).

Urination difficult, tightening sensation radiating into pain in the genital organs: *(DACH) yingu* (KI-10).

Pain and swelling of the genital organs: *(DACH) kunlun* (BL-60).

Inguinal neuralgia: *(JM) lidui* (ST-45).

Pain and swelling of the inguinal area: *(DACH) jimen* (SP-11).

Strangling pain below the umbilicus, flowing and coming into the genitals: *(DACH) guanyuan* (CV-4).

Pain in the genital organs responding in front and in back: *(DACH) huiyin* (CV-1).

Spasms and contractions of the genital organs in general:
Spasms of the genital organs: *(YXRM) chongmen* (SP-12).

Tightening of the genital organs: *(DACH) xuanzhong* (GB-39), *jiaoxin* (KI-8).

Urination difficult, tightening sensations radiating into pains of the genital organs: *(DACH) yingu* (KI-10).

Accumulations; contractions and pains going down to the feet; also, the knee is without action: *(YXRM) taixi* (KI-5, IS KI-3); genital organs contracted with internal swelling: *rangu* (KI-2).

Women — red or white discharge, interior contracted: *(DACH)* hip-*wushu* (GB-27).

Genital organs tightened, feet straight: *(YXRM, 9, ''Yinqiao mai''): zhaohai* (KI-3, IS KI-6).

Spasms of the genital organs: *(DACH) weiyang* (BL-53, IS BL-39).

Genital organs jerking or lifting up: *(DACH) zhaohai* (KI-3, IS KI-6).

Pruritis in general:
Pruritis of the genital organs: *(DACH) shaofu* (HT-8), *ququan* (LR-8).

Pruritis of the genital organs, heat, pain: *(DACH) zhongji* (CV-3).

Women — can no longer have children, pruritis of the genital organs: *(DACH)* abdomen-*yinjiao* (CV-7).

Genital organs — pruritis, sweat, humidity: abdomen-*yinjiao* (CV-7).

Pain and pruritis of the genital organs, spreading to the lower pelvis, can neither bend forward or backwards: *(YXRM) xialiao* (BL-34).

Pruritis and bad odor of the genital organs: disperse *shenmen* (HT-7) and *xingjian* (LR-2) *(YXRM)*.

Sweat, perspiration of the genital organs:
Too abundant perspiration of the genital organs: *(JM) huiyin* (CV-1).

Perspiration of the genital organs: *(DACH) jiaoxin* (KI-8), *(DACH) zhongji* (CV-3).

Dampness or sweating of the genital organs: *(DACH) heyang* (BL-55).

Genital organs, pruritis, sweating, dampness: *(JM, DACH)* abdomen-*yinjiao* (CV-7).

Odors:
Stinking and itching of the genital organs: *(DACH) shaochong* (HT-9).

(DACH XI, 11v) In rich people, a rancid stench; comes from the liver, from drinking too much wine: disperse *xingjian* (LR-2) and *shaochong* (HT-9).

II. Genitality, Sexual Pleasure, Frigidity, Impotence, Hyperexcitation, Fatigue

Orgasm:
Yin chao, ''tides of licentiousness''; luo chao, ''tides of pleasure.''

Orgasm slow in coming. If the condition is old, the point will not work: *(YIZ, 46v) wuyi* (ST-15).

Orgasm radiating into the vertebral column: *(DACH) weizhong* (BL-54, IS BL-40).

During orgasm, convulsions and paresis: *(DACH) chengman* (ST-20).

Chills on orgasm: *(DACH) qichong* (ST-30).

Acute pain and stoppage of function during orgasm: *(DACH) chongmen* (SP-12).

The four limbs numb during orgasm: *(DACH) jiaoxin* (KI-8).

The four limbs and knees fatigued during orgasm: *(DACH) shenshu* (BL-23).

Legs numb during orgasm: *(DACH) rangu* (KI-2), *guangming* (GB-37), *taichong* (LR-3); and vertigo: foot-*linqi* (GB-41).

Spasms of the genital organs during orgasm: *(DACH) chongmen* (SP-12).

Women: total loss of energy during orgasm: *(DACH) chongmen* (SP-12).

Women: during orgasm, upset in the kidney meridian and the four limbs: *(DACH) zhaohai* (KI-3, IS KI-6).

Women: paresis of the vagina during orgasm: *(DACH) zhiyang* (GV-8, IS GV-9).
Men: during the flow of sperm, limbs numb: *(DACH) rangu* (KI-2).

Sexual frigidity.

Produces and increases sexual pleasure: *(GSdeM) shimen* (CV-5) tonify with daily moxa (ten) to the desired level. The Chinese consider that a certain degree of pleasure is necessary in order to have children and that an excess prevents fertilization.

Constant coldness and illnesses of the genital organs: *(YXRM I, 46r) qihai* (CV-6).

Women — coldness of the genital organs; men — coldness of the testicular sack: *(YIZ, 4r) guilai* (ST-29).

Cold of the genital organs: *(YXRM) huiyin* (CV-1).

Severe coldness in lower pelvis: *(DACH)*. Zhongji (CV-3): emptiness and cold of the lower functions *(YXRM I, 46r)*.

Frigidity caused by the paralysis of the uterus: *(DACH X, 34r) sanyinjiao* (SP-6).

Extreme coldness of the uterus and of the opening to the vagina: *(JM) shuidao* (ST-28).

Extreme coldness of the uterus: *(JM) qichong* (ST-30), *guilai* (ST-29), *tianshu* (ST-25).

Does not know sexual pleasure: *(YXRM) lidui* (ST-25).

Frigidity of the sexual system, chills: *(DACH) xingjian* (LR-2).

Sexual energy insufficient: *(DACH, YXRM) diji* (SP-8).

Dreads sexual fatigue and cold food: *(DACH) changqiang* (GV-1).

Women — genital system cold, ovaries painful, also vaginismus: *dadun* (LR-1), *taichong* (LR-3), or *xiaxi* (GB-43), *rangu* (KI-2).

Opens coitus; excessive chastity: *(DACH) yaoshu* (GV-2).

Impotence:
Yin wei, ‘‘paralysis of the genital organs’’; yang wei, ‘‘paralysis of yang.’’

Insufficient or incomplete erections (*bu ji bu quan; ru xian,* ‘‘rope of milk’’):
(Europe) Lesion of the caudis equinus (third, fourth, fifth sacral and coccygeal nerves) causes genital impotence, the absence of erection, anaphrodisia.

> Cannot serve his wife; the same as **yang wei.** *(Ci Yuan, ‘‘Yin-wei’’)*

> Refers to the male reproductive organ having lost its power and strength for reproduction; comes either from weakening of the nerves or from exhaustion and loss of substance. *(Ci Yuan, ‘‘Yang-wei’’)*

The origin of this illness is in most cases onanism (*shou yin*).

> Uselessness of the genital organ . . . if there are internal problems, there are no more erections. If there are problems of cold, there is retraction of the genital organs, which go inside. If there are problems of heat, there is hyperexcitation and erection without control. The cure comes through flowing water and from pure food. *(DACH IX, 13r, ‘‘Liver’’)*

> **Ru xian shan qi,** ‘‘spasms of the cord of milk.’’ Comes from licentiousness and wine in excess. The water of the kidneys is dried up; from limitless coitus, the sexual energy is without strength, the erections without enthusiasm; even where there is stiffness, the sperm flows inappropriately or to the outside; when one enters the vagina, the sperm flows upon entry. *(DACH XI, 7v)*

(DACH) The left kidney *(ming men)* stores the male sexual energy and it must be full. *(GSdeM)* Massage causes sexual excitation, in men erection and ejaculation: *chongmen* (SP-12).

Europe: if there is anemia or overwork, tonify *gaohuangshu* (BL-38, IS BL-43) and moxa (ten daily) at leg-*sanli* (ST-36); tonify the left kidney at *yingu* (KI-10) and *fuliu* (KI-7).

Impotency *(yin wei): (YXRM I, 46r) yanggu* (SI-5); *(YIZ, 42) yangxi* (LI-5); *(DACH) yongquan* (KI-1), *(DACH) rangu* (KI-2); *(JM, DACH, YXRM) yingu* (KI-10); *(DACH, YXRM) qichong* (ST-30); *(JM) dahe* (KI-12), *fujie* (SP-14), *huiyang* (BL-35).

‘‘Rope of milk’’: *(DACH XI, 7v) guanyuan* (CV-4), *shuidao* (ST-28), *sanyinjiao* (SP-6); if not better, *huiyin* (CV-1), *guilai* (ST-29), *guanyuan* (CV-4), *sanyinjiao* (SP-6).

‘‘Illness of the wilted genital organ’’ *(yin wei xiu): (JM) shangliao* (BL-31), *zhongliao* (BL-33), *xialiao* (BL-34), 2 *fen, qugu* (CV-20), *guilai* (ST-29), 1 *fen;* moxa, from five to eight.

Tonify *mingmen* (GV-4) and *yaoshu* (GV-2), daily moxa. Also tonify the heart governor at *zhongchong* (PC-9) and daily moxa in order to raise the blood pressure; and abdomen-*yinjiao* (CV-7) and *xuehai* (SP-10), a herald point of the third warmer (genitourinary functions); tonification of the liver is very important: *ququan* (LR-8).

Sea of generation of energy for males: *(DACH) qihai* (CV-6).

Incomplete erections: *(JM) changqiang* (GV-1).

Loss of sexual energy: *(DACH) guanyuan* (CV-4).

Sexual energy insufficient: *(DACH, YXRM)* lack of fluids of sexual energy, fatigue: *(JM) diji* (SP-8), *rangu* (KI-2).

Sperm diminished: *(JM) dahe* (KI-12).

Excessive coitus: *(JM) ququan* (LR-8).

In young people, brothel fatigue: *(DACH) jiuwei* (CV-15).

Loss of sexual energy, dreads sexual fatigue and cold food: *(DACH) changqiang* (GV-1).

Diabetes, brothel fatigue, no longer responding to the ideas in the heart: *(DACH) taixi* (KI-5, IS KI-3).

Excessive genitality, priapism, nymphomania, sexual hyperexcitement: Jin shan, luan tui, ding chang, ding bang shu.

> **Jin shan,** *"spasms of the muscles." The penis* **(yin geng)** *is erect, stiff and cannot be retracted; sometimes it itches and is painful when the case is extreme; comes from excessive coitus.* (YXRM V, 5v)

> **Luan tui,** *"spasms of the testicles." The penis is swollen and hard causing a pain in the umbilicus. In serious cases, the penis does not retract; the limbs are cold, abscesses occur on the scrotum. If water comes out endlessly, death.* (YXRM V, 2r)

A lot of licentiousness: *(DACH) zhourong* (SP-20); *(GSdeM)* disperse *qichong* (ST-30).

Fluids of sexual energy (sperm) too abundant: *(JM) zhongfeng* (LR-4).

Penis (or clitoris, *yin geng*) swelling and rising too much: *(JM) zhaohai* (KI-3, IS KI-6).

Liver troubled by heat or inflammation, then an erection which does not obey: *(DACH IX, 13r) xingjian* (LR-2).

Prolonged erections: fullness of the secondary vessel, disperse: *(DACH) ligou* (LR-5); the same with fullness of liver and gallbladder, disperse. *(DACH IV, 12v)*

Painful erections: *(JM) qichong* (ST-30); *(JM) guilai* (ST-29).

Spasms of the genital organs: *(DACH) weiyang* (BL-53, IS BL-39).

Priapism *(jin shan)* from energy of the bladder: *(YXRM I, 40r)* bleed *taichong* (LR-3), disperse *dadun* (LR-1), disperse *xiaxi* (GB-43), disperse *rangu* (KI-2).

III. Men
(Seminal Loss, Testicles, Epididymis, etc.)

Seminal loss:
Yi jing, meng yi.

> *Loss of sexual energy; illnesses which consist of losing sperm unintentionally. Losses during dreams* **(meng yi)** *are differentiated from losses related to illnesses* **(bing yi)**. *The latter are easy to cure; the first are difficult.*
> *(Ci Yuan, "Yi-jing")*

Seminal loss *(yi jing)*:
(DACH, YXRM, Fuji) zhiyin (BL-67); *(YXRM I, 46v) rangu* (KI-2); *(YXRM) ququan* (LR-8); *(DACH) yinlingquan* (SP-9); *(YXRM) lougu* (SP-7); *(DACH) zhongfeng* (LR-4); *(YXRM) chengfu* (BL-50, IS BL-36); *(DACH IV, 7r) zhongji* (CV-3); *(YXRM I, 26r) guanyuan* (CV-4); *(DACH, YXRM, JM) qugu* (CV-2); *(DACH, JM) henggu* (KI-11); *(JM) gaohuangshu* (BL-38, IS BL-43); *(DACH) xinshu* (BL-15); *(YIZ, 40r; YIX I, 12v) shenshu* (BL-23); *(DACH) huiyang* (BL-35), *changqiang* (GV-1); *(YIX I, 5v) qihai* (CV-6), *sanyinjiao* (SP-6); *(JM; YXRM I, 46r) dahe* (KI-12).

Seminal loss from emptiness or tuberculosis: *(DACH; YXRM) dahe* (KI-12).

Seminal loss, no more children: *(DACH) zhongji* (CV-3).

Seminal loss during dreams *(meng yi)*:
Especially cures seminal losses during dreams: *(DACH X, 28r) guanyuan* (CV-4); *(YXRM I, 46v) zhishi* (BL-47, IS BL-52).

Seminal loss during dreams, energy in the upper body: *(JM; YXRM I, 46v; DACH X, 14v) gaohuangshu* (BL-38, IS BL-43).

Dreams, nightmares, succubus *(mo meng)*: *(DACH)* foot-*qiaoyin* (GB-44).

Union in dreams with ghosts: *(YIX I, 4v, 5v) xinshu* (BL-15), *baihuanshu* (BL-30), *qihai* (CV-6).

Seminal loss, union in dreams with ghosts: *(DACH VI, 34r) zhaohai* (KI-3, IS KI-6), *rangu* (KI-2), *zhongji* (CV-3), *gaohuangshu* (BL-38, IS BL-43), *xinshu* (BL-15), *shenshu* (BL-23).

Seminal losses in dreams, comes mainly from the joining of heat and humidity: *(DACH X, 35r)* moxa *zhongji* (CV-3), *qugu* (CV-2), *gaohuangshu* (BL-38, IS BL-43), *shenshu* (BL-23).

Penis:
Yin geng.

Men — pain in the penis *(yin geng): (DACH) sanyinjiao* (SP-9).

Pain in the penis *(yin geng)*, both testicles painful; *(DACH),* both testicles propelling the pain, patient can neither get up nor lie down: *(YXRM) qichong* (ST-30).

Pain in the penis on ejaculation: *(DACH) lieque* (LU-7).

Pain in the penis (or clitoris, *yin geng*): *(JM) dadun* (LR-1); *(DACH) ququan* (LR-8); *(YXRM) xingjian* (LI-2); *(DACH, YXRM) sanyinjiao* (SP-6); *(DACH, YXRM, JM) dahe* (KI-12), *guilai* (ST-29); *(DACH) quchong* (ST-30).

Pain in the penis (or clitoris, *yin geng*), pain in the lumbar area, cannot bend forward or get up again: *(DACH) xingjian* (LR-2).

In Japanese *kuatsu* massage at *gongsun* (SP-4) is used to revive one who has suffered a blow to the genitals.

Pain at the head of the genital organ: *(DACH, YXRM) dadun* (LR-1), *huiyin* (CV-1).

Pain at the head of the penis (or clitoris, *yin geng*): *(YIZ, 46v) dadun* (LR-1).

Heat in the meatus: *(DACH) huiyin* (CV-1).

Neuralgia of the spermatic canal: *(JM) qichong* (ST-30), *wushu* (GB-27), *chongmen* (SP-12).

Blenorrhagia: see Urethritis.

Testicles:
Gao wan, luan zi, wai shen, wan

> *A physiological term: male mobile beings have this organ; it is used for making sperm* (**jing zi**). *Their number is not fixed; the more evolved have two; the lower animals have a large number. (Ci Yuan, ''Gao-wan'')*

> *The exterior kidneys* (**wai shen**) *are called* **luan***. (Ci Yuan, ''Luan'')*

> *[*Wan*] used for* **luan***. (Ci Yuan, ''Wan'')*

> *When the liver meridian* (**zu jueyin**) *is emptied to the point of the retraction of the muscles, it causes a tiredness of the tongue and testicles. (Nan Jing)*

Illnesses of the testicles: *(JM) daimai* (GB-26).

Pains:
Testicular neuralgia: *(GSdeM) fuliu* (KI-7).

Counterflow of energy, then testicles suddenly painful: *(DACH) ligou* (LR-5).

Neuralgia of the spermatic canal: *(JM) qichong* (ST-30), *chongmen* (SP-12), hip-*wushu* (GB-27).

Pain (and inflammation) of the epididymis: *(JM) yangchi* (TW-4), *chongmen* (SP-12), *wushu* (GB-27), *shangliao* (BL-31).

In Japanese *kuatsu,* beating quickly or massaging *gongsun* (SP-4) will revive after a blow to the testicles.

Spasms:
Pain from spasms in both testicles: *(JM)* abdomen-*yinjiao* (CV-7).

Men — spasms, testicles going up and going into the lower abdomen, pain: *(DACH, YXRM)* hip-*wushu* (GB-27).

Testicles rising and entering the belly: *(DACH) guilai* (ST-29).

Genital organs going up into the lower pelvis: *(DACH) dadun* (LR-1).

Skin of the scrotum entering the abdomen: *(DACH) shimen* (CV-5).

Genital organs retracted: *(JM),* genital organs retracted, rising; *(YXRM)* men — genital organs retracted, bound; *(DACH)* scrotum retracted: *(JM) dahe* (KI-12).

Deficiency:
Both testicles smaller, deficient: *(DACH) taichong* (LR-3).

Relaxation under the genitals: *(DACH, YXRM)* thorax-*qimen* (LR-14).

Inflammation, swelling:
Inflammation of the spermatic canal: *(JM) chongmen* (SP-12).

Inflammation of the epididymis *(fu gao wan): (JM)* moxa at *yangchi* (TW-4), hip-*wushu* (GB-27), *chongmen* (SP-12), *shangliao* (BL-31).

Inflammation of testicles and epididymis: *(JM) yangchi* (LR-12, IS *jimai*).

Swelling of the scrotum: *(DACH) dadun* (LR-1).

Orchitis, inflammation of testicles *(gao wan yan, pian zhui, shan qi)*:

Name of an illness; a variety of **shan qi.** *The energy of the kidneys descends and falls; the testicles swell a lot or a little. It is also called* **shan qi.** *(Ci Yuan, "Pian-zhui")*

Among the **tui shan,** *there is* **pian zhui,** *falling to one side. There are great ones and small ones. Those of the left mostly come from repressed blood, (thickened) from energy, or from emptiness of energy of the kidneys. Those of the right come from humidity, mucus, or accumulation of food. (YXRM V, 25v)*

Orchitis and epididymis: origin — acute illnesses, urethritis, prostatitis, trauma, typhoid, malaria, contagious parotitis (mumps and related illnesses), syphilis, tuberculosis, etc. Symptoms: in acute cases, swelling and violent pain. Between acute and chronic cases the difference in pain is slight. (JO, 30)

Treatment with needles:

juliao *(GB-28, IS GB-29)*	8 *fen,*
qichong *(ST-30)*	6 *fen,*
daimai *(GB-26)*	5 *fen,*
qugu *(CV-2)*	1 *cun,*
dahe *(KI-12)*	1 *cun,*
jimen *(SP-11)*	5 *fen,*
sanyinjiao *(SP-6)*	5 *fen. (JO, 30)*

Treatment with moxa:

juliao *(GB-28, IS GB-29)*	10 *moxas,*
daimai *(GB-26)*	7 *moxas,*
sanyinjiao *(SP-6)*	7 *moxas. (JO, 30)*

Treatment with needles and moxa:

zhongzhu *(TW-3)*	1 to 3 **fen,** 7 to 10 *moxas,*
daimai *(GB-26)*	1 to 3 **fen,** 7 to 10 *moxas,*
wailing *(ST-26)*	1 to 3 **fen,** 7 to 10 *moxas,*
the four sacral hollows: **qihaishu** *(BL-24)*	2 **cun,** 7 to 10 *moxas,*
the four sacral hollows: **dachangshu** *(BL-25)*	2 **cun,** 7 to 10 *moxas. (JM, 320)*

Acute or chronic orchitis: *(JM)* moxa on the ill side at *yangxi* (LI-5).

Inflammation of testicle and epididymis: *(JM) yangshi* (LR-12, IS *jimai*).

Orchitis: *(DACH) shaofu* (HT-8); *(JM) taichong* (LR-3); *(YXRM I, 40r) xiaxi* (GB-43), *zhaohai* (KI-3, IS KI-6); *(JM) dadun* (LR-1), *zhongfeng* (LR-4), *heyang* (BL-55), *guanyuan* (CV-4), *guilai* (ST-29), *qichong* (ST-30), *shui-dao* (ST-28), the four sacral hollows, *baohuang* (BL-48, IS BL-53); *(YXRM I, 4r) daimai* (GB-26).

Also cures simple orchitis: *(YXRM I, 40r) xuehai* (SP-10). *(YXRM I, 46v)* Swollen genital sack; *(YXRM; DACH III, 32r)* orchitis; *(DACH)* one side of the genital organs big: *dadun* (LR-1).

Orchitis of children: *(YIX, I, 6r) guanyuan* (CV-4), three moxas, *dadun* (LR-1), seven moxas.

The testicles become as large as a bushel (enlarged to a frightening degree): *(DACH IV, 11r; YIX I, 4v) baihui* (GV-19, IS GV-20) moxa.

Hydrocele *(shui shan, shui tui shan):*

In **shui shan,** *either the scrotum swells like a rock crystal, or the scrotum itches and emits a yellow liquid flow; the genital organs sweat; pressed, the lower abdomen gives a watery sound. It comes just after drunken coitus. (YXRM V, 25r)*

In **tui shan,** *the testicles are swollen and big as bushels; no pain, no pruritis. It comes from humidity. (YXRM V, 25v)*

Testicles swollen as large as a bushel, red, painless: *(YIZ, 45) dadun* (LR-1), *sanyinjiao* (SP-6), *guilai* (ST-29), needles 2.5 *cun,* 7 moxas.

Can also be treated as with the "seven spasms," through *dadun* (LR-1) and *taichong* (LR-3) and general points of the genital organs.

IV. Women

Breasts:
ru zi.

In general:

All illness of the breast: *(DACH) zhongji* (CV-3).

Women: various breast illnesses: *(YXRM)*. Women: illnesses of the breast: *(DACH) huangmen* (BL-46, IS BL-51). The belt vessel *(dai mai)* cures diseases of lactation (and menses) in women. Its point of crossing and reunion: foot-*linqi* (GB-41).

Lactation *(ru, ru zhi):*

No milk: *(DACH XI, 8v; YIX I, 6r)* tonify *shaoze* (SI-1), *hegu* (LI-4) and *shanzhong* (CV-17), this last point towards the breasts on the right and left; women will feel the energy circulate up to the nipple, accelerating lactation.

Women who have delivered but have no milk: *(DACH)*. After delivery, milk blocked: *(JM) qiangu* (SI-2).

Women: weak lactation: *(DACH)*. Weak lactation: *(JM)* needles to the right and left and the milk will come while the needles are in: *shanzhong* (CV-17).

Difficulties of lactation: *(DACH) chongmen* (SP-12).

Insufficient milk, if tired or anemic: *(GSdeM)* tonify *gaohuangshu* (BL-38, IS BL-43).

Illnesses following lactation: *(YXRM) zhongji* (CV-3).

Women — milk does not come, the blood pours out: *(DACH VII, 33r) lieque* (LU-7), *shaoze* (SI-1), *taiyuan* (LU-9), *daling* (PC-7), *shanzhong* (CV-17), *guanchong* (TW-1).

Pain in the breasts:

Pain in the breast, difficult to dissipate: *(DACH IV, 6r) shaoze* (SI-1).

Pain in the breast: *(YXRM) liangqiu* (ST-34); *(DACH) rugen* (ST-18).

Pains of the nipple: *(JM) liangqiu* (ST-34).

Nursing mothers — swollen breasts, acute pain: *(YIX I, 5v)* 3 *fen* behind, tonify then disperse *shaoze* (SI-1).

Heat and pain of the breast rising to the subclavicular fossa: *(YXRM) rugen* (ST-18).

Spasms:

Spasms of the fibers of the breast, sometimes pain obstructing the heart: *(DACH VII, 34r) zhaohai* (KI-3, IS KI-6), *yongquan* (KI-1), *taixi* (KI-5, IS KI-3), *dadun* (LR-1), *daimai* (GB-26).

Swellings, inflammation of the breasts, breast abscess:

Swelling of the breast *(YXRM I, 46r) shaoze* (SI-1); *(DACH) liangqiu* (ST-34).

Inflammation of the mammary gland: *(JM) yuji* (LU-10), arm-*xialian* (LI-8), arm-*sanli* (LI-10), foot-*linqi* (GB-41), *diwuhui* (GB-42), *xiaxi* (GB-43), *chongmen* (SP-12), *shanzhong* (CV-17), *yingchuang* (ST-16), *rugen* (ST-18), *ruzhong* (ST-17), *huangmen* (BL-46, IS BL-51).

Inflammation of the cavity of the breast: *(JM) tianxi* (SP-18).

Swelling of the breast, putrefaction: *(YXRM) xiaxi* (GB-43).

Swelling of the cavity of the breast: *(JM) rugen* (ST-18).

Swelling of the breast: *(DACH III, 29r; Ju Ying) shaoze* (SI-1), *tongziliao* (GB-1).

The front of the chest and the two breasts red, swollen, painful: *(DACH VII, 32r) lieque* (LU-7), *shaoze* (SI-1), *daling* (PC-7), *shanzhong* (CV-17).

Ulceration, abscess of the breast:

Women: swelling of the breast, ulceration, deep abscess: *(DACH) tianxi* (SP-18).

Abscess of the breast: *(YIX I, 11v) lieque* (LU-7); *(DACH) yuji* (LU-10), arm-*xialian* (LI-8), leg-*sanli* (ST-36), *diwuhui* (GB-42); *(DACH I, 30v) liangqiu* (ST-34); *(DACH, YXRM)* leg-*xialian* (ST-39, IS *xiajuxu*); *(DACH III, 19r) jianjing* (GB-21); *(DACH; YXRM) yingchuang* (ST-16), *shengfeng* (KI-23).

Abscess in the breast, fullness of the last ribs and the limbs: *(DACH, YXRM)* foot-*linqi* (GB-41).

Nipples generating abscesses: called *du ru*, "jealousy-breast": *lieque* (LU-7), *shaoze* (SI-1), *tianjing* (GB-21), *rugen* (ST-18), *shanzhong* (CV-17).

Abscess of breast, swelling, pain, the baby rejects the milk: *(DACH VIII, 32v) lieque* (LU-7), *shaoze* (SI-1), *zhongfu* (LU-1), *shanzhong* (CV-17), *dadun* (LR-1).

Breast cancer *(nai yan):*

> *Energy of the spleen-pancreas shrunken, reduced; energy of the liver disturbed, in counterflow; consequently, there is a tubercle similar to a piece in a checkers game with neither pain nor pruritis. After ten years or more, this becomes a hollow abscess; it is called breast cancer. It has the form of an abscess, but similar to a ravine in a mountain, to a cliff with caves; it cannot cure itself. However, even at the point between life and death, one can make the root of this additional perversity shrink by clarifying the heart and appeasing the consciousness. Then, after that, the doctor can cure: disperse **wuyi** (ST-15). (DACH)*

The pulse of cancer is slow with interruptions.

Ovaries:
Luan chao.

> *Instrument of production of eggs; area of the female genital organ; analogous to the testicles in the male genital system. (Ci Yuan, ''Luan-chao'')*

In general:

Illnesses of the ovaries: *(JM) daimai* (GB-26); (Abrams) ninth thoracic vertebra (T9) *(jinsuo,* GV-7, IS GV-8).

Pain:

Pain of the ovaries, female genital organs cold: *dadun* (LR-1), *taichong* (LR-3), or *xiaxi* (GB-43), *rangu* (KI-2).

Ovaritis, inflammation of the ovaries *(luan chao yan):*

> *Many acute cases come from the microbe of urethritis; others come from fever and trouble with delivery, or from metritis or inflammation of the external membrane of the uterus, from peritonitis, etc. Chronic cases come from menses, metritis, localized peritonitis. The symptoms of acute cases are acute pains; in chronic cases the symptoms are swelling of the ovaries, sensations too strong, contracting pain in the area of the ovaries. From constipation and during menses the pains are greater, appetite is less, there is difficulty in sleeping peacefully, etc.*

Treatment with needles:

guanyuan (CV-4).........	*1 cun,*
zhongji (CV-3)	*8 fen,*
guilai (ST-29)...............	*8 fen,*
dahe (KI-12)	*1 cun,*
qichong (ST-30)...........	*5 fen,*
sanyinjiao (SP-6).........	*5 fen,*
pangguangshu (BL-28)	*6 fen. (JO, 65)*

Treatment with moxa:

guilai (ST-29)	*7 moxas,*
qichong (ST-30) .	*7 moxas,*
sanyinjiao (SP-6)	*7 moxas. (JO, 65)*

Inflammation of the ovaries: *(JM) qixue* (KI-13), *guilai* (ST-29), *qichong* (ST-30); salpingitis: *(GSdeM) qixue* (KI-13), *guilai* (St-29), *qichong* (ST-30).

Uterus:
Zi gong, bao.

> *An anatomical term; an important area of the female reproductive system; looks like a sack. It is located inside the lower pelvis; this is the area where the fetus is formed and is developed. (Ci Yuan, ''Zi-gong'')*

The word *bao,* which indicates the placenta, is sometimes used for the uterus.

In general:

Uterus: *(JM)* leg-*sanli* (ST-36), *tianshu* (ST-25), *siman* (KI-14), *qichong* (ST-30), *shangliao* (BL-31), *ciliao* (BL-32).

Chronic illnesses of the uterus: *(JM)* guanyuan (CV-4).

Illnesses of the uterus: *(JM)* qichong (ST-30), *guilai* (ST-29), *qixue* (KI-13), hip-*juliao* (GB-28, IS GB-29), *zhongwan* (CV-12), *tianshu* (ST-25), *yaoshu* (GV-2).

Illnesses and trouble of the uterus: *(JM) yangshi* (LR-12, IS *jimai*).

Displaced uterus, anteversion of the uterus, retroversion of the uterus:

Uterus not straight *(DACH);* and painful, swollen: *(YXRM) zhongji* (CV-3), *qichong* (ST-30).

> *Retroversion: from predisposition or from bad placement of the uterus after delivery, the ligaments are relaxed. Symptoms: difficult menses, painful, too abundant, pains extending into the bladder, sensation of pressure on the rectum and the neighboring organs. Half the difficulties of menstruation and sterility come from this.*

Treatment with needles:

qihai *(CV-6)*.........	*8 fen,*
guanyuan *(CV-4).*	*1 cun,*
dahe *(KI-12)*	*1 cun,*
shangliao *(BL-31)*	*1 cun,*
ciliao *(BL-32)*	*1 cun,*
jianshi *(PC-5)*......	*3 fen,*
sanyinjiao *(SP-6).*	*4 fen. (JO, 66)*

Treatment with moxa:

qihai *(CV-6)*........	*10 moxas,*
guanyuan *(CV-4)*	*10 moxas,*
dahe *(KI-12)*	*10 moxas,*
jianshi *(PC-5)*.....	*7 moxas,*
sanyinjiao *(SP-6)*	*7 moxas,*
xuehai *(SP-10)* ...	*7 moxas. (JO, 66)*

(JM) Retroversion of the uterus: yinlian (LR-11), *qugu* (CV-2).

Inflammation of the body of the uterus *(zi gong shi zhi yan):*

> *"It is differentiated from metritis. The uterus is swollen, enlarged and painful under pressure. Acute types: accompanied by pains in the abdomen; often loss of substance. Chronic types: lumbar pain, heaviness and pressure in the lumbar area, frequent impulse to urinate, menses too abundant, coming with pain, body fatigue.*

Treatment with needles:

guanyuan (CV-4)	*1 cun,*
qihai (CV-6)	*1 cun,*
guilai (ST-29)	*8 fen,*
*thorax-**qimen** (LR-14)*	*6 fen,*
huiyang *(BL-35)*........	*5 fen,*
sanyinjiao *(SP-6)*	*5 fen. (JO, 64)*

Treatment with moxa:

*thorax-**qimen** (LR-14)*	*7 moxas,*
huiyang *(BL-35)*........	*7 moxas,*
sanyinjiao *(SP-6)*	*7 moxas,*
guanyuan *(CV-4)*	*15 moxas. (JO, 64)*

Prolapsed uterus (Japan: *zi gong tuo chu;* China: *yin ting chu, yin tui shan*):

> *Name of an illness of the female organ; an object similar to a snake or mushroom comes out; it comes either from a problem or an exhaustion of the uterus (**bao**) or from excessive strain during delivery, or from an emptiness of energy digging downwards, or heat and humidity flowing downwards. (Ci Yuan, ''Yin-ting'')*

> **Yin tui shan:** *the door of the uterus protrudes. If cold dominates, there is pain. If there is serious heat, there is swelling hard as stone. When the uterus protrudes, there is cold and heat. The heat does not last. (YXRM V, 2v)*

Prolapsed uterus *(yin ting chu): (DACH)* and shivering: *shaofu* (HT-8); *(YXRM) zhaohai* (KI-3, IS KI-6); *(DACH, YXRM) shuiquan* (KI-4, IS KI-5); *(DACH) rangu* (KI-2), *jiaoxin* (KI-8), *dadun* (LR-1), *shangliao* (BL-31), *ciliao* (BL-32), *ququan* (LR-8).

Uterus not retracting completely after delivery: *(JM) qugu* (CV-2).

Uterus; interruption of continuity: *(DACH III, 31r) zhongji* (CV-3).

Door of the uterus closed: *(DACH)* causes the upper neck of the uterus to open: *(GSdeM) guanyuan* (CV-4).

Severe cold of the uterus: *(JM) tianshu* (ST-25), *guilai* (ST-29), *qichong* (ST-30).

Cold of the uterus: *(DACH, YXRM) chengfu* (BL-50, IS BL-36).

Severe cold of the uterus and of the opening to the vagina: *(JM) shuidao* (ST-28).

Paresis of the uterus causing coldness: *(DACH X, 34r)* moxa at *sanyinjiao* (SP-6).

Pain of the uterus, uterine neuralgia:
(See pains in the genital organs in general.)

Uterine neuralgia: *(JM) siman* (KI-14), *guilai* (ST-29), *qichong* (ST-30).

Spasms of the uterus, uterine contractions:
(See pain during menses.)

Spasms of uterus: *(JM) shenmai* (BL-62), *taixi* (KI-5, IS KI-3), *dazhong* (KI-6, IS KI-4), *yinshi* (ST-33), *shimen* (CV-5), *siman* (KI-14), hip-*wushu* (GB-27), *wailing* (ST-26), *daimai* (GB-26), *zhangmen* (LR-13), *shangqiu* (KI-17).

Pruritis and inflammation of the uterus:
(JM) Qugu (CV-2).

Congestion of the uterus:
(JM) jianshi (PC-5), *rangu* (KI-2), *diji* (SP-8), *shiguan* (KI-18), *shangqiu* (KI-17).

Women without children, bad blood in the uterus, unbearable strange pain: *(YXRM) yindu* (KI-19).

Accumulation of energy in the uterus: *(DACH) shuidao* (ST-28).

Vagina:
Ancient meaning: yin dao, zi men; Japan: zhi, sheng zhi kou.

> *Sexual passage,* **yin dao** *of women. At the upper end, communicates with the uterus,* **zi gong**. *It is also called* **sheng zhi kou**. *(Ci Yuan, ''Zhi'')*

Pain in the vagina:
Neuralgia in the interior part of the vagina: *(JM) shaofu* (HT-8); *(YIZ, 42) dadun* (LR-1); *(JM) huiyin* (CV-1).

Swelling and pain of the vagina: *(DACH) kunlun* (BL-60).

Spasms of the vagina, vaginismus *(han shan):*
(YXRM V, 25r): Han shan: the female genitals are cold, bound, hard as stone. The clitoris, *yin geng,* does not become erect. The ovaries are painful from cold or sexual excess; if prolonged, there will be sterility. *(DACH): taixi* (KI-5, IS KI-3), *xingjian* (LR-2), *huangshu* (KI-16); *(JM, YXRM I, 46r) ganshu* (BL-18).

Vaginismus, lumbar pain: *(YXRM) xingjian* (LR-2), *zhongfeng* (LR-4).

Vaginismus, heat in the lower pelvis and abdomen: *(YXRM) huangshu* (KI-16).

Vaginismus, pain in the side of the genitals: *(DACH) heyang* (BL-55).

Vaginismus, swelling of the lower pelvis rising and piercing the chest and sides: *(DACH, YXRM) rangu* (KI-2).

Sudden vaginismus: *(DACH) yinshi* (ST-33).

Vaginismus, pain in the lower pelvis: *(DACH) ganshu* (BL-18).

Vaginismus, cold and heat of the muscles, contraction of the leg muscles: *(DACH) ganshu* (BL-18).

Vaginismus, strangling pain: *(YXRM)* abdomen-*yinjiao* (CV-7).

Tightening of the genitals: *(DACH) xuanzhong* (GB-39).

Treated like the seven spasms: *(YXRM V, 25v) dadun* (LR-1), *taichong* (LR-3); or *guanyuan* (CV-4), *dadun* (LR-1); or *dadun* (LR-1), *sanyinjiao* (SP-6).

Inflammation of the vagina (vaginitis):
Pain and swelling of the vagina: *(DACH) kunlun* (BL-60).

Inflammation of the vagina: *(JM) yinlingquan* (SP-9), *yingu* (KI-10), *guilai* (ST-29), *huiyin* (CV-1).

Cold, paresis of the vagina (see sexual frigidity):
Extreme coldness of the uterus and vaginal opening: *(JM) shuidao* (ST-28).

At orgasm, paresis of the vagina: *(DACH) zhiyang* (GV-8, IS GV-9).

Discharges:

Flowing of clear fluid, pain in the sides of the lower pelvis: *(DACH) zhaohai* (KI-3, IS KI-6).
Fluid from sexual energy which is too abundant: *(JM) zhongfeng* (LR-4).

Vulva:

**Yin men, door of the genital organ; yin hu, gateway to the genital organ;
wai yin bu, external area of the genitals; yin chun, lips of the genitals.**

> *Anatomical term: in the external area of the female genital organ. There is a difference between the large lips, **da
> yin chun**, and the small lips, **xiao yin chun**. The large lips are on both external sides of the opening of the repro-
> ductive organ. The small ones are inside the large. (Ci Yuan, "Yin-chun")*

> *The clitoris, a small body in the shape of a sea anemone, is situated in the anterior part of the genital area, **yin bu**,
> of women. At the union of the two symmetrical sides there is a central point similar to the male penis, **yin geng**, but
> of minute dimensions; useless for reproduction. (Ci Yuan, "Yin-ting")*

(Sometimes referred to as *yin geng,* like the penis.)

Vulvar pain:

Acute vulvar *(yin men)* pain: *(JM) huiyin* (CV-1).
Pain and swelling of the vulva: *(JM) ququan* (LR-8), *kunlun* (BL-60), *(JM) zhishi* (BL-47, IS BL-52), *huiyin* (CV-1).
Pain of the clitoris (or penis, *yin geng*): *(JM) dadun* (LR-1); *(YXRM) xingjian* (LR-2), *sanyinjiao* (SP-6), *ququan*
(LR-8), *dahe* (KI-12) *qichong* (ST-30), *guilai* (ST-29), *huiyin* (CV-1).

Inflammation of the vulva:

See above — Pain and Swelling.
Inflammation of the vulva: *(JM) huiyang* (BL-35).
Inflammation of the large lips: *(JM) yingu* (KI-10), *rangu* (KI-2).
Congestion of the large lips: *(JM) rangu* (KI-2).
Vulva swollen, painful, not correct: *(DACH, YXRM) zhongji* (CV-3).

Vulvar pruritis:

(See Pruritis of the genital organs): *ququan* (LR-8), *rangu* (KI-2), *shaofu* (HT-8), *zhongji* (CV-3).
Pruritis of the vulva: *(JM) shaofu* (HT-8), *ququan* (LR-8), *yingu* (KI-10), *rangu* (KI-2), *huiyin* (CV-1).

Cold, heat:

Cold of vulva: *(DACH) shuidao* (ST-28).
Heat of the meatus: *(DACH) huiyin* (CV-1).

White or red discharges.

White or red discharges can have their sources either in the uterus (metritis) or in the vagina (vaginitis).

Metritis (inflammation of the uterus, *zi gong nei mo yan*):

> ***Zi gong nei mo yan,*** *inflammation of the internal membrane of the uterus. Origins: urethritis, delivery, suffering
> from delivery, lack of care during menses, onanism, typhoid, measles, scarletina, contagion. Symptoms: in acute
> metritis, bad cold, during the attack of fever one feels a heaviness of the bones with pain, pus coming out; there are
> foul-smelling discharges. In chronic metritis, there is an easy discharge of blood; blood is abundant during
> menses; there is pain in the lower pelvis. The external mouth of the uterus is surrounded by a pasty and disin-
> tegrated substance. White discharges are abundant, and if they are not stopped, blood discharge occurs.*

Treatment with needles:

ciliao (BL-32)	*8 fen,*
hip-wushu (GB-27) .	*6 fen,*
daimai (GB-26)	*7 fen,*
qihai (CV-6)	*8 fen,*
quanyuan (CV-4)	*1 cun,*
ligou (LR-5).............	*2 fen,*
sanyinjiao (SP-6)	*4 fen,*
baihuanshu (BL-30)	*5 fen. (JO, 63)*

Treatment with moxa:

qihai *(CV-6)*........ *10 moxas,*
guanyuan *(CV-4)* *10 moxas,*
daimai *(GB-26)...* *10 moxas,*
wushu *(GB-27)...* *10 moxas,*
sanyinjiao *(SP-6)* *7 moxas,*
ciliao *(BL-32)* ..... *15 moxas. (JO, 63)*

Inflammation of the internal membrane of the uterus (metritis): *(JM) shenmen* (HT-7), *yinxi* (HT-6), *jianshi* (PC-5), *xuehai* (SP-10), *heyang* (BL-55), *lougu* (SP-7), abdomen-*yinjiao* (CV-7), *qugu* (CV-2), *tianshu* (ST-25), *wushu* (GB-27), *daimai* (GB-26), *shangliao* (BL-31), *ciliao* (BL-32), *zhongliao* (BL-33), *xialiao* (BL-34), *xiaochangshu* (BL-27), *pangguangshu* (BL-28), *baihuanshu* (BL-30).

Chronic inflammation of the internal membrane of the uterus (chronic metritis): *(JM) dahe* (KI-12).

White or red discharges *(bai chi dai):*

White or red discharges: *(YXRM I, 46v) sanyinjiao* (SP-6); *(YXRM) xingjian* (LR-2); *(DACH) qihai* (CV-6), *guanyuan* (CV-4), *zhongji* (CV-3), *qugu* (CV-2), *daimai* (GB-26), hip-*wushu* (GB-27); *(YXRM I, 46r) shenshu* (BL-23).

White or red discharges with emptiness of heart and attacks of heat: *(DACH II, 29v) shaochong* (HT-9).

Red or white discharges, pains like a storm piercing the abdomen: *(DACH) ligou* (LR-5).

White or red discharges, interior contracted; tonify for white and disperse for red: hip-*wushu* (GB-27).

Red discharges *(chi dai xia)* (consider fibroma, or polyp, or chronic metritis): *(DACH)* discharge of blood, discharge of energy, discharge through blood; *(YXRM)* flow of blood *(xue liu xia): xuehai* (SP-10); *(DACH)* red discharges; *(YXRM)* of women: 30 moxas at *dahe* (KI-12).

White discharges (leukorrhea, *bai dai, bai dai xia*); chronic vaginitis *(man xing zhi yan):*

> White belt: name of an illness of women. In fact it is called **bai dai xia,** *"white descending from the belt."* Through the vaginal passage the patient has a flowing fluid with pus. When the color is white it is called **bai dai,** *"white belt."* When the color is scarlet, it is called **chi dai,** *"red belt."* If the discharges are abundant, the body will become weak. In Japan, it is called **man xing zhi yan,** *"chronic inflammation of the vagina."*
> *(Ci Yuan, "Bai-dai")*

Vaginitis, inflammation of the vagina *(zhi yan):*

(JM) Yinlingquan (SP-9), *yingu* (KI-10), *guilai* (ST-29), *huiyin* (CV-1).

White discharge *(bai dai, bai dai xia, dai xia, liu xia):*

White discharge, comes mainly from emptiness or weakness; tonify a lot and add moxa: *(DACH IV, 7r; YIX I, 5v) zhongji* (CV-3).

Discharges of women *(dai xia): (DACH; YXRM) xiaochangshu* (BL-27), *zhongliao* (BL-33); *(DACH) liu xia: xuehai* (SP-10); without stopping *(DACH) taichong* (LR-3); *(JM)* discharge *(dai xia)* too abundant: *zhongdu* (LR-6).

Discharge with a particular quality:

Flowing of clear fluid, pain in the side of the lower pelvis: *(DACH) zhaohai* (KI-3, IS KI-6).

Women — descent of genital fluid, cannot be controlled: *(YXRM) xialiao* (BL-34).

Fluid from sexual energy which is too abundant (?): *(DACH) zhongfeng* (LR-4).

Losses of a strange quality: *(JM) ligou* (LR-5).

Extraordinary discharges: *(JM) lougu* (SP-7), *qugu* (CV-2).

Gonorrhea: *(JM) yangchi* (TW-4), daily moxa.

Green-azure fluid through the lower [orifice]: *(DACH) xialiao* (BL-34) (gonorrhea).

Discharges after delivery:

(Tonify for white, disperse for red):

After delivery; foul, unremitting moisture: *(JM, DACH) zhongdu* (LR-6); *(DACH, YXRM)* and pain and cold around the umbilicus: abdomen-*yinjiao* (CV-7); *(DACH) qihai* (CV-6); *(DACH)* and forming lumps: *shimen* (CV-5); *(DACH, YXRM) guanyuan* (CV-4); *(DACH) zhongji* (CV-3), *(DACH) qugu* (CV-2).

After delivery, foul, unremitting moisture, followed by spasms and formation of accumulations; menses difficult, painful; blood accumulation forming lumps: *(YXRM) zhongji* (CV-3).

Metrorrhagia.

(China: *xue beng;* Japan: *zi gong chu xue*): disperse.

> *A female menstrual illness: menses arriving too abundantly and not stopping; popularly called* **xue beng,** *flowing of blood. (Ci Yuan, "Xue-beng")*

Warm the needles and leave them for a long time in order to tonify the energy and disperse the blood, and to harmonize blood and energy. (DACH II, 28r, ''Xue-beng'')

Zi gong chu xue, ''blood coming out of the uterus.'' *(JM)*

Metrorrhagia: *(JM, YXRM) sanyinjiao* (SP-6); *(JM) taichong* (LR-3); *(JM, DACH) xingjian* (LR-2); *(JM) jiaoxin* (KI-8); *(JM) ligou* (LR-5); *(JM) yingu* (KI-10), *heyang* (BL-55), *xuehai* (SP-10), *tongli* (HT-5).

Metrorrhagia which does not stop: *(DACH, YXRM) dadun* (LR-1).

Women — blood flowing without stopping: *(DACH) jiaoxin* (KI-8).

Flowing of blood which does not stop, descent of quantities of pasty substance; comes either from unruly eating and drinking or from fatigue which injures the form and the constitution, or from a habitual insufficiency of energy: *(DACH) xuehai* (SP-10), seven moxas.

Blood accumulation forming lumps: *(DACH) zhongji* (CV-3).

Women — blood accumulation forming lumps: *(DACH) jianshi* (PC-5).

Miscarriage, delivery and metrorrhagia *(beng chong dai xia):*

(DACH) Abdomen-*yinjiao* (CV-7), *shimen* (CV-5); *(GSdeM)* disperse *sanyinjiao* (SP-6).

Menses, menstruation, periods:
Yue jing, tian gui.

*Also called **tian gui,** ''water of the sky.'' Girls around fourteen years old notice their menses functioning. At around forty-nine years menses stop. **Jing** means constant (**chang**) because it is a constant rule. One time for each lunar cycle is the rule. They can neither be in advance or late, or come to be blocked. These deviations are illnesses. There are some which come in counterflow: one comes for three days, another for a year. During an entire lifetime, [there are cases where] the periods do not come; however, conception occurs. There are women who are pregnant and yet have their monthly menses and have the child. There are women who are pregnant and who suddenly have a great descent of blood without the fetus being injured. (Ci Yuan, ''Yue-jing'')*

Women are governed by the blood (yin). When the true energy (yin) descends and is united with the liquids, that is, when the energy of the kidneys is complete and abundant, then the blood vessels flow and act, and it is certain that, every three decades, it will be seen once. By following the phases of the waxing of the moon, the menses occur, whence comes the name ''menses of the moon'' [ovulation at the full moon, menses at the new moon].

*If, when the moment comes, the blood is in excess, or impure, or if there is an external trouble from the wind, cold, humidity, heat, or if there is an internal trouble bringing cold, or if the seven feelings cause repression and knots, a thickening mucus of the blood, or accumulations, are formed internally; this is called engorgement [stasis] of blood, **yu xue.***

*On the other hand, if after menses one strains, or has too much sex, or consumes drying foods, then the fire will become agitated. Perverse energy abounds and exhausts the blood, which declines. This is desiccation of the blood, **xue ku.** Engorgement or desiccation of blood can come from emptiness as well as heat.*

*Generally, it is said that menses are not harmonious (**bu tiao,** unregulated) when the case is slight; then we speak of emptiness or heat. For engorgements of blood, one must break down the blood. For desiccation, mostly through tiredness and worries, one must tonify and warm.*

However, the energy is always united with the blood. If the energy is warm, there is fever; if it is cold, there is cold; if it rises, the blood rises; if it descends, the blood descends; if it is blocked, the blood is blocked. Thus, if the energy is upset, harmonize it; if it is cold, warm it; if it is empty, tonify it. When the yang (energy) is produced, the yin (blood) grows by itself. When the energy declines, the blood is also frozen. So how can one regulate the energy? Following the discourses of [Wang] Shu-he, for the two meridians of the liver and lungs, it is necessary that the liver be more prosperous than the lungs; if the lungs are full (normal), then energy and blood are equal and harmonious and one can become pregnant. (YXRM VI, 1r)

*The dwelling place of the blood for women having their menses is the **chong mai,** attack vessel [point of crossing and reunion: **gongsun** (SP-4)]. (DACH, ''Chong Mai'')*

*The **dai mai,** belt vessel, also cures diseases of lactation and menses of women [point of crossing and reunion: foot-**linqi** (GB-41)]. (DACH, ''Dai Mai'')*

When the blood prospers and the energy is feeble, the menses occur. (DACH, ''Sanyinjiao'')

Sanyinjiao (SP-6) commands the blood, *hegu* (LI-4) commands the energy. The tonification of *sanyinjiao* (SP-6) and the dispersal of *hegu* (LI-4) makes the menstruation come, and allows conception. The contrary blocks conception and is recommended for easy delivery.

(JM) It is called the way of the blood from the uterus: *xuehai* (SP-10), the herald point of the third warmer

(genitourinary functions); *guanyuanshu* (BL-26).

(JM) Way of the blood: hip-*juliao* (GB-28, IS GB-29).

Menses no longer coming:

If the blood is prosperous and the energy weak, the menses will come. Distinguish: with malaise, disperse; without malaise, tonify.

(GSdeM) If there is anemia, exhaustion, or overwork, tonify *gaohuangshu* (BL-38, IS BL-43) and *sanyinjiao* (SP-6). If there is insufficiency of the liver and excess of the gallbladder, tonify *ququan* (LR-8) and disperse *yangfu* (GB-38). For ovarian insufficiency tonify *xuehai* (SP-10). Tonify *shuiquan* (KI-4, IS KI-5) for the kidneys; disperse the energy at *hegu* (LI-4).

Menses start under the needle: *(YXRM)* disperse *hegu* (LI-4). *(YXRM)* Makes the menses start: *hegu* (LI-4); *(JM)* menses blocked, stopped: *hegu* (LI-4); *(YXRM I, 40r)* in order to make the menstruation come, disperse *hegu* (LI-4), but if there is emptiness, tonify *hegu* (LI-4). However, it is said for pregnant women one can disperse this point, but not tonify; tonification causes the fetus to fall *(DACH)*.

In order to make the menses come: disperse *hegu* (LI-4), leg-*sanli* (ST-36), and *zhiyin* (BL-67). But if there is emptiness, tonify *hegu* (LI-4) *(YXRM I, 40r)*.

In order to make the menses come: tonify *sanyinjiao* (SP-6) *(YIZ, 40)*.

Menses not coming: *(JM, DACH, YXRM)* *shuiquan* (KI-4, IS KI-5), *jiaoxin* (KI-8); *(DACH)* *guanyuan* (CV-4); menses not coming: *(DACH)* *qichong* (ST-30); *(YXRM)* *qixue* (KI-13); *(DACH, YXRM, JM)* *huiyin* (CV-1).

Helps to make the menses come: *(YXRM I, 40r)* *zhiyin* (BL-67).

Blood blocked, not passing, with malaise: *(YXRM I, 40r)* disperse *xuehai* (SP-10); without malaise, tonify.

Women — vessels of menses not communicating: *(DACH)* *quchi* (LI-11).

Menses blocked, stopped: *(JM)* *hegu* (LI-4), *guilai* (ST-29), *qichong* (ST-30), *yaoshu* (GV-2).

(DACH XI, 8v; YIX I, 6r) Menses closed, stopped. Distinguish if there is fullness (disperse) or emptiness (tonify): *hegu* (LI-4), *sanyinjiao* (SP-6), *zhongji* (CV-3), *shenshu* (BL-23).

Menses no longer recurring *(bu zai chuan)*; menopause:

Menses no longer recurring, chest bound because of the blood; heat has entered into the home of blood: *(DACH III, 29r)* thorax-*qimen* (LR-14).

Hot flashes of menopause: *(GSdeM)* tonify *sanyinjiao* (SP-6), *xuehai* (SP-10), disperse *shenmai* (BL-62), *fengchi* (GB-20); excess of sympathetic system and the yang. For insufficiency of the parasympathetic system and the yin, tonify *tianzhu* (BL-10) and leg-*sanli* (ST-36).

Tides of heat; violent perspiration: *(YXRM I, 47r)* *xinshu* (BL-15).

Attacks of heat coming and going, entering and exiting: *shendao* (GV-10, IS GV-11).

Pruritis at menopause: see Vulva.

Getting fat at menopause (excess yin, insufficiency of yang): *(GSdeM)* insufficiency of the sympathetic system and the thyroid, excess of parasympathetic system: tonify *fengchi* (GB-20), *renying* (ST-9), *hegu* (LI-4); disperse *tianzhu* (BL-10), leg-*sanli* (ST-36) and *zhaohai* (KI-3, IS KI-6).

Before menses:

Menses come with a lot of melancholy and pain: *(DACH, YXRM)* *shuiquan* (KI-4, IS KI-5).

During the eight days preceding menses, either melancholy and tears (tonify), or irritability, violence (disperse): *(GSdeM)* *shuiquan* (KI-4, IS KI-5).

Pain and troubles during menses:

Pain from energy in the blood: *(DACH)* disperse *shenmai* (BL-62).

Pain during menses: *(JM)* *diji* (SP-8), *shuidao* (ST-28), *siman* (KI-14).

Menses painful, difficult, hard: *(JM)* *shuidao* (ST-28).

Menses difficult, tiring: *(JM)* *siman* (KI-14).

Counterflow during menses: *(DACH)* *zhaohai* (KI-3, IS KI-6); *(JM)* foot-*linqi* (GB-41), *xuehai* (SP-10); *(DACH, JM)* *qixue* (KI-13); *(JM)* *yinjiao* (CV-7), abdomen-*zhongzhu* (KI-15), *tianshu* (ST-25), *qimen* (LR-14); *(JM)* *shangliao* (BL-31), *ciliao* (BL-32), *zhongliao* (BL-33), *xialiao* (BL-34), *huiyin* (CV-1), *shenshu* (BL-23).

See Uterus: pains, spasms, congestion.

(DACH VII, 34r) Irregular menses in virgins, acute pain of the lower pelvis and umbilicus: *zhaohai* (KI-3, IS KI-6), *sanyinjiao* (SP-6), *guanyuan* (CV-4), *shenshu* (BL-23).

(DACH VII, 34r) Women whose menses come well, but with vertigo and pain of the lower pelvis: *zhaohai* (KI-3, IS KI-6), *neiting* (ST-44), *yangjiao* (GB-35), *hegu* (LI-4).

Irregular menses (not coming every twenty-eight days):
  1) Changing (sometimes late, sometimes early):
  Menses without date: *(DACH) tianshu* (ST-25).
  Menses like colds, coming without a fixed period: *(DACH X, 31r) guanyuan* (CV-4).
  Menses changing from the usual: *(DACH II, 19r; YIX I, 5r) xuehai* (SP-10), *diji* (SP-8).
  2) Spaced too far apart (more than 28 days):
  Menses coming late: *(DACH) qimen* (LR-14); *(GSdeM)* tonify foot-*linqi* (GB-41).
  3) Coming too soon (less than 28 days):
  Menses coming in advance: *(GSdeM)* disperse *sanyinjiao* (SP-6) and *xuehai* (SP-10).

Insufficient menses or with slight stoppages (not harmonious, *bu tiao*):
From engorging of blood or moral shock, disperse; from drying of blood, warm foods or sexual excess, tonify.
(JM, YXRM) Jianshi (PC-5), *quchi* (LI-11); *(GSdeM) ququan* (LR-8), *sanyinjiao* (SP-6); *(JM) xuehai* (SP-10); *(JM, DACH, YXRM) rangu* (KI-2), *yinbao* (LR-9); *(JM, DACH) ligou* (LR-5); *(YXRM)* abdomen-*yinjiao* (CV-7); *(JM, DACH) qihai* (CV-6); *(YXRM I, 46r) zhongji* (CV-3), abdomen-*zhongzhu* (KI-15); *(JM, DACH) siman* (KI-14); *(JM, DACH, YXRM) daimai* (GB-26); *(JM) ciliao* (BL-32); *(JM, DACH) zhongliao* (BL-33).

Insufficient menses or slight stoppage (not harmonious):
(DACH XI, 8r) zhongji (CV-3), *qihai* (CV-6), *shenshu* (BL-23), *sanyinjiao* (SP-6).
(DACH VII, 26r) Gongsun (SP-4), *sanyinjiao* (SP-6), *qihai* (CV-6), *guanyuan* (CV-4), *tianshu* (ST-25).

Insufficient menses (not productive, *bu li, bu zu*):
Diminished menses: *(JM) shuiquan* (KI-4, IS KI-5).
Insufficient menses (not productive): foot-*linqi* (GB-41).
To tonify during menses increases and prolongs them: *(GSdeM) hegu* (LI-4), leg-*sanli* (ST-36).
If there is anemia, tonify *gaohuangshu* (BL-38, IS BL-43).

Menses too abundant (see metrorrhagia).
Disperse: *(JM, DACH) tongli* (HT-5); *(JM) dadun* (LR-1), *(JM) xingjian* (LR-2), *(JM) sanyinjiao* (SP-6), *(JM) yinbai* (SP-1).
Menses for more than six days yet have not stopped: *(DACH VI, 26v) rugen* (ST-18).
Menses not stopping, blood flowing without stopping: *(DACH)* tonify *sanyinjiao* (SP-6).
Blood of menstruation too abundant and not stopping: *(DACH) xingjian* (LR-2).
Menses have not stopped: *(DACH)* abdomen-*yinjiao* (CV-7).
Menses passing their term: *(DACH VII, 19v; YIX I, 3v) tianshu* (ST-25) *shuiquan* (KI-4, IS KI-5).
(YIX I, 4r) Women: blood flowing: *jiaoxin* (KI-8), *heyang* (BL-55).

Fertility, sterility, miscarriages.

Excessive fertility:
(DACH, "Sanyinjiao") Blood weak, energy abundant: no conception. *Hegu* (LI-4) commands energy: tonify it; *sanyinjiao* (SP-6) commands the blood: disperse it. The commentaries explain that the energy is measured by sexual pleasure. The greater the pleasure, the less likelihood of infertility. A certain level of pleasure must occur in order to conceive. *Shimen* (CV-5), 15 daily moxas, increases the pleasure.
(DACH XI, 8r) Women who have many children: moxas at *hegu* (LI-4) increases the energy, needles at *sanyinjiao* (disperse) (SP-6).
(DACH II, 25v) In order to prevent conception 2 x 7 moxas, up to 100 at *shimen* (CV-5).
(DACH XI, 8r) Women who have many children: *shimen* (CV-5), tonify (increases the pleasure). *Sanyinjiao* (SP-6), disperse (weakens the blood).

Sterility (*wu zi*, "no children"; *jue zi*, "infertility"; Japan: *bu ren zheng* "illness of non-conception"):
  Europeans recognize a certain number of causes of sterility, among which are: defective ovulation, either by ovarian deficiency or by malformation of the fallopian tubes; contracture of the upper and lower neck of the uterus; displacement of the uterus; irritation of the internal membrane of the uterus. China and Japan add to this excessive sex- On the other hand, complete frigidity, which often causes sterility, is generally accompanied by a contracture of the neck of the uterus. It can be caused by the husband.
        weak energy: conception is possible; weakened blood, abundant energy: no conception.
        yinjiao")
        commands the energy, disperse it. *Sanyinjiao* commands the blood, tonify it. As the energy is measured pleasure, dispersing *shimen* (CV-5) will diminish the pleasure if it is excessive.

For uterine displacements, tonify *qichong* (ST-30), which tightens all the uterine ligaments; ten daily moxas at *yanglingquan* (GB-34) tightens the muscles.

Moreover, it is said that in order to become pregnant, it is necessary for the liver meridian to be more abundant than the lung meridian which must, however, be normally full.

> *Ming men* (heart governor) is the minister of unions; through it men form sperm and women detach the ovule. *(YXRM I, 17v)*

Thus, tonify *zhongchong* (PC-9).

Finally, "women draw out of the right kidney, thus called the 'door of destiny', the strength for knotting the germ."

The closure of the neck of the uterus is generally neutralized by dispersing *guanyuan* (CV-4); this has been observed in Paris. The Chinese describe it this way: *(YXRM)* passages of conception interrupted; *(DACH)* door of the uterus closed; *(YXRM I, 46r)* allows people to conceive. Moreover, this point acts on menses which do not come and on white or red discharges. *Zhongji* (CV-3) dispersed has the same power on the uterine passages. *(DACH III, 31r)* Uterus: interruption of continuity; *(JM)* no conception; *(YXRM)* infertility; *(DACH)* pass the needle and one can have a child (disperse); *(DACH III, 31r)* puncture four times and there will be conception; this gives harmony and tepidness to the uterus. *(YXRM I, 46r)* Moxas, three at a time, cause the conception of a child; also acts on menses which do not come or descend, and on discharges.

The most detailed indications are as follows:

> *Women not producing sons or daughters: disperse the energy of* **hegu** *(LI-4) through needles; disperse six times. Tonify the blood at* **sanyinjiao** *(SP-6) with needles; tonify nine times. In addition, on the day menses is expected, moxa at* **zigong** *(MP-35, IS M-CA-18). Increase the moxas and the person will become pregnant. There is no case on earth where conception has not been achieved in this way. (YIX I, 5r & 6r)*

(YIZ, 38r) Women who have not had children for a long time: *zigong* (MP-35, IS M-CA-18).

(YIZ, 34r) When menses have come, start the moxas during the three days following and stop; that can cause conception. Do not use too many moxas: *zigong* (MP-35, IS M-CA-18).

For women who do not yet have a child: three moxas and they will have one. Women: infertility *(DACH, YXRM)*. Non-conception *(JM)*. Also acts on retroversion of the uterus: *(JM) yinlian* (LR-11).

Women without children: *(DACH XI, 8r) zigong* (MP-35, IS M-CA-18), *zhongji* (CV-3).

No children: *(DACH II, 19r; YIX I, 4r; Ju Ying)* abdomen-*yinjiao* (CV-7), *shimen* (CV-5).

Uterus cold for a long time; does not become pregnant: *(DACH VII, 34v) zhaohai* (KI-3, IS KI-6) *sanyinjiao* (SP-6), *zhongji* (CV-3), *zigong* (MP-35, IS M-CA-18).

Illness of non-conception: *(JM),* women with no children: *(DACH) qichong* (ST-30) acts on the displaced uterus and amenorrhea.

Problems and anger about not having children: *(YXRM) qichong* (ST-30).

China: infertility, no children or progeny: *(DACH, YXRM) yinlian* (LR-11); *(DACH) guanyuan* (CV-4); *(YXRM) zhongji* (CV-3); *(DACH)* and with pruritis: abdomen-*yinjiao* (CV-7); *(JM, DACH, YXRM)* no children: *siman* (KI-14); *(DACH)* infertility: foot-*shanqiu* (SP-5), *rangu* (KI-2), *(YXRM) shangliao* (BL-31).

(JM) No conception; *(DACH) yongquan* (KI-1), *rangu* (KI-2), *qichong* (ST-30), *guilai* (ST-29), *huangshu* (KI-16), *shangliao* (BL-31), *ciliao* (BL-32).

No more male children: *(DACH III, 31r)* tonify *zhongji* (CV-3).

Many moxas can cause people to give birth to sons: *(YXRM I, 46r) qihai* (CV-6). If it is a question of masculine sterility without impotence, *qihai* (CV-6) is given as the ocean of energy for males.

Miscarriage *(xiao chan, liu chan, chan beng, beng zhong):*

> *Popularly called* **xiao chan** *— little delivery — when the term is at about three or four months of the pregnancy. It comes either from insufficient nutrition in the uterus, or from an internal trouble, or from syphilis of the father. (Ci Yuan, "Liu-chan")*

> *When the fetus is delivered before term at less than seven months, it is called* **xiao chan** *or* **liu chan,** *"sunken delivery." (Ci Yuan, "Xiao-chan")*

Also: *chan beng,* "flowing delivery," and *beng zhong,* "in the flow."

(GSdeM) When miscarriages are caused by hereditary syphilis, tonify *zhubin* (KI-9) and *jiuwei* (CV-15); it allows the child to be brought to term.

(GSdeM) When miscarriages are caused by the weakness of the uterine membrane, tonify *sanyinjiao* (SP-6) and the cure is assured.

Does not fulfill pregnancy: *(YXRM I, 36v) sanyinjiao* (SP-6).

Women with cold uterus for a long time and who are unable to keep the fetus when it is conceived: *(DACH VII, 34r)* *zhaohai* (KI-3, IS KI-6) or *zhongji* (CV-3), *sanyinjiao* (SP-6), *zigong* (MP-35, IS M-CA-18)

Can keep the fetus; it is of proven effectiveness: *(YIX, 7v)* *zigong* (MP-35, IS M-CA-18).

Miscarriages and discharges: *(YXRM)* abdomen-*yinjiao* (CV-7), *heyang* (BL-55).

Miscarriages: *zhongliao* (BL-33), *qihai* (CV-6); *(DACH)* *xingjian* (LR-2), leg-*zhongdu* (LR-6), *tongli* (HT-5).

Miscarriages: *(DACH)* *shimen* (CV-5); *(YXRM)* *taichong* (LR-3), *jiaoxin* (KI-8).

Miscarriage with foul, unremitting pink discharge: *(YXRM)* *zhongdu* (LR-6).

After premature delivery, extreme coldness of the lower limbs *(JM)*.

After the fetus has fallen, counterflow cold in the feet and hands: *(YXRM)* *jianjing* (GB-21).

Pregnancy.

False pregnancy:

Women — as if pregnant; men — like ascites: *(DACH)* *yingu* (KI-10), *yongquan* (KI-1).

Pregnancy *(yun)*:

Poisoning of the fetus from hereditary syphilis: *(JM)* *zhubin* (KI-9).

Acts on the syphilitic toxins, point of Weihe for Mercurius vivus: *(GSdeM)* *jiuwei* (CV-15).

Vomiting of pregnancy: *(JM)* *youmen* (KI-21), disperse.

Pregnant women: urination inconvenienced because of the position of the fetus: *(YIZ, 40)* *guanchong* (TW-1).

Pregnant women, the child rises and attacks the heart: *(DACH)* *chongmen* (SP-12), *qichong* (**ST**-30); *(DACH)* and trouble, melancholy: *juque* (CV-14).

Aerogastria, aerocolia, gas and eructations: *(GSdeM)* tonify *gongsun* (SP-4).

Needles and moxa forbidden to pregnant women after the fourth month: *(JM)* forbidden to pregnant women, by touching with needles the fetus will fall. If it does not come out, needles at *kunlun* (BL-60). *(DACH, YXRM)* disperse *guanyuan* (CV-4) (opens the lower part of the neck of the uterus: *GSdeM*).

Forbidden to pregnant women, to disperse causes the fetus to fall: *(DACH)* *sanyinjiao* (SP-6) acts on the blood.

Forbidden to pregnant women; by inserting the needle, the fetus falls; *(DACH)* disperse *kunlun* (BL-60).

Pains of delivery: *(YXRM)* disperse *qichong* (ST-30).

Delivery:
Chan; fen mian.

Before delivery:

Movements of the fetus towards an irregular birth: *(DACH)* tonify *sanyinjiao* (SP-6).

Dead fetus:

To make the dead child come out when it will not: *(YXRM I, 40v)* disperse *sanyinjiao* (SP-6).

Fetus dead and not coming out, cold in the diaphragm: *(DACH VII, 32v; YIX I, 11v)* *lieque* (LU-7).

Five moxas causes the dead fetus to descend: *(DACH, YIZ)* *duyin* (MP-44, IS M-LE-18a).

Dead fetus: *(DACH, 31r)* disperse *sanyinjiao* (SP-6) and *taichong* (LR-3).

Normal delivery:

(The points can be punctured repeatedly every quarter hour):

In order to facilitate and make delivery less painful: weak blood, strong energy facilitates delivery: disperse *(GSdeM)* *kunlun* (BL-60); tonify *hegu* (LI-4), disperse *sanyinjiao* (SP-6), disperse *guanyuan* (CV-4).

To tonify causes the fetus to fall: *(DACH)* *hegu* (LI-4).

Hastens the delivery: *(YXRM I, 40r)* disperse leg-*sanli* (ST-36); tonify *hegu* (LI-4) if empty, disperse if there is fullness and nervous tension; disperse *zhiyin* (BL-67). Relaxes the ligaments and muscles of the uterus and lower pelvis: *(GSdeM)* disperse *qichong* (ST-30), *guanyuan* (CV-4), *zhongji* (CV-3).

Weakness, fatigue during delivery: tonify the muscles. *(GSdeM)* Tonify *yanglingquan* (GB-34).

Difficult delivery:

(YXRM) I, 46r) Tonify *hegu* (LI-4), *qichong* (ST-30); *(DACH)* *jianjing* (GB-21); *(YXRM I, 41v)* *sanyinjiao* (SP-6).

Delivery, hand comes first: *(YIZ, 45)* *zhiyin* (BL-67).

Difficult delivery, panic, trouble, lumps from accumulations: *(DACH VII, 33v; YIX I, 11v)* *zhaohai* (KI-3, IS KI-6).

(JO, 73) Peaceful delivery: *shenshu* (BL-23), *dachangshu* (BL-25), *zhishi* (BL-47, IS BL-52), *ciliao* (BL-32), *yaoshu* (GV-2).

Placenta not coming:

(DACH, YXRM) Disperse *qichong* (ST-30); *(DACH) kunlun* (BL-60); *(YIX I, 9v; DACH VII, 25v; YXRM) gongsun* (SP-4), disperse; *(DACH, YIZ) duyin* (MP-44, IS M-LE-18a); *(YXRM I, 40r) zhaohai* (KI-3, IS KI-6), *neiguan* (PC-6); *(YIX I, 6r; DACH XI, 8r) zhongji* (CV-3), abdomen-*yinjiao* (CV-7); *(DACH X, 31v) zhongji* (CV-3), *tianjing* (TW-10).

During delivery:

Puerperal eclampsia: *(YIZ, 5v; YIX 4r, DACH VII, 26)* needles 3 *fen,* tonify; three moxas: *rangu* (KI-2).
Fainting during delivery: *(DACH)* leg-*sanli* (ST-36).

After the delivery:

All illnesses after delivery: *(DACH X, 31r) qimen* (LR-14); *(DACH XI, 31r) taichong* (LR-3), *sanyinjiao* (SP-6).
Puerperal fever (after delivery): *(DACH) ganshu* (BL-18).
After delivery the uterus does not completely retract: *(JM) qugu* (CV-2).
Abdominal swelling after delivery: *(YXRM I, 46r) shenque* (CV-8).
Metrorrhagia after delivery: *(GSdeM)* disperse *sanyinjiao* (SP-6); *(JM)* leg-*zhongdu* (LR-6).
After delivery, blood accumulation forming lumps, pains: *(DACH XI, 8r; YIX I, 5r) qihai* (CV-6), *sanyinjiao* (SP-6).
After delivery, vertigo from blood: *(DACH) zhigou* (TW-6); *(JM) shenmen* (HT-7), *(JM)* abdomen-*yinjiao* (CV-7).
Foul, unremitting pink discharges after delivery (white discharge, tonify): *(DACH, YXRM);* with pain and cold around the umbilicus: abdomen-*yinjiao* (CV-7); *(DACH) qihai* (CV-6); *(DACH)* and forming lumps: *shimen* (CV-5); *(DACH) guanyuan* (CV-4), *zhongji* (CV-3); *(JM) qugu* (CV-2); *(JM, DACH)* leg-*zhongdu* (LR-6).
After delivery, pain in the abdomen and umbilicus, dread of sexual relations, foul pink discharge: *(DACH VII, 34r) zhaohai* (KI-3, IS KI-6), *sanyinjiao* (SP-6), *shuifen* (CV-9), *guanyuan* (CV-4), *gaohuangshu* (BL-38, IS BL-43).
After delivery, palpitations, heat, problems of the head and eyes, eyes sunken; comes from fatigue before delivery: *(DACH XI, 8r)* tonify *hegu* (LI-4), *laogong* (PC-8), *bailao* (GV-13, IS GV-14, *dazhui*), *xinshu* (BL-15), *zhongji* (CV-3), *yongquan* (KI-1). If not better, *shaoshang* (LI-11), *quchi* (LU-11), *jianjing* (GB-21), *xinshu* (BL-15).
After delivery, hands and feet cold, frozen, collapsing: *(DACH X, 31r; YIZ, 45) jianjing* (GB-21).
Cerebral anemia after delivery: *(JM)* tonify *sanyinjiao* (SP-6).

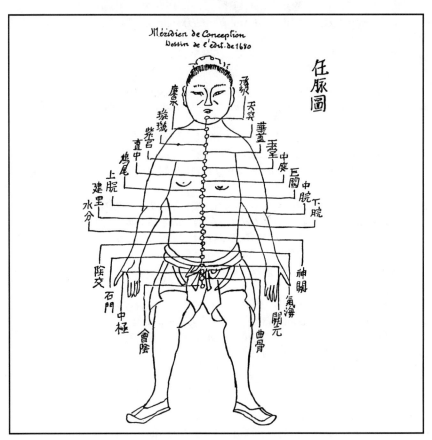

Conception vessel (DACH)

Chapter XII
Lower Pelvis *(Xiao-fu)*[1]

In general:

For the lower pelvis and throat: *(DACH)* zhaohai (KI-3, IS KI-6).

Cold; heat:

Bitter cold of the lower pelvis: *(DACH, YXRM)* zhongji (CV-3).

Heat of the lower pelvis: *(DACH, YXRM)* and pain of the sides: zhaohai (KI-3, IS KI-6); *(YXRM)* fuxi (BL-52, IS BL-38); *(YXRM)* and pain of the sides: weizhong (BL-54, IS BL-40); *(JM)* heat attacking the lower pelvis; *(DACH)* and desire to run: zhejin (GB-23) and riyue (GB-24).

Pain:

Acute pain of the lower abdomen: *(DACH X, 27v)* shenmai (BL-62).

Pain of the lower pelvis: *(DACH)* xiaohai (SI-8), *(DACH)* zhaohai (KI-3, IS KI-6); *(JM)* jinmen (BL-63); *(DACH)* yongquan (KI-1); *(DACH)* and central heat: dadun (LR-1); *(YXRM)* zhongfeng (LR-4); *(JM, YXRM, DACH)* leg-zhongdu (LR-6); *(DACH)* jingmen (GB-25); *(JM)* wailing (ST-26); *(DACH)* qichong (ST-30); *(JM)* pangguangshu (BL-28).

Women — pain in the lower pelvis: *(YXRM I, 46v)* neiting (ST-44); *(YXRM)* and hardness: daimai (GB-26).

Pain of the lower pelvis radiating to the throat: *(DACH)* ququan (LR-8); *(DACH)* radiating to the larynx: biguan (ST-31), zhaohai (KI-3, IS KI-6).

Pain in the lumbar area radiating to the lower pelvis: *(DACH)* taichong (LR-3).

Pain in the sides of the lower pelvis: *(DACH)* jiaoxin (KI-8).

Pain in the lower pelvis; central heat: *(DACH)* dadun (LR-1).

Swelling and pain:

Swelling and pain of the lower pelvis: *(DACH)* zhongfeng (LR-4), *(DACH X, 25v)* qihai (CV-6), *(DACH)* jimen (SP-11).

Spasms, contractions:

Spasms of the lower pelvis: *(JM)* arm-xialian (LI-8), wenliu (LI-7), xiaohai (SI-8), gongsun (SP-4), jinmen (BL-63), ligou (LR-5), weiyang (BL-53, IS BL-39), heyang (BL-55), jianli (CV-11), qugu (CV-2) pangguangshu (BL-28).

Sudden spasms in the lower pelvis, pain like a storm: *(DACH)* shimen (CV-5).

Strangling pain in the lower pelvis: *(DACH)* shimen (CV-5).

Contracting pain of the lower pelvis: *(JM)* leg-xialian (ST-39, IS xiajuxu).

Swelling:

Drum-swelling of the lower pelvis area: *(YXRM I, 46v)* leg-sanli (ST-36).

Swelling of the lower pelvis area: *(YXRM)* taichong (LR-3); *(DACH, YXRM)* xingjian (LR-2); *(YXRM)* zhongfeng (LR-4).

Swelling of the lower pelvic area, prolapsed uterus: *(YXRM)* ququan (LR-8).

Swelling of the lower pelvic area, heat, sighs, agitation: *(YXRM)* juque (CV-14).

Swelling and ballooning of the lower pelvic area: *(JM)* jiexi (ST-41), xingu (KI-10), back-yangguan (GV-3).

Fullness:

Fullness of the lower pelvis: *(JM, DACH)* arm-xialian (LI-8); *(DACH, YXRM)* daju (ST-27).

Fullness and swelling of the lower pelvis: *(DACH IV, 6v)* neiting (ST-44); *(JM)* weizhong (BL-54, IS BL-40), youmen (KI-21); *(DACH, YXRM)* qugu (CV-2); *(DACH, YXRM)* daju (ST-27).

Fullness and swelling, strangling pain: *(DACH)* xiaochangshu (BL-27).

Fullness of the lower pelvis, urine not passing: *(DACH)* henggu (KI-11).

Hardness of the lower pelvis:

(DACH) leg-sanli (ST-36), weizhong (BL-54, IS BL-40), *(DACH X, 31r)* daimai (GB-26).

Hardness of the lower pelvis, spasms, cold and heat: *(DACH)* qiuxu (GB-40).

Hardness and ballooning of the lower pelvis: *(DACH)* yinlingquan (SP-9).

Skin of lower pelvis resonant: *(DACH)* shimen (CV-5).

Note

[1] *Xiao-fu* is a technical term translated as ''smaller abdomen,'' ''lesser abdomen,'' or ''small hara.'' However, Soulie de Morant's choice, *bessin,* translates most directly to ''pelvis.'' — ed.

Chapter XIII
Urinary System

I. Kidney — II. Bladder — III. Prostate, Prostatitis — IV. Urethra, Urethritis — V. Urine

(DACH VIII, 18v) The flow of urine coming from the kidneys depends on the small intestine and the lower warmer.
(DACH) The herald point of the lower warmer (genitourinary function): *xuehai* (SP-10).
(JM) Illnesses of the genitourinary system: *qixue* (KI-13), *mingmen* (GV-4).

I. Kidney *(Shen)*

The kidney points also act on the ureters *(shou niao guan).*

> *The kidneys are the root of the original energy (yin), the home of the vitality. (Nei Jing, Ling Shu, Ch. 28)*

> *The kidneys are the storehouse of the sexual energy. . . . The left kidney is named* **shen,** *kidney. Males store their sexual energy here. (YXRM I, 77v)*

(It has been observed that the pulse of the left kidney is weak in impotent men and hard in those who are sexually hyperexcited.)

> *The right kidney is called* **ming men,** *the door of destiny. Through it women seal the seed.*

Ming men, the door of destiny, is also the name given to the part of the heart governor meridian corresponding to the sexual life.

> *Below,* **ming men** *is the prime minister of the kidney. Its vessels circulate in the intervals of the bladder . . . in fact,* **ming men** *is not a physical treasure organ in the same way as the triple warmer is not a physical workshop organ. . . .* **Ming men** *and its vessels descend between the anus and the genital organs and come out at the place of urination. This is the pathway outwards of the sexual energy.* **Ming men** *is the minister of unions; through it men form sperm and women detach the ovule. (YXRM I, 77v)*

> *The kidneys store the intent* **(zhi).** *They are the source of robustness and of male vitality, and for women of seductiveness (***zhi jiao:** *seductiveness, sex appeal). (DACH)*

> *Fear (which cures joy) injures (empties) the kidneys; their energy deflates and rises no longer. With excess fear the lower warmer swells and becomes full (the antidote to fear is sadness).*

> *The kidneys are stimulated in winter. They rule in autumn. (DACH)*

> *Renal congestion is more frequent in autumn and winter. (YXRM I, 21r)*

> *According to everyone, spasms come from the kidney; this is why we use this meridian in order to treat them. [The attack vessel,* **chong mai,** *is formed by the kidney points on the abdomen.] But Dan Xi considers that spasms come from the liver and have nothing to do with the kidney. (DACH VIII, 27v)*

The most effective points against spasms are the liver points *dadun* (LR-1) and *taichong* (LR-3); however, the best point against cramps is *chengshan* (BL-57).

> *The kidney responds to the energy of the earth, which generates water and fluids. (DACH I, 6v)*

> *Skin and body hair give life to the kidneys. The lungs give life to the skin and body hair. (DACH VIII, 2v)*

Europeans usually take into account three aspects of the urinary function relative to the kidney: filtration, excretion and secretion.

> *The superior renal nerves regulate the flow of water and the electrolytic disassociation of certain elements in the urine. The lower renal nerves rule the concentration of H-ions, the formation of ammonia and the elimination of acids and phosphates, which thus constitute the controlling agents for the internal function of the kidney. (Allinger and Hirt)*

Water and salts are separated from the blood by the glomeruli; the formation of the urine takes place in the other parts of the uriniferous tubes with the addition of other solid materials, such as urea.

The augmentation of filtration and secretion: 1) augmentation of the blood pressure in the renal artery either from an increase of the general blood pressure following excessive drinking or from an increase in the contraction of the heart; 2) dilation of the renal capillaries with the more active circulation of the blood, mostly in the glomeruli due to the relaxation (flaccidity) of the constricting motor fibers of the kidney and also of the splanchnic nerve (of the sympathetic system); 3) excess salt or sugar in the blood, generally from excess epinephrine, which blocks the production of insulin by the pancreas, which then stimulates the transformation of glucides into glycogen by the liver. Again, the epinephrine stimulates the transformation of the glycogen into sugar by the liver; 4) emotions, which often paralyze the sympathetic system, if repeated cause an increase in urination frequency and urgency: 5) cold.

Humans take in about three liters per day of liquid from drinks, vegetables, etc. They excrete one and a half liters through the urine, one liter through sweat and a half liter through the lungs. Humidity or dryness, cold or heat, exercise or rest cause these numbers to vary significantly.

Relation of organs:

The bladder is the yang workshop organ linked to the kidney (yin).

In illnesses of the kidney it is advisable to tonify the bladder and to harmonize the lower warmer (genitourinary function). (DACH XL, 10v)

The bladder precedes the kidney in the flow of energy. When the pulse of the kidney is deep, only slightly perceptible, which indicates abundant or frequent urine, disperse the bladder mainly at *jinggu* (BL-64), which gives amplitude and softness to the pulse of the kidney with diminished urine.

The heart, which is in danger when the kidney is ill, must be tonified. The tonification of the heart increases the urine but can elevate the blood pressure if the kidney is contracted (kidney pulse only slightly perceptible). The triple warmer must be harmonized if the kidneys are ill; the kidney must be tonified if the triple warmer is ill.

Lungs ill — slight problem for the kidney.

The water is the supreme yin; the kidneys are the root of accumulated water; the lungs are the branches of this. (DACH I, 6v)

In fact, it is advisable not to stop abundant urination too suddenly because this can cause congestive growths in the lungs. Reciprocally, in all congestive troubles of the lungs, positive results have been obtained by greatly increasing urination (tonify *fuliu*, KI-7, and *taixi*, KI-5, IS KI-3, and disperse *rangu*, KI-2, and *yongquan*, KI-1, according to the pulse).

The liver is also in slight danger when the kidneys are sick:

When the vessels of the five treasure organs are interrupted in the interior, the energy of kidney and liver is blocked in the interior (yin). Tonifying the kidneys and liver (yin) for an empty exterior (yang) fills up the full and empties the empty; it kills instead of cures. (DACH I, 14v)

The small intestine:

The flow of urine depending on the kidney depends on the small intestine and the lower warmer. (DACH VIII, 18v)

Paralysis of the nerves of the small intestine causes an afflux into it of liquid coming from the transudation of blood of the tissues.

The pancreas: we have seen reciprocal action of the adrenals and the pancreas. Insulin, when blocked by epinephrine, inhibits the adrenals.

In general:

Troubles and illnesses of the kidney (and bladder): *(JM) shenshu* (BL-23).
Kidney: *(JM, Fuji) sanjiaoshu* (BL-22), *tianshu* (ST-25).
The passage of the kidneys is *sanyinjiao* (SP-6): one puncture repeated six times. *(DACH I, 7v; Nei Jing)*
The action descending from the meridian of the kidney is obtained through *taichong* (LR-3). *(DACH)*
Keeps the humidity of the earth from seizing the kidney: *(DACH) taixi* (KI-5, IS KI-3).
Illnesses of the kidney, stomach, small intestine, liver: *(JM) weicang* (BL-45, IS BL-50).

The meridian of the kidney (zu shaoyin).

The kidneys are a yin treasure organ, the yang coupled workshop organ is the bladder. The meridian rises from the feet to the clavicle. The energy is at its maximum from 5 to 7 p.m.; it corresponds to the meridian of the large intestine, where the energy is at its maximum from 5 to 7 a.m.

Insufficiency of energy:

The pulse of the kidney is absent or without shape, soft, slightly perceptible (do not confuse it with the deep, "sunken" and tense pulse, without amplitude, which indicates an excess of energy). If the pulse is soft and without shape, but perceptible, the urine is uncolored and abundant. If it is soft but small, there is instability, either uncolored abundant urine or feeble urination, slightly abundant.

Physical symptoms: abundant urine, uncolored, frequent at night, sometimes with unusual odor; buzzing in the ears; headache at the vertex; heavy pain in the lumbar area and back; eyes without brightness; pale face, however the upper body energy abounds and the lower body is cold and empty; weakness; sensation of numbness of the bone and lack of suppleness.

Psychological symptoms: desire to close the door and stay alone, restlessness as if apprehensive or having forgotten an important duty; speech confused and troubled, energy chilled, yang paralyzed; dreams of floods, or trees and bushes in water, or being at the edge of a cliff, or emptiness.

Through the main meridian: tonify *fuliu* (KI-7) and *taixi* (KI-5, IS KI-3).

Through the herald point: *jingmen* (GB-25).

Through the circulation of energy: tonify the bladder (the mother nourishes) at *zhiyin* (BL-67) and the source point, *jinggu* (BL-64); tonify the heart governor (the child who suckles) at *zhongchong* (PC-9).

Through the coupled yang organ, tonify the bladder: *zhiyin* (BL-67).

Through the passage point: tonify *dazhong* (KI-6, IS KI-4).

Midday-midnight rule: kidney, maximum from 5 to 7 p.m. corresponds to the large intestine, maximum from 5 to 7 a.m. Tonify the latter at the hot, sunlit hours and in summer.

Husband-wife rule: governs the heart governor, *zhongchong* (PC-9) or *daling* (PC-7) according to the pulse.

Troubles from insufficiency of energy of the kidney:

Decline of the kidney, emptiness of the lumbar area, frequent need to urinate, wakes up at night, fatigue, consciousness tired: numerous moxa at *mingmen* (GV-4). *(DACH IV, 6r)*

(DACH III, 29v; Ju Ying) Decline of the kidney: a lot of moxa at *guanyuan* (CV-4).

(DACH IV, 2v; YIX I, 4v) Decline of the kidney: frequent urine, acute pain of the lumbar area: moxa *shenshu* (BL-23).

Weakness of the kidney, pain of the lumbar area: numerous moxas. *(YIX I, 5r)* Weakness of the kidney, extreme distress of the kidney which stops when walking: *shenshu* (BL-23). *(DACH IV, 7v)*

(DACH, YXRM) emptiness of the kidney; *(DACH X, 28r)* emptiness of the kidney, shivering in the sun: *shenshu* (BL-23); *(DACH)* emptiness of the kidney *zhonglüshu* (BL-29).

Old people — emptiness of the kidney, acute pain of the lumbar area: *(YXRM I, 46r)* *mingmen* (GV-4).

(DACH III, 29v; Ju Ying) emptiness and decline of the kidney: *daimai* (GB-26), *guanyuan* (CV-4), moxas in quantity.

Excess of energy of the kidney:

The pulse of the kidney will be hard and ample; or hard and contracted, deep, tense, slightly perceptible, "sunken"; or hard and small, contracted.

Physical symptoms: urine feeble, colored; anuria, pressing need; edema in the ankles; lower pelvis swollen; lumbar area and back contracted, stiff; pharynx painful, tongue dry, diarrhea during meals; cramps.

Psychological symptoms: as soon as one sits, there is a desire to stand up; dreams that it is difficult to undo one's belt or that the lumbar area and body are detached, not linked.

Through the main meridian: disperse *rangu* (KI-2) and *yongquan* (KI-1) and the source point, *taixi* (KI-5, IS KI-3).

Through the assent point: disperse *shenshu* (BL-23).

Assent point of the kidney, bladder, large intestine *(DACH)*: hip-*wushu* (GB-27).

Through the circulation of energy: disperse the bladder (the mother who nourishes) at *shugu* (BL-65), and the heart governor (the child who suckles) at *daling* (PC-7).

Through the linked yang organ: disperse the bladder at *shugu* (BL-65).

Through the passage point: disperse *dazhong* (KI-6, IS KI-4), or tonify *feiyang* (BL-58).

Midday-midnight rule: kidney, maximum from 5 to 7 p.m; corresponding to the large intestine, maximum from 5 to 7 a.m. Disperse the latter on sunlit, hot days, or in summer.

Husband-wife rule: disperse the heart governor at *daling* (PC-7).

Troubles from excess energy of the kidney:

Kidneys contracted, paralyzed: *(JM) dachangshu* (BL-25).

Congestion of the kidney: *(DACH) shenshu* (BL-23).

Accumulation of the kidney: *(DACH) yongquan* (KI-1); *(YXRM I, 46r) guanyuan* (CV-4).

A descending action of the kidney meridian is obtained through *taichong* (LR-3). *(DACH I, 7v)*

(DACH) Excess of the kidney, bladder, lower pelvis: *qihai* (CV-6).

Shock *(feng,* congestion) of the kidney, vertigo, blinded eyes see nothing. Under the eyes, red swelling called "water of shock," *feng shui*; can neither sleep nor eat. Coughing causes clear water to come out. Men: body heavy, cannot walk, yellowish urine; women: menses stopped, contractions. When there is abundance from shock, paresis and tightness of the knees and legs, cannot remain standing a long time: *rangu* (KI-2). *(YXRM I, 16v)*

Abscess from shock of the kidney: *(DACH XI, 8r) weizhong* (BL-54, IS BL-40), *sanyinjiao* (SP-6).

Pain of the kidney:

Energy of spasms and stiffness around the kidney: very frequent attacks. If the energy rises to the heart, death: *(DACH IV, 7r) guanyuan* (CV-4), *dadun* (LR-1).

Energy of the kidney attacking the heart: *(DACH IV, 7r) guanyuan* (CV-4), *daimai* (GB-26).

Nephritis, inflammation of the kidney.

Europe — acute nephritis: first oliguria, albuminuria, diminution of urea. Chronic nephritis (Bright's disease). Initial symptoms: frequent need to urinate, red cells or cylinders in the urine, pulse always rapid, sometimes facial edema, generally fingers numb, arm numb, jerks of the feet at night. Later, either interstitial chronic nephritis — small red contracted kidney, abundant uncolored urine, buzzings, nocturnal cramps, hypertension, dry skin, fetid breath, very slow development; or epithelial nephritis — big white kidney, smooth, begins with facial edema when awakened or pulmonary edema, dark diminished urine, pale skin, fetid breath.

> *Inflammation of the kidney (***shen zang yan***). Acute nephritis; origin: scarlet fever, measles, smallpox, chicken pox, purulent parotitis, typhoid fever, pneumonia, malaria, inflammation of the bladder, inflammation of the renal pelvis, influenza, burns, conception, intoxication.*

> *Symptoms: many have no fever; sometimes shivering and fever, acute pain in the area of the kidney, urinates blood, blood pressure increased, slight swelling, urine diminished going from scarlet to black, specific gravity increased (from 1020 to 1030); a lot of albumin (0.311; 5%), red cells in the urine; kidneys rounded.*

Treatment with needles:

shenshu (BL-23)	*8 fen,*
jingmen (GB-25)	*6 fen,*
sanjiaoshu (BL-22)	*8 fen,*
dachangshu (BL-25)	*1 cun,*
zhishi (BL-47, IS BL-52)	*8 fen,*
riyue (GB-24)	*5 fen,*
zhongwan (CV-12)	*8 fen,*
tianshu (ST-25)	*8 fen,*
guanyuan (CV-4)	*1 cun,*
sidu (TW-9)	*6 fen,*
xuanzhong (GB-39)	*6 fen. (JO, 26)*

Treatment with moxa:

shenshu (BL-23)	*10 moxas,*
sanjiaoshu (BL-22).	*10 moxas,*
jingmen (GB-25)	*10 moxas,*
riyue (GB-24)	*5 moxas,*
xuanzhong (GB-39)	*5 moxas. (JO, 26)*

Acute nephritis:

Treatment with needles and moxa:

tianshu (ST-25)	*.5 to 1 ***cun,*** 7 to 8 moxas,*
fujie (SP-14)	*.5 to 1 ***cun,*** 7 to 8 moxas,*
mingmen (GV-4)	*5 ***fen,*** 7 to 8 moxas,*
qihaishu (BL-24)	*1 to 2 ***cun,*** 7 to 8 moxas,*

dachangshu *(BL-25)*	*1 to 2* **cun**, *7 to 8 moxas,*
xiaochangshu *(BL-27)*	*1 to 2* **cun**, *7 to 8 moxas,*
zhibian *(BL-49, IS BL-54)*	*5* **fen**, *7 to 8 moxas,*
leg-**sanli** *(ST-36)*..............	*5* **fen**, *7 to 8 moxas,*
sanyinjiao *(P-6)*...............	*5* **fen**, *7 to 8 moxas.* *(JM, 318)*

Chronic nephritis: choose from among the points for acute nephritis. (JM, 319)

Inflammation of the kidney: *(JM)* guanyuan (CV-4), zhongwan (CV-12), *riyue* (GB-24), tianshu (ST-25), *jingmen* (GB-25), *qixue* (KI-13), *xuanzhong* (GB-39), senshu *(BL-23),* sanjiaoshu (BL-22), dachangshu (BL-25), zhishi (BL-47, IS BL-52).

Inflammation of the renal pelvis *(shen yu yan):*

*Origins: comes from small bacteria or from intoxication, influenza, or external lesion of the kidney; renal problems or illnesses, illnesses of heart, small pox, dysentery, exanthem **(dan du)**, pneumonia, typhoid, contagious illnesses, intoxication with carbon dioxide.*

Symptoms: acute inflammation — frequently the urinary passages give shooting pain, bad cold, headache, laziness of the whole body, frequent need to urinate, diminution of the quantity of urine which is troubled with traces of pus or blood; on the upper skin with small bubbles one can recognize blood cells or bleeding pieces or destroyed tissues. Chronic inflammation — acute pain from time to time, urination increased with symptoms analogous to those of acute inflammation. (JO, 27)

Treatment with needles:

shenshu *(BL-23)*......	*8* **fen,**
sanjiaoshu *(BL-22)*..	*8* **fen,**
dachangshu *(BL-25)*	*1* **cun,**
zhangmen *(LR-13)*...	*6* **fen,**
jingmen *(GB-25)*	*6* **fen,**
riyue *(GB-24)*	*6* **fen,**
daimai *(GB-26)*........	*6* **fen,**
shuidao *(ST-28)*.......	*8* **cun.** *(JO, 27)*

II. Bladder *(Pang Guang)*

The *Nei Jing* calls the bladder the Minister of the Rivers, the Treasury of the Excreted Liquids. The flow of urine coming from the kidney depends on the lower warmer and the small intestine *(DACH VIII, 18v)* (see pancreas). The kidney and bladder are stimulated in the winter *(YXRM I, 7v)*. The bladder is the yang workshop organ of the kidney (yin treasure organ). The bladder (left wrist) dominates the triple warmer (right wrist) but is put in danger by it; the bladder responds to nervous tension.

In illnesses of the bladder, it is advisable to clarify the energy of the lungs, which is the master *(DACH XI, 10r; Li Gao)* (midday-midnight rule). The bladder is not only considered as a reservoir; it activates or inhibits the renal function; emptiness of energy (soft pulse, slightly perceptible) — the bladder stops or slows down the filtration; to disperse it diminishes the urine. Fullness of energy (tense pulse) — it activates excretion and filtration; to tonify it makes one urinate.

(Europe) The lumbar sympathetic hypogastric nerves innervate the transverse fibers and the sphincter, which retains the urine. The sacral nerves innervate the vertical fibers, which expel the urine.

In general:
All illnesses of the bladder (and kidney): *(JM)* shenshu (BL-23).
Bladder: *(JM)* shenshu (BL-23).
Illnesses of the bladder: *(JM)* yaoshu (GV-2).

The meridian (shou taiyang).

Goes down the back and the external face of the lower limb. Energy at its maximum from 3 to 5 p.m.; corresponds to the lung, the maximum of which is from 3 to 5 a.m.

Insufficiency of energy of the bladder:

The pulse of the bladder abolished or soft, weak, without amplitude, without shape, proximal.

Physical symptoms: urine a little abundant and frequent, difficult to bend forward or backward; muscles of the feet contracted, hard of hearing to the point of deafness; sexual impotence; children have a lot of intestinal worms.

Psychological symptoms: habitual fear, decline, brain problems, lack of decision, of cleverness, of character.
Through the main meridian: tonify *zhiyin* (BL-67) and the source point *jinggu* (BL-64).
Through the circulation of energy: tonify the small intestine (the mother who nourishes) at *houxi* (SI-3) and the kidney (the child who suckles) at *fuliu* (KI-7).
Through the herald point: *zhongji* (CV-3).
For the coupled yin organ: tonify *fuliu* (KI-7).
Through the passage point: tonify *feiyang* (BL-58) and *weiyang* (BL-53, IS BL-39), secondary vessel of the bladder.
Midday-midnight rule: bladder, maximum from 3 to 5 p.m., corresponds to the lung, maximum from 3 to 5 a.m.
Husband-wife rule: tonify the triple warmer: hand-*zhongzhu* (TW-3).

Troubles from insufficiency of energy:

Cold of bladder: *(DACH, YXRM) shuidao* (ST-28).

Paralysis of bladder *(pang guang ma bi)*:

The paralyses of the bladder are anuria or cold micturition with pain in the belly and at the umbilicus. *(YXRM V, 28r)*

> **Pang guang ma bi.** *Origins: neurasthenia, illnesses or troubles of the spinal cord or of the brain; hysteria, intestinal typhus, pneumonia, cystitis, prostatitis, shortening of the urethra.*
>
> *Symptoms: urine does not flow at will, there are interruptions of flow without stopping. It comes either from a paralysis of the sphincter or from spasms of the muscles releasing the urine. In addition to total paralysis of the muscles releasing the urine, the urine is blocked; can either come from the production or emission of urine. (JO, 51)*

Treatment with needles:

mingmen *(GV-4)*	*4 fen,*
shenshu *(BL-23)*	*5 fen,*
tianshu *(ST-25)*	*8 fen,*
qihai *(CV-6)*	*8 fen,*
guanyuan *(CV-4)*	*1 cun,*
pangguangshu *(BL-28)*	*8 fen,*
qugu *(CV-2)*	*8 fen,*
zhongji *(CV-3)*	*8 fen. (JO, 51)*

Treatment with moxa:

qihai *(CV-6)*	*10 moxas,*
guanyuan *(CV-4)*	*10 moxas,*
zhongji *(CV-3)*	*10 moxas,*
pangguangshu *(BL-28)*	*10 moxas,*
dadun *(LR-1)*	*5 moxas. (JO, 51)*

> *Paralysis of the bladder: with needles —* **xiaochangshu** *(BL-27),* **dachangshu** *(BL-25),* **pangguangshu** *(BL-28), the four sacral hollows (***baliao***, BL-31 to BL-34),* **zhongzhu** *(TW-3),* **fujie** *(SP-14),* **zhibian** *(BL-49, IS BL-54). With moxa — twelve each at the same points. Or alternatively:* **chengfu** *(BL-50, IS BL-36),* **huiyang** *(BL-35),* **changqiang** *(GV-1),* **yinmen** *(BL-51, IS BL-37), the four sacral hollows (***baliao***, BL-31 to 34), and if of a nervous nature add:* **tianshu** *(ST-25),* **fengchi** *(GB-20),* **mingmen** *(GV-4),* **sanyinjiao** *(SP-6). With moxa: eight moxas on the same points. (JM, 319)*

Paralysis of the bladder: *(JM) tianyuan* (LU-9), arm-*xialian* (LI-8), arm-*shanglian* (LI-9), *chize* (LU-5), *jiquan* (HT-1), *dabao* (SP-21), *qihai* (CV-6), *zhongji* (CV-3), *qixue* (KI-13), *henggu* (KI-11).

Excess energy of the bladder:

The pulse of the bladder is hard, ample, long, big. If hard and small, there is an urgent and frequent need to urinate. If hard and round, there are stones. If like a wire, hard and without amplitude in old people: prostatitis. If hard, ample and contracted in women: cystitis and general colibacillus.
Physical symptoms: urine troubled, particles, urgent or abundant micturition, or difficult with little result. In excess, there is retention or incontinence.

Psychological symptoms: oppressiveness, agitation, fullness, desire for sleep, not eating, excessive decision making, cleverness of character.

Through the main meridian: disperse *shugu* (BL-65) and the source point, *jinggu* (BL-65).

Through the assent point: *pangguangshu* (BL-28).

Through the circulation of energy: disperse the small intestine (the mother who nourishes) at *xiaohai* (SI-8), and the kidney (the child who suckles) at *rangu* (KI-2) and *yongquan* (KI-1).

Through the passage point: tonify *dazhong* (KI-6, IS KI-4).

Through the coupled organ: disperse the kidney at *rangu* (KI-2) and *yongquan* (KI-1).

Midday-midnight rule: the bladder, maximum from 3 to 5 p.m., corresponds to the lung, maximum from 3 to 5 a.m.

Husband-wife rule: disperse the wife, triple warmer, at *tianjing* (TW-10).

Problems from excess energy:

Heat:

Heat of the bladder meridian: *(YXRM) fuxi* (BL-52, IS BL-38).

Heat of the meatus: *(DACH) huiyin* (CV-1).

Heat, occlusion, cannot urinate; *(DACH, YXRM)* thigh-*wuli* (LR-10).

Energy:

Energy from the bladder: disperse *rangu* (KI-2), *xiaxi* (GB-43).

Pain from energy of the bladder: *(DACH VII, 33r) zhaohai* (KI-3, IS KI-6).

Spasms:

Spasms of the bladder: *(JM) henggu* (KI-11); *(YXRM I, 40r) rangu* (KI-2), *xiaxi* (GB-43); *(JM) shenshu* (BL-23).

Bladder twisted, cannot urinate: *(DACH) zhongji* (CV-3), *yongquan* (KI-1).

Bladder twisted, urine not passing, occlusion: *(YXRM) guanyuan* (CV-4).

Cystitis, inflammation or catarrh of the bladder (pang guang yan, bai zhuo):

Bai zhuo, "white impurities": name of an illness which starts with an inflammation of the bladder. Distinguish the acute from the chronic types. 1) Acute: bad cold, attack of heat; slow, very difficult urination. There is a mixture of pus, white fluid and blood. 2) Chronic: the illness is comparatively light but also comparatively difficult to cure completely. (Ci Yuan, "Bai-zhuo")

Cystitis *(bai zhuo): (DACH) guanyuan* (CV-4); *(YXRM) xingjian* (LR-2); *(DACH) rangu* (KI-2), *xinshu* (BL-15).

Pang guang yan: inflammation of the bladder. Origin: urethritis, prostatitis, intestinal typhus, dysentery, pneumonia, inflammation of the spinal cord, tuberculosis of the spinal cord, stones in the bladder, intestinal worms, swelling and pruritis, tuberculosis or inflammation of the neighboring organs.

Symptoms: in acute inflammation of the bladder the area is very painful; frequent need to urinate accompanied with heat; urine troubled or even bloody, acid. Threads of the superficial skin of the bladder and small traces of pus are floating in the urine. We notice red blood cells. In chronic inflammation of the bladder there are the same symptoms but reduced. If there is inflammation of the pelvis with decomposed skin in the pus, the prognosis is serious. (JO, 29)

Treatment with needles:

qihai (CV-6)	*8 fen,*
guanyuan (CV-4)	*1 cun,*
pangguangshu (BL-28)	*8 fen,*
shenshu (BL-23)	*8 fen,*
dachangshu (BL-25)....	*1 cun,*
dahe (KI-12)	*1 cun,*
sanyinjiao (SP-6)	*6 fen,*
ciliao (BL-32)	*8 fen,*
shuidao (ST-28)	*1 cun,*
leg-sanli (ST-36)	*1 cun. (JO, 29)*

Treatment with moxa:

guanyuan (CV-4)	*10 moxas,*
dahe (KI-12)	*10 moxas,*

shuidao (ST-28)..	*10 moxas,*
shenshu (BL-23).	*7 moxas,*
ciliao (BL-32)	*7 moxas,*
leg-sanli (ST-36)	*7 moxas. (JO, 29)*

Catarrh of the bladder *(pang guang jia da er):*

Treatment with needles and moxa:

*the four sacral hollows **baliao**, (BL-31 to BL-34)*	*2 **cun**, 15 moxas,*
***dachangshu** (BL-25)*	*2 **cun**,*
***pangguangshu** (BL-28)*	*5 **fen**,*
***yaoyan** (guiyan,* MP-29b)...................................	*5 **fen**,*
***chengfu** (BL-50, IS BL-36)*...............................	*3 to 6 **fen**,*
***huiyang** (BL-35)*	*3 to 6 **fen**,*
***yinmen** (BL-51, IS BL-37)*................................	*3 to 6 **fen**,*
*leg-**sanli** (ST-36)*	*3 to 6 **fen**,*
***daheng** (SP-15)*	*1 to 1.5 **cun**. (JM)*

Catarrh of the bladder (cystitis):

(JM) qugu (CV-2); *(GSdeM) zhongji* (CV-3); *(JM) qihai* (CV-6), *henggu* (KI-11), *shuidao* (ST-28), hip-*juliao* (GB-28, IS GB-29), *zhangmen* (LR-13), *rangu* (KI-2), *zhongfeng* (LR-4), *pangguangshu* (BL-28), *zhibian* (BL-49, IS BL-54).

Feeble urination, inflamed, blood, swelling: *(YXRM) qugu* (CV-2).

Stones, lithiasis *(shi lin, sha lin).*

The distinction between kidney or gallbladder lithiasis is not clearly indicated. Hematuria is divided into "beginning" (urethritis), "finishing" (gallbladder) and "total" (kidney).

> **Shi lin,** *"stone urethritis." One of the five urethrites, has stones and sand in the urine. The penis is stiff and painful. (YXRM V, 28r)*

Sha lin, "sand urethritis." The more frequently used term for urine which leaves a deposit of brick-colored sand.
It is first treated through the general points for the five types of urethritis: *xuehai* (SP-10), *qihai* (CV-6), *rangu* (KI-2), *qugu* (CV-2). The pain is lessened through *kunlun* (BL-60), *shenshu* (BL-23), *zhongji* (CV-3).
Stone urethritis: *(DACH) guanyuan* (CV-4).
Urine stones: *(YXRM) guanyuan* (CV-4); *(DACH, YXRM) qichong* (ST-30).

Sand urethritis: *(YXRM I, 40r)* disperse *yinlingquan* (SP-9), leg-*sanli* (ST-36); *(GSdeM)* tonify *fuliu* (KI-7), *taixi* (KI-5, IS KI-3), disperse *qichong* (ST-30).

Sand urethritis, spasms from energy of the bladder: *xiaxi* (GB-43), *rangu* (KI-2).

Colic nephritis *(shen shi shan tong):*

Treatment with needles and moxa:

***pangguangshu** (BL-28)*	*1.5 to 2 **cun**, 10 moxas,*
***xiaochangshu** (BL-27)*.....................	*1.5 to 2 **cun**, 10 moxas,*
***baohuang** (BL-48, IS BL-53)*	*1.5 to 2 **cun**, 10 moxas,*
***zhibian** (BL-49, IS BL-54)*.................	*1.5 to 2 **cun**, 10 moxas,*
***fujie** (SP-14)*	*2 **cun**, 10 moxas,*
*leg-**sanli** (ST-36)*	*5 **fen**, 10 moxas,*
*leg-**shanglian** (ST-37, IS **shangjuxu**)*	*5 **fen**, 10 moxas. (JM, 319)*

Colic nephritis: *(GSdeM)* ten moxas hourly at *yongquan* (KI-1), *taixi* (KI-5, IS KI-3), *kunlun* (BL-60), leg-*sanli* (ST-36).

III. Prostate, Prostatitis *(She-Hu-Xian Yan)*

Origin: urethritis, external lesion, inflammation of the neighboring organs, inflammation of the bladder, narrowing of the ureters **(niao dao),** *excess coitus, onanism, etc.*

Symptoms: 1) Acute prostatitis: scrotal area weighted down, heavy with pruritis, troubles from heat, pain when sitting or kneeling. A little after the urge to urinate, heaviness comes, the urine is blocked and if it arrives it is accompanied by heat. 2) Chronic prostatitis: pain and heaviness of the scrotal area, feeling of pruritis, slight pain when urinating, urine troubled and milky; the prostatic fluid flows and comes out. (JO, 31)

Treatment with needles:

guanyuan *(CV-4)...*	1 **cun,**
dahe *(KI-12)*..........	1 **cun,**
changqiang *(GV-1)*	6 **fen,**
fuliu *(KI-7)*............	3 **fen,**
dadun *(LR-1)*.........	2 **fen.** *(JO, 31)*

Treatment with moxa:

qugu *(CV-2)*...........	10 *moxas,*
dahe *(KI-12)*	10 *moxas,*
changqiang *(GV-1)*	15 *moxas,*
dadun *(LR-1)*	5 *moxas. (JO, 31)*

Prostatitis: *(JM, Dr. Nakayama)* moxa at *yangchi* (TW-4); *(JM) guanyuan* (CV-4). *(GSdeM)* Disperse *guanyuan* (CV-4), *zhongji* (CV-3) and *qugu* (CV-2); tonify *yangchi* (TW-4); disperse *xuehai* (SP-10).
Urethritis from energy *(qi lin),* urine slowed down, rough, there is always a little left, flows in drops: *(YXRM I, 40r) xuehai* (SP-10); *(DACH X, 8r) yinlingquan* (SP-9); *(DACH) jiaoxin* (KI-8), *shimen* (CV-5), *guanyuan* (CV-4); *(DACH)* with abdominal pain: *shiguan* (KI-18).

IV. Urethra, Urethritis *(Niao Dao),* ''Route of Urine''

It is the passageway for the emission of the urine. Communicates with the bladder. (Ci Yuan, ''Niao-dao'')

The ureter, **niao guan,** *must not be confused with the urethra,* **niao dao.** *(Ci Yuan, ''Niao-guan'')*

In general:
Urethra: *(JM) shenshu* (BL-23).

Pains:
Pains of the urethra: *(YXRM) zhongji* (CV-3).

Paralysis:
Paralysis of the urethra: *(JM) shenmen* (HT-7).

Urethritis, inflammation of the urethra *(lin, niao dao yan):*

Name of an illness of the reproductive system. There is poisoning from pathogenic microbes which can be transmitted. The urethra is injured, damaged; pus is mixed with the urine and comes out. (Ci Yuan, ''Lin'')

Also called **lin.** *In those who are attacked, the urethra* **(niao dao)** *is swollen and inflamed. The urine is difficult and rough, and comes out mixed with pus. It comes from unclean sexual union. The chronic form is not very painful and the pus is only slightly present, scant, not very thick. In the acute form, pus abounds with a yellow-green color; if serious, it contains blood. During micturition, there is violent pain. In the past, five types of urethritis were described. The cases where the urine was difficult and rough were called urethritis from energy* **(qi lin);** *there is always something left (prostatitis?). Stone urethritis* **(shi lin)** *or sand urethritis* **(sha lin):** *pain in the middle of the penis, the urine cannot come out quickly (lithiasis, gallstones). Fatty urethritis* **(gao lin):** *urine like grease and coming out by itself. Urethritis from tuberculosis* **(lao lin):** *exhaustion from tuberculosis and pain leading the energy to attack the bottom. Bloody urethritis* **(xue lin):** *heat comes by attacks; if serious, blood is urinated. (Ci Yuan, ''Lin'')*

There is added:

> *Urethritis from heat (re lin), with extreme pain and painful contractions; urethritis from cold (leng lin), which comes after a cold. The urine is rough, the meatus is swollen and painful. For all patients, stop wine and meat. When there is thirst and anuria . . . the heat is in the upper warmer; it depends on the energy. When there is no thirst with anuria . . . the heat is in the lower warmer; it depends on the blood. (YXRM V, 28r)*

> **Lin ji,** *illness of urethritis. Origin: the cause is a contagion from "poisonous spherical microbes from urethritis" (staphylococcus, gonococcus).*

> *Symptoms:*

> *1) Acute urethritis in men: the orifice of the urethra is attacked from time to time by pruritis. Between micturitions, pus comes out from the meatus; frequent desire to urinate with acute pain on urination.*

> *2) Chronic urethritis in men: same symptoms as for acute urthritis, but the pain is less. On urinating, a pasty fluid is emitted. The urine is troubled with threads from urethritis.*

> *3) Acute urethritis in women: from the meatus or the [lower] external orifice of the uterus a pasty material with pus is emitted; the mucosa of the vagina and of the vulvar lips is scarlet and swollen. A pasty material with pus is emitted. There is pruritis and extreme pain.*

> *4) Chronic urethritis in women: the neck of the uterus is pasty and oozes. There are attacks of pain in the lower pelvic area.*

Treatment with needles:

qihai (CV-6)	*1 cun,*
shimen (CV-5)	*1 cun,*
qugu (CV-2)	*8 fen,*
dahe (KI-12)	*1 cun,*
yinlingquan (SP-9)	*5 fen,*
dadun (LR-1)	*2 fen. (JO, 28)*

Treatment with moxa:

zhongji (CV-3)	*7 times,*
qugu (CV-2) ...	*7 times,*
dadun (LR-1) ..	*5 times. (JO, 28)*

Urethritis *(lin qi):*

Treatment with needles and moxa:

tianshu (ST-25)	*5 fen, 5 to 8 moxas,*
the four sacral hollows: **baliao** *(BL-31 to BL-34)*	*2 cun, 5 to 8 moxas,*
daheng (SP-15)	*1.5 cun, 5 to 8 moxas,*
pangguangshu (BL-28)	*5 fen, 5 to 8 moxas,*
yaoshu (CV-20)	*5 fen, 5 to 8 moxas,*
chengfu (BL-50, IS BL-36)	*5 fen, 5 to 8 moxas,*
sanyinjiao (SP-6)	*5 fen 5 to 8 moxas. (JM, 319)*

The five types of urethritis: *(DACH, YXRM) dadun* (LR-1); *(YXRM) xuanzhong* (GB-39); *(DACH XI, 12r; X, 34r) sanyinjiao* (SP-6); *(YXRM I, 40r)* men and women: *xuehai* (SP-10); *(DACH)* and cannot urinate: *zhongfeng* (LR-4); *(DACH III, 26v) qihai* (CV-6); *(DACH, YXRM) guanyuan* (CV-4); *(DACH) henggu* (KI-11); *(DACH II, 32r) qihai* (CV-6), *xuehai* (SP-10); *(DACH II, 19r; YIX I, 4r; Ju Ying) henggu* (KI-11), *huangshu* (KI-16). *(DACH XI, 12r)* For the five types of urethritis: fill the umbilicus with powdered salt and burn seven large moxas on it, or moxas on *sanyinjiao* (SP-6). *(YXRM)* The five types of urethritis, micturition like fire: *fuliu* (KI-7).

Catarrh of the urethra:

(JM) rangu (KI-2); *(JM)* women: abdomen-*yinjiao* (CV-7).

Urethritis:

(JM) Arm-*shanglian* (LI-9), *dazhong* (KI-6, IS KI-4) *jiaoxin* (KI-8); *(YXRM) jinggu* (BL-64); *(DACH)* urethritis, *(YXRM)* women, urethritis: *zhaohai* (KI-3, IS KI-6); *DACH, YXRM) shuiquan* (KI-4, IS KI-5); *(JM) yingu* (KI-10);

(DACH, YXRM, JM) jimen (SP-11); *(JM) guangming* (GB-37), *lougu* (SP-7), *chengshan* (BL-57), *shenshu* (BL-23), *dachangshu* (BL-25); *(DACH, YXRM, JM) xiaochangshu* (BL-27), *ciliao* (BL-32); *(DACH) zhongliao* (BL-33); *(YXRM) zhongji* (CV-3); *(JM) henggu* (KI-11), *qugu* (CV-2).

Chronic urethritis: *(JM) changqiang* (GV-1).

Urethritis, fullness of abdomen, cannot urinate: *(YXRM) qichong* (ST-30).

Urethritis, rough urine, does not pass: *(YXRM) qugu* (CV-2).

Urethritis, pain in the lumbar area: *(YXRM) weiyang* (BL-53, IS BL-39).

Urethritis, urination rough: *(DACH VII, 33v) zhaohai* (KI-3, IS KI-6).

Urethritis, urinates blood without stopping, pain of the genitals: *(DACH VII, 34r) zhaohai* (KI-3, IS KI-6), *yingu* (KI-10), *yongquan* (KI-1), *sanyinjiao* (SP-6).

Rough urethritis, the urine does not pass: *(DACH VII, 33v) zhaohai* (KI-3, IS KI-6), *yinlingquan* (SP-9), *sanyinjiao* (SP-6), *guanchong* (TW-1), *hegu* (LI-4).

Blenorrhagia, gonorrhea (*xue lin*, "blood urethritis"):

> *Burning micturition. At the extreme, there is blood. (Ci Yuan, "Xue-lin")*

> *Urethritis of blood is painful and rough. There are sudden emissions of whitish material; at the end, thready or reddish matter. When the color is like bean curd, there is then inflammation of the bladder and kidney. When the color is clear, there is emptiness and heat of the heart. (YXRM V, 28r)*

Blood urethritis: *(YXRM I, 40r) yinlingquan* (SP-9), leg-*sanli* (ST-36); *(YXRM I, 46v) yongquan* (KI-1); *(YXRM I, 40r) xuehai* (SP-10); *(DACH) shimen* (CV-5), *(DACH III, 31r) zhongji* (CV-3).

Urethritis of blood, micturition like fire: *(DACH) fuliu* (KI-7).

Gonorrhea: *(JM, Dr. Nakayama)* moxa *yangchi* (TW-4).

Flow in the morning; *(JM) sanyinjiao* (SP-6), *dahe* (KI-12), *zhishi* (BL-47, IS BL-52).

V. Urine *(Niao, Ni)*

Quality, color, problems.

Uncolored, abundant:

Pulse of the kidney soft and without amplitude: *(GSdeM)* if usual, tonify *fuliu* (KI-7) and *taixi* (KI-5, IS KI-3). If in crisis, nervous discharges: tonify *taixi* (KI-5, IS KI-3) and *lieque* (LU-7).

Abundant urine in old people: *mingmen* (GV-4), *shenshu* (BL-23).

Relaxed and numerous urinations (nervousness): *(DACH)* disperse *lieque* (LU-7).

Frequent urination, gets up at night, decline of the kidney: *(DACH) mingmen* (GV-4).

Numerous urinations, decline of the kidney: *(DACH) shenshu* (BL-23).

Dark, not very abundant:

Pulse of the kidney hard, pointed, contracted: disperse *rangu* (KI-2) and *taixi* (KI-5, IS KI-3); tonify *shaochong* (HT-9); disperse *tianjing* (TW-10) if the pulse of the triple warmer is tight. Or use ten daily moxas at *yongquan* (KI-1).

Yellow urine (i.e., dark, orange):

Urine of a yellow color, illness of excess of the stomach meridian: *(DACH)* disperse *lidui* (ST-45).

Yellow urine: *(DACH) duiduan* (GV-26, IS GV-27), *taixi* (KI-5, IS KI-3), *geguan* (BL-41, IS BL-46), *hunmen* (BL-42, IS BL-47).

Yellow urine, swollen abdomen, fullness, cannot breathe: *(DACH) yingu* (KI-10).

Scarlet-yellow urine: *(DACH)* head-*wangu* (GB-17, IS GB-12), *zhibian* (BL-49, IS BL-54), *yishe* (BL-44, IS BL-49), *yaoshu* (GV-2).

Scarlet urine:

(DACH) qiangu (SI-2), *laogong* (PC-8), *xiawan* (CV-10), *qihai* (CV-6), *zhongji* (CV-3), *ciliao* (BL-32), *zhibian* (BL-49, IS BL-54), *pangguangshu* (BL-58).

Scarlet urine, disfluent: *(DACH) xiaochangshu* (BL-27).

Scarlet, difficult urine: *(YXRM) weizhong* (BL-54, IS BL-40).

Blue-black urine:

Blue-black urine: *(DACH) weishu* (BL-21).

Changing:

The color of the urine is transformed by acridity: *(DACH) taiyuan* (LU-9).

Problems:

See Cystitis: *(GSdeM)* disperse *zhongji* (CV-3), *qugu* (CV-2).

Phosphaturia: *(GSdeM)* tonify *xuanzhong* (GB-39), *zhongting* (CV-16), *gaohuang* (BL-38, IS BL-43).

Urine with many cloudy problems: *(DACH) zhangmen* (LR-13).

Urine not clear: *(DACH) shenshu* (BL-23).

Urine not clear with white clouds, difficult, painful: *(YXRM) zhongfeng* (LR-4).

Women — urine with white foam: *(DACH) xingjian* (LR-2).

Urethritis from fat *(gao lin),* "fatty urine," frequent urination: *(DACH XI, 6r) zhongji* (CV-3), *shenshu* (BL-23), *yinlingquan* (SP-9).

Bloody (hematuria, *ni xue*):

(DACH VIII, 35r) lieque (LU-7); *(DACH) xialian* (LI-8); *(JM, DACH) shenshu* (BL-23), *daling* (PC-7), *laogong* (PC-8), *xiawan* (CV-10), *guanyuan* (CV-4).

Blood in urine and stools: *(DACH) laogong* (PC-8).

Urine and blood in the intestines: *(DACH) guanyuan* (CV-4).

Urea — diminished: insufficiency of the liver; increased: insufficiency of the pancreas.

Problems upon urination:

Urine hot and painful: *(DACH, YXRM) lieque* (LU-7).

Micturition like fire, bloody urethritis (blenorrhagia): *(DACH) fuliu* (KI-7).

Urination difficult and painful with white foam: *(YXRM) xingjian* (LR-2).

Heat with urination *(DACH) fuxi* (BL-52, IS BL-38).

Insufficiency of urine (retention, anuria, oliguria).

Retention:

The bladder does not allow the evacuation of collected urine; swelling and pain from the lower pelvis and lower abdomen to the umbilicus; the urine which passes is not very different from normal. There is contracture of the sphincter or paralysis of the vertical muscles of the bladder (innervated by sacral nerves III, IV and V) which govern the expulsion, or contracture of the transverse muscles (lumbar sympathetic) which retain the urine, or prostatitis, etc. The vagus nerve (which relaxes the sphincter of the bladder and which activates intestinal peristalsis) can, because of its insufficiency, cause the sphincter not to relax, causing retention.

In summary: there will be either passive retention and excess repletion due to weakness of the expulsor muscles, resulting in excess urine flow; or active retention from spasms of the sphincter, allowing nothing to pass; the pain is intense; there is excess energy.

Need to urinate with no result; nothing passes; lower pelvis hard and full: disperse leg-*sanli* (ST-36).

Urge to urinate with no result; from perverse energy in the bladder, the liquid does not release. Either excess fatigue or energy from unhappiness have injured the bladder, then the energy is closed off and held. All twisted bladders in women come from this: *(DACH XI, 6r) qihai* (CV-6), *yinlingquan* (SP-9), *sanyinjiao* (SP-6); in addition, disperse *yingu* (KI-10) and *daling* (PC-7).

Twisted bladder *(zhuan bao);* cannot urinate: *(DACH)* disperse *zhongji* (CV-3), *yongquan* (KI-1).

(DACH) Bladder twisted, closed, blocked, urine does not pass; *(DACH)* occlusion, urine not passing; *(YXRM) guanyuan* (CV-4).

Water not passing; women: pain, hardness and fullness of the lower pelvis *(YXRM)*; energy of the bladder: *(YXRM I, 40r)* disperse *xiaxi* (GB-43) and *rangu* (KI-2).

Lower pelvis hard and full, need to urinate with no result; urine not passing: *(DACH)* disperse leg-*sanli* (ST-36).

Swelling of the belly radiating to the back; cannot breathe; the waterway is disfluent: *(YXRM) jingmen* (GB-25).

Difficult urination *(xiao bian nan):*

> *Paralysis of the bladder brings difficult urination with pain in the abdomen and umbilicus. (YXRM V, 28r)*

(DACH IV, 11r; YIX I, 11v*) lieque* (LU-7); *(DACH)* arm-*shanglian* (LI-9), *ququan* (LR-8), *yinbao* (LR-9), leg-*shanglian* (ST-37, IS *shangjuxu*), *weizhong* (BL-54, IS BL-40); *(YXRM) xingjian* (LR-2); *(YXRM)* leg-*xialian* (ST-39, IS *xiajuxu*), *qugu* (CV-2). With abdominal pain: *henggu* (KI-11), *daju* (ST-27); *(DACH, YXRM) guanyuanshu* (BL-26); with red urine: *(YXRM) pangguangshu* (BL-28).

Urine not passing; fullness of the secondary vessel from the kidney to the bladder: *(DACH) dazhong* (KI-6, IS KI-4).

Urine not passing: *(YXRM I, 46r) shenque* (CV-8); *(YIX I, 5v) daling* (PC-7), *yingu* (KI-10), *yinlingquan* (SP-9), *sanyinjiao* (SP-6), *qihai* (CV-6); *(DACH XI 9r) yinlingquan* (SP-9), *yingu* (KI-10); *(DACH VII, 33v) yinlingquan* (SP-9), *sanyinjiao* (SP-6), *hegu* (LI-4), *guanchong* (TW-1), *zhaohai* (KI-3, IS KI-6).

Anuria, oliguria:

The kidney no longer filters (see Kidney); little urine, darkened or stopped, kidney and lumbar area painful, abundant sweat. Tonifying the bladder activates the filtration of the kidney. (See above: Scarlet urine, useless, difficult).

> *Urine not passing; at the root, fullness and heat. The Classic says: The bladder is useless; this means a stoppage of functions* **(long).** *If the top of the nose is yellow, surely the urination is difficult. There is a binding from emptiness, from mucus, from energy. Emptiness, exhaustion, old illnesses have sweating without reason; the five interiors are dry. Mucus and saliva block and congest; the way of the energy no longer communicates . . . anger, unhappiness, energy, binding, closure . . . the kidney responds to the heart; if in the heart the fire abounds, then from heat the small intestine is bound and micturition is difficult. (YXRM V, 28v)*

Secretion is slowed down with a drop in the blood-pressure that stops at about 40 mm. Hg.

Particularly cures disfluent urination (and scarlet and rough urine): *(DACH XI, 5r) qihai* (CV-6).

Disfluent urination: *(DACH, YXRM) yinlingquan* (SP-9), *diji* (SP-8), *lougu* (SP-7), *sanyinjiao* (SP-6), *zhiyin* (BL-67), *yongquan* (KI-1); *(YXRM) ligou* (LR-5); *(DACH, YXRM)* leg-*sanli* (ST-36), *shaofu* (HT-8); *(YXRM) zhongji* (CV-3); and scarlet urine: *(DACH) xiaochangshu* (BL-27).

Little secretion passing from the bladder and the lower warmer: *(DACH) xiaochangshu* (BL-27).

Diminution of the urine: *(JM) dabao* (SP-21).

The six illnesses of the stoppage of urination: *(YXRM) guanyuan* (CV-4).

Stoppage of urination: *(YXRM) shimen* (CV-5).

Stoppage of the function *(long bi)* of urination: *(YXRM) ligou* (LR-5).

Chills, bound water: *(DACH) chengshan* (BL-57), *erjian* (LI-2).

Heat, occlusion, cannot urinate: *(DACH, YXRM)* thigh-*wuli* (LR-10). *ligou* (LR-5).

Urine closed off *(niao bi):*

Urine closed off *(niao bi)* to the excess; not passing: *(DACH)*

(DACH, YXRM) shaofu (HT-8), *ligou* (LR-5); *(JM) jiaoxin* (KI-8), *zhiyin* (BL-67), *yinbao* (LR-9); *(YXRM) dazhong* (KI-6, IS KI-4); *(JM) jimen* (SP-11), *houxi* (SI-3), *guanyuan* (CV-4), *shuidao* (ST-28), *daju* (ST-27), *shangliao* (BL-31), *ciliao* (BL-32), *xialiao* (BL-34), *baohuang* (BL-48, IS BL-53), *baihuanshu* (BL-30), *huiyin* (CV-1).

Water blocked, swelling, panting, hardness and pain under the ribs: *(YXRM) zhongwan* (CV-12).

Swelling of abdomen radiating into the back; cannot breathe; waterway disfluent: *(YXRM) jingmen* (GB-25).

Urine dark yellow; abdomen swollen; fullness, cannot breathe: *(DACH) yingu* (KI-10).

Urination or defecation insufficient or stopped: (see Blockage of function).

The frequency and abundance of urine can be caused either by an elevation of the blood-pressure, or increase of the volume of the blood from excess drinking, or from an insufficiency of energy of the kidney from paralysis, or insufficiency of the bladder, or from an irritation of the bladder, or from insufficiency of the energy of the small intestine, or from an excess of energy of the lung, or from prostatitis, or from insufficiency and inflammation of the pancreas, or from excess of pituitary gland, or from an irritation of the large intestine (intestinal worms).

Excess urination to the point of incontinence.

Excess quantity (volume):

Do not forget that the balance consists of 1500 ml. of urine each twenty-four hours for men (about 1200 ml. for women) with about one liter of sweat excreted through the skin and a half liter exhaled through the lungs. The sweat-urine ratio inevitably varies from summer to winter, from dry to humid countries, from central heating to a fire in the hearth. The average quantity of liquid drunk for this result is about one liter and must vary with the seasons and dry or humid climate.

The causes of excess urine are numerous:

1) Excess general arterial blood-pressure: disperse *shenmen* (HT-7) and *daling* (PC-7). Diminish the amount drunk. The urine is abundant and tends to be a little colored. Urination can be frequent but is not necessarily urgent except after a prolonged wait. There is excess filtration (hydruria) with normal excretion and secretion. There is excess of the blood volume from excess drinking or from excess cardiac energy.

2)   Relaxation of the renal capillaries from which comes an insufficiency of pressure and blood velocity into the renal vessels: renal stasis. Under the dependence of the vasomotor system of the kidney, the lumbar sympathetic system. The symptoms are the same as number 1. Tonify *shenshu* (BL-23) and *mingmen* (GV-4). *Fengchi* (GB-20) acts on the general sympathetic.

3)   Insufficiency of the function of the pancreas from inflammation or weakness. From insufficiency, the pulse of the pancreas is almost abolished; from inflammation it is big, long, hard and ample. There is often hypertension due to an excess of the adrenals or pituitary glands. The patient has an acid stomach mostly after jams and cakes; he digests chestnuts and beans poorly, and fats and meats as well, without noticing a problem. The quantity of lightly colored urine can be great. Disperse *yamen* (GV-14, IS GV-15) and if that is not enough, *fengfu* (GV-15, IS GV-16). For the pituitary disperse the interval between C6 and C7.

4)   ˙ The kidneys, as indicated by the pulse, which is soft, weak, without amplitude and without shape, are excessive in relation to the filtration function. That is, the renal capillaries are relaxed and in reality the energy of the kidney is insufficient. However, in such cases tonification of the kidney will increase the urine more. Moreover, it is necessary to clearly understand whether or not one kidney is in excess while the other is insufficient (see both sides of the kidney pulse). Disperse *taixi* (KI-5, IS KI-3).

5)   The excess of the pituitary can be translated into an excess of urine: disperse the interval of C6 and C7.

6)   Excess energy of the lung can cause an excitation of the kidney with frequent urination and a lot of urine. The pulse of the lungs is hard and ample or contracted. Disperse *chize* (LU-5), *lieque* (LU-7), *taiyuan* (LU-9).

7)   The ends of nervous crises generally translate themselves into a strong emission of uncolored urine. Tonify *lieque* (LU-7) and *yangchi* (TW-4).

8)   Irritation of the bladder can cause a summons to the kidneys and provoke abundant and colored urine. The pulse of the bladder is hard, large and tense. Disperse *zhongji* (CV-3) and *shugu* (BL-65), *jinggu* (BL-64) and *pangguangshu* (BL-28).

9)   "The flow of urine coming from the kidneys depends on the small intestine and the lower warmer." The sugars from the small intestine indeed have an important stimulating effect on the pancreas, the insulin of which blocks the adrenals (and the lumbar sympathetic system?). Insufficiency of the small intestine gives bluish lips with white edges and dry skin. Tonify *houxi* (SI-3) and *wangu* (SI-4).

10) Nervous people often have a heavy need to urinate just as they get ready to get into bed at the beginning of night. There is excess yang at the yin time. Tonify *lieque* (LU-7).

Frequency of urination.
(The frequency is generally linked to the urgency.)

1)   Inflammation of the bladder, cystitis (bladder catarrh). The need to urinate is constant but with very little quantity. The urine is colored and often cloudy; it holds threads in suspension which appear when a glass of the urine is held against a light. When the disease is serious there is an emission of blood mixed with the urine (no blood before or after urination). Colibacillosis is generally the cause. Disperse *zhongji* (CV-3), *qugu* (CV-2), and daily ten moxas.

2)   Irritation of the large intestine, often by worms, particularly oxyurids. For the large intestine disperse *sanjian* (LI-3), *hegu* (LI-4) and *erjian* (LI-2). For the intestinal worms tonify *zhiyin* (BL-67), *jinggu* (BL-64) and *qugu* (CV-2).

3)   In men, by congestion (or tumor) of the prostate. This usually occurs in the middle of the night. Disperse *guanyuan* (CV-4), *zhongji* (CV-3) and *qugu* (CV-2).

Chinese treatments:
Urine descending in torrents: tonify *yinlingquan* (SP-9), leg-*sanli* (ST-36).
Relaxed and numerous urinations: *(DACH)* *lieque* (LU-7).
Numerous small urinations of old people: *(DACH II, 29r)* *mingmen* (GV-4), *shenshu* (BL-23).
Abundant urinations from fullness of the lungs: *chize* (LU-5), *feishu* (BL-13).
Many small urinations: *(YXRM)* *guanyuan* (CV-4); *(DACH, YXRM)* *dadun* (LR-1), *chize* (LU-5).
Frequent and numerous urinations; emptiness of the lumbar area; decline of the kidneys; gets up at night, extreme oppressiveness tiring the consciousness: *(DACH IV, 6v)* *mingmen* (GV-4), a gold needle helps; moxas at *shenshu* (BL-23).

Frequent and numerous urinations, lower pelvic area cold and painful: *(DACH VII, 33r) zhaohai* (KI-3, IS KI-6), *sanyinjiao* (SP-6), *qihai* (CV-6), *guanyuan* (CV-4), *shenshu* (BL-23).

Thoughts of urination pressing and numerous: *(JM) zhongji* (CV-3).

Urination pressing and numerous: *(DACH) zhongji* (CV-3).

Frequent and numerous urination, seminal losses, cystitis: *(DACH VII, 34v) zhaohai* (KI-3, IS KI-6), *sanyinjiao* (SP-6), *taixi* (KI-5, IS KI-3), *guanyuan* (CV-4), *baihuanshu* (BL-30).

Frequent and numerous urinations, comes from cold of the bladder, urine cold and painful: *(DACH XI, 6r) zhongji* (CV-3), *shenshu* (BL-23), *yinlingquan* (SP-9); if not better *sanyinjiao* (SP-6), *qihai* (CV-6).

Incontinence of urine, enuresis.

The involuntary loss of urine, either in the day or at night, which is called incontinence, presents under different types and is attributed to various causes. The Chinese texts relating to these troubles are as follows:

> *Loss of perception of the bladder. It can come from intestinal worms causing an irritation. It is a frequent illness in children. Adults whose constitutions are declining and weakened are sometimes attacked.*
> *(Ci Yuan, "Yi-niao" [relaxation of the urine])*

> **Yi ni:** *this is* **yi niao.** *" (Chi Yuan, "Yi-ni")*

> *One no longer feels [the urination]. If there is fullness, then there is heat; the fire of the bladder is in movement; red [urine] is from heat. If there is emptiness, the energy of the kidney and bladder is empty; white [urine] is from emptiness. At night, when yin abounds, there is sometimes perspiration without reason. If there is internal empti-ness, there is humidity and heat (an excess of yang). If there is emptiness at the bottom and exhaustion of the inte-rior (both emptiness of yin) the bladder does not bind itself (does not close) and the urine flows by itself, or after urinating there is still some left. If there is always an abundance of fire, the water cannot remain peaceful. Those with fatigue of the heart or the spleen-pancreas have frequent and small urinations. One must either tonify the bladder and blood, or dissipate the fire. (YXRM V, 29v, "Xiao bian bu jin [uncontrolled urination]"*

Moreover, it is advisable to differentiate:

1) Losses of urine in daytime when laughing, coughing or having waited too long. They generally indicate a weakness of the sphincter and of the transverse fibers (see 6 below).

2) Continuous daytime losses; flaccid paralysis of the sphincter or lesion of the terminal cones: tonification of the sphincter can cure this (see 6 below).

3) Nocturnal incontinence in children (enuresis). Most often from intestinal worms (see 5 below), or from fear of the dark and nervousness (see 8 below), or muscular weakness of the sphincter (see 6 below). However, the insufficiency of the pancreas from the abuse of sugar is frequent as well as excessive drinking. Drink only a total of a half liter and keep from drinking in the afternoon.

For Europeans, the causes of incontinence can be:

1) The lesion of the terminal cone of the spinal cord (sacral nerves III, IV and V), for which acupuncture can only attempt to awaken some supplementary energy through tonification of *zhibian* (BL-49, IS BL-54), *baohuang* (BL-48, IS BL-53), and *baihuanshu* (BL-30).

2) Excess consumption of liquids (more than a liter daily, less in winter, a little more in summer or very dry coun-tries).

3) General hypertension: disperse *shenmen* (HT-7), *daling* (PC-7).

4) Dilation and relaxation of the renal capillaries, which depend on the lumbar sympathetic nerves: tonify *san-jiaoshu* (BL-22) and *shenshu* (BL-23).

5) Irritation from intestinal worms, particularly oxyurids. Give a vermifuge for three days after the new moon. Tonify *zhiyin* (BL-67), *jinggu* (BL-64) and *quchi* (LI-11), twenty moxas daily.

6) Relaxation of the transverse fibers and of the sphincter of the bladder, which retains the urine and which depends upon the lumbar sympathetic nerves: tonify *sanjiaoshu* (BL-22), *shenshu* (BL-23), and *yanglingquan* (GB-34).

Excess energy or spasm of the vertical fibers, which expel and which depend on sacral nerves III, IV and V: disperse *pangguangshu* (BL-28), *zhonglüshu* (BL-29), *baihuanshu* (BL-30), *zhongliao* (BL-33), *xialiao* (BL-34), *dadun* (LR-1).

7) Insufficiency of the pancreas, either from inflammation (disperse *yamen,* GV-14, IS GV-15) and *fengfu* (GV-15, IS GV-16); or from weakness: tonify *dadu* (SP-2) of the right foot and *taibai* (SP-3) of the right foot.

8) Fear of the night. The child awakens from emotional distress and the bladder empties: tonify *zhongchong* (PC-9) and *baihui* (GV-19, IS GV-20). Also, the child often cries at night.

Nervous, emotional children generally wet their beds in the beginning of the night; a small light calms them.

9) Weakness of the sphincter can come from a lymphatic condition or general weakness: tonify foot-*linqi* (GB-41), *gaohuang* (BL-38, IS BL-43), leg-*sanli* (ST-36), *yanglingquan* (GB-34) and *sanyinjiao* (SP-6), with twenty daily moxas at leg-*sanli* (ST-36), foot-*linqi* (GB-41) and *yanglingquan* (GB-34).

The treatments indicated in the Far East are as follows:

Illness of urinating at night, small children: *(JM, 319) huiyin* (CV-1) and *huiyang* (BL-35), 1 to 3 *fen.* With moxa: *sanyinjiao* (SP-6) and *pangguangshu* (BL-28), five moxas.

Incontinence of urine in children: *(JM) sanyinjiao* (SP-6).

Loss of urine, loss of control: *(YXRM I, 46r)* disperse (tonify?) *hegu* (LI-4) and *taichong* (LR-3).

Urination uncontrolled without the patient knowing it: *(DACH) yinlingquan* (SP-9), tonify.

Uncontrolled urination: *(DACH X, 34r) yanglingquan* (GB-34) and *yinlingquan* (SP-9).

Uncontrolled loss of urine *(YXRM);* loss of urine *(DACH): yinbao* (LR-9).

Incontinence and loss of urine without measure: *taiyuan* (LU-9).

Uncontrolled urination: *(DACH)* leg-*sanli* (ST-36); *(DACH) yinbao* (LR-9), *quanyuan* (CV-4).

Loss of urine: *(DACH, YXRM) tongli* (HT-5), *shaofu* (HT-8); *(DACH) jimen* (SP-11), *weizhong* (BL-54, IS BL-40), *sanyinjiao* (SP-6), *zhongfeng* (LR-4), *taichong* (LR-3); *(JM) guanmen* (ST-22), *dachangshu* (BL-25), *xiaochangshu* (BL-27), *pangguangshu* (BL-28), *changqiang* (GV-1).

Nocturnal spasms, urinates at night, insufficiency of yin: *(GSdeM) zhaohai* (KI-3, IS KI-6).

Incontinence of urine (Dabry): *yinlingquan* (SP-9), *weizhong* (BL-54, IS BL-40), *chengshan* (BL-57) *pangguangshu* (BL-28).

Involuntary evacuation of urine (Dabry): *yinlingquan* (SP-9), *taichong* (LR-3), *dadun* (LR-1), *xingjian* (LR-2), *yangfu* (GB-38), *chengshan* (BL-57), *yuji* (LU-10), *shimen* (CV-5).

Chapter XIV

The Form

I. Height — II. Thinness — III. Obesity — IV. Bone Marrow — V. Bone — VI. Vertebral Column — VII. Muscles — VIII. Hair, Nails, Body Hair

I. Height

Height, for Europeans, is directly related to pituitary activity. In order to cause growth, tonify the C7-C6 interval. According to the Chinese: tonify *dadu* (SP-2). Insufficiency of the spleen-pancreas meridian retards growth and development. Tonify it in order to attain the normal height.

(DACH) The spleen-pancreas meridian commands the form and flesh; *(GSdeM)* mostly the pancreas, right meridian.

(DACH) Feet and hands particularly small: *guangming* (GB-37).

II. Thinness

(DACH) Thinness: leg-*sanli* (ST-36), *weishu* (BL-21), *qihai* (CV-6); *(JM) zhiyang* (GV-8, IS GV-9); *(YXRM) naokong* (GB-19); *(JM) shenshu* (BL-23).

(DACH) Illness of thinness: *naokong* (GB-19).

(DACH) Progressive thinness: *xiawan* (CV-10); *(DACH III, 30v)* the same during cold days: *shenshu* (BL-23).

(DACH) Thinness in abundance; eats a lot and becomes thin; makes neither flesh nor skin: *lougu* (SP-7), *tianshu* (ST-25), *weishu* (BL-21), *pishu* (BL-20), *shenshu* (BL-23), *dachangshu* (BL-25).

(DACH) Thinness, can neither eat nor drink: *sanjiaoshu* (BL-22).

(DACH) Children, thinness, do not form flesh: *weishu* (BL-21).

(DACH) Children, thinness, big abdomen, shoulders and back without strength, four limbs lazy: moxa at *zhangmen* (LR-13).

(GSdeM) Thinness, emptiness, worn out: tonify *gaohuangshu* (BL-38, IS BL-43) and leg-*sanli* (ST-36).

(DACH) Thinness and exhaustion from shivering: leg-*sanli* (ST-36).

(DACH III, 29r) Thinness, oppressed panting: *xuanji* (CV-21).

(DACH) Thinness and tuberculosis: *shenshu* (BL-23); thinness and fatigue of the five types of tuberculosis; emptiness and fatigue from their seven lesions: leg-*sanli* (ST-36).

(DACH) Extraordinary thinness from *ge qi* (esophagospasm?): *shanzhong* (CV-17) and *qihai* (CV-6), tonify and moxas.

(DACH) Thinness of women after coitus near their menses: *qihai* (CV-6). From coitus near menses, thinness, cold and heat: *zhongji* (CV-3); from coitus near menses, thinness. *Zheng* and *jia* accumulations: *sanyinjiao* (SP-6).

(GSdeM) From excess pituitary, which activates dehydration and takes off fat: disperse C7, upper edge of the vertebra and *guangming* (GB-37).

(GSdeM) Thinness from non-retention of water: tonify *lougu* (SP-7).

III. Obesity

According to the Europeans, the hydration of fats and tissues is in inverse relation with pituitary activity: tonify C7. Take note of the rapid diminutions and augmentations of weight and volume; there are people who get fat while resting, and those who get thin from rest. The effects on these are weak and transitory.

(See metabolism of fatty emulsified substances operating in the capillaries through the internal function of the lungs.)

(GSdeM) Dispersing leg-*sanli* (ST-36) each evening can cause the loss of about a pound per week, but is very tiring; it diminishes the weight more than the volume.

(DACH) Swelling of the skin: leg-*sanli* (ST-36), disperse each morning.

(DACH) Obesity: *shaoshang* (LU-11).

(DACH) Causes the flesh to melt: moxa *zhangmen* (LR-13) a little, herald point of the spleen-pancreas; *(GSdeM)* deflates the abdomen, mostly by dispersing the right point.

(YXRM) Beware of the arms and hands becoming thin due to abuse of moxa at *jianyu* (LI-15).

(DACH) For thinness of the calf: disperse *chengjin* (BL-56).

(DACH) Rules the fat of the lower abdomen: *neiting* (ST-44) and foot-*linqi* (GB-41).

(DACH) Swelling obesity of the belly: *dachangshu* (BL-25).

(DACH) Either fattens or thins: *taiyuan* (LU-9), *juque* (CV-14), *chengman* (ST-20), *geshu* (BL-17).

(GSdeM) Women who become fat because the menses stop: tonify *fengchi* (GB-20, sympathetic system), *renying* (ST-9, thyroid), *hegu* (LI-4); disperse *tianzhu* (BL-10, parasympathetic), leg-*sanli* (ST-36), *zhaohai* (KI-3, IS KI-6); or tonify *shuiquan* (KI-4, IS KI-5), *sanyinjiao* (SP-6), *xuehai* (SP-10).

(DACH) Water energy acting in the skin: *shuifen* (CV-9), abdomen-*yinjiao* (CV-7), *shimen* (CV-5; *(GSdeM)* for all, thirty daily moxas.

Obesity of the breasts: insufficient pituitary gland, tonify C7.

IV. Bone Marrow

(DACH) Bone marrow cold: *shanglian* (LI-9); *(DACH)* with pain: arm-*shanglian* (LI-9) and leg-*shanglian* (ST-37, IS *shangjuxu*), *lingdao* (HT-4).

V. Bone

In general:

(DACH) The kidneys support the bone.

(DACH) Reunion of the bones: all illnesses of the bones are cured here: *dazhu* (BL-11).

(YXRM) Bones: *xuanzhong* (GB-39).

(JM) Illnesses of the bone: *shangliao* (BL-31).

Weakness:

(YXRM) Weakening of the bone: foot-*shangqiu* (SP-5).

Localized bony rarification, insufficient parathyroids: tonify at the C5 and C6 interval.

Cold:

(DACH) Cold of the bones: *fuliu* (KI-7).

(DACH IV, 11v; YIX I, 4v) Cold in the bone, ice cold in the bone marrow, patient goes to get warm near the fire: *lingdao* (HT-4).

(DACH) Cold in the bone marrow: arm-*shanglian* (LI-9).

Heat:

(DACH) Heat of the bones, energy from food: *bailao* (GV-13, IS GV-14 *dazhui*).

Pain, rheumatism:

(DACH VIII, 15v) Pain from energy or rheumatism *(bi)* of the bone, joint pain: *shangqiu* (SP-5).

Bone pain: *(DACH)* foot-*dadu* (SP-2), *taibai* (SP-3).

(YXRM) Bone pain, cold and heat: *geshu* (BL-17); the same with fever: *pangguangshu* (BL-28).

(YXRM) Bone pain, hot convulsions: *pishu* (BL-20), *pangguangshu* (BL-28).

(DACH III, 25r) Muscles in contracture *(luan)*, painful bones: *hunmen* (BL-42, IS BL-47); *(YXRM)* numbness of the bones, vomiting: *tinghui* (GB-2).

Pain of the bone of the lateral face of the calf (fibula): *(YXRM) fuyang* (BL-59).

(DACH) Acute pain of the bone of the lower limbs: *huantiao* (GB-29, IS GB-30), *fengshi* (GB-31), *yinshi* (ST-33).

Inflammation of bone or periosteum:

Periostitis: *(GSdeM) shangqiu* (SP-5).

Exostosis of the tarsal bone: *(GSdeM)* tonify *fuliu* (KI-7), disperse *shangqiu* (SP-5), *taichong* (LR-3), *kunlun* (BL-60).

Lateral malleolus red and swollen: *(GSdeM) shenmai* (BL-62).

Internal malleolus inflamed: *(GSdeM) zhaohai* (KI-3, IS KI-6).

(DACH IV, 11v) Acute pain of muscle and bone: *chize* (LU-5).

Abscess of bone:

(DACH) Serious attack of tubercular abscess of the bone: head-*qiaoyin* (GB-18, IS GB-11).

(DACH VIII, 13r) Abscess eroding the bone: foot-*shangqiu* (SP-5).

(DACH) Superficial abscess from energy of the bone: foot-*shangqiu* (SP-5).

Hot abscess in the calf reappearing from year to year: *xuehai* (SP-10) (osteomyelitis?).

(DACH XI, 18r) Tubercular abscess of the arm: *quchi* (LI-11).

Gu zheng (*zheng*, ''bone caries''): ''Diseases of the bone with rheumatic pain. *Gu zheng* is a sort of syphilitic cachexia.'' *(Wells Williams Dictionary)*

(DACH X, 24v) *Gu zheng* transmitted from a cadaver, paresis of the lungs: *gaohuangshu* (BL-38, IS BL-43), *feishu* (BL-13), *ganshu* (BL-18), *danshu* (BL-19).

(DACH) Gu zheng, heat from tuberculosis: *danshu* (BL-19).

(DACH XI, 14v) The seven lesions of the five types of tuberculosis; emptiness of energy, weakness of the blood, *gu zheng:* tides of heat, cough, mucus, thinness: *geshu* (BL-17), *ganshu* (BL-18), *gaohuangshu* (BL-38, IS BL-43).

Gu zheng: (DACH, YXRM) peishu (BL-13), *geshu* (BL-17), *danshu* (BL-18), *lidui* (ST-45), *shenshu* (BL-23).

(DACH II, 25v) Gu zheng in children: *yinxi* (HT-6).

(DACH) Gu zheng transmitted from a cadaver: *gaohuangshu* (BL-38, IS BL-43).

Deformations:

(DACH) Tortoise-chest in children: *waiqiu* (GB-36).

VI. Vertebral Column *(Ji Zhu)*

Acts on the cervical vertebrae: *(GSdeM) qianding* (GV-20, IS GV-21).

Acts on the dorsal vertebrae: *(GSdeM)* head-*wuchu* (BL-5).

Acts on the lumbar and sacral vertebrae: *(GSdeM) weizhong* (BL-54, IS BL-40).

Deviations:

Illness of curvature of the vertebral column. (Ci Yuan, ''Yu-liu'')

Yu: scoliosis; *liu:* kyphosis.

(YXRM VI, 16r) Comes from birth, or having been made to sit up too early, etc.

(DACH VI, 11v) Puncture at *lianquan* (CV-23), *quanliao* (SI-19) or *ruzhong* (ST-17) risks causing deviations. *Yuji* (LU-10) brings them back.

(DACH III, 29r) Deviations *(yu liu): fengchi* (GB-20), *xuanzhong* (GB-39), *feishu* (BL-13).

(JM) Illness of deviation of the spine: *kunlun* (BL-60), *jinggu* (BL-64).

(YXRM) Deviation of the spine *(yu liu),* nape and back; *(DACH)* deviation of the spine *(yu liu)* with weakness of the muscles; does not come back: *fengchi* (GB-20).

(JM) Deviation of the spine in children: *waiqiu* (GB-36).

(DACH X, 29v) Deviation of the spine *(yu liu),* lumbar and back: *fengchi* (GB-20), *feishu* (BL-13).

(DACH III, 29r) Deviation *(yu,* scoliosis) and paralysis *(wei): quchi* (LI-11), *shuigou* (GV-25, IS GV-26, *renzhong)* disperse; *(DACH IV, 44r)* cannot lie face down.

(DACH IV, 4r) Deviation *(liu,* kyphosis): *fengchi* (GB-20), *xuanzhong* (GB-39).

(YIX I, 5r) Deviation *(liu,* kyphosis), cannot straighten: tonify *quchi* (LI-11), disperse *xuanzhong* (GB-39).

(DACH IX, 15r; YXRM I, 46r) Tortoise back *(gui bei)* in children: *feishu* (BL-13); *(YXRM VI, 16r) feishu* (BL-13), *geshu* (BL-17) from three to five large moxas.

(GSdeM) Lumbar vertebrae deviated forwards: curved (lordosis); think of the greater psoas muscle: disperse the point *yangshi* (LR-12, IS *jimai).*

(YIZ, 43v) Lumbar area curved, cannot straighten: *shuigou* (GV-25, IS GV-26 *renzhong).*

Vertebral pain (ji):

In general:

(DACH II, 29r) Vertebral pain: *shenzhu* (GV-11, IS GV-12); *(YIZ, 45r) shuigou* (GV-25, IS GV-26 *renzhong); (JM) zhangmen* (LR-13).

(DACH II, 29r) Vertebral and shoulder pain; *(JM)* neuralgia of the lumbar area, back and scapula: hip-*wushu* (GB-27).

(DACH) Vertebral pain, muscles in contracture: *weishu* (BL-21).

(YXRM) Vertebral pain, abdominal pain: *chengshan* (BL-57).

(DACH VI, 15v) Acute pain in the vertebrae behind the heart: *guanchong* (TW-1).

(DACH III, 32r) Intervals between the vertebrae behind the heart: hand-*zhongzhu* (TW-3).

Cervical vertebrae:

Pain of the seventh cervical vertebra: *(DACH) shuigou* (GV-25, IS GV-26 *renzhong); (GSdeM) houxi* (SI-3).

Dorsal vertebrae:

(JM) Neuralgia of the dorsal vertebrae: head-*wuchu* (BL-5), *jinsuo* (GV-7, IS GV-8), *weizhong* (BL-45, IS BL-50).

Lumbar vertebrae:

(JM) Neuralgia of the lumbar vertebrae: *shangliao* (BL-31), *zhibian* (BL-49, IS BL-54), *baohuang* (BL-48, IS BL-53); *(YXRM I, 46r) dachangshu* (BL-25); *(DACH) zhiyang* (GV-8, IS GV-9).

(DACH III, 30v) Pain of the bottom of the lumbar vertebrae: *kunlun* (BL-60).

(DACH) Rheumatism *(bi)* from cold in the lumbar vertebrae: *shenmai* (BL-62).

(DACH) Acute pain and cold of the lumbar vertebrae: *zhangmen* (LR-13), and cannot rest for a long time: *baihuanshu* (BL-30).

(DACH) Pain in the lumbar area radiating into the vertebrae, can neither bend nor straighten, cannot sit or stand up: *fuliu* (KI-7).

(YXRM) Pain and stiffness of the lumbar vertebrae radiating into the abdomen: *heyang* (BL-55); *(DACH) chize* (LU-5).

(YXRM, DACH) Pain and stiffness of the lumbar vertebrae, can neither bend forward nor straighten: *sanjiaoshu* (BL-22).

Sacrum:

(JM) Acute pain of the sacral area, neuralgia of the sacrum: *baihuanshu* (BL-30), *xiaochangshu* (BL-27), *pangguangshu* (BL-28).

Stiffness, contracture of the vertebrae:

(DACH) Stiffness of the vertebral column, whole body painful, cannot twist: *yamen* (GV-14, IS GV-15).

Stiffness of the vertebral column: *feishu* (BL-13); *(YXRM) shiguan* (KI-18), *geguan* (BL-41, IS BL-46).

(DACH III, 30v) Pain and stiffness of the vertebrae: *shuigou* (GV-25, IS GV-26 *renzhong*).

(YXRM) Stiffness and tightening of the lumbar vertebrae: *shendao* (GV-10, IS GV-11), *pishu* (BL-20), *geshu* (BL-17), *pangguangshu* (BL-28), *zhishi* (BL-47, IS BL-52), *yinmen* (BL-51, IS BL-37).

(DACH) Stiffness and tightness of the dorsal and lumbar vertebrae, can neither bend forward nor straighten: *shentang* (BL-39, IS BL-44).

(YXRM) Women — tightened vertebrae: *zhigou* (TW-6).

(YIX I, 4r) Stiffness of the spine: *shuidao* (ST-28), *yanglingquan* (GB-34) (it is surely *shuigou*, GV-26, IS *renzhong*, which is meant here).

(DACH) When the secondary vessel from the governor to the conception vessel is full, there is stiffness of the spine: disperse *changqiang* (GV-1).

Displaced vertebrae:

(GSdeM) Disperse the contracted muscle at the edge of the transverse process which pulls the vertebra out of alignment; tonify the relaxed muscle on the opposite side.

VII. Muscles *(Jin)*

For each of the muscles, see Parts of the Body, either for pains, rheumatism, spasm, contractures or paralysis, etc.

> *Wei (paresis of muscles) depends on the* **yangming** *(LI-ST), which is the reunion of all the muscles. When the* **yangming** *is full (but not in excess), the muscles are soft. (YXRM I, 38r)*

> *The cause of* **wei** *is internal and from emptiness of the blood. (YXRM I, 15r)*

(DACH) Reunion of the muscles; all the illnesses of the muscles are cured here: *yanglingquan* (GB-34); the same for myelitis.

(DACH) Illnesses of the skin, flesh, muscles, blood and bone: leg-*sanli* (ST-36).

Pain:

(YIX I, 4r) Acute pain from tight, bound muscles: *jigou* (TW-6).

(DACH IV, 11v) Acute pain of the muscles and bones: *chize* (LU-5); *(YXRM) jianyu* (LI-15) (see Muscular Rheumatism).

Contractures:

(DACH) Muscles and bones contracted, painful: *xuanzhong* (GB-39), *hunmen* (BL-42, IS BL-47).

(DACH) Muscles tight and painful: *chengshan* (BL-57).

(YXRM, DACH) Muscles tight, body hot: *weiyang* (BL-53, IS BL-39).

(YXRM) Muscles and vessels in contracture, tightened: *weishu* (BL-21), *sanjiaoshu* (BL-22).

(DACH) Muscles contracted: *dazhu* (BL-11).

Cold:

(DACH) Energy from cold lodged in the intervals between the muscles *(fen rou,* divisions of the flesh), pain attacking at the top and bottom: *zhongdu* (GB-32).

Tendons:

(DACH) All the joints relaxed: tonify *dabao* (SP-21); disperse *zhizheng* (SI-7).

VIII. Hair, Nails, Body Hair

Hair.

The absence of a beard in women comes from the fact that the *ren mai* and the *chong mai* are not linked at the lips. In eunuchs the communication is cut from the beginning. Excess body hair is caused by excess energy and the absence of blood in the conception vessel.

Hypertrichosis (ovarian insufficiency, adrenal troubles):

> *The lungs, which feed the kidneys, give life to the skin and body hair. (DACH VIII, 2v)*

> *The kidneys flourish in the hair. (DACH VIII, 2v)*

Seborrhea and alopecia depend on the genital glands (in excess); hypertrichosis depends on the adrenals.
(DACH) Great shock; falling of hair and eyebrows: bleed *weizhong* (BL-54, IS BL-40).
(DACH) Body hair and hair dried, falling from inside: leg-*xialian* (ST-39, IS *xiajuxu*).
(YIZ, 40r) Hair and body hair dry and falling: leg-*xialian* (ST-39, IS *xiajuxu*).

Alopecia? Tinea? *(lai la, la la, bai tou feng, bai xian, bai yun tou):*

> *Also called **bai tou feng, bai xian,** or **bai yun tou;** caused by a variety of tiny, contagious fungi. It always starts on the top of the head. It looks like white colored coins. Serious cases can spread over the entire head. (Ci Yuan, ''Lai'')*

> *Also written **lai,** popularly called **la,** ulcers of the head, and **fa tou,** baldness. (Ci Yuan, ''Lai-la'')*

(GSdeM) Darkens the hair: tonify and daily moxas at *weizhong* (BL-54, IS BL-40).
Dandruff: *xinhui* (GV-21, IS GV-22).

Nails.

> *The liver flourishes in the nails. (DACH)*

(GSdeM) Nails falling or breaking in flakes; soft nails: tonify *ququan* (LR-8).

Felon *(jia ju):*

> *It is a poisonous energy of the fingers or toes. Acute pain of the nails, which exude blood; there are microbes in the abscesses. (YXRM VI, 37r)*

(GSdeM) Felon: disperse *shenmai* (BL-62).
    Felon around the nails *(dai zhi):*

> *The fingers swell. Breaking and burning pain. At times, pus forms at the edge of the nail and it falls. (YXRM VI, 37r)*

(GSdeM) Dai zhi: weizhong (BL-54, IS BL-40) *shenmai* (BL-62), *ququan* (LR-8).
(GSdeM) Nailbiting: tonify *ququan* (LR-8) and disperse *tianjing* (TW-10); if serious, add *taichong* (LR-3), tonify.

Body hair.

> *The lungs give life to the body hair and skin. ... Body hair and skin give life to the kidneys. ... Heat and oppressiveness injure the skin and body hair. (DACH III, 2v)*

> *The excess of body hair is caused by an excess of energy and an absence of blood in the conception vessel. (DACH III, 2v)*

> *When only the blood abounds in the conception vessel, the skin is slippery and produces body hair. Disperse lieque (LU-7). (DACH III, 2v)*

Chapter XV

Complexion — Skin

I. Complexion — II. Skin

The skin and blood depend on the lung and the heart. (DACH)

The skin and body hair receive life from the lung and nourish and feed the kidney. (DACH VIII, 2v)

(DACH) The skin is made healthy by the spleen-pancreas. *(GSdeM)* The spleen produces the mononuclear leukocytes which are very numerous in many types of dermatosis: pemphigus, eczema, erysipelas, etc: tonify foot-*dadu* (SP-2).

The red bone marrow produces polynuclear leukocytes, which are abundant in illnesses with pus and inflamed mucosa.

Insufficiency of the liver is the cause of most skin troubles: eczema, intertrigo, acne, psoriasis; then microbes develop. Stomach troubles also produce skin problems. The large intestine acts on the skin, particularly of the face.

Adrenal insufficiency causes dark skin.

Heat and oppressiveness injure the skin and body hair. (DACH VIII, 2v)

I. Complexion

Without color:
Insufficient energy in the small intestine: arm-*xialian* (LI-8), leg-*xialian* (ST-39, IS *xiajuxu*).

Changing:
(DACH) Insufficiency of the lungs: tonify *taiyuan* (LU-9).

Red:
(GSdeM) At meals, with cold feet (insufficiency of stomach): tonify *jiexi* (ST-41).
(GSdeM) From emotiveness, reddens easily: tonify *tongli* (HT-5), *dazhong* (KI-6, IS KI-4).
(DACH) With nosebleeds, congestion: disperse *xinhui* (GV-21, IS GV-22), *shangxing* (GV-22, IS GV-23).
(YIZ, 39r) With heat of the skull and under the chin, and pain of the temples: hand-*zhongzhu* (TW-3).
(DACH X, 34v) With cough and fever: *zhigou* (TW-6).
(DACH) With yellow eyes: *naohu* (GV-16, IS GV-17).
(DACH) Scarlet face: *shenshu* (BL-23).
(JM) Congestion of the face: *zhizheng* (SI-7), *qianding* (GV-20, IS GV-21), *tiantu* (CV-22), *xuanlu* (GB-5), *xuanli* (GB-6).
(DACH) Skin of the face scarlet: *xuanlu* (GB-5), *xuanli* (GB-6).

Acne rosacea:
(YXRM) I, 46r) Face becoming red with plaques: *ganshu* (BL-18).

Heat:
(DACH) Heat of the skin of the face: *tiantu* (CV-22); without sweat: *tongli* (HT-5).

Black:
(DACH) Black around the eyes and even to the top of the forehead: *ganshu* (BL-18).
(DACH) Dusty black: *taichong* (LR-3).
(DACH) Face the color of cinders; easy to purify: *yangfu* (GB-38).
(YIZ, 39r) Blue-black; *(YXRM)* blue-black, chest and back pain; *(DACH)* blue-black as if dead, heart and liver pain, dusty face without color: *xingjian* (LR-2).
(DACH) Black, long and unclean teeth: *tongli* (HT-5).
(YXRM) From shock, face black, swollen: *jiexi* (ST-41).
(DACH) Black-yellow without color: *tianyou* (TW-16).

Bluish-white:
(JM, DACH) Bluish-white, vertigo: *xinhui* (GV-21, IS GV-22).

Burnt:
(DACH) Burnt, dry complexion: *jianyu* (LI-15).

II. Skin.

General command points.

(JM) Illnesses of the skin: *quchi* (LI-11).
(JM) Illnesses of the skin (and vessels, blood, muscles and bone): leg-*sanli* (ST-36).
(YIX I, 10r) Illnesses of the skin from shock or rheumatism: *waiguan* (TW-5).
(DACH) All persistent skin illnesses: *weizhong* (BL-54, IS BL-40).

Pain of the skin.

(DACH, YXRM, JM) Acute pain of the skin: *huizong* (TW-7); *(DACH) huiyin* (CV-1).
(DACH) Pain of the skin, pruritis, thinness: *feishu* (BL-13).
(DACH, YXRM) Pain of the skin, cannot bear clothes: *chengman* (ST-20).
(DACH) Pain of the skin, swollen face: *zhongfu* (LU-1).

Various problems.

Humidity:
(DACH) Skin of the body always wet: *geshu* (BL-17). *(YIZ, 46v)* Skin usually wet: gallbladder meridian; *(GSdeM)* vagotonia.

Dryness:
(DACH) Dry skin if one does not drink, but if one drinks, there is sweating: *quchi* (LI-11).
(DACH) Dry skin: leg-*xialian* (ST-39, IS *xiajuxu*).
(GSdeM) Sign of interstitial chronic nephritis with hypertension and abundant urine; also a sign of sympathetico-tonia.
(GSdeM) Skin drying and peeling here and there: tonify *jiuwei* (CV-15).

Paralysis:
(DACH) Paralysis of the skin, pulse slowed down: *taibai* (SP-3), *shaoshang* (LU-11).
(YIZ, 46v) Paralysis of the skin: *taiyuan* (LU-9) and *hegu* (LI-4).

Thinness:
(DACH) Thinness of the skin: *feishu* (BL-13).

Relaxed pores:
(DACH) fengmen (BL-12).

Perversity in the skin:
(DACH) taiyuan (LU-9), *quchi* (LI-11).

Swelling of the skin.

All swellings: *(DACH)* tonify *taichong* (LR-3).
(DACH) Illnesses with swelling: *dadun* (LR-1).
(YXRM) Problems of swelling: foot-*linqi* (GB-41).
(DACH) Multiple swellings, pain of the heart: *juque* (CV-14).
(DACH) Pain from swellings: *naohu* (GV-16, IS GV-17), *xiaochangshu* (BL-27).
(DACH) Swellings from energy: *lidui* (ST-45).
(YXRM I, 46v) Swelling from wind and water: leg-*sanli* (ST-36).

Skin:
(DACH) Swelling of the skin: leg-*sanli* (ST-36).
(YIZ, 40) Energy of water acting in the skin: *yinjiao* (CV-7), *shimen* (CV-5).

Face:
Quincke's edema (insufficiency of the liver): tonify *taichong* (LR-3), *ququan* (LR-8).
(JM) Swelling of the tissues of the face: *yingxiang* (LI-20).
(DACH) Swelling or abscess of face or eyes, or of the four limbs: *lieque* (LU-7).
(JM) Swelling of the face or acne: *shanglian* (LI-1).

(DACH) Swelling and redness of the skin and of the face: *xuanlu* (GB-5), *xuanli* (GB-6).
(JM) Facial swellings like grains of millet: *zhizheng* (SI-7).
(DACH) Swelling of the skin, causing white particles: *xinhui* (GV-21, IS GV-22).

The entire body:
Swelling of the entire body: *(DACH VII, 27v)* and sweating of the head: *shenmai* (BL-62); *(JM, Fuji) wuyi* (ST-15), *guanmen* (ST-22); *(YXRM) zhangmen* (LR-13); *(DACH)* with pain: *geshu* (BL-17).
Body as if swollen with water: *(DACH X, 27r) jiexi* (ST-41).
Swelling of the abdomen, of the body: *(DACH) jianli* (CV-11).

Edema (shui zhong, gu zhang).

Gu zhang, "deep poisonous swelling." Simple *(dan gu zhang)*:

> The whole body is swollen and generates water; insufficient urination, insufficient energy of the stomach. *(YXRM I, 46v)*

> Double *(xuang gu zhang)*:

> The kidneys are in decline, very difficult to cure. *(YXRM I, 46v)*

> **Shui zhong,** *"swelling from water"*: excess yin, insufficient yang; tonify and daily moxas. *(DACH)*

> An illness either of the spleen-pancreas or of the kidneys, lungs, heart, or of all together; can also come from the genital system. *(YXRM V)*

> Only the benign cases can be cured with the needles. *(DACH)*

Shui zhong, swelling from water:
(GSdeM) Tonify *shaochong* (HT-9), *fuliu* (KI-7).
(DACH) The five types of illnesses from water: *fuliu* (KI-7); blue type: *yongquan* (KI-1); red type: *rangu* (KI-2); yellow type: *taixi* (KI-5, IS KI-3); white type: *fuliu* (KI-7); black type: *yingu* (KI-10).
(DACH) Body as if swollen from water: *shenshu* (BL-23). *(JM)* An important and special point in order to improve the water; *(YXRM I, 46r)* separates and improves the way of the water; *(DACH IV, 14v)* all water [problems], use moxa; illnesses from swelling from water *(YXRM I, 39v)*
Swelling from water, puncture deeply and bring back to the middle level, then tonify again deeply, then take out slowly. *(DACH III, 32r)* Swelling from water: moxa at *shuifen* (CV-9).
(JM) Illness from swelling from water; *(DACH III, 31r)* swelling from water: *zhongji* (CV-3).
(JM) Swelling from water: *jianli* (CV-11); *(JM) shimen* (CV-5), *guanyuan* (CV-4); *(Fuji) guanmen* (ST-22); *(JM, DACH) tianshu* (ST-25); *(DACH, YXRM, JM) huantiao* (GB-29, IS GB-30); *(YXRM)* leg-*sanli* (ST-36); *(JM) jiaoxin* (KI-8), *xiangu* (ST-43); *(JM, DACH) lidui* (ST-45); *(YXRM) diji* (SP-8); *(YXRM I, 46v) hegu* (LI-4).
(YIZ, 40v) Energy from water acting in the skin: *yinjiao* (CV-7), *shimen* (CV-5).

Gu zhang, "poisoned swelling":
(YXRM I, 46v) Poisoned swelling (simple edema) of the whole body: *xingjian* (LR-2); *qihai* (CV-6) and *xingjian* (LR-2); *yinjiao* (CV-7) and leg-*sanli* (ST-36); *neiting* (ST-44), *shuifen* (CV-9) and *shimen* (CV-5).
Double poisoned swelling *(xuang gu zhang)*: *hegu* (LI-4), *zhigou* (TW-6), *quchi* (LI-11) and *shuifen* (CV-9). If not: leg-*sanli* (ST-36), *sanyinjiao* (SP-6), *xingjian* (LR-2), *neiting* (ST-44).

See also Ascites, Quincke's Edema, Edema of the Glottis.

Pruritis, itching (yang).

> The skin likes to be scratched. Very slight irritations of the skin cause this feeling. *(Ci Yuan, "Yang")*

> Pruritis is caused by emptiness, it is yang; therefore, one must puncture superficially. *(DACH VI, 9r)*

The blood and skin depend on the heart and lungs.

In fact, most pruritis comes from an insufficiency of the liver (thus insufficiency of yin, excess yang) and stops quickly with *ququan* (LR-8) and *ligou* (LR-5), tonified and thirty daily moxas. If there is retention of biliary salts in the blood, disperse *yangfu* (GB-38) and *weizhong* (BL-54, IS BL-40).

(DACH IX, 12r) When the secondary vessel from the liver to the gallbladder is empty, one scratches: tonify *ligou* (LR-5).

(DACH IX, 12r) When the secondary vessel from the conception to the governor vessel is empty, there is pruritis and scratching: tonify *huiyin* (CV-1). (In fact, this acts wonderfully on anal and vulvar pruritis.)

Pruritis (from emptiness of the conception vessel): tonify *lieque* (LU-7).

(DACH VII, 31r) Pruritis and scratching from superficial shock: foot-*linqi* (GB-41).

(DACH) Pruritis of the skin, pain of the skin: *feishu* (BL-13).

(DACH VIII, 5v) Pruritis as if gnawed by insects, skin coming off, leaving sores: *quchi* (LI-11).

(DACH X, 31v) Children — pruritis, swelling, trembling: *shaohai* (HT-3).

(DACH) Pruritis, swelling, shivering: *xiaohai* (SI-8).

(DACH) Pruritis of the whole body: *xuanzhong* (GB-39), *fengshi* (GB-31).

(YIZ 47; DACH II, 19v) Pruritis of the skin of the whole body: *zhiyin* (BL-67) and *wuyi* (ST-15). *(DACH)* Pruritis of the skin: *wuyi* (ST-15). *(GSdeM)* Urticaria, pruritis: *wuyi* (ST-15).

(DACH VII, 31r) Pruritis of the whole body from superficial shock: foot-*linqi* (GB-41), *fengshi* (GB-31), *xuehai* (SP-10), *weizhong* (BL-54, IS BL-40), *xuanzhong* (GB-39), *baihui* (GV-19, IS GV-20), *bailao* (GV-13 IS GV-14 *dazhui*), *mingmen* (GV-4), *quchi* (LI-11), *shuifen* (CV-9), *qihai* (CV-6), *tongziliao* (GB-1).

(DACH) Skin painful, cannot wear clothes: *wuyi* (ST-15).

Illnesses of the skin (dermatosis).

(GSdeM) Tonify *ququan* (LR-8), *xuanzhong* (GB-39), *dadu* (SP-2), *weizhong* (BL-54, IS BL-40).

Acne, pimples *(ding, ding du):*

> *A small elevation with a round shape, about the size of a pea. They always start on the epidermis in the little sack of the hair or sweat gland. At the beginning, the skin generates a small head which itches; then there is hardness and a little pus: called **ding du** if there is fever, shivering or stiffness. (Ci Yuan, "Ding")*

(YIZ, 48) Acne coming on the face or corners of the mouth: moxa at *hegu* (LI-4).

(YIZ, 39r) Face and chin swollen generating acne: *hegu* (LI-4), *lieque* (LU-7), *dicang* (ST-7, IS ST-4).

(JM) Acne of the face: *shangyang* (LI-1), *jiache* (ST-3, IS ST-6).

(DACH) Acne or superficial swelling of the face: *lieque* (LU-7).

Furuncles, abscess *(chuang, yong, ju):*

> *General name for all **yong** or **ju** abscesses; swelling of the skin forming pus and rotting. (Ci Yuan, "Chuang")*

> **Yong** *is a large and superficial abscess; in the past it was the name given to swollen and scarlet abscesses: redness, swelling, pain, and pus. The surrounding skin is purplish.* **Ju** *is a deep abscess (anthrax). In the past it was the name given to abscesses which were not scarlet. (Ci Yuan, "Yong-ju")*

> *See "Gu-zao-feng" article. (Ci Yuan, "Ya-gan")*

> **Gu zao feng,** *"wind of deathly encounter," or* **zhu sai feng,** *"pig-cheek wind," are popular names given to abscesses of babies' cheeks. Both cheeks are red and engender abscesses.*

> *(Ci Yuan, "Gu-zao-feng" See also DACH XI, 3v.)*

(YIZ, 40) All furuncles and abscesses: *shenmai* (BL-62). *(GSdeM)* Dispersal of *shenmai* (BL-62) aborts furuncles not yet formed and stops furunculosis. It speeds the expulsion of the pus and scar formation.

(YXRM I, 46v) All abscesses: *taichong* (LR-3).

(JM) Furunculosis: *shenmai* (BL-62), *rangu* (KI-2), *xinshu* (BL-15), foot-*qiaoyin* (GB-44).

(DACH VIII; DACH IX, 16r) All blood illnesses and abscesses: *xuehai* (SP-10). All abscesses, furuncles: *shugu* (BL-65), *fengmen* (BL-12).

(JM) Bad abscess: *geshu* (BL-17), *weishu* (BL-21), *dadu* (SP-2); *(YXRM)* *fengshi* (GB-31). *(JM)* Bad swelling, abscess, furuncles, acne: fifty moxas at *geshu* (BL-17), seven at *wenliu* (LI-7) and *hegu* (LI-4).

(DACH) Face — facial abscess of children *(ya gan),* persists a long time without being cured: gum-*yinjiao* (GV-27, IS GV-28).

(YXRM I, 40r) Sycosis, abscess in the moustache, stomach trouble: choose from among: *lidui* (ST-45), *neiting* (ST-44), *xiangu* (ST-43), *chongyang* (ST-42), *jiexi* (ST-41). Abscess in the beard, gallbladder problems: choose from among: *xiaxi* (GB-43), foot-*linqi* (GB-41), *yangfu* (GB-38), *yanglingquan* (GB-34).

(YXRM) Abscess of nose: *yinjiao* (GV-27, IS GV-28); *(DACH)* *tongtian* (BL-7), nose-*heliao* (LI-19), *suliao* (GV-24, IS GV-25); *(JM)* *qucha* (BL-4).

(DACH) The whole body, children: *quchi* (LI-11).

(YIX I, 5v; DACH XIII, 8v) Abscess and swelling of the whole body: *quchi* (LI-11), *hegu* (LI-4), *xingjian* (LR-2), leg-*sanli* (ST-36), or *neiting* (ST-44).

Warts:
(DACH) zhizheng (SI-7), *zhongkui* (MP-21).

Ulcers *(You, zhui you, hou zi):*
(DACH) taichong (LR-3).

>*The smallest are the same as **jia jie** (illnesses with crusts). (DACH)*

Jia jie: (DACH) hegu (LI-4), *yangxi* (LI-5), *houxi* (SI-3), *quchi* (LI-11).

Urticaria *(tan ma zhen, tan zao zhen, zhong you du):*

>*Due to ingestion of poison fish, there are plaques and points on the skin: **hegu (LI-4), 4 fen, zhongwan (CV-12), 8 fen, sanyinjiao (SP-6), 4 fen, yanggu (SI-5), 3 fen.** (JO, 76)*

(GSdeM) Disperse *wuyi* (ST-15).

Flaking skin (*bai xie*, "white bits"):
(YIZ, 39r) Formation of white bits; *(DACH)* swollen face forming white bits: *xinhui* (GV-21, IS GV-22).

Freckles (*jiao ban*, "marks of little birds"; *han ban*, "spots from sweat"; *dian lao*, "points from burning"; same as *dian ge*): "spots from sweat"; *dian lao*, "points from burning"; same as *dian ge*):
(DACH) Points from burning *(dian ge):* gum-*yinjiao* (GV-27, IS GV-28).

Chilblains (*dong chuang*, "freezing abscess":

>"These are not true abscesses."

(DACH) Red swelling of the back of the hand: *yemen* (TW-2), hand-*shangdu* (MP-16) 1 *fen*, seven moxas.
(YIZ, 43v) Red and swollen heels from chilblains: needles 3 *fen* on the toes and at the white and pink flesh under the bones: 2 x 7 moxas.

Scabies *(xie chuang, xie xian):*

>*Originates from the scabies insect: contagious. On the hands the patients have small bubbles similar to millet grains. Two types: dry or wet. (Ci Yuan, "Xie-chuang")*

(DACH) Scabies *(xie xian): daling* (PC-7); *(JM)* (LI-4), *zhigou* (TW-6).
(DACH) Xie chuang: lidui (ST-45); *(JM) zhigou* (TW-6).

Eruptions *(yin zhen):*
Purpura (see especially anemia): tonify *gaohuangshu* (BL-38, IS BL-43), *xuanhong* (GB-39).
(DACH) All constant eruptions: *weizhong* (BL-54, IS BL-40).

>*The skin itches with neither swelling nor pain. The eruption **(zhen)** is formed by grains with heads like millet or like a puncture. A hidden redness invades the skin and seems to come out without coming out; it itches with neither swelling nor pain. Also called **yin chuang**.*

>*When the face produces these purple or scarlet eruptions either with spots similar to bird's eggs or with freckles, it is slow.*

>*In the past, **yin zhen** were divided into many types. Today they are grouped together because their treatment is the same. Thus **ban, zhen, yin zhen, dan zhen, dian,** and **xian** illnesses have many similarities and few differences. The remedies used for one are the same as for the others. (YXRM V, 15v)*

(YXRM) All the *yin zhen* from heat or wind: *jianyu* (LI-15).
(DACH IV, 15) Yin zhen and tonsillitis: *tianjing* (TW-10).
(DACH) Yin zhen: neiting (ST-44); of the whole body: thigh-*futu* (ST-32); from shock: *quchi* (LI-11).

Ban:

>*Spots like a piebald horse; that which is of various colors. (Ci Yuan, "Ban")*

>***Ban** depends on the triple warmer. It is fire without roots. The serious cases are red like a brocade, blotching mostly the chest and abdomen; [patient has] sore throat, delirium; sees blood. From an internal cause, coated with spots like mosquito bites. When they are mostly on the hands and feet and there is neither headache nor fever, it is an emptiness of the stomach. (YXRM V, 15v)*

(DACH IV, 15v) Scarlet *ban* on the face: *danshu* (BL-19).

Ban feng:

> Small points start to appear, then spread and form spots. (Ci Yuan, ''Ban-feng'')

(DACH XI, 14v) Marks forming blotches on the skin during a hot wind: *zhongkui* (MP-21, IS M-UE-16).

Han zhen or *fei:*

> During summer, small elevations produced on the skin, called **han zhen** or **fei**; comes from prolonged sweating. Like grains of sand, first red, then later there is sometimes a little pus; appears mainly on the chest, abdomen and axilla. (Ci Yuan, ''Fei'')

(GSdeM) Tonify *ququan* (LR-8).

Chi zhen, bai zhen:

> **Zhen** which come out like grains of rice are divided into white (**bai zhen**) or scarlet (**chi zhen**). The scarlet type (**chi zhen**) comes from burning energy during hot weather. The white type (**bai zhen**) comes from cold weather or from chilled energy. There are others that are similar, but there is a little yellow hidden between the epidermis and dermis. The four limbs are heavy. They come from wind heat or humidity. Many also come from cold after a bath or after taking off the clothes when sweating. (YXRM V, 15v)

(GSdeM) Disperse *weizhong* (BL-54, IS BL-40).

Dan ju; tong mian hong zhong zheng ("red swelling of the entire face):

> An evil inflammation which causes itching of the head; illness of swelling and redness of the whole face. (Ci Yuan, ''Dan-ju'')

Huo dan:

> An illness of children. Red and hot skin. Creates spots and points which coat the skin. (Ci Yuan, ''Huo-dan'')

Chi you feng; chi dian; tian hou, dan du:

> An illness which is also called **chi you feng** or **tian hou**. It comes from a bite or lesion of the mouth which has taken in a pathogenic bacteria. It is produced more easily on the face and at the side of the nose. At the affected point, there are tides of redness with acute pain in the body; bad cold with attack of fever. It easily becomes chronic. (Ci Yuan, ''Dan-du'')

> The skin of the face, neck, nape and body change color and become scarlet. Also called **chi dian**. It depends on the blood. When this illness persists, harmonize and nourish blood and energy; then the fire will be calmed. The pruritis will stop. When pruritis from emptiness does not stop, it is difficult to improve the blood; the blood circulates poorly. (YXRM V, 16r, ''Chi-you-feng'')

(DACH XI, 9r; YIX I, 6r) Chi you feng of small children: *weizhong* (BL-54, IS BL-40) and *baihui* (GV-19, IS GV-20).

Dian; chi dian feng:

> An illness of the skin. First, some small violet bumps come out which, after an extended time, coat the skin. Popularly called **chi dian feng**. (Ci Yuan, ''Dian'')

(DACH XI, 14v) Skin illness *(dian feng):* points appearing on the skin and coating it: *zhongkui* (MP-21, IS M-UE-16).

Vitiligo *(bai you feng, bai dian):*

> The skin of the face, nape, neck or body change color and become white. Also called **bai dian**; depends on energy. Harmonize and nourish blood and energy. (YXRM V, 16r)

> A skin illness. First, little white points erupt, which after a long time spread and coat the skin. (Ci Yuan, ''Dian'')

(DACH XI, 14r) Moxa *zhongkui* (MP-21, IS M-UE-16).
Eczema *(she zhen):* tonify *ququan* (LR-8).

Eruptive illnesses (zhen; dan zhen).

> When the **zhen** are scarlet colored, they are called **dan zhen**. (YXRM V, 15v)

> Name of [various] illnesses. From heat of boiling blood which flows backwards; the skin produces some small red points. Some are contagious, such as measles (**ma zhen**), or slight like rubella (**feng zhen**). (Ci Yuan, ''Zhen'')

Scarlet fever *(xing hong zhen):*

(JM) quchi (LI-11).

(DACH XI, 9r) Attack of vermillion-red over the entire body: *weizhong* (BL-54, IS BL-40), *quchi* (LI-11), leg-*sanli* (ST-36), *baihui* (GV-19, IS GV-20).

Measles *(ma zhen, ma zheng, sha zi):*

(JM) weizhong (BL-54, IS BL-40), *daling* (PC-7), *bailao* (GV-13, IS GV-14 *dazhui*), *shuifen* (CV-9).

Rubella *(feng zhen, feng sha):*

(JM) hegu (LI-4), *quze* (PC-3), *huantiao* (GB-29, IS GB-30), *yongquan* (KI-1).

Purulent illnesses:

> *Tian pao chuang:* On the skin or mucosa there appear water bubbles. The skin is slightly raised; red in color. Inside is found a transparent fluid; large bubbles like peas with round shape. It occurs anywhere on the body, or on the bronchial mucosa, or in the stomach or intestines. Rarely in the hair, on the palms, or the soles of the feet. Sometimes there are attacks of fever with acute pain. Cured after some months. (Ci Yuan, "Tian-pao-chuang")

> *E zhang feng:* A variety of pustules from the poison of syphilis. If, after several years, it is not cured, **laogong** (PC-8) and **neiguan** (PC-6) will cut the root. (YXRM V, 1r)

> *Gua zhang:* An illness which is produced in the middle of the palm. Both hands touch, and it starts. It begins with pustules of yellowish pus. Pruritis and intermittent pain, extreme fatigue, peevish; difficult to cure. (Ci Yuan, "Gua-zhang")

(DACH VIII, 29v) Gua zhang: daling (PC-7).

Sycosis *(xu fa cheng du,* **"hair or beard generating poison"**)**:**

(DACH VIII, 28r) Sycosis: *shenmai* (BL-62), *taixi* (KI-5, IS KI-3), *hegu* (LI-4), *waiguan* (TW-5), *tongziliao* (GB-1). (See Facial Abscess.)

Papulous and squamous illnesses, with crusts:

> *Xian:* A skin illness similar to scabies; it collects in one place and then spreads slowly. (Ci Yuan, "Xian")

Jia jie: crusts, scabies (see also Ulcers); *(DACH) jia jie: yangxi* (LI-5), *hegu* (LI-4), *quchi* (LI-11), *houxi* (SI-3). *Feng xian lai: (YIZ I, 7v) quchi* (LI-11).

Purulent illnesses (see abscesses); *chuang jie,* **"abscess-scabies":**

(DACH) Chuang jie: xuehai (SP-10), *lidui* (ST-45), *daling* (PC-7), *zhigou* (TW-6), *yangxi* (LI-5).

Herpes: *(GSdeM)* at the base of the back, tonify *jiuwei* (CV-15); generalized: *weizhong* (BL-54, IS BL-40).

Tumors, cysts (ying; liu).

Tumors *(ying):*

Five varieties: 1) Stone *ying (shi ying):* hard like stone; 2) Energy *ying (qi ying):* soft like a silk purse; 3) Blood *ying (xue ying):* like a net of swollen or red vessels (varicosities); 4) Muscle *ying (jin ying):* like muscles without bone; 5) Flesh *ying (rou ying):* like a sack.

Ying tumors: *(DACH) fengchi* (GB-20), moxa at *jianyu* (LI-15) or *tianfu* (LU-3), or *chongyang* (ST-42), or *tianrong* (SI-17).

Energy from *ying* tumors: *tianfu* (LU-3), *jianyu* (LI-15); *(DACH) yunmen* (LU-2); *(YXRM I, 46) shanzhong* (CV-17); *(DACH) feishu* (BL-13).

Ying from energy: *fubai* (GB-16, IS GB-10).

Liu tumors:

"Blood which accumulates forms *liu*" (varicosities?).

Liu tumors: *(DACH)* foot-*shangqiu* (SP-5), *naohui* (TW-13).

Swelling from *liu* tumors: *naohu* (GV-16, IS GV-17).

Ying and liu tumors:

(DACH VI, 16v) Foot-*qiaoyin* (GB-44), *naohu* (GV-16, IS GV-17), *tongtian* (BL-7), *fubai* (GB-16, IS GB-10), *qishe* (ST-11), *tiantu* (CV-22), *zhongfu* (LU-1).

Ying and *liu* tumors contracted from flying cadavers (plague, buboes?): *zhongfu* (LU-1).

Cancer (yan).

Of the breast: *wuyi* (ST-15).

Of the stomach: *zhongwan* (CV-12), *burong* (ST-19), *weishu* (BL-21), *geshu* (BL-17).

Chapter XVI

Head, Limbs, Trunk

I. Head and Face — II. Neck and Nape — III. Nape, Nape and Shoulders — IV. Shoulders — V. Upper Limb — VI. Lower Limbs — VII. The Four Limbs — VIII. Anterior Trunk — IX. Posterior Trunk, Back, Lumbar, Vertebral Column

I. Head and Face

General command points.

Head:
(DACH) The hundred illnesses of the head: *fengfu* (GV-15, IS GV-16).
(YXRM I, 46r) All types of illnesses of the head: *hegu* (LI-4).
(DACH II, 32v) Head area: *lieque* (LU-7).
(YIX I, 7r) Forehead and nape: *lieque* (LU-7).
(DACH) The front of the head: *zhiyin* (BL-67).
(DACH VI, 10r) Vertex: *fengchi* (GB-20), *touwei* (ST-1, IS ST-8).
(DACH) Vertex and nape: *fengmen* (BL-12).
(DACH) All which concerns the head, vertex and nape: *houxi* (SI-3), *lieque* (LU-7).
(YXRM I, 46v) All illnesses of head, face, arm, wrist: *wangu* (SI-4).

Face:
(DACH IV, 10v; YIX I, 7v) Illnesses of the face: *quchi* (LI-11), *zhiyin* (BL-67).
(YIX I, 5r) All illnesses of the face; *(DACH)* all that concerns the face: *chize* (LU-5).
(YXRM I, 46v) Region of the face, upper part: *jiache* (ST-3, IS ST-6).
(YXRM I, 39r) Illnesses of the face, nose, mouth, ears, eyes, pharynx, teeth: *hegu* (LI-4) and *quchi* (LI-11).
(YXRM I, 46v) Illnesses of the face, arm and hands: *yanggu* (SI-5).

Headaches, pains of head and face (migraines, neuralgias, cephalalgia, etc.).

There is extreme confusion in both ordinary and medical language concerning the exact meaning of the existing terms for the different pains of the head and face. One term is used constantly for another, to the point where the ideas themselves have lost their clarity. "Migraine" is used for all headaches, while it in fact indicates pains on one side of the head (hemicrania). "Neuralgia" is used for congestive headaches as well as for pains of an exterior nerve. "Cephalalgy" and "cephalalgia" are not differentiated. It is useful to define these terms by recalling their exact meaning:
Cephalalgy *(Larousse):* temporary pain of the head.
Cephalalgia *(Larousse):* chronic or periodic headache.
Migraine *(Larousse):* pain which affects only one side of the head.
Neuralgia *(Larousse):* pain along the pathway of a nerve.

From antiquity, the Chinese have started from reality to derive their theories and vocabulary. They differentiate three groups of head pains:
Internal congestive headaches *(tou tong).*
External headaches, pains of the nerves *(tou feng).*
Pains on one side of the head *(bian tou tong, bian tou feng),* either internal or external.
(See also Cerebral Congestion, Cerebral Anemia, Encephalitis, Meningitis).

In fact, the localization of headaches (or one-sided headaches) indicates their origin:
On the temples (migraine), the pain can extend to the middle of the skull; it comes from excess energy of the gallbladder, often with an insufficiency of the liver. They are removed by dispersing *yangfu* (GB-38) and tonifying *ququan* (LR-8).
On the top of the head (vertex) to the nape (congestive): these come mostly from excess energy of the kidneys and are removed completely by dispersing *rangu* (KI-2) and *taixi* (KI-5, IS KI-3). It is sometimes necessary to additionally disperse *jiaoxin* (KI-8), or add seven daily moxas at *yongquan* (KI-1).
On the edges of the eyebrows: these come from excess energy of the bladder and stomach, and are stopped by dispersing *shenmai* (BL-62), or by tonifying *touwei* (ST-1, IS ST-8) or *jiexi* (ST-41).

The whole head becomes heavy during stormy weather: disperse *waiguan* (TW-5).

Following drinking excessively: disperse *shuaigu* (GB-8).

Internal pains of the whole head (congestive): disperse *shenmai* (BL-62).

Pains of head and forehead (ophthalmic neuralgia): disperse *yuzhen* (BL-9).

Internal and external headaches:

Some points act on both congestive headaches and external neuralgias. They are:

(DACH) baihui (GV-19, IS GV-20), *xinhui* (GV-21, IS GV-22), *qianding* (GV-20, IS GV-21), *sizhukong* (TW-21, IS TW-23), *tongziliao* (GB-1), *quchi* (LI-11), arm-*xialian* (LI-8), *shenmai* (BL-62), *jinmen* (BL-63).

From changing of weather or wind: *waiguan* (TW-5).

In general it is advisable to disperse according to the affected meridian.

Internal congestive headaches (tou tong):

*In **tou tong**, the pain radiates primarily to the vertex and to the epicranium.*

If everything is painful, if the feet and hands are cold up to the articulations, it means death. If there is counterflow, the perverse energy rises in the yang meridians and causes the pain; if serious, there is syncope. One must cure according to the external and internal cause:

From external excitation (wind, cold, etc.) there is surely cold and heat. If wind and cold have entered the brain and even the teeth are painful, there are problems from wind. If the hair is painful, there are problems from cold. If the pain starts in the ear, there are problems from heat or humidity.

From internal excitation (emptiness of energy or blood):

*1) From emptiness of energy (yang, excess yin and blood) there are buzzings in the ears; the points of the two **taiyang** meridians (BL-SI) are painful. This sometimes occurs after a major illness leading to painful emptiness of energy, or from insufficiency of energy after the seven emotions; the epigastrium is full, with vomiting of acid water. In loss from mucus the head spins, the eyes are black, there is confused speech, nausea, closed eyes and cold limbs. There are also headaches from accumulations and painful contractions (**ji ju**).*

2) From emptiness of blood (yin, excess yang and nerves) there is irascibility and anger, emptiness of the kidney; the lower body is empty and the upper body abounds (heat above, cold below); the vertex is very painful; the pulses are like a rope and hard on pressure. (YXRM V, 9v)

There is also a type which causes death, called "true headache," *zhen tou tong*, described as follows:

In the true pain of the head, attack in the morning, death in the evening; attack in the evening, death in the morning. (DACH XI, 1v)

The practical treatment of congestive headaches, which attack primarily the top of the head with a sensation of swollen or hot brain, consists of first removing the congestion by dispersing *shenmai* (BL-62), which acts on the brain, and leg-*sanli* (ST-36), which acts against the excess yin compressing the yang; that is usually enough. If there is emptiness of energy (weak, superficial pulses), tonify *qihai* (CV-6) and *hegu* (LI-4), and disperse *daling* (PC-7), especially if there is high blood pressure. If there is emptiness of blood (yin, weak deep pulses) and excess energy, disperse *tianjing* (TW-10) and tonify *neiguan* (PC-6).

(YIX I, 10v) Tou tong during thunder; edge of the eyebrows painful: *shenmai* (BL-62).

(YXRM I, 46r) All varieties of *tou tong*: *hegu* (LI-4).

(DACH III, 30v) Unbearable *tou tong*: *sizhukong* (TW-21, IS TW-23).

(DACH) Tou tong: qiangu (SI-2), *houxi* (SI-3), *tongli* (HT-5), *yangchi* (TW-4), *yinxi* (HT-6), *yanggu* (SI-5), *shaoze* (SI-1), *xialian* (LI-8), *tianjing* (TW-10), *qingling* (HT-2), *xiaoluo* (TW-12), leg-*sanli* (ST-36), *kunlun* (BL-60), *zhiyin* (BL-67), *chengshan* (BL-57), *feiyang* (BL-58), foot-*qiaoyin* (GB-44), *fengchi* (GB-20), *hanyan* (GB-4), *xuanlu* (GB-5), *xuanli* (GB-6), ear-*heliao* (TW-22, IS TW-21 *ermen* by location), *taodao* (GV-12, IS GV-13), *touwei* (ST-1, IS ST-8), *tianchong* (GB-15, IS GB-9), *naohu* (GV-16, IS GV-17), *mingmen* (GV-4), *sanjiaoshu* (BL-22), *shendao* (GV-10, IS GV-11).

(DACH IV, 4r; YIX I, 5r) Internal headache on the top or side; difficult to cure: *sizhukong* (TW-21, IS TW-23) under the skin toward *shuaigu* (GB-8) (towards the back); if with mucus: *fengchi* (GB-20) 1.5 *cun* towards *fengfu* (GV-15, IS GV-16) (i.e., towards the medial line); first tonify then disperse and eleven moxas. When the mucus has not come yet: *hegu* (LI-4), 5 *fen* towards *laogong* (PC-8) (middle of the palm) and 2 x 7 moxas.

(DACH III, 32v) Internal headaches, shivering from the exterior: *waiguan* (TW-5).

(DACH VII, 28r) Internal headaches, difficulty bending forward: *shenmai* (BL-62), *jinmen* (BL-63).

Headaches and vertigo *(xuan yuan): (DACH IV, 7r)* needles at *baihui* (GV-19, IS GV-20); *(JM) shenmai* (BL-62), *tianzhu* (BL-10), *jiaxi* (ST-41).

(DACH II, 29r) Internal headaches, acute pain of the eyes; *(DACH IV, 4r)* the same with foggy vision, acute pain between the eyebrows that is difficult to bear: disperse *zanzhu* (BL-2) disperse 1 *fen* under the skin towards the frontal eminences. If there is pain, disperse, if vertigo *(xuan yuan),* tonify *touwei* (ST-1, IS ST-8).

(YIX I, 4r) Internal headache at the vertex, eyes not opening: *yongquan* (KI-1).

(DACH) Internal headaches, red and swollen eyes: *tongziliao* (GB-1), *sibai* (ST-5, IS ST-2).

(DACH) Internal headaches, buzzing: *qimai* (TW-18).

(DACH) Internal headaches, swollen face: *wenliu* (LI-7), *fenglong* (ST-40), foot-*linqi* (GB-41).

(DACH) With nose blocked: *meichong* (BL-3).

(DACH) With head as if broken, eyes as if gouged out: *touwei* (ST-1, IS ST-8), *jinggu* (BL-64).

(DACH) Like the blows of a hammer: head-*qiaoyin* (GB-18, IS GB-11).

(YXRM I, 46v) Women — internal headaches along the stomach meridian (cheeks and forehead): *neiting* (ST-44)).

(DACH) Of the vertex: *yuzhen* (BL-9).

(DACH) From the vertex and lateral side radiating to the cervical vertebrae: *hegu* (LI-4).

(DACH) With pain at the two frontal eminences, brings depression; becomes a weakness of the eyes *(YIZ, 38v)* from emptiness or counterflow: *qubin* (GB-7).

(YIZ, 38v) From emptiness of the kidney: *guanyuan* (CV-4), 100 moxas, *yongquan* (KI-1), 3 *fen,* agitate the needle.

(DACH) From cold and heat: *wenliu* (LI-7), *xiaoluo* (TW-12).

(DACH) Coming and going: *guanyuan* (CV-4).

(DACH) When defecating: *shugu* (BL-65).

(DACH) With dry heaves: *shenzhu* (GV-11, IS GV-12).

(YIZ, 38v) With vomiting; *shenting* (GV-23, IS GV-24), *yintang* (GV-23a, IS M-HN-3), first under the skin to the left and tonify for three inhalations, then under the skin to the right and tonify for three inhalations.

(JM) With spasms of all the parietal muscles: *binao* (LI-14).

(JM) With pains of the occiput: *yamen* (GV-14, IS GV-15).

(YXRM) With heat of the head: *kunlun* (BL-60).

(DACH) With darkened eyes, head spinning, nausea, vomiting of saliva: *qiangjian* (GV-17, IS GV-18).

(DACH) From hemorrhoids: *xiaochangshu* (BL-27).

(YIZ, 38v) And if there is no cure: fifty moxas at *jiaxi* (ST-41), leg-*sanli* (ST-36), *zhongwan* (CV-12).

(DACH) Internal headaches, dazzling: *tongli* (HT-5), foot-*tonggu* (BL-66).

(DACH) Internal headaches from drunkenness: *fengmen* (BL-12).

(DACH) After drunkenness: *shuaigu* (GB-8), *yintang* (GV-23a, IS M-HN-3), *zanzhu* (BL-2).

(GSdeM) From cerebral fatigue: tonify arm-*shanglian* (LI-9).

(DACH) From lack of sleep: *yuzhen* (BL-9), ear-*heliao* (TW-22, IS TW-21 *ermen* by location), *taodao* (GV-12, IS GV-13), and foggy vision.

(DACH) Pain of temples, heaviness of head: *fuyang* (BL-59).

(DACH) Pain increases from bending the head: *tongtian* (BL-7).

(DACH) After drinking wine, scarlet face, brain on fire: *baihui* (GV-19, IS GV-20).

External headaches, neuralgia (tou feng):

In **tou feng,** *the nape is stiff; one must differentiate between the frontal types (**zheng**) and the lateral types (**pian**). (YXRM V, 9v)*

Pain at the vertex of the head is called **zheng tou feng,** *frontal. (DACH VII, 32v)*

Zheng tou feng: *there are those in which the skin of the skull is painful, those in which the mouth and tongue cannot taste, those in which there is deafness, those in which there is pain in the eyes, those in which there is boring pain above and under the eyebrows, those in which there is hypersensitivity to odors, those in which there is yawning or vertigo. In serious cases the nape is stiff and hard and the back contracted. (YXRM V, 9r)*

Tou feng *patients, during the attack, want to be covered with cotton-soft clothing, they have repression of heat; it is necessary to cool their blood.*

When there is repression of heat of the three yang [hand: small intestine, large intestine, triple warmer; foot: bladder, gallbladder, stomach], with aversion to light and desire for ice on the head, it is necessary to cool with bitter taste and cause perspiration and vomiting.

Tou feng *which has persisted for years, with hot urine, red eyes and vertigo, are from a repression of the energy of the liver which bothers the lungs.*

In **tou feng** *from external causes, from evil cold, the head and face have a lot of sweat. There is also pain of the eyebrows, and the eyes cannot open. There is calm in the daytime with acute pain at night (excess yang); the body feels heavy. (YXRM V, 9v)*

(DACH XI, 1v) External headaches of the frontal or lateral vertex: *sizhukong* (TW-21, IS TW-23), *fengchi* (GB-20), *hegu* (LI-4). If these points do not improve the case, there is mucus bearing down on the diaphragm and chest. If vertex or lateral *tou feng* is accompanied by pains on the medial side of the arm, if the feet and hands are cold, and if it is not cured for a long time, it changes into hemiplegia of the left or right (it is a question here of internal *tou tong*).

(DACH) External headaches: *shangxing* (GV-22, IS GV-23), thigh-*futu* (ST-32), *quchi* (LI-11), *tianjing* (TW-10), arm-*xialian* (LI-8), *tongli* (HT-5).

(YIZ, 38v) Tou feng during thunder: *xinhui* (GV-21, IS GV-22), *baihui* (GV-19, IS GV-20), *fengchi* (GB-20).

(YIX I, 3v; DACH I, 11v; DACH II, 18v) toufeng: *xinhui* (GV-21, IS GV-22) and *yuzhen* (BL-9), gold *(jin)* needle.

(YXRM I, 39v) tou feng — dizziness, nape stiff and as if ripped out: *shenmai* (BL-62), *jinmen* (BL-63), arm-*sanli* (LI-10). For external headaches with swelling of the nape or radiating into the shoulder, puncture these three points. If there is dazzling, tonify *shenmai* (BL-62) and *jinmen* (BL-63); for external headaches during thunder, these points also help. In order to tonify emptiness: *shangxing* (GV-22, IS GV-23).

(YXRM I, 39v) External headaches, pain of the nape and brain. If one tonifies a lot and disperses a little, the problem will return: use *baihui* (GV-19, IS GV-20), *shangxing* (GV-22, IS GV-23), *hegu* (LI-4).

(YIZ, 38v) External headaches, swelling of the face, stiffness of the nape, cannot turn to look backwards: *tianyou* (TW-16) 5 *fen,* leave for six exhalations. It must not be tonified, and no moxas used because these would cause swelling of the face. At the same time, *yixi* (BL-40, is BL-45) must be stimulated (6 *fen*); leave for three exhalations and disperse for five inhalations. Afterwards: *tianyou* (TW-16), *fengchi* (GB-20) and the patient will be cured. This is a method which comes from antiquity.

Facial neuralgia (trigeminal neuralgia, san cha shen jing tong:

Distal points: *(JM)* trigeminal neuralgia: *shaohai* (HT-3), *quchi* (LI-11), *fuyang* (BL-59). Disperse leg-*sanli* (ST-36), *naohu* (GV-16, IS GV-17), *wangu* (GB-17, IS GB-12), *tongtian* (BL-7), *yuzhen* (BL-9), head-*qiaoyin* (GB-18, IS GB-11).

Local points: *(YIZ 38v)* pain of the nerves, face, temples, vertex, nape: *qubin* (GB-7). Trigeminal neuralgia: *quanliao* (SI-18), *juliao* (ST-6, IS ST-3), *kezhuren* (GB-3, IS *shangguan*), *xiaguan* (ST-2, IS ST-7), *jiache* (ST-3, IS ST-6), *daying* (ST-8, IS ST-5), *dicang* (ST-7, IS ST-4).

Various pains of the head:

Pain of the vertex: *(DACH)* pain of the flesh of the skull: *neiting* (ST-44); *(DACH)* pains of the vertex: *lieque* (LU-7), foot-*linqi* (GB-41), *yongquan* (KI-1), *qucha* (BL-4), *qianding* (GV-20, IS GV-21), *xuanlu* (GB-5), *changqiang* (GV-1).

Vertex or laterally: *(DACH)* *xinhui* (GV-21, IS GV-22), *fengchi* (GB-20).

Vertex and nape: *(DACH III, 32r)* *houxi* (SI-3), *fengmen* (BL-12).

Vertex, temple, nape: *(JM)* *qubin* (GB-7); *(DACH)* *shugu* (BL-65).

From eyebrows to nape: *(DACH)* *waiguan* (TW-5).

Occiput: *(DACH)* pain of the mastoid process, occiput, temples: *linqi* (GB-41). Occiput and temples: *(DACH)* head-*linqi* (GB-11, IS GB-15), *yangfu* (GB-38), *tianzhu* (BL-10), *yuzhen* (BL-9), *yamen* (GV-14, IS GV-15).

Parietal: *(DACH)* acute pain of the parietal area: *shuaigu* (GB-8).

Face: *(DACH)* *naohu* (GV-16, IS GV-17), head-*wangu* (GB-17, IS GB-12), *quchi* (LI-11) and *hegu* (LI-4).

Eyebrows and forehead (depends on the bladder and stomach):

Edge of eyebrows: *shenmai* (BL-62); between the eyebrows: *zanzhu* (BL-2), *touwei* (ST-1, IS ST-8). Eyebrows pierced through, face red: *jiexi* (ST-41).

Forehead — anterior of face: *yangbai* (GB-10, IS GB-14).

Middle of the forehead and root of the nose: *touwei* (ST-1, IS ST-8), gum-*yinjiao* (GV-27, IS GV-28).

Top of the forehead: *houding* (GV-18, IS GV-19).

Pain at the frontal eminences and under the chin: *yangfu* (GB-38).

Eyes — headaches, inflamed eyes, flowery vision: *shenting* (GV-23, IS GV-24).

Acute pain in the head, inflamed eyes with tears flowing *houxi* (SI-3). (See also Sense Organs: Eyes).

Cheeks — *(DACH)* pain in the middle of the cheeks: gum-*yinjiao* (GV-27, IS GV-28).

Pain and stiffness of the cheeks, nape and head: *shugu* (BL-65).

(GSdeM) Pain of the cheekbones: *tongtian* (BL-7).

Temples — *(DACH)* pain of the temples, heavy head: *fuyang* (BL-59).

Pain of the temples and occiput: *yangfu* (GB-38), head-*linqi* (GB-11, IS GB-15).

In front of the ear — *(DACH)* pain in front of the ear: *shaoshang* (LU-1), *quchi* (LI-11).

Behind the ears — *(DACH)* *tianjing* (TW-10), foot-*linqi* (GB-41), *wangu* (GB-17, IS GB-12).

Jaw — *(DACH)* pain of the face and jaw: *zanzhu* (BL-2).

Pain of the maxilla: *xiaxi* (GB-43), arm-*shanglian* (LI-9), *tianchuang* (SI-16).

Maxilla and below the chin: *tianzong* (SI-11).
Chin: *yanggu* (SI-5).
Below the chin: *jianzhen* (SI-9).
Below the chin and frontal eminences: *yangfu* (GB-38).

Various pains of the head:
(DACH) Head as if pierced with needles: *qiangjian* (GV-17, IS GV-18).
(DACH) Pain of the head as if from blows of a hammer: head-*qiaoyin* (GB-18, IS GB-11).
(DACH) Headache pulling from all sides: *yongquan* (KI-1).
(DACH) Children — internal headaches at mealtime: *yixi* (BL-40, IS BL-45).
(DACH) Pain of the head and back: *feiyang* (BL-58).

Heaviness:
(DACH) Head heavy like a stone: *yintang* (MP-23a, IS M-HN-3), *naokong* (GB-19), ear-*heliao* (TW-22, IS TW-21 *ermen* by location); heaviness of the head: *taibai* (SP-3), thigh-*futu* (ST-32).
(DACH) Heaviness of the head, foggy vision: *taodao* (GV-12, IS GV-13), *luxi* (TW-19).
(DACH) Heaviness of the head, pain of the temples: *fuyang* (BL-59).

Migraines (pain of one side of the head, pian tou feng):

When the pain is on the left (yin) it is generally an emptiness of blood (yin), either fire or heat (excess yang). It increases at night. (YXRM V, 9v)

The Japanese call this *pian tou tong:*

An illness sometimes existing by itself. In general, it attacks patients with a nervous constitution or comes from heredity. Women, mostly between twenty and thirty years old, begin to suffer from it either from excess fatigue of body or mind, from onanism, or from drinking wine, etc.

Symptoms: acute pain on the side of the head; lasts from one half to one day; comes one or two at a time and stops. Women often have them at the time of menses. The attack is accompanied by stomachaches. Often there is trouble of the motor nerves of the vessels; the face is full of redness, burning and dryness; the pupils are changed. In the fifteen or twenty minutes before the attack, there are spots and dark places in front of the eyes with attacks of flowers-in-front-of-eyes. Hemianopia is rare. (JO, 35)

Treatment with needles:

naokong (GB-19)	3 *fen,*
fengchi (GB-20)	6 *fen,*
shangxing (GV-22, IS GV-23)	2 *fen,*
shenting (GV-23, IS GV-24)	6 *fen,*
shuaigu (GB-8)	3 *fen,*
taichong (GB-15, IS GB-9)	2 *fen,*
baihui (GV-19, IS GV-20)	3 *fen,*
xuanlu (GB-5)	3 *fen,*
sizhukong (TW-21, IS TW-23)	1 *fen,*
hegu (LI-4)	4 *fen. (JO, 35)*

Treatment with moxa:

shuaigu (GB-8)	5 *moxas,*
fengchi (GB-20)	7 *moxas,*
luxi (TW-19)	5 *moxas,*
tianchong (GB-15, IS GB-9)	5 *moxas,*
hegu (LI-4)	5 *moxas. (JO, 35)*

With both needles and moxa, stimulate the side which is ill. (JO, 35)

Pian tou tong, *migraines — on the side which is ill:*

Treatment with needles:

tianzhu (BL-10)	5 *fen,*
fengchi (GB-20)	5 *fen,*

kezhuren (GB-3, IS shangguan)	*3 fen,*
xuanlu (GB-5)	*2 fen,*
xuanli (GB-6)	*2 fen,*
sizhukong (TW-21, IS TW-23) ...	*2 fen. (JM, 320)*

Treatment with moxa:

bailao *(GV-13, IS GV-14 **dazhui**)*	*10 moxas,*
shenzhu *(GV-11, IS GV-12)*........	*10 moxas,*
*leg-**sanli** (ST-36)*	*8 moxas,*
fengchi (GB-20)	*8 moxas. (JM, 320)*

For migraines, it is usual in the center of China to cut a circle of mustard plaster about three centimeters in diameter and to place this on the temple at the level of the eyebrows on the side which is ill, leaving it there until relief comes (consequently, on the points *hanyan,* GB-4, and *xuanlu,* GB-5).

The very great majority of one-sided migraines come from an excess energy of the gallbladder (the pulse is hard, tense and ample) with insufficiency of the liver (the pulse of which is either nonexistent, or soft, small and without amplitude). The pains in this case are mostly on the temple (beginning point of the gallbladder meridian) and mostly on the right. Tonify *ququan* (LR-8) and the insufficient yin will be tonified at the expense of the yang; then disperse *yangfu* (GB-38). If the pain does not stop almost immediately, tonify *guangming* (GB-37) during the first six months of the year (thus helping the yang to rise) or tonify *ligou* (LR-5) during the last six months of the year (thus helping the yin to rise).

(YXRM I, 39r) Acute pains of the head, either vertex or lateral. If the pain is on the left, disperse on the right. If the pain is on the right, disperse on the left. Pain on both the right and the left, disperse on the right and left: *lieque* (LU-7); if not better, disperse: *taiyuan* (LU-9). *(YXRM I, 39r)* Acute pain on the side of the head: if there is fullness, disperse; if there is emptiness, tonify *lieque* (LU-7).

(YIX I, 4r) Migraines: *xuanlu* (GB-5), *hanyan* (GB-4).

(JM) Migraines: *touwei* (ST-1, IS ST-8) 1 *fen* under the skin towards the frontal eminences. If there is pain, disperse; if there is vertigo, tonify.

(JM) Migraines: *hegu* (LI-4), *baihui* (GV-19, IS GV-20), *touwei* (ST-1, IS ST-8), *hanyan* (GB-4), *xuanlu* (GB-5), *xuanli* (GB-6), *sizhukong* (TW-21, IS TW-23), *shangguan* (GB-3), *wangu* (GB-17, IS GB-12), *qubin* (GB-7), *houding* (GV-18, IS GV-19), *tianchong* (GB-15, IS GB-9).

(DACH) Lateral pain of the head and nape: *zhengying* (GB-13, IS GB-17).

Internal headaches on one side: *(JM) qubin* (GB-7); *(DACH) jiuwei* (CV-15).

Intermittent contractions of the head and face (spasms, tics).

Head:

(JM) Spasms *(jing luan)* of all the muscles of the head: *jianyu* (LI-15).

(JM) Spasms *(jing luan)* of the parietal muscles: *binao* (LI-14).

(JM) Spasms *(jing luan)* of the occipital and trapezius muscles: *luoque* (BL-8); of the occiput and neck: *shuaigu* (GB-8); of the area of the nape: *daying* (ST-8, IS ST-5).

Face:

(JM) Spasms *(jing luan)* of the facial nerve: *daying* (ST-8, IS ST-5), cheek-*juliao* (ST-6, IS ST-3), *quanliao* (SI-18), *xiaguan* (ST-2, IS ST-7), *sibai* (ST-5, IS ST-2).

(JM) Spasms *(jing luan)* of the face: *lieque* (LU-7), ear-*heliao* (TW-22, IS TW-21 *ermen* by location), *yangbai* (GB-10, IS GB-14), *shuigou* (GV-25, IS GV-26 *renzhong*), *daying* (ST-8, IS ST-5).

(JM) Spasms *(jing luan)* of all muscles of mouth and eyes: *shuigou* (GV-25, IS GV-26 *renzhong*), *dicang* (ST-7, IS ST-4).

(DACH) Face moving like leaves; *(DACH)* eyes blinking and moving, nape and mouth reacting: *chengqi* (ST-4, IS ST-1).

(DACH) Tic of upper part of face: gum-*yinjiao* (GV-27, IS GV-28).

(JM) Spasms of all the muscles of the corners of the mouth: *kezhuren* (GB-3, IS *shangguan*).

Prolonged contractures of the head and face.

Head:

Stiffness of the head: *(DACH IX, 11v)* tonify *neiguan* (PC-6); *(DACH, YXRM) jianzhen* (SI-9); head and neck stiff and contracted: *(YIX I, 4r) chengjiang* (CV-24).

Mouth:

(JM) Contraction of all the muscles of the mouth: *tongtian* (BL-7).

(DACH) Stiffness of the corners of the lips; *(JM)* and hardness: *jiaosun* (TW-20), *ermen* (TW-23, IS TW-21), *kezhuren* (GB-3, IS *shangguan*).

Contracture of masseter muscles, trismus, mouth tightened — *(JM)* contracture of masseter muscles (spasms, *jing luan*): (ST-3, IS ST-6).

(DACH, YXRM) Mouth tightened; *(DACH)* when chewing, teeth tighten and jaw does not open, cannot speak: *yifeng* (TW-17).

(DACH) Mouth tightened: *kezhuren* (GB-3, IS *shangguan*).

(YIX I, 7v) Mouth tightened, cannot open in order to speak; *(DACH)* mouth tightened, cannot open the mouth; *(YXRM)* mouth tightened: *hegu* (LI-4).

(YIX I, 8r; DACH IV, 11v) Mouth tightened, not opening; *(YXRM)* mouth tightened: *lieque* (LU-7).

(YXRM) Mouth tightened: *neiting* (ST-44).

(YXRM) Mouth tightened: *lidui* (ST-45).

(DACH) Mouth tightened, not opening; *(YXRM)* mouth tightened: *zhigou* (TW-6); *(DACH, YXRM)* nose-*heliao* (LI-19).

(DACH) Jaw tightened, cannot chew things; *(YXRM)* mouth tightened, jaw tight and painful: *tinghui* (GB-2).

(YXRM) Mouth tightened: *tinggong* (SI-19).

(YXRM) Mouth tightened, no longer speaks; *(DACH)* mouth tightened, not opening: *daying* (ST-8, IS ST-5).

(YXRM) Jaws tightened: ear-*heliao* (TW-22, IS TW-21 *ermen* by location).

(JM) Jaw tightened; *(YXRM)* mouth tightened, maxillary muscles tight and painful; *(DACH)* mouth tightened, cannot speak; *(DACH)* swelling of the jaw, and under the chin which cannot open, tightened and painful: *qubin* (GB-7).

(YXRM) Shock of face, mouth not opening: *chengjiang* (CV-24).

(DACH) Mouth tightened; *(YIZ, 40r)* mouth with corners not opening, cannot speak; *(DACH)* apoplexy, mouth tightened; *(DACH, YXRM)* barrier of the teeth not opening: *shuigou* (GV-25, IS GV-26 *renzhong*).

(DACH) Mouth tightened, epilepsy from shock: *kunlun* (BL-60).

Eyes:

(See Sense organs.)

Flaccid paralysis; facial paralysis (mian feng; yan mian shen jing ma bi); paralysis of the facial nerves.

Disperse the healthy, retracted side and tonify the paralyzed, flaccid side.

*Origin: chills (**gan mao**); external problems, leprosy, syphilis, lead poisoning; injury of a prominent bone, swelling of the parotid gland, injury to the base of the brain, meningitis, typhoid fever. Often there is first shoulder pain or swelling of the face; suddenly, half of the face loses its mobility, folds and cannot move. The eyelids always remain open; the corners of the mouth fall; nose and lips are awry. There is difficulty in speaking and chewing. Even the tip of the tongue is deviated and disturbed. (JO, 45)*

Treatment with needles:

juliao (ST-6, IS ST-3)	*3 fen,*
dicang (ST-7, IS ST-4)............	*3 fen,*
jiache (ST-3, IS ST-6)............	*3 fen,*
daying (ST-8, IS ST-5)............	*5 fen,*
yangbai (GB-10, IS GB-14)....	*2 fen,*
sizhukong (TW-21, IS TW-23)	*1 fen,*
zanzhu (BL-2)	*1 fen,*
chengjiang (CV-24)	*3 fen,*
hegu (LI-4)	*4 fen,*
leg-sanli (ST-36)	*1 cun. JO, 45)*

Treatment with moxa:

dicang (ST-7, IS ST-4)	*7 moxas,*
chengjiang (CV-24)...	*7 moxas,*
jianwai (SI-14)..........	*7 moxas,*
leg-sanli (ST-36)........	*7 moxas,*
hegu (LI-4)	*5 moxas. (JO, 45)*

(JM) Paralysis of the facial nerve: *lieque* (LU-7) arm-*sanli* (LI-10), *chongyang* (ST-42), *neiting* (ST-44), *shuigou* (GV-25, IS GV-26 *renzhong*), *ermen* (TW-23, IS TW-21), ear-*heliao* (TW-22, IS TW-21 *ermen* by location), *yangbai* (GB-10, IS GB-14), *kezhuren* (GB-3, IS *shangguan*), *yingxiang* (LI-20), *hanyan* (GB-4), *sibai* (ST-5, IS ST-2), *sizhukong* (TW-21, IS TW-23), *xiaguan* (ST-2, IS ST-7), *daying* (ST-8, IS ST-5), *jiache* (ST-3, IS ST-6), *juliao* (ST-6, IS ST-3), *tinghui* (GB-2), *chengjiang* (CV-24), *quanliao* (SI-18), *qucha* (BL-4), *yifeng* (TW-17).

(DACH XI, 3v) Mouth and eyes awry; comes from sleeping exposed to the wind after drunkenness, or from unhappiness which injures the liver, or from excess sex: *jiache* (ST-3, IS ST-6), *dicang* (ST-7, IS ST-4), *shuigou* (GV-25, IS GV-26 *renzhong*), *hegu* (LI-4). If not better, *baihui* (GV-19, IS GV-20), *tongziliao* (GB-1), *dicang* (ST-7, IS ST-4), *chengjiang* (CV-24).

Mouth and eyes awry: *(DACH)* *chengjiang* (CV-24), head-*wangu* (GB-17, IS GB-12), *chengqi* (ST-4, IS ST-1), *chongyang* (ST-42), *dicang* (ST-7, IS ST-4), *jiache* (ST-3, IS ST-6).

(DACH X, 32v) Mouth and eye awry; towards the left side, moxa on right; towards the right side, moxa on the left; moxa two times seven, repeated until realignment occurs: *tinghui* (GB-2), *jiache* (ST-3, IS ST-6), *dicang* (ST-7, IS ST-4).

(YIX I, 14v) On the paralyzed side, opposite to the elevated side: *dicang* (ST-7, IS ST-4), *jiache* (ST-3, IS ST-6), *tongziliao* (GB-1), *shuigou* (GV-25, IS GV-26 *renzhong*), *chengjiang* (CV-24), *hegu* (LI-4).

(DACH) Mouth and eye awry. Large moxas cause the mouth to turn opposite to the moxa. With needle, under the skin towards the back. When the energy is obtained, disperse. For illness on the right, treat on the left; for illness on the left, treat on the right. *(JM)* Paralysis or pain of the facial nerve: *dicang* (ST-7, IS ST-4). (Tonify the paralyzed, relaxed side; disperse the healthy, retracted side.)

(DACH) Eyes cannot be closed, mouth awry: *daying* (ST-8, IS ST-5).

(DACH II, 19r; YIX I, 5r) Lips awry: *taichong* (LR-3).

(YXRM I, 39r) Mouth awry, abundant flow of saliva; deviation on the left (left paralysis) disperse on the right (healthy side); deviation on the right, disperse on the left.

(DACH) Eyes cannot be closed; *dicang* (ST-7, IS ST-4).

(DACH) Corners of the lips unequal; will not retract, without control: *hegu* (LI-4).

(DACH) Mouth to the side, contracted; food not passing: *erjian* (LI-2).

(GSdeM) Motor point of the eyebrows: *sizhukong* (TW-21, IS TW-23).

(GSdeM) Canine muscle, elevator of the upper lip and the zygomatic muscles: *tongtian* (BL-7), *juliao* (ST-6, IS ST-3).

(JM) Risorius and orbicularis of the lips: *lidui* (ST-45); paralysis of the risorius muscle: *yifeng* (TW-17).

(JM) Yamen (GV-14, IS GV-15) is close to the center for closing the eyelids.

(GSdeM) Eyes not closing; peripheral paralysis, not central. This comes from flaccidity of the depressor muscle (orbicular muscle moved by the facial nerve) or from contracture of the elevator muscle (moved by the third cranial nerve). Tonify the facial nerve at the opposite arm-*sanli* (LI-10), opposite *lieque* (LU-7) and opposite *quchi* (LI-11). For the contracted elevator muscle, disperse at *xuanlu* (GB-5), *kezhuren* (GB-3, IS *shangguan*), *zanzhu* (BL-2), *yuzhen* (BL-9).

(GSdeM) Cheek-*juliao* (ST-6, IS ST-3) acts on the lower eyelids.

(GSdeM) Yangbai (GB-10, IS GB-14) acts on the frontal nerve.

Cold or heat of the head; congestions of the face.

Cold:
(YXRM) Pain from cold in half of the head: opposite *yuzhen* (BL-9).

(DACH) Shock and cold of the face: ear-*heliao* (TW-22, IS TW-21 *ermen* by location).

(DACH) Cold of the eyes: hand-*wangu* (SI-4).

Heat:
(YXRM) Heat of the head, yellow eyes: *zhongwan* (CV-12).

(YXRM) Heat of the head, dazzling *(mu xuan)*: *jinggu* (BL-64).

(JM) Movements of heat in the head, pressure of burning heat to the vertex: *qucha* (BL-4).

(DACH) Puncturing with a fine triangular needle (dispersing a lot) disperses all the energy (yang) heat and does not allow it to rise for attacking the head and eyes. *(JM)* Congestion of the face, dazzling; *(YXRM I, 46r)* redness of the face; *(DACH)* scarlet, swollen: *shangxing* (GV-22, IS GV-23).

(YIZ, 39r) Heat of the face; *(DACH)* heat of the skin of the face: *tiantu* (CV-22), *tianchuang* (SI-16).

(JM) Face becoming congested: *zhizheng* (SI-7).

(DACH) After a temporary unhappiness, if there has been great cold, heat in front of the ear; if there has been great heat, only on the shoulder: leg-*xialian* (ST-39, IS *xiajuxu*).

Redness of the face:
(YXRM I, 46r) Redness of the face: *shangxing* (GV-22, IS GV-23).

(DACH) Scarlet face: *shenshu* (BL-23).

(YXRM) Heat, scarlet face: *neiguan* (PC-6).

(JM) Attacks of redness and heat of the cheeks and lips: *juliao* (ST-6, IS ST-3).

(YIZ, 39r) Face scarlet and painful: *xuanli* (GB-6).

(DACH, YXRM) Redness and swelling of the skin of the face; *(JM)* congestion of the face: *xuanlu* (GB-5), *xuanli* (GB-6).

(YXRM) Face scarlet, nosebleeds; *(JM)* congestion of the face: *xinhui* (GV-21, IS GV-22).

Swelling of the head and face.

Head:
Swelling of the head: *(DACH X, 34v)* needle *quchi* (LI-11); *(YXRM) qiuxu* (GB-40); *(DACH) naohu* (GV-16, IS GV-17); *(YXRM) shangxing* (GV-22, IS GV-23).

Beriberi — head swollen: *(DACH)* thigh-*futu* (ST-32).

Swelling of head, heat and pain, headache, swelling of top of the head: *(DACH) qianding* (GV-20, IS GV-21).

Face: (sometimes the sign of beginning of chronic nephritis; see Quincke's edema).
Swelling of face: *(JM, YXRM, DACH) yanglingquan* (GB-34), *lidui* (ST-45); *(JM) jiexi* (ST-41); *(YXRM)* with mouth and eye awry: *xiangu* (ST-43), *chongyang* (ST-42); *(DACH) hegu* (LI-4), *tianfu* (LU-3); *(JM, DACH) muchuang* (GB-12, IS GB-16); *(DACH)* head-*wangu* (GB-17, IS GB-12); *(JM, YXRM, DACH) chengjiang* (CV-24); *(YXRM) tianshu* (ST-25); *(DACH X, 29v)* moxa at *shuifen* (CV-9).

Inflammation of the tissue of the face: *(JM) yingxiang* (LI-20), *shangyang* (LI-1), *shaoshang* (LU-11).

(YXRM) Swelling of the face and eyes, abscess; *(YIZ, 39v)* swelling of the face, swelling and compression of the eyes: bleed *xiangu* (ST-43).

(DACH) Swelling or abscess of the face or eyes: *lieque* (LU-7).

(DACH) Swelling of face and head, pain in heart: *gongsun* (SP-4).

Skin of the face swollen, red: *(DACH, YXRM) xuanlu* (GB-5); *(DACH) xuanli* (GB-6).

Skin of face swollen and painful: *(DACH) zhongfu* (LU-1).

Swelling and pruritis of the face: *shangyang* (LI-1); *(DACH) yingxiang* (LI-20); *(JM)* head-*wangu* (GB-17, IS GB-12).

Quincke's (angioneurotic) edema, lips and eyes suddenly swollen (insufficiency of liver — *GSdeM*): tonify *ququan* (LR-8) and *taichong* (LR-3).

Forehead:
Swelling of the forehead: *(YXRM) jiache* (ST-3, IS ST-6).

Nose:
(YXRM) Swelling and pain of the tip of the nose; *(DACH)* shock of the face; swelling of nose and cheeks: *juliao* (ST-6, IS ST-3).

(DACH) Swelling of the tip of the nose: ear-*heliao* (TW-22, IS TW-21 *ermen* by location).

Fatty inflammation of the nose: *(JM) hegu* (LI-4), *yingxiang* (LI-10), *qucha* (BL-4).

Lips:
(YXRM I, 39v) Swelling of the lips so that one cannot open them: disperse; "donkey's-mouth shock": swelling of the labial corners, cannot open the lips: disperse arm-*sanli* (LI-10).

(DACH, YXRM) Swelling of the lips: *taichong* (LR-3), *yingchuang* (ST-16).

(DACH III, 30r; DACH X, 29v; DACH) Lips swollen, painful: *yingxiang* (LI-20).

Cheeks and cheekbones:
(From dental caries: see Fluxions, Teeth.)
(YIZ, 4r) Swelling of the cheeks in false croup *(chan hou feng): shangxing* (GV-22, IS GV-23).

Cheeks and chin:
(JM) Swelling of the cheek and tissue of the chin: arm-*sanli* (LI-10).

(JM) Swelling of the bottom of the cheek and of the chin: *shangyang* (LI-1), *jiache* (ST-3, IS ST-6).

Cheek and jaw:
(JM) Swelling of the jaw and cheek: *jiache* (ST-3, IS ST-6).

Jaw:
Swelling and pain of the jaw: *tianjing* (TW-10); *(YXRM) tianchuang* (SI-16).

(DACH) Habitual swelling of the jaw, mastoid and teeth: foot-*linqi* (GB-41).
(DACH) Jaw swollen, pain radiating behind the ear: head-*wangu* (GB-17, IS GB-12).
(JM) Inflammation of the tissues of the jaw and below the chin: *yifeng* (TW-17).

Chin:
(JM) Swelling of the tissue of the chin: *shaoshang* (LU-11).
(DACH) Swelling of the chin: *qiangu* (SI-2).
(DACH IV, 7v) Chin and throat swollen: *shaoshang* (LU-11), *yanggu* (SI-5), hand-*wangu* (SI-4).
Swelling below the chin: *(DACH) shaoze* (SI-1), *zhizheng* (SI-7).

Jaw and below the chin:
Inflammation of the tissues of the jaw and below the chin: *(JM) yanggu* (SI-5), *yifeng* (TW-17).
Swelling of the jaw and below the chin: *(DACH) xiaxi* (GB-43), ear-*heliao* (TW-22, IS TW-21 *ermen* by location), *tianzong* (SI-11), *qubin* (GB-7).

Complexion, acne: see Skin.

Dislocation of the jaw.

(DACH) Dislocation of the jaw when yawning: *sanyinjiao* (SP-6).
(DACH) Dislocation of the jaw: *yifeng* (TW-17), *tinghui* (GB-2), *jiache* (ST-3, IS ST-6), *xiaguan* (ST-2, IS ST-7).

II. Neck and Nape *(Jing-Xiang)*

In general.

Illnesses of the face, neck and nape: *(DACH) houxi* (SI-3).

Pain.

Anterior neck *(jing):*
Pain of the front of the neck: *(DACH) yongquan* (KI-1), *naoshu* (SI-10), *hanyan* (GB-4), *daying* (ST-8, IS ST-5), *tianchuang* (SI-16).
(JM) Pain of all the nerves and muscles of the front of the neck: *jiache* (ST-3, IS ST-6).
(DACH) Pain of the front of the neck below the chin and of the shoulder: *xiaohai* (SI-8).
(JM) Neuralgia or inflammation of all the muscles of the neck and scapula: *quepen* (ST-12).
(GSdeM) Sternoclavicular arthritis: *qiche* (ST-11), *yufu* (KI-27).

Front of the neck and nape:
Pain of front of neck and nape: *(DACH) qiangu* (SI-2), *tianjing* (TW-10), *xuanzhong* (GB-39), *feiyang* (BL-58), *waiqiu* (GB-36), *zhizheng* (SI-7), *xiaohai* (SI-8), *tianrong* (SI-17), gum-*yinjiao* (GV-27, IS GV-28), *qiangjian* (GV-17, IS GV-18), *fengfu* (GV-15, IS GV-16), head-*wangu* (GB-17, IS GB-12).
Stiffness and pain of the front of the neck and nape: *(DACH) jianjing* (GB-21), foot-*qiaoyin* (GB-44).
Pain like a necklace, tightness of shoulder and back: *shangyang* (LI-1).

Intermittent contractions, spasms.

Front of the neck:
Spasms of the front of the neck: *(DACH) fufen* (BL-36, IS BL-41).

Front of neck and nape:
Spasms of the front of the neck and nape: *(DACH) qiangu* (SI-2), *shaoze* (SI-1), *xiaoluo* (TW-12), *tianliao* (TW-15), *jianliao* (TW-14), *jianzhen* (SI-9), *bailao* (GV-13, IS GV-14 *dazhui*), *baihui* (GV-19, IS GV-20), *tianzhu* (BL-10), head-*wangu* (GB-17, IS GB-12), *tianyou* (TW-16), *benshen* (GB-9, IS GB-13), *tiantu* (CV-22), *lingxu* (KI-24).

Contracture, stiffness; torticollis.

Anterior neck:
Stiffness of the anterior neck: *(DACH) jiache* (ST-3, IS ST-6), foot-*qiaoyin* (GB-44).

Torticollis (*xie jing*, "wry neck"; *jing li*, "twisting of neck"):

1)   Wry neck: *(JM) tianchuang* (SI-16), *qishe* (ST-11).

2)   Twisting of neck: *(YXRM, DACH) sanjian* (LI-3), *xiaohai* (SI-8), *lidui* (ST-45); *(DACH)* head-*linqi* (GB-11, IS GB-15); *(YXRM) tianchuang* (SI-16), *tianjing* (TW-10).

Contracture of sternocleidomastoidius muscle (innervated by the spinal nerves): neck-*futu* (LI-18), *qishe* (ST-11), *fufen* (BL-36, IS BL-41).

Front of neck and nape:
(DACH) Front of neck and nape stiff: *qishe* (ST-11).
Difficulty turning nape and front of neck: *tianjing* (TW-10), *tongtian* (BL-7).
(DACH VII, 28r) houxi (SI-3), *hegu* (LI-4), *chengjiang* (CV-24).
Nape and front of neck stiff and tightened, cannot turn: *shaoze* (SI-1), gum-*yinjiao* (GV-27, IS GV-28).
Stiffness and pain of the front of the neck and nape: *jinggu* (BL-64).

Cold and heat of the front of the neck and nape.

Cold:
(JM) Extreme coldness of the front of the neck and nape: *tianliao* (TW-15).

Heat:
(JM) Heat invading the area of the neck and scapula: *quepen* (ST-12).

Swelling of the front of the neck and nape; abscess.

Neck:
(DACH) Swelling of the neck: *qiuxu* (GB-40), *lidui* (ST-45); *(YXRM) jiaosun* (TW-20).
(YXRM) Swelling of the front of the neck, pain of the nape: *tianrong* (SI-17).

Front of neck and nape:
(JM) Inflammation of the front of the neck and nape: *fubai* (GB-16, IS GB-10).
(JM) Inflammation of the tissues of the neck and nape: *xiaohai* (SI-8), *qiangu* (SI-2), *naohui* (TW-13), head-*wangu* (GB-17, IS GB-12), *fubai* (GB-16, IS GB-10).
(DACH) Swelling of the front of the neck and nape: *qiangu* (SI-2); *(JM) naohui* (TW-13), head-*wangu* (GB-17, IS GB-12).
(DACH) Swelling of the front of the neck and nape, abscess, tumors: *fubai* (GB-16, IS GB-10).

Subclavicular fossa:
(DACH) Swelling of the subclavicular fossa of the axilla, pruritis, lesions: foot-*linqi* (GB-41).
(DACH) Swelling and pain of the subclavicular fossa: *yangfu* (GB-38).
(DACH) Abscess of the neck and nape: *tianrong* (SI-17); *(DACH VII, 28r) waiguan* (TW-5), *jianjing* (GB-21), *fengfu* (GV-15, IS GV-16), *chengjiang* (CV-24); *(DACH) fubai* (GB-16, IS GB-10).

Goiter.

(GSdeM) Disperse *renying* (ST-9), *shuitu* (ST-10), *tiantu* (CV-22), *qishe* (ST-11).
(GSdeM) Swelling of the thyroid: *renying* (ST-9), disperse the C6-C7 interval.
(DACH) Neck and nape — swelling, abscess, *ying* tumors: *fubai* (GB-16, IS GB-10).

III. Nape; Nape and Shoulder

In general.

Illnesses of the face, neck and nape: *(DACH) houxi* (SI-3).

Pains.

Nape *(xiang):*
(GSdeM) Pain of the cervical vertebra: *qianding* (GV-20, IS GV-21).
(GSdeM) Pain of the seventh cervical vertebra: *shuigou* (GV-25, IS GV-26 *renzhong*).
Pain of the nape: *(DACH) xiaoluo* (TW-12), *taibai* (SP-3), *qianding* (GV-20, IS GV-21), *jiaosun* (TW-20).

Pain and swelling of nape: *(DACH) lidui* (ST-45).

Nape as if torn out: *(DACH) taodao* (GV-12, IS GV-13), *tianzhu* (BL-10), *yuzhen* (BL-9), gum-*yinjiao* (GV-27, IS GV-28); and the neck with energy: *xiaoluo* (TW-12).

Stiffness and pain of nape: *(DACH) houxi* (SI-3), *lieque* (LU-7), *qiangjian* (GV-17, IS GV-18); *(GSdeM) jian-zhongshu* (SI-15).

Pain of the nape, swelling of the front of the neck: *tianrong* (SI-17).

Occipital neuralgia: *(JM) tianzhu* (BL-10), *yamen* (GV-14, IS GV-15); *(GSdeM) yuzhen* (BL-9).

Nape and shoulder pain: *(DACH) tianchuang* (SI-16), *ganshu* (BL-18).

Nape and body pain: *(DACH) yongquan* (KI-1).

Head and nape pain: *houxi* (SI-3); *(DACH) qucha* (BL-4), *shugu* (BL-65).

Spasms.

Spasms of nape and occiput: *(DACH). shuaigu* (GB-8)

Spasms of nape and shoulder: *(DACH) dazhu* (BL-11), *tianzong* (SI-11), *bingfeng* (SI-12).

Nape:

Spasms of the nape: *daying* (ST-8, IS ST-5).

Spasms of occipital and trapezius muscles: *luoque* (BL-8).

Spasms of the front of neck, nape and scapula: *taodao* (GV-12, GV-13).

Spasms of neck and scapula: *tianchuang* (SI-16).

Stiffness, contracture.

Nape:

Stiff nape, cannot turn to look backwards: *houxi* (SI-1), *tianzhu* (BL-10).

Stiff nape: *(DACH) lieque* (LU-7), *chize* (LU-5), foot-*tonggu* (BL-66), *jinggu* (BL-64), *fufen* (BL-36, IS BL-41), *pohu* (BL-37, IS BL-42), *jianjing* (BL-21), *naokong* (GB-19), *fengfu* (GV-15, IS GV-16), *qiangjian* (GV-17, IS GV-18).

Cannot turn nape: *shaohai* (HT-3).

Cannot look back: *(DACH)* leg-*sanli* (ST-36), *xiaohai* (SI-8), *bailao* (GV-13, IS GV-14 *dazhui*), *tianzhu* (BL-10), *fengchi* (GB-20), *tianchuang* (SI-16), *tianyou* (TW-16), *tianrong* (SI-17).

Nape, back and abdomen contracted: *bailao* (GV-13, IS GV-14 *dazhui*).

Head stiff: tonify *neiguan* (PC-6).

Swelling of the nape.

(DACH) Swelling and pain of the nape: *lidui* (ST-45).

Tumors of the nape.

Blood tumors *(liu)* of the front of neck and nape: *(DACH) naohui* (TW-13).

Energy of tumors *(ying)* at the nape: *(DACH) naohui* (TW-13).

Neck and nape, swelling, abscess, tumors: *(DACH) fubai* (GB-16, IS GB-10).

IV. Shoulder

In general.

Shoulder: *jianjing* (GB-21); shoulder and back: *(YIX I, 4v)* hand-*zhongzhu* (TW-3).

Pains, arthritis.

Shoulder:

Shoulder pains: *(YXRM) yanglao* (SI-6), *quchi* (LI-11); *(DACH, YXRM)* cannot lift the arm: *bingfeng* (SI-12); *(GSdeM) jianshugu* (MP-10); *(DACH III, 29r)* pain of the shoulder: *jianjing* (GB-21); *(YXRM) shentang* (BL-39, IS BL-44); *(DACH X, 28v)* acute pain: *ganshu* (BL-18).

Shoulder pain, the arm cannot be lifted: *yunmen* (LU-2).

Shoulder arthritis (inflammation of the shoulder joint): *(JM) fubai* (GB-16, IS GB-10), *binao* (LI-14), *jugu* (LI-16), *jianzhen* (SI-9); *(JM)* inflammation of the scapulohumeral articulation: *naoshu* (SI-10).

Acromioclavicular arthritis: *(GSdeM) jugu* (LI-16), *tianyou* (LI-15).

Scapulohumeral arthritis: *(GSdeM) jianliao* (TW-14), *xianzhen* (SI-9), *binao* (LI-14), *jianliu* (LI-15), *jianshugu* (MP-10).

(DACH) Shoulder on the verge of breaking: *yanglao* (SI-6).

(DACH IX, 27r; DACH III, 29r) Pain of the shoulder linked with umbilicus: arm-*sanli* (LI-10).

(DACH) Pain and heat in the subclavicular fossa and shoulder: *jianzhen* (SI-9).

Shoulder and arm:

(JM) Shoulder and arm pain: *erjian* (LI-2), *lieque* (LU-7); *(DACH, YXRM)* cannot lift the arm: *yangchi* (TW-4); *(DACH) chize* (LU-5); *(DACH)* acute pain: *jianyu* (LI-15); *(JM) jianzhen* (SI-9); *(JM)* acute pain: *shentang* (BL-39, IS BL-44); *(DACH)* cannot lift the arm: *binao* (LI-14).

(YXRM I, 39r) Acute pain of the shoulder, back, arm and elbow: *hegu* (LI-4) and *quchi* (LI-11).

(YXRM I, 46v) Acute pain of shoulder and arm connected to the back: hand-*zhongzhu* (TW-3).

(DACH) Pain and numbness of the shoulder and arm: *zhigou* (TW-6), *tianliao* (TW-15), *tianzong* (SI-11), *guanchong* (TW-1); *(DACH)* shoulder on the verge of breaking, arm as if torn out: *yanglao* (SI-6).

(JM) Rheumatism of the shoulder-arm articulation: *zhouliao* (LI-12).

(JM) Arthritis of the shoulder-scapular articulation: *jugu* (LI-16), *binao* (LI-14).

(JM) Pain of the shoulder and elbow joints: *neiguan* (PC-6), *quze* (PC-3).

(JM) Pain of the nerves of the scapula and top of the arm: *naoshu* (SI-10).

(DACH) Pain behind the ear, in the shoulder, arm and elbow: *tianjing* (TW-10).

(JM) Pain of the nerves of the shoulder, elbow and finger joints: *guanchong* (TW-1).

(DACH) Pain and heat of the shoulder and arm, energy flowing into a seized and tightened scapula, pain, melancholy: *quyuan* (SI-13).

Shoulder and sides:

(DACH) Pain of shoulder and sides: *burong* (SI-19).

Shoulder and back:

(DACH) Pain under the chin, front of the neck, back and shoulder: *erjian* (LI-2).

(DACH, YXRM) Pain of the shoulder and back radiating to the nape: *tianchuang* (SI-16); *(GSdeM) jianzhongshu* (SI-15).

(JM) Pain of the nerves of the shoulder and back: *sanjian* (LI-3); *(DACH VI, 14v)* acute pain of the shoulder and back from panting or cough: *shaoshang* (LU-11); *(YXRM I, 39r, YIX, 43r)* pain of the shoulder and back after a prolonged cold: hand-*zhongzhu* (TW-3); *(DACH, YXRM)* pain of the shoulder and back, shivering: *erjian* (LI-2); *(DACH) taiyuan* (LU-9); *(JM) yunmen* (LU-2); *(JM) gaohuangshu* (BL-38, IS BL-43); *(YXRM) zhongfu* (LU-1); *(JM) pohu* (BL-37, IS BL-42); *(YXRM) fubai* (GB-16, IS GB-10).

Problems of the shoulder and back: *(DACH III, 32r)* arm-*sanli* (LI-10); *(YIX I, 4v; DACH IV, 11v) zhongzhu* (TW-3).

(DACH, YXRM) Shoulder pain, back and body on the verge of breaking: *tianzhu* (BL-10).

(DACH III, 29r) Pain of the shoulder and vertebral column: *wushu* (GB-27).

(JM) Pain of the nerves, shoulder and scapula: *hegu* (LI-4), *lougu* (SP-7).

(DACH) Pain of the shoulder radiating to the scapula; *(YXRM)* from cold and heat swelling of the shoulder, bringing pain in the scapula: *naoshu* (SI-10).

(DACH, YXRM) Severe coldness, tightening of the shoulder and back, pain radiating to the subclavicular fossa: *shangyang* (LI-1).

(GSdeM) Pain like suspenders: *yangfu* (GB-38), *jianjing* (GB-21).

(JM) Pain to the point of paralysis of shoulder and back: arm-*shanglian* (LI-9).

Shoulder and chest:

Spasms of all the muscles of the shoulder and chest: *burong* (ST-19).

Spasms of the shoulder, contractures.

Spasms:

Spasms of the trapezius muscle (innervated by the spinal nerves): *(JM) naokong* (GB-19), *fufen* (BL-36, IS BL-41).

Spasms of the occipital and trapezius muscles: *luoque* (BL-8).

Spasms of all the muscles of shoulder and scapula: *xiaoluo* (TW-12).

Spasms of the shoulder and back: *(JM) gaohuangshu* (BL-38, IS BL-43), *fufen* (BL-36, IS BL-41), *pohu* (BL-37, IS BL-42).

Spasms or contractures of the shoulder and back: *kunlun* (BL-60).
Contractions from cold of the shoulder and back: *(DACH, YXRM) jingmen* (GB-25).

Contractures of the shoulder:
(YXRM) Shoulder cannot be lifted: *wenliu* (LI-7).
(YXRM, DACH) Contracture *(luan)* and tightening *(ji)* of the shoulder, radiating to the arm and chest: *juliao* (GB-28, IS GB-29).
(GSdeM) Contracture of the trapezius muscle: *jianjing* (GB-21), *quyuan* (SI-13).
(DACH) Contracture of the shoulder, armpit; *(YXRM)* and hand: *shaofu* (HT-8).
(GSdeM) Contracture of the infraspinatus muscle: *quyuan* (SI-13).

Shoulder and back:
(YXRM) Shoulder and back impossible to bend forward or backward: *geshu* (BL-17).
(DACH, YXRM) Tightening of the shoulder and back: *sanjiaoshu* (BL-22).
(YXRM) Shoulder and scapula seized, tightened with acute pain and melancholy: *quyuan* (SI-13).

Shoulder and elbow:
(DACH) Shoulder and elbow contracted *(luan),* arm and hand not lifting: *chize* (LU-5).
Armpit painful, contracted: *(DACH) naohui* (TW-13).

Cold, heat.

Cold:
Extreme coldness of the shoulder and back: *(JM) dazhu* (BL-11).
Frozen shoulder: *(JM) naoshu* (SI-10), *jugu* (LI-16), *jianwaishu* (SI-14), *jianzhongshu* (SI-15), *tianliao* (TW-15), *jueyinshu* (BL-14).

Heat:
(DACH) Heat in the shoulder: *jianyu* (LI-15).

Numbness.

Numbness and pain of the shoulder and arm: *(DACH) tianzong* (SI-11), *tianliao* (TW-15), *yanglao* (SI-6).
Numbness and pain of the shoulder, arm, elbow and wrist: *pianli* (LI-6).

Flaccidity, flaccid paralysis.

(JM) Paralysis *(ma bi)* of the shoulder area: *bingfeng* (SI-12).
(JM) Paralysis *(ma bi)* of the nape and shoulder: *tianzong* (SI-11).
(YXRM) Shoulder not rising: *qinglengyuan* (TW-11), *wenliu* (LI-7); *(DACH)* heavy shoulder, cannot lift it: *jianliao* (TW-14); *(YXRM)* shoulder cannot be lifted; *(DACH)* shoulder and arm not lifting: *qingling* (HT-2).
(JM) Paralysis *(ma bi)* of the shoulder and arm: *erjian* (LI-2), *yanglao* (SI-6).
(GSdeM) Weakness of the trapezius and infraspinatus muscle: *quyuan* (SI-13).

Swelling of the shoulder.

Swelling of the shoulder: *(DACH) taichong* (LR-3), *naoshu* (SI-10), *jianyu* (LI-15).
Swelling of the shoulder radiating into pain of the scapula: *naohui* (TW-13).

V. Upper Limb

General command points.

(YXRM I, 46v) All illnesses of arm and hand: *jianyu* (LI-15), *quchi* (LI-11).
(DACH) All illnesses of the head, face, arm and hand: *wangu* (SI-4), *yanggu* (SI-5).

Pain, arthritis, rheumatism.

Nerves:
(JM) Neuralgia of the brachial plexus: *quepen* (ST-12); *(GSdeM)* C6 to T2.
(JM) Pain of all the nerves of the arm: *tianding* (LI-17), *tianfu* (LU-3).
(JM) Illness or trouble of the radial nerve: *jingqu* (LU-8).
(JM) Pain of the radial nerve (which innervates the extensors): *lieque* (LU-7).

(JM) Pain of the cubital nerve: *yanggu* (SI-5), *yanglao* (SI-6), *xiaohai* (SI-8).

(JM) Trouble or pain of the medial nerve: arm-*ximen* (PC-4).

(GSdeM) Pain of the circumflex nerve: *naohui* (TW-13).

The entire upper limb:

(JM) Pain of the nerves of the upper limb: *zhigou* (TW-6), *sanyangluo* (TW-8), *tianzong* (SI-11), *tinggong* (SI-19), *jianliao* (TW-14), *pohu* (BL-37, IS BL-42).

(DACH) Pain in the arm, elbow and hand: *chize* (LU-5), *quze* (PC-3).

(DACH) Pain in the small intestine meridian; shoulder, arm, little finger: *xiabai* (SI-8).

(JM) Arthritis of the upper limb: *yangchi* (TW-4), hand-*wangu* (SI-4), *hanyan* (GB-4), *jugu* (LI-16).

Arm and humerus:

(JM) Pain of the nerves of the arm: *sanjian* (LI-3), *quchi* (LI-11), *tianfu* (LU-3), *jianyu* (LI-15), *bingfeng* (SI-12), *tianzong* (SI-11), *quyuan* (SI-13), *tinggong* (SI-19).

(DACH) Rheumatism of the arm: *jianyu* (LI-15).

(JM) Pain of all the muscles of the arm: *xiaohai* (SI-8).

(YXRM) Pain of the lateral surface of the arm; elbow painful, hand no longer reaches the head; cannot dress oneself: *guanchong* (TW-1).

(DACH) Pain of the lateral surface of the arm; cannot lift it: *yanggu* (SI-5).

(YXRM) Pain of the medial surface of the arm, scapula, back and chest: *tianquan* (PC-2); *(DACH X, 30r)* pain of the medial surface of the arm: *taiyuan* (LU-9).

(DACH) Pain of the posteromedial surface of the arm: *shaochong* (HT-9).

(DACH) Pain tightening both arms: *tianjing* (TW-10), *jianjing* (GB-21).

Arm and elbow:

(JM) Pain of the nerves of the arm and elbow: *lingdao* (HT-4), *quchi* (LI-11).

(YXRM) Pain of the arm and elbow: arm-*xialian* (LI-8), *zhongzhu* (TW-3).

(YXRM) Pain of the arm and elbow: *lieque* (LU-7), arm-*wuli* (LI-13).

(YXRM) Pain and lack of strength of arm and elbow, cannot reach the head; *(DACH)* the same with difficulty in extension or flexion: *kongzui* (LU-6).

(DACH) Pain of arm and elbow: cannot lift them: *guanchong* (TW-1).

Elbow:

(DACH III, 30v) Acute pain of the elbow: *chize* (LU-5).

(JM) Pain of the nerves of the elbow: *zhongzhu* (TW-3).

(JM) Arthritis of the elbow: *yemen* (TW-2), *quchi* (LI-11).

(DACH VI, 15v) Elbow pain: *guanchong* (TW-1), head-*wangu* (GB-17, IS GB-12).

(YXRM) Elbow pain, difficulty in flexion or extension: *naohui* (TW-13).

(DACH, YXRM) Elbow pain, posterior surface: *tianzong* (SI-11).

(DACH) Elbow pain, cannot extend it: *shaochong* (HT-9).

(YXRM) Elbow pain from a bad cold: leg-*sanli* (ST-36).

(DACH) Apoplexy, with elbow pain: *tongli* (HT-5).

Elbow and axilla:

(DACH) Pain and swelling of the elbow and axilla: *xiaohai* (SI-8).

Elbow and forearm:

(JM) Arthritis of the elbow, forearm, wrist and hand: hand-*wangu* (SI-4).

Forearm:

(JM) Pain of the nerves of the forearm: *shaoze* (SI-1), *qiangu* (SI-2), *taiyuan* (LU-9), *sidu* (TW-9), arm-*wuli* (LI-13), *jianjing* (GB-21), *tianchi* (PC-1).

(GSdeM) Pain of the medial surface of the forearm (cubital side): *xiaohai* (SI-8).

(GSdeM) Pain of the forearm, lateral surface (radial): *taiyuan* (LU-9).

(GSdeM) Pain and weakness of the radial muscles; cannot serve from a heavy pitcher: arm-*xialian* (LI-8).

(DACH, YXRM) Pain of the forearm and hand; cannot raise or lower by themselves: *yemen* (TW-2).

(DACH X, 32v) Pain and numbness of the elbow and wrist: *tongli* (HT-5).

Wrist:

(DACH IV, 5r) Wrist without strength, painful; great difficulty holding or moving objects: neither tonify nor disperse — leave the needle: hand-*wangu* (SI-4).

(DACH) Pain of the wrist: *quchi* (LI-1), *yanggu* (SI-5).

(DACH IV, 5v) Pain of the wrist, forearm and hand red and swollen: *yemen* (TW-2).
(JM) Arthritis of the elbow, wrist and fingers: hand-*wangu* (SI-4).
(JM) Arthritis of the wrist: *taiyuan* (LU-9); *(GSdeM) waiguan* (TW-5).

Hand, fingers:
(DACH X, 5r) Acute pain of the five fingers: *(DACH)* pain of the five fingers, cannot hold objects; *(YXRM)* fingers of the hand are all painful; *(YXRM I, 46v)* pain and impossibility of extending and flexing the fingers: *waiguan* (TW-5).
(DACH) All ten fingers are painful; *(JM)* acute pain of the fingers: *zhizheng* (SI-7).
(DACH) Fingers painful, palm hot: *shaoshang* (LU-11).
(JM) Arthritis of fingers. *(DACH, YXRM)* The five fingers can neither be flexed nor extended; *(DACH III, 32r)* the five fingers cannot be extended: hand-*zhongzhu* (TW-3).
(JM) Inflammation of the bony joints of the fingers; *(DACH)* fingers do not take hold: *kongzui* (LU-6).

Spasms of the upper limb.

The whole upper limb:
Spasms: *(JM)* spasms *(jing luan)* of the upper limb: *shaochong* (HT-9), *tongli* (HT-5), *pianli* (LI-6), *qinglengyuan* (TW-11), *quepen* (ST-12), *pohu* (BL-37, IS BL-42) *rugen* (ST-18), hip-*juliao* (GB-28, IS GB-29) and at level of C5, C6, C7.

Upper limb and elbow:
Upper limb and elbow: *(JM) houxi* (SI-3), *yemen* (TW-2), *zhizheng* (SI-7), *quchi* (LI-11).

Upper limb and scapula:
Upper limb and scapula: *(JM) jianliao* (TW-14).

Arm:
Spasms of all the muscles of the arm: *(JM) quepen* (ST-12).
Spasms of the arm and shoulder: *(JM) yanglao* (SI-6).
Spasms of the arm and elbow: *(JM) yemen* (TW-2), *zhizheng* (SI-7). See also: Trembling.
(DACH) Arm, elbow and hand agitated, cannot be stopped: *quze* (PC-3).

Hands:
(DACH VII, 31v) Both hands agitated, cannot take hold of objects: trembling of the head and face: foot-*linqi* (GB-41), *quze* (PC-3), hand-*wangu* (SI-4), *hegu* (LI-4), *zhongzhu* (TW-3).
(DACH VII, 27r) Hands and feet are all trembling, cannot walk, unable to take hold of objects: *houxi* (SI-3), hand-*wangu* (SI-4), *yangxi* (LI-5), *quchi* (LI-11), *taichong* (LR-3), *gongsun* (SP-4), *yanglingquan* (GB-34).
(DACH II, 32r) Hands trembling, pain in the heart: *shaohai* (HT-3).
(DACH) Hands and face trembling: *houxi* (SI-3).

Writer's cramp *(shou jing):*

> Origins: this illness occurs mainly in those who write a lot: bad brush, bad posture of the scribe or trauma to the wrist; osteitis, neuritis, etc. Symptoms are of a progressive nature. The movements of writing are bothered by the muscles, mainly by the "interosseous vermiform muscles," the extensors of the forearm and the flexors. This then extends to the arm, elbow and shoulder; it happens when one is writing. Distinguish: 1) the contractile type; 2) the trembling type; 3) the flaccid type; 4) the neuralgic type. (JO, 50)

Treatment with needles:

***gaohuangshu** (BL-38, IS BL-43)*	*4 fen,*
***jugu** (LI-16)*	*6 fen,*
***tianzong** (SI-11)*	*3 fen,*
***bingfeng** (SI-12)*	*3 fen,*
***naoshu** (SI-10)*	*8 fen,*
***jianyu** (LI-15)*	*8 fen,*
***binao** (LI-14)*	*5 fen,*
***tianjing** (TW-10)*	*5 fen,*
***quchi** (LI-11)*	*8 fen,*
***arm-sanli** (LI-10)*	*6 fen,*
***yangxi** (LI-5)*	*3 fen. (JO, 50)*

Treatment with moxa:

tianzong (SI-11) .	*7 moxas,*
jianyu (LI-15).....	*7 moxas,*
binao (LI-14)......	*7 moxas,*
tianjing (TW-10)	*7 moxas,*
quchi (LI-11)......	*7 moxas,*
arm-sanli (LI-10)	*7 moxas,*
yangxi (LI-5)......	*7 moxas. (JO, 50)*

(JM) Writer's cramp: *laogong* (PC-8), hand-*wangu* (SI-4), *tianzhu* (BL-10), *yuzhen* (BL-9).

(DACH VI, 15r) Hand contracted: *zhongchong* (PC-9); *(YXRM)* *daling* (PC-7).

(DACH X, 32v) Hand contracted *(jing luan)* without strength, cannot extend: arm-*sanli* (LI-10). (On the extensor muscles, tonify.)

(GSdeM) Spasms or contracture of the flexor pollicis longus muscle: *erbai* (MP-12, IS M-UE-29).

Contractures of the upper limb.

Muscles:

(GSdeM) Contracture of the biceps: *jianyu* (LI-15), *tianfu* (LU-3).

(GSdeM) Coracobrachialis muscle: *tianquan* (PC-2), *yunmen* (LU-2).

(GSdeM) Extensor muscles (innervated by the radial nerve): *lieque* (LU-7), *jingqu* (LU-8), arm-*sanli* (LI-10); tonify *waiguan* (TW-5).

(GSdeM) Flexors: *waiguan* (TW-5), *zhizheng* (SI-7); tonify arm-*sanli* (LI-10).

(GSdeM) Pronator muscles: *quze* (PC-3).

(GSdeM) Supinator muscles: *quchi* (LI-11).

(GSdeM) Flexor pollicis longus: *erbai* (MP-12, IS M-UE-29).

The entire upper limb:

(YXRM) Arm, elbow, hand contracted, cannot be extended (on the extensors, tonify): arm-*sanli* (LI-10); *(YXRM I, 46v)* *zhizheng* (SI-7) (on the flexors, disperse).

(DACH IV, 10v) Arm and hand contractures *(ju luan); (DACH)* arm and hand contracted, tightened: *jianyu* (LI-15).

(YIX I, 4r) Contracture *(ju luan)* of the arm and back, without action: *chize* (LU-5), *bailao* (GV-13, IS GV-14 *dazhui*).

(YIZ, 44r) Contracture *(ju luan)* of the upper limb: *sanjian* (LI-3), 1 *fen,* and moxa; *qiangu* (SI-2), 1 *fen,* and moxa.

(DACH XI, 4v) Contracture *(ju luan)* of arm and hands, muscles of the hands not opening by themselves, comes from sleeping outside or in a humid area: *yangchi* (TW-4), *zhongshu* (TW-3), *hegu* (LI-4), *quchi* (LI-11), *chize* (LU-5); if not better, *jianyu* (LI-15), arm-*sanli* (LI-10), hand-*zhongzhu* (TW-3), *shaoshang* (LU-11).

(YXRM) Contracture of the shoulder, axilla, hand: *shaofu* (HT-8).

(YXRM) Pain and tightness *(ji)* of the axilla, elbow and palm: *shaochong* (HT-9).

(YXRM) Arm and hands, contracted, folded: *shenmen* (HT-7).

(YXRM) Pain in the arm, contracture, tightening *(ji); (DACH, YXRM)* arm paralyzed *(ma mu),* tightened *(ji),* without action, contractures *(luan): zhouliao* (LI-12).

(DACH) Arm and elbow cannot be extended or flexed: *waiguan* (TW-5).

Elbow:

(DACH, YXRM) Elbow contractures: *lingdao* (HT-4); *(YXRM)* *qiangu* (LI-2), *shaohai* (HT-3); *(YIZ, 45r; DACH IV, 15v; DACH III, 30v)* *quchi* (LI-11), arm-*sanli* (LI-10), *waiguan* (TW-5); *(DACH X, 24r, DACH)* hand-*wangu* (SI-4); *(DACH X, 32v)* *lieque* (LU-7); and fullness of the limbs: *neiguan* (PC-6); *(DACH, YXRM)* and swelling of the axilla: *jianshi* (PC-5).

Hands:

(DACH X, 30r) Hand contractures *(luan); (YIX I, 4v)* finger contractures: *shaoshang* (LU-11); *(YXRM)* *daling* (PC-7); five fingers impossible to extend or flex: *(DACH)* five fingers contracted *(liu):* hand-*wangu* (SI-4); *(YXRM)* hand contractures: *yanglao* (SI-6), *waiguan* (TW-5).

(YIZ, 45v) Elbow numb, hand in an arc: *chize* (LU-5), 5 *fen,* first tonify, then disperse.

(YIX I, 4v) Contracture like a bow, cannot open: *quchi* (LI-11).

(DACH VI, 15r) Hand contractures: *zhongchong* (PC-9).

(DACH) Hand flexed, cannot be extended: *shaofu* (HT-8).

(GSdeM) Retraction of the palmar aponeurosis (Dupuytren's Contracture): disperse *shaofu* (HT-8) and *laogong* (PC-8).

(YIZ, 37v) Contracture *(ju luan)* of the five fingers; *wuhu* (MP-19 to 23, IS M-UE-45).

Cold and heat of the upper limb.

Cold (insufficiency: tonify):
(JM) Extreme coldness of the upper limb: *jiquan* (HT-1), *jianwaishu* (SI-14).

(DACH) Coldness and insufficiency of the arm and elbow: *jiquan* (HT-1).

(DACH) Cold up to the elbow: *jianwaishu* (SI-14).

(DACH VII, 27v) Cold of the arms: *shenmai* (BL-62), *chize* (LU-5).

(DACH) Cold of the arms and hands: *shenmen* (HT-7).

(JM) Cold and insufficiency of the fingers: *shaohai* (HT-3).

(DACH) Can remove cold as well as heat: *shenmai* (BL-62).

Heat (excess, disperse):
(DACH) Can remove heat as well as cold: *shenmai* (BL-62).

(DACH) Heat and apoplexy of the hands: *neiguan* (PC-6).

(DACH) Heat of the palm, pain radiating to the subclavicular fossa, a lot of yawning: *taiyuan* (LU-9).

(DACH) Heat in the palms: *jingqu* (LU-8).

(DACH VI, 14) Attack of heat in the hands, painful fingers: foot-*linqi* (GB-41), *hegu* (LI-4), *yemen* (TW-2), *yangchi* (TW-4).

Numbness (suan) of the upper limb.

Shoulder and arm:
Numbness and pain of the shoulder and arm: *(DACH)* *yanglao* (SI-6), *tianzong* (SI-11), *tianliao* (TW-15), *zhigou* (TW-6).

(DACH) Numbness of the shoulder, arm, elbow and wrist: *pianli* (LI-6).

(DACH, YXRM) Arm numb, without strength: *naoshu* (SI-10).

(DACH) Arm numb, painful, without strength, pain to the point of not being able to lift it: *naohui* (TW-13).

(YXRM) Numbness and pain of the arm and elbow, cannot lift: *quchi* (LI-11).

(YXRM) Numbness or paralysis *(bi)* of the arm and elbow: *zhigou* (TW-6).

(DACH X, 32v) Numbness and pain of the elbow and wrist, sadness: needles and moxa at *tongli* (HT-5).

(YXRM) Numbness and heaviness of the elbow and wrist, cannot extend or flex: *waiguan* (TW-5).

(DACH III, 30v; DACH VII, 5v) Elbow numb, cold and heat, restlessness from mucus and cough: *lieque* (LU-7).

Weakness of the upper limb.

(DACH) Arm without strength, cannot lift it to the head; *(YXRM)* arm thin, without strength: *jianyu* (LI-15).

(DACH, YXRM) Arm numb, without strength: *naoshu* (SI-10).

(YXRM I, 46v) Excessive weakness of the forearm: *waiguan* (TW-5).

(GSdeM) In order to increase the strength of the flexor muscles which close the hand, tonify arm-*shanglian* (LI-9).

(DACH, YXRM) Hand not able to grip from a fracture or lesion; *(DACH X, 32v)* apoplexy, and cannot lift; *(DACH)* hand cannot grasp objects: *yangchi* (TW-4), needles and moxa.

(DACH) Hand cannot grip: *zhizheng* (SI-7).

(DACH) Cannot grasp objects: *tianjing* (TW-10).

(DACH) Hand cannot be lifted or dropped by itself: *yanglao* (SI-6).

(DACH) Fingers not grasping: *kongzui* (LU-6).

(YXRM) Lassitude of the hand, fatigue; *(DACH II, 27r)* apoplexy, hand weak, cannot be tightened or extended: arm-*sanli* (LI-10), needles and moxa.

(DACH) Awkward hands: *lieque* (LU-7).

(GSdeM) For the thumb and index finger: *pianli* (LI-6).

Flaccid paralysis, flaccidity of the upper limb.

Nerves:
(JM) Paralysis of the brachial plexus: *quepen* (ST-12).

(JM) Paralysis *(ma bi)* of the radial nerve: arm-*sanli* (LI-10), *lieque* (LU-7), *jingqu* (LU-8). (The radial nerve innervates the extensor muscles.)

All problems or illnesses of the medial nerve: arm-*ximen* (PC-4). (The medial nerve innervates the flexors.)

(JM) Pain (and paralysis?) of the cubital nerve: *yanglao* (SI-6), *yanggu* (SI-5). (The cubital nerve innervates the flexors.)

(JM) Paralysis of the circumflex nerve: *jianyu* (LI-15).

Muscles:

(JM) Paralysis of the latissimus dorsi muscle: *yuanye* (GB-22).

(JM) Paralysis *(ma bi)* of all the muscles of the forearm: *naohui* (TW-13).

The entire upper limb:

(JM) Paralysis *(ma bi)* of the upper limb: *pianli* (LI-6), *zhouliao* (LI-12), *qinglengyuan* (TW-11), *sanyangluo* (TW-8), arm-*sanli* (LI-10), *jugu* (LI-16), *jianzhen* (SI-9), *tianzong* (SI-11), *jianwaishu* (SI-14), *zhourong* (SP-20).

(DACH VI, 14v) Arm weak, pain in the side: *shaochong* (HT-9).

(DACH) Arm not lifting: *yuanye* (GB-22) (paralysis of the latissimus dorsi muscle).

(DACH) Cold and insufficiency of the upper limb: *jiquan* (HT-1).

(YXRM) Paresis of the arm *(wei)* without action; *(DACH)* arm not retracting: *waiguan* (TW-5).

(DACH) Arm and hand without action; elbow cannot be extended: arm-*sanli* (LI-10).

Elbow:

(YXRM) Arm and hand not lifting, pain of the abdomen: *juque* (CV-14).

(DACH, YXRM) Elbow cannot be lifted: foot-*qiaoyin* (GB-44).

(DACH) Arm and elbow no longer lift (from emotional shock): *yangxi* (LI-5).

(DACH) Elbow without action: *fufen* (BL-36, IS BL-41).

Forearm:

(JM) Paralysis of the forearm *(ma pi): sidu* (TW-9).

Hand:

(YIZ, 37v) Unable to raise the hand: *jianzhukou* (MP-10).

(DACH) Unable to raise or lower the hand by themselves: *yanglao* (SI-6).

(DACH; YXRM) The two hands cannot stretch to the head: *jianjing* (GB-21).

(DACH) Loose muscles, unable to grasp objects; *(YXRM)* loose muscles, unable to spread or flex; *(DACH)* both hands do not obey: *quchi* (LI-11).

(GSdeM) Hand grasps without strength: arm-*shanglian* (LI-9).

(DACH) Fingers do not grip: *kongzui* (LU-6).

(DACH) Unable to grip objects: *tianjing* (TW-10).

(DACH) Hand does not grip: *zhizheng* (SI-7).

(YXRM) Hand paralyzed *(pi): laogong* (PC-8).

(YXRM) Hand without movement: *shaoshang* (LU-11).

(YXRM) Impossible to spread or flex the five fingers: hand-*wangu* (SI-4).

(YXRM) Little finger without movement: *shaoze* (SI-1).

Abscesses of arms and hands.

Upper limb:

(DACH XI, 18r) Abscess on the arm: *quchi* (LI-11).

(DACH X, 31v) Abscess on the hand: *quchi* (LI-11), moxa.

(DACH) Painful abscess on the hand: *laogong* (PC-8).

(YXRM I, 46v) Poison from abscess on the back of the hand: hand-*zhongzhu* (TW-3).

(YIX I, 4v) Abscesses all over the hand, energy attacking the heart and chest: disperse *daling* (PC-7) and *laogong* (PC-8).

(YXRM I, 46v) "Goose-palm wind" (retraction of the palmar aponeurosis? Pemphigus?): *laogong* (PC-8), and *neiguan* (PC-6).

VI. Lower Limb

General command points.

All troubles or illnesses of the lower limbs: *(DACH) yanglingquan* (GB-34), *yinmen* (BL-51, IS BL-37); *(DACH X, 34v) kuangu* (MP-38b).

(DACH IV, 11v; YIX I, 4v) Illnesses of the lower limb and feet: *fengfu* (GV-15, IS GV-16).

Pain, arthritis, rheumatism, neuralgia.

Nerves:

(GSdeM) The four sacral hollows (*shangliao, ciliao, zhongliao, xialiao* — BL-31 to 34) act on the roots of the sacral plexus and on all the nerves of the lower limb.

(JM) Pain of the crural nerve: *jimen* (SP-11).

(JM) Pain of the inguinal nerve: *lidui* (ST-45).

(JM) Pain of the femerocutaneous nerve (anterolateral surface of the thigh): *futu* (ST-32).

(JM) Pain of the obturator nerve (rotation of the thigh): *biguan* (ST-31), *yinmen* (BL-51, IS BL-37), *yinbao* (LR-9).

(JM) Sciatic nerve; the four sacral hollows: *xiaochangshu* (BL-27), *pangguangshu* (BL-28), *zhonglushu* (BL-29), *baihuanshu* (BL-30), *yanglingquan* (GB-34).

(JM) Pain of the tibial and peroneal nerves: *guangming* (GB-37).

(JM) Pain of the posterior tibial nerve: *taixi* (KI-5, IS KI-3).

Groin:

Pain and swelling of the groin: *jimen* (SP-11).

(JM) Inguinal neuralgia: *lidui* (ST-45); *(GSdeM) jiaoxin* (KI-8).

The whole lower limb:

(JM) Pain of the nerves of the lower limb: *shenmai* (BL-62), *fuyang* (BL-59), *fuxi* (BL-52, IS BL-38), *taibai* (SP-3), *shangqiu* (SP-5), *sanyinjiao* (SP-6), *lougu* (SP-7), *diji* (SP-8), foot-*linqi* (GB-41), *xuanzhong* (GB-39), *yangfu* (GB-38), *chongyang* (ST-42), *tiaokou* (ST-38), *kuangu* (MP-38b).

(YXRM) Pain with impossibility of lifting from the foot and lower leg to the pivot of the hip; *(DACH)* hip joint cannot be bent: *shugu* (BL-65).

(YIX I, 10v; DACH VII, 31r) Acute pain of the lower limb, swelling of the sides: foot-*linqi* (GB-41).

(JM) All trouble or malaise of the lower limb: *yanglingquan* (GB-34), *yinmen* (BL-51, IS BL-37).

(DACH III, 30v) Acute pain of the lower limb and foot; *(DACH X, 31r)* illnesses of the lower limb: *quangu* (MP-38b).

(DACH IV, 8v) Pain of the lumbar area and lower limb: tonify hand-*wangu* (SI-4) and disperse leg-*sanli* (ST-36).

(DACH IV, 11v) Pain of the lumbar area and lower limb for years: *dadu* (SP-2).

(JM) Acute pain of the medial side of the lower limb: *yingu* (KI-10).

(DACH) Pain of the chest, sides, hip joints and external side of the lower limb: *yangfu* (GB-38).

Hip:

(YXRM) Pain of the pivot of the hip: *(YIX I, 8r)* pain from the groin to the calf; *(DACH IV, 11r)* pain of the groin, lower limb and calf: *huantiao* (GB-29, IS GB-30).

(DACH) Pain in the hip joint: foot-*linqi* (GB-41): *jinggu* (BL-64), *qiuxu* (GB-40), *jiaoxin* (KI-8), *weizhong* (BL-54, IS BL-40).

(JM) Arthritis of the hip: *weizhong* (BL-54, IS BL-40), *yanglingquan* (GB-34).

(YXRM) Pain and impossibility of lifting from the foot and lower leg up to the hip; *(DACH)* hip joint not bendable; *(DACH)* lumbar and back painful, cannot bend the hip: *shugu* (BL-65).

(DACH III, 27r) Pain of lumbar area and hip joint: disperse once, tonify three times — leg-*sanli* (ST-36).

(DACH) Pain of hip joint, thigh and lower leg: *fuyang* (BL-59).

Sciatica (*tun gu shen jing tong*, "pain of the ischial nerve"; *tun gu jie zhi tong*, "pain of the ischial tendons"; *tui feng*, "shock of the lower limb"; in Japan, *zuo gu shen jing tong*, "pain of the ischial nerves"):

Sciatica is most often caused by arthritis of the sacroiliac joint (see below). For simple sciatica, it is sometimes enough to disperse *yanglingquan* (GB-34). If not better, add *kunlun* (BL-60), *xuanzhong* (GB-39), *fengshi* (GB-31) or *zhongdu* (GB-32), *huantiao* (GB-29, IS GB-30). If there are cramps: *chengshan* (BL-57).

(JM) kunlun (BL-60), *yaoyangguan* (GV-3), *xiyangguan* (GB-33), *yangjiao* (GB-35), *yinmen* (BL-51, IS BL-37), *weizhong* (BL-54, IS BL-40), *baohuang* (BL-48, IS BL-53), *huantiao* (GB-29, IS GB-30), *zhibian* (BL-49, IS BL-54), *shangliao* (BL-31), *ciliao* (BL-32), *zhongliao* (BL-33), *xialiao* (BL-34), *huiyang* (BL-35).

(DACH III, 29v) Shock of the lower limb: hip-*juliao* (GB-28, IS GB-29), *huantiao* (GB-29, IS GB-30), *weizhong* (BL-54, IS BL-40).

(YIZ, 44v) Pain of the ischial nerves, of the lower limb; foot slow and without action; acute pain of the calf, knee cold on the lateral side, cannot bend or extend; without movement in humid weather, with swelling: *fengshi* (GB-31), *xiadu* (GB-32, IS *zhongdu*), *xiaguan* (GB-33), *xuanzhong* (GB-39).

(DACH XI, 22r) Shock of the lower limb, pain from the lower limb into the foot: *huantiao* (GB-29, IS GB-30), *xuanzhong* (GB-39), *fengshi* (GB-31), *yanglingquan* (GB-34), *kunlun* (BL-60).

(YIX I, 84) Pain of the hip joint and thigh connected with the calf: *huantiao* (GB-29, IS GB-30), 2 *fen,* five moxa.

Sacroiliac arthritis:

Arthritis causes pain and swelling along the sacrum at one or many points. Puncture the sacral hollows and the point just beside the sacrum corresponding to the pain and swelling, at about one centimeter depth. But first puncture *guanyuanshu* (BL-26), then either *shangliao* (BL-31) and *xiaochangshu* (BL-27) if the pain extends also into the anterolateral surface of the thigh (femoral-cutaneous nerve) or to the anteromedial side (crural or obturator nerve gives pain on rotation of the thigh); or *ciliao* (BL-32) and *pangguangshu* (BL-28), or *zhongliao* (BL-33) and *zhonglushu* (BL-29) (at the level of the third and fourth sacral hollows); or *xialiao* (BL-34) and *baihuanshu* (BL-30) when the pain is mostly at the bottom of the leg.

In difficult cases, it is good to recommend 15 to 20 moxas, morning and evening, on the painful edge of the sacrum. Generally, several days are necessary before the material deposit in the joint is expelled. It is sometimes possible to perceive a large grain of sand caught in the joint or coming out. As long as the joint is swollen, the pain will continue.

(JM) Pain of the nerve of the sacral area: *xiaochangshu* (BL-27), *baihuanshu* (BL-30), *pangguangshu* (BL-28).

Thigh:

(JM) Subcutaneous pain of the lateral part of the thigh: *futu* (ST-32).

(DACH, YXRM) Pain of the medial surface of the thigh: *yingu* (KI-10), *ququan* (LR-8); *(JM)* pain of the nerves of the medial part of the thigh: *jiaoxin* (KI-8); *(DACH)* pain on the medial surface of the thigh: foot-*shangqiu* (SP-5), *jimen* (SP-11).

(JM) Rheumatism of the thigh: *xiadu* (GB-32, IS *zhongdu*).

(JM) Inflammation of the thigh; *(DACH, YXRM)* lateral swelling of the thigh: *yinmen* (BL-51, IS BL-37).

(DACH) Women — accumulations *(zheng jia)*. When palpated, strange bubbling sensations radiate down the medial thigh to the knee; *(YXRM)* women — accumulations *(jia)* of blood. When palpated, strange bubbling sensations; the thighs, knees and genital organs are all painful: *diji* (SP-8). *(DACH, YXRM)* Women — accumulations *(jia)* of blood; when palpated, it feels as if bubbling water were overflowing the interior of the thigh: *ququan* (LR-8).

Thigh and knee:

(DACH III, 30v) Thigh and knee pain: *yinshi* (ST-33).

Knee:

(DACH) Simple knee pain: *xingjian* (LR-2); *(JM)* pain in the knee area: *yinshi* (ST-33), *fengshi* (GB-31). *(DACH)* Knee pain: disperse *guangming* (GB-37); *(DACH)* *tiaokou* (ST-38), *weizhong* (BL-54, IS BL-40).

(JM) Pain of the nerves in the area of the knee: *liangqiu* (ST-34).

(JM) Pain of the nerves in the area of the patella: *dubi* (ST-35).

(DACH) Knee painful, cannot flex or extend it: *dazhu* (BL-11).

Arthritis of the knee: *(JM)* *pucan* (BL-61), *yangfu* (GB-38), *tiaokou* (ST-38), leg-*zhongdu* (LR-6), *xiyan* (MP-37a & 38a, IS M-LE-16), *weizhong* (BL-54, IS BL-40), *xiguan* (LR-7), *yanglingquan* (GB-34), *yinlingquan* (SP-9), *liangqiu* (ST-34), *xiyangguan* (GB-33), *yingu* (KI-10), *dubi* (ST-35), back-*yangguan* (GV-3).

(GSdeM) Overflowing of the synovial fluid: tonify *xiyan* (MP-37a & 38a, IS M-LE-16).

(DACH) Pain and swelling of the patella and knee: *lidui* (ST-45).

(JM) Pain of the nerves of the popliteal fossa: *weiyang* (BL-53, IS BL-39).

(DACH) Pain of the medial surface of the knee: *sanyinjiao* (SP-6), *xiguan* (LR-7); medial surface: knee-*yangguan* (GB-33).

(DACH) Acute pain of the knee, can neither kneel nor get up: *dubi* (ST-35).

(YXRM) Pain of the knee, muscles contracted: *ququan* (LR-8).

(YXRM, DACH) Pain of the knee as if pierced by an awl; *(YIZ, 45v)* pain as if the knee were dislocated: *rangu* (KI-2).

Pain and cold of the knee: *(DACH)* *shangliao* (BL-31).

Knee and lower leg:

(YIZ, 40v) Leg-*sanli* (ST-36); *(YXRM, DACH)* *xuanzhong* (GB-39).

Knee and foot:

(YIZ, 40r) Apoplexy — knee and foot painful: *chengshan* (BL-57).

(DACH) All that concerns the knee and foot: *yingu* (KI-10).

Lower leg:

Pain of the lower leg: *(JM)* *shenmai* (BL-62), *huantiao* (GB-29, IS GB-30).

Pain of the tibial and peroneal nerves: *guangming* (GB-37).

All old rheumatisms of the leg: *(YXRM)* *chengshan* (BL-57).

(DACH X, 30v) Articular rheumatism *(li jie feng),* knee swollen, cannot get out of bed, muscles of the feet shortened and tightened, feet heavy, sunken, attacks of shock, severe swelling: *fengshi* (GB-31).
(DACH) Prolonged illnesses of the lower leg and foot: *jinmen* (BL-63).

Malleolae and feet:
Sprain of the medial malleolus: moxa *neihuaijian* (MP-42, IS M-LE-17).
Sprain of the lateral malleolus: *(DACH) shenmai* (BL-62), *waihuaijian* (MP-41, IS M-LE-22).
(JM) Arthritis of the malleolus and heel: *kunlun* (BL-60).
(DACH) Pain of the lateral malleolus: *xiaxi* (GB-43).
(DACH) Pain in front of the medial malleolus: *taichong* (LR-3).
Pain of the malleolus and feet: *(DACH) zhubin* (KI-9); lateral malleolus: *xiaxi* (GB-43).

Feet:
(DACH) When the energy is in the feet: *neiting* (ST-44) and *xiangu* (ST-43).
(DACH) Pain of the feet: *shenmai* (BL-62), *xiaxi* (GB-43); *(DACH VI, 14r) lidui* (ST-45); *(DACH) tiaokou* (ST-38).
(DACH IV, 11v) When punctured, the feet are improved; *(YXRM)* cannot place the foot to the ground: *yongquan* (KI-1).
Arthritis of the foot: *(JM) yinshi* (ST-33).
Pain of the arch of the foot: *(DACH II, 5r; YIX I, 4r) shangqiu* (SP-5); *(YXRM) fuliu* (KI-7); *(DACH) xingjian* (LR-2).
Arthritis of the arch of the foot: *(JM) chongyang* (ST-42), *jiexi* (ST-41), *kunlun* (BL-60).
(DACH) Cannot place the foot to the ground: leg-*xialian* (ST-39, IS *xiajuxu*).
(GSdeM) Metatarso-phalangeal arthritis: *neiting* (ST-44), *taichong* (LR-3), *xiaxi* (GB-43).

Heel:
Pain of the heel: *(DACH) chengshan* (BL-57), leg-*xialian* (ST-39, IS *xiajuxu*).
Acute pain of the heel; cannot press against the ground: *(DACH) pucan* (BL-61).
Pain of the heel, tightening: *(DACH) chengjin* (BL-56); *(YXRM) chengshan* (BL-57).

Soles of the feet:
(DACH) Acute pain of the soles of the feet: *kunlun* (BL-60), *neiting* (ST-44); *(JM)* plantar neuralgia: *fengshi* (GB-31).

Gout:
(YIZ, 45v) Feet painful and broken, cracking heat: bleed *weizhong* (BL-54, IS BL-40) to disperse.
(DACH IV, 7r) Gout *(jiao feng): weizhong* (BL-54, IS BL-40); *(GSdeM) taichong* (LR-3).

Heat of the lower limb.

Thigh:
(DACH, YXRM) Heat of the thigh and knee: *heyang* (BL-55).

Lower leg:
(YXRM) Lower leg and feet warm: *guangming* (GB-37).

Foot:
(DACH, YXRM) One foot warm, the other foot cold: *rangu* (KI-2).
(YXRM) Heat of the feet: leg-*sanli* (ST-36).
(YXRM) Feet hot and painful: *lougu* (SP-7).
(DACH) Feet hot when walking: *guangming* (GB-37).
(DACH) Hot syncope; heat of the feet: *yongquan* (KI-1).
(YXRM) Feet — heat and insufficiency in counterflow: *weizhong* (BL-54, IS BL-40).
Heat on the soles of the feet: *(DACH, YXRM) zhiyin* (BL-67); *(YXRM I, 46v) rangu* (KI-2), *yongquan* (KI-1); *(DACH) tiaokou* (ST-38); *(YXRM)* leg-*zhongdu* (LR-6), *chengshan* (BL-57).

Swelling of the lower limb.

Lower limb swollen: *(DACH III, 27v) shenmai* (BL-62).
Swelling and redness of the lower limb and foot: *(YXRM I, 46v) kunlun* (BL-60).
Inflammation of the lumbar area, thigh knee: *(JM) huantiao* (GB-29, IS GB-30).

Thigh:
(DACH) Swelling; *(JM)* inflammation of the thigh: *yinmen* (BL-51, IS BL-37).
(DACH) Swelling of the thigh from shock: *fengshi* (GB-31) and *yinshi* (ST-33).

Thigh and knee:

(DACH IV, 11r) Thigh and knee swollen: *taichong* (LR-3).

(DACH) Thigh, knee and lower leg swollen: *jiexi* (ST-41).

Knee:

From rheumatism, (see Pains, Arthritis of the knee).

From synovial swelling: *(GSdeM)* tonify *xiyan* (MP-37a & 38a, IS M-LE-16).

(DACH III, 30r; YIX I, 4r) Swelling of the knees: *xingjian* (LR-2); *(YXRM) zhongfeng* (LR-4).

(DACH IV, 10r; YIX I, 8r) Swelling of the knee, beriberi: *chengshan* (BL-57).

(DACH) Swelling of the knee from wind and water: leg-*shanglian* (ST-37, IS *shangjuxu*).

(DACH) Knee swollen without reason: tonify leg-*sanli* (ST-36) and *dubi* (ST-35).

(DACH) Bones of the knee swollen: disperse *taichong* (LR-3).

(DACH) Knee swollen, difficult to cure: *yanglingquan* (GB-34) and *yinlingquan* (SP-9).

(DACH) Swelling of the patella; if there is pus, it cannot be cured: *dubi* (ST-35), *lidui* (ST-45).

(DACH III, 27v) Swelling of the knee, pain of the foot: leg-*sanli* (ST-36); *(DACH)* swelling under the knee: *yangfu* (GB-38).

(DACH) Top of the knee swollen and painful: *yangqu* (ST-34), *xiguan* (LR-7), *chize* (LU-5), *quchi* (LI-11), *fengfu* (GV-15, IS GV-16).

Lower leg:

Swelling of the lower leg: *(DACH IV, 10v)* leg-*sanli* (ST-36); *(DACH) ququan* (LR-8).

Swelling of the lower leg and attack of cold: *(YXRM) taichong* (LR-3).

(YXRM) Swelling of the calf and heel, cannot place the foot to the ground: *kunlun* (BL-60).

Lower leg and feet:

(GSdeM) Swelling of the legs and feet: tonify the heart at *shaochong* (HT-9) and disperse the kidneys at *rangu* (KI-2).

Abscess in the lower limb.

Lower limb: *(YIX I, 4v)* Abscess on the lower leg: *xuehai* (SP-10).

(DACH) Abscess of the foot: foot-*qiaoyin* (GB-44).

(DACH VII, 28r) Poison in the arch of the foot, called *fa bei: shenmai* (BL-62), *weizhong* (BL-54, IS BL-40), *neiting* (ST-44), *xiaxi* (GB-43), *xingjian* (LR-2).

Trembling, spasms and intermittent contractions of the lower limb.

Spasms *(qing luan)*:

Spasms of the lower limb: *(JM) yinbao* (LR-9), *yanglingquan* (GB-34), *fen* (ST-40), thigh-*futu* (ST-32), *zhongdu* (GB-32).

Spasms of the lumbar area and knees: *(JM)* abdomen-*yinjiao* (CV-7).

Spasms of the medial side of the thigh: *(JM) ququan* (LR-8).

Spasms of the vastus lateralis: *(JM) biguan* (ST-31).

Spasms of the gastrocnemius muscle: *(JM) shugu* (BL-65), *qiuxu* (GB-40), *zhubin* (KI-9), *chengshan* (BL-57), *chengjin* (BL-56), *weiyang* (BL-53, IS BL-39).

Spasms of the soleus muscle: *(JM) zhubin* (KI-9), *feiyang* (BL-58).

Cramps:

(YXRM I, 40r) Cramping of the feet to the point of flowery vision: *rangu* (KI-2) and *chengshan* (BL-57).

(DACH) Cramps of the feet, lateral side: *waihuaijian* (MP-41, IS M-LE-22).

(DACH) Cramps of the feet, medial side: *neihuaijian* (MP-42, IS M-LE-17).

(DACH VI, 15v) Cramps of the soles of the feet: *yongquan* (KI-1).

Trembling:

Hands and feet: see Four Limbs.

(YXRM) Agitation of the feet: foot-*qiaoyin* (GB-44).

(DACH VII, 31r) Both feet agitated, cannot move them or walk: foot-*linqi* (GB-41), *taichong* (LR-3), *kunlun* (BL-60), *yanglingquan* (GB-34).

(DACH) Knee, leg, foot without control: *yangjiao* (GB-35).

Continuous contracture of the lower limb.

All illnesses of the lower limb: *yanglingquan* (GB-34), *yinmen* (BL-51, IS BL-37), *kuangu* (MP-38b).

Muscles:

Semitendinosis and semimembranosus: *kuangu* (MP-38b) *(GSdeM)*.

Contracture of posterior muscles of the thigh: *weizhong* (BL-54, IS BL-40).

Vastus lateralis and medialis: *biguan* (ST-31).

Vastus lateralis: *fuxi* (BL-52, IS BL-38).

Adductor magnus: *xuehai* (SP-10).

Adductor longus: *jimen* (SP-11).

Adductor brevis: *yinlian* (LR-11).

Knee:

(DACH IV, 10v; YIX I, 7v) Top of the knee, difficulty in extension or flexion: needle 5 *fen* and moxa at *weizhong* (BL-54, IS BL-40).

(DACH) Pain at the barrier of the knee, muscles contracted, can neither flex nor extend: *ququan* (LR-8).

(YIZ, 47r) Muscles of the knee contracted, not opening: 2 x 7 moxas at *weiyang* (BL-53, IS BL-39).

(YXRM I, 46v) Apoplexy from humidity, pain and contracture of the thigh and knee: *huantiao* (GB-29, IS GB-30).

(YXRM) Paralysis *(bi)* (or rheumatism, *bi*) of the knee, contracture of the muscles, can neither extend nor flex: *liangqiu* (ST-34).

(DACH) Popliteal fossa as if bound, calf as if torn: *shugu* (BL-65).

Feet:

(YXRM) Contracted feet: *chengshan* (BL-57).

(GSdeM) Contracture of the small plantar muscles (foot dropped and turned medially, fifth toe flexed): disperse *weizhong* (BL-54, IS BL-40).

(DACH) Hands and feet turned laterally: *guangming* (GB-37).

(GSdeM) Big toe flexed: disperse *yangjiao* (GB-35), which acts on the flexor hallucis longus.

(GSdeM) Big toe lifted: disperse *yangfu* (GB-38), which acts on the extensor hallucis longus.

(GSdeM) Four smaller toes flexed: disperse *lougu* (SP-7) and *diji* (SP-8), insertion of the extensor digitorum longus; *yongquan* (KI-1), flexor digiti minimi brevis.

(GSdeM) Four small toes lifted: disperse *yanglingquan* (GB-34), insertion of the extensor digitorum longus; *chongyang* (ST-42), extensors.

(DACH) Posterior edge of the foot contracted, bound, cannot walk: *jiaoxin* (KI-8).

Numbness, heaviness of the lower limb.

The whole lower limb:

(DACH X, 30v) Heaviness of the lower limb, thigh and lower leg: *fuyang* (BL-59).

(DACH, YXRM) Numbness of the lower limb or lower leg: *qiuxu* (GB-40).

(DACH) Numbness of the thigh, knee and lower leg: *taibai* (SP-3).

(DACH) Lower limb and knee numb, difficulty flexing or extending: *fenglong* (ST-40).

Lower leg:

(DACH) Numbness of the lower leg, cannot stand up for a long time: *rangu* (KI-2).

(YXRM) Knees and lower leg without strength, numb, painful: tonify *guangming* (GB-37).

(DACH) Numbness of the knee and lower leg: *yanggu* (GB-38), *jinmen* (BL-63).

(DACH) Knee and foot numb, slow, weak: *tiaokou* (ST-38).

(DACH, YXRM) Numbness of the lower leg: *zhiyang* (GV-8, IS GV-9); *(YXRM) taichong* (LR-3).

(DACH) Numbness of the calf: *chengjin* (BL-56).

(DACH) Numbness and swelling of the calf and foot: *feiyang* (BL-58).

(DACH) Numbness and pain of the lower leg and foot, difficulty in flexing and extending the foot, cannot remain standing for a long time: leg-*shanglian* (ST-37, IS *shangjuxu*).

(DACH) Lower leg and foot cold, numb; difficulty in extending or flexing: *ligou* (LR-5).

(DACH) Numbness of the lower leg and foot: *jinmen* (BL-63).

Feet:

(YXRM I, 40r) Both feet numb, paralyzed *(ma mu)*: *taixi* (KI-5, IS KI-3).

(YXRM) Paresis *(wei)* of the feet: *chongyang* (ST-42), *kunlun* (BL-60).

(DACH) Paresis of the feet, cannot keep one's shoes on: *fuliu* (KI-7).

(DACH) Paresis of the feet, cannot walk: *sanyinjiao* (SP-6).

Cold of the lower limb.

Lower limb:
(JM) Extreme coldness of the lower limb: *yinbai* (SP-1), *zhongfeng* (LR-4).
(JM) Extreme coldness of the lower limb after a premature delivery: *jianjing* (GB-21).
(YXRM) Lower limb cold, paralyzed *(ma bi)* without action: *lougu* (SP-7).

Knee, lower leg:
(DACH) Knee cold, not able to get warm: thigh-*futu* (ST-32).
(JM) Cold and insufficiency of the area of the patella: *ciliao* (BL-32).
(JM) Cold and insufficiency of the knee, extreme coldness in the area of the patella: *shangliao* (BL-31).
(DACH) Cold and pain of the knee and lower leg: *ququan* (LR-8).
(DACH) Cold of the lower legs, cannot get warm by themselves: *fuliu* (KI-7).
(YXRM) Cold of the lower leg; *(DACH VI, 11v)* lower legs and feet cold: *lidui* (ST-45).

Foot:
(DACH, YXRM) One foot hot, one foot cold: *rangu* (KI-2).
(YXRM) Counterflow cold of the feet: *yinbai* (SP-1).
(DACH) Cold and insufficiency of the feet: *dadu* (SP-2).
(DACH, YXRM) Feet cold without the color given by blood: *yanglingquan* (GB-34).
(DACH) Cold of the feet: *liangqiu* (ST-34), *tiaokou* (ST-38), *taichong* (LR-3), *yongquan* (KI-1), *shenshu* (BL-23).
(DACH) Cold from underside of the foot up to the knee: *yongquan* (KI-1).

Flaccid paralysis, flaccidity of lower limb.

The whole lower limb:
(JM) Flaccidity *(ma bi)* of the lower limb: *biguan* (ST-31), thigh-*futu* (ST-32), thigh-*xiadu* (GB-32, IS *zhongdu*), thigh-*yangguan* (GB-33), *fenglong* (ST-40), *tiaokou* (ST-38), *ligou* (LR-5), leg-*zhongdu* (LR-6), *sanyinjiao* (SP-6), *fuyang* (BL-59), *xiaxi* (GB-43), *fuliu* (KI-7), *wangu* (GB-17, IS GB-12), *chongyang* (ST-42).
(DACH X, 32v) Flaccidity *(ma mu)* of the lower limb and foot: *yanglingquan* (GB-34).
(DACH, YXRM) No action from the lumbar area to the feet: *ciliao* (BL-32).
(JM) Cold and insufficiency of the lower limb: thigh-*futu* (ST-32).
(YXRM) Flaccidity *(ma bi)* without action, cold of the lower limb: *lougu* (SP-7).
(DACH) Paresis *(wei),* limping: *guangming* (GB-37).
(JM) Flaccidity *(ma bi)* of the lateral side of the lower limb: *fuxi* (BL-52, IS BL-38).

Thigh:
(DACH) Medial, lateral sides of the thigh and feet without action: *yanglingquan* (GB-34).
(DACH) Paralysis, insufficiency, pain of the thigh, posteromedial surface: *yongquan* (KI-1).
(GSdeM) Flaccidity of the rectus femoris muscle: thigh-*futu* (ST-32); of the vastus intermedius: thigh-*yangguan* (GB-33).

Knee:
(YXRM) Paralysis of the knee: *huantiao* (GB-29, IS GB-30). *Wei:* leg-*sanli* (ST-36); *(DACH) lougu* (SP-7).
(JM) Paralysis *(ma bi)* of the area of the knee: *yinshi* (ST-33), *liangqiu* (ST-34).
(DACH) Knee paralyzed *(wai bie)* from cold, without action, cannot flex or extend: *yinshi* (ST-33).
(DACH, YXRM) When the knee is extended, it cannot be flexed: *yanglingquan* (GB-34).
(JM) Cold and insufficiency of the knee; *(DACH)* knee cold without action: *biguan* (ST-31).

Knee, lower leg and foot:
(DACH, YXRM) Rheumatism from cold; knee and leg not bending back: *yangjiao* (GB-35).
(DACH) Paresis *(wei)* of the knee and foot: leg-*sanli* (ST-36).
(DACH) Knee and foot not following: *baihuanshu* (BL-30).
(YXRM) Knee and foot without action: *taixi* (KI-5, IS KI-3).

Lower leg:
(YXRM) Lower leg paralyzed *(bi)* without action: *yaoyangguan* (GV-3).
(JM) Flaccidity *(ma bi)* of the lower leg: *shenmai* (BL-62).

Foot:
(DACH) Flaccidity *(ma mu)* of the feet: *biguan* (ST-31), *tiaokou* (ST-38).
(DACH, YXRM) Feet paralyzed without action: *yaoshu* (GV-2).

(YXRM I, 40r) Difficulty moving either foot; *(DACH, YXRM)* feet not bending: *xuanzhong* (GB-39).

(DACH) Feet slow, not bending: *chongyang* (ST-42), *tiaokou* (ST-38).

(DACH) Feet not bending, atrophied legs: *fenglong* (ST-40).

(DACH) Feet not able to walk: *fengshi* (GB-31), *fubai* (GB-16, IS GB-10), *lougu* (SP-7).

(DACH IV, 10v; YIX I, 8r) Neither foot able to walk; *(YIX I, 4 & 5r)* difficulty walking: *taichong* (LR-3).

(DACH) Feet without action: *tianzhu* (BL-10).

(YIX I, 8r) Feet not able to be lifted: *yanglingquan* (GB-34).

(YXRM) Paresis of the feet, which do not bend: *feiyang* (BL-58).

(DACH, YXRM) Toes not able to extend or flex: *feiyang* (BL-58).

(DACH) Paresis *(wai)* of the feet, one loses his shoes, feet not bending: head-*wangu* (GB-17, IS GB-12).

(DACH) Heel paralyzed: *yanglingquan* (GB-34).

(JM) Apoplexy, paralysis *(ma bi)* under the feet: *fengshi* (GB-31).

(YIZ, 40r) Great cure for feet which do not function: leg-*sanli* (ST-36).

VII. The Four Limbs

(DACH) Illnesses of the four limbs: foot-*linqi* (GB-41).

Pain of the four limbs.

(DACH VII, 26r) Pain of the four limbs from shock (wind): *gongsun* (SP-4), *quchi* (LI-11), *fengchi* (GB-20), *waiguan* (TW-5), *yanglingquan* (GB-34), *sanyinjiao* (SP-6), arm-*sanli* (LI-10).

(DACH VII, 31r) Pain in the four limbs when walking; ''wind-stopping-walking'': foot-*linqi* (GB-41), *quchi* (LI-11), leg-*sanli* (ST-36), *weizhong* (BL-54, IS BL-40). If not better: *waiguan* (TW-5), *mingmen* (GV-4).

(JM) Neuralgia of the four limbs: *fubai* (GB-16, IS GB-10), leg-*sanli* (ST-36).

Spasms, intermittent contractions, trembling.

Spasms:
(JM) Spasms of the four limbs: head-*qiaoyin* (GB-18, IS GB-11), *daheng* (SP-15), *zhiyin* (GB-23).

Trembling:
(DACH VII, 27r) Feet and hands trembling, cannot grasp objects, cannot walk: *houxi* (SI-3), *yanggu* (SI-5), *quchi* (LI-11), *wangu* (SI-4), *taichong* (LR-3), *xuanzhong* (GB-39), *gongsun* (SP-4), *yanglingquan* (GB-34).

(DACH VII, 27v) Four limbs trembling, joints painful, acute pain of the lumbar area and feet: *shenmai* (BL-62), *kunlun* (BL-60), *yanglingquan* (GB-34), *jianyu* (LI-15), *quchi* (LI-11).

(DACH) Hands and feet agitated and hot: foot-*qiaoyin* (GB-44), head-*qiaoyin* (GB-18, IS GB-11).

(DACH VII, 27r) Trembling and contractures *(luan)* of feet and hands; *(YIX I, 10r)*: *houxi* (SI-3).

(DACH VII, 27v) Four limbs trembling: *neiguan* (PC-6), *tongli* (HT-5), foot-*linqi* (GB-41), *danshu* (BL-19).

Prolonged contractures.

(DACH VII, 27r; YIX I, 10r) Contracture and trembling of hands and feet: *houxi* (SI-3).

(DACH VII, 27v; YIX I, 10v) Feet and hands contracted *(ma luan)*: *shenmai* (BL-62); *(DACH VII, 27v; YIX I, 10v)* evil shock of the four limbs.

(DACH IV, 11v) Four limbs twisted; if cold, tonify; if hot, disperse: *xuanzhong* (GB-39).

Fatigue, exhaustion, sluggishness.

(DACH, YXRM) Four limbs heavy, painful; *(JM)* four limbs sluggish, tired: *fuliu* (KI-7).

(JM) Sluggishness of the four limbs: leg-*sanli* (ST-36); *(DACH, YXRM)* *zhangmen* (LR-13). *(JM)* Heaviness and sluggishness of the four limbs: *daju* (ST-27). *(DACH)* Sluggishness of the four limbs: *geshu* (BL-17).

(DACH III, 30v) Sluggishness and slowness of the four limbs: *zhaohai* (KI-3, IS KI-6).

(DACH, YXRM) Heaviness of the body, four limbs cannot be lifted: *sanyinjiao* (SP-6).

(DACH) Four limbs empty and weak: *zhizheng* (SI-7).

Flaccidity, flaccid paralysis.

Flaccidity *(ma bi)* of the four limbs: *(JM)* *wuli* (LI-13); *(YXRM, ''wei-bi'')* *hegu* (LI-4); *(JM)* *chize* (LU-5), *jianzhen* (SI-9), leg-*sanli* (ST-36), leg-*shanglian* (ST-37, IS *shangjuxu*), *fuyang* (BL-59), *baihuanshu* (BL-30), *fubai* (GB-16, IS GB-10).

Four limbs cannot respond: *(DACH, YXRM)* *jiquan* (HT-1); *(DACH)* *daju* (ST-27), *riyue* (GB-24), *zhejin* (GB-23).

Four limbs cannot be lifted: *(DACH)* *zhigou* (TW-6), *xiaohai* (SI-8); *(DACH)* *shaohai* (HT-3), *tianchi* (PC-1); *(YXRM)* *ququan* (LR-8), *fuyang* (BL-59); *(YXRM)* *xuanzhong* (GB-39); *(YIX, 10)* foot-*linqi* (GB-41).

Four limbs can no longer move: *(YXRM)* *sanyangluo* (TW-8), arm-*wuli* (LI-13), *daheng* (SP-15), thigh-*wuli* (LR-10).

Hands and feet paralyzed: *(YIX I, 11r)* paralyzed *(ma)* and hot: *waiguan* (TW-5); *(YIX I, 10r)* paralyzed *(ma mu);* pliant tetanus: *houxi* (SI-3).

Hands and feet without action: *(DACH)* *shanglian* (LI-9); *(DACH)* *baihuanshu* (BL-30).

(YXRM I, 46v) Hand and foot flaccid *(ma mu)* or tightened or agitated, contracted or folded: hand-*zhongzhu* (TW-3).

(DACH IV, 10v) Insufficiency of the four limbs: *neiting* (ST-44).

(DACH) Feet and hands not obeying: *xuanzhong* (GB-39), *tinghui* (GB-2).

(DACH) Paralysis from shock, hands and feet flaccid *(ma mu),* not lifting: *jianzhen* (SI-9).

(YXRM) Relaxation of hands, slowness of the feet: *fubai* (GB-16, IS GB-10).

Cold of the four limbs.

Counterflow cold of the four limbs: *(DACH, YXRM)* *xingjian* (LR-2).

Four limbs insufficient, cold: *(JM)* *sanyinjiao* (SP-6); *(DACH)* *taixi* (KI-5, IS KI-3).

Counterflow cold of the four limbs: *sanyinjiao* (SP-6).

Heat of the four limbs.

(DACH) Shivering; endless heat of the four limbs: *yunmen* (LU-2), *yaoshu* (GV-2).

Swelling of the four limbs.

(DACH) Swelling of the four limbs: *lieque* (LU-7); *(YXRM)* swelling like a storm of the four limbs: *chize* (LU-5); *(JM, DACH)* four limbs swollen: *zhongfu* (LU-1), *fuliu* (KI-7), *chengjin* (BL-56).

(DACH) *sanyinjiao* (SP-6) and *yinlingquan* (SP-9), *hegu* (LI-4), *yemen* (TW-2), hand-*zhongzhu* (TW-3), *tongli* (HT-5), *quchi* (LI-11) leg-*sanli* (ST-36), *sanyinjiao* (SP-6), or *hegu* (LI-4), *yemen* (TW-2), *xingjian* (LR-2), *neiting* (ST-44).

(DACH) Four limbs and abdomen swollen: *chize* (LU-5).

(DACH) Swollen ''stork-knee'': *chize* (LU-5).

(DACH) Swelling from emptiness and fullness of the limbs: *geshu* (BL-17).

(DACH) Swelling of the four limbs, endless cold and heat: *chengshan* (BL-57).

VIII. Anterior Trunk

Pains.

In general:

(DACH) Pain in the front of the body: *chongyang* (ST-42).

(DACH) Acute pain of the front of the thorax; *(YXRM)* pain of the sternum: *yutang* (CV-18).

(JM) Pain of the nerves of the pectoral region: *taiyuan* (LU-9).

Upper part:

(YXRM) Pain of the medial side of the subclavicular fossa; *(DACH)* pain radiating to the subclavicular fossa, hot palms, a lot of yawning: *taiyuan* (LU-9).

(DACH) Pain and swelling of the subclavicular fossa: *yangfu* (GB-38).

(GSdeM) Sternoclavicular arthritis: disperse *qishe* (ST-11).

Sternum:

Pain of the sternum: *(YXRM)* *yutang* (CV-18), *zigong* (CV-19).

Armpit:

(YXRM) Pain of the armpit: *zhigou* (TW-6), *quchi* (LI-11); *(JM, YXRM)* *qiuxu* (GB-40); *(DACH)* *diwuhui* (GB-42).

(YXRM) Pains of the armpit and ribs, internal headaches: *wangu* (SI-4).

(DACH) Pain of the armpit and bottom of the ribs: *shaohai* (HT-3).

(YIX I, 7r) Pain of the armpit, ribs and front of the knee: *huantiao* (GB-29, IS GB-30).

Chest: (see also Respiratory System)

(DACH III, 32r) Energy piercing both breasts: *taiyuan* (LU-9).

(DACH) Pain of the chest, energy at the top not descending: *rugen* (ST-18).

Pain of the chest: *(DACH) shanglian* (LI-9); *(JM) xiabai* (LU-4), *taiyuan* (LU-9); *(YXRM) yinbai* (SP-1); *(DACH) fubai* (GB-16, IS GB-10), head-*qiaoyin* (GB-18, IS GB-11).

Pain in the chest: *(DACH) youmen* (KI-21), *shaohai* (HT-3), *shufu* (KI-27); *(DACH)* unbearable pain: *qimen* (LR-14).

Pain of the membrane of the ribs (pleurisy): *(JM) shufu* (KI-27), *yuzhong* (KI-26), *shencang* (KI-25).

(DACH) Pain of the chest radiating to the lumbar area and seizing the axilla: *yixi* (BL-40, IS BL-45).

Neuralgia in the front of the chest, cannot turn or bend to one side: *xiaxi* (GB-43).

(JM) Rheumatism of the muscles of the chest: *lieque* (LU-7), *tianquan* (PC-2).

Chest and ribs:

Intercostal neuralgia: *(JM) shaochong* (HT-9), *yanggu* (SI-5), *shaofu* (HT-8), *taiyuan* (LU-9), *daling* (PC-7), *shaohai* (HT-3), *qingling* (HT-2), *xiaxi* (GB-43), leg-*xialian* (ST-39, IS *xiajuxu*), *yuanye* (GB-22), *zhangmen* (LR-13), *xuanji* (CV-21), *zigong* (CV-19), *bulang* (KI-22), *shanzhong* (CV-17), *shufu* (KI-27), *yuzhong* (KI-26), *shentang* (BL-39, IS BL-44), *lingxu* (KI-24), *shenfeng* (KI-23), *youmen* (KI-21), *qihu* (ST-13), *jinquan* (HT-1), *dabao* (SP-21), *shidou* (SP-17), *ganshu* (BL-18), *shenshu* (BL-23).

(DACH) Pain like a belt surrounding the chest without fixed location: *zhiyin* (BL-67), *huantiao* (GB-29, IS GB-30).

(DACH) Pain in the middle of the ribs and chest: *dabao* (SP-21).

Pain of the chest and ribs; *(YXRM)* acute: *gongsun* (SP-4); *(DACH) xingjian* (LR-2); *(DACH)* with fullness of the limbs: *qimen* (LR-14).

Ribs:

Pain of the ribs: *(DACH) yanggu* (SI-5), *yunmen* (LU-2); *(YXRM I, 46v) xuanzhong* (**GB-39**); *(YXRM I, 39r) yanglingquan* (GB-34), *weizhong* (BL-54, IS BL-40); from energy: *xingjian* (LR-2).

Pain of ribs and sides: *(DACH IV, 25v) zhigou* (TW-6); *(DACH) chize* (LU-5); *(JM) dushu* (BL-**16**).

(YXRM I, 39v) Pain of the ribs and sides, desire to die, leading to swelling of the face is especially cured by *yanglingquan* (GB-34).

(DACH IV, 11r) Pain of the sides, ribs and lower limbs: *houxi* (SI-3).

(DACH) Pain at the bottom of the ribs, cannot breathe: hand-*wangu* (SI-4).

(DACH) Pain of the rib, cannot sleep: *zhangmen* (LR-13).

(DACH, YXRM) Pain of the ribs, paresis *(bi)* of the chest, pain of the heart: head-*linqi* (GB-11, IS GB-15).

(DACH) Pain and fullness of the ribs: *jiquan* (HT-1).

(DACH) Both sides tightened, painful: *zhishi* (BL-47, IS BL-52).

(DACH) Pain of the ribs and heart: *yangfu* (GB-38).

(DACH, YXRM) Pain of the ribs and back: *yunmen* (LU-2).

(DACH IX, 29r; DACH IV, 5v) Pain of the ribs radiating into the vertebrae: *ganshu* (BL-18).

(YXRM) Pain of the ribs, heat of lower pelvis; *(DACH)* pain and swelling at the bottom of the ribs; *weizhong* (BL-54, IS BL-40).

(DACH, YXRM) Pain of the ribs, pain of the abdomen as if pierced: *burong* (ST-19).

(YXRM) Pain of the epigastrium and ribs: *fushe* (SP-13).

(DACH) Pain of the chest and ribs: *xingjian* (LR-2); *(YXRM)* acute: *gongsun* (SP-4).

(DACH) Pain of shoulder and ribs: *burong* (ST-19).

(DACH) Pain at the bottom of the ribs and in the axilla: *shaohai* (HT-3).

(DACH) Fullness under the ribs: *yinlingquan* (SP-9).

(See also Epigastrium, Abdomen, Lower Pelvis, Genital System.)

Spasms, contractures of the anterior trunk.

Chest:

(GSdeM) Spasms of the pectoralis major muscle: *wuyi* (ST-15).

(GSdeM) Spasms of the pectoralis minor muscle: *yunmen* (LU-2) or *zhongfu* (LU-1).

(JM) Spasms of the muscles of the chest and abdomen: *zhangmen* (LR-13); *(JM) ququan* (LR-8).

(JM) Spasms of all the muscles of the chest and shoulder: *burong* (ST-19).

(JM) Spasms of all the muscles of the chest and back: *fengmen* (BL-12).

Hiccoughs, spasms of the diaphragm: see Digestive System.

Knotted chest (*jie xiong*):

(DACH II, 30v) Chest bound, body yellow: *yongquan* (KI-1).

(DACH VII, 26r) Women — chest bound, tightened, difficult to bear: *neiguan* (PC-6).

(DACH X, 33r) Women — chest bound because blood has entered into the chamber of blood: *qimen* (LR-14).

(YIX I, 9v) Chest contracted: *gongsun* (SP-4).

(DACH) Both chest and back are tightened: *jingqu* (LU-8).

See also: Epigastrium and Abdomen.

Axilla:

(DACH) Axilla contracted, painful: *naohui* (TW-13).

Heat of the anterior trunk.

(YXRM) Chest hot, mouth dry; *(YIZ, 37)* masters the heat of the chest; *(DACH)* heat of the chest: *shenshu* (GV-11, IS GV-12).

(DACH) Heat of the chest: *yinlingquan* (SP-9), *qimen* (LR-14), *yinbai* (SP-1), *zhongchong* (PC-9).

(YXRM) Shivering, heat in the chest: *zhongfu* (LU-1).

See also: Epigastrium, Abdomen.

Cold of the anterior thorax.

(DACH X, 29v) Cold in the chest: *shanzhong* (CV-17), *rangu* (KI-2).

(YXRM) Cold in the chest as if from wind: *xiaxi* (GB-43).

Paralysis of the anterior trunk.

(JM) Intercostal paralysis *(ma bi): rugen* (ST-18).

(GSdeM) Causes one to breathe deeply, activates the respiratory muscles: *shanzhong* (CV-17).

(JM) Paralysis of the latissimus dorsi: *yuanye* (GB-22).

Swelling of the front of the trunk.

Chest:

(DACH) Pain and swelling of the subclavicular fossa: *yangfu* (GB-38).

(DACH) All swelling of the chest: *rugen* (ST-18).

See also: Breast, Epigastrium, Abdomen, Belly, Lower Pelvis, Groin, Genital System.

Axilla:

Swelling of the axilla: *(DACH) weiyang* (BL-53, IS BL-39), *qiuxu* (GB-40), *taichong* (LR-3), head-*linqi* (GB-11, IS GB-15), *tianchi* (PC-1).

Swelling under the axilla (see also Adenitis): *zhongchong* (PC-9).

(YXRM) Swelling and pain of the axilla: *weiyang* (BL-53, IS BL-39), *qiuxu* (GB-40).

Sides:

(DACH) Swelling of the sides: leg-*sanli* (ST-36).

(DACH) Swelling of the sides and limbs, pain of the lower limbs: foot-*linqi* (GB-41).

(DACH) Swelling of the ribs, pain of the heart: *qimen* (LR-14).

Abscesses of the front of the trunk.

Chest:

(DACH XI, 35r) Abscess *(chuang)* on the chest: *xuanzhong* (GB-39).

See also: Breast and Lungs.

IX. Posterior Trunk, Back, Lumbar Area, Vertebral Column

Pains.

In general:

(YIX I, 4v) Illnesses of the shoulder and back: hand-*zhongzhu* (TW-3).

(GSdeM) All problems of the lumbar area: *weizhong* (BL-54, IS BL-40).

Back:

(DACH IV, 7v) Pain of the back: hand-*zhongzhu* (TW-3); *(YXRM) geguan* (BL-41, IS BL-46).

(DACH III, 43r) Pain in the intervals between the vertebrae behind the heart: hand-*zhongzhu* (TW-3), *guanzhong* (TW-1).

(JM) Pain of the nerves of the back: *zhongshu* (GV-6a, IS GV-7); Japanese point: *(JM) geguan* (BL-41, IS BL-46).

(DACH) Pain of the back, bad cold: *geguan* (BL-41, IS BL-46).

(YIZ, 43v; YIX I, 2v) Pain of the back from tiredness or coitus: *gaohuangshu* (BL-38, IS BL-43).

(DACH) Pain with mutual onslaught from the heart and back: *tiantu* (CV-22).

(DACH) Pain of the chest and back to the point of not being able to breathe: *yuji* (LU-10).

(DACH, YXRM) Pain of the back radiating into the chest: *xiongxiang* (SP-19).

(YXRM I, 46v) Pain of the back and arm, acute: arm-*sanli* (LI-10); *(DACH) pohu* (BL-37, IS BL-42).

(DACH, YXRM) Pain of the back and sides: *yunmen* (LU-2).

(JM) Rheumatism *(luo ma zhi si)* of the muscles of the back: *fufen* (BL-36, IS BL-41).

(YXRM I, 46v) Acute pain of the bottom of the back: arm-*sanli* (LI-10).

(GSdeM) Sacrovertebral arthritis: *guanyuanshu* (BL-26).

Vertebrae:

(YXRM I, 39v) Pain of the vertebrae *(ji liu); (DACH III, 30v)* pain and stiffness of the vertebrae: *shuigou* (GV-25, IS GV-26 *renzhong*).

(DACH III, 29r) Can remove the heaviness of the vertebrae: *shenshu* (GV-11, IS GV-12); *(JM)* neuralgia of the vertebrae: *zhangmen* (LR-13).

(DACH) Pain of the seventh cervical vertebra: *shuigou* (GV-25, IS GV-26 *renzhong*).

(GSdeM) Pain of the cervical vertebrae: *wuchu* (BL-5).

(JM) Pain of the dorsal vertebrae: *weicang* (BL-45, IS BL-50), *wuchu* (BL-5), *jinsuo* (GV-7, IS GV-8).

Pain of the lumbar vertebrae: *(DACH) dazhu* (BL-11), *zhiyang* (GV-8, IS GV-9); *(YXRM I, 46r) dachangshu* (BL-25); *(JM) shangliao* (BL-31); *(YXRM) qixue* (KI-13), *(YXRM)* as if broken: *shugu* (BL-65).

Pain of the nerves of the lumbar vertebrae: *(JM) zhibian* (BL-49, IS BL-54).

Acute pain and cold of the lumbar vertebrae, cannot rest for an extended time: *baihuanshu* (BL-30).

Pain and stiffness of the lumbar vertebrae: *(DACH III, 30v) kunlun* (BL-60).

Rheumatism from cold of the lumbar vertebrae: *shenmai* (BL-62).

Lumbar vertebrae mutually radiating as if linked: *(DACH) chengfu* (BL-50, IS BL-36).

Sacral area — nerve pain: *(JM) dachangshu* (BL-25), *pangguangshu* (BL-28), *baihuanshu* (BL-30).

Scapula:

(JM) Rheumatism of the muscles of the scapula: *jianjing* (GB-21); *(JM) jianliao* (TW-14).

(DACH IV, 5v) Acute pain of the scapula: *jianjing* (GB-21), *jianwaishu* (SI-14).

(DACH IV, 7v) Acute pain of the scapula; *(YIZ, 41v)* both scapulae painful: *tianjing* (TW-10), 2.5 *cun* (do not leave needle for a long time).

(JM) Pain of the nerves of the scapula: *quchi* (LI-11), *jingmen* (GB-25).

(DACH, YXRM) Pain of the medial side (medial angle) of the scapula; can neither bend nor straighten: *yixi* (BL-40, IS BL-45).

(JM) Painful attacks on the scapula: *naohui* (TW-13).

(JM) Pain of the nerves, or inflammation of all the muscles of the scapula or of the neck: *quepen* (ST-12).

(YXRM) Pain of the scapula down to the elbow, radiating to the nape which is tightened: *jianwaishu* (SI-14).

Pain of the shoulder and scapula: *lougu* (SP-7), *naoshu* (SI-10), *hegu* (LI-4).

(JM) Pain of the nerves of the scapula and top of the arm: *naoshu* (SI-10).

(JM) Arthritis of the scapula and arm (scapulohumeral): *naoshu* (SI-10), *binao* (LI-14), *fubai* (GB-16, IS GB-10), *jianzhen* (SI-9); *(GSdeM) jianliao* (TW-14).

(JM) Pain of the lumbar area, scapula and back: *wushu* (GB-27).

Lumbar area, lumbago *(yao tong):*

Under the name lumbago, or lumbar pain, the public and many doctors refer to several kinds of pain: 1) pain of the lumbar muscles, generally represented by contractures of the muscles in reaction to the pain of movement; 2) pain of the vertebrae, displaced vertebrae or rheumatism with or without osteophytes (''parrot beaks''); 3) true neuralgia, pain of the lumbar nerves; 4) pain coming from one or both kidneys (generally congested or blocked). Japan clearly differentiates these types. In China they seem to think that what cures one type will also cure another. This has not appeared to be exactly the case in the experiments conducted in Paris.

Japanese treatments:

1) Rheumatism or strain of the lumbar muscles:

> *Origin: generally rheumatism, arthritis, chronic constipation, bending forward too much, flu, sudden attack or blow. Symptoms: the muscles of those who have a sudden attack are hard. By pressing a little, or on movement, there is an acute pain. Sometimes there is swelling, paresis and violent pain. Loss of the freedom to stand after*

lying down. Treatment, with needles: **dachangshu** *(BL-25), 1* **cun;** **zhishi** *(BL-47, IS BL-52), 1* **cun;** **mingmen**
(GV-4), 5 **fen;** **shenshu** *(BL-23), 1* **cun;** **ciliao** *(BL-32), 1* **cun;** **zhongliao** *(BL-33), 1* **cun;** **xialiao** *(BL-34), 1* **cun.**
(JO, 48)

Rheumatism of the lumbar muscles:

> **Xuanshu** *(GV-5),* **mingmen** *(GV-4),* **sanjiaoshu** *(BL-22),* **dachangshu** *(BL-25),* **qihaishu** *(BL-24),* **huangmen**
> *(BL-46, IS BL-51),* **zhishi** *(BL-47, IS BL-52), [needle] from 3 to 7* **fen** *and ten moxas. (JM, 320)*

(GSdeM) Painful contractures of the lumbar muscles: *guanyuanshu* (BL-26), *shenshu* (BL-23).
"Back strain" (lumbago): disperse *yinmen* (BL-51, IS BL-37).

2) Pains of the lumbar vertebrae: see Vertebrae.

3) Lumbar neuralgia: *(JM) yaoyangguan* (GV-3), *pangguangshu* (BL-28), *guanyuanshu* (BL-26), *sanjiaoshu*
(BL-22), *weizhong* (BL-54, IS BL-40), *taichong* (LR-3), *dadun* (LR-1), *yangfu* (GB-38), *diji* (SP-8), *jinggu* (BL-64),
fuyang (BL-59).

4) Congested kidneys: disperse *rangu* (KI-2), *yongquan* (KI-1), *taixi* (KI-5, IS KI-3).

Chinese treatments:
(DACH III, 32r) The five types of pain of the lumbar area; *(YIX I, 7r)* for the lumbar area and back; *(DACH IV, 10v;*
YIX I, 7v) acute pain of the lumbar area, cannot lift anything, pain radiates into the vertebral column, fatigue, numbness, muscles not relaxing; *(YXRM)* pain of the lumbar area pinching the vertebrae, all of them painful up to the head;
(YIX, 4r) pain and stiffness of the lumbar area and spine; *(DACH I, 4v)* pain of the lumbar area and spine; *(DACH I,*
4v) pain of the lumbar area (from the *chong mai*), cannot bend or straighten, fears falling; *(YIZ, 44)* lifting a weight
causes pain in the lumbar area: *yinmen* (BL-51, IS BL-37), 7 *fen*, bleed three times. Great emptiness in lumbar area;
pain returns after improvement with the needles: *weizhong* (BL-54, IS BL-40).

Pain of the lumbar area:
(YXRM I, 40r; YIX I, 7v; DACH IV, 8v):

1) Slight cases: bleed *weizhong* (BL-54, IS BL-40); cures immediately.

2) Serious cases: disperse *weizhong* (BL-54, IS BL-40), tonify *huantiao* (GB-29, IS GB-30).

3) Old cases: tonify *weizhong* (BL-54, IS BL-40), *huantiao* (GB-29 IS GB-30) and *kunlun* (BL-60).

(DACH X, 34r) Pain of the lumbar area from emptiness of energy, emptiness of blood, illness of kidneys, wind and
humidity, humidity and heat, heat accumulating, blockage from cold, blood blocked in the bottom: bleed (i.e.,
disperse) *weizhong* (BL-54, IS BL-40); moxa (i.e., tonify) at *kunlun* (BL-60) and *shenshu* (BL-23).
Acute pain of the lumbar area: *(DACH III, 30v; YXRM I, 46v) shenshu* (BL-23); *(JM) mingmen* (GV-4); *(DACH IV,*
10v) chengshan (BL-57).
Pain of the lumbar area: *(DACH, YXRM) guanyuanshu* (BL-26), *pangguangshu* (BL-28); *(JM)* foot-*dadu* (SP-2),
taibai (SP-3), *diji* (SP-8), leg-*sanli* (ST-36), *yinlingquan* (SP-9), *yinmen* (BL-51, IS BL-37).
(DACH I, 4v) Pain in the lumbar area from the gallbladder, like needles poking the skin, can neither bend forward
nor straighten, nor turn: bleed (disperse) except in summer at *yanglingquan* (GB-34).
(YIZ, 43v) Lumbar area curved, cannot straighten: *shuigou* (GV-25, IS GV-26 *renzhong*).
(DACH XI, 4v; JM) Cures the lightning-like pains which come upon sitting: *yanglingquan* (GB-34); *(DACH,*
YXRM) pain in the lumbar area when sitting or squatting: *shenshu* (BL-23).
(DACH) When lying down, can neither straighten nor bend to one side: *xinshu* (BL-15).
(YIX I, 7v) Pain when turning: *chengshan* (BL-57), *huantiao* (GB-29, IS GB-30).
(DACH) Pain in the lumbar area, cannot remain standing for a long time; when seated cannot get up: *fuyang*
(BL-59).
(DACH X, 30v) Pain in the lumbar area; cannot lift: *pucan* (BL-61).
(YIZ, 43v) Lightning pain in the lumbar area: tonify *qihai* (CV-6) three times, disperse three times during thirty
respirations; during each interval of twenty-five respirations press heavily on the point.
(DACH VII, 31v) Pain in the lumbar area coming like lightning; great difficulty geting up or sitting down: *weizhong*
(BL-54, IS BL-40), *shenshu* (BL-23), *jizhong* (GV-6), *yaoshu* (GV-2), foot-*linqi* (GB-41).
(YIZ, 43v; YIX I, 5v; DACH XI, 5v) Sudden pain like lightning in the lumbar area: *shuigou* (GV-25, IS GV-26 *ren-*
zhong), *weizhong* (BL-54, IS BL-40), *chize* (LU-5); if not better: *kunlun* (BL-60), *shugu* (BL-65), *yanglingquan*
(GB-34), *xialiao* (BL-34).

(DACH IV, 5v; YIX I, 4v) Acute pain in the lumbar area; frequent urine; decline of the kidneys: many moxas at *shenshu* (BL-23).

(DACH) Lumbar area cold like water: *shenshu* (BL-23). *(DACH IX, 10v)* Lumbar area frozen as if patient were seated in water: foot-*linqi* (GB-41).

(YXRM I, 46r) Old people — acute pain of the lumbar area from emptiness of the kidney: *mingmen* (GV-4).

Pain in the lumbar area through the meridians:

(DACH IX, 20):

   Bladder meridian (pain in the lumbar area, spine, coccyx): bleed *zhiyin* (BL-67).

   Kidney meridian (pain of the anterior face of the spine): *fuliu* (KI-7), two times.

   Gallbladder meridian (like needles piercing, cannot move): bleed *yanglingquan* (GB-34).

   Liver meridian (lumbar contractures): *ligou* (LR-5); if talkative, three times.

   Yangwei mai (slight swelling): *chengshan* (BL-57).

   Yinwei mai (boiling pain; if serious, there is chagrin and fear): *fuliu* (KI-7), *zhubin* (KI-9).

Lumbar area and back:

(YIX I, 7r) For the lumbar area and back: *weizhong* (BL-54, IS BL-40).

(DACH X, 10v) Extreme pain in the lumbar area and back: *weizhong* (BL-54, IS BL-40), *fuliu* (KI-7); *(YXRM I, 40r; YIX I, 7v)* *weizhong* (BL-54, IS BL-40), *kunlun* (BL-60). *(DACH II, 19r; YIX I, 4r)* Pain in the lumbar area linked to the back: *weizhong* (BL-54, IS BL-40), *baihuanshu* (BL-30). *(JM)* Neuralgia or spasms of the back of lumbar area: *yinmen* (BL-51, IS BL-37).

(YIZ, 43v) Pain in the lumbar area and behind the body: *jinggu* (BL-64).

Pain in the lumbar area and back: *(JM)* *weiyang* (BL-53, IS BL-39), *heyang* (BL-55) *shugu* (BL-65); *(DACH)* *fengshi* (GB-20); *(YXRM)* *shuidao* (ST-28).

(DACH) Malaise of the lumbar area and back: *baihuanshu* (BL-30).

(DACH) Acute pain of the lumbar area and back when coughing: *shenshu* (GV-11, IS GV-12).

(DACH) Neuralgia of the lumbar area, back and scapula: hip-*wushu* (GB-27).

Lumbar area and spine:

(YIZ, 43r) Interior pain of the lumbar area and spine to the point of not being able to straighten or bend forward. If the pain is at the top: *hegu* (LI-4); if the pain is close to the bottom: *kunlun* (BL-60), *fuliu* (KI-7).

(YIZ, 44) Pain in the lumbar area and spine: *kunlun* (BL-60).

(DACH I, 4v) Pain in the anterior surface of the lumbar area and spine: *fuliu* (KI-7) *feiyang* (BL-58).

(DACH) Pain in the lumbar area going along the spine to the nape when pressing: *zhonglushu* (BL-29) moxa.

(DACH) Lumbar area and spine exchanging the pain as if linked: *chengfu* (BL-50, IS BL-36).

(YXRM) Pain in the lumbar area pinching the vertebrae; all vertebrae painful up to the head: *weizhong* (BL-54 IS BL-40).

(DACH) Pain in the lumbar area and spine from accumulations in the kidney: *qixue* (KI-13).

Lumbar area and coccyx:

(DACH IV, 10v; YIX I, 8r) Cramps and pain in the lumbar area and coccyx: *kunlun* (BL-60) and lower pelvis: *yinbao* (LR-9).

Lumbar area and sides:

(YIZ) Pain of the lumbar area and sides: *qiuxu* (GB-40).

(DACH) Pain in the lumbar area and hip; injury from a blow: *tianjing* (TW-10).

(YXRM) Lumbar area and sides exchanging pain from tightening: *huantiao* (GB-29, IS GB-30).

(YIX I, 5r; DACH XI, 5r) When sitting there is lightning pain in the lumbar area and sides; comes from an excess energy penetrating the kidney meridian and drying up the blood and sperm; or, the person has come a long way carrying a heavy load: first, *chize* (LU-5), *weizhong* (BL-54, IS BL-40), *shuigou* (GV-25, IS GV-26 *renzhong*), then *kunlun* (BL-60), *shugu* (BL-65), *zhigou* (TW-6) and *yanglingquan* (GB-34).

Lumbar area and hip:

(DACH III, 27r) Pain of the lumbar area and hip joint: leg-*sanli* (ST-36); *(DACH)* cannot get up: *qiuxu* (GB-40).

Lumbar area and abdomen:

Pain in the lumbar area and abdomen: *(JM)* *zhongfeng* (LR-4); *(YXRM, DACH)* *heyang* (BL-55). *(DACH, YXRM)* Cannot bend down, straighten up or remain standing for a long time: *jingmen* (GB-25). *(YXRM)* Lumbar area and abdomen exchanging the pain. *(DACH)* Lumbar area and abdomen responding to each other: *mingmen* (GV-4).

Lumbar area and lower abdomen:

Pain in the lumbar area and lower abdomen: *(DACH, YXRM)* *taichong* (LR-3), hip-*juliao* (GB-28, IS GB-29), *xialiao* (BL-34).

Lumbar area and groin:

(DACH II, 27v) Pain in the lumbar area and groin, vaginismus: leg-*sanli* (ST-36), disperse one time, tonify three times.

Lumbar area and ischium:

(DACH) Baihuanshu (BL-30).

Lumbar area and lower limb:

(DACH IV, 8v; YXRM I, 40r) Pain in the lumbar area and lower limb: tonify hand-*wangu* (SI-4), disperse leg-*sanli* (ST-36); *(DACH IV, 11v)* foot-*dadu* (SP-2), moxa *huantiao* (GB-29, IS GB-30) and *fengshi* (GB-31).

(YIZ, 44) Pain in the lumbar area; heaviness of thigh, knee and legs, the four limbs weighed down, cannot stand for a long time: *fuyang* (BL-59).

Pain of the lumbar area and thigh: *biguan* (ST-31); *(JM)* lumbar area, thigh and knee: *jiaoxin* (KI-8); lumbar area, knee and foot: *liangqiu* (ST-34); lumbar area and feet: hand-*wangu* (SI-4), *diji* (SP-8), *ciliao* (BL-32); *(YIZ, 44)* *weizhong* (BL-54, IS BL-40), *kunlun* (BL-60), *shuigou* (GV-25, IS GV-26 *renzhong*).

Spasms of the posterior thorax, back and lumbar area.

Back:

(JM) Spasms of the back: *xiongxiang* (SP-19) *zhourong* (SP-20), *geguan* (BL-41, IS BL-46).

(JM) Spasms of the thoracic longissimus: *shentang* (BL-39, IS BL-44).

(JM) Spasms of all the muscles of the back and chest: *fengmen* (BL-12).

Shoulder and back:

(JM) Spasms of the shoulder and back: *gaohuangshu* (BL-38, IS BL-43), *fufen* (BL-36, IS BL-41), *pohu* (BL-37, IS BL-42), *kunlun* (BL-60).

(JM) Spasms of the scapula: *(DACH, YXRM)* contractions from cold in the shoulder and back: *jingmen* (GB-25).

Back and lumbar area:

(JM) Spasms of the back and lumbar area: *feishu* (BL-13), *xuanshu* (GV-5), *xiaochangshu* (BL-27), *zhejin* (GB-23).

(DACH) Lumbar and back seized and tightened: *yinmen* (BL-51, IS BL-37), *weiyang* (BL-53, IS BL-39), *qiuxu* (KI-13), *shuifen* (CV-9).

Lumbar area:

Spasms of the lumbar muscles: *(JM)* *fuliu* (KI-7), *biguan* (ST-31), *dachangshu* (BL-25), *guanyuanshu* (BL-26); spasms of the lumbar area: *biguan* (ST-31).

Spasms of the lumbar area and buttock: *(JM)* *yinbao* (LR-9).

Sacrum:

Spasms of the sacrum: *(JM)* *baihuanshu* (BL-30).

Spasms of the anus: *(JM)* *baihuanshu* (BL-30).

Lumbar area and knees:

(JM) Abdomen-*yinjiao* (CV-7).

Lumbar area and lower pelvis:

(JM) Hip-*juliao* (GB-28, IS GB-29).

Contractures, stiffness of the posterior part of the trunk.

Stiffness of the spine:

Taodao (GV-12, IS GV-13), *weiyang* (BL-53, IS BL-39), *feishu* (BL-13), *pangguangshu* (BL-28).

(YIZ, 43) Stiffness and pain of the spine: *weizhong* (BL-54, IS BL-40).

(YXRM) Stiffness of the spine; *(DACH)* spine stiff, useless: *shiguan* (KI-18).

(YIZ, 43) Vertebral column stiff; the whole body is painful and cannot be turned: *yamen* (GV-14, IS GV-15).

(DACH) Stiffness of the spine; difficulty bending or straightening: *geguan* (BL-41, IS BL-46), *weicang* (BL-45 IS BL-50); from cold and heat: *taodao* (GV-12, IS GV-13).

(DACH IV, 4v) Back and spine stiff and painful: *shuigou* (GV-25, IS GV-26 *renzhong*), *weizhong* (BL-54, IS BL-40); back and lumbar area stiff: *shenmai* (BL-62), *weizhong* (BL-54, IS BL-40).

(DACH X, 29r) Back, abdomen and nape contracted: *bailao* (GV-13, IS GV-14 *dazhui*).

Contracture:

(DACH) Back curved, cannot straighten it: *shuigou* (GV-25, IS GV-26 *renzhong*).

(DACH) Back, nape, neck curved: *fengchi* (GB-20).

(YIZ, 43v) Back contracted, back and chest tightened all together: *jingqu* (LU-8).

(YXRM) Women — vertebrae tightened: *zhigou* (TW-6).

(DACH, YXRM) Back bound: *jianjing* (GB-21).

(DACH) On turning to one side, difficulty turning back: *ganshu* (BL-18).

(DACH) Back, vertebrae: difficulty bending forward or backwards: *jingqu* (BL-64).

(YXRM) Stiffness and tightening of the lumbar vertebrae: *shendao* (GV-10, IS GV-11), *pishu* (BL-20), *sanjiaoshu* (BL-22), *zhishi* (BL-47, IS BL-52), *yaoshu* (GV-2).

(DACH, YXRM) Lumbar vertebrae cannot fold or straighten: *yinmen* (BL-51, IS BL-37).

(DACH I, 4v) Lumbar area tightened like the string of a crossbow: *ligou* (LR-5); *(DACH I, 4v)* lumbar tightened, cannot bend forward or backward.

(YIX I, 4v) Lumbar area and arm contractures: *quchi* (LI-11).

Cold of the posterior trunk, back and lumbar area.

Shoulder and back:

(JM) Extreme coldness of the shoulder and back: *dazhu* (BL-11).

(DACH, YXRM) Contractions from cold in the shoulder and back: *jingmen* (GB-25).

Back:

(YXRM) Cold in the back; *(DACH)* shivering from cold in the pores of the back, same with thick clothing, cannot get warm: *yangbai* (GB-10, IS GB-14).

(DACH) Cold in the areola of the back: *ciliao* (BL-32).

Lumbar area:

(DACH IX, 10v) Lumbar area frozen as if in water: foot-*linqi* (GB-41), *yangfu* (GB-38), *shenshu* (BL-23).

(JM) Extreme coldness of the lumbar area: *yangfu* (GB-38).

(YXRM) Cold like ice in the lumbar area; pain so that one cannot see: *yinshi* (ST-33).

Flaccidity, flaccid paralysis of the back and lumbar area.

Shoulder and nape:

(JM) Flaccidity *(ma bi)* of the shoulder and nape: *tianzong* (SI-11).

Scapula:

(JM) Flaccidity *(ma bi)* of the nerves of the scapula: *tianzong* (SI-11).

Swelling of the posterior part of the trunk.

All illnesses of the shoulder and back: *zhongzhu* (TW-3).

(YXRM) Swelling of the lumbar area and coccyx: *kunlun* (BL-60).

(YXRM) Swelling and heaviness of the lumbar area and feet: *weizhong* (BL-54, IS BL-40).

(DACH) Area of the buttocks swollen: *chengfu* (BL-50, IS BL-36).

(DACH) Swelling of the scrotum: *dadun* (LR-1).

Abscess of the posterior part of the trunk.

Back:

(DACH) If one punctures frequently, there will never be abscesses on the back: *fengmen* (BL-12), which also controls abscesses of the back. Abscess of the back: *shugu* (BL-65).

(DACH X, 32r) Abscess appearing on the back: *weizhong* (BL-54, IS BL-40), leg-*sanli* (ST-36), *jianjing* (GB-21); *(DACH XI, 8v)* *weizhong* (BL-54, IS BL-40), *huiyin* (CV-1).

Chapter XVII

Children

I. In General — II. Emotional — III. Nervous System — IV. Sense Organs — V. Digestive Apparatus — VI. Respiratory System — VII. Circulatory System — VIII. Various Ailments — IX. Bones

I. In General

Special point for all problems or illnesses of children: *(JM) shenzhu* (GV-11, IS GV-12).
All emptinesses of yin or yang in children: *(YXRM I, 47r) xinshu* (BL-15).

II. Emotional

Nighttime tears in children: *(DACH X, 31v; YIX I, 5v) baihui* (GV-19, IS GV-20); *(JM) zhongchong* (PC-9).
The hundred illnesses from tears at night: *(YXRM I, 46r) baihui* (GV-19, IS GV-20).
Illnesses from terror at night: *(JM) zhongchong* (PC-9).
Children not speaking, up to several years old; insufficiency of mental energy: *(DACH) xinshu* (BL-15).

Restive, contrary children *(ke wu)*:

> *An illness of children. If there is a sudden emotional shock, or he meets a visitor **(ke)** or an unaccustomed object, then there will be intractability **(wu)**. A lot of tears at night, no pain, cold from the spleen-pancreas. Sometimes it appears to be epilepsy, but the eyes are not dazed; there is saliva, or convulsions or pain in the abdomen, or panting: tonify the spleen. (YXRM VI, 15r)*

Restive, contrary children *(ke wu): (DACH)* foot-*dadu* (SP-2), *yinbai* (SP-1), *sanyinjiao* (SP-6), *jianshi* (PC-5).
Likes to move: *(YXRM) jianshi* (PC-5).
Acute emotional agitation in children: *(YXRM I, 46r) hegu* (LI-4).
In children — emotional agitation, deranged mind, disquietude; caused by an emptiness of the heart: *(DACH XI, 24) shaochong* (HT-9).

III. Nervous System

Children bending backwards: *(DACH X, 31v) baihui* (GV-19, IS GV-20).
Children, head loose, body bent backwards: *(DACH) mingmen* (GV-4).
Children, mouth open wide, head loose, body bent backwards, as if broken: *(DACH)* moxa the size of a grain of wheat at *jinmen* (BL-63).
Children bent backwards, eyes looking up: *(DACH) ganshu* (BL-18).
Children beating their heads on the wall, the furniture, or the floor: *(GSdeM) jinmen* (BL-63).
Spasms of children: *(DACH) jinmen* (BL-63), *taichong* (LR-3), *hegu* (LI-4), *chize* (LU-5), *jugu* (LI-16), *qiangjian* (GV-17, IS GV-18), *yintang* (GV-23a, IS M-HN-3), *qianding* (GV-20, IS GV-21).
Convulsions or spasms of children: *(JM) hanyan* (GB-4).
Chronic convulsions of children: *(DACH) yanggu* (SI-5), *kunlun* (BL-60), foot-*shangqiu* (SP-5), *jinmen* (BL-63), *xingjian* (LR-2), foot-*dadu* (SP-2), *yinbai* (SP-1), *jiuwei* (CV-14), *sizhukong* (TW-21, IS TW-23), *qimai* (TW-18), *shenzhu* (GV-11, IS GV-12).
Chronic convulsions of babies: tongue stiff, no longer suckles: *(DACH) yanggu* (SI-5).
Stiff spasms of small children: *(JM) rangu* (KI-2).

Meningitis of children:
Acute or chronic meningitis of children: *(DACH) shaoshang* (LU-11), *baihui* (GV-19, IS GV-20), *shuigou* (GV-25, IS GV-26 *renzhong), jianjing* (GB-21), *mingmen* (GV-4), *dadun* (LR-1).
Acute or chronic meningitis of children; if there are screams, disperse; if there are no screams, tonify: *yintang* (GV-23a, IS M-HN-3).
Meningitis of children: *zhongchong* (PC-9), *shaohai* (HT-3), *chengjiang* (CV-24), *mingmen* (GV-4).
Meningitis of children: *xingjian* (LR-2).
Chronic meningitis of children: *chize* (LU-5), *yinbai* (SP-1), foot-*shangqiu* (SP-5).

Meningitis of children, diarrhea and vomiting; for boys who are vomiting puncture on the right; if they have diarrhea, puncture on the left; for girls, do the opposite: *(DACH) yongquan* (KI-1).
Children — sudden death from meningitis: *(DACH) hegu* (LI-4).

Epilepsy of children:
Epilepsy from milk in babies: *(DACH) guiyan* (MP-29b).
Epilepsy of children: *(DACH) yintang* (GV-23a, IS M-HN-3), *qianding* (GV-20, IS GV-21), *guiyan* (MP-29b).
The five epilepsies of adults and children: *(DACH) shenmen* (HT-7).
Children — epilepsy with contraction: *(DACH) gezhuren* (GB-3, IS *shangguan*).
Children — epilepsy with hyperexcitation: *(DACH) shenzhu* (GV-11, IS GV-12).

IV. Sense Organs

Children from two to three years: corners of the eyes protruding: *hegu* (LI-4).
Hemeralopia of children: *zhongchong* (PC-9), *weishu* (BL-21), *pishu* (BL-20).

V. Digestive System

Children teething: *(GSdeM) kunlun* (BL-60).
Lack of appetite of children: *(DACH)* leg-*sanli* (ST-36), *xuanzhong* (GB-39).
Children regurgitating their milk: *(DACH) zhongting* (CV-16), *shanzhong* (CV-17), *shenmai* (BL-62), *weishu* (BL-21).
Vomiting in small children: *(DACH) luxi* (TW-19), and for saliva of babies.
Children who cannot suckle: *yangchi* (TW-4).
Children who always yawn: *yifeng* (TW-17).
Children who do not digest their milk: *(GSdeM)* tonify *ququan* (LR-8).
Diarrhea from milk in babies: *shenque* (CV-8).
Babies with big abdomen and thinness: *zhangmen* (LR-13); from emptiness of the pancreas, the food is not digested: leg-*sanli* (ST-36).
Children; headache when they eat: *yixi* (BL-40, IS BL-45).
Prolapsed rectum in children: *baihui* (GV-19, IS GV-20), *shenque* (CV-8), *changqiang* (GV-1).
Children: intestines falling to the knees: *jizhong* (GV-6).

Inflammation of the mouth:
Children — rotten teeth with cavities, fetid breath: *laogong* (PC-8).
Children — abscesses in the mouth: *laogong* (PC-8), *mingmen* (GV-4).

Noma? Infantile scurvy? *(ya gan; kou zao feng)*:

> It begins in front of the ear, and reaches the cheeks and jaws. A dull, hidden pain of the bones and muscles. After a while, putrefaction and rottenness. Pus often crosses the cheek and comes out; that is why it is also called **chuan sai feng**, shock crossing the cheek. (Ci Yuan, "Kou-zao-feng")

> Illnesses of accumulation and tuberculosis of children are of this type: rotten teeth, rotting on the surface, rotten blood. They are called **ya gan** or **zou ma ya gan**. (Ci Yuan, "Gan")

(YIX I, 6r) Ya gan (gnawing): moxas at *changqiang* (GV-1), gum-*yinjiao* (GV-27, IS GV-28).
(DACH XI, 3v) Both cheeks red and swollen, generating abscesses; called *gu zao feng* or *zhu sai feng* (pork-cheek wind), comes from inflammation of the blood, the three warmers being blocked: *hegu* (LI-4), *lieque* (LU-7), *dicang* (ST-7, IS ST-4), *jiache* (ST-3, IS ST-6). If not better: *chengjiang* (CV-24), arm-*sanli* (LI-10), *jinjin* (MP-6, IS M-HN-20a), *yuye* (MP-7, IS M-HN-20b).

VI. Respiratory System

Tuberculosis of children (*xiao er gan chong*, "microbes of tuberculosis in children" or *pi gan*, "tuberculosis of the spleen"):
(JM) Shaoze (SI-1), *shaoshang* (LU-11), *guanchong* (TW-1), *laogong* (PC-8), *zhongchong* (PC-9), *qiangu* (SI-2), hand-*wangu* (SI-4), *yangxi* (LI-5), *xinhui* (GV-21, IS GV-22), *shenzhu* (GV-11, IS GV-12), *wuyi* (ST-15), *zhongshu* (GV-6a, IS GV-7), abdomen-*yinjiao* (CV-7), *shuifen* (CV-9).
Bony tuberculosis of children: *yinxi* (HT-6).

VII. Circulatory System

Infantile anemia: food is difficult to assimilate; complexion is grey-white; comes from bad food and hygiene, or from intestinal worms. (Ci Yuan, "Gan-ji" [tuberculosis accumulation])

(GSdeM) Gaohuang (BL-38, IS BL-43).

VIII. Various Ailments

Swelling of the umbilicus in babies: *(DACH) taixi* (KI-5, IS KI-3).
Children — swelling, pruritis and trembling: *(DACH) shaohai* (HT-3).

> *An illness of children; the five treasure organs in the interior are in pain from pulling and tension. The origin of this is found in the emotions of the fetus and movements from shock of the fetus. The muscles of the eyes are reddened, with spots of blood; the body is arched, black lips. When lying down, they cry. Swelling of the testicles, vomiting, diarrhea, then convulsions; inner and outer fullness to the point of causing fear. In meningitis and **nei diao,** extreme pain inside the abdomen; when lying down they cry, the face is blue, limbs cold; urine like rice water. Resembles intestinal pain, but with copious tears. Resembles symptoms of worms, but these attack the heart. There is sobbing, closed eyes, vomiting of clear saliva, thinness of the four limbs, yellow and blue complexion. (YXRM V, 16r, "Nei-diao" or "Diao-chang-qi" [taken with a fishhook])*

> *An illness of children; depends on the yang. It comes from the milk when the mother has eaten too much cured meat, or acid foods, or too much wine. The poison goes into the milk and from there into the heart and lungs of the child, where it generates heat. If there is external shock, then the eyes are suddenly fixed, the body is stiff like a fish taken with the hook, thus the name. The appearance is that of the tonic convulsions of meningitis — eyes rolled back, or with tears or laughing as in "evil influences." If serious, the nails are blue; sometimes the abdomen is swollen and hard; during sleep there are spasms in the abdomen; there is foul-smelling diarrhea. Harmonize the spleen and the stomach. This must not be confused with meningitis.*
> *(Ci Yuan, "Tian-diao" [heavenly fishing line])*

IX. Bones

Babies — fontanelles do not join: *(DACH) yinjiao* (CV-7), *qihai* (CV-6), *shuifen* (CV-9), *changqiang* (GV-1).
Children — tortoise back (kyphosis): *feishu* (BL-15).
Deviations of the spine in children: *waiqiu* (GB-36), *feishu* (BL-15).
Children — tortoise chest: *waiqiu* (GB-36), *rugen* (ST-18).

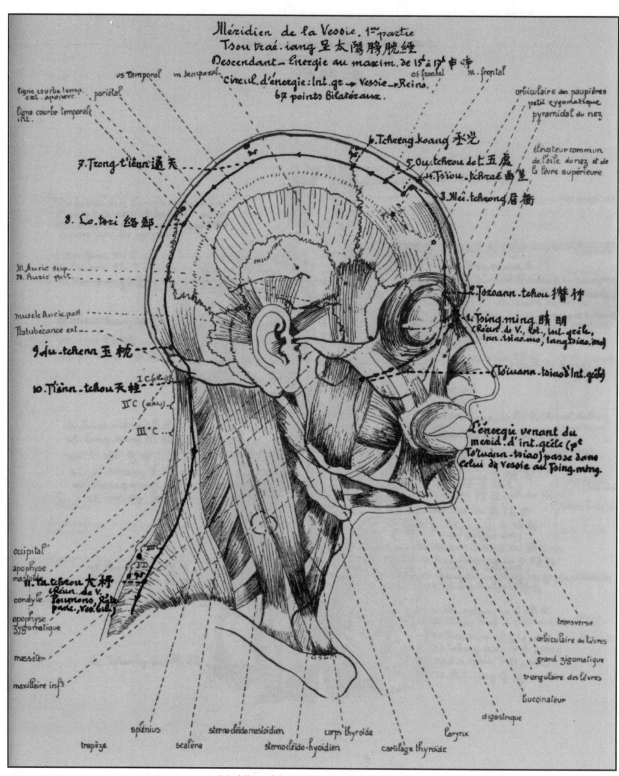

Meridian of the bladder (part 1) (GSDM)

Bibliography

Specialized Chinese Books on Acupuncture[1]

High Antiquity

Before the third century B.C., books were written either on white silk with a wooden twig dipped in black varnish, or engraved on bamboo slats. Paper and brush date from the third century B.C.

The emperor Shi Huang Di, of the Qin dynasty (fourth century B.C.), apparently burnt all the philosophical and sociological books whose precepts contradicted his, but he saved the books on medicine and science. The works of Confucius (Kong-zi), burnt completely at that time, were reconstituted a century later by transcribing the memories of old literati; these memories were later confirmed by the discovery, some decades later, of inscriptions on bamboo slats.

Whether authentic, or orally transmitted, or more or less expanded with interpolations, all the ancient texts were put into writing in several manuscripts during the second and first centuries before our era. Regarding acupuncture, the *Su Wen* and the *Ling Shu* (together forming the *Nei Jing*) and the *Nan Jing* remain from this ancient period.

The *Nei Jing,* or "Internal Meridians" (the title can also be translated as "Rule of the Interior" or "The Classic of the Interior"), is the name given to two books: *Su Wen* and *Ling Shu.* Both of these were supposed to have been compiled under the direction of the Yellow Emperor Huang Di (2697-2596 B.C.) by his medical advisors Qi Bo, Lei Gong, Dong Jun,[2] Yu Fu, and Shao Yu.

The bibliography in the *History of the Former Han,* written at the beginning of the Christian era, mentions the *Nei Jing* as having a total of eighteen *juan,* or rolls (the chapters or sections being written on a long strip of rolled paper imitating, or more likely imitated by, the Romans. Now there are said to be thirteen rolls for the *Su Wen* and eighty-one for the *Ling Shu,* all of which are very short. Were they previously grouped into sections, or were there later additions?

Critics discuss the two parts separately:

(1) *Su Wen, "Questions on White Silk,"* thirteen *juan.*

The thirteen *juan* of the *Su Wen:* tradition says that it is a book of questions and answers of Huang Di and Qi Bo, but upon examining its aim and imagery we find that its language is not that of a single epoch; it has not been composed by the hand of one person.

Liu Xiang (first century B.C.) shows that it was compiled by Han Gong-zi. Cheng-zi (Cheng Yi, A.D. 1033-1070) writes that it was orally transmitted, like the words of Confucius (Kong-zi) and his disciple, Zi Si. The remainder, a large part, was an invention of Han dynasty writers (from the second century B.C. to the third century A.D.), as was the *Li Ji,* "Memorial of the Rites." Finally, it was probably recast in the Warring States period *(YIX I, 1r; DACH I, 1r).*

The bibliography of the *History of the Western Han* (written at the beginning of the Christian era) says: *Nei Jing,* eighteen rolls. Bian Que (fifth century B.C.) and Master Bo write that the *Nei Jing* had five authors.[3] "the name *Su Wen* is not mentioned" *(DACH I, 1r).*

In the bibliography of the *History of the Sui* (written in the sixth century A.D.) the name *Su Wen* begins to appear, and it is indicated as being the *Nei Jing.* In fact, in the bibliography of the *History of the Eastern Han* (written in 95 B.C.), there is listed the *Nei Jing,* in eighteen rolls.

Wang Bing, of the Tang dynasty (eighth century A.D.), in his "Nine Immaterials," corrected the number of Han dynasty books, and said that this book (*Su Wen*) had been compiled by Master Zhang.[4] "During the Song dynasty (tenth to twelfth centuries A.D.), Lin Yi, Gao Ruo Na, and others corrected textual errors and added missing passages" *(DACH; YIX).*

In summary, it is reasonable to suppose that the *Su Wen,* taken as a whole, was perhaps composed by several authors around the twenty-eighth century B.C., that it was set down, perhaps with corrections, around the third century B.C., and was finally revised and appended during the Song dynasty, around the eleventh century A.D. It is constantly cited, studied, and commented on by all the masters of acupuncture, the masters of yin and yang.

(2) *Ling Shu, "Immaterial Axis."* Also called *Zhen Jing, "Needle Classic."* Eighty-one *juan* (chapters).

An ancient medical book on needles and moxa. Together with the *Su Wen*, it goes under the name *Nei Jing*. Since the Southern Song dynasty (thirteenth century A.D.) this book has spread throughout the world.

"It is questionable upon what Wang Bing (eighth century A.D.) based his evidence. He suggests that this book consists of twelve *juan*" *(Ci Yuan)*.

"Wang Bing (eighth century A.D.) asserts that this book formed nine of the eighteen rolls of the *Nei Jing* mentioned in the *Bibliography of the Former Han* (95 B.C.). However, skeptics suggest that when Huang-fu Mi (fl. A.D. 265 to 316) compiled the *Nei Jing*, Cang Gong, at that time, promoted the book as being from antiquity. The matter is unclear" *(Wen Xian Tong Kao, juan XVIII, 114,* a thirteenth century encyclopedia).

In summary, opinions about the *Ling Shu* are less clear than those about the *Su Wen*. However, although its popularity dates from the thirteenth century, a glorious epoch for acupuncture, even skeptics themselves attribute it to the third century after Christ, while the illustrious critic Wang Bing, of the eighth century, thought that it formed part of the ancient *Nei Jing*. It is reasonable to assume that a large part of it is very old.

The "twelve rolls" mentioned in the *Ci Yuan* encyclopedia are probably distributed among the current eighty-one chapters.

In any case, this book contains the essentials of the doctrine of needles and moxa. Acupuncture doctors in Japan and China consult it constantly; its title, *Classic of Needles,* demonstrates its importance. It contains more practical advice than the *Su Wen*.

I have made a draught translation, which needs revision and is still in manuscript form.

(3) *Nan Jing, "Classic (or Rules) of Difficulties."* Now in two "rolls" or *juan* (three according to *DACH I, 10*).

The *Nan Jing* is attributed to Qin Yue Ren (Bian Que), who is said to have lived during the fifth century B.C., although some critics suggest that he lived during the Qin dynasty of the third century B.C. Through questions and answers, he explains and comments on the whole of the *Nei Jing*. The famous thirteenth century physician Hua Shou republished this book with commentaries, stating, "The judgements of this book are well proven and very conscientious."

The *Da Cheng I, 1r* indicates that the texts of the *Su Wen* and *Ling Shu* referred to by Bian Que are not all the same as those which are incorporated into the *Nei Jing*. They are apparently original texts, unchanged during the course of the centuries.

The thirteenth century encyclopedia *Wen Xian Tong Kao (juan XIX, 124)* states that during the Han dynasty (second century B.C. to third century A.D.), Bian Que was only known from the *Nei Sai Jing, "Rule of the Internal Limits,"* which no longer exists. Was this the *Nan Jing*? There is no doubt about this among writers on acupuncture. Moreover, the book is mentioned in the *History of Sui* (fourth century A.D.).

"During the Sui dynasty, a commentary was written by Lu Bo Wang, but it has not come down to us."

"In the Tang dynasty (seventh to tenth century), Wang Wei Yi, along with five other authors, discusses it in a volume."

"In our dynasty (the Ming, fourteenth to seventeenth centuries), the critic Wang Shao Qing declares it to be a redoubled obscurity, which does nothing to clarify the confusion of the ancient writers."

"Hua Shou [Song, twelfth and thirteenth centuries] left what was long and cut what was short, editing it according to his own ideas to create the *Nan Jing Ben Yi, "Explanation of the Roots of the Classic of Difficulties"* " *(DACH I, 1r).*

In our own time, besides the *Nan Jing,* there are three other extant works attributed to Bian Que. They are admittedly apocryphal, but very useful:

(1) *Zi-Wu Jing, "Book of Midnight and Midday,"* in one *juan*. This work, in rhythmic songs, gives the essentials of the method *(DACH I, 1r),* but by showing the relations between morning and evening, yin and yang, and between the yin and yang meridians. "Earlier people attributed it to Bian Que" *(YIX I, 1r).*

(2) *Bian Que Xin Shu, "Book of Bian Que's Mind,"* by Dou Cai, published in A.D. 1146. It contains everything that is attributed to Bian Que.

(3) *Yu Long Fu, "Song of the Jade Dragon."* A rhythmic therapeutic repertory. Reproduced in the *Da Cheng* as being by Bian Que.[5]

From the Third Century B.C. to the Sixth Century A.D.
The Han, Jin and Wei Dynasties

It is strange that the two Han dynasties, which produced so many great literary works, only created (if we are to believe the bibliographies) a single work on acupuncture, which, moreover, is lost:

Jin Gui Yao Lue, "*Important Summary of the Golden Chest,*" by Zhang Ji[6] (cited by the *Ci Yuan,* "*Shang-han*" and "*Shang-han Lun*" articles). It was during this period that the famous Hua Tuo lived (A.D. 125-220).

Under the Jin, a short dynasty which followed (A.D. 265-420), there appeared a very important book:

Jia Yi Jing, "*Rule of One and Five,*" referring to the correspondences of points and meridians between one half-day and the other half-day (i.e., yin and yang), by Huang-fu Mi (Shi An, Yuan Yan), who lived from 215 to 282. The book was published between 265 and 280, in twelve *juan.* It is also known as *Zhen Jing,* "*Book of Truth.*"

Dr. Fang *(Jin Zhen Bi Zhuan, 7)* indicates that it is thanks to the *Jia Yi Jing* that in our time the number and locations of the points of each meridian are known exactly. The ancient books did not give this information in such an organized fashion. Besides the rules which it gives, this book is also important because it refers to and summarizes works which have disappeared. It is the basis for modern studies on acupuncture.

In the same period, a work was published that summarized and perfected the most important discoveries for diagnosis and the differentiation between fullness and emptiness of energy (of function) of each internal organ:

Mo Xue, "*Pulse Traditions,*" also known as the *Mo Jing,* "*Rule of the Pulse,*" by Wang Shu He, whose life is placed, imprecisely, during the Jin dynasty (265-420).

"Born during the Jin dynasty, Wang Shu He, author of the *Mo Xue,* decided to use the radial pulses *(cun kou)* in the same way as the left and right carotid pulses had been used" *(DACH VIII, 8r).*

The *Ci Yuan,* referring to a thirteenth century author, makes the attribution of the book to Wang Shu He doubtful. It has been suggested that it is one of a number of fabrications produced during the Song period (tenth to thirteenth centuries). Its attribution to Wang Shu He, however, emphasizes its reputation in this special science.

One might also cite:

Zhou Hou Fang, "*Prescriptions Behind the Elbow,*" by Ge Hong (fourth century), which contains many acupuncture treatments which are still referred to in our day.

From the Sixth to the Tenth Centuries
The Sui and Tang Dynasties

The acupuncture literature from this period of great national prosperity is rather prolific.

Qian Jin Fang, or *Qian Jin Yao Fang, [Important] Treatments Worth a Thousand Ounces of Gold,*" for needles and moxa, in thirty *juan.* By Sun Simo (585-682), one of the great names in acupuncture.

"It was said that Sun was venerated. One of his treatments was enough to cure. They were valued at a thousand ounces of gold. He used needles and moxas, determining the points through the pulses. As well as the rules for conducting the energy, he discussed at length the reasons for not puncturing or burning certain points" *(DACH I, 1v).*

Sun Simo is also the author of a second work, "added like wings" to the former:

Qian Jin Yi Fang, "*Wings to the Treatments Worth a Thousand Ounces of Gold,*" in thirty *juan.*

"He begins with a register of medicines. Then he gives treatments for cold damage, women's diseases, children, nourishing the character, various illnesses, needles and moxa, and finally, forbidden methods" *(DACH I, 1v).*

Su Wen Ci Zhu, "*Successive Commentaries on the Su Wen,*" by Wang Bing, who was named Court Physician in 762. Its studies of the form and essence, the origin and value of the *Su Wen* are still respectfully reiterated and discussed in detail.

Wai Tai Bi Yao, "*Important Secrets From the Tower,*" thirty *juan,* by Wang Dao, Governor of Da Ming from 742 to 755.

This book, always very popular, deals more with medicines than with acupuncture. For twenty years, Wang Dao was the Secretary of the "Tower Pavilion," where the ancient books were kept. There he found thousands of volumes of prescriptions and treatments. From them he compiled 1104 treatments, both with medicines and acupuncture *(q.v. DACH I, 1v).*

"Wang Dao knew the art of medicine. He published this book while he was Governor of the Garrison at Ye (now called Da Ming). First there are discussions, then prescriptions. The secret rules, transmitted from antiquity, are taken from there" *(Ci Yuan).*[7]

From the Tenth to the Thirteenth Centuries
Song Dynasty

By the end of the Tang dynasty, the entire north of China was occupied by the nomads of Mongolia and Manchuria. Then, at the beginning of the eleventh century, the Song dynasty succeeded in reconquering the north of China. Prosperity returned with peace.

Consequently, the Song emperors took a personal interest in acupuncture studies. Under their rule, the ancient books were investigated. Since the payment was high, skeptics accuse this period (which, moreover, was said to have received writings from Heaven) of fabricating or falsifying many works. Printing was becoming available, and many ancient and contemporary books were published.

Engravings made by Zhang Shu Gong, representing the meridians and the points, were printed. A bronze lifesize bronze statue, which had all the points with their depths, was cast. Many reproductions, 40 cm. high, were made for the libraries of different palaces. I possess one from the Winter Palace in Peking. An acupuncture school was opened in this palace.

For the first time, this method spread widely, and at the same time there was an immense effort at making more precise the exact location and effects of each point.

The most notable books of this period, which are still extant, are:

Tong-Ren Zhen-Jiu Jing, "Book of Needles and Moxa of the Bronze Man," three *juan,* by Wang Wei De [more commonly known as Wang Wei Yi — ed.], during the reign of Ren Zong (1023-1064).

The *Si Ku* catalogue refers to this book as having seven *juan,* without the author's name. It has been asked whether Wang is the true author.

"Wang Wei De wrote *Tong-Ren Shu-Xue Zhen-Jiu Jing, "Book of Needles and Moxa and the Points of the Bronze Man,"* in three *juan.* See *Du Shu Hou Zhi, "Register After Reading,"* by Yao Gongwu. Yao wrote that the Emperor Ren Zong asked Wang Wei De to study the method of needles and moxa and to have a statue cast as a model. In order to fix what is known abut the points, he also made boards on which to print drawings. The *Yu Hai* says almost the same thing" *(Ci Yuan).*

The *Da Cheng I, 1* comments that many of the points do not correspond exactly to the indications of the *Ling Shu* and other works. It gives this volume the title *Tong-Ren Zhen-Jiu Tu, "Drawings of the Needles and Moxas from the Bronze Man."*

Cun Zhen Tu, "Drawings For Preserving the Truth," one *juan,* by Yang Jie (Ji Lao, fl. 1102-1107).

"The Governor delivered to him criminals who were to be executed. Surrounded by draughtsmen, he dissected them alive and studied the relationships of the points" *(DACH I, 1v).*

Zhen Jing Zhi-Nan, "Compass to the Needles and Meridians," by Dou Han Qing (Tai Shi, of Gu-Fei; the *Yi Xue, 32v,* has "from He-Fei").

"In the beginning it explains obscure texts. Then it establishes the rules for entering the points. There are many disagreements with the *Su Wen" (DACH I, 2r).*

Nan Jing Ben Yi, "Explanations of the Roots of the Book of Difficulties," by Hua Shou (Bo Ren, from Ying-Ning-Cheng),[8] thirteenth and fourteenth centuries. One of the most accomplished physicians China has ever known.

"Hua Shou Bo Ren "left what was long and cut what was short," editing according to his ideas in order to create the *Nan Jing Ben Yi" (DACH I, 1v).*

Shi-Si Jing Fa Hui, "Explanations of the Fourteen Meridians," three *juan,* by Hua Shou.

"He received his method from Gao Dong Yang: to open and close, to make flow and stop, to join and separate. He differentiated the *ren mai,* "conception vessel," and the *du mai,* "governor vessel," from the eight marvellous vessels and joined them to the twelve meridians, pointing out that they had their own special points. He used 657 points" *(DACH I, 2r).*

Xiao-Er An-Mo Jing, "Massage of the Meridians for Children," by Chen Wen Zhong (Wen Xu, from Si-Ming in Xu Zhou), twelfth and thirteenth centuries *(DACH I, 2r).*

A short, remarkable work, partially reproduced in the *Da Cheng.* Chen also published a book on illnesses of children, which is now lost.

Zi Sheng Jing, "Classic of Native Disposition," seven *juan,* by Wang Shi Zhong of the Song dynasty.

"It describes 360 points with their depths, differences and relationship to illnesses. It is in agreement with the *Tong-Ren,* the *Qian Jin,* the *Ming Tang,* and other books." *(DACH I, 2r).*

Pi Wei Lun, "Discussion of the Spleen and Stomach," and *Lan Shi Bi Cang, "Secret Treasure of the Orchid Lodge,"* both by Li Gao (Dong Yuan), end of the thirteenth century (died during the Yuan dynasty). Contains indications to which reference is constantly made.

Late Thirteenth to Mid-Fourteenth Centuries
Yuan Dynasty

Under the domination of the Mongols of the Yuan dynasty, an important work, still referred to today, was published:

Ba Cui, or *Ji Sheng Ba Cui, "Graded Lessons Which Aid Living,"* nineteen *juan,* by Du Si Jing, published between 1314 and 1321. *"Ba Cui"* was a title given during the Tang dynasty to authors named by selection, without examination.

"First volume: the more important meridians and needles. Second volume: clarification of the ancient needling methods and of the "flowing and blocking" *(liu-zhu)* method of Diu Gui Fang, etc." *(DACH I, 1v).*

Some other less important but useful books appeared during this dynasty:

Jin Lan Xun Jing, "The Book Beside the Golden Orchids," by Wu-Tai Bi Lie, a Mongol member of the Hanlin Academy. Published by his son, with a preface dated 1303 and signed Shao Wen Long.

"A description of the organs and the fourteen meridians, and of the rule "to make flow and to block" *(liu-zhu),* with plates" *(DACH I, 1r).*

Xiao-Er Ming Tang, "Audience Hall for Children," by Dou Gui Fang, of Jian-An, late thirteenth, early fourteenth centuries.

Dou Gui Fang is the author of the "flowing and blocking" rule discussed and commented upon in the first two books cited in this section.

Zhen-Jiu Za Shuo, "Various Talks on Needles and Moxa," by Dou Gui Fang.

"It explains human consciousness, and that which must be avoided in the *Qian Jin [Fang]* (by Sun Simo, of the seventh century). It separates the good from the bad, but does not exhaust what is admirable about needles and moxas" *(DACH I, 2r).*

Ming Tang Zhen-Jiu Tu, "Drawings for Needles and Moxa from the Audience Hall," also called *Huang Di Ming Tang Jiu Jing, "Rules for Moxa from Huang Di's Audience Hall,"* by Dou Gui Fang.

"The preface says: "Discussions of Huang Di on the points of the body and the arguments for moxas" " *(DACH I, 1v).*

Late Fourteenth to Mid-Seventeenth Centuries
Ming Dynasty

National peace and prosperity, brought by the Ming dynasty, allowed a renaissance of acupuncture. In fact, this period produced some of the most important compilations that exist on the subject.

Shen Ying Jing, "Rules for the Response of the Consciousness," one *juan* (according to the *Da Cheng I, 2r,* two *juan*), by Chen Hui (Shan Tong, of Hong-Gang). Revised by his student, Liu Jin (from Nan-Cheng) and published in 1425-26 (Hong-Si period). (See *Tu Jie Jing Xue Xue,* by Dr. Tatse-i, Tokyo, 1931, page 357.)

"Chen Hui first wrote *Guang Ai Shu, "The Book of Extended Love,"* in twelve *juan.* Then, in order to respond to the critics, and so that students could follow the rules, he took only 119 points, and with them composed the *Shen Ying Jing.* Liu Jing of Nan-Cheng revised it" *(YIX I, 1v).* The *Da Cheng I, 2r,* says: ". . . 119 points with songs and drawings."

Ju Ying, "Collection of Blossoms," or *Zhen-Jiu Ju Ying, "Collection of Blossoms for Needles and Moxa,"* by Gao Wu (Mei Hu, of Si-Ming), published during the Jia-Jing period (1522-1562). See *Jin Zhen Bi Zhuan, 10; DACH I, 2r;* Dr. Tatse-i, 1931, page 337. Very often cited.

Zhen-Jiu Da Quan, "Great Completion of Needles and Moxas," by Yang Ji Shi (Ji Zhou), physician of the Supreme Court of Medicine. Published during the Wan-Li period (1573-1620). An important work.

"During the Yuan and Ming periods, there was a very secret book on acupuncture. Those who could consult it considered it to be a rare treasure. It was entitled *Wei Sheng Zhen-Jiu Yuan* (or *Xuan) Ji Bi Yao, "Important Secrets on the Original (or Mysterious) Powers of Needles and Moxas for the Protection of Life."* During the Wan-Li period, Yang Ji Shi, feeling the book should be published, completed and corrected it, and had it printed, changing its name to *Zhen-Jiu Da Quan" (Jin Zhen Bi Zhuan, 10).* It is frequently cited in the *Da Cheng.*

Xuan Ji Bi Yao San Ju, "The Three Important and Secret Ways of the Subtle Powers," by Yang Ji Shi. Wan-Li period (1573-1620).

"Published according to family traditions" *(YIX I, 1v).*

Is this the same book as the previous entry, with a slightly different title, or is it a commentary or extract from a secret book perfected by Yang Ji Shi? Some references are made to it in the *Da Cheng* (particularly volume VI).

Zhen-Jiu Da Cheng, "Great Perfection of Needles and Moxa," ten *juan,* by Yang Ge Xian[9] (from Wei-Jin or from Du-Men). Wan-Li period (1573-1620).

A very important work. It reproduces the most useful passages of all the known books from the *Nei Jing* up to the *Zhen-Jiu Da Quan,* published a short time before it.[10] It has some not very precise diagrams; explanations; symptoms of illnesses cured by each point; numerous treatments, etc.

I own a large edition with a preface from 1680, another large edition printed between 1798 and 1826, and a small edition in which the second and fourth *juan* are each divided in two, giving twelve *juan* for the entire work. The edition I own was printed in 1900. There are some recent reimpressions (1928, etc.).

At the end of the sixteenth century, under the same title, there appeared an abridged version of the same work in six *juan,* by Xu Fong (Ting Hui).[11]

Qi Jing Ba Mo Kao, "Explanations of the Eight Vessels of the Marvellous Meridians," by Li Shi Zhen (Dong Pi) from Ji-Zhou. Wan-Li period (1573-1620).

In 1590, Li Shi Zhen, who was First Sacrificer for the King of Shu, also published a materia medica in fifty-two volumes, entitled *Ben-Cao Gang Mu.*

From the Seventeenth Century to Modern Times
Qing Dynasty and the Republic

The Qing dynasty is singularly poor in books on acupuncture. Truly, the work done under the previous dynasty satisfied all their requirements, and it was thanks to them that acupuncture continued to develop. As it was still considered useful to give the essentials of the doctrine and its methods in summary, only one work was published under the Qing:

Zhen Jiu Yi Xue, "Easy Studies of Needles and Moxa," in three *juan,* by Li Shou Xian (Shan Shu). First edition in 1798, republished in 1897, 1918, etc.

An abridged text for the use of acupuncture in the home. It gives the general rules of use. It is a memory aid with not very exact drawings, and without symptoms for the points, but with somewhat precise indications of their locations.

The Republic (since 1911) has seen the publication of two works, the latter of which is the more important:

Zhen Jiu Yi Zhi, "Easy Knowledge of Needles and Moxa." Compiled by a group of physicians for the Wen Ming Shu Ju Publishing Company of Shanghai in 1919. Republished in 1927. 47 pages.

Similar to the preceding book, but better presented and better arranged, although the drawings are still very imprecise.

Jin Zhen Bi Zhuan, "Important Secrets of the Golden Needles," 338 pages, the first volume bound in the Western fashion, by Dr. Fang Zun'an (northern pronunciation: Fang Shen'an) of He-Fei. Xian Dai Yin Shua Gong Ci edition, Shanghai, 1937.

This very important work researches and discusses all the traditions of acupuncture. It contains passages taken from lost books and a discursive bibliography. The new drawings are far superior to all those previously published. It also gives symptoms for the points taken from the author's experience, etc.

A collection published in Shanghai in 1936, entitled *Huang Han Yi Xue Zong Shu,* *"General Books for the Imperial Chinese Medical Studies,"* consists of four works:

Jing Xue Cuan Yao, "Important Groupings of the Meridians and Points."
Zhen Xue Tong Lun, "General Discussion of the Study of the Points."
Zhen Jiu Xue Gang Yao, "The Important Essentials for the Study of Needles and Moxa."
Xuan Zhen San Yao Ji, "Review of the Three Importances for the Choice of Needles."

China: General Medical Works

The first great reviews of medicine date from the Ming dynasty:

Gu Jin Yi Tong, "Ancient and Modern Medical Generalities," 100 *juan,* by Xu Chun Fu from Xin-An, 1556.

A large medical encyclopedia, of which two large volumes are given to acupuncture.

Yi Xue Ru Men, "Gate of Entry to Medical Studies," eight *juan,* by Li Chan (from Nan-Feng), 1575.

A highly respected work, containing all the essential information for all forms of treatment. One volume is devoted entirely to acupuncture.

Korean Works

Tong Yi Bao Jian, "Precious Mirror of Oriental Medicine," by Xu Zun.

Chao Xian Guo Zhen Jiu Jing Mian Fang, "Verified Prescriptions from the Classic of Needles and Moxa of Korea," by Xu Ren.

Japanese Works

(Pronunciation Given in Chinese)

Zhen Jiu Jing Xue Yi Dian, "Repertory of Medicine for the Points, Meridians, Needles and Moxas," by Dr. Tamamori Minosuke, Tokyo, 1930. Bound in the western style.

An important work, showing the meridians and points through overlays on photographs of people, symptoms of each point, treatments, etc.

Tu Jie Jing Xue Xue, "Drawings and Explanations for the Study of the Meridians and the Points," by Dr. Tatse-i, Tokyo, 1931.

A book constructed along the same lines as the preceding, but with more numerous and less precise drawings. Also contains symptoms and treatments.

Jian Ming Zhen Jiu Yi Xue, "Medical Studies of Needles and Moxa, Clarified and Selected," by Dr. Tatse-i, seventh edition, 1937.

Han Fang Yi Xue Xin Bian Jiu, "A New Examination of Medical Studies and of Chinese Treatments," one volume, by Dr. Nakayama Tyotuko, Bao Wen Guan, Tokyo, 1931.

A comparison of European and Chinese methods. Descriptions of laboratory experiments with moxas. Comparisons of the meridians. Translated by George Soulié de Morant and Dr. Sakurazawa as *L'acuponcture chinoise vérifiée au Japon,* Editions du Trianon, Paris, 1935.

Jiu Fa Shi Yi Xue De Bian Jiu, "Examination of Medical Studies and the Method of Moxa," one volume, by Dr. Hara, Tokyo, 1930.

This book gives the results of laboratory experiments on the effects of moxa on the blood.

Documented, Serious European Works

Specimen medicinae sinicae, Sive opuscula medica ad mentem sinensium, cum figuris, by A. Cleyer, Frankfurt, Zubrodt, 1682.

On the whole, an interesting book, with thirty plates and many texts translated from Chinese by Reverend Father Boym, published by Cleyer.

La Médecine chez les Chinois, by Dabry, consul in Han-Kou, Plon, Paris, 1853; 576 pages with plates (one chapter on acupuncture).

A very serious presentation of Chinese texts on medicine dictated to the author. Contains a well-done chapter on acupuncture with symptoms for each point and treatments.

La Médecine des chinoise, by Dr. J. Regnault, Hanoi, 1902, 230 pages. Some pages on acupuncture.

A short but precise work containing an excellent list of identified Chinese medicines. Contains a general but very well done passage on acupuncture.

Die Chinesische Medezin zu Begin. Verlag der Asia Major, by Fr. Hubötter D. Bruno Schendler, Leipzig, 1929.

Précis de la vraie Acuponcture chinoise, by George Soulié de Morant, Editions du Mercure de France, 1935, one volume; 201 pages with plates.

The first completely practical book giving the overall principles with symptoms for the seventy-five most important points. Some treatments; complete illustrations.

L'Acuponcture chinoise vérifiée au Japon, Paris, 1936.

An abridged translation of Dr. Nakayama's book (q.v. above) by G. Soulié de Morant and Dr. Sakurazawa. Le Francois, 1934; 88 pages.

L'Acuponcture chinoise, by Dr. Nguyen Van-quan, Paris, 1936.

A doctoral thesis, copied almost verbatim from *Précis de la vraie Acuponcture chinoise,* from which even the illustrations have been borrowed. With some medical observations by Dr. Martiny and G. Soulié de Morant.

L'Acuponcture chinoise et les dermalgies, echo des douleurs viscérales, by Dr. Jean-Louis Verheggen, Imprimerie du Progress, 1937; 206 pages.

A very interesting work, taken from a doctoral thesis. It borrows from the presentations given above, but also includes personal observations and discussions, studying the effects of the needles through the eyes of modern science.

Aide-mémoire des indications de l'Acuponcture chinoise, by Dr. Borrey, Lyon, 1936.

The author has substituted numbers for the Chinese names; he has also taken the symptoms as given by G. Soulié de Morant for each point and isolated them in alphabetical order, thus divorcing them from their complete syndromes.

Acuponcture chinoise appliquée, by Dr. Bonnet-Lemaire, Maloine, Paris, 1940.

Serious Medical Articles and Reports

''L'Acuponcture en Chine,'' by G. Soulié de Morant and Dr. Ferreyrolles, *Homéopathie francaise,* June, 1929.

''Les Aiguilles et les Moxas en Chine,'' by G. Soulié de Morant and Dr. Ferreyrolles, *Science Médicale Pratique,* June, 1931.

''L'Acuponcture chinoise,'' by G. Soulié de Morant, *Annales de l'Hôpital Saint-Jacques,* June, 1932.

''Valeur d'une piqûre d'aiguille pour le treatment des arthrites,'' by Dr. Ferreyrolles, *Bulletin et Mémoires de la Société de Médecine de Paris,* meeting of May 13th, 1932.

''L'Acuponcture chinoise,'' by G. Soulié de Morant. Mercure de France, June 1, 1932.

''La méthode chinoise de l'Acuponcture,'' by Dr. Ferreyrolles, *Science Médicale Pratique,* June, 1933.

''Les Pouls chinois,'' by G. Soulié de Morant, *Mercure de France,* January 1, 1933.

''Traitement des algies par l'Acuponcture chinoise,'' by Drs. Flandin, Ferreyrolles, Macé de Lépinay, *Bulletin de la Société Médicale des Hôpitaux,* May 3, 1933.

''L'Acuponcture chinoise,'' by Dr. Thérèse Martiny, *Vie Médicale,* November 10, 1933.

''L'Acuponcture chinoise,'' by the surgeon, Dr. Flandin, *Progrès Médical,* December 6, 1933.

''Curiosités de la médecine chinoise et Acuponcture,'' by Dr. J. Regnault, *Lettre Médicale,* January, 1934.

''L'Acuponcture chinoise,'' by Dr. Bonnet-Lemaire, *France du Centre,* May 15th and June 1st, 1934; also in a brochure, édition Ayar, 1934.

''Qu'est-ce que l'Acuponcture?'' by Dr. Marcel Lavergne, *Monde Médical,* May 15, 1934.

''L'Acuponcture,'' by G. Soulié de Morant, special issue of *Médecine,* May 26, 1934.

''L'Acuponcture chinoise contre les vomissements habituels,'' by Dr. Marcel Lavergne, *Le Formulaire,* September, 1934.

''Quelques notions pratiques d'Acuponcture,'' by Dr. Ferreyrolles, *Bulletin de la Société des Hôpitaux libres,* July, 1934.

''Que penser actuellement de l'Acuponcture?'' by Dr. Ferreyrolles, *Archives des Hôpitaux,* May, 1935.

''Acuponcture et glandes endocrines,'' by Dr. Bonnet-Lemaire, *Guérir,* May 1, 1935.

''Quelques précisions sur l'Acuponcture chinoise,'' by Dr. Marcel Lavergne, *Paris Médicale,* July 13, 1935.

''Dans quelle mesure l'étude des pouls chinoise est-elle utile pour pratiquer l'Acuponcture?'' by Dr. Marcel Lavergne, *Paris Médicale,* July 13th, 1935.

''Quelques précisions sur les indications de l'Acuponcture chinoise, by Dr. Marcel Lavergne, *Paris Médicale,* April 13, 1935.

''Traitement de l'anorexie des nourissons par l'Acuponcture chinoise,'' by Dr. Marcel Lavergne, *Le Nourrisson,* May, 1935.

''L'Acuponcture chinoise,'' by Dr. Thérèse Martiny of Leopold-Bellan Hospital. *Vie Médicale,* August 25, 1935.

''Note sur les phénomènes électriques que se manifest dans l'Acuponcture,'' by Ponillet, 1936.

''L'Acuponcture chinoise,'' by Dr. Bonnet-Lemaire of Hahnemann Hospital, *Revue Franco-chinoise et Politique de Pékin,* December 1, 1938.

''An Unknown System of Nerves,'' by Sir Thomas Lewis, *British Medical Journal,* February, 1937.

Accounts of Travelers, Second-Hand Accounts

Dissertation de acupunctura, by V. Ten-Rhyne, Londini, 1683.

Amaenitatum exoticarum, by Kaempfer, Paris, 1712.

Histoire et description du Japon, by Kaempfer, Lemgovia, 1779.

A Description of Surgical Operations Peculiar to Japanese and Chinese, by J.M. Churchill, London, 1821.

Médecins et médecine en Chine, by C. Daumas, Grasse, 1858.

Pharmacie et matière médicale chinoises, by Debeaux, Paris, 1865.

La Matière médicale ches les Chinois, by Dr. Soubeyran, Paris, 1873. A serious work from information furnished by Consul Dabry.

Superstitions, crime, misère en Chine, by Dr. Matignon, Lyon, 1899. A very odd book, mostly anecdotal and somewhat biased, as the title indicates.

Pratique médical en Chine, by Jeanselme, Paris, 1901.

Dix ans au pays du dragon, by Dr. Matignon, Paris, 1910.

La médecine en Chine, by Dr. Vincent, Paris, 1915. A book with neither references nor documentation; mostly denigration and ridicule.

The Medical Missionary in China, by Lockhart.

''La médecine chinoise,'' by R.P. Weiger, *Bulletin Médical Franco-chinoise,* number 1, July-October, 1920.

''Four Milleniums of Chinese Medicine,'' by K.C. Wong, *The Lancet,* July 20 and 27, August 3, 1929. An article based on European texts, by a person educated in the English colleges of Hongkong, and who does not read Chinese.

History of Chinese Medicine, by K.C. Wong and Wu Lien-teh, Tien-tsin Press, Tianjin, 1930. Actually a history of European medicine in China. The authors, who studied in English colleges in Hong Kong, have studied neither Chinese literature nor language. Chinese medicine is briefly described in this book through references to English journals from the Far East.

The False Chinese Acupuncture in Paris from 1820 to 1830

During the nineteenth century, a method was developed in France that had nothing to do with Chinese acupuncture. Since it was intended to imitate the Chinese method, and since it employed needles, it caused confusion among the uninformed. The principal works to which these experiments were consigned are:

Mémoire sur les maladies, chronique, les évacuations sanguines et l'acuponcture, by Dr. Berlioz, Paris, 1825.

Traité de l'Acuponcture, after to the observations of Dr. J. Cloquet, by Dr. Dantu, Paris, 1826.

Mémoire sur l'électroponcture, by Dr. Sarlandiere, Paris, 1825.

Notes

[1] Books published after 1940 are not included in this bibliography, because it was prepared for the first edition of *L'Acuponcture chinoise.* — ed.

[2] We are unable to confirm this name. — ed.

[3] We were unable to check the Chinese source for this information. — ed.

[4] We were unable to check the Chinese source for this information. — ed.

[5] According to Dr. Fang (*Jin Zhen Bi Zhuan, 13),* in great antiquity there were two other important works from the famous Bo, both lost, but mentioned in the Han bibliographies:

   (1) *Bo Shi Nei Jing,* "Master Bo's Book of the Interior," in thirty-eight *juan* (before the fourth century B.C.).

   (2) *Pang Bian,* "Asides," by the same Master Bo, in twenty-five *juan* (also before the fourth century B.C.).

[6] The *Jin Gui Yao Lue* of Zhang Ji was originally part of his *Shang Han Za Bing Lun,* "Discussion of Cold Damage and Miscellaneous Disorders." It is an herbal text that has little or no information about acupuncture. It remains extant to the present day. — ed.

[7] According to Dr. Fang (*Jin Zhen Bi Zhuan, 6),* the lost books dating from this period are:

Huang Di Nei Jing Ming Tang Lei Cheng, "Perfections Chosen for the Audience Hall, from the Nei Jing of Huang Di," by Yang Shang Shan (Sui, sixth century).

Nei Jing Tai Su, "Great White Silk of the Nei Jing," twenty *juan,* also by Yang Shangshan.

Zhen Fang, "Needle Treatments," by Zhen Quan of Xu Zhou (Tang dynasty). This book is mentioned in the bliography (336) of Dr. Tatse-i's book. Does it still exist in Japan?

Mo Jing, "Book of the Pulses," also by Zhen Quan.

Ming Tang Tu, "Drawings for the Audience Hall," also by Zhen Quan. Also mentioned in the Dr. Tatse-i's bibliography. Perhaps it also still exists in Japan.

Ming Tang Kong Xue Tu, "Drawings of the Points Made for the Audience Hall," three *juan.* Mentioned in the Sui bibliography. Is it the same as the preceding title?

Ming Tang Kong Xue, "Drawings for the Audience Hall," five *juan* (Sui bibliography).

Gaohuang Jiu Fa, "Method of Moxas at the Point Gaohuang," two *juan,* by Chuo Jiyu, from Qing-Yuan-Zhuang, Tang period.

Zi-Wu Liu-Zhu Zhen Jing, "Book of Needles and Commentaries Flowing from Midnight and Midday," one *juan,* by He Ruo Yu of the Southern Tang (937-975).

Huang Di Nei Jing Ming Tang, "Audience Hall, Nei Jing of Huang Di," thirteen *juan.*

Huang Di Shi-Er Jing-Mo Ming Tang Wu Zang Tu, "Drawings of the Five Treasure Organs and the Twelve Meridians from Huang Di's Audience Hall," one *juan.*

Huang Di Shi-Er Jing Ming Yan, Zuo Ren Tu, "Drawings of a Man from the Front and Side from Huang Di's Audience Hall, with the Twelve Meridians," twelve *juan.*

Huang di Ming Tang, "Huang Di's Audience Hall," four *juan.*

The last four books are mentioned in the bibliography of the Tang dynasty.

[8] We were unable to verify the Chinese place name. — ed.

[9] Actually by Yang Jishi (Ji Zhou). The author's contention that the *Zhen Jiu Da Cheng* was written by a "Yang Gexian" comes from a misreading of the last line of the first chapter of that book, which should read, "The *Zhen Jiu Da Cheng* was compiled and corrected under the direction of Jin Xian from Jinyang." Jin Xian was an editor for the first publisher of this book, Zhou Wenbing, but the text itself is credited to Yang Jishi (Jizhou). — ed.

[10] Actually, the *Zhen-Jiu Da Quan* was published over 150 years before the *Da Cheng.* — ed.

[11] Xu Fong was actually the fifteenth century author of the *Zhen-Jiu Da Quan.* — ed.

Index

Usage

The first three volumes of *l'Acuponcture Chinoise* contain literally thousands of useful references to ideas, concepts and principles. Hence the indexing has been accomplished so as to make these most accessible; for example, biomedical labels and Chinese medical principles. Acupoints are also referenced, as are books and authors of historical significance. To create visual distinction, names of books or periodicals are in italic type. Proper names, including the pinyin transliteration of Chinese proper names, are set in the standard font. As each of the many quotations and paraphrases contain a reference, the index refers only to prose that describes or discusses, rather than merely cites, a book or author. Conditions, principles and practical instructions are indexed to the page level. For example, several entire charts of relationships are indicated by a single reference to the "insufficiency-excess" of each organ.

Volume IV, "Meridians, Points and Their Treatment," and *Volume V, "Illnesses and Their Treatment,"* are mutually cross-referenced compilations of data concerning acupuncture treatment. Indexing every one of these references would thus produce a third ordering of these two sections. That would accomplish little by way of reference speed or simplicity, because it would require an unwieldy index of several hundred pages. Thus the indexing strategy in the two final volumes has been to select references in each of these major sections according to the author's principal purpose, and thus the most likely use for the index. *Volume IV* is referenced using all three nomenclatures: alphanumeric, pinyin and English. Entries have been merged into a single list for easier access. Knowing any part of the acupoint nomenclature allows the other parts to be found in a single search without reference to the text itself. English acupoint names are enclosed in quotes, the pinyin transliterations are set in italics, and alphanumerics are capitalized. The pinyin and English acupoint index entries note only the page number of the *Volume IV* summary. The alphanumeric record identifies this summary by enclosing the volume and page in square brackets (e.g.: [IV: 422]). However, the alphanumeric record also lists every page reference in all parts of the text. Points that are not mentioned in the treatment section are listed but without page references.

Volume V is indexed to the lowest level of treatment heading, or to a single page, whichever produces the smallest entry. For example, where treatments for multiple but related conditions are found on a single page, the index entry is generalized by category. For example, the entry, "physical problems of sight" leads to several treatment differentiations and options. On the other hand, where there are multiple distinct entries on different pages, each is listed individually. For example, the many scattered references to specific pain conditions are each listed. Where distinct but related topics are few enough to permit, a single combined entry has been provided, for example, "physiology: 27; of energy: 179; of points: 216". In sets of references to large topics, there are both summarized and detailed references. For example, paralysis is noted both under a general heading and in individual references to specific paralytic problems.

Pinyin terms have been treated as a special case as these provide the most direct access to the set of terms Soulié de Morant saw as having a fixed meaning in Chinese traditional medicine. The approximately one thousand references to fixed terms included in the index are those where a definition is provided or may be reasonably taken from context. As the pinyin is not toned, there are instances where more than one search will be required to find a specific term discussion. English words that could be mistaken for pinyin transliterations are identified by font and topic qualifiers. For example, "sun (solar/sunny)" is distinguished from *sun*.

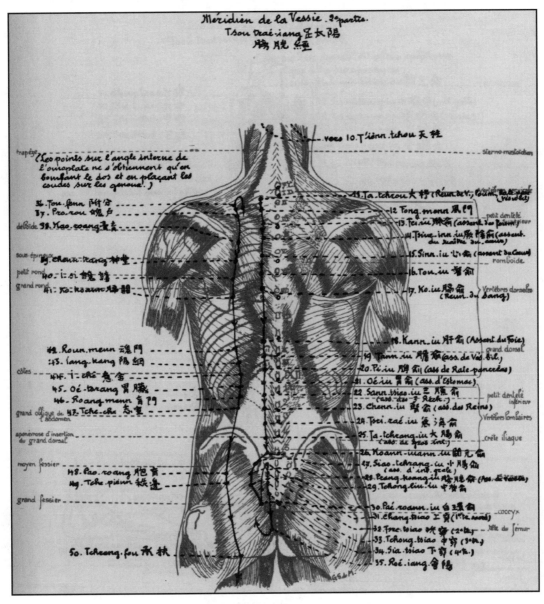

Meridian of the bladder (part 2) (GSDM)

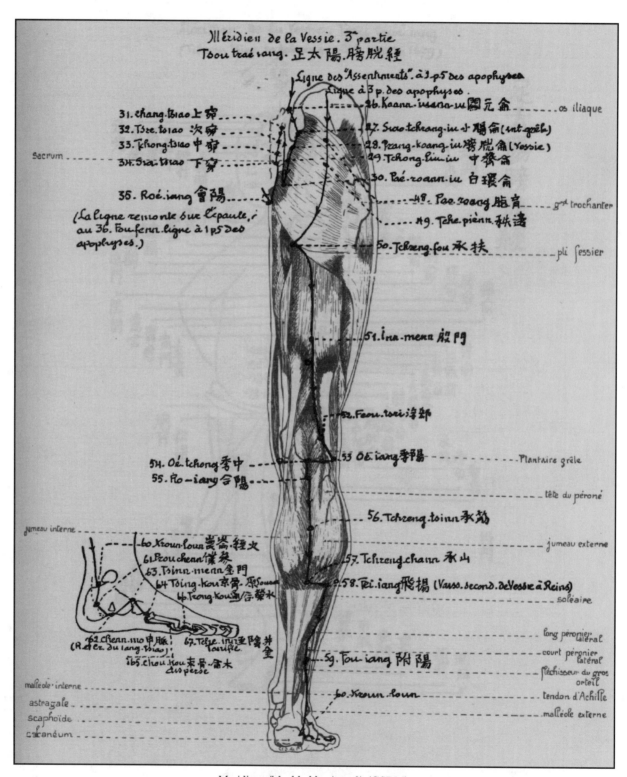

Meridian of the bladder (part 3) (GSDM)

Conception vessel (GSDM)

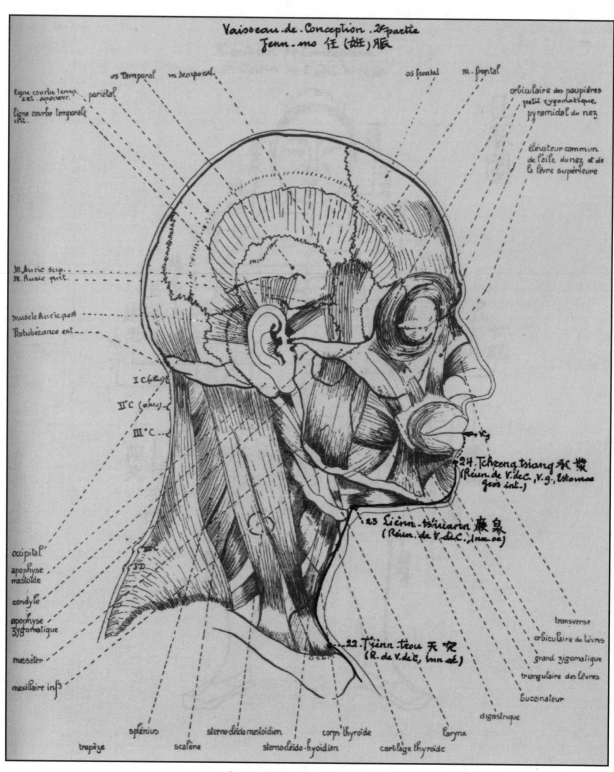

Conception vessel (part 2) (GSDM)

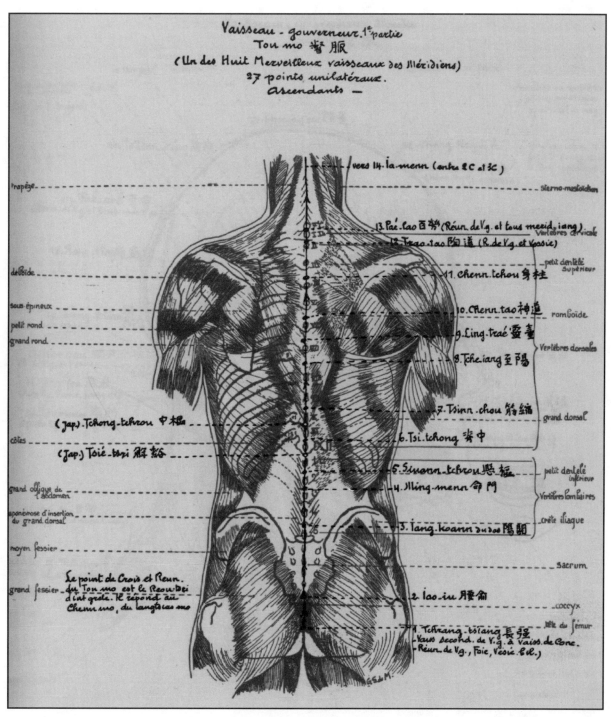

Governor vessel (part 1) (GSDM)

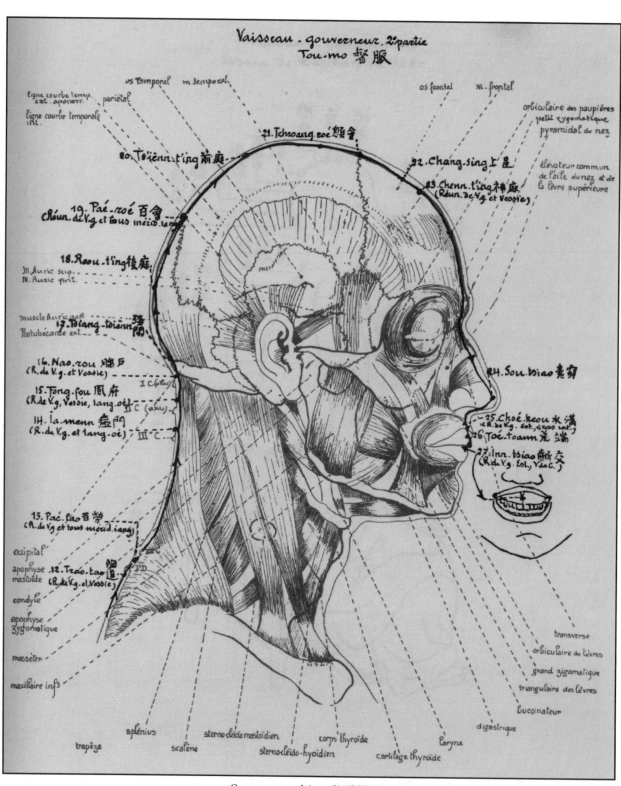

Governor vessel (part 2) (GSDM)

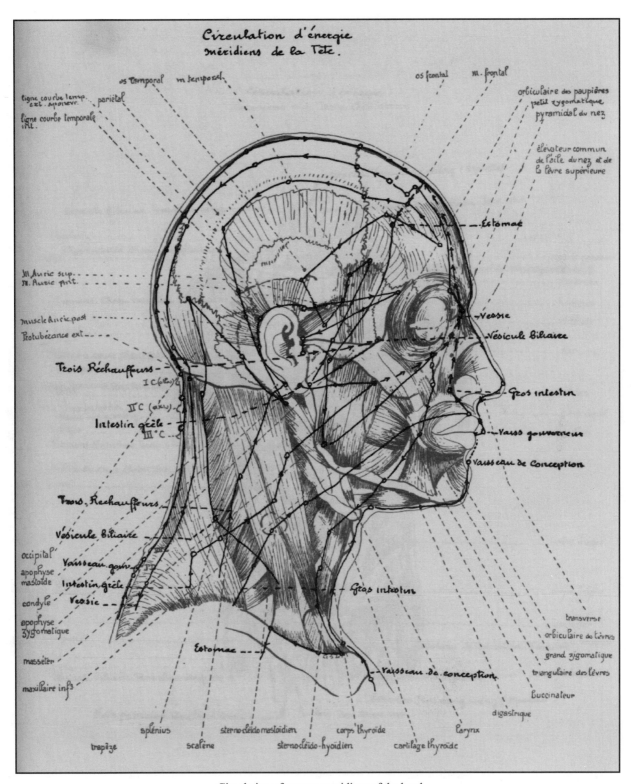

Circulation of energy, meridians of the head

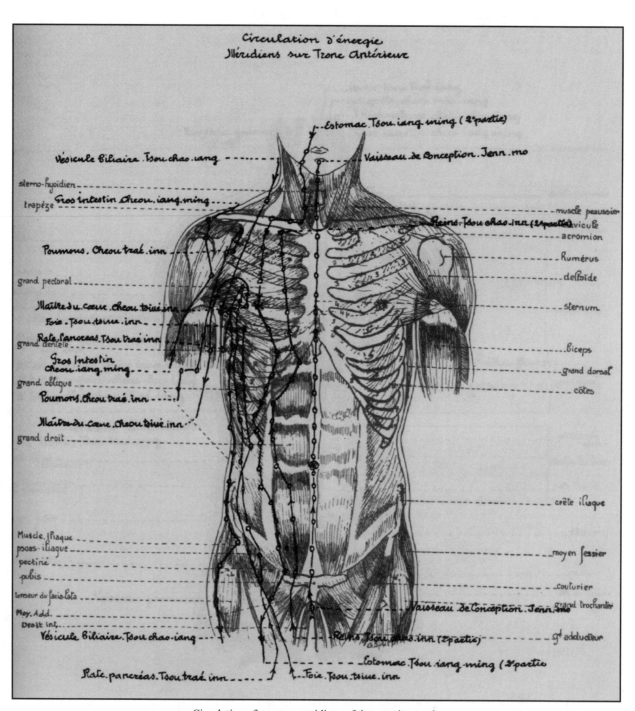

Circulation of energy, meridians of the anterior trunk

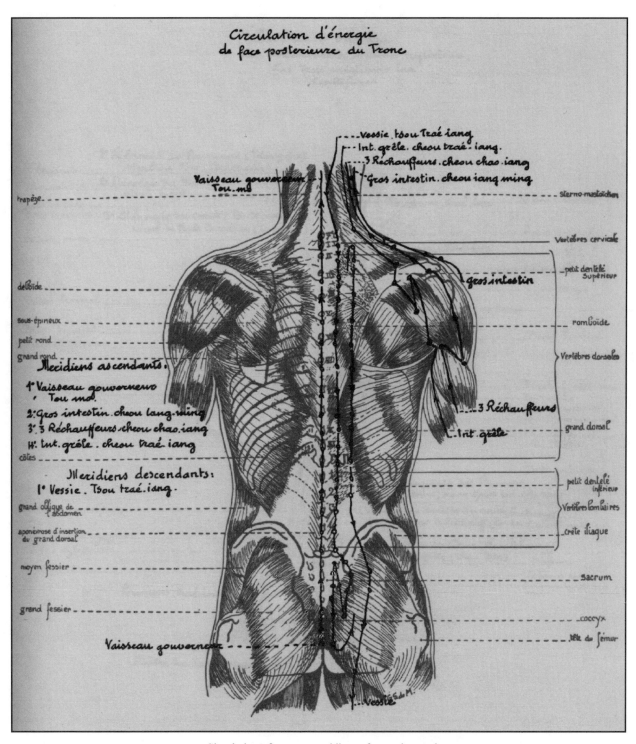

Circulation of energy, meridians of posterior trunk

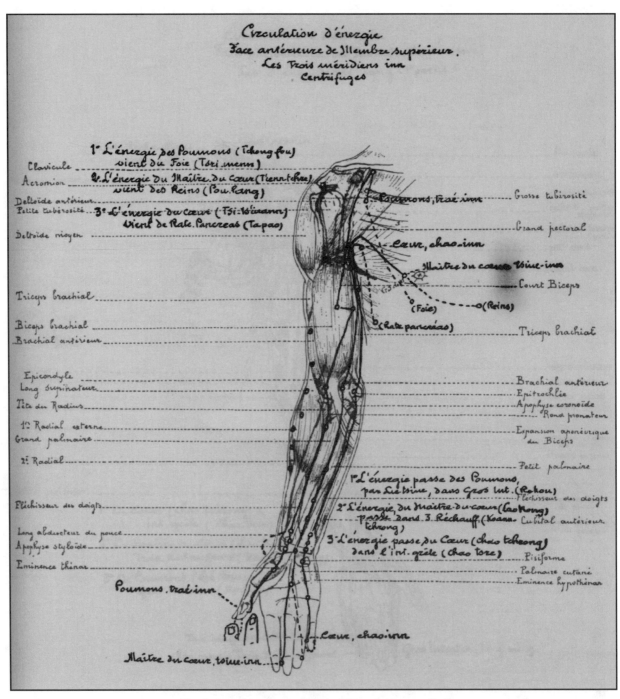

Circulation of energy, meridians of the anterior upper limb

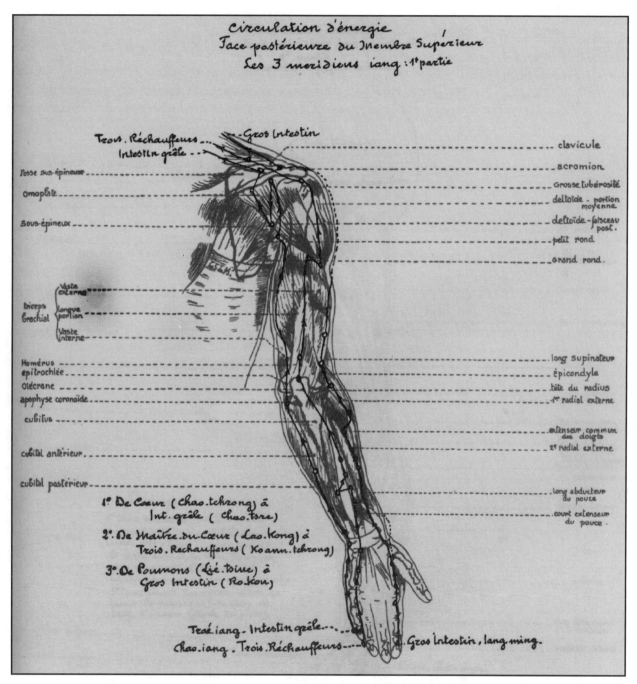

Circulation of energy, meridians of the posterior upper limb

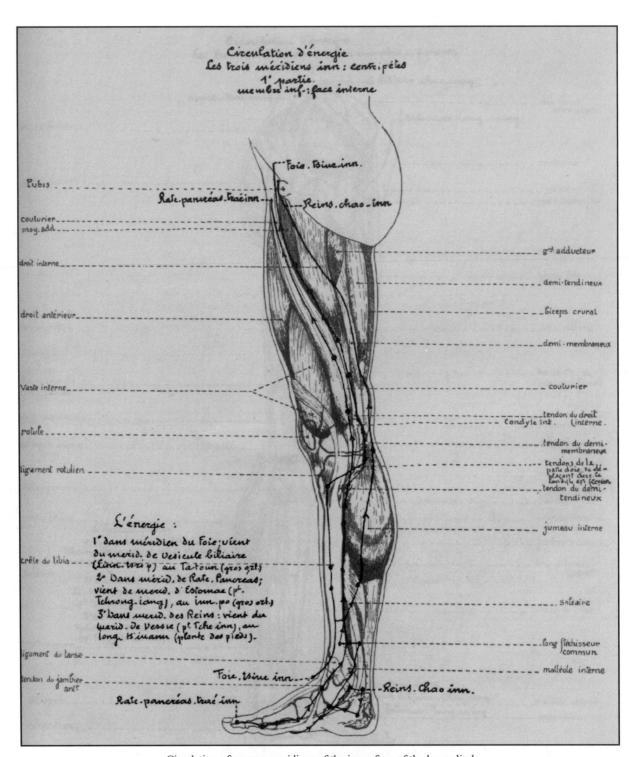

Circulation of energy, meridians of the inner face of the lower limb

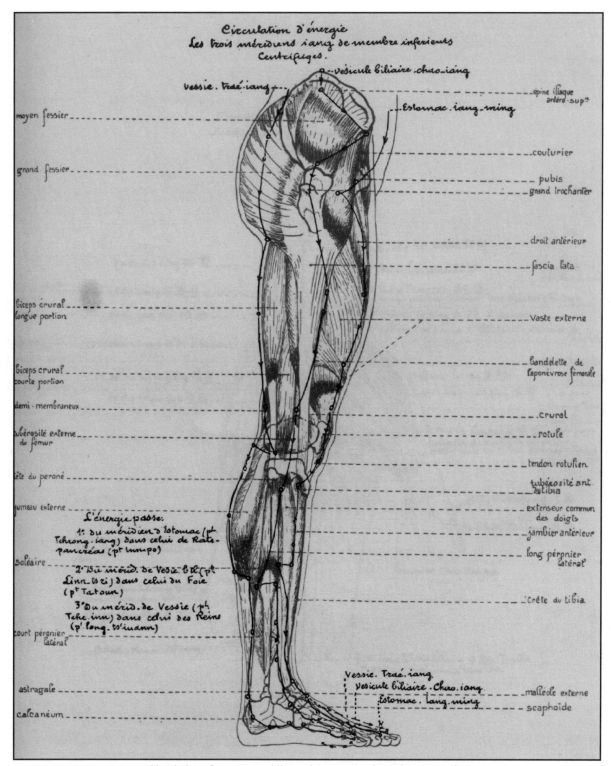

Circulation of energy, meridians of the exterior face of the lower limb

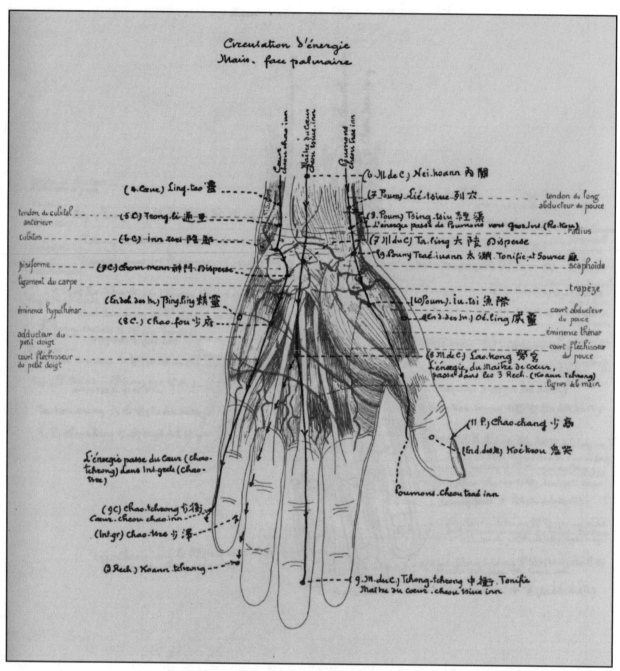

Circulation of energy, meridians of the palmar suface of the hand

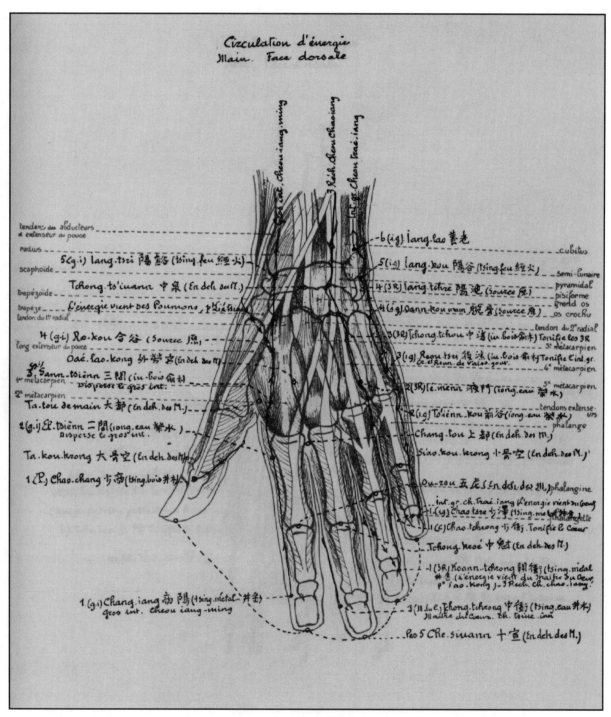

Circulation of energy, meridians of the dorsal surface of the hand

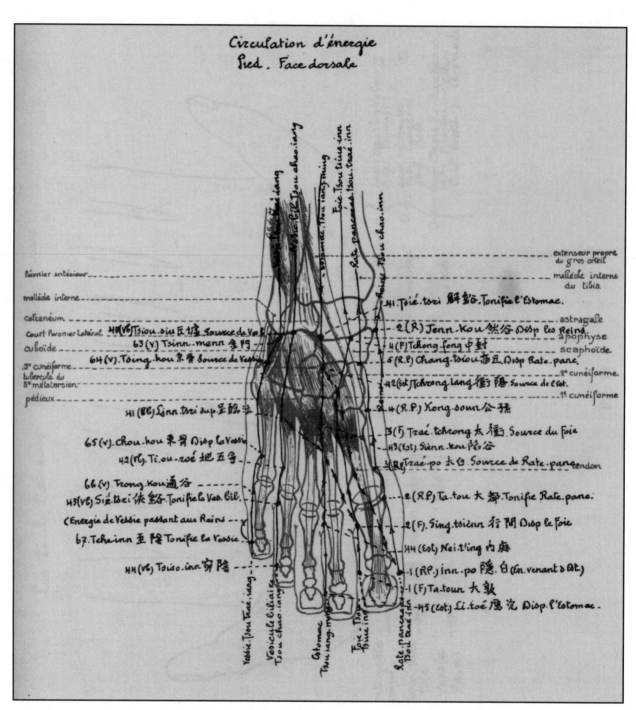

Circulation of energy, meridians of the dorsal surface of the foot